# *Lippincott's*
# *State Board Review for*
# *NCLEX-RN*

# Lippincott's
# State Board Review for
# NCLEX-RN
## FOURTH EDITION

### Edwina A. McConnell, RN, PhD
Independent Nurse Consultant
Madison, Wisconsin

### LuVerne Wolff Lewis, RN, MA
Formerly Consultant, College of Nursing
Arizona State University, Tempe, Arizona;
Research Associate, Institute of Research
 and Service in Nursing Education
Teachers College, Columbia University
New York, New York

J.B. LIPPINCOTT COMPANY
Philadelphia

Grand Rapids    New York    St. Louis    San Francisco
London    Sydney    Tokyo

**Acquisitions Editor:** *Donna Hilton*
**Copy Editor:** *Wendy Walker*
**Project Editor:** *Kathy Crown*
**Art Director:** *Susan Hess Blaker*
**Designer:** *Doug Smock*
**Design Coordinator:** *Doug Smock*
**Production Manager:** *Carol A. Florence*
**Production Coordinator:** *Barney Fernandes*
**Compositor:** *Circle Graphics*
**Text Printer/Binder:** *The Murray Printing Company*
**Cover Printer:** *New England Book Components*

Fourth Edition

6  5  4  3  2  1

**Library of Congress Cataloging-in-Publication Data**

McConnell, Edwina A.
    Lippincott's State board review for NCLEX-RN/
Edwina A. McConnell, LuVerne Wolff Lewis.—4th ed.
    p.      cm.
    Rev. ed. of: Lippincott's State board review for
NCLEX-RN/LuVerne Wolff Lewis. 3rd ed. c1986.
    Includes bibliographical references.
    ISBN 0-397-54722-6
    1. Nursing—Examinations, questions, etc.   I. Lewis,
LuVerne Wolff.   II. Lewis, LuVerne Wolff. Lippincott's State
board review for NCLEX-RN.   III. Title.   IV. Title: State
board review of NCLEX-RN.
    [DNLM:   1. Nursing—examination questions. WY 18
M47755L]
RT55.M29 1989
610.73'076—dc20
DNLM/DLC
for Library of Congress

Any procedure or practice described in this book should be
applied by the health-care practitioner under appropriate
supervision in accordance with professional standards of
care used with regard to the unique circumstances that apply in each practice situation. Care has been taken to confirm the accuracy of information presented and to describe
generally accepted practices. However, the authors, editors
and publisher cannot accept any responsibility for errors or
omissions or for consequences from application of the information in this book and make no warranty, express or implied, with respect to the contents of the book.

The authors and publisher have exerted every effort to ensure that drug selection and dosage set forth in this text
are in accord with current recommendations and practice at
the time of publication. However, in view of ongoing research, changes in government regulations, and the constant
flow of information relating to drug therapy and drug reactions, the reader is urged to check the package insert of
each drug for any change in indications and dosage and for
added warnings and precautions. This is particularly important when the recommended agent is a new or infrequently
used drug.

# SECTION COORDINATORS

**Linda Brown,** RN, PhD

Formerly, Assistant Professor
Yale University
School of Nursing
New Haven, Connecticut

**Lola J. Gould,** RNC, MSN

Assistant Professor
University of Mississippi
School of Nursing
Jackson, Mississippi

**Yondell Masten,** RNC, PhD

Texas Tech University Health Sciences Center
School of Nursing
Lubbock, Texas

**Linda Denise Oakley,** RN, PhD

Robert Wood Johnson Clinical Scholar
University of California
School of Nursing
San Francisco, California

**Judith K. Sands,** RN, EdD

Assistant Professor
University of Virginia
School of Nursing
Charlottesville, Virginia

# CONTRIBUTORS

**Janice R. Anderzon,** RN, BSN MS

Clinical Professor
Adult Medical-Surgical Nursing
University of Wisconsin—Madison
School of Nursing
Madison, Wisconsin

**Deborah Chyun,** RN, BSN, MSN

Lecturer, Cardiovascular Specialty
Medical-Surgical Nursing Program
Yale University
School of Nursing
New Haven, Connecticut

**Joanne R. Conger,** RN, BSN, MS

Clinical Associate Professor
Adult Medical-Surgical Nursing
University of Wisconsin—Madison
School of Nursing
Madison, Wisconsin

**Suzanne Saunders Cooke,** RN, MSN, CS

Medical-Surgical Nursing
Texas Tech University Health Sciences Center
School of Nursing
Lubbock, Texas

**Richard Creager,** RN, BSN

Meriter/Madison General Hospital
Madison, Wisconsin

**Catherine Gray Deering,** RN, MSN, CS

Psychiatric Nursing
Yale University
School of Nursing
New Haven, Connecticut

**Patricia E. Downing,** RN, MN

Nursing Education Consultant
Formerly with School of Nursing
University of California
San Francisco, California

**James A. Fain,** RN, PhD

Assistant Professor and Chair, Master's Program
for Non-Nurse College Graduates
Yale University
School of Nursing
New Haven, Connecticut

**Pamela Billings Farley,** RN, MSN

Assistant Professor
Berea College
Department of Nursing
Berea, Kentucky

**Sarah P. Farrell,** RN, MSN, CS

Assistant Professor
Yale University
School of Nursing
Clinical Nurse Specialist
Connecticut Mental Health Center Day Hospital
New Haven, Connecticut

**Kathleen A. Furitano,** RN, BSN, MSN

Pediatric Clinical Nurse Specialist
University of Illinois Hospital
Adjunct Assistant Professor
University of Illinois
College of Nursing
Chicago, Illinois

**Diane Hamilton,** RN, PhD

Medical University of South Carolina
Charleston, South Carolina

**Brenda Hanson-Smith,** RNC, MSN

OB/GYN Nurse Practitioner in Private Practice
Co-Director of Heartwork
Long Beach, California

**Marsha L. Heims,** RN, MS

Associate Professor
Department of Family Nursing
Oregon Health Sciences University
School of Nursing
Portland, Oregon

**Cindy Peterson Helstad,** RN, BSN

> Head Nurse
> Eating Disorders
> Meriter/Methodist Hospital
> Madison, Wisconsin

**Louise Juliani,** RN, BSN, MS

> Medical-Surgical Nursing
> Canon City, Colorado

**Kathryn R. Kolar,** RN, MSN

> Nursing Care of Children
> University of Mississippi
> School of Nursing
> Jackson, Mississippi

**Sara E. Kolb,** RN, PhD

> Associate Professor
> Incarnate Word College
> San Antonio, Texas

**Nancy A. Smyth Markin,** RN, MSN, PNA

> Associate Professor
> Oakton College
> School of Nursing
> Des Plaines, Illinois

**Marlene L. McClure,** RN, MSN

> Associate Professor, Pediatric Nursing
> Pittsburg State University
> Department of Nursing
> Pittsburg, Kansas

**Ellen K. Murphy,** RN, MS, JD

> Associate Professor
> University of Wisconsin—Milwaukee
> School of Nursing
> Milwaukee, Wisconsin

**Susan A. Nitzke,** RD, PhD

> Assistant Professor
> Nutritional Sciences
> University of Wisconsin—Madison
> Madison, Wisconsin

**Joyce M. Olson,** RN, MSN

> Pediatric Clinical Specialist
> University of Kansas Medical Center
> Department of Nursing Services
> Kansas City, Kansas

**Carol J. Pederson,** RN, MS

> Pediatric Nursing
> University of Minnesota
> School of Nursing
> Minneapolis, Minnesota

**Colleen Pfeiffer,** RN, PhD, CCRN

> Assistant Professor
> Critical Care
> University of Colorado, Health Science Center
> Denver, Colorado

**Diane Matousek Propper,** RN, MSN, OCN

> Oncology Clinical Nursing Specialist
> Program Instructor
> Yale University
> School of Nursing
> New Haven, Connecticut

**Cheryl V. Ratliff,** RN, MS, MN

> Director of Clinical Services
> Child Health Corporation of America
> Shawnee Mission, Kansas

**Carol Freeman Rosenkranz,** RN, MN

> Associate Professor
> Maternal-Newborn Nursing
> University of Mississippi
> School of Nursing
> Jackson, Mississippi

**M. Lisa Sinacore,** RN, MSN

> Instructor, Nursing of Children
> West Virginia University
> School of Nursing
> Morgantown, West Virginia

**Susanne Smith,** RN, MSN

> Psychiatric/Mental Health Nursing
> Winona State University
> College of Nursing and Health Sciences
> Winona, Minnesota

**Kathryn Lee Sridaromont**, RNC, MSN
: Asssistant Professor of Clinical Nursing
Pediatric Clinical Nurse Specialist
Texas Tech University Health Sciences Center
School of Nursing
Lubbock, Texas

**Jo Stejskal**, RN, MSN
: Associate Professor
Winona State University
College of Nursing and Health Sciences
Winona, Minnesota

**Barbara Romano Teague**, RN, MSN, CPNA
: Pediatrics
University of Kentucky
College of Nursing
Lexington, Kentucky

**Bridget Thompson**, RN, MS
: Assistant Professor
Parent-Child Nursing
University of North Dakota
Grand Forks, North Dakota

**Kay Weinkam**, RN, BS, MS
: Maternal-Child Health
Meriter/Madison General Hospital
Madison, Wisconsin

**Lynnda Zibell**, RN, MSN
: Psychiatric Mental Health Nursing
Meriter/Methodist Hospital
Madison, Wisconsin

## CONTRIBUTORS TO PREVIOUS EDITIONS

**Ola Burns Allen**, RN, MS

**Carolyn M. Bolter Feller**, RN, PhD

**June E. Lawrence**, RN, PhD

**Norma Beggerly Reed**, RN, EdD

**Penny J. Starkey**, RN, MSN

**Jimmye M. Stephenson**, RN, PhD

# FOREWORD

*He who knows not and knows not that he knows not is a fool. Shun him.*
*He who knows not and knows that he knows not is simple. Teach him.*
*He who knows and knows not that he knows is asleep. Waken him.*
*He who knows and knows that he knows is wise. Follow him.*

*Arabic Apothegm*

This book provides an opportunity for the reader to become a wise person. It does this in three ways. First, it provides a framework, paradigm, and model within which the reader can organize knowledge already possessed. Many new graduates find that knowledge as organized and taught in schools of nursing is different from the way knowledge is organized in the work world. Curricula and courses in most schools are designed to promote inquiry, critical thinking, and discussion of general principles. In the work world, however, immediate recall and application of knowledge is demanded. The nurse confronted with a clinical situation must know how to select, from the total array of knowledge she possesses, those facts, principles, and rationales relevant to the particular situation. The nurse must learn to weigh and criticize the alternatives, to hold some in abeyance, to discard some, and to implement others as the situation dictates. Such use of knowledge requires a different organizational framework from that used in school.

*Lippincott's State Board Review for NCLEX-RN* is superb in its organization. Following the State Board paradigm, this review presents the reader with patient care situations commonly encountered by registered nurses. The questions following the clinical situations cover all five phases of the nursing process—assessment, analysis, planning, implementation, and evaluation—and represent realistic avenues for resolving the patient's needs for a safe, effective care environment, for physiological integrity, for psychosocial integrity, and for health promotion and maintenance. The questions given in the test situations are in the same proportion as in the State Board examination.

A second way in which this review promotes wisdom is by validating knowledge the reader already possesses. Unless one's knowledge is tested and validated consistently and methodically, one runs the risk

of being simple or foolish. Knowing whether one knows or does not know enables the reader to choose to build upon her knowledge base.

The rationales provided in this text are excellent and will help the reader assess that personal knowledge base. Provided at the end of each section, the rationales not only provide scientific background and clinical information that supports the correct answer, but they also invalidate those answers that are incorrect. It is just as important to know why some information or nursing intervention is incorrect or inappropriate as it is to know why an appropriate action is selected from the vast repertoire of knowledge a nurse possesses. These rationales, along with the reference section at the end of each of the five major sections (new to this edition), comprise one of the strongest features of this review by Dr. McConnell and colleagues. Another strong feature is the addition of a fourth comprehensive test.

A third way in which this book promotes wisdom is by helping the reader update knowledge. It may well have been several years since the reader first studied some of the facts and concepts presented through the test questions in this book. Although the reader might have been up-to-date when actually studying a given area, this may not be so now. Knowledge doubles and triples at an alarming rate, and unless one stays current, one cannot be a safe practitioner of nursing. Conscientious study and use of the suggested practices and procedures in this book will enable the reader to determine his or her level of currency in the field. Toward this end, not only have all items in this fourth edition been reviewed and revised from the third edition, but more than 500 new items have been added for a grand total of 3,057 questions.

In any health care organization, the nursing department is the *raison d'etre*. The hospital staff nurse is vitally important because she is the person that has the most contact and interaction with the primary consumer, the patient. As such, the staff nurse *directly controls* the quality of patient care. It stands to reason, therefore, that the quality of patient care is directly related to the knowledge level of the staff nurse. Research has continually demonstrated that autonomous nursing practice leads to quality patient care. The basis of autonomy is knowledge and competence. Autonomy means the freedom to act upon that which one knows. Unless the nurse knows and knows that she knows, she cannot be competent or autonomous and hence will not be able to give the patient high quality nursing care. The very first step in becoming a successful, competent, and autonomous staff nurse is for the student to know and know that she knows. This will enable the student to pass the State Board Exam, which gives the student the legal right to practice nursing. The positive self-concept and self-esteem associated with this wisdom and with passing State Boards will provide the nurse with the psychological lift that comes from establishing knowledge and competence in one's own eyes.

If I were to identify the points that best illustrate the value of this book, I would emphasize its integrated perspective on the nursing care of patients and the rationales it provides for both correct and incorrect answers. By providing an opportunity for verifying and validating nursing knowledge, *Lippincott's State Board Review for NCLEX-RN* sets the stage for expanding and discovering new knowledge. In this way, the wisdom of knowing and knowing that one knows is fostered in all nurses.

Marlene Kramer, RN, PhD, FAAN

# PREFACE

Passing the National Council Licensure Examination for Registered Nurses (NCLEX-RN) marks the beginning of a nurse's professional career. *Lippincott's State Board Review for the NCLEX-RN* was developed to help students write this examination successfully, although they have been preparing for it since entering nursing school. The same examination is presently used in all 50 states, the District of Columbia, and the possessions of the United States. Students graduated from baccalaureate, diploma, and associate degree programs in nursing must pass this examination to meet licensure requirements in the United States.

The National Council of State Boards of Nursing, Inc., is an organization with representation from all state boards of nursing. This organization prepares the test plan used to develop the licensure examination. The test plan is formulated on health care situations that registered nurses commonly encounter, and the plan addresses two components: (1) phases of the nursing process and (2) client needs. Representative items test knowledge of these components as they relate to specific health care situations.

The major features of this book include the following:

- The introduction explains how the licensure examination is prepared, how to review for it, strategies to help write it successfully, how it is scored, and ways in which to use this book most effectively.
- The test plan developed for the state licensure examination by the National Council of State Boards of Nursing, Inc., was used to prepare this book.
- Students can enter their choice for correct answers directly in this book. There are no answer sheets, which is also true of the licensure examination.
- This book is divided into five major sections. The first four sections represent the four main clinical areas of nursing, and the fifth section is composed of four comprehensive tests. This format enables candidates to review one or more clinical areas and/ or to write one or more comprehensive tests, which are designed to resemble NCLEX-RN.
- Each test presents a variety of situations commonly encountered in nursing practice. Just as NCLEX-RN is comprehensive, so are the tests in this book.

- The items in this book total 3,057. Twenty-nine review tests contain 2,697 items, and 4 comprehensive tests contain 360 items. The test items are objective and accompanied by typical health care situations that require the knowledge and skills of a registered nurse. Each item offers four alternatives from which to select the best answer. This is also true of NCLEX-RN.
- Hundreds of items are new to this edition of the book. Items used from the previous edition have been carefully reviewed and in some instances extensively revised before being included in this edition. Outdated items have been discarded.
- Each of the 29 review tests contains approximately 90 items, which is similar to each of the four tests on the licensure examination.
- The review tests are grouped according to clinical disciplines so that candidates can review one clinical area at a time.
- The topics tested in all clinical disciplines have been expanded.
- The four comprehensive tests resemble NCLEX-RN. Just as the licensure examination samples all clinical disciplines, so do each of the comprehensive tests.
- Candidates using this book can evaluate their success on the comprehensive tests. Directions for interpreting self-evaluative results direct the candidates review.
- Correct answers and rationales are given for all items in this book. The rationales explain why the correct answer is correct, as well as why the distractors are incorrect.
- References are provided for each item. Candidates can verify correct answers, clarify subject matter, or increase knowledge about a specific content area by consulting these references.
- The references used in preparing this book are listed for each of the five major sections. Books published no more than 5 years ago have been listed, except when a book is a classic in its field.
- Contributors to the book were selected for their expertise in specific content areas. A national perspective, rather than regional policies and practices, is represented.
- The address and telephone number of the National

Council of State Boards of Nursing, Inc., and for each state board of nursing are listed in the Appendix.

• While the target audience of this book is the student preparing to write the licensure examination for registered nurses, other nurses will find it helpful. These nurses include those preparing for challenge examinations, inactive nurses preparing to return to practice, practicing nurses transferring to a different clinical area, and nursing faculty.

Certain policies have been observed in the book for consistency and clarity:

• The word *patient* refers to people who receive health care, although in some agencies the term *client* is used.

• The registered nurse is usually referred to as "she," keeping in mind that not all nurses are women.

• The word *sign* is used to describe observations made by health care personnel, while the word *symptom* is used to describe observations made by patients.

• Generic drug names are used. Common brand or trade names are given in parentheses following the generic names when they first appear in a situation.

A "thank you!" to Alice M. Bradee, Robert Horowitz, "the corner apothecary," Abbie McConnell, Sherry VanGorder, James F. Welch, and Mary F. Zimmerman for their friendship, kind words, and sense of humor. And a very special "thank you!" to Patricia Downing, Peggy T. Ford, Chris (Daphne) Ludwig, and Louise Juliani for their help in preparing the manuscript.

Edwina A. McConnell, RN, PhD

# CONTENTS

INTRODUCTION     *xix*

**PART I**
**THE NURSING CARE
OF PATIENTS WITH
PSYCHOSOCIAL ALTERATIONS**     **1**

**Test 1**     **3**

The Patient with a Major Mood Disorder     3
The Patient with Bipolar Disorder, Manic
    Phase     4
The Patient Who is Depressed     7
The Patient with Depressive Disorder and
    Suicidal Ideation     9
The Patient Who Attempts Suicide     11
The Patient in Crisis     12
*Correct Answers and Rationales*     *15*

**Test 2**     **25**

The Patient Who is Paranoid     25
The Patient with Catatonic Schizophrenia     27
The Patient with Chronic Mental Illness     28
The Patient with an Obsessive-Compulsive
    Disorder     30
The Patient with Organic Brain Syndrome     32
Using a Therapeutic Milieu     34
*Correct Answers and Rationales*     *36*

**Test 3**     **43**

The Patient with a Personality Disorder     43
The Patient Who Abuses Alcohol     45
The Patient with Alcohol Withdrawal     47
The Patient Who is Dependent on Narcotics     48
The Patient Who Abuses Barbiturates     50
The Patient with an Eating Disorder     51
*Correct Answers and Rationales*     *54*

**Test 4**     **63**

The Patient with Anxiety     63
The Patient with Maladaptive Behavior
    Patterns     64
The Patient with Problems with Expression
    of Anger     67

The Patient with Family Abuse and Violence     68
The Patient with a Psychophysiological
    Disorder     70
The Patient with a Terminal Illness     72
*Correct Answers and Rationales*     *75*

**PART II**
**THE NURSING CARE OF
MATERNITY PATIENTS
AND NEWBORNS**     **83**

**Test 1**     **85**

The Pregnant Patient Receiving Prenatal
    Care     85
The Pregnant Patient in Childbirth
    Preparation Class     89
The Preconception Patient     90
The Patient with a Spontaneous Abortion     93
*Correct Answers and Rationales*     *94*

**Test 2**     **101**

The Teenaged Patient with Pregnancy-
    Induced Hypertension (PIH)     101
The Pregnant Patient with Third-Trimester
    Bleeding     104
The Pregnant Patient with Premature
    Labor     105
The Pregnant Patient with Diabetes
    Mellitus     107
The Patient with an Ectopic Pregnancy     108
The Pregnant Patient with a Hydatidiform
    Mole     108
*Correct Answers and Rationales*     *110*

**Test 3**     **117**

The Primigravid Patient in Labor     117
The Intrapartal Patient with Single-Room
    Maternity Care     118
The Intrapartal Patient with Risk Factors     120
*Correct Answers and Rationales*     *126*

Contents

## Test 4                                                 133

The Postpartal Patient with a Vaginal Birth      133
The Postpartal Patient Who Breast-Feeds          136
The Postpartal Patient Who Bottle-Feeds          138
The Postpartal Patient with a Cesarean
  Birth                                          138
The Postpartal Patient with Risk Factors         140

*Correct Answers and Rationales*                 *143*

## Test 5                                                 151

The Neonatal-Patient                             151
Physical Assessment of the Neonatal
  Patient                                        152
The Postterm Neonatal Patient                    154
The Neonatal Patient with Risk Factors           155

*Correct Answers and Rationales*                 *160*

## PART III
## THE NURSING CARE
## OF CHILDREN                                            167

## Test 1                                                 169

Health Promotion of the Infant and Family        169
Health Promotion of the Toddler
  and Family                                     170
Health Promotion of the Preschooler
  and Family                                     172
Health Promotion of the School-Aged
  Child and Family                               173
Health Promotion of the Adolescent
  and Family                                     174
Meetings to Discuss Common Childhood
  and Adolescent Health Problems                 175

*Correct Answers and Rationales*                 *179*

## Test 2                                                 187

The Patient with Tonsillitis                     187
The Patient with Chronic Otitis Media            188
The Patient with Aspiration of a
  Foreign Body                                   189
The Patient with Bronchial Asthma                190
The Patient with Cystic Fibrosis and
  Bronchopneumonia                               191
The Patient with Sudden Infant Death
  Syndrome                                       192
The Patient Requiring Cardiopulmonary
  Resuscitation                                  193

*Correct Answers and Rationales*                 *195*

## Test 3                                                 203

The Patient with a Ventricular Septal
  Defect                                         203
The Patient with Tetralogy of Fallot             204
The Patient with Down Syndrome                   205
The Patient with Rheumatic Fever                 206
The Patient with Sickle-Cell Anemia              208
The Patient with Iron-Deficiency Anemia          208
The Patient with Hemophilia and Acquired
  Immune Deficiency Syndrome                     209
The Patient with Leukemia                        210

*Correct Answers and Rationales*                 *213*

## Test 4                                                 223

The Patient with Cleft Lip and Palate            223
The Patient with Tracheoesophageal Fistula       224
The Patient with Imperforate Anus                225
The Patient with Pyloric Stenosis                227
The Patient with Intussusception                 228
The Patient with Inguinal Hernia                 229
The Patient with Hirschsprung's Disease          230

*Correct Answers and Rationales*                 *232*

## Test 5                                                 241

The Patient with Diarrhea/Gastroenteritis        241
The Patient with Appendicitis                    243
The Patient with Ingestion of Toxic
  Substances                                     245
The Patient with Celiac Disease                  246
The Patient with Phenylketonuria                 247
The Patient with Colic                           248
The Patient with Obesity                         248
The Patient with Cow's Milk Sensitivity          249

*Correct Answers and Rationales*                 *251*

## Test 6                                                 259

The Patient with Cryptorchidism                  259
The Patient with Hydrocele                        260
The Patient with Hypospadias                      260
The Patient with a Urinary Tract Infection       261
The Patient with Acute/Chronic
  Glomerulonephritis                             262
The Patient with Nephrotic Syndrome              264
The Patient with Acute/Chronic Renal
  Failure                                        265
The Patient with Wilms' Tumor                    266

*Correct Answers and Rationales*                 *268*

**Test 7**                                                   **275**

The Patient with Myelomeningocele                           275
The Patient with Hydrocephalus                              276
The Patient with a Seizure Disorder                         277
The Patient with Meningitis                                 279
The Patient with Reye Syndrome                              280
The Patient with Infectious Polyneuritis
    (Guillain-Barré Syndrome)                               281
The Patient with a Head Injury                              282
The Patient with a Brain Tumor                              282
The Patient with a Spinal Cord Injury                       283
*Correct Answers and Rationales*                            285

**Test 8**                                                   **293**

Screening Patients for Musculoskeletal
    Dysfunction                                              293
The Patient with Cerebral Palsy                             294
The Patient with Muscular Dystrophy                         295
The Patient with Congenital Hip Dysplasia                   296
The Patient with Congenital Clubfoot                        297
The Patient with Juvenile Rheumatoid
    Arthritis                                                298
The Patient with a Fracture                                 299
The Patient with Osteomyelitis                              302
*Correct Answers and Rationales*                            303

**Test 9**                                                   **313**

The Patient Who is Preterm                                  313
The Patient with Sepsis                                     314
The Patient with Failure to Thrive                          315
The Patient with Atopic Dermatitis
    (Eczema)                                                 316
The Patient with Burns                                      316
The Patient with Hypothyroidism                             319
The Patient with Insulin-Dependent
    Diabetes Mellitus                                        319
The Patient Who is Abused                                   321
*Correct Answers and Rationales*                            324

**PART IV
THE NURSING CARE OF ADULTS
WITH MEDICAL/SURGICAL
DISORDERS**                                                 **335**

**Test 1**                                                   **337**

The Patient with Pneumonia                                  337
The Patient with Tuberculosis                               338

The Patient with Chronic Obstructive
    Pulmonary Disease                                        340
The Patient with Lung Cancer                                341
The Patient with Chest Trauma                               344
*Correct Answers and Rationales*                            346

**Test 2**                                                   **353**

The Patient with Myocardial Infarction                      353
The Patient with Congestive Heart Failure                   355
The Patient with Valvular Heart Disease                     356
The Patient with Hypertension                               358
The Patient with Angina                                     360
*Correct Answers and Rationales*                            362

**Test 3**                                                   **369**

The Patient with Peptic Ulcer Disease                       369
The Patient with Cholecystitis                              371
The Patient with Cancer of the Stomach                      372
The Patient with Pancreatitis                               375
The Patient with a Hiatal Hernia                            376
*Correct Answers and Rationales*                            378

**Test 4**                                                   **385**

The Patient with Cancer of the Colon                        385
The Patient with Hepatitis A                                386
The Patient with Hemorrhoids                                387
The Patient with Inflammatory Bowel
    Disease                                                  389
The Patient with an Intestinal Obstruction                  390
The Patient with Cirrhosis                                  391
*Correct Answers and Rationales*                            395

**Test 5**                                                   **401**

The Patient with Hyperthyroidism                            401
The Patient with Diabetes Mellitus                          403
The Patient with Pituitary Adenoma                          405
The Patient with Addison's Disease                          406
The Patient with Cushing's Disease                          407
*Correct Answers and Rationales*                            410

**Test 6**                                                   **417**

The Patient with Cancer of the Bladder                      417
The Patient with Renal Calculi                              418
The Patient with Acute Renal Failure                        420
The Patient with Cystitis                                   421
The Patient with Chronic Renal Failure                      423
*Correct Answers and Rationales*                            426

Contents

**Test 7**                                              **433**

   The Patient with Uterine Fibroids         433
   The Patient with Breast Cancer            434
   The Patient with Benign Prostatic
     Hypertrophy                        436
   The Patient with a Sexually Transmitted
     Disease                            438
   The Patient with Cancer of the Cervix     439
   The Patient with Testicular Cancer        441
*Correct Answers and Rationales*                         *443*

**Test 8**                                              **451**

   The Patient with a Head Injury            451
   The Patient with Seizures                 452
   The Patient with a Cerebrovascular
     Accident                           454
   The Patient with Parkinson's Disease      456
   The Patient with Multiple Sclerosis       457
   The Unconscious Patient                   458
*Correct Answers and Rationales*                         *460*

**Test 9**                                              **467**

   The Patient with Rheumatoid Arthritis     467
   The Patient with a Hip Fracture           468
   The Patient with a Herniated Disc         470
   The Patient with Peripheral Vascular
     Disease                            471
   The Patient with a Femoral Fracture       472
   The Patient with a Spinal Cord Injury     474
*Correct Answers and Rationales*                         *476*

**Test 10**                                             **483**

   The Patient with Cataracts                483
   The Patient with Glaucoma                 484

   The Patient with a Retinal Detachment     486
   The Patient Undergoing Rhinoplasty        487
   The Patient with Ménière's Disease        488
   The Patient with Cancer of the Larynx     490
*Correct Answers and Rationales*                         *492*

**Test 11**                                             **499**

   The Patient in Pain                       499
   The Patient with Pernicious Anemia        500
   The Patient with Hodgkin's Disease        502
   The Patient Requiring Cardiopulmonary
     Resuscitation                      503
   The Patient with Burns                    505
   The Patient in Shock                      506
*Correct Answers and Rationales*                         *508*

**PART V
COMPREHENSIVE TESTS**                                   **515**

**Comprehensive Test 1**                                **517**
*Correct Answers and Rationales*                         *527*

**Comprehensive Test 2**                                **535**
*Correct Answers and Rationales*                         *545*

**Comprehensive Test 3**                                **553**
*Correct Answers and Rationales*                         *562*

**Comprehensive Test 4**                                **571**
*Correct Answers and Rationales*                         *581*

**APPENDIX
STATE BOARDS OF NURSING**                               **589**

# INTRODUCTION

*"We are the engineers of our lives."*
*—Marion Dolan*

Your license as a registered nurse is your key to the future. Nursing offers myriad career opportunities, and they all begin with a license to practice as a registered nurse. Thus, the purpose of *Lippincott's State Board Review for NCLEX-RN* is to help you prepare to write NCLEX-RN successfully.

## NCLEX-RN

The National Council Licensure Examination for Registered Nurses (NCLEX-RN) is developed by the National Council of State Boards of Nursing, Inc. The test plan or framework of the examination, which is based on the results of an analysis of the entry-level performance of registered nurses, was used to prepare this book. The test plan is formulated on health care situations that registered nurses commonly encounter and addresses two components: (1) phases of the nursing process and (2) patient needs.

## NURSING PROCESS

There are five phases of the nursing process: (1) assessment, (2) analysis, (3) planning, (4) implementation, and (5) evaluation.

**Assessment.** Assessment involves establishing a data base. The nurse gathers objective and subjective information about the patient. She verifies the data and communicates information gained from the assessment.

**Analysis.** Analysis involves the identification of actual or potential health care needs/problems based on assessment data. The nurse interprets the data, collects additional data as indicated, and identifies and communicates the patient's nursing diagnoses. The nurse also determines the congruency between the patient's needs/problems and ability of the health team members to meet these needs.

**Planning.** Planning is the setting of goals for meeting the patient's needs and designing strategies to attain these goals. The nurse determines the goals of care, develops and modifies the plan, collaborates with other health team members for delivery of the patient's care, and formulates expected outcomes of nursing interventions.

**Implementation.** Implementation involves initiating and completing actions necessary to accomplish the defined goals. The nurse organizes and manages the patient's care, performs or assists the patient in performing activities of daily living, counsels and teaches the patient, significant others, and health team members, and provides care to attain the established patient goals. The nurse also provides care to optimize the achievement of the patient's health care goals; she supervises, coordinates, and evaluates the delivery of the patient's care provided by nursing staff; and she records and exchanges information.

**Evaluation.** Evaluation determines goal achievement. The nurse compares actual with expected outcomes of therapy. She evaluates compliance with prescribed and/or proscribed therapy, and records and describes the patient's response to therapy and/or care. The nurse also modifies the plan as indicated, and reorders priorities.

The five phases of the nursing process are equally important. Therefore, each is represented by an equal number of items on NCLEX-RN.[1]

## CLIENT NEEDS

The health needs of patients are grouped under four broad categories: (1) safe, effective care environment, (2) physiological integrity, (3) psychosocial integrity, and (4) health promotion/maintenance.

**Safe, effective care environment.** The nurse meets the patient's needs for a safe and effective environment by providing and directing nursing care

---

[1]*National Council of State Boards of Nursing, Inc. NCLEX-RN Test Plan for the National Council Licensure Examination for Registered Nurses. Chicago: The National Council of State Boards of Nursing, Inc., 1987*

that promotes attainment of patient needs. These needs include coordinated care, environmental safety, preparation for treatments and procedures, and safe and effective treatments and procedures.

**Physiological integrity.** The nurse meets the physiological integrity of patients with potentially life-threatening and/or recurring physiological conditions, and of patients at risk for the development of complications or untoward effects of treatments or management of modalities. The nurse meets the physiological integrity of these patients by providing and directing nursing care that promotes achievement of such needs as physiological adaptation, mobility, comfort, and provision of basic care.

**Psychosocial integrity.** The nurse meets the patient's needs for psychosocial integrity in stress and crisis-related situations throughout the life cycle. The nurse does this by providing and directing nursing care that promotes achievement of the patient's needs for psychosocial adaptation and coping/adaptation.

**Health promotion/maintenance.** The nurse meets the patient's needs for health promotion/maintenance throughout the life cycle by providing and directing nursing care that promotes achievement, within patients and their significant others, of such needs as continued growth and development, self-care, integrity of support systems, and prevention and early treatment of disease.

Each category of patient need is represented on NCLEX-RN as follows:

1. Safe, effective care
   environment                    25 to 31 percent
2. Physiological integrity        42 to 48 percent
3. Psychosocial integrity          9 to 15 percent
4. Health promotion and
   maintenance                   12 to 18 percent[1]

For further information about NCLEX-RN, write to the National Council of State Boards of Nursing, Inc. For information about the dates, requirements, and specifics of writing the examination in your state, contact the appropriate state board of nursing. The addresses and telephone numbers of the National Council of State Boards of Nursing, Inc. and of each state board of nursing are provided in the appendix.

## FORMAT AND USE OF THIS BOOK AND TEST-TAKING STRATEGIES

This book has been developed to help you prepare to write NCLEX-RN successfully. The format of the book and its organization reflect this purpose. The ef-

fectiveness of your review and success on the examination may be enhanced by following these suggestions:

**1.** Make plans to review over a period of time. Plan your review so that you finish a few days before you are to write NCLEX-RN. Plan to spend most of your review time studying areas about which you feel least confident.

This book is divided into five major sections. The first four sections represent the four main clinical areas of nursing: psychiatric nursing, obstetrical nursing, pediatric nursing, and medical-surgical nursing. The fifth section is composed of four comprehensive tests. This format enables you to review content in a variety of ways, depending on your needs and time constraints.

You can simulate the state board examination by completing each of the four comprehensive tests within 90 minutes. This approach would enable you to determine your areas of strengths and limitations. Once you have identified the areas in which you need more concentrated review, you can complete the questions in the section devoted to that clinical area. Or you can complete tests in each of the first four sections, and culminate your review by completing the comprehensive tests.

NCLEX-RN is comprehensive; that is, each test presents a variety of situations commonly encountered in nursing practice and across all clinical disciplines. Underlying knowledge related to the basic physiopsychosocial sciences, fundamentals of nursing, pharmacology and other therapeutic measures, communicable diseases, legal and ethical considerations, and nutrition, is included in items as applied to a particular patient. This is also true of tests in this book.

**2.** Pace yourself when writing the tests in this book. Plan to answer at least one item per minute. Each test contains approximately 90 items, which is similar to NCLEX-RN. NCLEX-RN is composed of four tests, each containing approximately 90 items. Therefore, on NCLEX-RN you will be expected to answer approximately 90 items in 90 minutes.

The total number of items in this book, 3,057, is much greater than the total number of items on NCLEX-RN (approximately 360). No examination is able to test all knowledge related to a particular course of study. Therefore, the tests in this book, like NCLEX-RN, sample relevant material, but more generously than NCLEX-RN can. The tests in this book will help you review nursing knowledge in preparation for your writing NCLEX-RN from a very broad sampling of knowledge related to nursing practice. Because of this large sampling, more items accompany each health care situation than could be used on NCLEX-RN with its smaller sampling.

**3.** Read each situation with its accompanying choices *carefully* before selecting the correct answer. Be alert for key words, such as *best, least, usually, rarely, highest, lowest, primarily,* and *contra-indicated.* Similarly, be alert to priority items; that is, items that ask what the nurse should do *first* or *next* in a given situation.

Each test item in this book is composed of two parts, a stem and options, which is also true of items on NCLEX-RN. The stem presents the problem and is stated either as a question or as an incomplete sentence. The options in the item present alternatives from which you are asked to select the correct answer. There are four options in each item. Only one option is the *correct* or *best* answer, which is also true of the licensure examination. The other three options are incorrect answers and are called distractors.

On NCLEX-RN the options for the correct answers are selected randomly; there is no pattern of responses for NCLEX-RN. This is also true of this book.

**4.** Focus on the item you are answering and concentrate on understanding the information being tested. Do not let your thoughts wander or return to previous items. Do not search for clues to correct answers among the items.

**5.** Use only the information given in the item when answering the question. Do not read into the question. Read the stem carefully, identifying the specific problem. Try to state the correct answer in your mind and then read the options to find the correct response.

**6.** Select the *one* option you believe to be the *best* or *correct* response for each item. At times you may find the options do not include what you believe to be the best possible response in a particular situation. In such cases, select the *best* answer from the options presented, even though you may believe the best possible choice has not been given.

**7.** Apply basic principles to new or unfamiliar health care situations when you have had little or no experience with the situation given.

**8.** Narrow your choices if you are unsure of the correct answer. In many instances, you may be able to rule out one or two options as incorrect. Eliminating the incorrect options sharpens your thinking. Narrowing your choices helps focus your attention on options that you have identified as being reasonably correct. This increases the chance that you will select the correct answer, even if you are unsure of the correct response. Guessing is not penalized, either in this book or on NCLEX-RN. It is to your advantage to answer *all* questions on NCLEX-RN.

Your NCLEX-RN score, which is reported as pass/fail, is based on the number of correct responses. That score is converted to a standardized score. The percentage of correct responses that equals a passing standardized score is not known to candidates.

**9.** Be prepared to find that some patients described in this book, and on NCLEX-RN, may have health problems not directly related to their reason for seeking health care. For example, a patient who has had a heart attack may have glaucoma. A patient who requires surgery may have diabetes mellitus. This book, like NCLEX-RN, is based on the philosophy that people, not diseases, require care.

**10.** Indicate your choice for the correct answer directly in the book. There are no answer sheets, which is also true of the licensure examination.

**11.** Note on scrap paper any item you find particularly difficult. Skip the item and continue with the examination. This technique enables you to complete all items of which you are certain. After completing all questions in the section, return to the skipped items. Use this approach on NCLEX-RN.

**12.** Look at the correct answers *after* completing the tests in this book. Looking at the correct answers before completing the tests defeats part of the reason for your review and self-evaluation.

**13.** Refer to the section entitled "Correct Answers and Rationales" *after* you have completed each test. Make a check mark next to items you answered incorrectly. After you have completed checking your answers, you can determine the items you answered correctly and those you answered incorrectly. Neither correct answers nor rationales for items on NCLEX-RN are distributed at the examination. Test results are sent to applicants in the mail.

**14.** Study the rationale for each item carefully. Review the answer rationale for *every* question, regardless of whether or not you answered the question correctly. The rationales are comprehensive. They explain why the correct answer is correct, as well as why the distractors are incorrect. To validate an answer, clarify subject matter, or increase your knowledge about a specific content area, consult the references provided for each answer.

**15.** Evaluate your results after completing the tests. Determine the percentage of items you answered correctly in each test. To do so, divide the number of your correct responses by the total number of questions in the test and multiply by 100. For example, if you answered 72 of 90 items correctly in a particular test, divide 72 by 90 and multiply by 100. The result is 80%. If you answered more than 75% of the items correctly, you are most likely prepared to write NCLEX-RN. If, however, you answered less than 75% of the items correctly, examine the items that you answered incorrectly. Did you answer incorrectly because of lack of content knowledge or because you did not read carefully? Lack of knowledge indicates the need for further review in that content area. Errors attributable to not reading carefully indicate the need to do so. Do not sacrifice accuracy in an attempt to answer all of the questions.

**16.** Use relaxation techniques if you experience tension. Use techniques that have worked well for you in the past. Use the same techniques during NCLEX-RN.

Your career begins with passing NCLEX-RN, but learning is a life-long process. As Solon wrote, "I grow old ever learning many things."

# Lippincott's
# State Board Review for
# NCLEX-RN

# PART I

## The Nursing Care of Patients with Psychosocial Alterations

# test 1

*The Patient with a Major Mood Disorder*

*The Patient with Bipolar Disorder, Manic Phase*

*The Patient Who Is Depressed*

*The Patient with Depressive Disorder and Suicidal Ideation*

*The Patient Who Attempts Suicide*

*The Patient in Crisis*

*Correct Answers and Rationales*

Select the one *best* or *correct* answer and indicate your choice by filling in the circle with a pencil in front of the option you have chosen. If the answer you would prefer is not given, select the one you think is *most appropriate.*

## THE PATIENT WITH A MAJOR MOOD DISORDER

Mr. Ned Packard, 62, is admitted to the psychiatric unit of the hospital 1 month after retiring involuntarily. Ms. Frank, a registered nurse, is assigned to care for him. She notes that he keeps his head bowed in a dejected manner and that his facial expression is sad.

1. Ms. Frank visualizes Mr. Packard's depression from a holistic framework. According to holistic theory, Mr. Packard's depression should be viewed as a
   - ○ 1. reaction to a stressful event.
   - ○ 2. symptom of high intake of sugar.
   - ○ 3. disturbance caused by numerous factors.
   - ○ 4. disturbance caused by destructive environmental influences.

2. When Ms. Frank uses the holistic framework in her one-to-one interactions with Mr. Packard, she should plan to focus *primarily* on the patient's
   - ○ 1. dreams and free associations.
   - ○ 2. childhood and past life history.
   - ○ 3. current feelings and experiences.
   - ○ 4. underlying conflicts and defense mechanisms.

3. After a few minutes of conversation, Mr. Packard warily asks the nurse, "Why pick me to talk to when there are so many other people here?" Which of the following replies by the nurse would be *best?*
   - ○ 1. "I am assigned to care for you today, if you will let me."
   - ○ 2. "You have a lot of potential, and I would like to help you."
   - ○ 3. "Why shouldn't I want to talk to you, as well as the others?"
   - ○ 4. "You're wondering why I am interested in you, and not the others?"

4. Ms. Frank meets with Mr. Packard daily. He stays mostly in his room and speaks only when addressed, answering briefly and abruptly while keeping his eyes on the floor. At this stage of their relationship, it would be *best* for Ms. Frank to focus on the ability of the patient to
   - ○ 1. make decisions.
   - ○ 2. relate to other patients.
   - ○ 3. function independently.
   - ○ 4. express himself verbally.

5. Which of the following behaviors of Mr. Packard would *best* indicate to Ms. Frank that her relationship with the patient is in a *working* phase?
   - ○ 1. The patient attempts to familiarize himself with the nurse.
   - ○ 2. The patient makes an effort to describe his problems in detail.
   - ○ 3. The patient tries to summarize his progress in the relationship.
   - ○ 4. The patient starts to challenge the boundaries or outer limits of the relationship.

6. Ms. Frank consciously works to become *aware* of Mr. Packard's feelings and emotions. This practice of trying to comprehend the psychological state of another or of trying to perceive how he feels is called
   - ○ 1. empathy.
   - ○ 2. climate.
   - ○ 3. rapport.
   - ○ 4. sympathy.

7. Mr. Packard is concerned that the information he gives the nurse remain confidential. Which of the following comments would be *best* for the nurse to make in this situation?
   - ○ 1. "We can keep the information just between the two of us if you prefer."
   - ○ 2. "I will share the information with staff members only with your approval."

**3**

○ 3. "You can decide whether your physician needs this information for your care."

○ 4. "If the information you share with me is important in relation to your care, I shall need to share it with the staff."

**8.** On the day following an interview during which Mr. Packard talked at length and tearfully about feeling useless and unmanly since his retirement, he fails to keep an appointment with the nurse. Which of the following actions would it be *best* for the nurse to take next?

○ 1. Assume that he had a good reason for not coming and let him make the next move.

○ 2. Confront him with his behavior and ask him to explain the reason for his absence.

○ 3. Seek him out at the end of the scheduled interview time and tell him he was missed today.

○ 4. Arrange for another session with him later the same day and say nothing about his absence.

**9.** Mr. Packard speaks in an enthusiastic, seemingly sincere manner about his former employer, who was responsible for suddenly replacing him with a younger man: "He surely was a swell fellow. Best boss I ever had. It was a privilege to know him." Which of the following defense mechanisms is Mr. Packard *most probably* using?

○ 1. Sublimation.

○ 2. Suppression.

○ 3. Repression.

○ 4. Reaction formation.

**10.** Mr. Packard begins to attend group therapy daily. He explains to the group how he lost his job after 20 years with the company. Which of the following responses by a group member is *most therapeutic* for the patient?

○ 1. "Tell us about what you did on your job."

○ 2. "It must have been very upsetting for you."

○ 3. "With your skills, finding another job should be easy."

○ 4. "The company must have had some reason for letting you go."

**11.** The physician orders a different drug when Mr. Packard does not respond positively to a tricyclic antidepressant. While the patient is taking the newly prescribed drug, tranylcypromine sulfate (Parnate), which of the following reactions is likely to occur if the patient's diet includes foods containing tyramine?

○ 1. Heart block.

○ 2. Grand mal seizure.

○ 3. Respiratory arrest.

○ 4. Hypertensive crisis.

**12.** While Mr. Packard is taking tranylcypromine sulfate (Parnate), one type of food he should *most* *certainly* be taught to *avoid* because of its high tyramine content is

○ 1. nuts.

○ 2. aged cheeses.

○ 3. grain cereals.

○ 4. reconstituted milk.

**13.** Mr. Packard obtains permission for a 24-hour pass to go home. Which of the following suggestions concerning how his family can prepare for the visit indicates the *best* understanding of the patient's needs?

○ 1. Planning to encourage the patient to do some job hunting.

○ 2. Limiting friends' visiting so that the patient can rest during the day.

○ 3. Scheduling a day of interesting activities for the patient outside of the home.

○ 4. Planning to involve the patient in usual at-home pursuits of the immediate family.

**14.** Which of the following subjects would be *most helpful* to discuss when preparing to terminate the nurse-patient relationship between Ms. Frank and Mr. Packard?

○ 1. The gains the patient has made during therapy.

○ 2. The plans the patient should make to find a job.

○ 3. The knowledge that the patient's daughter is divorcing her husband.

○ 4. The conflicts the patient has had with another staff member.

**15.** Ms. Frank reviews the counseling sessions she had with Mr. Packard with the clinical nurse specialist (CNS) on the unit. Consulting the CNS serves many purposes, but the overall *primary* purpose is to

○ 1. increase nurse awareness of patient behavior.

○ 2. increase nurse awareness of patient thoughts.

○ 3. evaluate nursing practice.

○ 4. evaluate nursing style.

**16.** Which of the following possible reactions of Mr. Packard to termination of his relationship with Ms. Frank should be considered the *most* healthy?

○ 1. A lack of response.

○ 2. A display of anger.

○ 3. An attempt at humor.

○ 4. An expression of grief.

## THE PATIENT WITH BIPOLAR DISORDER, MANIC PHASE

Mrs. Stephanie Jamet, 56, insists on being taken to her room immediately upon admission to the hospital. She orders one nurse to unpack her clothes, another to bring her some coffee, and a third to get her agent on the phone for her. She states, "I am the greatest actress since Sarah Bernhardt. I will take my meals in my room. You may prepare my bath now." Mr. Jamet says his wife has not slept for three nights and has spent her days writing checks to charitable institutions, which they can ill afford to do. Mrs. Jamet has bipolar disorder, manic phase.

17. For which of the following qualities would the nursing staff *most likely* look when deciding in which room to house Mrs. Jamet?
    ○ 1. A cordial roommate.
    ○ 2. A quiet atmosphere.
    ○ 3. A view of the hospital grounds.
    ○ 4. A large amount of storage space.

18. Mr. Jamet apologizes to the nurse for his wife's demanding behavior. Which of the following possible replies would be *best* for the nurse to make?
    ○ 1. "I am sure she is doing the best she can."
    ○ 2. "It's all right. We have been treated worse."
    ○ 3. "It must be hard for you to see her like this."
    ○ 4. "I understand. What happened to set her off like this?"

19. Mrs. Jamet puts out her hand and says to the nurse, "Watch out! Here I come." She then puts her hand down and sits in a chair. At this time, after the nurse determines that the patient is not about to harm anyone, it would be *best* for the nurse to intervene by
    ○ 1. giving the patient a book of her choice to read.
    ○ 2. placing the patient in isolation to work out her aggression in private.
    ○ 3. taking the patient to a punching bag for exercise to release excess energy.
    ○ 4. having the patient continue to sit while holding her hands to help her gain control of herself.

20. Mrs. Jamet is scheduled to go to the radiology department. Before taking the patient for her x-ray examination, which of the following actions should the nurse take?
    ○ 1. Explain the x-ray procedure to her in simple terms.
    ○ 2. Give her a detailed explanation of the x-ray procedure.
    ○ 3. Say nothing to the patient before taking her to the x-ray department.
    ○ 4. Bring another staff member along in case she resists going to the x-ray department.

21. The nurse notes that Mrs. Jamet is too busy investigating the unit and overseeing the activities of other patients to eat much dinner. To help Mrs. Jamet obtain sufficient nourishment, which of the following plans would be *best* for the nurses to implement?

○ 1. Serve foods that she can carry with her.
○ 2. Allow her to send out for her favorite foods.
○ 3. Serve food in small, attractively arranged portions.
○ 4. Allow her in the unit kitchen for extra food as necessary.

22. Later the same evening, Mrs. Jamet appears at the nurses' station with brightly rouged cheeks, ornaments in her hair, and three pairs of false eyelashes. She is wearing a sheer nightgown, high heels, and bracelets up to her elbows. Which of the following actions should the nurse take in relation to the patient's attire?
    ○ 1. Redirect the patient to her room and assist her to put on proper apparel.
    ○ 2. Allow the patient to wear what she likes and get her involved in a unit activity.
    ○ 3. Remind the patient that she agreed to wear slacks and a shirt when out of her room.
    ○ 4. Ask the patient to put on hospital pajamas since she has not earned the privilege of wearing her own clothing.

23. While watching television in a lounge, Mrs. Jamet says quickly and abruptly to the nurse, "The sun is shining. My son is in Virginia. Who's afraid of Virginia Woolf?" Which of the following disorders is the patient displaying?
    ○ 1. Concreteness.
    ○ 2. Flight of ideas.
    ○ 3. Depersonalization.
    ○ 4. Use of neologisms.

24. The speech pattern (described in the previous item) that Mrs. Jamet is using is *chiefly* due to
    ○ 1. feelings of anxiety.
    ○ 2. loose ego boundaries.
    ○ 3. underlying hostilities.
    ○ 4. distortions in the self-concept.

25. Which of the following responses would be the *most therapeutic* for the nurse to make when Mrs. Jamet says, "The sun is shining. My son is in Virginia. Who's afraid of Virginia Woolf?"
    ○ 1. "Let's talk about what you did today instead."
    ○ 2. "How does the sun shining relate to your son being in Virginia?"
    ○ 3. "You are talking nonsense. Why don't you try to stay on one subject?"
    ○ 4. "I cannot follow you. It would help me if you would speak a little slower."

26. If the following activities are available, which would be *most therapeutic* for channeling Mrs. Jamet's hyperactive behavior?
    ○ 1. Allowing the patient to lead some group activities.

○ 2. Allowing the patient to clean her room and the dayroom.

○ 3. Allowing the patient to read to patients who are depressed.

○ 4. Allowing the patient to exercise and move about as much as possible.

**27.** Which of the following feeling states does Mrs. Jamet's behavior during a manic episode reflect?

○ 1. Guilt, projected onto others.

○ 2. Anger, turned against the self.

○ 3. Distrust, focused on the family.

○ 4. Hostility, directed against the environment.

**28.** Mrs. Jamet sometimes makes inappropriate requests. For example, she calls a department store to order several dresses and pairs of shoes and charges them to her husband's account. Which of the following nursing interventions would be *best* in this situation?

○ 1. Tell the patient that her request will be filled.

○ 2. Explain to the patient that her request is denied.

○ 3. Suggest to the patient that part of her request can be met.

○ 4. Call the store to cancel the request without telling the patient.

**29.** The nurse evaluates Mrs. Jamet's physical condition daily. During the patient's period of euphoria, for which of these conditions should the nurse be *especially* alert?

○ 1. Gastritis and vertigo.

○ 2. Exhaustion and infections.

○ 3. Convulsions and dermatitis.

○ 4. Bradycardia and palpitations.

**30.** The drug regimen for the management of Mrs. Jamet's hyperactivity includes the administration of lithium carbonate (Lithane). While Mrs. Jamet is taking this drug, the nurse should make certain that the patient has an adequate intake of

○ 1. sodium.

○ 2. iron.

○ 3. iodine.

○ 4. calcium.

**31.** Which of the following clinical manifestations would alert the nurse to lithium carbonate (Lithane) toxicity?

○ 1. Increasingly agitated behavior.

○ 2. Markedly increased food intake.

○ 3. Sudden increase in blood pressure.

○ 4. Anorexia with nausea and vomiting.

**32.** After 10 days of treatment with lithium carbonate (Lithane), Mrs. Jamet's lithium level is 1.0 mEq/L. The nurse knows that this indicates which of the following?

○ 1. A laboratory error.

○ 2. An anticipated therapeutic blood level of the drug.

○ 3. An atypical patient response to the drug.

○ 4. An idiosyncratic reaction to the drug.

**33.** Mrs. Jamet expresses the belief that she was born out of wedlock to a famous woman. When dealing with this delusion of grandeur, the nurse should *first* try to

○ 1. get the patient to discuss another topic.

○ 2. involve the patient in a simple group project.

○ 3. convince the patient that she is wrong in her belief.

○ 4. satisfy the implied need of the patient to feel important.

**34.** Mrs. Jamet becomes angry and utters a stream of profanities when her charmingly delivered request for a pass is refused by the physician. Which of the following statements describes the *best* evaluation of the patient's behavior?

○ 1. The patient's anger is usually not intended personally.

○ 2. The patient's anger is usually a reliable sign of serious pathology.

○ 3. The patient's anger is usually an intended attack on the physician's skills.

○ 4. The patient's anger is usually a sign that the patient's condition is improving.

**35.** A goal in Mrs. Jamet's treatment plan is to reduce her activity and aggression. Which of the following comments the nurse could make when the patient's anger escalates would *best* help the patient move toward her treatment goal?

○ 1. "You must go to your room or into seclusion now."

○ 2. "You are disturbing other patients. If you do not stop, you will need to go into seclusion."

○ 3. "You have a choice of going to your room now voluntarily or being escorted to your room."

○ 4. "Your behavior is disrupting the unit. Let's find a quiet place and talk about what is happening."

**36.** Mrs. Jamet improves with the help of drug and relationship therapy. She appears less often at the nurses' station and makes fewer demands. In relation to her prognosis, when this particular illness has abated, it is *most likely* that the symptoms of her mood disorder will

○ 1. not occur again.

○ 2. recur periodically.

○ 3. prove ultimately fatal.

○ 4. increase in occurrence with age.

**37.** Mr. Jamet asks the nurse what he can do to help his wife when she goes home from the hospital. Of the following actions, which would probably be *least helpful* for the family members to take on behalf of the patient?

○ 1. Try to keep the patient free from worry and anxiety.

○ 2. Relieve the patient of some home responsibilities she had.

○ 3. Develop effective communication techniques with the patient at home.

○ 4. Learn to recognize when the patient is showing signs of drug toxicity.

**38.** To which of the following factors is Mrs. Jamet's illness *most likely* related?

○ 1. Having been molested as a preschool child.

○ 2. Having a family history of manic depression.

○ 3. Building up high serotonin levels in the brain.

○ 4. Drinking alcoholic beverages more frequently than usual.

## THE PATIENT WHO IS DEPRESSED

Mrs. Mary Bullen, 49, is admitted involuntarily to a psychiatric hospital. Her admission is for 30 days by court order. Documents sent with her cite, among other things, that she will not eat because she feels her stomach "is missing" and her bowels have "turned to jelly," and she views this as "just punishment for my past wickedness and for the evil I have brought on my family."

**39.** To be evaluated as being legally committable, which of the following criteria did Mrs. Bullen *most likely* have to meet?

○ 1. The patient had to be psychotic.

○ 2. The patient must have tried to harm herself or others.

○ 3. The patient must have been unable to afford private treatment.

○ 4. The patient must have made threatening remarks to friends or relatives.

**40.** Which of the following rights did Mrs. Bullen lose by virtue of being admitted involuntarily to a psychiatric hospital?

○ 1. The right to send and receive mail.

○ 2. The right to vote in a national election.

○ 3. The right to make a will or legally binding contract.

○ 4. The right to sign out of the hospital against medical advice.

**41.** Through which of the following legal methods could Mrs. Bullen seek release from the psychiatric hospital if she believes she is being improperly detained?

○ 1. A malpractice suit.

○ 2. A guardianship hearing.

○ 3. A writ of habeas corpus.

○ 4. A lien of property petition.

**42.** When Mrs. Bullen expresses feelings of unworthiness, it would be *best* for the nurse to respond by saying,

○ 1. "Your family loves you even if you feel unworthy."

○ 2. "Your idea of being unworthy is just your imagination."

○ 3. "It would be best for you to try to forget the idea that you are unworthy."

○ 4. "As you begin to feel better, your ideas of unworthiness will begin to disappear."

**43.** Mrs. Bullen has not been eating. After serving the patient her tray, which of the following actions by the nurse is *most likely* to encourage Mrs. Bullen to eat?

○ 1. Leave the patient's room without comment.

○ 2. Sit beside the patient and place the fork in her hand.

○ 3. Tell the patient that she will not recover unless she eats.

○ 4. Comment on how good the food looks.

**44.** Mrs. Bullen is to receive tube feedings because she continues to refuse food in any form. Gastric gavage is usually used as a *last* resort with the suspicious patient because the feedings are *very likely* to

○ 1. be aspirated by the person.

○ 2. arouse fears of dying in the person.

○ 3. be viewed as an attack on the person.

○ 4. increase the irritability of the person.

**45.** Mrs. Bullen becomes restless and increasingly incoherent at night. Besides administering a prescribed antipsychotic medication, which of the following actions by the nurse would be *most helpful* for the patient at this time?

○ 1. Encourage the patient to talk about her family.

○ 2. Read to the patient with the lights turned down low.

○ 3. Help the patient take a cool shower before retiring.

○ 4. Sit quietly with the patient until the medication takes effect.

**46.** Mrs. Bullen demands to be left alone to die. "If you try to cheat the avenger, you will suffer," Mrs. Bullen tells the nurse. Which of the following possible replies by the nurse would be *best?*

○ 1. "I will not let anything harm you."

○ 2. "It sounds like you are trying to frighten me."

○ 3. "I'm not trying to cheat anyone. What do you mean by that?"

○ 4. "I'll leave you alone for 15 minutes. Then I will be back to see how you are doing."

47. Mrs. Bullen repeatedly tells the nurse that she has accepted suffering as a fact of life and that the nurse should stop trying to change her life. The nurse would correctly assess that Mrs. Bullen's depression includes which of the following thought patterns?

○ 1. Manipulation.
○ 2. Agitation.
○ 3. Delusions.
○ 4. Hallucinations.

48. The nurse also assesses that Mrs. Bullen has been under a significant amount of stress recently. Which of the following stressors is *most likely* to be occurring in Mrs. Bullen's life at this time?

○ 1. Social role changes.
○ 2. Fear of pregnancy.
○ 3. Peer pressure.
○ 4. Old age.

49. Which of the following factors *most likely* has the greatest impact on Mrs. Bullen's ability to handle stress at this time?

○ 1. Her grooming and appearance.
○ 2. Her family's attitude toward her.
○ 3. The weather.
○ 4. Her weight.

50. After expressing much concern about his wife's welfare, Mr. Bullen asks the nurse if Mrs. Bullen would be better off if he were out of her life. The nurse should base her reply on knowledge that

○ 1. Mr. Bullen probably feels at fault.
○ 2. Mr. Bullen is hard to get along with.
○ 3. Mr. Bullen wants a divorce.
○ 4. depression affects significant relationships.

51. Mrs. Bullen tells the nurse that she and her husband have not had sexual intercourse since her husband had a heart attack 6 months ago. When counseling Mr. and Mrs. Bullen, the nurse should point out that sexual intercourse following a myocardial infarction can be safely resumed after Mr. Bullen is able to

○ 1. run around the block.
○ 2. play a game of tennis.
○ 3. walk up two flights of stairs.
○ 4. maintain an erection for 5 minutes.

52. The goal of nursing care that should have *highest* priority when Mrs. Bullen demonstrates suicidal tendencies is to

○ 1. provide contact between the patient and her husband.
○ 2. use measures to protect the patient from harming herself.

○ 3. reassure the patient of her worthiness in a gentle manner.
○ 4. maintain a calm environment in which the patient can express her feelings and thoughts.

53. Nortriptyline hydrochloride (Aventyl) is ordered for Mrs. Bullen. After the nurse explains the purpose of the medication to Mr. and Mrs. Bullen, Mr. Bullen asks, "If she starts taking the pills, she will have to take them the rest of her life, won't she?" Which of the following would be the *most accurate* and *therapeutic* reply for the nurse to make?

○ 1. "Her condition determines the need for continued medication."
○ 2. "The medication prescribed is safe and routine."
○ 3. "After the symptoms decrease, the need for medication will be re-evaluated."
○ 4. "Are you concerned about her taking the medication?"

54. Which of the following health status assessments must be completed before Mrs. Bullen starts taking nortriptyline hydrochloride (Aventyl)?

○ 1. An electrocardiogram (EKG).
○ 2. A urine sample for protein.
○ 3. A thyroid scan.
○ 4. A creatinine clearance test.

55. One of the nurses strongly believes that all psychiatric medication is a form of "chemical mind control." When Mrs. Bullen's daughter asks about the efficacy of antidepressant medications, which of the following courses of action would be *best* for the nurse to take?

○ 1. Give her an honest opinion of the treatment.
○ 2. Refer her to another knowledgeable person for information about the treatment.
○ 3. Explain that she does not have the most current statistics about the efficacy of the treatment.
○ 4. Give her a photocopy of the package insert.

56. The nurse develops a medication teaching plan for Mrs. Bullen. *All* of the following are essential components of the teaching plan *except*

○ 1. a description of possible side effects.
○ 2. an opportunity for Mrs. Bullen to express her fears and concerns about the therapy.
○ 3. a description of the current research about antidepressant therapy.
○ 4. an explanation of why the first dose of medication is less than a full dose.

57. Mrs. Bullen has been taking nortriptyline hydrochloride (Aventyl) 150 mg at bedtime for 5 days. The nurse *correctly* judges that the medication is beginning to produce therapeutic effects when the patient

○ 1. asks for a snack of cookies.
○ 2. sleeps 12 to 14 hours a night.
○ 3. states that she can feel her stomach growing back.
○ 4. asks to take the medication in the morning.

**58.** Mrs. Bullen says that the medication is helping her feel less depressed, but she is very upset about the side effects. Of the following side effects of tricyclic antidepressant medications, which is the *most* common?
○ 1. Urticaria.
○ 2. Dry mouth.
○ 3. Rash.
○ 4. Diaphoresis.

**59.** Mrs. Bullen's condition improves, but she still remains alone in her room most of the time. Which of the following statements by the nurse is *most likely* to help Mrs. Bullen become involved with a unit activity?
○ 1. "Mrs. Bullen, would you like to go to the movie with me today?"
○ 2. "Mrs. Bullen, I will be back at 4 p.m. to take you to the movie."
○ 3. "Mrs. Bullen, I hope you go to the movie this afternoon. It will cheer you up."
○ 4. "Mrs. Bullen, you might want to go to the movie in the dayroom this afternoon."

**60.** Which of the following adaptive actions is *most likely* to improve Mrs. Bullen's ability to cope with the stress in her life?
○ 1. Being involved with people she enjoys.
○ 2. Continuing to take mild tranquilizers at home.
○ 3. Attending marital therapy sessions with her husband.
○ 4. Developing crisis intervention techniques.

## THE PATIENT WITH DEPRESSIVE DISORDER AND SUICIDAL IDEATION

A nurse who makes weekly rounds of area boarding homes observes a patient who was discharged from a psychiatric hospital. The patient, Ms. Rachel Cory, 65, is irritable and walks about her room slowly and morosely.

**61.** After 10 minutes the nurse prepares to leave, since Ms. Cory seems to have nothing to say. But each time the nurse tries to leave, Ms. Cory plucks at her sleeve and quickly asks for help in rearranging her belongings or moving small articles of furniture she could easily have moved herself. She also anxiously makes inconsequential remarks to keep the nurse with her. Which of the following statements provides the *most likely* explanation for the patient's behavior?
○ 1. The patient is lonely and looking for a way to pass the time.
○ 2. The patient is self-centered and possessive of the nurse's time.
○ 3. The patient needs attention paid to some as yet unknown concern.
○ 4. The patient desires assistance to improve the appearance of her room.

**62.** The nurse is careful not to act rushed or impatient with Ms. Cory and gradually learns that the patient is very "down" and feels worthless and unloved. In view of the fact that Ms. Cory made a suicidal gesture previously when unhappy, which of the following interventions by the nurse is indicated at this time?
○ 1. She should ask the patient frankly if she has thoughts of or plans for committing suicide.
○ 2. She should avoid bringing up the subject of suicide to prevent giving the patient ideas of self-harm.
○ 3. She should outline some alternative measures to suicide for the patient to use during periods of sadness.
○ 4. She should mention others she has known who have felt like the patient and attempted suicide, to draw her out.

**63.** The nurse evaluates Ms. Cory's depression and is *most* concerned about the depression when Ms. Cory tells her that she
○ 1. feels more tired than usual.
○ 2. has difficulty falling asleep and wakes up early in the morning.
○ 3. no longer watches her favorite television programs.
○ 4. is gaining weight.

**64.** A friend of Ms. Cory asks the nurse, "What is the best way to act around her since she's been so blue?" When the nurse considers therapeutic ways to behave with Ms. Cory, it would be *best* for her to recommend that the friend *avoid* behaving in a way that is
○ 1. firm.
○ 2. serious.
○ 3. cheerful.
○ 4. spontaneous.

**65.** Ms. Cory is to receive amitriptyline hydrochloride (Elavil). How long after Ms. Cory begins taking the medication can the nurse expect that it will *most likely* achieve the desired effect of lifting the patient's depression?
○ 1. Almost immediately.
○ 2. Within a few days.

○ 3. In 2 to 4 weeks.

○ 4. After about 6 to 7 weeks.

66. The nurse begins visiting Ms. Cory daily to evaluate her condition and progress. The *main* focus of a planned activity program for Ms. Cory at this time is to improve her

    ○ 1. mobilization.

    ○ 2. socialization.

    ○ 3. nutrition.

    ○ 4. rest.

67. As the nurse helps Ms. Cory plan an activity program, which action by the nurse is likely to be *most helpful* for Ms. Cory?

    ○ 1. Finding a volunteer to visit regularly at the boarding home.

    ○ 2. Arranging for Meals-on-Wheels.

    ○ 3. Arranging transportation to a senior citizens' social group that meets near the boarding home.

    ○ 4. Asking a friend of the patient to spend more time with her.

68. It is difficult to maintain effective relationships with depressed persons such as Ms. Cory because their

    ○ 1. pessimism arouses frustration and anger in others.

    ○ 2. poor personal grooming invites disgust and ridicule from others.

    ○ 3. independence prevents them from asking for any kind of assistance.

    ○ 4. laziness keeps them from putting forth the necessary effort to get well.

69. Ms. Cory complains that her mouth feels dry after she takes amitriptyline hydrochloride (Elavil) for about a week. Which of the following measures would be *least* desirable to relieve the dryness in the patient's mouth?

    ○ 1. Chew sugarless gum.

    ○ 2. Suck on hard candies.

    ○ 3. Drink plenty of fluids.

    ○ 4. Rinse the mouth with water.

70. The nurse judges *correctly* that Ms. Cory is experiencing an adverse effect from amitriptyline hydrochloride (Elavil) when Ms. Cory demonstrates having

    ○ 1. diarrhea.

    ○ 2. insomnia.

    ○ 3. hypertension.

    ○ 4. urinary retention.

71. Ms. Cory continues to stress her faults in conversations with the nurse even though her insomnia improves and her poverty of thought diminishes. When Ms. Cory starts to point out the things she cannot do, which of the following responses by the nurse would provide the *best* intervention?

    ○ 1. "You can do anything you put your mind to."

    ○ 2. "Try to think more positively about yourself."

    ○ 3. "Let's talk about your plans for the weekend."

    ○ 4. "You were able to write a letter to your friend today."

72. The nurse has important business to attend to elsewhere, so she tells Ms. Cory that she will spend more time with her at their next weekly meeting. When the nurse arrives as planned, Ms. Cory is taciturn and sits staring angrily at her. When dealing with this situation, which of the following actions that the nurse could take would probably be the *least helpful?*

    ○ 1. Commenting that the patient looks angry.

    ○ 2. Remaining silent until the patient decides to talk.

    ○ 3. Asking the patient what her thoughts are at the moment.

    ○ 4. Apologizing for not being more available to the patient the previous week.

73. Before the nurse decides which strategy she will use with the patient, Ms. Cory blurts out, "You hate me, don't you?" Which of the following replies that the nurse could make would be the *most therapeutic?*

    ○ 1. "You are imagining things."

    ○ 2. "I could never hate anyone."

    ○ 3. "What did I do or say to give you that impression?"

    ○ 4. "You are unhappy with me for not staying last week, aren't you?"

74. Ms. Cory would like to have someone comfort her. At the same time she dreads the questions it may raise and the explanations she may be required to make. The nurse judges that the patient is *most likely* exhibiting a phenomenon called

    ○ 1. a conflict.

    ○ 2. an impulse.

    ○ 3. a regression.

    ○ 4. an ego break.

75. Although Ms. Cory would like comfort, she isolates herself from others because of her anger and pessimism. Which of the following interventions by the nurse would be *most therapeutic* in helping Ms. Cory deal with her feelings?

    ○ 1. Ignore the angry behavior and focus on the patient's needs for comfort.

    ○ 2. Confront the angry behavior and help the patient learn more positive behaviors.

    ○ 3. Listen to the patient's angry statements and help her plan a schedule to keep occupied.

○ 4. Acknowledge the angry behavior and deal with the feeling content of the patient's behavior.

**76.** Which of the following events has *most likely* been experienced recently when people like Ms. Cory become depressed?
○ 1. Financial upset.
○ 2. Physical injury.
○ 3. Real or imagined loss of a loved object.
○ 4. Increased personal or social responsibility.

**77.** The nurse makes a *correct* judgment when she concludes that the danger of a suicide attempt is *greatest* when Ms. Cory's behavior indicates that she
○ 1. resumes her former life-style.
○ 2. has a return in her energy level.
○ 3. is at a point of deepest despair.
○ 4. agrees to visit with an estranged brother.

**78.** Which of the following variables should the nurse judge as *least likely* to indicate high risk when she assesses Ms. Cory's potential for suicide?
○ 1. The patient's age.
○ 2. The patient's angry behavior.
○ 3. The patient's home environment.
○ 4. The patient's previous suicidal gesture.

**79.** Which of the following defense mechanisms would Ms. Cory be using if she adopts the nurse's ideas and attitudes as her own?
○ 1. Introjection.
○ 2. Restitution.
○ 3. Conversion.
○ 4. Substitution.

## THE PATIENT WHO ATTEMPTS SUICIDE

Jenny Kline, 16, is brought to the emergency room of the hospital in a state of unconsciousness after having swallowed "a bottle of red pills" 45 minutes earlier. The pills are identified as secobarbital (Seconal). A suicide note is found that asks for forgiveness and states, "I can't live without my boyfriend. He has left me because I'm no good."

**80.** Which of the following measures should the nurse be prepared to carry out when Jenny is admitted?
○ 1. Forcing fluids.
○ 2. Giving a diuretic.
○ 3. Inducing vomiting.
○ 4. Lavaging the stomach.

**81.** Which of the following interventions should be of *primary* concern to the nurse after Jenny's physical condition is no longer critical?
○ 1. Providing the patient with a safe environment.
○ 2. Ensuring that the patient's diet is high in fiber.
○ 3. Providing the patient with quiet periods for reflection.
○ 4. Ensuring that the patient's fluid intake is generous.

**82.** After Jenny regains consciousness, she says to the nurse, "I can't even kill myself. I can't even do that right." Which of the following responses would be *most therapeutic* for the nurse to make at this time?
○ 1. "These feelings will pass."
○ 2. "Is that how you are feeling?"
○ 3. "Why would you feel that way?"
○ 4. "You have a great deal to live for."

**83.** When the nurse evaluates the effectiveness of Jenny's therapy, the nurse can judge that progress is being made when the patient's behavior illustrates an improvement in her
○ 1. appetite.
○ 2. self-concept.
○ 3. activity level.
○ 4. gender identity conflict.

**84.** Family therapy sessions are initiated for Jenny, her parents, and her older brother. Which of the following statements reflects the *most important* reason why family therapy is initiated in this situation?
○ 1. The parents need guidance to deal with the dysfunctional adolescent.
○ 2. A dysfunctional parent-child relationship affects everyone in the family.
○ 3. Overpermissive or overrestrictive parenting causes dysfunctioning in the adolescent.
○ 4. The parents feel a strong sense of failure in the rearing of the dysfunctional adolescent.

**85.** Jenny goes to her room and slams the door immediately after the first family therapy session. Jenny says to the nurse, "I'm so mad. The therapist did not let me tell my side of the story. He just agreed with everything my parents said." Which of the following actions by the nurse would be *most therapeutic* in this situation?
○ 1. Consider terminating the therapy because it upsets the patient.
○ 2. Redirect the patient to the therapist to tell him how she feels.
○ 3. Allow the patient to continue to ventilate her feelings to the nurse.
○ 4. Suggest to the therapist that he allow the patient to tell her side of the story.

86. Jenny tells the nurse that before her admission she had one homosexual experience with a classmate and is feeling confused about this encounter. Which of the following statements *best* describes *most* homosexual experiences during adolescence?
    ○ 1. A homosexual experience often leads to sexual dysfunctioning.
    ○ 2. A homosexual experience is not an unusual occurrence during adolescence.
    ○ 3. A homosexual experience often indicates fear of the opposite sex.
    ○ 4. A homosexual experience will increase gender identity confusion.

87. The adolescent unit where Jenny is housed uses behavior modification to encourage appropriate patient behaviors. Which of the following statements *best* describes the theory on which behavior modification has been developed?
    ○ 1. Behavior is learned.
    ○ 2. Behavior is related to intrapsychic conflicts.
    ○ 3. Behavioral changes result from stress on the individual and his body systems.
    ○ 4. Behavior is a result of interaction between an individual and the environment.

## THE PATIENT IN CRISIS

Ms. George, Ms. Salter, and Mr. Victor are nurse counselors at a crisis shelter. The length of their experience in crisis counseling ranges from 3 weeks to 2 years. Several patients arrive at the shelter one evening simultaneously.

88. Ms. George brings Cari, an anxious-looking, pretty blonde teenager, to an interviewing room. The girl sobs and says that she thinks she is pregnant but does not know what to do. Which of the following possible interventions would be the *most appropriate* at this time?
    ○ 1. Ask the patient what she had thought of doing.
    ○ 2. Give the patient some ideas about what to do next.
    ○ 3. Summarize what the nurse heard and ask the patient to confirm the nurse's perceptions.
    ○ 4. Question the patient in more detail about her feelings and about what her parents' reactions are likely to be.

89. Cari says that she and her boyfriend have engaged in "mostly heavy petting and necking." Which of the following responses would be *best* for the nurse to make to Cari's comment?
    ○ 1. "You mean you have had sexual intercourse?"

○ 2. "You will need to describe what heavy petting and necking means."
○ 3. "I think we need to talk about what is involved in sexual intercourse."
○ 4. "All you have been doing with your boyfriend is heavy petting and necking?"

90. Cari says she would rather die than be pregnant. Which of the following responses would be *most helpful* for the nurse to make?
    ○ 1. "Try not to worry until after the pregnancy test."
    ○ 2. "Pregnancy is normal."
    ○ 3. "Why are you so upset?"
    ○ 4. "You are very upset now; it will be easier for you to talk about this if you can relax."

91. Ms. George teaches Cari about sexual intercourse, contraception, and the like. For which of the following behaviors will the nurse *most probably* be indirectly responsible for increasing in Cari?
    ○ 1. The patient's promiscuity.
    ○ 2. The patient's antagonism toward men.
    ○ 3. The patient's rejection of the female role.
    ○ 4. The patient's responsibility for sexual encounters.

92. Cari states that although she is grateful for the information she has received from Ms. George, she does not believe she needs it. "No more fooling around for me!" she states. Which of the following replies by the somewhat skeptical nurse would be *best*?
    ○ 1. "Just in case, why don't you try the pills for a while?"
    ○ 2. "The last person who said that ended up having a baby."
    ○ 3. "It's up to you, but if you should change your mind, come back and we'll try to help you."
    ○ 4. "Aren't you being a little bit overconfident about it, as attractive as you must be to the fellows?"

93. Mr. Victor talks to two 11-year-old boys on the telephone who think a friend sniffs glue. They say his breath sometimes smells like glue and he acts "drunk." They ask if they should tell their parents about the friend. When the nurse formulates a reply, he should be guided by the knowledge that
    ○ 1. the boys probably fear punishment.
    ○ 2. sniffing glue is illegal.
    ○ 3. the boys' observations could be wrong.
    ○ 4. glue-sniffing is a minor form of substance abuse.

94. Mr. Victor urges the boys to seek help for their friend and warns them that delayed treatment could result in the boy's death. A person who

inhales noxious substances is *most likely* to die from

- ○ 1. brain lesions.
- ○ 2. malnutrition.
- ○ 3. cardiac failure.
- ○ 4. kidney damage.

**95.** Ms. Salter is caring for Fred Seymour, a 19-year-old patient who came to the crisis shelter with friends. Fred is frightened and behaving aggressively. The nurse learns that he has smoked cocaine for the last 3 hours. The name for smoked cocaine is

- ○ 1. p-dope.
- ○ 2. dope.
- ○ 3. stuff.
- ○ 4. crack.

**96.** Fred is having a severe reaction to the cocaine. He is very suspicious of his friends who came with him and he does not want to talk to the nurse. He seems to have lost touch with reality. Suddenly he yells out, "I'll kill you before I'll let you take me." The nurse should base his intervention on knowledge that Fred's primary need is

- ○ 1. physical contact with his friends.
- ○ 2. isolation from other patients.
- ○ 3. reassurance from the staff.
- ○ 4. protection from his own behavior.

**97.** Which of the following comments would be *most useful* for the nurse to make to Fred to help him re-establish his self-control and orientation?

- ○ 1. "You have no need to be concerned. You are going to be all right."
- ○ 2. "You have taken a drug you should not have and it is making you sick."
- ○ 3. "You are reacting to the cocaine and will soon be past the main drug reaction. You are safe here."
- ○ 4. "You have a temporary psychosis from taking a psychedelic. Let's watch some television while we wait for it to pass."

**98.** The use of tranquilizing drugs, such as chlorpromazine hydrochloride (Thorazine), to shorten the drug reaction Fred experienced, should be *avoided* because

- ○ 1. the major tranquilizers can cause a reuptake of the drug in the brain.
- ○ 2. flashbacks increase in severity when mediating drugs are used to treat the initial reaction.
- ○ 3. the emotions might stem from a source entirely different from the cocaine.
- ○ 4. other incompatible drugs may have been combined with the cocaine that, together with the tranquilizer, might be fatal.

**99.** If Fred describes the following effects from using

cocaine, the nurse should be *skeptical* if the patient says cocaine helps

- ○ 1. give him energy.
- ○ 2. him focus on his work.
- ○ 3. him need less sleep.
- ○ 4. cope more effectively in social situations.

**100.** If Fred continues to use cocaine on a long-term basis, it is *very likely* that he might

- ○ 1. develop a tolerance for the drug.
- ○ 2. become psychologically addicted.
- ○ 3. become physically addicted.
- ○ 4. have children with birth defects.

Sheila Boone, 17, has come to the crisis shelter because she wants to "ask someone a question." Matter-of-factly she asks, "How would you feel if your girlfriend had been raped?"

**101.** Mr. Victor suspects that Sheila may have been sexually assaulted. Which would be the nurse's *best* reply to Sheila's question?

- ○ 1. "Before I answer, tell me what's really on your mind, okay?"
- ○ 2. "I have not thought about it. How would you expect me to feel?"
- ○ 3. "Probably I'd be upset and angry. Do you have a special reason for asking?"
- ○ 4. "It would bother me. But don't you think there is too much violence these days?"

**102.** Sheila has been ambivalent about telling anyone of a recent sexual assault on her. Which of the following beliefs about the rape experience is probably the *most widely* held in this society and no doubt has contributed to the patient's reluctance to speak about being raped?

- ○ 1. The woman is somehow to blame for the rape.
- ○ 2. The woman is probably out to "get" the man involved.
- ○ 3. The woman must show physical injury to prove her innocence.
- ○ 4. The woman gets more enjoyment than pain from the experience.

**103.** Sheila has constantly sought out brightly lit places and the company of friendly people since the rape. She also plans to move to another part of the city. When the nurse analyzes Sheila's behavior, the nurse *correctly* identifies the patient's *most likely* goal for her maneuvers as being

- ○ 1. self-defense.
- ○ 2. self-assertion.
- ○ 3. self-deception.
- ○ 4. self-gratification.

**104.** In which of the following instances can the nurse anticipate that Sheila will have future adjustment problems and a need for additional counseling in relation to being sexually assaulted?
○ 1. When she becomes upset when talking about the rape to anyone.
○ 2. When she seeks support from formerly ignored relatives and friends.
○ 3. When her parents show shame and suspicion about her part in the rape.
○ 4. When her life becomes focused on helping other rape victims like herself.

**105.** When a rape victim arrives at an emergency room for treatment, which of the following measures should the nursing staff be *especially* sure to carry out for its own and the patient's legal protection?
○ 1. Keep prying, insensitive personnel away from the victim.
○ 2. Record the victim's account of the assault in her own words.
○ 3. Arrange for the victim to be escorted home by a trustworthy person.
○ 4. Hand-carry any evidence from the victim's person to the pathology laboratory.

**106.** Mr. Victor tells Sheila that even if she was protected against pregnancy by a contraceptive and has no intention of taking any legal action against her assailant, she should still be checked by a physician. This postrape physical examination is recommended for the early detection of
○ 1. venereal disease.
○ 2. neurotic reaction.
○ 3. periurethral tears.
○ 4. menstrual difficulties.

**107.** A nurse at the clinic has been invited to lecture about rape prevention. The nurse would include *all* of the following information in the lecture *except*
○ 1. the assault is rarely caused by the victim.
○ 2. the assailant is often known to the victim.
○ 3. the best response to an attack is to resist.
○ 4. rape remains an underreported crime in this country.

# CORRECT ANSWERS AND RATIONALES

Numbers appear in parentheses following the rationales. The numbers identify textbooks listed in the references at the end of Part I, where correct answers can be verified.

## The Patient with a Major Mood Disorder

**1.** 3. The holistic approach to health care takes into account the whole person and recognizes that many factors can cause poor health. Holistic theory believes that all elements of disruption should be examined and eliminated or minimized to allow the person to attain a state of well-being. Reacting to a stressful event, having a high sugar intake, and destructive environmental influences describe specific causes of a disruption in health rather than numerous factors influencing the life of a patient as a whole. (2, 12)

**2.** 3. A holistic approach is used when a nurse focuses on current life experiences to help a patient identify disruptions in his life that are currently occurring and causing ill health. Focusing on dreams and free associations, childhood and past life history, and underlying conflicts and defense mechanisms describe psychoanalytically based therapy. (2, 5)

**3.** 4. The nurse is using a therapeutic technique of restatement when she reiterates the patient's comment in the form of a question. This technique best helps the patient continue the conversation with an expression of his feelings. Telling the patient that the nurse is assigned to care for him and that is why she is there is impersonal and implies that the patient is being uncooperative. Telling the patient that the nurse is there because the patient has potential implies that other patients perhaps do not have potential for improvement. Asking the patient a question with the use of the word "why" challenges the patient and asks him for an explanation. None of these latter approaches is as effective as using the technique of restatement. (2, 5)

**4.** 4. When working with a patient who speaks little, answers briefly, and looks at the floor, the nurse should focus on the simplest type of behavior (that is, behavior that requires the least effort for the patient). The relationship described in this item is in an early exploratory stage, when self-expression and verbalization are more appropriate goals than decision making, relating to others, and functioning independently. (2, 5)

**5.** 2. The relationship between the nurse and the pa-tient described in this item is most probably in the working phase when the patient makes an effort to describe his problems to the nurse. It illustrates that the patient has gone beyond testing and acquainting himself with a new relationship and is now working on his problems. The relationship is in an exploratory, or initial, phase when the patient attempts to familiarize himself with the nurse and challenges boundaries of the relationship. The relationship is in a termination phase when the patient summarizes and evaluates his progress. (2, 5)

**6.** 1. Empathy is the quality of being aware of the feelings and emotions of another and perceiving how he feels. Climate refers to environmental conditions characterizing a relationship. Rapport is described as the harmonious feeling experienced by two people who hold one another in mutual respect. Sympathy implies a warmth toward, or urge to act to alleviate the distress of, another. (2, 5)

**7.** 4. A nurse should make sure that the patient understands she will need to discuss information given by the patient when, in her judgment, the information is necessary in relation to his therapy. This is a judgment the patient is unable to make with safety. Telling a patient that the nurse can keep information confidential and that she will not share it with anyone places her in a difficult position. If the patient tells her something that she considers vital information for others on the health team, she would need to break a promise she made to the patient if she feels that she must share the information. (2, 12)

**8.** 3. The responsibility for maintaining a relationship with a patient rests with the nurse. If a patient misses a scheduled interview, the nurse is assuming responsibility for the relationship when she seeks him out at the end of the scheduled interview time and tells him he was missed. To confront the patient with his absence and ask him to explain it is non-therapeutic and threatening. To arrange another session with the patient and to say nothing about the missed appointment does not keep to the terms of the nurse-patient contract and offers little help to the patient. The nurse makes an assumption without knowing the facts if she believes the patient has good reason for not keeping his appointment. She is not assuming responsibility when she waits for the patient to make the next move in this situation. (5, 12)

**9.** 4. Reaction formation is a defense mechanism that is present when a person expresses an attitude or feeling opposite from his unconscious feelings or attitudes. The patient described in this item is complimentary of his employer when, unconsciously, he most probably does not like his employer because he fired the patient from his job. Sublimation is directing unacceptable impulses into constructive channels. Suppression is a conscious effort to overcome unacceptable thoughts or desires. Repression is a defense mechanism that is present when a person excludes or bars painful experiences and thoughts from his state of consciousness. (2, 12)

**10.** 2. It is most therapeutic when patients in group therapy help each other explore feelings further and when they demonstrate understanding of each other. In the situation described in this item, asking the patient to describe his work and indicating that the company must have had a reason for retiring the patient avoid discussing the patient's feelings. Suggesting to the patient that he will have no trouble finding another job offers false hope without knowing the situation completely. (2, 12)

**11.** 4. Tranylcypromine sulfate (Parnate) is a monoamine oxidase (MAO) inhibitor. If this drug is taken in combination with foods or beverages rich in tyramine, the patient is likely to have a hypertensive crisis. The medication should be discontinued and the physician notified if the patient presents symptoms related to an impending hypertensive crisis, such as headaches, diaphoresis, palpitations, pallor, nausea and vomiting, and chest pains. (5, 11)

**12.** 2. Aged and strong cheeses are tyramine-rich foods and, when ingested in combination with MAO inhibitors, can cause a severe hypertensive crisis. The crisis is often referred to as a "Parnate-cheese reaction"; Parnate is an MAO inhibitor. Other foods and beverages rich in tyramine include aged meat and other meat that is not fresh, liver, dried fish, any fermented high-protein food (i.e., yeast extracts and concentrates), Italian broad beans (pods), green bean pods, wine, beer, and ale. In many instances, the following caffeine-containing foods and beverages are also restricted: coffee, tea, cocoa, chocolate, and caffeine-containing soft drinks. (11, 12)

**13.** 4. Planning to involve the patient in usual at-home pursuits of the immediate family is best when the patient described in this item is to go home for a 24-hour pass. There are no indications that this patient requires extra rest or unusual activities. It is too early for the patient to start looking for employment. (2, 12)

**14.** 1. Terminating a nurse-patient relationship is a weaning process. Subjects such as plans for finding employment, divorce plans of a family member, and a discussion of conflicts the patient has had while hospitalized do not provide for weaning. A discussion of the gains the patient has made during therapy does promote a weaning process. The content focuses on gains made in therapy, feelings about terminations, and saying goodbye. Introduction of new material at the time of termination may be a distraction and stall termination. (2, 12)

**15.** 3. The overall purpose of the nurse's reviewing the patient's counseling sessions with the clinical nurse specialist is to evaluate nursing practice. Awareness of patient behavior and patient thoughts and evaluation of nursing style are parts of nursing practice. (2, 12)

**16.** 4. Grief is a direct and appropriate response to termination of a positive relationship and indicates acceptance of termination. Anger is healthy when openly expressed but is a less healthy reaction than grief. A lack of response may be interpreted as indifference but it represents a profound emotional reaction that the patient is unable to express. Humor may be a defense against feelings of loss. (2, 12)

## The Patient with Bipolar Disorder, Manic Phase

**17.** 2. The very active patient is usually best placed in a quiet atmosphere to help decrease stimuli for activity. (2, 5, 12)

**18.** 3. When the husband of the patient described in this item apologizes for his wife's behavior, it is best to focus on the husband's feelings and be supportive of him. To say that the patient is doing the best she can and that the nurse is used to being treated worse by patients ignores the husband's feelings. To ask what caused the patient's behavior suggests criticism of the patient and asks the husband for a judgment that he may not be able to make accurately. (2, 12)

**19.** 3. If a patient with overactive behavior acts aggressively, the nurse must *first* use measures to protect her and others from harm. However, when the aggression subsides, as described in this item, efforts should be made to provide activity that is most likely to decrease tension and energy, such as using a punching bag. Reading a book, holding the patient's hands, or placing her in isolation to work out aggression in private will not meet the patient's needs to reduce energy and tension. However, when selecting an activity for a hyperactive patient, care should be taken so that the activity does not overstimulate an already overactive patient. (2, 5, 12)

**20.** 1. It is best to explain the x-ray procedure to the

patient described in this situation in simple terms. Saying nothing to the patient or giving her detailed explanations is inappropriate; the patient needs some explanation but details are unnecessary. There is no indication that additional help is needed for this patient. (2, 5, 12)

**21.** 1. Because the patient described in this situation is very active, it would be best to give her food she can carry with her and eat as she moves. Allowing the patient in the unit kitchen is an impractical measure, and the patient would most probably be too busy to eat anyway. Allowing the patient to send out for her favorite foods and serving food in small, attractively arranged portions do not meet the problem of ensuring that the patient has proper nourishment while being very active. (2, 12)

**22.** 1. Explanations are unlikely to be of value for helping the patient described in this situation. It is best to assist her into proper attire in a matter-of-fact way. At this point, the nurse needs to assist the patient in setting limits on her behavior. (2, 5, 12)

**23.** 2. The patient is demonstrating flight of ideas in this situation. Concreteness is interpreting another person's words literally. Depersonalization refers to feelings of strangeness concerning the environment or the self. A neologism is a word coined by a patient. (2, 12)

**24.** 1. The anxiety the patient feels gives rise to the distorted thinking displayed in speech patterns such as flight of ideas. Loose ego boundaries, underlying hostilities, and distortions in the self-concept have little, if any, relation to the thought disorder described here. (2, 5, 12)

**25.** 4. The nurse takes responsibility for not being able to understand the patient with flight of ideas when she asks the patient to speak more slowly in order to follow her train of thought. This is least likely to arouse anxiety in the patient. Although helping the patient make adequate connections between events is desirable, the manner in which it is being done when the nurse asks how the sun shining relates to her son being in Virginia offers a threat by requiring that the patient analyze thoughts and by describing why they occur. Changing the subject by suggesting that the patient talk about what she did yesterday is not helpful and does not focus on the patient's needs. Reprimanding the patient by indicating that she is talking in a nonsensical manner is also not helpful for the patient in this situation. (2, 5)

**26.** 2. Channeling activities through constructive tasks, such as cleaning, allows for the expression of aggressive behavior. During periods of hyperactivity, it is generally advisable not to involve the patient in activities with other patients because the technique tends not to be therapeutic for anyone. Allowing the patient to exercise and move about as much as possible is likely to lead to exhaustion of a hyperactive patient. (2, 12)

**27.** 4. During a manic phase, the patient is unlikely to show evidence of feelings of guilt, anger, or distrust. Hostility is a more characteristic feeling. (2)

**28.** 2. In the situation described in this item, when the patient orders a large amount of clothing from a department store, the nurse has a responsibility to deny the patient's request because it is inappropriate and the patient is not being financially responsible. Limit-setting is also an important part of working with patients, especially those who are in a very hyperactive phase of their illness. (5, 12)

**29.** 2. The patient should be observed for physical exhaustion, which predisposes to infections when a hyperactive patient experiences euphoria and engages in extreme activity. (2, 5, 12)

**30.** 1. Sodium is necessary for the renal excretion of lithium carbonate (Lithane). A low sodium intake results in the retention of lithium and lithium toxicity. (2, 5, 11)

**31.** 4. Clinical manifestations of lithium carbonate (Lithane) toxicity include anorexia, nausea and vomiting, diarrhea, coarse hand tremors, twitching, lethargy, decreased urine output, decreased blood pressure, and impaired consciousness. (11, 12)

**32.** 2. The therapeutic blood level range for lithium carbonate (Lithane) is between 0.6 and 1.4 mEq/L for adults. A level of 1.0 is an anticipated level after 10 days of treatment. (2, 11, 12)

**33.** 4. Behavior is caused. When a patient has delusions of grandeur, it is not helpful to change the patient's topic of discussion, involve the patient in a group project, or try to convince the patient that her thoughts are erroneous. It is far better to try to satisfy the implied need of the patient to feel important, because this recognizes the cause of the patient's behavior and helps make the patient feel important. (2, 5, 12)

**34.** 1. Staff members sometimes are the recipients of a patient's angry behavior because they are "safe" and are available for attack. The display of anger is rarely intended personally. Nor is such behavior necessarily a sign of serious pathology, an attack on a physician's skills, or a sign that the patient's condition is improving. (2, 12)

**35.** 3. Whenever possible, the patient should first be given choices when action must be taken because of behavior. In the situation described in this item, this is best accomplished by telling the patient that she has a choice of going to her room voluntarily or being escorted to her room. The patient's room should be used first and, if this does not help, then seclusion may be indicated. Because the patient's anger is increasing, the situation is beyond discussion. (2, 12)

**36.** 2. Research has shown that patients with a bipolar disorder are likely to have recurrences periodically. (2, 5)

**37.** 1. For the patient going home, it is best to suggest that, if possible, she be relieved of some home responsibilities she had previously, that better communications be developed, and that family members learn to recognize signs of toxicity while the patient is on drug therapy. It is unrealistic and impractical to attempt to eliminate worry and anxiety from a patient's environment. (2, 5)

**38.** 2. A family history of bipolar disorder is often present. Having been molested as a child, building up high serotonin levels in the brain, and drinking alcoholic beverages have not been found to be of etiologic significance for this illness. (2, 5)

## *The Patient Who Is Depressed*

**39.** 2. A patient is legally committable when she tries to harm herself or others. (2, 5)

**40.** 4. A person who has had to be committed to a hospital for the mentally ill loses the right to leave the hospital of his own accord. He does not necessarily lose rights to vote, make a will or contract, or send and receive mail. (2, 5)

**41.** 3. A writ of habeas corpus is defined as an order requiring that a prisoner (in this case, the patient) be brought before a judge or into court to decide whether he is being held lawfully. Its purpose is to obtain liberation of a person held without just cause. (5, 12)

**42.** 4. When the patient feels unworthiness, she reflects low self-esteem. Presenting another set of facts in a manner that is accepting of the patient, but avoids a power struggle, is necessary. Telling the patient that her feelings are imaginary, that her family still loves her, and that she should try to forget ideas of unworthiness disregard the feelings and may be perceived as rejection. (2)

**43.** 2. Sitting beside the patient and placing the fork in the patient's hand are techniques that are likely to stimulate the depressed patient to eat. Sitting with the patient also conveys a message of having time for her and of caring. Leaving the patient alone, telling the patient she must eat to recover, and trying to encourage the patient by saying the food looks good are techniques that are less likely to interest the patient in eating. (2, 12)

**44.** 3. The suspicious person characteristically views others as wishing to attack him. Attempting to feed the patient by gavage is likely to be interpreted as an attack. A gavage feeding is no more likely to be aspirated by the patient described in this item than by any other patient. Gavaging a patient is safe when proper technique is used. Patients are unlikely to view gavage as a sign of approaching death or to become increasingly irritable toward others. (5, 9)

**45.** 4. Doing something with or to the patient described in this situation is unlikely to help restlessness and incoherence. It is best to sit quietly with the patient until the medication takes effect. A warm bath might be helpful, but not a cool shower. (2, 5)

**46.** 4. When the patient described in this situation wants to be left alone to die, it is best to leave the patient for a few minutes but return to see how the patient is getting along. This response acknowledges the patient's request and also lets the patient know that the nurse will be back shortly. It responds to reality. Telling the patient that the nurse will not allow anything to hurt the patient, that the nurse is not trying to cheat the patient, and that the patient may be trying to frighten the nurse is to respond to delusional material. (5, 12)

**47.** 2. Depression can make daily interactions with others trying and, typically, patients become irritated and uncooperative. In an extreme case, the irritation frequently becomes agitation. (2, 12)

**48.** 1. The social roles for younger women are more positive and have greater social rewards than the roles for middle-aged women. In the past, women's distress with this loss in social status was incorrectly attributed to fear of old age. (2, 12)

**49.** 2. Social support has been demonstrated to have a stress reduction effect, particularly within the context of significant relationships with relatives. In the past, individual characteristics such as appearance and weight were incorrectly identified as the major source of positive and negative feelings among women. While weather can be a stressor, it has not been shown to be a major factor influencing the ability to manage stress. (2, 12)

**50.** 4. The sad and angry feelings common to depression make it difficult for the patient to interact positively with significant others. At this point in the situation described, the nurse has no information to suggest the presence of marital conflict or to assume that there is a single cause for the feelings of depression. (2, 12)

**51.** 3. Exercise tolerance is the best measure to determine whether a patient is ready for sexual intercourse following a myocardial infarction. If the patient can climb two flights of stairs and walk a treadmill at 3 to 4 miles per hour without an increase in the target pulse rate or blood pressure, the heart is most probably also able to tolerate sexual intercourse. (9)

**52.** 2. Whenever a patient is suicidal, steps must be taken to prevent the patient from harming herself. Other goals of care are less important than being sure the patient does not carry out the threat of suicide. All threats of suicide should be taken seriously and proper precautions should be taken to protect the patient from self-harm. (2, 5, 12)

**53.** 3. This response provides the most complete information about both the current and future treatment plan and answers the question asked by the patient's husband. (2, 12)

**54.** 1. Because tricyclic antidepressants such as nortriptyline hydrochloride (Aventyl) cause tachycardias and EKG changes, an electrocardiogram should be done before the patient takes the medication. Other side effects include urinary retention, constipation, and drowsiness. Nortriptyline hydrochloride is administered cautiously to patients receiving thyroid medication. (2, 11)

**55.** 2. When strongly opposed to a type of therapy, it is best for the nurse to refer people who ask her about the therapy to another knowledgeable person for information. If the nurse gives the patient and family an honest opinion, she may cause the patient and family to lose confidence in prescribed therapy. It would be dishonest to tell the patient and family that she does not know enough about the treatment to be of help. Giving a copy of the package insert is impersonal and is likely to be of little help. (2, 5)

**56.** 3. A medication teaching plan includes information relevant to the patient's care. A description of current research about antidepressant therapy is not essential unless the patient is participating in a research protocol. (2, 12)

**57.** 1. Improved appetite and improved sleep patterns indicate that the medication is having a therapeutic effect. Sleeping too much could indicate oversedation. (2, 11)

**58.** 2. Dry mouth is the most common side effect of tricyclic antidepressant medications. Other side effects include urticaria, rash, and diaphoresis. (2, 11)

**59.** 2. Depressed patients are often ambivalent; that is, they want to and do not want to carry out an activity. They should not be given choices that allow them to say no. Their disinterest may not really indicate a wish to be left alone. Making an appointment to take a patient to a unit activity is more

helpful than allowing the patient to say he does not wish to go or leaving it up to the patient to decide on his own. (2, 5)

**60.** 1. Maintaining a system of social support helps avoid the social isolation that often precedes depression. There is no indication in this item that continued therapy in the form of medication or psychotherapy will improve this patient's ability to cope. (2, 12)

## The Patient with Depressive Disorder and Suicidal Ideation

**61.** 3. The patient described in this item, who appears not to want the nurse to leave, most probably needs attention paid to some unknown concern. Her behavior should be considered meaningful but not as yet fully understood. The patient is also showing signs of agitated depression. Judging that the patient is lonely and looking for a way to pass time, that she is self-centered and possessive of the nurse's time, or that she desires assistance to improve the appearance of her room describes conclusions or value judgments based on insufficient data in this situation. (2, 5)

**62.** 1. Bringing up the subject of suicide when there is reason to suspect the patient may be considering it has not harmed anyone and has helped a great many. To avoid the subject when a patient appears suicidal is unwise; the safest procedure is to investigate. It would be premature in the situation described in this item to outline alternative measures to suicide or to describe other patients the nurse has known who have attempted suicide. (2, 5)

**63.** 2. Sleep disturbances are markers of the biologic changes associated with depression and indicate increased severity. Feelings of fatigue, decreased interest in usual activity, and changes in appetite are common symptoms of depressed mood. (2, 12)

**64.** 3. Cheerfulness and gaiety have a tendency to make a depressed person feel more guilty and unworthy. It is helpful to be firm and businesslike or serious with depressed persons and to behave naturally and spontaneously. (2, 5)

**65.** 3. It ordinarily takes 2 to 4 weeks before amitriptyline hydrochloride (Elavil) can be expected to have a favorable effect on the patient. This is important for the nurse to keep in mind because the patient described in this item is likely to continue to be suicidal until the drug takes effect. (2, 5)

**66.** 1. Mobilization is important to decrease depressed thinking and behaviors in the patient described in this situation. Mobilization may also help to accomplish other goals, such as socializing and attending to nutrition and rest. (2, 12)

**67.** 3. Arranging for a volunteer visitor, a friend to visit, and Meals-on-Wheels all increase the patient's activity but do not get her out of the house and increase her social resources as transportation to the senior group does. (2, 5, 12)

**68.** 1. Depressed patients are difficult to relate to because of their expressed feelings of hopelessness and general apathy. The concomitant feelings of hopelessness and lack of success experienced by the nurse with these patients may lead her to withdraw or to feel angry with the patient. Poor personal grooming by the patient may describe a factor in this situation but can be easily and directly managed by the nurse. Depressed persons are typically dependent on others. They are not motivated by laziness and are usually conscientious and dependable. (2, 5)

**69.** 2. Such measures as chewing sugarless gum, drinking generous amounts of fluid, and rinsing the mouth with water help overcome feelings of thirst and of having a dry mouth. Sucking hard candies will increase thirst and also predisposes to dental caries. (2, 3, 5)

**70.** 4. Depressed patients have sleep disturbances, and hence the property of sedation in a drug is a valuable one. Often, the patient is treated with antipsychotic, antidepressant, and antiparkinsonism agents simultaneously. An additive effect may cause urinary retention and paralytic ileus, both of which are serious problems and should be reported promptly. Insomnia, diarrhea, and hypertension are not associated with amitriptyline hydrochloride (Elavil) therapy. (2, 5, 12)

**71.** 4. Pointing out to the patient who is depressed, has been suicidal, and complains of not being able to do much that she has made progress by describing what she now is able to do is therapeutic. Telling the patient that she can do anything she puts her mind to, encouraging her to think more positively about herself, and talking about weekend plans may prove more frustrating than helpful for a patient who is already finding fault with herself. Also, by suggesting that the patient and nurse make plans for the patient's weekend changes the subject that the patient introduced in the conversation. (2, 5, 12)

**72.** 2. When the nurse is unable to keep an appointment for the allotted time with the patient described in this item and the patient appears angry about it when the nurse next visits, it is best for the nurse to comment that the patient looks angry, ask the patient what her thoughts are at the moment, and apologize for having to leave early on the pre-

vious visit. In this situation, it would be least helpful to remain silent until the patient chooses to speak. The nurse should take the initiative and give the patient every opportunity to ventilate her anger and other feelings and thoughts she may have. (2, 5)

**73.** 3. A good rule of thumb is to let the patient bring up his own topics for discussion and to explore given clues more fully, especially if they relate to the patient's feelings about the nurse. If the nurse states that the patient is unhappy because the nurse cut the previous visit short, she is reading the patient's mind. It would be impersonal for the nurse to say that she could not hate anyone. Telling the patient that she is imagining things is not therapeutic and is belittling to the patient. (2, 5)

**74.** 1. The patient described in this situation is exhibiting a conflict when she wants comfort but dreads the questions it may raise and explanations she will be expected to offer. An impulse is a sudden inclination to take some unpremeditated action. Regression is a return to earlier, more satisfying ways of behaving. An ego break would be manifested as a severe personality disturbance. (2, 5)

**75.** 4. Helping the depressed patient learn to express feelings instead of turning the negative ones inward is an important goal of therapy. Confronting the angry behavior and helping the patient learn more positive behaviors are more likely to be useful for a patient who is more active than depressed. To ignore the patient's behavior and to plan a schedule to keep while the patient expresses anger avoids the feelings of the patient. (2, 5)

**76.** 3. Loss is of most importance in the depressive syndromes. Financial upset, physical injury, and increased personal or social responsibility may lead to feelings of depression, but noting a real or imagined loss in the history of a depressed person is a broad concept and universally applicable. (2, 5)

**77.** 2. Suicide attempts are more likely to occur soon after the depression lifts and the patient has more energy to act on her thoughts and impulses. The patient does not have the energy to commit suicide during times of greatest depression. The energy level of the patient, rather than her status, is related to the danger involved. (2, 12)

**78.** 2. Anger is a low risk factor for suicide, certainly less than such factors as the patient's age, home environment, and previous suicidal gestures. Anger turned outward is usually more positive than anger turned inward. (2, 12)

**79.** 1. Introjection is the adoption of another's attitudes, values, and feelings as one's own. Conversion occurs when repressed ideas are converted into a variety of somatic symptoms. Restitution is a coping mechanism whereby an individual atones for his unacceptable ideas, feelings, or actions. When substitution is present, an unacceptable or unattainable goal is replaced by one that is more acceptable or attainable. (5, 12)

## *The Patient Who Attempts Suicide*

80. 4. Stomach contents should be removed to prevent further absorption of the secobarbital (Seconal) the patient has taken in this situation. Lavaging is preferred to inducing vomiting in an unconscious patient to prevent aspiration of stomach contents. Forcing fluids and giving a diuretic are inappropriate measures in this situation. (3, 9)

81. 1. The primary nursing responsibility when caring for a patient who is suicidal is to provide a safe environment and to protect the patient from harming himself or herself. (5, 12)

82. 2. When the patient described in this item criticizes herself for not being able to commit suicide successfully, it is most therapeutic when the nurse makes a comment that helps the patient elaborate and ventilate her feelings, such as, "Is that how you feel?" To tell the patient that her feelings will pass or that she has a great deal to live for discounts the patient's feelings. A comment that includes the word "why" asks the patient to defend her feelings and tends not to be therapeutic. (2, 5)

83. 2. An improved self-concept indicates that the patient's therapy is effective. A poor self-concept is a very common sign of depression and is almost always present in the suicidal patient. Appetite and activity level are not necessarily decreased in depression. Gender identity conflict is common in adolescence, but is not a sign of depression. (2, 5)

84. 2. Adolescents will show signs of dysfunction and acting-out behaviors when they live in an unhealthy family environment. The inner conflicts will not be resolved if the system they came from and will return to remains unchanged. The family's need for guidance on how to deal with a dysfunctional adolescent, parenting that is either overpermissive or overrestrictive, and a strong sense of failure on the part of the parents in rearing a dysfunctioning adolescent describe part of the total family's dysfunctioning, but are not the primary reasons for family therapy. (2, 5)

85. 2. Because self-responsibility is part of the focus of family therapy, direct communication between the persons involved in the situation is encouraged. Learning to express oneself clearly and to give direct feedback is part of healthy communication. In the situation described in this item, terminating the therapy because it upsets the patient and suggesting to the therapist that the patient be allowed to speak do not allow the patient to deal directly with the person with whom the patient is angry and discourage the patient from taking responsibility for her own feelings. It is satisfactory to allow a patient to ventilate to a nurse, but in this situation it would be best for the patient to open communication with her therapist. (2, 12)

86. 2. Homosexual and heterosexual experimentation occurs during adolescence. This does not necessarily indicate a preference for a specific life-style or acceptance or rejection of sexual relations with either sex. The literature describes a fear of the opposite sex and gender identity difficulties in adolescent homosexual experiences. However, in the situation described in this item, especially because it was a one-time encounter, a better evaluation of the situation is not to consider the encounter unusual. (5, 12)

87. 1. Behavior modification originates from learning theories that state that behavior is learned or determined by its consequences and can be reinforced or extinguished. The psychodynamic model of behavior is reflected in the theory that behavior is related to intrapsychic conflicts. The interpersonal model of behavior is reflected in the theory that behavioral changes result from stress on the individual and his body systems. The systems model is reflected in the theory that behavior is the result of interaction between an individual and the environment. (5, 12)

## *The Patient in Crisis*

88. 3. For the patient described in this item who believes she is pregnant and comes to a crisis center for help, it would be best for the nurse first to summarize the patient's comments and ask the patient to confirm the nurse's perceptions. The first step in the nursing process is assessment, which includes obtaining accurate information about the patient. Other types of intervention then follow. (2, 12)

89. 2. When the patient describes what she has been doing in sexually oriented encounters with her boyfriend, the best and initial response to the patient's comments in the situation described in this item is to gather data that will help the nurse determine meanings of terms used by the patient. Other comments at this time are less effective because they would assume an understanding of what the patient has said. (2, 12)

**90.** 4. Because individuals in the midst of emotional crisis find it difficult to focus their thinking, the goal of the nursing intervention is to return the individual to noncrisis functioning. Pointing out the level of distress the person is actually experiencing is the first step in attaining this goal. (2, 5, 12)

**91.** 4. Sex education has the goal of increasing one's knowledge about sex, and this ordinarily leads to the person's taking more responsibility for his or her sexual behavior. (5, 12)

**92.** 3. When the patient described in this item says she needs no more help because she is going to stop "fooling around," it is best for the nurse to make a comment that lets the patient know the door is open for the patient to return. The nurse leaves the decision to the patient, but does not threaten or push the nurse's point of view. Nor does the nurse put the patient down or ridicule her. (5, 12)

**93.** 1. Telephoning the crisis shelter indicates that the boys are alarmed, but are reluctant to talk with their parents. The nurse should focus on assisting the boys to talk with their parents. Because of their ages and the involved problem, the boys may fear that their parents will assume they have been sniffing glue. (2, 5, 12)

**94.** 3. Persons who inhale noxious substances, such as glue, risk cardiac failure because of overexertion when under the influence of the substance. Respiratory failure is also a cause of death from inhalants. Liver and kidney damage may occur with prolonged use, but are not the most common cause of death. (11, 12)

**95.** 4. Crack is the well-established street name for smoked cocaine. (5, 12)

**96.** 4. The patient in this situation may be experiencing delirium or delusions secondary to cocaine intoxication. Both processes diminish reality testing, while making the person fearful. Because the patient is a potential danger to himself and to others, he should be protected from his own behavior. (5, 11, 12)

**97.** 3. To help the patient described in this item reestablish self-control and orientation, it would be best for the nurse to make a truthful statement about what is happening to the patient and prepare the patient for what to expect. To tell the patient he has no need for concern offers false assurance. It is not helpful to "moralize" by stating that the patient should not have done what he did. A statement consisting of technical terms the patient may not understand is futile. Television is generally contraindicated when a patient is suffering from ill effects after using cocaine. (11, 12)

**98.** 4. Major tranquilizers should not be given to shorten the drug reaction because of the danger, possibly fatal, of drug incompatibility. Street drugs are often combined with other substances; atropine has been present in a few cases in which death has occurred. (11)

**99.** 2. Cocaine is a stimulant that increases activity and causes sleeplessness. The use of cocaine may make the user feel more comfortable in social situations. Cocaine does not improve concentration or work performance. (2, 11)

**100.** 2. Cocaine users do not become physically dependent on the drug, nor do they develop a physical tolerance. Strong psychological dependency is common. Birth defects have not been associated with use of cocaine. (11)

**101.** 3. When the patient described in this item asks how the nurse would feel if his girlfriend had been raped, and the nurse believes that the question is most probably personal, it would be best for the nurse to be straightforward in his response while focusing on the patient. It is better not to respond to the patient's question with a question that probes. If the nurse asks the patient how she thinks the nurse should feel if his girlfriend had been raped, he is asking the patient to analyze the nurse's feelings rather than her own. The patient's problem is ignored if the nurse changes the subject of conversation. (2, 5)

**102.** 1. Many people still believe that the woman who has been raped is responsible for being raped. Less often do people assume that a raped women was out to "get" the man involved or that the woman enjoyed the experience. A woman does not have to show physical injury to prove her innocence when she has been raped. (5, 12)

**103.** 1. When a patient who has been raped seeks out brightly lit places and the company of friends and plans to move to another part of the city, she is exhibiting self-defense to help avoid being raped again. (5, 12)

**104.** 3. The potential for problems and difficulty in adjusting after rape will be increased when those around the victim treat her as though she is to blame for the rape, especially when she already may feel some guilt and shame about it. A rape victim is very likely showing adjustment to her experience when she is upset about her experience, when she seeks out formerly ignored relatives and friends for support, and when she attempts to help other rape victims. (5)

**105.** 2. It is most important to have an account of the person's description of the assault when rape has occurred. It may be desirable but is not necessarily a legal requirement to hand-carry evidence following a rape to a pathology laboratory, keep prying persons away from a rape victim, and have a patient escorted home. (3, 5)

**106.** 1. Venereal diseases can be spread through the act of rape. If the victim or the rapist was not using a contraceptive, postcoital contraceptive methods should be discussed. (5, 9)

**107.** 3. Studies of rape have shown that victims do not cause the attack and that the attacker is often known to the victim. Response to the attack should be based on the situation. Resisting is not always the best response. Rape continues to be an under-reported crime in the United States. (4, 12)

# test 2

The Patient Who is Paranoid

The Patient with Catatonic Schizophrenia

The Patient with Chronic Mental Illness

The Patient with an Obsessive-Compulsive Disorder

The Patient with Organic Brain Syndrome

Using a Therapeutic Milieu

Correct Answers and Rationales

Select the one *best* or *correct* answer and indicate your choice by filling in the circle with a pencil in front of the option you have chosen. If the answer you would prefer is not given, select the one you think is *most appropriate*.

## THE PATIENT WHO IS PARANOID

Mr. Jerry Rand, a slender man in his early forties, glances disdainfully around the adult inpatient unit on his arrival at the hospital. He is neatly and attractively dressed and clutches a leather briefcase tightly in his arms.

1. Mr. Rand refuses to let the nurse who admits him touch his briefcase or check it for valuables or contraband. The plan that would be *most appropriate* in this situation is for the nurse to learn of the briefcase's contents by
   - ○ 1. obtaining help to take the briefcase away from the patient.
   - ○ 2. asking the patient to open the briefcase while he describes its contents.
   - ○ 3. inspecting the briefcase when the patient is temporarily out of the room.
   - ○ 4. telling the patient it is necessary to observe hospital policy if he wishes to stay.

2. The nurse stands near the window in Mr. Rand's room while explaining how the bed operates. The patient shouts, "Come away from the window! They'll see you!" Which of the following responses would be *best* for the nurse to make?
   - ○ 1. "Who are 'they,' Mr. Rand?"
   - ○ 2. "No one will see me, Mr. Rand."
   - ○ 3. "You have no reason to be afraid, Mr. Rand."
   - ○ 4. "What will happen if they do see me, Mr. Rand?"

3. The nurse should recognize that moving away from the window quickly, as Mr. Rand requested, is *contraindicated* because moving away would
   - ○ 1. reveal a lack of poise in the nurse.
   - ○ 2. make the patient feel the nurse is only humoring him.

   - ○ 3. indicate nonverbal agreement with the patient's false ideas.
   - ○ 4. let the patient think he will have his way when he wishes.

4. Mr. Rand thinks he is being followed by foreign agents who are after secret papers in his briefcase. The thought disorder from which he is suffering is called
   - ○ 1. an idea of reference.
   - ○ 2. an idea of influence.
   - ○ 3. a delusion of grandeur.
   - ○ 4. a delusion of persecution.

5. Mr. Rand's refusal to eat because he fears something has been placed in his food is delusional thinking that *most clearly* demonstrates that the patient is
   - ○ 1. aware of his dependency on others.
   - ○ 2. sensitive to the thoughts and feelings of others.
   - ○ 3. making excuses for refusing to cooperate with the staff.
   - ○ 4. unable to differentiate between thoughts and external reality.

6. The team leader overhears a nursing assistant respond to Mr. Rand's statement that he is the only person alive who has the answer to the world food shortage with, "How can that be? Tell me more, Mr. Rand." On which of the following statements about the effects of questioning a patient closely about his false ideas should the team leader base her subsequent comments to the nursing assistant?
   - ○ 1. This questioning leads the patient to reverse his thinking.
   - ○ 2. This questioning leads the patient to defend his thinking.
   - ○ 3. This questioning leads the patient to share more of his thinking.

○ 4. This questioning leads the patient to clarify some of his thinking.

7. To help establish a therapeutic relationship with Mr. Rand, which of the following plans would be *best* for the nurse to implement?
○ 1. Initiate conversations with the patient whenever he becomes agitated.
○ 2. Set aside specific times each day for conversations with the patient.
○ 3. Allow the patient to initiate conversations when he feels ready for them.
○ 4. Plan conversations with the patient at frequent but unspecified times during the day.

8. During a conversation with the nurse, Mr. Rand suddenly jumps up, begins pacing, and wrings his hands. In this situation, the *best* course of action for the nurse to follow is to
○ 1. take the patient for a walk to help overcome his restlessness.
○ 2. change the subject of conversation she is having with the patient.
○ 3. share her observations with the patient and comment that he appears anxious.
○ 4. suggest to the patient that the nurse leave and point out to him that he does not appear to want to talk now.

9. Which of the following characteristics of a suspicious patient makes it *especially* difficult for the nurse to establish and maintain a therapeutic relationship with him?
○ 1. The patient's tendency to question the motives of others.
○ 2. The patient's tendency to ridicule and belittle other persons.
○ 3. The patient's tendency to believe he is right and others are wrong.
○ 4. The patient's tendency to see others as part of the conspiracy against him.

10. Mr. Rand is ordered to receive chlorpromazine (Thorazine). To avoid the problem of Mr. Rand's possibly "cheeking" the medication, in which of the following forms would it initially be *best* to plan to give the patient the medication?
○ 1. In liquid form.
○ 2. In capsule form.
○ 3. In suppository form.
○ 4. In an intramuscular injection.

11. After 3 days of taking chlorpromazine (Thorazine), Mr. Rand shows an inability to sit still; he has motor restlessness, fidgets, and tends to pace around the unit. Of the following extrapyramidal adverse reactions, the patient is showing signs of
○ 1. dystonia.
○ 2. akathisia.

○ 3. parkinsonism.
○ 4. tardive dyskinesia.

12. Which of the following medications can the nurse anticipate will be prescribed to treat Mr. Rand's extrapyramidal side effects?
○ 1. Chlordiazepoxide (Librium).
○ 2. Benztropine mesylate (Cogentin).
○ 3. Imipramine hydrochloride (Tofranil).
○ 4. Thioridazine hydrochloride (Mellaril).

13. Which of the following observations about Mr. Rand warrants the *most prompt* reporting and the nurse's use of safety precautions for him?
○ 1. The patient cries when he talks about his divorce.
○ 2. The patient starts a petition to end the curfew hour.
○ 3. The patient declines to attend a daily group therapy session.
○ 4. The patient names another patient who he says is his adversary.

14. When a psychoanalytic approach is used, the *best* interpretation of Mr. Rand's behavior would be that beneath his air of arrogance and superiority lie deep-seated feelings of inferiority and inadequacy. Which of the following defense mechanisms is Mr. Rand using to protect his self-esteem?
○ 1. Denial.
○ 2. Introjection.
○ 3. Idealization.
○ 4. Reaction formation.

15. The nursing assistant assigned to care for Mr. Rand comments to the nurse, "That Mr. Rand! He surely gets on my nerves. Just who does he think he is?" Which of the following replies would be *best* for the nurse to make?
○ 1. "It sounds as though you are angry with him."
○ 2. "You should not talk about a patient that way."
○ 3. "I wonder if you might try to consider his feelings."
○ 4. "We can consider changing your patient assignment."

16. For which of the following reasons should the nurse *avoid* the use of touch with Mr. Rand?
○ 1. Touch may be misinterpreted by the patient.
○ 2. Touch may arouse transference feelings in the patient.
○ 3. Touch may lead to dependency on the part of the patient.
○ 4. Touch may inhibit development of trust in the relationship.

17. The secure atmosphere of the hospital eventually helps effect a decrease in Mr. Rand's paranoid ideation. *All* of the following activities of the nurse

*very likely* contributed to the patient's recovery *except*

   ○ 1. encouraging the patient to take responsibility for his actions.

   ○ 2. acting as a role model for the patient in everyday social situations.

   ○ 3. minimizing making promises to the patient but keeping those that are made.

   ○ 4. letting the patient see the nurse talking with other patients outside of his hearing range.

**18.** Plans are made for Mr. Rand's discharge from the hospital. The nurse should use remaining interactions with the patient *primarily* to

   ○ 1. explain to the patient possible causes of his illness.

   ○ 2. discuss the termination of the nurse-patient relationship.

   ○ 3. teach the patient about the administration of medications he will use at home.

   ○ 4. give the patient advice on how to handle possible future problems.

## THE PATIENT WITH CATATONIC SCHIZOPHRENIA

Mrs. Dinah Wallace, 43, is brought to the hospital by her husband. She wears sandals, revealing dirty and swollen feet, and is wearing a wrinkled dress with a stain down the front. She moves slowly and looks confused.

**19.** The *initial* goal of the nurse who admits Mrs. Wallace should be focused on

   ○ 1. making the patient feel safe and accepted.

   ○ 2. helping the patient get acquainted with others.

   ○ 3. giving the patient information about the program.

   ○ 4. providing the patient with clean and comfortable clothes.

**20.** When asked about herself during the admission interview, Mrs. Wallace stares blankly at the nurse and mutters unintelligibly to herself. This behavior is *best* charted as

   ○ 1. "not able to answer questions at this time."

   ○ 2. "uncooperative during admission procedure."

   ○ 3. "responded to questions with a blank look and incomprehensible mumble."

   ○ 4. "stared at the nurse when asked questions and was disoriented and incoherent."

**21.** Fluphenazine decanoate (Prolixin Decanoate) is prescribed for Mrs. Wallace. The outstanding characteristic of this drug is that it

   ○ 1. is inexpensive and can be self-administered.

   ○ 2. relieves the patient's symptoms quickly.

   ○ 3. needs to be administered only once every 2 to 4 weeks.

   ○ 4. has fewer side effects than the other major tranquilizers.

**22.** In order to evaluate the effects of fluphenazine decanoate (Prolixin Decanoate) on Mrs. Wallace, it is *least* important for the nurse to regularly monitor Mrs. Wallace's

   ○ 1. weight.

   ○ 2. white blood cell count.

   ○ 3. blood pressure.

   ○ 4. pulmonary function.

**23.** Mrs. Wallace begins to express herself verbally occasionally. Which of the following nursing actions should be credited with helping a mute patient express herself verbally?

   ○ 1. Asking questions that draw the patient out.

   ○ 2. Using hand signals to entice the patient to communicate.

   ○ 3. Making open-ended statements that are followed with a silence.

   ○ 4. Saying out loud what the nurse thinks the patient is experiencing.

**24.** Mrs. Wallace often does the opposite of what she is requested to do. For example, if asked to stand up, she sits down; if asked to dress, she undresses. In view of the patient's negativism, which of the following actions would be *best* for the nurse to take to get Mrs. Wallace to the dining room for meals?

   ○ 1. Ask her to eat in her room away from the other patients.

   ○ 2. Wait for her to get hungry enough to come to the dining room by herself.

   ○ 3. Tell her it is time for lunch and lead her firmly by the arm to the dining room.

   ○ 4. Promise her a reward if she eats in the dining room and get help to take her there if she refuses.

**25.** Mrs. Wallace curls into a fetal position in bed when she is upset. Which of the following defense mechanisms is she using when she displays behavior reminiscent of an earlier level of emotional development?

   ○ 1. Fixation.

   ○ 2. Regression.

   ○ 3. Substitution.

   ○ 4. Symbolization.

**26.** To help evaluate Mrs. Wallace's progress, the nurse pays close attention to nonverbal communications whenever conversing with the patient. Which of the following statements *best* describes why the nurse's observations of nonverbal messages are important?

○ 1. Nonverbal communications convey feelings more accurately than do verbal communications.

○ 2. Nonverbal communications reveal inner defects in a person better than do verbal communications.

○ 3. Nonverbal communications allow for a healthier expression of negative emotions than do verbal communications.

○ 4. Nonverbal communications provide better concealment for the true feelings of a person than do verbal communications.

27. Psychotic patients may suddenly behave in an impulsive, hyperactive, and unpredictable manner. Which of the following approaches would be *best* for the nurse to use *first* if Mrs. Wallace becomes violent?

○ 1. Provide a physical outlet for her energies.

○ 2. Let her know her behavior is not acceptable.

○ 3. Get enough help to handle the situation safely.

○ 4. Use heavy sedation to keep the patient calm.

28. Restraints are ordered for Mrs. Wallace, to be used according to the nurse's discretion. With which of the following offenses could the nurse be charged in the event she uses the restraints on the patient without good cause and a legal suit develops?

○ 1. Fraud.

○ 2. Assault.

○ 3. False imprisonment.

○ 4. Invasion of privacy.

29. Although Mrs. Wallace shows signs of progress daily, her husband complains to the nurse, "Why isn't she well yet? She's been here over 2 weeks already. Aren't you people doing your job?" Which of the following replies by the nurse would be the *most* therapeutic in this situation?

○ 1. "You are anxious for your wife to get better. Shall we talk about it for a while?"

○ 2. "She is really doing a lot better than you think. It won't be long before she will be home again."

○ 3. "We are doing the best we can. She has deep-seated conflicts which cannot be cured overnight."

○ 4. "I know it is difficult for you. But you wouldn't want to rush her and have her get worse again, would you?"

30. Mrs. Wallace's children are being cared for by her mother-in-law. One day after a visit with her children, Mrs. Wallace becomes agitated and shaky and whispers to the nurse, "That woman has turned my children against me." Which of the following interventions would be *best* for the nurse to make *first?*

○ 1. Arrange for a social service consultation.

○ 2. Ask family members to limit their visiting with the patient.

○ 3. Determine the identity of the woman to whom the patient is referring.

○ 4. Assign a staff member to watch the patient carefully for the rest of the day.

## THE PATIENT WITH CHRONIC MENTAL ILLNESS

31. Ms. Jakes, a nurse, is interested in working with the chronically mentally ill. She knows the needs of this large patient population include *all* of the following *except*

○ 1. community-based treatment programs.

○ 2. psychosocial rehabilitation.

○ 3. employment opportunities.

○ 4. better custodial care in long-term hospitals.

32. Ms. Jakes is offered a position as a psychiatric nurse in a psychosocial rehabilitation program. She knows as a nurse in the program that her role will include *all* the following functions *except*

○ 1. teaching independent living skills.

○ 2. assisting patients with living arrangements.

○ 3. avoiding insight-oriented therapy.

○ 4. linking patients with community resources.

33. Susan Terry, a 35-year-old woman in the program, has worked as a hotel maid for the last 3 years. She tells Ms. Jakes she is thinking of quitting her job because voices on television are talking about her. The *most important* thing for Ms. Jakes to do *first* is to

○ 1. get information about the patient's medication compliance.

○ 2. remind the patient that hearing voices is a symptom of her illness with which she can cope.

○ 3. check with the patient's employer about her work performance.

○ 4. arrange for the patient to be admitted to a psychiatric hospital for a short stay.

34. Ms. Terry tells Ms. Jakes she stopped taking her chlorpromazine hydrochloride (Thorazine) 2 weeks ago because she is better again and wants "to make it on my own without this damned medicine." Which of the following is the *most therapeutic* response for Ms. Jakes to make?

○ 1. "You've told me about other times like this when you stopped taking your meds and got sick again. Please don't do it again this time."

○ 2. "You're a smart girl, Susan. You know what will

happen if you don't take your meds. Why do you want to be so bad to yourself?"

○ 3. "I know you get tired of taking the meds—especially when you're doing well. Is there any special reason you decided to stop right now?"

○ 4. "Maybe you are ready for a short holiday from the Thorazine. I'll talk it over with Dr. Poll. But you need to take it until I talk with him."

35. Ms. Jakes has been asked to develop a medication education program for patients in the rehabilitation program. When developing the course outline, Ms. Jakes should plan to include *all* of the following topics *except*

○ 1. a categorization of a wide variety of psychotropic drugs.

○ 2. intervention for common side effects of psychotropic drugs.

○ 3. the role of medication in the treatment of chronic illness.

○ 4. the effect of using common street drugs with psychotropic medication.

36. Ms. Jakes has been asked to orient a new nurse to the psychosocial rehabilitation program. In planning the nurse's orientation, Ms. Jakes wants to be sure that the nurse understands the concept of chronic mental illness. Ms. Jakes would include *all* of the following information in the orientation program *except*

○ 1. the chronically mentally ill have been labeled deviant by society and much of their behavior is related to this role identity.

○ 2. while care of the chronically mentally ill is an important goal, the ultimate goal of long-term treatment is cure of the psychiatric disorder.

○ 3. the chronically mentally ill have both primary and secondary symptoms of psychiatric illness.

○ 4. the development of chronic mental illness follows a common, predictable pattern.

37. Mr. Toll, another nurse at the mental health center, has been asked to develop an in-service program for the staff about young adult chronically mentally ill patients since more patients in this group are being seen at the center. Which of the following characteristics is Mr. Toll *most likely* to find common to this group of patients?

○ 1. They have minimal experience with lengthy periods of hospitalization.

○ 2. They accept the role of patient easily.

○ 3. They have a low incidence of substance abuse.

○ 4. They have lower expectations of achieving social goals of employment and relationships than older chronically mentally ill patients.

38. Mr. Toll receives a telephone call from the mother of one of the patients who lives at home. The patient, 23-year-old Emily Hoff, refuses to go to the sheltered workshop where she has worked for the last year. Ms. Hoff's mother reports that the patient has been taking her medication. What should Mr. Toll do *first?*

○ 1. Call the director of the sheltered workshop for information about the patient.

○ 2. Reserve an inpatient bed.

○ 3. Reserve a place in the day hospital program.

○ 4. Make an appointment to see the patient.

39. Ms. John, director of the sheltered workshop, tells Mr. Toll that Ms. Hoff had done well until last week when a new patient started at the workshop. This new patient worked faster than Ms. Hoff and took her place as leader of the group. Which of the following is the *most appropriate* intervention for Mr. Toll to implement?

○ 1. Make a home visit and tell Ms. Hoff that if she does not return to the workshop, she will lose her place there.

○ 2. Ask Ms. John to assign Ms. Hoff to another work group when she returns to the workshop.

○ 3. Make an appointment to meet Ms. Hoff at the mental health center and ask her about the situation.

○ 4. Arrange placement for Ms. Hoff in a skill training program.

40. Ms. Hoff tells Mr. Toll that she quit going to the workshop because "the job doesn't pay enough." Her sister just finished school and has been able to buy a car. Ms. Hoff plans to look for an office job like her sister. Which of the following characteristics of a young adult chronically mentally ill patient *best* explains Ms. Hoff's behavior?

○ 1. Difficulty accepting the role of patient.

○ 2. Low self-esteem.

○ 3. Lack of coping resources.

○ 4. High expectations of self in achieving social goals.

41. The mental health center has a psychoeducational program for families of the chronically mentally ill. Mr. Toll invites Ms. Hoff's parents to attend the program. His actions are based on the knowledge that the desired outcomes of psychoeducational programs for families of the chronically mentally ill include *all* of the following *except* helping the families

○ 1. feel less guilty about the patient's illness.

○ 2. develop a support network with other families.

○ 3. improve their conflicted relationship.

○ 4. recognize the patient's strengths more accurately.

42. A 52-year-old woman who has not left the bus station for 3 days is brought to the mental health

center by a police officer because she had been "bothering people." She denies this, will not give her name, and holds tightly to her purse. She refuses to talk to anyone except to say, "You have no right to keep me here. I have money and I can take care of myself." The police can hold her for disturbing the peace but think she needs psychiatric evaluation. Which of the following factors is *most relevant* to a decision about her disposition?

○ 1. The woman's ability to care for herself.
○ 2. The woman has no known family.
○ 3. The woman is not known to the mental health center.
○ 4. The woman has $500 in cash and says she will go to a hotel.

43. The decision is made to admit the woman involuntarily on an emergency basis. Ms. Mather, the nurse on the inpatient unit, explains the involuntary hospitalization process to the woman, who listens quietly. Which of the following statements made by Ms. Mather is *inaccurate?*

○ 1. "You are in the hospital because the psychiatrist who saw you earlier thought you were unable to care for yourself right now."
○ 2. "You are free to talk to a lawyer if you would like to do so."
○ 3. "You cannot leave the hospital until the doctor or a judge thinks you can take care of yourself."
○ 4. "You cannot have any visitors while you are here involuntarily."

44. During the 3 days of involuntary hospitalization, the patient has refused to give any information except her name and the fact that she is a visitor to the city. She has been able to care for herself, has eaten well, and has shown no evidence of psychotic symptoms. In a staff meeting, the patient's doctor argues that the hospital should ask the court to extend the hospitalization order because he has a feeling she is very sick. The nursing staff believes it would be paternalistic and unethical to keep the patient any longer against her will. Which of the following statements *most accurately* describes a paternalistic act?

○ 1. The act is taken in the belief that one knows what is best for the patient and is qualified to act on the patient's behalf.
○ 2. The act is taken based on careful consideration among the staff of what is best for the patient.
○ 3. The act is taken after careful consideration of what the patient would want if she were capable of making an informed decision.
○ 4. The act is taken after careful consideration of what the patient says she would like to have done.

45. As the nurse helps the patient prepare for discharge, the patient says, "You know, I've been in lots of hospitals and I know when I'm sick enough to be there. I'm not that sick now. You don't need to worry about me." Which of the following would be the *most therapeutic* response for the nurse to make?

○ 1. "We are worried about you. Is there any way we can help you now?"
○ 2. "We could have helped you more if you had told us more."
○ 3. "You told us you were a visitor here. Is there any information you need before you leave the hospital?"
○ 4. "How do you know when you need to be in the hospital?"

## THE PATIENT WITH AN OBSESSIVE-COMPULSIVE DISORDER

Jay Bonner, 18, was released from a psychiatric hospital 1 year ago and has been seeing a nurse for outpatient follow-up care. He arrives late for an appointment. During the interview, he fidgets restlessly, has trouble remembering what topic is being discussed, and says he thinks he is "going crazy."

46. Which of the following statements that the nurse could make would *best* deal with Jay's feeling about "going crazy"?

○ 1. "I see that is a concern to you, but what does 'crazy' mean to you?"
○ 2. "Most people feel that way occasionally. You are no different from anyone else."
○ 3. "I don't know enough about you to judge. Why don't you tell me more about yourself?"
○ 4. "You sound perfectly sane to me. Maybe your perception of the word 'crazy' is different from mine."

47. Jay reveals that he was late for his appointment because of "my dumb habit. I have to take off my socks and put them back on 41 times! I can't stop until I do it just right." The nurse judges *correctly* that Jay's behavior is *most likely* representing an effort by the patient to

○ 1. relieve his anxiety.
○ 2. control his thoughts.
○ 3. gain attention from others.
○ 4. express hostility toward his mother.

48. A decision is made not to hospitalize Jay. Of the following abilities Jay has demonstrated, the one

that probably *most* influenced the decision not to hospitalize him is that the patient is able to

- ○ 1. hold a job.
- ○ 2. relate to his peers.
- ○ 3. perform activities of daily living.
- ○ 4. behave in an outwardly normal manner.

**49.** Diazepam (Valium) is prescribed for Jay to help control his anxiety. Of the following considerations, the one that represents the *most serious* problem associated with the regular use of most antianxiety agents is the potential for the drug to

- ○ 1. be abused.
- ○ 2. be lethal.
- ○ 3. cause hypotension.
- ○ 4. cause excessive sleepiness.

**50.** The patient reports that before he leaves home to go anywhere, he counts the money in his wallet as many as 12 times. The *best* explanation for the patient's motives when performing this particular ritual is that he is attempting to

- ○ 1. channel excessive sexual energy into an appropriate habit.
- ○ 2. compensate for not having enough money to spend as a child.
- ○ 3. avoid the embarrassment of having a shortage of funds on hand.
- ○ 4. substitute emotions unacceptable to him with a relatively acceptable activity.

**51.** Which of the following defense mechanisms is Jay using when he overengages in ritualistic behavior?

- ○ 1. Fixation.
- ○ 2. Projection.
- ○ 3. Conversion.
- ○ 4. Displacement.

**52.** In addition to Jay's urge to perform repetitive acts, he is afflicted with the persistent, unwanted thought of doing harm to his brother. This latter disturbance is called

- ○ 1. a phobia.
- ○ 2. an obsession.
- ○ 3. a compulsion.
- ○ 4. a dissociation.

**53.** Jay's mother asks if her son will ever get over "those awful habits of his." Which of the following replies would be *most therapeutic* for the nurse to make?

- ○ 1. "With long-term psychotherapy, he can definitely be helped."
- ○ 2. "It's not always possible to free a person from his symptoms."
- ○ 3. "He is most likely to show improvement with family and individual therapy."
- ○ 4. "That goal is within his reach, although it will require a lot of hard work on his part."

**54.** Which of the following actions would be *best* for the nurse to take when she observes Jay in a ritualistic pattern of behavior?

- ○ 1. Isolate the patient so that he will not disturb others.
- ○ 2. Observe the patient closely for marked changes in behavior.
- ○ 3. Remind the patient he can control his behavior if he wishes.
- ○ 4. Enable the patient to continue so that he will not become more agitated.

**55.** Which of the following qualities is *most important* for the nurse to possess if she is to work successfully with neurotic patients such as Jay?

- ○ 1. Patience.
- ○ 2. Compassion.
- ○ 3. Friendliness.
- ○ 4. Self-confidence.

**56.** Jay is introduced to the other day-care patients, who shortly begin to include him as part of their group. Which of the following factors is probably *most influential* in bringing about the group's positive behavior toward Jay?

- ○ 1. The patient's acceptance of the staff.
- ○ 2. The patient's self-effacing mannerisms.
- ○ 3. The patient's ability to tell funny stories.
- ○ 4. The patient's wardrobe of expensive clothes.

**57.** The staff considers it important to decrease Jay's dependence on others. To meet that goal, when Jay says, "What time is it?" which of the following replies would be the *most effective* for a staff member to make?

- ○ 1. "My watch says 10 o'clock."
- ○ 2. "What time do you think it is?"
- ○ 3. "Has anyone else got the time?"
- ○ 4. "There is a clock behind you on the wall."

**58.** Jay eats slowly and is always the last to finish lunch, which makes it difficult for the group to start its 1 p.m. outing. Which of the following approaches constitutes the *best* plan of action for this problem?

- ○ 1. Change the time of the outing to accommodate the patient.
- ○ 2. Arrange for the patient to start eating earlier than the other patients.
- ○ 3. Plan to go without the patient so that he will have ample time for his lunch.
- ○ 4. Inform the patient he will have to eat faster so that the group can leave on time.

**59.** Jay wants to take up a hobby and asks the day-care nurse for some suggestions. From a therapeutic standpoint, which of the following activities would be the *most desirable* for Jay?

- ○ 1. Swimming.

○ 2. Solo flying.

○ 3. Drama club.

○ 4. Photography.

## THE PATIENT WITH ORGANIC BRAIN SYNDROME

Mrs. Mary Silver, a 72-year-old widow, is brought by ambulance to the psychiatric hospital from a nursing home where she has been a patient for 3 months. Transfer data indicate that she has become increasingly confused and disoriented and has become a "management problem." Mrs. Silver's illness is diagnosed as organic brain syndrome.

**60.** In which of the following ways should the hospital admission routine be modified for an older, confused person like Mrs. Silver?

○ 1. The patient should be left alone to promote recovery of her faculties and composure.

○ 2. The patient should be medicated to ensure her calm cooperation during the admission procedure.

○ 3. The patient should be allowed sufficient extra time in which to gain an understanding of what is happening to her.

○ 4. The patient should be given a tour of the unit to acquaint her with the new environment in which she will live.

**61.** Chronic organic brain syndrome, from which Mrs. Silver suffers, differs from acute organic brain syndrome in that chronic organic brain syndrome is a

○ 1. painful condition.

○ 2. reversible condition.

○ 3. permanent condition.

○ 4. potentially terminal condition.

**62.** If Mrs. Silver experienced a typical onset of her illness, the onset was *most probably*

○ 1. abrupt, with no forewarning.

○ 2. rapid, with many precursory signs.

○ 3. slow, with obvious symptomatology.

○ 4. gradual, with lucid intervals interspersed throughout.

**63.** Mrs. Silver is to undergo a series of diagnostic tests to determine whether or not her organic brain disorder is treatable. Treatable forms of dementia (those with symptoms that can be arrested or reversed) include *all* of the following disorders *except* those caused by

○ 1. cerebral abscess.

○ 2. multiple sclerosis.

○ 3. syphilitic meningitis.

○ 4. electrolyte imbalance.

**64.** An electroencephalogram (EEG) is ordered for Mrs. Silver. The procedure is *most accurately* described as one that

○ 1. is somewhat painful but short.

○ 2. does not involve the use of electrical shock.

○ 3. tests the patient's intelligence but not her sanity.

○ 4. enables the examiner to know what the patient is thinking.

**65.** The night before her EEG, which of the following preparations will *most probably* be required for Mrs. Silver?

○ 1. Washing her hair.

○ 2. Taking a laxative.

○ 3. Going to bed early.

○ 4. Providing a sample of her handwriting.

**66.** After the diagnostic tests are completed, Mrs. Silver's organic condition is found to be due to cerebral arteriosclerosis. Because no known cure exists for this disorder, which of the following attitudes should the nursing staff try to influence the patient (and each other) to adopt?

○ 1. A hopeful attitude.

○ 2. A resigned attitude.

○ 3. A concerned attitude.

○ 4. A nonchalant attitude.

**67.** Which of the following factors has the *most* bearing on the present severity of Mrs. Silver's mental symptoms?

○ 1. Her age and socioeconomic level.

○ 2. The specific areas of her brain that are damaged.

○ 3. Her psychological response to the organic changes.

○ 4. The amount of brain damage inflicted by the causative illness.

**68.** In addition to disturbances in her mental awareness and in her orientation to reality, Mrs. Silver is also likely to show loss of ability in her

○ 1. hearing, vocalizing, and seeing.

○ 2. learning, creativity, and judgment.

○ 3. endurance, strength, and mobility.

○ 4. balance, flexibility, and coordination.

**69.** Of the following comments the nurse could make, which would provide the *best* reality orientation for Mrs. Silver when the patient first awakens in the morning?

○ 1. "Do you remember who I am, Mrs. Silver, or what day it is today?"

○ 2. "Hello, Mrs. Silver, did you sleep well? Which dress would you like to wear today, the yellow or the green one?"

○ 3. "Here I am again, Mrs. Silver, your favorite nurse. Today is Tuesday, so there will be pancakes for breakfast this morning."

○ 4. "Good morning, Mrs. Silver. This is your second day in Memorial Hospital and I am your nurse for today. My name is Ms. Daly."

**70.** Because of Mrs. Silver's age and organic impairment, which of the following courses of action should *most certainly* be included in the plan of care for her?

○ 1. Have two people accompany the patient when she is up and about.

○ 2. Make sure objects the patient may trip over are removed from her path.

○ 3. Put the patient's favorite belongings in a safe place so that she will not lose them.

○ 4. Give the patient her medications in liquid form to make certain that she swallows them.

**71.** Mrs. Silver roams about the hospital unit at night, disturbing the sleep of other patients. When asked why she walks about, she complains of being lost and unable to sleep. A large sign is posted on the door of her room to help her locate it. Which of the following programs would be *best* for dealing with the patient's insomnia?

○ 1. A daily afternoon nap to prevent overtiredness at night.

○ 2. The administration of a hypnotic drug at bedtime.

○ 3. Enough active exercise daily so she will be comfortably tired at night.

○ 4. A cup of hot tea with lemon before bed to promote a feeling of well-being.

**72.** Phenothiazines rather than barbiturates may occasionally be prescribed to treat severe insomnia for Mrs. Silver *primarily* because barbiturates tend to cause

○ 1. eventual kidney damage.

○ 2. respiratory and cardiac depression.

○ 3. delirium and paradoxical excitement.

○ 4. loss of rapid-eye-movement stages during sleep.

**73.** Mrs. Silver's daughter says that her mother wore the same dirty, worn-out undergarments for weeks at home. Of the following techniques, which would be *best* for the nursing staff to follow with Mrs. Silver while she is hospitalized to prevent further regression in her personal hygiene habits?

○ 1. Accept her need to go without bathing if she so desires.

○ 2. Make her assume responsibility for her own physical care.

○ 3. Encourage her to do as much self-care as she is capable of doing.

○ 4. Do most of her physical care while letting her think she did it herself.

**74.** A 35-year-old nurse on the unit often avoids Mrs. Silver's company, preferring to associate with patients of her own age group or younger. Which of the following factors is *most likely* responsible for the nurse's extreme discomfort with older patients and her unconscious avoidance of them?

○ 1. Her own fears and conflicts about aging.

○ 2. Her dislike of physical contact with older people.

○ 3. Her desire to be surrounded by beauty and perfection.

○ 4. Her recent experiences with her mother's elderly friends.

**75.** Mrs. Silver asks the nurse to help her make out her will one day when she is more alert than usual. Which of the following possible responses by the nurse would be *best* in this situation?

○ 1. "I'm not a lawyer, but I will do what I can for you."

○ 2. "You have a long way to go before you will need to do that. Let's wait on it a while, shall we?"

○ 3. "I don't believe in getting involved in legal matters, but maybe I can find another nurse who will help you."

○ 4. "You need to consult an attorney because I am not trained in such matters. Is there a family lawyer I could call for you?"

**76.** Mrs. Silver is allowed to reminisce about her past life. What effect can reminiscing by an elderly patient be expected to have on the patient's functioning in the hospital?

○ 1. Increase the patient's confusion and disorientation.

○ 2. Subject the patient to the impatient responses of others.

○ 3. Decrease the patient's feelings of isolation and loneliness.

○ 4. Keep the patient from participating in therapeutic activities.

**77.** Mrs. Silver's daughter brings an article about Alzheimer's disease to the nurse and says, "This sounds just like Mother. Are you sure she doesn't have Alzheimer's? Maybe she should be in a special treatment program." Which of the following responses by the nurse would be *inaccurate?*

○ 1. "The symptoms that your mother has are common to a number of brain disorders."

○ 2. "You may be right. I'll talk with the physician about doing more tests so we can know for sure."

○ 3. "Even if we were certain that she has Alzheimer's, the treatment that will help her is the same as she is getting."

○ 4. "As we learn more about how the brain ages, it is possible to diagnose these problems more accurately."

78. A clinical manifestation *uncommon* to patients with organic brain syndrome including Alzheimer's disease is

○ 1. agnosia.

○ 2. sleep disturbances.

○ 3. problems with long-term memory retrieval.

○ 4. elevated mood.

79. Mrs. Silver's daughter is convinced that her mother has Alzheimer's disease and asks the nurse, "Does this disease run in families? Will this happen to me when I get old?" The nurse bases her response on knowledge that which of the following factors is *not* associated with increased incidence of Alzheimer's disease?

○ 1. Excessive alcohol consumption.

○ 2. Head trauma.

○ 3. A family history of Alzheimer's disease.

○ 4. Old age.

## USING A THERAPEUTIC MILIEU

Ms. Jones is a nurse employed in a psychiatric hospital, where she works toward providing a therapeutic milieu for patients.

80. The *primary* purpose of managing the milieu on a psychiatric unit is to ensure that the environment will

○ 1. help the patients meet treatment goals.

○ 2. meet the comfort needs of the patients and staff.

○ 3. allow the staff to observe and evaluate the patients.

○ 4. facilitate the implementation of the physicians' orders.

81. Mr. Thomas, a patient for whom Ms. Jones is caring, asks for a medication because he is "feeling nervous." In terms of a therapeutic milieu, it would be *best* for the nurse to respond to the patient's request by saying,

○ 1. "Let's sit down and talk about your feeling nervous."

○ 2. "Why don't you play some ping-pong with Mr. Smith?"

○ 3. "Try lying down awhile and thinking about something else."

○ 4. "I'll call your doctor and get an order for some medication."

82. For which of the following patients for whom Ms. Jones is caring is it *least important* to take steps to set limits?

○ 1. For Ms. Warner, who uses the telephone most of the day.

○ 2. For Mr. Jacobs, whose behavior is disturbing other patients.

○ 3. For Ms. Carney, whose attire is offensive to the nursing staff.

○ 4. For Ms. Frank, whose behavior indicates she may harm herself.

83. Several adolescents are playing the stereo loudly in a common recreation area, and the adult patients complain about the loud music. Which of the following steps should the nurse plan to take as a *first* step in setting limits in this situation?

○ 1. The nurse should set limits on permissible volume while the stereo is being used.

○ 2. The nurse should set limits by denying the use of the stereo in the recreation area.

○ 3. The nurse should set limits by turning down the volume while the stereo is being used.

○ 4. The nurse should set limits by explaining to the adults that the adolescents are in need of recreational activity.

84. Ms. Knight, an elderly patient, is diagnosed as having organic mental disorder and is showing signs of confusion, short attention span, and mood swings. Which of the following activities is *best* suited for Ms. Knight?

○ 1. Having the patient join others going on a field trip.

○ 2. Having the patient become a member in group therapy.

○ 3. Having the patient meet with the assertiveness training group.

○ 4. Having the patient participate in a reality-orientation group.

85. Ms. Knight is transferred to a nursing home from the hospital. The nurse should prepare the patient's family for this move by explaining that Ms. Knight's behavior after moving to the nursing home is *most likely* to demonstrate increased

○ 1. social activity.

○ 2. physical activity.

○ 3. anorexia and sleeplessness.

○ 4. disorientation and forgetfulness.

86. Alice Locker, a hyperkinetic 5-year-old, exhibits signs of extreme restlessness, short attention span, and impulsiveness. Which of the following ways in which the nurse could alter Alice's milieu is likely to be *most therapeutic* for Alice?

○ 1. Increase the child's sensory stimulation and activity.

○ 2. Limit the child's opportunities to display her anger and frustration.

○ 3. Define behaviors of the child that will be acceptable and those that will be unacceptable.

○ 4. Allow the child freedom to choose activities in which to participate and others with whom to associate.

**87.** Jim Barter, age 15, shows signs of mild intoxication. When questioned, he states that another patient, whom he refuses to name, gave him beer. Courses of action are discussed by the staff. The *best* one to initiate at this time is to

○ 1. search the patient's room for beer.

○ 2. call a community meeting to deal with the problem.

○ 3. try to persuade the patient to tell who gave him the beer.

○ 4. call the physician to obtain additional orders for the patient.

**88.** Two adolescents, who do not have smoking privileges, are discovered smoking cigarettes in a patient's room. Of the following courses of action the nurse could take in this situation, it would be *best* for her to plan to restate the limits about cigarette smoking clearly to these patients and

○ 1. restrict their television privileges.

○ 2. send them to separate rooms.

○ 3. discuss their behavior with them.

○ 4. report the incident to their physician.

**89.** Which of the following abilities that the nurse may possess is *best* suited to help provide a therapeutic milieu for patients?

○ 1. The ability to display leadership and persuasiveness.

○ 2. The ability to set goals for the patients' final recovery.

○ 3. The ability to accept behavior as meaningful and motivated.

○ 4. The ability to meet her own needs while helping patients to meet theirs.

**90.** Patient government is often an important component in a therapeutic milieu. The *most important* advantage of this activity is that it

○ 1. saves time for the nursing and auxiliary staff.

○ 2. fosters better planning and implementation of social activities.

○ 3. bridges the gap between the hospital and community environments.

○ 4. promotes better organization for changing hospital unit policies and rules.

**91.** When patients fail to clean the recreation room after using it, a patient-government meeting is held to discuss the problem. In this situation, it is *best* when staff members assume a role of

○ 1. offering their view but agreeing to the group's decision.

○ 2. co-leading the meeting with assistance from any one of the patients.

○ 3. remaining silent while observing the group's process of decision making.

○ 4. allowing a patient the leadership role but requiring staff approval of the group's decision.

# CORRECT ANSWERS AND RATIONALES

Numbers appear in parentheses following the rationales. The numbers identify textbooks listed in the references at the end of Part I, where correct answers can be verified.

## The Patient Who Is Paranoid

1. 2. When a patient refuses to have his belongings checked for valuables or contraband according to hospital policy, the least threatening course of action is for the nurse to ask the patient to open his briefcase while he describes its contents. Obtaining help to take the briefcase away from the patient is a threatening maneuver. Inspecting the briefcase while the patient is out of his room involves secrecy and is less desirable than an open discussion with the patient. Telling the patient he must observe hospital policy to stay is threatening and very probably an inaccurate statement as well. (2, 12)

2. 1. Asking the patient described in this item who "they" are when he is fearful that someone will see the nurse through the window allows the nurse to understand his behavior and is least demanding of the patient. The patient is very unlikely to accept statements that indicate no one will see the nurse and that there is no reason to be afraid. Asking the patient what will happen if someone sees the nurse is also unlikely to be acceptable to the patient. (5, 12)

3. 3. The behavior of the patient described in this item is likely to be reinforced when the nurse takes steps to agree with the false ideas he holds. The nurse's action of moving away from the window as requested by the patient is less likely to be interpreted as a lack of poise, an effort to humor the patient, or an admission of giving in to the patient's wishes. (2, 5)

4. 4. The patient's thought process, as described in this item, is best defined as a delusion of persecution. A delusion of grandeur involves an exaggerated idea of one's importance or identity. An idea of reference assumes that the remarks and behavior of others apply to oneself. (2, 5)

5. 4. Delusional thinking is a belief that is not validated by reality and is maintained even when proof is given to the contrary. In this item, the patient is unable to differentiate between his thoughts and external reality. Some suspicious patients demonstrate sensitivity to the thoughts and feelings of others, but this is not evidence of delusional thinking. (2, 12)

6. 2. The effect of questioning a patient closely about his false ideas is to place him on the defensive, and he will most likely continue to defend his unrealistic point of view even more rigorously. Close questioning is unlikely to lead the patient to reverse, share, or clarify his thinking. (2, 5)

7. 2. To promote a therapeutic relationship with a suspicious patient, it is best to set aside periods for conversation with the patient at the same time each day. During the working phase of a therapeutic relationship, the nurse should be as consistent as possible. It is less satisfactory to use unspecified times or to allow the patient to initiate meetings with the nurse. It is difficult to have meaningful conversations that promote a therapeutic relationship when meetings occur only when the patient is agitated, although the nurse may need to use intervention measures at those times as well. (2, 12)

8. 3. When the patient becomes restless during a conversation with the nurse, as described in this item, the best course of action for the nurse is to help the patient recognize and acknowledge his feelings and to share her observations with him. Other courses of action, such as changing the subject, taking the patient for a walk, and leaving the patient, do not encourage him to express his anxiety. (2, 12)

9. 4. The suspicious patient characteristically considers others part of a conspiracy against him. Questioning the motives of others, ridiculing and belittling others, and believing he is right and others are wrong are more easily managed and are not central to the core problem of suspicion. (2, 12)

10. 1. It is generally best to try giving a medication in its liquid form if the patient is "fighting" taking the medication. If he refuses to swallow or expectorates the medication, the intramuscular route then can be used, although it too will probably meet with resistance from the patient. (2, 12)

11. 2. The patient's behavior described in this item is best defined as akathisia, also sometimes spelled acathisia. Dyskinesia is characterized by twitching or involuntary muscular movement. Dystonia is characterized by uncoordinated spasmodic movements. (2, 5, 12)

12. 2. The drug of choice when a patient is experiencing extrapyramidal side effects to chlorpromazine (Thorazine) is benztropine mesylate (Cogentin) because of its anticholinergic properties. Chlordiazepoxide (Librium) is a minor tranquilizer, or antianxiety agent. Imipramine hydrochloride (Tofranil) is an antidepressant. Thioridazine hydrochloride (Mellaril) is a major tranquilizer, or antipsychotic agent. (5, 11)

**13.** 4. The patient described in this item shows aggression against his perceived adversary when he names another patient as his adversary. The staff will need to watch him carefully for signs of impending violent behavior that may cause injury to others. Crying about a divorce describes appropriate, rather than pathologic, behavior. A petition to end the curfew hour describes a positive, direct action aimed at a bothersome situation. Declining to attend group therapy needs follow-up but may be due to any number of unknown reasons. (2, 12)

**14.** 4. Reaction formation uses the defense of substituting the opposite behavior or beliefs for the true feelings the individual holds. Denial involves a refusal to accept some aspect of reality. Introjection means turning feelings and responses inward against the self. Idealization prevents the patient from seeing another person's faults. (2, 12)

**15.** 1. Like patients, health personnel have feelings and rights. The nurse described in this item permits the assistant her rights by making a statement that allows the assistant to be angry without scolding her or dismissing her feelings. (2, 5)

**16.** 1. Touch should be used cautiously with patients, especially paranoid patients who have poor reality testing and who project their own feelings and impulses. These patients may easily misinterpret the use of touch. (2, 12)

**17.** 4. The suspicious patient is likely to begin paranoid ideation when he sees his nurse talking with other patients outside of his hearing range. Taking actions that encourage the patient to take responsibility for his own actions, having nurses as role models, and minimizing promises while keeping those that are made are unlikely to arouse feelings of suspicion and conspiracy. (2, 12)

**18.** 2. In preparation for discharging the patient from the hospital, it is best for the nurse to work toward ending the relationship and exploring reactions to the separation. Advice is not recommended. Health teaching is important, but during final interactions with the patient it is of primary importance to work toward ending the nurse-patient relationship. Furthermore, the health teaching should not be left until the last minute. (2, 12)

## *The Patient with Catatonic Schizophrenia*

**19.** 1. It is important to help make the patient described in this situation feel safe and accepted. Helping the patient get acquainted with others and giving her information about the program are important but have lesser priority at the time of ad-

mission. Providing the patient with clean c̦ desirable but less important than conveyi̧ņ ings of safety and trust. (2, 5)

**20.** 3. The best charting describes exactly what ᵥ patient did and said in a particular situation. Noting that the patient was unable to answer questions, was uncooperative, and was disoriented and incoherent do not follow this basic principle of documenting and are not objective descriptions. (2, 5)

**21.** 3. An outstanding characteristic of fluphenazine decanoate (Prolixin Decanoate) is that it can be used effectively while being administered relatively infrequently. (5, 11, 12)

**22.** 4. It is least important to check the results of pulmonary function tests for the patient receiving fluphenazine decanoate (Prolixin Decanoate). Weight checks are indicated because a side effect of this drug is edema with weight changes. The patient should be monitored for blood dyscrasias. Blood pressure may fluctuate while the drug is being used and should be monitored. (2, 11, 12)

**23.** 3. The best approach when the patient has difficulty expressing herself verbally is to use a nondemanding, open-ended statement. When the patient is ready to talk, the silences following the statement will give the patient the opportunity to do so. Asking the patient questions, using hand signals, and saying what the nurse thinks the patient is experiencing are ineffective when a patient has a verbal communication problem. (2, 5)

**24.** 3. Punishment and reward are likely to be of little value when a patient does the opposite of what she is requested to do. The patient simply may not eat if allowed to decide when to go to the dining room. The best course of action is to lead the patient described in this item firmly to the dining room. This type of positive and firm approach is also needed to help increase the patient's socialization. (2, 12)

**25.** 2. A patient's behavior is best described as regression when it is typical of an earlier stage of development. Fixation means not progressing beyond a given level of development. Substitution means replacing unacceptable ideas with more acceptable ones. Symbolization occurs when one idea or object comes to stand for another. (2, 12)

**26.** 1. It has been shown that nonverbal communication usually conveys feelings more accurately than spoken words. Words very often are used to cover feelings, while nonverbal communication offers less opportunity to hide true feelings. (2, 12)

**27.** 3. The recommended first course of action is to prevent accidents and injuries when a patient becomes violent. In the situation described in this item, it would be best to call for help to handle the situation safely. Other courses of action may be followed later, after safety is ensured. (5, 12)

**28.** 3. The indiscriminate use of restraints can lead to charges of false imprisonment, which is defined as unjustifiable retention without proper consent. Fraud is willful and purposeful misrepresentation that could cause or has caused harm. Assault refers to a threat or an attempt to make bodily contact with another person without consent. Invasion of privacy is a wrong that invades the right of a person to be left alone. (2, 12)

**29.** 1. The nurse demonstrates her interest in the feelings the husband expresses about his wife, as described in this item, and provides an opportunity to discuss them when she acknowledges his anxiety and offers to converse with him. Statements to the husband that indicate the staff is doing the best it can, that the patient is better than the husband thinks, and that rushing through treatment may make matters worse give the husband no reassurance and ignore his feelings. (2, 5)

**30.** 3. The nurse needs to know to whom the patient is referring in the situation described in this item and should try to obtain this information from the patient. Such plans as arranging for a social service consultation and assigning someone to watch the patient are premature, although they may be indicated later. Asking the family to limit visits would not be helpful in gaining an understanding of the situation. (2, 5)

## The Patient with Chronic Mental Illness

**31.** 4. Among the needs of the chronically mentally ill are community-based treatment programs, psychosocial rehabilitation programs, and appropriate employment opportunities. During necessary periods of hospitalization, active treatment rather than custodial care is needed. (2, 12)

**32.** 3. The role of a nurse in a psychosocial rehabilitation program involves teaching the patient to live independently by using interpersonal skills and community resources. Insight-oriented psychotherapy is a program goal. (2, 12)

**33.** 1. Symptom exacerbation is most often related to medication noncompliance. Therefore, obtaining information about the patient's compliance with medication is the first priority. Helping the patient recognize the symptoms and her ability to manage them, and checking with her employer are appropriate, but not the first priority. Hospitalization is

not indicated because the patient is still working and can talk about the symptoms. (2, 5, 12)

**34.** 3. Recognizing the patient's feeling and her progress while obtaining more information is the most therapeutic response. Reminding the patient of her previous related experience is also appropriate but could be done more therapeutically. To suggest the possibility of a drug holiday when symptoms are recurring is clinically unsound. (2, 5, 12)

**35.** 1. The psychotropic drug categories used in the treatment of chronic mental illness are more appropriate for inclusion in the teaching plan than a variety of psychotropic drug categories. Teaching should be focused on the needs and interests of the target audience. Interventions for common side effects of psychotropic drugs, the role of medication in the treatment of chronic mental illness, and the effects of using common street drugs with psychotropic medication are topics that should be included in the teaching program. (2, 5, 12)

**36.** 2. Care rather than cure is the treatment focus with the chronically mentally ill. This group has been labeled deviant and many of the secondary symptoms develop in response to the deviant role assigned to them. Primary symptoms are those associated with the psychiatric illness such as hallucinations and delusion. While individual variation exists, the development of chronic mental illness follows a predictable pattern. (2, 12)

**37.** 1. Young adult chronically mentally ill patients are between the ages of 18 and 35. Due to deinstitutionalization they did not experience long periods of hospitalization in which to learn a patient role and decreased self-expectations that accompany the chronic patient role in older chronically mentally ill patients. Substance abuse is very common in the young adult chronically mentally ill patient. (2, 12)

**38.** 1. Getting information from the director of the sheltered workshop is the most efficient first step in planning appropriate intervention. This information will help the nurse decide if inpatient or day hospital treatment is indicated. The nurse will meet with the patient before implementing more intensive treatment. (2, 12)

**39.** 3. An appointment with the patient at the mental health center to explore her feelings and behavior acknowledges the patient's importance and makes her a partner in resolving the problem. Threatening the patient with loss of a position at the workshop, asking for a new assignment for the patient at the workshop, or changing the patient's program are premature actions. (2, 12)

**40.** 4. Because young adult chronically mentally ill patients have not been hospitalized for long periods, they have not learned or accepted lower role expectations and continue to expect to achieve the same social goals as non-mentally ill peers. While low self-esteem and lack of coping resources are common in this patient group, the patient's present behavior does not demonstrate these characteristics. (12)

**41.** 3. Psychoeducational groups for families have the following goals: education about the biochemical etiology of psychiatric disease to reduce family guilt; education about symptoms and symptom management; education about medication; family networking; and ways of coping with a mentally ill family member. (2, 5, 12)

**42.** 1. The ability of the woman described in this situation to care for herself is most relevant to a decision about her disposition. If she is gravely disabled or needs treatment in order to care for herself, involuntary hospitalization is indicated whether or not the woman is known to the mental health center. Having monetary resources does not mean the woman will be able to use them to care for herself. (2, 12)

**43.** 4. Patients have a right to see visitors regardless of admission status. Involuntary hospitalization requires a psychiatrist state-of-need. Release requires medical and/or legal approval. Any patient admitted involuntarily has the right to legal counsel. (2, 12)

**44.** 1. A paternalistic act is characterized by a belief that one is qualified to act on the patient's behalf for his own good and is justified in this act whether or not the patient has ever or will ever give consent. The act may frequently involve violating a moral rule, such as breaking a promise. (12)

**45.** 1. It is most therapeutic to let the patient know of continued staff concern and to ask her what might be useful to her. Making the point that she did not use the hospital well is not therapeutic on discharge. Offering information and reviewing patient symptom recognition are both therapeutic responses. (2, 5, 12)

## The Patient with an Obsessive-Compulsive Disorder

**46.** 1. When the patient in this item says he thinks he is "going crazy," it is best for the nurse to ask him what "crazy" means to him. Before the nurse can move toward consensual validation, she must have a clear idea of what the patient means by his words and action. (2, 12)

**47.** 1. The patient who is experiencing an obsessive-compulsive type of behavior is attempting to con-trol his anxiety. The compulsive part of the behavior is an act that is performed by the individual to relieve or avoid anxiety. (5, 12)

**48.** 3. A patient who is able to take care of his basic nutritional and hygiene needs is probably not sufficiently incapacitated by his illness that he requires hospitalization. The ability to behave normally is of lesser importance in this decision, depending on the tolerance of the patient's family or significant others for the behavior. The patient's abilities to hold a job and relate to his peers may be considered in making the decision but are not valid criteria for hospitalization. (2, 5, 12)

**49.** 1. Antianxiety agents are among the most often prescribed and abused drugs in the United States, and diazepam (Valium) is one of them. Only very high dosages are likely to be lethal or cause sleepiness when mixed with depressant drugs or alcohol. Hypotension is not associated with the use of antianxiety medications. (2, 9, 12)

**50.** 4. The dynamics of compulsive activity involve a defense against anxiety by persistently doing something else (that is, a substitution activity). This behavior occurs each time threatening thoughts or impulses appear. Channeling excessive sexual energy into an appropriate habit describes a defense mechanism that is almost always healthy (sublimation). The judgments that the patient described in this item counts money repeatedly to compensate for not having enough money to spend as a child or to avoid the embarrassment of running short of money are based on insufficient data and oversimplification of the problem the patient presents. (2, 5)

**51.** 4. Displacement is the mechanism employed when a patient overengages in ritualistic behavior. Fixation is the arrest of psychosocial maturation. Projection occurs when emotionally unacceptable self-traits are unconsciously rejected and attributed to others. Conversion occurs when repressed ideas or impulses are converted into a variety of somatic symptoms. (2, 12)

**52.** 2. The disturbance described in this item (that is, having a persistent unwanted thought of harming another) is an obsession. A phobia is a persistent, unrealistic fear of an external object or situation through the mechanism of displacement. A compulsion is an unwanted urge to perform an act. Dissociation is an unconscious process of separating and detaching emotional significance from an idea, situation, or effect. (2, 5, 12)

**53.** 3. When the mother of a young man with an obsessive-compulsive disorder asks if her son's behavior will eventually return to normal, it is best for the nurse to point out that the patient is most likely to show improvement with family and individual therapy. Because a neurosis is believed to stem from disturbances rooted in childhood, family and individual therapy will be important for the patient's recovery. (2, 5)

**54.** 4. It is best to accept compulsive behavior in a comparatively permissive manner. The patient may become restless and anxious if the ritualistic activity is denied him. Isolating the patient, observing the patient for marked changes in behavior, and reminding the patient that he can control his behavior if he wishes describe unwarranted or inappropriate measures in this situation. (2, 5)

**55.** 1. While compassion, friendliness, and self-confidence may be desirable to some degree in caring for a patient with an obsessive-compulsive disorder, it is considered most important that the nurse demonstrate patience. It takes the patient a long time to complete necessary tasks. Unless the nurse is patient, she can easily become frustrated, upset, or angry. The obsessive-compulsive patient cannot be hurried. (2, 5)

**56.** 1. Patients use the staff as role models. A new patient in the group is likely to be accepted more readily when he demonstrates accepting the staff as other members of the group have done. An established group is likely to devalue a new member in the group when he uses self-effacing mannerisms. Also, they are likely to resent an expensive wardrobe. Telling stories is unlikely to be sustained as a basis for acceptance and may irritate depressed patients. (2, 12)

**57.** 4. To decrease a patient's dependence on others, when the patient described in this item asks what time it is, it is best for a staff member to point out where the clock is for the patient to use. Telling the patient the time or asking someone else the time increases the patient's dependence. It is belittling to the patient described in this item to be asked what time he thinks it is. (2, 12)

**58.** 2. Letting the patient described in this item eat earlier meets both his needs for more time and the group's need for prompt departure on an outing. It also protects the patient from being resented by others and lets him be included in group activity. Changing the time of an activity to meet the needs of one patient is undesirable and may be impractical as well. (2, 12)

**59.** 3. Drama clubs are good for their social and self-expressive qualities. Patients such as the one described in this situation need outlets that are creative and oriented toward others. Swimming, solo flying, and photography are hobbies with few social and other-oriented qualities. (2, 12)

## The Patient with Organic Brain Syndrome

**60.** 3. When admitting an elderly patient, especially one who is confused and disoriented, it is best to give the patient extra time in which to gain an understanding of what is happening to her. This will help her get her bearings and adjust to a new environment. In the situation described in this item, it would be less desirable to leave the patient alone, medicate her, or try to orient her to the new environment. (2, 5, 12)

**61.** 3. Chronic organic brain syndrome is considered a permanent and irreversible condition. Acute organic brain syndrome is usually a temporary and reversible condition and is not necessarily painful or fatal. (2, 12)

**62.** 4. Chronic organic brain disorder characteristically produces symptoms gradually, and lucid moments may be interspersed throughout the course of the disease. (2, 12)

**63.** 2. Multiple sclerosis is a progressive chronic disease; its course cannot be reversed, although patients may experience periods of remission. A cerebral abscess, syphilitic meningitis, and an electrolyte imbalance are treatable, and cure is possible. (9)

**64.** 2. Electroencephalography records the electrical activity in the brain. It does not involve the use of electrical shock, is not painful, does not test the patient's intelligence, and does not enable others to know what the patient is thinking. (9)

**65.** 1. The patient's hair should be free of oils, sprays, and lotion prior to an EEG; hence, preparation of the patient includes a shampoo. Preparations such as giving the patient a laxative, going to bed early, and providing a sample of her handwriting are not indicated for an EEG. (9)

**66.** 1. People of all ages need to sense a future for well-being. They must have hope of things to come and believe in growth and change to live life to its fullest. Health personnel need to foster this feeling of hopefulness and subscribe to it to help people attain well-being, even when the prognosis appears poor. (5, 12)

**67.** 3. Symptoms vary widely among patients with chronic organic brain syndrome. However, the patient's age, socioeconomic level, areas of the brain damaged, and amount of brain damage are not necessarily related to the severity of symptoms. It is the manner in which the patient responds psychologically that will have the most bearing on the patient's symptoms. (2, 5)

**68.** 2. Basic symptomatology demonstrates that patients with chronic organic brain disorders experience defects in memory, orientation, and intellectual functions, such as judgment and discrimination. Loss of other abilities is less typical. (2, 5)

69. 4. To promote reality orientation, the nurse should be as specific as possible when addressing a confused and disoriented patient. Such comments as indicating what day it is, where the patient is, and the nurse's name help the patient. Asking the patient questions about her environment is likely to be challenging and may decrease the patient's self-esteem. Stereotyped comments give the patient no basic information. Nor is it helpful when the nurse gives the patient mostly irrelevant information. (2, 5)

70. 2. When caring for a patient with organic brain impairment, it *may* be necessary to have two people accompany the patient when she ambulates, place the patient's favorite things in safekeeping, and give medications in a liquid form to be sure they are swallowed. However, it is most essential to remove objects in the patient's path of ambulation to help prevent falls. (2, 12)

71. 3. A patient with insomnia is more likely to sleep well if she feels tired at bedtime, which is likely if she had enough daily exercise so that she is comfortably tired at night. Having the patient take a daily afternoon nap is likely to interfere with nighttime sleep. Offering the patient tea at bedtime is unlikely to promote sleep, especially since it contains caffeine, which may lead to further wakefulness. Sedatives should be used only as a last resort because they are likely to be habit-forming. (9)

72. 3. Delirium, confusion, and excitement are signs of barbiturate toxicity, and therefore barbiturates are less preferable than other sedatives for a patient who is often confused and disoriented. (11)

73. 3. The best procedure for helping the patient remain independent and observe good habits of hygiene is to encourage her to do as much self-care as she is capable of doing. For the patient described in this item, it would be inappropriate to accept her poor personal hygiene habits. It would be impractical and unrealistic to expect the patient to start taking care of all her hygiene needs. To do all of the patient's hygienic care would further cause the patient to become dependent, and it would be dishonest to care for the patient while letting her think she did it herself. (2, 12)

74. 1. The most likely reason for a nurse's discomfort with the elderly is that she has not examined her own fears and conflicts about aging. Until she does, it is unlikely that she will feel comfortable with elderly patients. (5, 12)

75. 4. A will is an important legal document, and it is best to have one prepared with the help of an attorney. It would be unsafe for the nurse to help the patient described in this item because a nurse is not a lawyer. Asking the patient to delay preparing the will avoids the problem. It is also not helpful for the nurse to seek out another nurse to help the patient prepare a will. (2, 12)

76. 3. Reminiscing can help reduce depression in an elderly person and lessens feelings of isolation and loneliness. It gives the person permission to be old. (2, 12)

77. 2. The cluster of symptoms, including increased confusion and disorientation, that led to the patient's admission are common to a number of brain disorders for which the treatment is similar. Although medical science is rapidly learning more about the aging brain, no definitive test for Alzheimer's exists. Changes found at autopsy are the most definitive markers known at this time.(7)

78. 4. Elevated mood states are uncommon among patients with organic brain disorders. Irritability, anxiety, and depression are more common mood states. Agnosia (the decreased ability to recognize both people and objects), sleep disturbances, and problems with long-term memory retrieval are common. (7, 10)

79. 1. Alcohol consumption among individuals with Alzheimer's disease has not been found to be greater than that in individuals without Alzheimer's disease. A family history of the disease, a history of head trauma, and old age have all been shown to be associated with increased incidence of the disease. (7)

## Using a Therapeutic Milieu

80. 1. A therapeutic milieu is described as an environment that helps patients meet treatment goals. Meeting the comfort needs of the patients and staff, allowing the staff to observe and evaluate the patients, and facilitating the implementation of physicians' orders are significant but do not describe the primary purpose of managing the patient's environment, or milieu. (12)

81. 1. The nurse should take the time to listen to the patient to discover more about his feelings before making an assessment or intervening. Calling the physician describes an intervention made without complete data. Giving advice by suggesting that the patient rest or play a game with another patient would not be considered therapeutic in this situation. (5)

82. 3. The nurse should judge a patient's behavior in relation to the milieu and clarify the behavior's effect on the milieu, not on personal values held by

staff members. Overuse of the telephone, behavior that disturbs other patients, and the presence of behavior that may harm the patient describe situations requiring a degree of limit setting. (5, 12)

**83.** 1. The nurse should state the limits clearly to patients who are disturbing others. The limits should be objective and fair and should reflect the situation at hand. When possible, the patients should be included in decision making, but the nurse is ultimately responsible. (5, 12)

**84.** 4. Since the patient described in this item has impaired memory, attention, and concentration, a reality-orientation group is recommended to assist her to maintain an optimal level of functioning. Becoming a member in group therapy, going on a field trip, and meeting with an assertiveness training group are likely to be too stressful or stimulating to the patient in this situation and may increase her frustration and decrease her sense of accomplishment. (5, 12)

**85.** 4. Patients with organic mental disorders are sometimes placed in nursing homes where care tends to be routinized and sensory stimuli are minimal. As a result, disorientation and an inability to recall and retain information are further aggravated. Increased physical and social activity, anorexia, and sleeplessness are less likely to occur when a patient with organic mental disorder is moved to a nursing home. (5, 12)

**86.** 3. Children need to know what types of behavior will be acceptable and what types will be unacceptable. They feel more secure when boundaries are clear and when policies concerning their behavior are consistently enforced. Increasing sensory stimulation and activity, limiting opportunities to display anger and frustration, and allowing freedom to choose activities are types of interventions that would tend to increase stress and a sense of frustration for the hyperkinetic patient. (5, 12)

**87.** 2. The milieu should be used to increase peer support and handle confrontation when necessary. Peer pressure on adolescents is generally more effective to help change behavior than the staff's influence. Searching the patient's room and trying to persuade a patient who was involved to tell on his friends are authoritarian actions and may increase

mistrust of the staff. Calling a physician is not necessary at this time in the situation described in this item. (5, 12)

**88.** 3. Adolescents tend to test the limits of their surroundings as an expression of inner conflicts. The relationship between limit setting and inner conflicts needs to be explored through discussion to increase self-awareness in the situation described in this item. Sending the patients to separate rooms or reporting the situation to their physician may be used if necessary after discussion has occurred. Restricting television privileges has no relationship to the abused privilege. (5, 12)

**89.** 3. The milieu should provide an atmosphere that fosters growth, change, and self-responsibility. The staff needs to accept behavior as meaningful and motivated. Staff interventions should also be flexible and open and should encourage patients to achieve their own potential. Displaying leadership and persuasiveness, setting goals for patients, and meeting one's own needs while helping patients meet their needs are not well-suited for a therapeutic milieu. (5, 12)

**90.** 3. Patients are helped to bridge the gap between the hospital and community environments when they learn to function in leadership, membership, and decision-making positions in an activity that increases their awareness of the democratic process. Saving staff time, planning better social activities, and promoting better organization for changing policies and rules describe possible outcomes of patient government, but none of these is the *main* advantage of the activity described in this item. (5, 12)

**91.** 1. The milieu should foster relationship development and decision-making abilities among patients. Staff members need to encourage patient discussion and decision making by offering their view but agreeing to abide by the group's decision concerning unit (but not hospital) policies and issues. Co-leading a patient-government meeting, remaining silent during a meeting, and requiring staff approval of the group's decision are not the most therapeutic roles for staff members in the milieu setting and may hinder effective patient government. (5, 12)

# *test* 3

*The Patient with a Personality Disorder*

*The Patient Who Abuses Alcohol*

*The Patient with Alcohol Withdrawal*

*The Patient Who is Dependent on Narcotics*

*The Patient Who Abuses Barbiturates*

*The Patient with an Eating Disorder*

*Correct Answers and Rationales*

Select the one *best* or *correct* answer and indicate your choice by filling in the circle with a pencil in front of the option you have chosen. If the answer you would prefer is not given, select the one you think is *most appropriate*.

## THE PATIENT WITH A PERSONALITY DISORDER

Monica Moore, 14, is readmitted to the adolescent unit of the psychiatric hospital. She recently ran away from home for the fifth time this year and while hitchhiking in a state of drug-induced euphoria on a freeway was picked up by the police. She is accompanied to the unit by her juvenile worker.

1. "Hi, gang, I'm back," Monica says cheerfully to the unit at large. Which of the following statements that Monica could make about her readmission would show the *best* prospects for her eventual success in therapy?
   ○ 1. "I'm here because my parents were bugging me again."
   ○ 2. "I'm here because my shrink thought it would be best."
   ○ 3. "I'm here because I made a mess of it on the outside."
   ○ 4. "I'm here because I missed all the fun we had together."

2. Monica is called a "manipulator" by a nurse because in the past, Monica played one staff member against another for favors and made them angry with each other. When the staff analyzes the nurse's comment, it *correctly* judges that labeling Monica as a manipulator is *most likely* to function by
   ○ 1. preventing the staff from expecting too much of the patient.
   ○ 2. preventing the staff from seeing the patient as she really is.
   ○ 3. helping the staff find ways to prevent the patient from mocking them.

   ○ 4. helping the staff identify approaches for appropriate therapy for the patient.

3. An attitude on the part of the nurse that would *most likely* foster a therapeutic relationship between the nurse and Monica, who tries to manipulate people, is an attitude of
   ○ 1. sympathy.
   ○ 2. aloofness.
   ○ 3. strictness.
   ○ 4. consistency.

4. Monica is assigned to the care of an overweight nurse on the evening shift. The nurse recalls that after finding Monica in bed with a young male patient during her last admission, she became the butt of some of Monica's jokes. Which of the following courses of action would be *best* for the nurse to take concerning such previous negative experiences with a patient?
   ○ 1. Forget them as quickly as possible.
   ○ 2. Accept them as unpleasant but past experiences.
   ○ 3. Excuse them as part of the patient's poor upbringing.
   ○ 4. Remember them as significant examples of the patient's present capacity for mischief.

5. The nurse initiates a conversation with Monica. Monica tries to put the nurse at ease, graciously telling her to sit down and inquiring what she could do for her. Monica leads the discussion and informs the nurse how much time she can spend with her. Which of the following phenomena is *best* illustrated by this interaction?
   ○ 1. Denial.
   ○ 2. Incongruency.
   ○ 3. Role reversal.
   ○ 4. Self-fulfilling prophecy.

6. The nurse recognizes that she is having difficulty

**43**

maintaining control in her relationship with Monica. Which of the following actions would be *best* for the nurse to take in relation to being outmaneuvered by this patient?

○ 1. Seek help from the other staff members.
○ 2. Request to be assigned to a different patient.
○ 3. Discuss feelings of frustration with the patient.
○ 4. Focus attention on the patient's nonadaptive behavior.

7. In the course of their conversation, Monica tells the nurse bitterly, "My parents are mean. They don't care about me at all." Which of the following responses by the nurse would be the *least* therapeutic?

○ 1. "You feel your parents don't care about you."
○ 2. "What would be a sign to you that your parents cared?"
○ 3. "I am sure your parents have your best interests at heart."
○ 4. "Tell me more about your parents being mean and not caring."

8. Monica is quick to learn about the problems of other people and to use this knowledge for her own amusement. She makes a target of a 15-year-old withdrawn girl and has the other patients tease and play tricks on her. Of the following people, who would probably have the *most* influence in helping Monica change her behavior?

○ 1. Her physician.
○ 2. Her peer group.
○ 3. Her juvenile worker.
○ 4. Her religious counselor.

9. It did not bother Monica that her trick playing, teasing, and running away from home may have caused others to suffer. According to psychoanalytic theory, this lack of remorse is due to a defect in the functioning of the

○ 1. id.
○ 2. ego.
○ 3. superego.
○ 4. self-concept.

10. When the nurses plan Monica's nursing care, which of the following traits that Monica would also be *most likely* to display should be taken into account?

○ 1. Poor judgment.
○ 2. Faulty memory.
○ 3. Low intelligence.
○ 4. Disordered thinking.

11. Susan Twill, 32, is in treatment at the day hospital. This is her seventh admission since age 18. She has been unable to hold part-time jobs and has had four abortions in the last four years. She is now living with her family after being evicted from her apartment. She complains of feeling empty and lonely. Her arms are scarred from frequent episodes of self-mutilation. Which of the following personality disorders does Ms. Twill exhibit?

○ 1. Antisocial personality disorder.
○ 2. Avoidant personality disorder.
○ 3. Borderline personality disorder.
○ 4. Compulsive personality disorder.

12. Ms. Twill has become attached to Ms. Brill, a part-time nurse, and frequently refuses to share her history with any other staff members. She tells Ms. Brill that other staff members mistreat her, that she can trust only her and fears for her safety during Ms. Brill's absence. This common defense mechanism is known as

○ 1. reaction formation.
○ 2. splitting.
○ 3. projection.
○ 4. denial.

13. Ms. Twill repeatedly states she is not like the other patients and asks the staff for special privileges. She does not follow the rules about the use of the telephone or television. The nurse develops a care plan related to this behavior. An immediate and major focus of the plan would be to

○ 1. enforce the unit rules consistently.
○ 2. limit the patient's contact with others.
○ 3. obtain vocational training for the patient.
○ 4. ignore the patient's behavior.

14. Ms. Twill describes her personal history with sadness. Her mother died when Ms. Twill was two years old, and Ms. Twill's life after that was chaotic and disorganized. She lived with a number of relatives and in foster homes. In planning Ms. Twill's care, the nurse attempts to promote completion of the developmental task on which the patient would most likely have been working when her mother died. According to Erikson, this basic task is the achievement of

○ 1. trust.
○ 2. independence.
○ 3. safety.
○ 4. autonomy.

15. As Ms. Twill's discharge date approaches, she asks to stay in the program and makes threats to "do something" to herself if discharged. The staff remains firm on the discharge date. Which of the following interventions would be *most important* to ensure Ms. Twill's safety?

○ 1. Request an immediate extension for the patient.
○ 2. Ask the patient to leave early.
○ 3. Transfer the patient to another hospital.
○ 4. Assess the seriousness of the patient's threats.

## THE PATIENT WHO ABUSES ALCOHOL

A friend accompanies Mr. Peter Willard to the substance abuse unit of the hospital, where he is to be admitted for detoxification from alcohol.

16. Mr. Willard consumes about 6 ounces of alcohol just before coming to the hospital. Which of the following methods would be *best* for the nursing staff to use to promote the rate of alcohol destruction in the patient's body?
    ○ 1. Give the patient black coffee to drink.
    ○ 2. Walk the patient around the unit following a cold shower.
    ○ 3. Have the patient breathe pure oxygen through a face mask.
    ○ 4. Provide the patient with a restful room so that he can sleep off the effects of alcohol.

17. Hospital policy requires that the patient's belongings be searched for contraband on admission. In view of Mr. Willard's drinking problem, which of his possessions is *most likely* to be confiscated by the nursing staff?
    ○ 1. Hair dressing.
    ○ 2. Electric razor.
    ○ 3. Shaving cream.
    ○ 4. Antiseptic mouthwash.

18. While obtaining a nursing history, the nurse questions Mr. Willard about the amount of alcohol he consumes daily. The nurse can expect that Mr. Willard will *most probably* answer the question by
    ○ 1. exaggerating the amount.
    ○ 2. underestimating the amount.
    ○ 3. indicating he does not know the amount.
    ○ 4. expressing uncertainty about the amount.

19. The *most important* reason for investigating the amount of alcohol Mr. Willard has consumed during the 24 to 48 hours before admission is to help determine
    ○ 1. how far the disease has progressed.
    ○ 2. the degree of severity of withdrawal.
    ○ 3. whether the patient will experience delirium tremens.
    ○ 4. whether the patient should be considered an alcoholic.

20. Which two of Mr. Willard's basic needs will probably require the *most* attention from the nursing staff during the early detoxification period?
    ○ 1. Rest and nutrition.
    ○ 2. Safety and security.
    ○ 3. Comfort and hygiene.
    ○ 4. Aeration and elimination.

21. The nurse who could probably relate *most effectively* with Mr. Willard is one who has an attitude of
    ○ 1. morality.
    ○ 2. optimism.
    ○ 3. acceptance.
    ○ 4. indulgence.

22. Of the following medications, the one *most likely* to be prescribed for Mr. Willard to provide sedation and to ease some of the anxiety and discomfort of the alcohol withdrawal process is
    ○ 1. paraldehyde (Paral).
    ○ 2. chlordiazepoxide (Librium).
    ○ 3. phenytoin sodium (Dilantin).
    ○ 4. phenobarbital sodium (Luminal).

23. Mr. Willard could not remember the events of the past weekend, although he had receipts in his pockets from several shops where he made purchases on Saturday. This problem is illustrative of a condition known as
    ○ 1. a blackout.
    ○ 2. a hangover.
    ○ 3. a dry drunk syndrome.
    ○ 4. an alcoholic hallucinosis.

24. After a day of abstinence, Mr. Willard has coarse tremors of the hands, which make it hard for him to feed himself. He asks the nurse how long it will be before his "shakes" go away. On which of the following statements should the nurse base her response?
    ○ 1. The tremors can only be relieved by a further intake of alcohol.
    ○ 2. The tremors usually disappear after about 2 days of abstinence.
    ○ 3. The tremors may persist for several days or even longer after alcohol intake has stopped.
    ○ 4. The tremors are a permanent condition due to irreversible central nervous system damage.

25. Mr. Willard starts to crave a drink while withdrawing from the alcohol. Which of the following measures is the *best* way to help him resist the urge to drink?
    ○ 1. A locked-door policy.
    ○ 2. A routine search of visitors.
    ○ 3. One-to-one supervision by the staff.
    ○ 4. Support from other alcoholic patients.

26. Mr. Willard ashamedly tells the nurse that he hit his wife during a recent argument and asks the nurse if she thinks his wife will ever forgive him. Which of the following replies would it be *best* for the nurse to make in this situation?
    ○ 1. "Perhaps you could call her up and find out."
    ○ 2. "That is something you can explore in family therapy."

○ 3. "It would depend on how much she really cares for you."

○ 4. "You seem to have some feelings about hitting your wife."

27. Mr. Willard's wife agrees to meet with her husband's therapist but says she has "about had it" with her husband's "foolishness and bad temper." Which of the following organizations would probably be the *most helpful* to her in obtaining additional assistance and support in coping with her alcoholic spouse?

○ 1. Alateen.

○ 2. Al-Anon.

○ 3. The Salvation Army.

○ 4. Alcoholics Anonymous.

28. Mr. Willard begins to attend daily group therapy sessions. Which of the following statements *best* describes people who are "typical" victims of alcoholism?

○ 1. Victims of alcoholism are typically from a low socioeconomic class.

○ 2. Victims of alcoholism are typically members of evangelistic religions.

○ 3. Victims of alcoholism are typically persons with male or mannish characteristics.

○ 4. Victims of alcoholism are typically individuals representative of the general adult population.

29. The nurse is teaching members of Mr. Willard's group how to give each other constructive feedback. Which of the following statements by the nurse *best* illustrates constructive feedback?

○ 1. "I think you are a real con artist."

○ 2. "You are dominating the conversation."

○ 3. "You interrupted John twice in 4 minutes."

○ 4. "You don't give anyone a chance to finish talking."

30. Toward which of the following ends would it be *best* to gear an inpatient alcoholism program to assist a chemically dependent individual, such as Mr. Willard, toward a state of health?

○ 1. Change the family interaction and communication patterns.

○ 2. Determine the underlying intrapsychic problem of the person.

○ 3. Rebuild the person's life around satisfying substitutes for alcohol.

○ 4. Withdraw the person from alcohol to a plateau of physiologic stability.

31. Mr. Willard is started on a regimen of disulfiram (Antabuse). A valuable and expected result of successful disulfiram therapy is that it

○ 1. decreases the need for alcohol.

○ 2. acts to deter alcohol consumption.

○ 3. improves the capacity of the alcoholic for drinking limited amounts.

○ 4. creates a nerve block so that the effects of alcohol are not felt.

32. While on disulfiram (Antabuse) therapy, Mr. Willard becomes nauseated and vomits severely. The nurse is justified in judging that the patient has *most probably*

○ 1. developed an allergy to disulfiram.

○ 2. been given an overdose of disulfiram accidentally.

○ 3. been drinking alcohol while on disulfiram therapy.

○ 4. developed gastritis as a result of disulfiram therapy.

33. A daily lecture series on alcoholism is conducted by the therapists on the substance-abuse unit where Mr. Willard is housed. The therapists should explain that the patient will *most likely* experience which of the following symptoms of alcoholism during the chronic stage of the disease?

○ 1. Increased alcohol tolerance.

○ 2. Vague feelings of apprehension and doom.

○ 3. Feelings of grandiosity and increasing combativeness.

○ 4. The desire to switch to a different form of alcoholic beverage.

34. Which of the following suggestions would be *most appropriate* for the nurse to make to members of Mr. Willard's family concerning how they can *best* help promote a supportive environment for him at home?

○ 1. Suggest that family members follow a program offered by Al-Anon.

○ 2. Suggest that family members obtain counseling in a mental-health clinic.

○ 3. Suggest that family members refrain from discussing alcoholism in their home.

○ 4. Suggest that family members make sure that no alcoholic beverages are served in the home.

35. Which of the following remarks that Mr. Willard might make before his discharge would show the *most* realistic analysis of his situation in relation to avoiding future drinking problems?

○ 1. "I promise I will never get drunk again."

○ 2. "I am going to try hard to stay away from that first drink."

○ 3. "I will just have one or two drinks at the most, now and then."

○ 4. "I can whip this drinking business if my wife keeps off my back."

## THE PATIENT WITH ALCOHOL WITHDRAWAL

Mrs. Gina Baxter, a 44-year-old homemaker, enters the hospital for treatment of cirrhosis of the liver. She is accompanied by her husband.

36. The nurse who admitted Mrs. Baxter comments to another nurse, "Cirrhosis. She must be an alcoholic." The practice of automatically attributing an overindulgence in alcohol to people with cirrhosis is an example of
   ○ 1. an ideology.
   ○ 2. a stereotype.
   ○ 3. a mental set.
   ○ 4. a halo effect.

37. By which of the following methods can nurses *best avoid* developing premature, biased views of patients, such as Mrs. Baxter?
   ○ 1. By reading about the person's illness.
   ○ 2. By asking others for their opinions of the person.
   ○ 3. By acquainting oneself with others of the person's kind.
   ○ 4. By personally getting to know what the person is really like.

38. The physician noted on the medical record that Mrs. Baxter has a 7-year history of drinking a 6-pack of beer and some wine every day. In which of the following ways did the cirrhosis *most likely* result from the consumption of alcohol?
   ○ 1. Directly from the effects of alcohol on the release of glycogen.
   ○ 2. Directly from the dilating effects of alcohol on arteries and veins in the portal circulation.
   ○ 3. Indirectly from deficiencies in nutrients and vitamin intake over a long period of time.
   ○ 4. Indirectly from the buildup of glycogen in the liver from excess carbohydrate ingestion.

39. The unit secretary reads the physician's notes about Mrs. Baxter's drinking habits and exclaims, "I have a friend who drinks more than that! Would he be considered an alcoholic?" Which of the following possible replies by the nurse shows the *best* understanding of alcoholism as a social disease?
   ○ 1. "Not if he drinks with others and not alone."
   ○ 2. "Not if he sticks to beer and avoids the hard liquor."
   ○ 3. "Not if he drinks only in the evening or on weekends."
   ○ 4. "Not if he is able to get along well at work and at home."

40. Most of the information about Mrs. Baxter has come from her husband, who says his wife sees no connection between her liver disorder and her alcohol intake. He reports that she believes she drinks very little and that her family is making something out of nothing. Which of the following defense mechanisms is the patient using?
   ○ 1. Denial.
   ○ 2. Displacement.
   ○ 3. Rationalization.
   ○ 4. Reaction formation.

41. Attempts by health team members to force Mrs. Baxter to face the fact that she is an alcoholic and to break her defenses would *most likely* lead to
   ○ 1. insight and rehabilitation.
   ○ 2. hallucinations and psychosis.
   ○ 3. restlessness and psychosis.
   ○ 4. disorganization and depression.

42. Medications for Mrs. Baxter include a B-complex vitamin. Mrs. Baxter wants to know why she must take this vitamin. The nurse's *best* response would be
   ○ 1. "The beer you have been drinking has caused you to become vitamin depleted."
   ○ 2. "Your daily alcohol consumption causes malnutrition."
   ○ 3. "The B vitamins help reduce the long-term effects of alcohol withdrawal."
   ○ 4. "The amount of vitamins in the wine you drink is very low."

43. The nurse teaches Mrs. Baxter about the value of good nutrition and the B vitamins. Which of the following statements is Mrs. Baxter *most likely* to make in response to the teaching?
   ○ 1. "This is all so complicated. Maybe I'll feel better after a good night's sleep."
   ○ 2. "I've been wondering why I felt so bad. I just need vitamins."
   ○ 3. "I don't know why you're telling me all of this. I don't drink enough to cause these problems."
   ○ 4. "I don't see what this has to do with me."

44. Besides her cirrhosis, Mrs. Baxter suffers from numbness, itching, and pain in her extremities and is prone to footdrop. This disorder of the nervous system is termed
   ○ 1. neuralgia.
   ○ 2. Bell's palsy.
   ○ 3. neurasthenia.
   ○ 4. peripheral neuritis.

45. Mrs. Baxter has neurologic damage. A precautionary measure is for the nurse to be *especially* careful when giving nursing care that includes
   ○ 1. cleansing the patient's skin.

○ 2. massaging the patient's feet.

○ 3. turning the patient from side to side.

○ 4. applying heat to the patient's lower legs.

46. A noncaffeinated beverage is substituted for Mrs. Baxter's usual morning coffee. This measure is taken because

○ 1. patients transfer their oral dependency needs symbolically to coffee.

○ 2. regular coffee aggravates tremors and interferes with sleep.

○ 3. patients tend to abuse coffee in the same way they once abused alcohol.

○ 4. regular coffee has a diuretic effect that interferes with the hydration of the patient.

47. Mrs. Baxter receives the appropriate medical and nursing treatment for her liver disorder and neurologic ailments, and her condition improves slightly. However, after 5 days in the hospital, she begins to thrash about in bed, pulling the sheets and yelling, "Go away, bugs, go away!" Several times she is overheard asking, "What? What did you say?" when alone in her room. Which of the following nursing notes *best* sums up Mrs. Baxter's behavior?

○ 1. Restless and disoriented; hallucinating.

○ 2. Agitated; having auditory and visual hallucinations.

○ 3. Fidgety; out of contact with reality; overheard talking to herself in her room.

○ 4. Seeing "bugs" in her bedclothes and slapping at them; responding to unseen voices with "What?"

48. Which of the following measures should be included in Mrs. Baxter's nursing care plan when the patient has delirium tremens?

○ 1. Restrain her and keep the room quiet.

○ 2. Touch her before saying anything and tell her where she is.

○ 3. Have someone stay with her and keep a light on in the room.

○ 4. Tell her she is having nightmares and that she will be better soon.

49. When the nurse develops a one-to-one relationship with Mrs. Baxter, it is *best* to use the first or early meetings to determine the patient's

○ 1. healthy coping mechanisms.

○ 2. most probable reasons for alcohol abuse.

○ 3. knowledge concerning Alcoholics Anonymous.

○ 4. childhood experiences that predispose to alcoholism.

50. Mrs. Baxter's husband tells the nurse that he also drinks heavily in the evenings and would like to stop. The nurse suggests that he attend Alcoholics Anonymous, but he says, "I went to one men's meeting and all they did was swear and brag about how drunk they got." Which of the following responses would be *best* for the nurse to make?

○ 1. "That's too bad. I can see how you might have been turned off by the experience."

○ 2. "Not everyone finds Alcoholics Anonymous helpful. There are other therapies available."

○ 3. "The Alcoholics Anonymous meetings vary from group to group. Have you thought about giving it another try?"

○ 4. "If you really want to stop your drinking, you would go back to Alcoholics Anonymous whether you liked it or not."

51. Mr. Baxter is unsure what requirements he must meet to be a member of Alcoholics Anonymous. To become a member of the organization, the alcoholic must *first*

○ 1. resolve to abstain from alcohol and help others to do so.

○ 2. admit he is powerless over alcohol and that he needs help.

○ 3. analyze the wrongs he has done while drinking and try to make amends for them.

○ 4. turn his life over to the care of a greater power and seek to improve contact with that power through meditation.

52. If Mrs. Baxter continues drinking and refuses treatment, the nurse can expect that eventually the patient is *most likely* to develop what type of mental disturbance?

○ 1. Alcoholic stupor.

○ 2. Alcoholic hallucinations.

○ 3. Organic brain disorder.

○ 4. Pathologic intoxication.

53. Mrs. Baxter is to be discharged from the hospital. What information is likely to be *most helpful* in her efforts to stop drinking?

○ 1. The process of alcohol metabolism.

○ 2. The disease concept of alcoholism.

○ 3. The stages of alcoholism.

○ 4. The importance of perseverance in her efforts to change her behavior.

## THE PATIENT WHO IS DEPENDENT ON NARCOTICS

Ms. Alice Choate, 22, is brought in her parents' limousine from a cold-water flat, where she has been living with several other drug addicts, to the emergency room of a psychiatric hospital. Ms. Choate is a known heroin user.

**54.** Ms. Choate had given herself her usual dose of heroin earlier in the day. However, it came from a purer-than-usual supply of heroin and caused the patient to fall into a light coma. A narcotic antagonist, naloxone (Narcan), is administered to Ms. Choate. When compared with the narcotic antagonists N-allylnormorphine (Nalline) and levallorphan (Lorfan), the duration of the action of naloxone is
- ○ 1. much shorter.
- ○ 2. about the same length of time.
- ○ 3. about twice as long.
- ○ 4. about five times as long.

**55.** After administering naloxone (Narcan), the nurse should *most certainly* monitor the patient carefully for signs of
- ○ 1. cerebral edema.
- ○ 2. kidney failure.
- ○ 3. seizure activity.
- ○ 4. respiratory depression.

**56.** In the past, Ms. Choate occasionally used cocaine. For which of the following telltale signs should the nurse look to help detect whether the patient has recently abused this drug?
- ○ 1. Red, excoriated nostrils.
- ○ 2. Clear, constricted pupils.
- ○ 3. White patchy areas on the tongue.
- ○ 4. Lumpy abscesses in intramuscular areas.

**57.** Ms. Choate is transferred to the chemical dependency unit when her condition becomes stable. Twelve hours later, she develops signs of heroin withdrawal. Of the following signs/symptoms of opiate withdrawal, which occur *late*, rather than early, in the course of withdrawal?

- ○ 1. Vomiting and diarrhea.   *Late signs*
- ○ 2. Yawning and diaphoresis.
- ○ 3. Lacrimation and rhinorrhea.
- ○ 4. Restlessness and nervousness.

**58.** Ms. Choate has numerous complaints of discomfort while abstaining from heroin. Which of the following nursing orders that appears on the patient's care plan would be the *least* advisable and effective?
- ○ 1. Be empathetic but firm with the patient's complaints.
- ○ 2. Promise to reevaluate the patient's withdrawal plan to ease her discomfort.
- ○ 3. Prepare the patient in advance for the minor discomforts that might occur.
- ○ 4. Inform the patient of alternative methods, such as warm baths, for dealing with aches and pains.

**59.** Knowing Ms. Choate's history, the nursing staff on the chemical dependency unit is concerned about her potential for acquired immune deficiency syndrome (AIDS). They suggest that she be tested for the human immunodeficiency virus (HIV) but she refuses, stating, "No way! I never share needles. None of my friends have it. And anyway, I'm straight." When teaching Ms. Choate about AIDS, the nurse should include *all* of the following information *except*
- ○ 1. people can be infected with the virus without having symptoms of the disease.
- ○ 2. the virus can be transmitted through heterosexual intercourse.
- ○ 3. people cannot transmit the infection when they are asymptomatic.
- ○ 4. due to the patient's high-risk life-style, testing is especially important.

**60.** The nursing staff is concerned about possible HIV exposure among other patients on the unit and themselves. Which is the *least important* of the following precautionary measures?
- ○ 1. Strict handwashing procedures.
- ○ 2. A private room for the patient.
- ○ 3. Wearing gloves when handling body fluids.
- ○ 4. Increased caution in disposal of needles and syringes.

**61.** Although Ms. Choate feels she was forced into the hospital, she reluctantly says she will give the chemical dependency program a try. Which of the following comments the nurse could make *most clearly* illustrates that she has a good understanding of the patient's condition?
- ○ 1. "You have hurt your mother and now is your chance to make it up to her."
- ○ 2. "Because you are thinking of staying, you must have a desire to give up the drugs."
- ○ 3. "Now that you are feeling better, you need to think more clearly about your health."
- ○ 4. "Perhaps there are some other things about your life you would like to change along with drug use."

**62.** Ms. Choate starts methadone therapy. If Ms. Choate experiences acute toxicity from the methadone, the nurse is *most likely* to note that the patient displays signs of
- ○ 1. fever.
- ○ 2. colitis.
- ○ 3. renal shutdown.
- ○ 4. respiratory depression.

**63.** Which of the following characteristics of methadone offers the *most potential* for its *abuse?*
- ○ 1. Methadone blunts the craving for heroin.
- ○ 2. Methadone blocks the pleasurable effects of heroin.

○ 3. Methadone is equally effective at low or high doses.

○ 4. Methadone lessens the severity of withdrawal symptoms.

**64.** Which of the following measures would be the *most feasible* to ensure the therapeutic use of methadone and to prevent Ms. Choate from abusing it?

○ 1. Monitor the patient's urine for drug levels.

○ 2. Administer the methadone in injection form.

○ 3. Supervise the patient when administering liquid methadone.

○ 4. Use methadone for the patient only while she is hospitalized.

**65.** In relation to Ms. Choate's drug habit, the *primary* reason she will need to learn new living and social skills from the health team members is that she formerly lived in a world dominated by

○ 1. false sensory data.

○ 2. fear of the authorities.

○ 3. minimal contact with family and friends.

○ 4. preoccupation with obtaining and taking drugs.

**66.** Ms. Choate attends meetings of Narcotics Anonymous as part of her rehabilitation program. To join this organization, an individual agrees to

○ 1. stay drug-free one day at a time.

○ 2. be "clean" of drugs at the meetings.

○ 3. abstain from drugs for the rest of his life.

○ 4. commit a certain amount of time to the organization.

**67.** Ms. Choate's eventual success or progress when out of the hospital can probably *best* be measured by the

○ 1. kinds of friends she makes.

○ 2. number of drug-free days she has.

○ 3. way she gets along with her parents.

○ 4. degree of responsibility her job entails.

**68.** Which of the following physical disorders is the heroin addict *least likely* to develop as a result of heroin addiction?

○ 1. Hepatitis.

○ 2. Pneumonia.

○ 3. Tuberculosis.

○ 4. Cholelithiasis.

## THE PATIENT WHO ABUSES BARBITURATES

Ms. Lola Albert, a 36-year-old mother of two children, is brought by ambulance to the emergency room of the hospital after taking an overdose of barbiturates. A male friend arrives a short time later, carrying some of her personal belongings.

**69.** Ms. Albert went into shock at home and is semi-comatose on admission. If death occurs shortly, the cause of death would *most likely* be

○ 1. kidney failure.

○ 2. cardiac standstill.

○ 3. internal hemorrhaging.

○ 4. respiratory depression.

**70.** Ms. Albert's acquaintance says Ms. Albert has been taking about eight "reds" (800 mg of secobarbital [Seconal]) daily, besides drinking more alcohol than she usually does. Which of the following terms *best* describes the interaction of barbiturates and alcohol?

○ 1. Additive.

○ 2. Suppressive.

○ 3. Potentiating.

○ 4. Antagonistic.

**71.** Ms. Albert's friend asks anxiously, "Do you think she will live?" Which of the following replies would it be *best* for the nurse to make?

○ 1. "We can only wait and see."

○ 2. "Do you know Ms. Albert well?"

○ 3. "Ms. Albert is very ill and may not live."

○ 4. "Ms. Albert's condition is serious. You are worried, aren't you?"

**72.** The nurse talks further with Ms. Albert's friend and tries to determine the nature of their relationship. Which of the following motivations provides the *best* justification for the nurse's inquiries?

○ 1. To ascertain the friend's capabilities as a source of support for the patient.

○ 2. To encourage the friend to realize the seriousness of the patient's condition.

○ 3. To determine whether the friend can be trusted with confidential information about the patient.

○ 4. To learn whether the patient's relationship with the friend may have caused the suicide attempt.

**73.** Before her hospitalization, Ms. Albert needed increasingly larger doses of barbiturates to achieve the same euphoric effect she initially realized from their use. From this information, the nurse should plan care while taking into account that Ms. Albert is *most probably* suffering from a drug

○ 1. tolerance.

○ 2. addiction.

○ 3. habituation.

○ 4. dependence.

**74.** By which of the following symptoms could Ms. Albert probably have been identified as a chronic user of barbiturates in the days before her hospitalization?

○ 1. Drooling, fainting, and illusions.

○ 2. Sluggishness, ataxia, and irritability.

○ 3. Diaphoresis, twitching, and sneezing.

○ 4. Suspiciousness, tachycardia, and edema.

**75.** After gastric gavage, Ms. Albert's vital signs stabilize and she later awakens in a confused state. Which of the following measures would be *least appropriate* for the nurse to take while Ms. Albert is recovering from the overdose of sedatives?

○ 1. Maintain seizure precautions for the patient.

○ 2. Close the windows in the vicinity of the patient.

○ 3. Use a p.r.n. order for a medication for anxiety and agitation.

○ 4. Use short, complete sentences when speaking to the patient.

**76.** Following a dose-response test, Ms. Albert receives pentobarbital sodium (Nembutal) at a non-intoxicating maintenance level for 2 days, and at decreasing doses thereafter. This regimen is prescribed for the patient *primarily* to help prevent the possibly fatal occurrence of

○ 1. psychosis.

○ 2. convulsions.

○ 3. hypotension.

○ 4. hypothermia.

**77.** In view of Ms. Albert's barbiturate dependency, toward which of the following ends *in particular* should her nursing care be directed during her first few days on the mental health unit?

○ 1. Increasing the patient's level of physical activity.

○ 2. Renewing the patient's optimism and faith in herself.

○ 3. Correcting the patient's fluid and electrolyte imbalance.

○ 4. Getting the patient's legal entanglements, if any, straightened out.

**78.** Which of the following items of information will Ms. Albert's nurse probably be *most concerned* about obtaining during the initial interview sessions with the patient?

○ 1. The effects of her drug dependency on her children.

○ 2. The personal and social drives that led to her drug dependency.

○ 3. The positive and negative ways she views her drug dependency.

○ 4. The length of time she thinks she will need to recover from her drug dependency.

**79.** The opinion of one staff member is that Ms. Albert is rich, pampered, and spoiled. Which of the following comments that the nurse could make would *best* influence the staff member to perceive the patient in a more positive light?

○ 1. "Are you possibly a bit jealous of her?"

○ 2. "It sounds as though you've already made up your mind about her."

○ 3. "I find her to be a frightened and lonely woman beneath that indulged exterior."

○ 4. "If you knew all the trouble she has had, you would probably be more understanding."

**80.** The staff notices that Ms. Albert spends most of her time with the young adult patients, most of whom have also misused drugs. This group of patients is a dominant force on the unit, keeping the non-drug users entertained with stories of their "highs." In which of the following ways is this problem *best* dealt with by the staff?

○ 1. By providing additional recreation for the patients.

○ 2. By breaking up drug-oriented discussions whenever possible.

○ 3. By speaking with the patients individually about their behavior.

○ 4. By bringing up for discussion staff observations of the patients' drug-oriented conversations at the weekly patient group meetings.

**81.** If Ms. Albert had been abusing amphetamines, which of the following disadvantages associated with a continuous high intake of the drugs would pose the *greatest* danger for her?

○ 1. She might become psychologically dependent on the drug.

○ 2. She might become paranoid and violent from taking the drug.

○ 3. She might develop an infection from self-administration of the drug.

○ 4. She might become depressed and suicidal between doses of the drug.

## THE PATIENT WITH AN EATING DISORDER

A nurse and a nutritionist are co-leaders of a therapy group for overweight women. The group meets once a week and is directed toward helping the eight members help themselves lose weight. The members decide to address each other by first names.

**82.** By the fourth meeting, the members are able to start sessions by themselves and are relating to each other in a warm, considerate manner. They are proud of each others' successful dieting attempts and able to cope supportively with an occasional member's feelings of discouragement. This unity and spirit illustrates a group quality known as

○ 1. mutuality.
○ 2. dependency.
○ 3. genuineness.
○ 4. cohesiveness.

83. It is desirable for group members to use functional roles in the group to obtain the most benefit from the group. In which of the following instances is a group role (versus an individual role) being used by one of the members?
   ○ 1. Jill shows the group the latest pictures of her child.
   ○ 2. Grace insists that everyone try her favorite reducing recipe.
   ○ 3. Lucille makes quiet comments to the person sitting next to her.
   ○ 4. Molly proposes an alternate task to keep from thinking about food.

84. The members of the group learn that many people in the American culture have difficulty with weight control because they unconsciously equate food with
   ○ 1. love and affection.
   ○ 2. power and control.
   ○ 3. status and prestige.
   ○ 4. survival and growth.

85. Jill says that her sister has been using amphetamines for weight control for a long period of time. If the sister is described as having the following symptoms, the one *least likely* to be related to prolonged use of amphetamines is
   ○ 1. gastritis.
   ○ 2. drug dependency.
   ○ 3. emotional lability.
   ○ 4. depression between doses.

86. The nurse teaches that, from a psychological viewpoint, obesity is *most often* associated with
   ○ 1. an unrealistic wish to be important.
   ○ 2. a lack of motivation to change behavior.
   ○ 3. an unconscious desire to gain attention.
   ○ 4. a maladaptive method to cope with stress.

87. The nutritionist correctly teaches that the *most common* direct cause of obesity is usually
   ○ 1. faulty nutritional information.
   ○ 2. the intake of more calories than are expended.
   ○ 3. a disturbance in the functioning of endocrine glands.
   ○ 4. the resistance of the body to metabolizing thyroid hormone.

Sue Girdler, 14, is admitted to the pediatric unit for weight loss associated with anorexia nervosa. She weighs 70 pounds and is 5-foot-2.

88. Physical manifestations *most likely* to be found during the nursing assessment include
   ○ 1. tachycardia, hypertension, and hyperthyroidism.
   ○ 2. tachycardia, hypertension, and iron deficiency anemia.
   ○ 3. hypotension, elevated serum potassium, and vitamin C deficiency.
   ○ 4. bradycardia, hypotension, and cold sensitivity.

89. A behavioral program for weight gain is instituted as part of the nursing care plan. Which of the following nursing interventions would be *most* specific to attainment of the program goal?
   ○ 1. Provide emotional support and active listening.
   ○ 2. Give positive rewards for gradual weight gain.
   ○ 3. Help the patient identify her problematic eating behaviors.
   ○ 4. Initiate intravenous hyperalimentation.

90. The nurse enters Sue's room and finds her doing sit-ups. What would be the nurse's *best* approach?
   ○ 1. Wait until she finishes and ask her why she feels the need to exercise.
   ○ 2. Remind her that if her weight decreases she will lose privileges.
   ○ 3. Ask her to stop doing the sit-ups and direct her to a quiet activity.
   ○ 4. Leave the room and allow her to exercise in private.

91. What would be the *most appropriate* and realistic outcome for Sue for this hospitalization?
   ○ 1. Her weight is stable and she is willing to begin outpatient psychotherapy.
   ○ 2. Her weight is normal and she no longer feels the need to diet.
   ○ 3. Her discharge weight is 15% more than her admission weight.
   ○ 4. Her eating behaviors have changed and she feels better.

Carol Wang is a 20-year-old college student who was admitted to a psychiatric unit with a four-year history of severe bulimia.

92. The nurse anticipates that Ms. Wang's current signs and symptoms will *most likely* include
   ○ 1. amenorrhea, bingeing, vomiting, and high serum potassium.
   ○ 2. normal weight, bingeing, vomiting, and low serum potassium.
   ○ 3. severe weight loss, vomiting, compulsive exercise, and tachycardia.

4. amenorrhea, laxative abuse, diet pill abuse, and vomiting.

**93.** Ms. Wang binges twice a day. These binges are *most likely* to involve

1. feelings of euphoria, excitement, and gratification.
2. feeling out of control, frightened, and disgusted with self.
3. leaving traces of food around to attract attention.
4. eating larger and larger amounts of food, resulting in substantial weight gain.

**94.** During hospitalization, Ms. Wang stops vomiting but becomes fearful that she will gain weight. She tells the nurse, "I can't gain weight. I'm fat enough as it is. I'll be really disgusting if I get fatter." When responding to Ms. Wang, it would be *most therapeutic* for the nurse to

1. explain that the number of calories prescribed in her diet is not enough to cause weight gain.
2. tell her that she is not fat and encourage her to negotiate a calorie change with the nutritionist.

3. validate her feelings and help her identify positive aspects of herself other than appearance.
4. reassure her that the staff will take complete control of her eating and will prevent her from gaining weight in the hospital.

**95.** After hearing Ms. Wang talk about her bizarre eating binges of raw pancake batter and bowls of whipped cream, the nurse feels disgusted. She finds it hard to understand how Ms. Wang can do this and feels like telling her to "snap out of it." At this point, it would be *best* for the nurse to

1. share her feelings with the patient and point out that her behavior alienates people.
2. ask the patient to talk more about her eating habits, and try harder to understand her underlying problem.
3. suggest that another nurse work with the patient because this relationship is no longer therapeutic.
4. discuss her feelings with another nurse and try to resolve them.

# CORRECT ANSWERS AND RATIONALES

Numbers appear in parentheses following the rationales. The numbers identify textbooks listed in the references at the end of Part I, where correct answers can be verified.

## The Patient with a Personality Disorder

1. 3. The patient described in this item, who is being readmitted to a psychiatric hospital, is likely to have the best prospects for eventual success in her therapy when she recognizes and admits to her failure to get along outside of the hospital. This shows that the patient has insight into her behavior. The patient appears to be blaming others when she says her parents annoyed her and when she says her physician advised readmission. If the patient says she has returned to the hospital because she missed being with the patients, the patient appears to be dependent on the hospital environment and still unable to understand her own behavior. (2, 12)

2. 2. Labels may cause staff to make assumptions about the patient, discount the patient's point of view, and cause the patient to live up to the label in a self-fulfilling prophecy. (2, 5)

3. 4. It is most important for the nurse to maintain an attitude of consistency when dealing with the patient who manipulates others, as described in this situation. The nurse should set limits on the patient's behavior and then be consistent to help prevent manipulation. Strictness for its own sake is not appropriate with this patient, nor is sympathy or aloofness. (2, 12)

4. 2. Previous negative experiences with a patient should not be suppressed by trying to forget them, be excused on the basis of the patient's past, or constitute a basis for present intervention with the patient. Past experiences should be reviewed and accepted as unpleasant in this case, but should be considered past experiences. A new relationship should be initiated with the patient based on present behavior and concerns. (4, 12)

5. 3. Role reversal is illustrated when the patient described in this item appears to be taking over the nurse's responsibilities. Incongruency is inconsistency in thinking, feeling, and acting. Denial is a mechanism by which the mind refuses to acknowledge a reality factor. Self-fulfilling prophecy is the tendency to behave according to the views and expectations significant others have of one and according to one's own views of the self. (2, 12)

6. 1. When a nurse is having problems dealing with a patient, it is best for her to admit to the need for help and seek the assistance of other staff who can help her. (2, 5)

7. 3. When the patient described in this item makes a derogatory comment about her parents, a good technique is to help the patient discuss her feelings more and to be more specific about her sweeping conclusion. It would be *least* therapeutic to tell this patient that the nurse is sure the parents have the patient's best interests at heart, because this accuses the patient of being unfeeling or wrong about her parents. (2, 5)

8. 2. Most teenagers respond best to their peers and less well to persons of authority, such as a physician, a juvenile worker, or a religious counselor. (5, 12)

9. 3. A lack of remorse is due to a defect in the functioning of the superego, the conscience of the person, according to psychoanalytic theory. The id strives to satisfy basic instinctual needs; the ego mediates in a reasonable way between the other components of the personality and the realities of the external world. Self-concept refers to a person's feelings about himself and is unrelated to psychoanalytic theory. (2, 12)

10. 1. The person with antisocial attitudes frequently uses extremely poor judgment. The person is often above average in intelligence, has an intact memory, and is usually a clever rather than a disordered thinker. (2, 12)

11. 3. This patient's primary diagnosis is borderline personality disorder. This is characterized by impulsive, often self-mutilating behavior and unstable, intense personal relationships. Antisocial personality disorder is characterized by failure to accept social norms, which often results in unlawful behavior. The avoidant personality demonstrates social withdrawal and hypersensitivity to criticism. The compulsive personality is preoccupied with details and rules, to the exclusion of other life activities. (1)

12. 2. Splitting refers to a primitive defense mechanism, as well as learned behavior, in which manipulation becomes an adaptive style. Reaction formation is a defense in which one replaces negative feelings with positive ones. Projection involves attributing one's own negative traits to someone else. Denial is a defense mechanism used to resolve emotional conflict and allay anxiety by disavowing thoughts or external reality that are consciously intolerable. (2, 4)

13. 1. Consistent enforcement of unit rules will help

the borderline patient control his or her behavior. Ignoring behavior leads to an increase in the behavior in order to evoke a response from the staff. If the staff assumes control of the behavior, the patient has little opportunity to learn increased responsibility for the behavior. While vocational plans will be important for discharge planning, they are not an immediate priority. (2, 12)

**14.** 4. The achievement of autonomy is the basic task of two-year-olds. Developing a sense of trust is a task for infants, while becoming independent more appropriately describes adolescent tasks. Safety is not a developmental task. (2)

**15.** 4. Assessment is an ongoing process throughout treatment. Any suicidal statement must be assessed. Extending the hospital stay would encourage dependency and manipulation. Early discharge is not indicated and may be seen as a punitive staff response to a patient threat. Transfer without careful assessment of need would also encourage dependency. (2, 5, 12)

## *The Patient Who Abuses Alcohol*

**16.** 4. The rate of alcohol destruction is not influenced by giving a patient black coffee to drink, having him walk after taking a cold shower, or having him breathe pure oxygen. Alcohol is destroyed and oxidized in the body at a slow, steady rate. Therefore, it would be best to have the patient described in this item sleep off the effects of the alcohol. (3, 5, 11)

**17.** 4. Antiseptic mouthwashes often contain alcohol and should be taken from patients entering a substance-abuse unit, unless labeling clearly indicates the solution does not contain alcohol. Such personal-care items as hair dressing and shaving cream do not contain alcohol. An electric razor should present no problems for a patient who is being admitted for the treatment of alcoholism as long as it is in good working order. (5, 12)

**18.** 2. The alcoholic usually underestimates the amount of alcohol consumed. He may be unaware of how much he really drinks or he may fail to admit, even to himself, how much he really consumes. (2, 12)

**19.** 2. The amount of alcohol consumed in the last 24 to 48 hours helps determine how much medication the patient requires to relieve the severity of withdrawal symptoms when a patient is admitted for the treatment of alcoholism. The amount of alcohol a patient has consumed during the day or two prior to admission will not help determine how far the disease has progressed or whether the patient should be considered an alcoholic. It is difficult to predict

delirium tremens during withdrawal, but if the patient has had them previously, he may likely have them again. (5)

**20.** 1. Some patients may be in need of safety, security, and comfort measures; hygienic care; aeration; and attention to elimination when admitted for care for alcoholism. However, most alcoholics are undernourished and are primarily in need of extra nourishment and rest. Alcoholism disrupts both eating and sleeping habits. (2, 3, 11)

**21.** 3. The best way to deal with the alcoholic is to be accepting and understanding. An attitude of morality, optimism, or indulgence has not been shown to be effective when caring for alcoholics. (5, 11)

**22.** 2. Tranquilizers, such as chlordiazepoxide (Librium) and diazepam (Valium), are frequently used to ease symptoms during alcohol withdrawal. The anticonvulsant phenytoin sodium (Dilantin) does not relieve anxiety, nor does paraldehyde (Paral), which is used primarily for its hypnotic and sedative effects. (3, 5)

**23.** 1. A patient is said to be suffering from a blackout when he cannot recall what he has been doing while under the influence of alcohol. Common symptoms of a hangover, including headaches and gastrointestinal distress, typically follow heavy consumption of alcohol. Dry drunk syndrome means the patient has not been drinking but acts grandiose, impatient, and uses many defense mechanisms. (5)

**24.** 3. The patient suffering with alcoholism may experience tremors for several days or even longer after alcohol intake has stopped. (5)

**25.** 4. Group support has proven to be more successful than individual attention from the staff in influencing positive behavior in alcoholics. Locked doors do not help patients change behavior or develop their own controls. Searching visitors is impractical and externally oriented. (5, 12)

**26.** 4. The patient described in this item is feeling remorse about hitting his wife. In this situation, it would be best to make a comment that will help him focus on his feelings and ventilate them. Reflecting what the patient has said is a good technique to accomplish these goals. Comments that give advice to the patient or hedge the issue are less satisfactory. (2, 5)

**27.** 2. Al-Anon is for the mates of alcoholics. Alateen is for the children of alcoholics. The Salvation Army does not have a program for alcoholics. Alcoholics Anonymous is for the alcoholic. (2, 5)

**28.** 4. Alcoholics are representative of the general public. No one group is likely to have a more-than-average number of alcoholics. (2, 5)

**29.** 3. When a nurse is using group therapy with patients, she is giving constructive feedback to the group when she describes specifically what was seen and heard in a descriptive, rather than judgmental, manner. The nurse described in this item is following this principle when she tells a patient how often he has interrupted the group within a set period of time. (2, 5)

**30.** 3. Although other methods have been tried, it has been found that the best and most practical way to help the alcoholic is by assisting him to rebuild his life around substitutes for alcohol. (5, 12)

**31.** 2. Disulfiram (Antabuse) helps curb the impulsiveness of the problem drinker. Any disulfiram in the body reacts with the alcohol to produce marked discomfort. (11)

**32.** 3. Disulfiram (Antabuse) is used to sensitize a person to alcohol because the drug brings on a most unpleasant disulfiram-alcohol reaction. Nausea with severe vomiting is common when the patient drinks alcohol. Other typical signs and symptoms of a disulfiram-alcohol reaction include vasodilatation of the upper part of the body, palpitations, hyperventilation, headache, and dyspnea. The reaction can be sufficiently severe to threaten life. (11)

**33.** 2. Vague feelings of apprehension and doom appear during the chronic phase of alcohol addiction. Such symptoms as an increased alcohol tolerance, feelings of grandiosity and combativeness, and a desire to switch to a different form of alcoholic beverage usually appear at an earlier stage of the disease. (5, 12)

**34.** 1. Alcoholism involves the entire family. The organization Al-Anon has helped family members understand and live comfortably with a person who is alcoholic and learn to deal with his behavior. Counseling in a mental-health program is not ordinarily recommended. Behavior in the home such as avoiding the subject of alcoholism in the patient's presence and making sure that alcohol is not served in the patient's home puts the onus of responsibility for helping the alcoholic on family members, whereas it is the patient who must take responsibility for maintaining sobriety after a course of treatment. (5, 12)

**35.** 2. The most realistic analysis in relation to avoiding future drinking problems in the alcoholic patient who has completed a course of therapy occurs when the patient says he is going to try hard to stay away from his first drink. The alcoholic must understand that he cannot take even one drink without returning to his old habits of drinking. It is unwise for the alcoholic to promise he will never drink again and almost tempts the alcoholic to return to drinking. The alcoholic who believes he will do fine

if his "wife keeps off my back" has a doubtful future in terms of abstinence; he is placing the responsibility for his behavior onto his wife rather than onto himself. (5, 12)

## The Patient with Alcohol Withdrawal

**36.** 2. Stereotype refers to the concept of labeling that categorizes persons into common groups. To say that a patient is an alcoholic because the person has cirrhosis of the liver is an example of stereotyping. Ideology is a manner of thinking that is characteristic of an individual. A mental set is a readiness to organize an individual's perceptions in a particular way. The halo effect is a tendency to be influenced by one's general impression of a person (favorable or unfavorable) when rating one of his specific traits. (2, 12)

**37.** 4. The best way to learn to know a person is to get to know the individual personally. Depending on others and books are poor substitutes. (2, 5)

**38.** 3. The pathology of cirrhosis of the liver due to alcohol primarily involves deficiencies in nutrients and vitamin intake. Alcohol is used in place of food. Although nutritional factors are involved, recent studies also show that the alcohol itself damages liver cells to cause pathologic results. (9)

**39.** 4. The alcoholic is usually differentiated from the person who consumes more-than-average quantities of alcohol by his inability to get along in his social relationships at work and at home. Behaviors such as drinking alone, drinking only beer and wine, and drinking only in the evenings and on weekends do not differentiate alcoholics from nonalcoholics. (5, 12)

**40.** 1. The person using denial as a defense mechanism refuses to acknowledge an aspect of reality. The patient described in this item is using denial when refusing to acknowledge that she has a problem with alcohol. Displacement is the transfer of a feeling to a more acceptable substitute object. Rationalization is substituting one reason for a behavior for the real one motivating the behavior. Reaction formation is when an opposite attitude takes the place of the real attitudes or impulses the individual harbors. (2, 5)

**41.** 4. When health team members attempt to break down a person's defense mechanism, the person is very likely to become disorganized and depressed. Authorities agree that the defense should not be attacked directly, for it may lead to complete disorganization in the face of a crisis, or it may give way to depression. (2, 12)

**42.** 3. Denial is a major symptom of alcohol dependence and it is helpful if confrontation can be avoided during the first few days of withdrawal. This response gives accurate information with minimal confrontation. (2, 12)

**43.** 3. Denial is a major factor in the patient's response to treatment at this time. This response best demonstrates her denial. (2, 12)

**44.** 4. Typical symptoms of peripheral neuritis include numbness, itching, and pain in the extremities, and the patient is often prone to footdrop. Neurasthenia is neurotic behavior in which the main pattern is motor and mental fatigue. Neuralgia is severe pain along the course of a nerve. Bell's palsy is a type of facial paralysis involving the seventh cranial nerve. (9)

**45.** 4. Patients often require help with keeping the skin clean. Also, massaging the feet may be important in some instances, and turning the patient from side to side is an essential nursing measure for many patients. However, a patient with neurologic disorders is likely to have sensory changes. Therefore, it is particularly important to guard against burns, because the patient may be unaware of the amount of heat present. (9)

**46.** 2. Regular coffee contains caffeine, which acts as a psychomotor stimulant. Hence, serving coffee to the alcoholic patient described in this item may add to her tremors and wakefulness. (11)

**47.** 4. Nursing notes most helpful to others are those that describe exactly what the patient did and said. Technical terms used to describe behavior may be misinterpreted by others. (2, 5)

**48.** 3. The patient with delirium tremens should not be left unattended. Unintentional suicide is a possibility when the patient attempts to get away from hallucinations. Shadows created by dim lights are likely to cause illusions. Such measures as restraining the patient, touching her before saying anything, and telling her where she is are likely to add to the patient's agitation. Explaining to the patient that she is having a nightmare and that she will soon be better are untruthful statements and offer the patient false assurance. (3, 5)

**49.** 1. In early one-to-one helping relationships with the patient described in this item, focusing on the positive aspects and on healthy coping mechanisms usually helps increase the patient's self-esteem. Seeking out reasons for alcohol abuse and delving into childhood experiences that predispose to alcoholism describe more traditional mental health therapies that have not been very successful. An alcoholic should have a good understanding of Alcoholics Anonymous, but this should not be the focus in early meetings with this patient. (2, 5)

**50.** 3. The man described in this item complains about the nature of an Alcoholics Anonymous meeting he attended. It would be best for the nurse to support AA without threatening the man and encourage him not to judge the group on the basis of one meeting. Offering sympathy and making judgments about the meeting are not recommended. Because this is the first meeting with the man, it would be inappropriate to suggest that he give up on AA and look at other therapies. (2, 12)

**51.** 2. Alcoholics Anonymous requires that the alcoholic admit that he is powerless over alcohol and that he needs help. Eligibility for membership in Alcoholics Anonymous does not require that the applicant resolve to abstain from drinking, help others to do so, analyze the wrongs he has done, make amends for wrongs committed, or turn his life over to a greater power. (5, 12)

**52.** 3. The person who abuses alcohol chronically is most likely to develop an organic brain disorder. Pathologic intoxication and alcohol stupor are the result of alcohol intoxication. Alcoholic hallucinosis is classified as an abstinence or withdrawal syndrome. (5, 12)

**53.** 4. Information about the importance of continued efforts to change her behavior takes into account the fact that alcohol dependence is a difficult problem but that the patient can conquer the problem. This approach is nonjudgmental but does not ignore the patient's responsibility. (2, 10)

## The Patient Who is Dependent on Narcotics

**54.** 1. The action of naloxone (Narcan) is much shorter than the action of *N*-allylnormorphine (Nalline) and levallorphan (Lorfan). This characteristic of naloxone is important to remember because the patient may lapse into respiratory depression after the effects of this drug have ended. (11)

**55.** 4. After administering naloxone (Narcan), the nurse should monitor the patient's respiratory status carefully. The drug is short-acting and the patient may fall back into a coma with respiratory depression again after the effects of naloxone have worn off. (11)

**56.** 1. Cocaine is usually sniffed through the nostrils. This procedure is likely to cause red, excoriated nostrils due to local irritation. (9)

**57.** 1. Vomiting and diarrhea are usually late, rather than early, signs of heroin withdrawal. (2, 11, 12)

**58.** 2. When a patient complains of discomfort while abstaining from the use of heroin, it would be least desirable for the nurse to tell the patient that she will reevaluate the patient's withdrawal plan for easing the patient's discomforts. Such a course of action "waffles" on the plan of therapy and may also aggravate the situation. Better courses of action for the patient described in this item include being empathetic but firm and telling the patient of alternative methods, such as warm baths, to deal with her discomfort. Also, it is important in the situation described to have prepared the patient in advance for the discomfort she is likely to experience as heroin is withdrawn. (2, 12)

**59.** 3. Patients who test positive for human immunodeficiency virus (HIV) can transmit the infection when they experience no symptoms or only mild nonspecific symptoms. Given the life-style of the patient described in this item, the probability of exposure to the virus is high. Thus, testing is important. The long incubation period of the virus means that individuals can be infected without exhibiting symptoms of the disease. The virus can be transmitted through heterosexual intercourse, if one partner is infected. (14)

**60.** 2. A private room is not indicated unless necessitated by the presence of another infection. Protection from human immunodeficiency virus (HIV) infection includes wearing gloves before touching mucous membranes and blood or other body fluids. Needles should not be broken or recapped; rather, the syringe and needle should be placed in a puncture-resistant container. Handwashing is the foundation of infection control. (14)

**61.** 4. It is usually not just the desire to want help with drug abuse that motivates a patient; ordinarily, there also are outside pressures, stresses, and problems associated with drug dependency. When the patient described in this item says she will try a chemical dependency program, it is helpful for the nurse to encourage her by saying that there may be other things in her life that she might like to change, along with drug use. Telling the patient that she has hurt her mother and that she needs to give up drugs because of this is unlikely to be supportive of her trying a chemical dependency program for help. This does not describe a personally motivated reason for giving up drug abuse and entering a therapy program. Because a patient says she wants to give a therapy program a try does not necessarily mean that she actually has a desire to give up drugs. (2, 5, 12)

**62.** 4. A typical sign of toxicity when methadone is used is respiratory depression. Fever, colitis, and renal shutdown are not associated with methadone toxicity. (11)

**63.** 3. Methadone is equally effective for a patient at a low dose or a high dose. The danger is that patients may take small doses and sell the excess to drug abusers. (11)

**64.** 3. The best method of keeping the methadone out of the illicit drug market is to administer the liquid form under direct supervision. (11)

**65.** 4. Obtaining and taking drugs is a full-time job for a drug addict, and therefore the person using a therapy program to overcome drug abuse needs help to learn new skills and interests. It may be true that a drug addict lives with false sensory data, fears authorities, and avoids family and friends, but these factors are not the main reason a patient needs to learn a new life-style while learning to live without drugs. (5, 11)

**66.** 1. Narcotics Anonymous suggests that the person plan only one day at a time. It is too frightening and unrealistic for the individual to agree to being "clean" of drugs at meetings of NA and abstain from drugs the rest of his life. Members of NA do not have to commit a certain amount of time to the organization, although members free of drug use for a period of time often voluntarily work with the organization. (2)

**67.** 2. The best judgment concerning progress made by a person who has been abusing drugs is based on the number of drug-free days the patient has. The longer one is free of drugs, the better the prognosis. The kinds of friends the patient has, the way she gets along with her parents, and the degree of responsibility her job requires could possibly influence the patient's success, but judgments concerning success are best based on the number of days the patient is free of drug use. (2, 5)

**68.** 4. The heroin addict is least likely to develop cholelithiasis as a result of drug abuse. Drug addicts are prone to develop such illnesses as hepatitis, pneumonia, and tuberculosis, primarily due to using poor sanitation measures and following an unhealthful life-style. (2, 12)

## The Patient Who Abuses Barbiturates

**69.** 4. The most likely cause of death when a patient has taken an overdose of barbiturates is respiratory failure. Cardiac arrest is not common. Circulatory depression may occur. (3, 11)

**70.** 1. It is the combination of barbiturates and alcohol that becomes dangerous because the two are depressants. An additive effect results. The agents do not enhance the effects of each other, nor do they suppress or act as antagonists. (11)

**71.** 4. When a friend asks if a seriously ill patient will live, it is best for the nurse to respond by admitting to the seriousness of the patient's condition and acknowledging the friend's concern. This type of comment does not offer false hope. It is stereotypical to say that one can only wait and see if the patient dies while offering no support. If the friend is asked to describe his relationship with the patient, the nurse is not focusing on the main problem present at the time. Simply to say that the patient is very ill and may not live is harsh and nonsupportive. (2, 4, 12)

**72.** 1. In the situation described in this item, the nurse should focus on the patient and her needs for support. The nurse inquires about the relationship between the friend and the patient to learn whether the friend is a source of support for the patient. The focus of attention at this time is not centered on the seriousness of the patient's condition. It is irrelevant to attempt to learn whether the relationship may be a factor in the patient's suicide attempt and whether the friend can be trusted with confidential information at this time. (2, 12)

**73.** 1. Tolerance for a drug is described when a patient requires increasingly large doses to obtain the desired effect. Addiction is the highest degree of physical and psychological dependence, and withdrawal is accompanied by severe physical symptoms. The drug-dependent person cannot keep drug intake under control and finds it hard to function without its effects. Habituation is defined as a mild degree of dependence. (11)

**74.** 2. Typical signs and symptoms of barbiturate abuse include sluggishness, difficulty in walking, and irritability. Judgment and understanding are impaired, and speech is slurred and confused. The patient acts drunk as from alcohol but does not have the odor of alcohol on his breath. (11)

**75.** 3. For the patient who is confused when she begins to awaken after taking a large dose of barbiturates, the nurse should plan to maintain seizure precautions, close windows near the patient to prevent her from falling from the window, and use short, complete sentences when speaking to the patient. Giving a medication for anxiety and agitation would be inappropriate because it may add to the depressant effects of the barbiturates that the patient took. (3, 9)

**76.** 2. Generalized convulsions may appear on the second or third day of withdrawal from barbiturates. Without treatment, as described in this item, the convulsions may be fatal. Postural hypotension and psychoses are possibilities but are unlikely to be fatal; they are unrelated to the pentobarbital sodium regimen. Hyperthermia, rather than hypothermia, occurs during withdrawal. (3, 9)

**77.** 3. The patient's associated medical problems, commonly sequelae of poor nutrition and the self-administration of drugs, are of primary concern during the first few days in caring for the patient who suffers with a barbiturate dependency. The patient should be allowed to sleep if she desires. When the toxic syndrome subsides, renewing the patient's optimism and faith in herself and helping with legal problems that may need attending to become more important in the care of the patient. (3, 9)

**78.** 2. Before planning nursing care for the patient, the nurse should obtain baseline information, which will include what possibly brought the patient to a stage of drug dependency. Obtaining information is part of assessment in the nursing process. As therapy proceeds, it may become important to determine the effects of drug dependency on such things as the patient's children, the positive and negative ways she views her health problem, and the length of time she thinks she will need to recover from her health problem. (2, 12)

**79.** 3. When a staff member is critical of the patient described in this item, it is best for a nurse to offer the member a new viewpoint to consider by a comment concerning why the nurse feels the patient is the type of person she is. Suggesting that the staff member may be jealous of the patient or that the member has already made up her mind puts the staff member on the defensive. Defending the patient's behavior is unlikely to help in this situation. (2, 12)

**80.** 4. This item points out a problem concerning how a group of patients may be having an undesirable influence on another patient. It would probably be best for a nurse who becomes aware of this situation to discuss her observations with the group of patients at one of their regular therapy sessions. The problem involves all the patients in the group, and discussing it with them gives the members an opportunity to offer suggestions. It is likely to be futile to try to break up the drug-oriented discussions the group described in this item is having. Providing additional recreation and speaking to patients on an individual basis do not attack the problem in a direct manner. (2, 5, 12)

**81.** 2. The greatest danger to self and others is believed to be posed by the patient's tendencies to act out violently and aggressively when the patient has a continuous high intake of amphetamines. It is recommended that this type of drug abuser be treated in an inpatient unit where appropriate sedation and restraint can be provided. (2, 3)

## The Patient with an Eating Disorder

**82.** 4. The quality of group cohesiveness is present when members are relating to each other warmly, are proud of their progress, and are supportive of a member who becomes discouraged. Mutuality is having the same or reciprocal feelings for the other person. Dependency is relying on another for emotional or physical support. Genuineness is being true to one's character and expressing oneself sincerely and honestly. (2, 5, 12)

**83.** 4. A member of the group working to lose weight is assuming a functional role when she proposes an alternate task to keep from thinking about food. She is in the role of a contributor to the group. Showing pictures of children, insisting that everyone try a favorite reducing diet, and making comments to a member sitting next to her are examples of individual role behavior that are irrelevant to the group task. Showing pictures of one's children in a group is an example of a "blocker." The person who insists everyone try her recipe is an illustration of a special-interest pleader. The person making comments to another group member is withdrawing from the group. (5, 12)

**84.** 1. Through the ages, communication has occurred around food. Honor is extended through food and punishment is given by withholding food. Food is recognized as giving comfort, because it often serves this purpose during childhood. Hence, food is very often equated with love and affection in the American culture. (2, 5)

**85.** 1. Adverse effects associated with amphetamine use include drug dependency, emotional lability, and depression between doses. Gastritis is not associated with the use of amphetamines. (2, 12)

**86.** 4. Overeating is most often associated with a maladaptive method of coping with stress. From a psychological viewpoint, obesity is not ordinarily associated with a lack of motivation to change behavior, a desire for attention, or a wish to be important. (2, 5)

**87.** 2. Obesity most often is the result of taking in more calories than the body uses. (2, 5)

**88.** 4. Bradycardia, hypotension, and cold sensitivity reflect the slowed metabolism that occurs with severe weight loss. Tachycardia and hypertension would reflect increased metabolic rate, which is inconsistent with anorexia nervosa. Hyperthyroidism and elevated serum potassium are atypical with anorexia. Vitamin C deficiency and anemia may occur, but they are not hallmark symptoms of the disorder. (2, 9, 12)

**89.** 2. Behavioral programs consist of rewards and punishments designed to elicit specific behavioral responses. Emotional support and listening is a general intervention that is not specific to the program goal. Identification of problematic eating behaviors is a general intervention related to behavioral programs, but is not specific to a behavioral program for weight gain. Hyperalimentation may be used as a last resort but is a physiologic, not a behavioral, intervention. Rapid weight gain is psychologically intolerable and physically dangerous for the patient. (8)

**90.** 3. The primary goal with severe anorexia is to promote weight gain through behavior modification. This involves actively monitoring and interrupting undesirable behaviors, even against the patient's protests. Waiting for the patient to finish exercising may be polite but exacerbates weight loss as calories are burned. Threatening future loss of privileges does not motivate a patient who is in the middle of a compulsion. Active intervention is required to prevent the patient from continuing to lose weight. (2, 5, 12)

**91.** 1. The goal of hospitalization for anorexia is to stabilize the patient's weight and facilitate entry into psychotherapy. Weight gain in the hospital may not be sustained unless the patient receives psychiatric help for the underlying problem. Most patients do not achieve a normal weight in the hospital and require continued follow-up. The urge to diet often continues for years following hospitalization. A change in eating behaviors does not address the central issue of dangerous weight loss and psychiatric disturbance. (8)

**92.** 2. Manifestations of bulimia always include eating binges, usually include vomiting, and often include low serum potassium secondary to the vomiting. Amenorrhea, severe weight loss, and compulsive exercise are symptoms of anorexia. Laxative abuse and diet pill abuse are sometimes present with bulimia. (4)

**93.** 2. Contrary to popular myth, binges are not enjoyable for the bulimic. They are frightening experiences that result in thoughts of self-deprecation. Binges are done secretively and there is no desire to attract attention. Because of the purging, substantial weight gain usually does not occur, although weight may fluctuate. (4)

**94.** 3. Bulimia involves low self-esteem and a belief

that one's appearance is the only attractive aspect of oneself. Thus, patients need to change their self-concept and challenge negative self-perceptions. Reassurance about weight gain misses the point and probably will be rejected. Changing calories perpetuates the need to focus on eating and weight. Emphasizing the staff's control detracts from the patient's sense of responsibility and capability to heal oneself. (4)

**95.** 4. This is a countertransference reaction that can only be resolved by self-reflection and discussion with other professionals. It is inappropriate for the nurse to tell the patient about her feelings and it might perpetuate the patient's low self-esteem. Continuing to struggle with the problem without analyzing her own reactions is counterproductive for the nurse. Asking another nurse to work with the patient may solve the problem momentarily, but the nurse will encounter similar problems and patients, and the patient may feel rejected. (5)

# test 4

*The Patient with Anxiety*

*The Patient with Maladaptive Behavior Patterns*

*The Patient with Problems with Expression of Anger*

*The Patient with Family Abuse and Violence*

*The Patient with a Psychophysiological Disorder*

*The Patient with a Terminal Illness*

*Correct Answers and Rationales*

Select the one *best* or *correct* answer and indicate your choice by filling in the circle with a pencil in front of the option you have chosen. If the answer you would prefer is not given, select the one you think is *most appropriate*.

## THE PATIENT WITH ANXIETY

Mr. Archie Rowland, 52, is driven to the emergency room of the hospital by his brother. On admission, Mr. Rowland is perspiring profusely, breathing rapidly, and complaining of dizziness and palpitations. Problems of a cardiovascular nature are ruled out. Mr. Rowland's diagnosis is tentatively listed as acute anxiety reaction.

1. The emergency department staff observes that Mr. Rowland is hyperventilating. Which of the following electrolyte imbalances is *most likely* to occur when a patient hyperventilates?
   ○ 1. Metabolic acidosis.
   ○ 2. Respiratory acidosis.
   ○ 3. Metabolic alkalosis.
   ○ 4. Respiratory alkalosis.

2. To ease the symptoms caused by hyperventilation, which of the following measures would be *best* for the nurse to try *first* with Mr. Rowland?
   ○ 1. Have him rebreathe into a paper bag.
   ○ 2. Instruct him to put his head between his knees.
   ○ 3. Give him a low concentration of oxygen via nasal cannula.
   ○ 4. Tell him to take several deep, slow breaths and exhale normally.

3. Mr. Rowland's episode of severe anxiety lasted for approximately 30 minutes. He was then admitted to the inpatient psychiatric unit for further evaluation and treatment, based on his urgent plea for definitive help. Mr. Rowland is aware that his anxiety is of neurotic origin. Neurotic anxiety differs from normal anxiety in that neurotic anxiety is
   ○ 1. out of proportion to the cause.
   ○ 2. lessened with the passage of time.
   ○ 3. a rational response to an objective danger.
   ○ 4. easily traceable to a consciously recognized stimulus.

4. The nursing staff learns that Mr. Rowland was recently promoted at work although he had not yet assumed his new duties and was ambivalent about doing so. To which of the following underlying feelings are the patient's present anxiety reactions to his promotion and his chronic anxiety neurosis *most likely* related?
   ○ 1. Feelings of distrust.
   ○ 2. Feelings of alienation.
   ○ 3. Feelings of inadequacy.
   ○ 4. Feelings of superiority.

5. The main coping method used by persons with an anxiety neurosis involves excluding unacceptable self-knowledge from awareness. The term used to describe this type of behavior is
   ○ 1. repression.
   ○ 2. projection.
   ○ 3. regression.
   ○ 4. sublimation.

6. Mr. Rowland often jumps when spoken to and complains of feeling uneasy. "It's as though something bad is going to happen," he says. *All* of the following nursing measures are likely to reassure Mr. Rowland *except* the nurse's
   ○ 1. being physically present.
   ○ 2. being technically competent.
   ○ 3. conveying optimistic verbalizations.
   ○ 4. communicating a respectful attitude.

7. Which of the following sympathetic nervous system responses should suggest to the nurse that Mr. Rowland is feeling anxious?
   ○ 1. Tachycardia.
   ○ 2. Bradycardia.
   ○ 3. Constricted pupils.
   ○ 4. Excessive salivation.

8. Mr. Rowland's feelings of distress are communicated to the nurse during the counseling session. The nurse perceives his distress and begins to feel

distressed as well. Which of the following statements of intent would be *best* for the nurse to make?
○ 1. "I need to leave for a few minutes to deal with my feelings but I will return shortly."
○ 2. "I wish I could stay to talk with you but I just remembered something I have to take care of."
○ 3. "I hate to cut you off but I think we should talk about something less upsetting to both of us."
○ 4. "I am feeling anxious about what you have told me but I will try to stay with you despite my feelings."

9. The *main* reason the activities planned for Mr. Rowland are directed toward increasing his contact with other people is to
○ 1. relieve his boredom.
○ 2. lessen his egocentricity.
○ 3. keep him safely occupied.
○ 4. prevent him from regressing.

10. Mr. Rowland is married but states that he cannot talk to his wife. He says he does not make sexual advances toward her because he is sure she would turn him down. Which of the following tendencies of neurotic patients is Mr. Rowland displaying in this situation?
○ 1. The tendency to set excessively high goals for oneself.
○ 2. The tendency to anticipate negative reactions from others.
○ 3. The tendency to use ineffective ways to satisfy a selfish need.
○ 4. The tendency to convert emotional conflicts into physical complaints.

11. Chlordiazepoxide (Librium) is prescribed for Mr. Rowland. Many therapists prefer that neurotic patients *not* receive antianxiety agents while in psychotherapy, the *primary* reason being that these agents tend to
○ 1. be habit-forming.
○ 2. decrease muscular tension.
○ 3. reduce motivation for change.
○ 4. have little effect on anxiety of panic proportions.

12. While Mr. Rowland is taking chlordiazepoxide (Librium), he should be taught to avoid ingesting
○ 1. coffee.
○ 2. cheese.
○ 3. alcohol.
○ 4. shellfish.

13. Mr. Rowland attends a psychodrama session twice weekly. Two major goals of psychodrama are to help patients to
○ 1. decrease emotional spontaneity and obtain attention from others.
○ 2. relive unpleasant situations and learn about the problems of others.
○ 3. gain new self-perception and develop more adequate responses to situations.
○ 4. confront individuals with unacceptable behaviors and increase group productivity.

14. Mr. Rowland progresses in this therapy and is soon discharged. He is referred to the outpatient clinic for follow-up. Which of the following hospital-learned abilities is probably *most important* for the continued alleviation of Mr. Rowland's neurotic symptoms?
○ 1. The patient recognizes when he is feeling anxious.
○ 2. The patient understands the reasons for his anxiety.
○ 3. The patient can alter his methods of handling anxiety.
○ 4. The patient is able to describe the situations preceding his feelings of anxiety.

15. If the physician in the outpatient clinic tells the nurse that he is prescribing a minor tranquilizer (antianxiety agent) for Mr. Rowland, the nurse should question the order *unless* the physician prescribes a medication such as
○ 1. oxazepam (Serax) or hydroxyzine pamoate (Vistaril).
○ 2. thiothixene (Navane) or thioridazine hydrochloride (Mellaril).
○ 3. biperiden hydrochloride (Akineton) or procyclidine hydrochloride (Kemadrin).
○ 4. desipramine hydrochloride (Pertofrane) or protriptyline hydrochloride (Vivactil).

16. A minor tranquilizer, rather than a major tranquilizer or a barbiturate, is *most probably* prescribed for Mr. Rowland to relieve his anxiety symptoms because minor tranquilizers tend to
○ 1. induce sleep more readily.
○ 2. cause fewer undesirable side effects.
○ 3. be excreted from the body more quickly.
○ 4. evoke a more rapid sensitization response.

17. Some anxiety is an asset to a person because it helps to
○ 1. slow down one's physiological functioning.
○ 2. lead to one's use of ego defense mechanisms.
○ 3. increase one's alertness to the environment.
○ 4. mobilize one's automatic behavior responses.

## THE PATIENT WITH MALADAPTIVE BEHAVIOR PATTERNS

Gary Ord, 19, is admitted to a psychiatric unit with a nonspecific diagnosis of personality disorder. He is accompanied by his mother and by a lawyer who tells the nurse he hopes his client will "stay out of mischief until we get this crank phone call business straightened out."

**18.** According to Gary's mother, Gary "always was a mean little boy, forever playing pranks on people and teasing the small animals in the neighborhood. Now he's just a bigger prankster and less easy to control." In view of Gary's history, which of the following courses of action would likely be the *most effective* for the nursing staff to follow initially?
  ○ 1. Let the patient know the staff has the authority to subdue him if he gets unruly.
  ○ 2. Keep the patient isolated from the other patients until he is better known by the staff.
  ○ 3. Provide the patient with a list of rules while emphasizing that he will have to pay for any damage he causes.
  ○ 4. Observe the patient's behavior on the unit closely to establish a baseline pattern of physical and social functioning.

**19.** Gary's parents have repeatedly told him that he was a bad, stupid person who would never amount to anything. When Gary confirmed their opinion by dropping out of school and behaving antisocially, which of the following phenomena is he acting out?
  ○ 1. Congruency.
  ○ 2. Double-bind.
  ○ 3. Consensual validation.
  ○ 4. Self-fulfilling prophecy.

**20.** After Gary has been on the unit for a few days, the nurses notice that he uses his shortness and unattractiveness as an excuse for not attending various social functions, such as the weekly dance. Which of the following interventions would be *best* for the nursing staff to plan to take *first* to deal with his avoidance of social functions?
  ○ 1. Tell the patient he will need a better excuse than his appearance for not participating.
  ○ 2. Explain to the patient that everyone's cooperation is necessary to make the program a success.
  ○ 3. Confront the patient with the fact that he is using his appearance as an excuse to avoid socializing.
  ○ 4. Insist that the patient come up with some alternative ways to spend the time when he should be socializing.

**21.** Gary often takes pleasure in startling people. His favorite trick is to belch loudly when in a group and laugh at the discomfort it causes others. In the American culture, belching loudly in public is considered to violate a cultural

  ○ 1. norm.
  ○ 2. more.
  ○ 3. folkway.
  ○ 4. proscription.

**22.** A staff member asks Gary after one of his loud belches, "Do you wonder that people find you repulsive?" The *most likely* possible effect of the nurse's comment on Gary is that it will make him feel
  ○ 1. defensive and defiant.
  ○ 2. insulted and indignant.
  ○ 3. ashamed and remorseful.
  ○ 4. embarrassed and unhappy.

**23.** Gary's past history of cruelty and present crass behavior arouse feelings of anxiety and antagonism in staff and patients. Of the following reasons for these responses in others, the one that *most probably* causes others to react as they do to Gary is that the patient's behavior is
  ○ 1. beyond comprehension.
  ○ 2. viewed as alien to their value system.
  ○ 3. easily misinterpreted as to its meaning.
  ○ 4. seen as only too understandable by others.

**24.** The staff member to whom Gary relates best is Mr. Dant, a registered nurse. Even so, Gary sometimes attempts to provoke Mr. Dant by yelling down the hall, "Hey nursie, where's your hat and purse?" In relation to being baited by the patient, which of the following actions is *best* for the nurse to take?
  ○ 1. Ignore the patient's kidding to avoid reinforcing it.
  ○ 2. Smilingly shake the head no at the patient to stop his teasing.
  ○ 3. Use feminine gestures to indicate acceptance of the patient's ribbing.
  ○ 4. Challenge the patient to an arm-wrestling match to prove the nurse's masculinity.

**25.** Gary tells the nurse that he likes to call hospitals and make bomb threats. He laughs because, he says, he enjoys watching the patients being evacuated and the police running in and out of the buildings. Which of the following replies that the nurse could make would be *least helpful* in encouraging Gary to examine the meaning and effects of such messages?
  ○ 1. "What does it do for you to tell me that?"
  ○ 2. "You could be sent to jail for that, you know."
  ○ 3. "You make bomb threats and everybody hops, is that right?"
  ○ 4. "You expect me to be shocked by what you are saying?"

**26.** One evening, Gary takes Mr. Dant aside and whispers, "Don't tell anybody, but I'm going to call in a bomb threat to this hospital tonight." Of the following actions the nurse could take, which would *best* preserve Gary's trust in the nurse and provide the *best* protection for all concerned parties?

○ 1. Warn the patient that his phone privileges will be taken away if he abuses them.

○ 2. Offer to disregard the patient's plan for wrongdoing if he does not go through with it.

○ 3. Say nothing to anyone until the patient has actually completed the call and notify the proper authorities.

○ 4. Explain to the patient that this information will have to be shared immediately with the staff and with his doctor.

27. Constructive discipline is taken each time Gary behaves in a foolhardy or cruel manner. At those times, which of the following ideas is the *most basic* and *most important* for the staff to convey to the patient?

○ 1. The patient is accepted although his behavior may not be.

○ 2. Everyone must cope with some restrictions on his actions.

○ 3. No one would bother with the patient if the staff did not care about him.

○ 4. If the patient cannot control his behavior, others will have to control it for him.

28. The nursing staff tries to provide Gary with corrective emotional experiences that will influence his present behavior positively. Which of the following possible interventions would constitute a corrective emotional experience for Gary?

○ 1. The staff gives the patient gifts to make up for his earlier suffering.

○ 2. The staff treats the patient's behavior more objectively than others have in his past.

○ 3. The staff promises the patient material rewards and extra privileges for good behavior.

○ 4. The staff allows the patient complete freedom in deciding what available therapies he will use.

29. Which of the following statements made by Gary's mother offers the *best* clue as to why Gary developed into a young adult with impulsive, antisocial tendencies?

○ 1. "He is just like his father, that no-good bum."

○ 2. "I guess I've always been a little afraid to say 'no' to him."

○ 3. "His birth entailed a difficult pregnancy for me with a very long labor."

○ 4. "We lived in a poor neighborhood and that's why he turned out so bad."

30. Gary and the nurse's relationship develops so that they are able to delineate and concentrate on a goal to help Gary increase his social skills. The nurse is talking with Gary about being able to socialize at mealtime without being disruptive. While discussing this topic, it would be *best* for the nurse to focus the discussion on the patient's

○ 1. strengths and responsibilities in the situation.

○ 2. manipulation and disruption in similar situations.

○ 3. explanations concerning his behavior at mealtimes in the past.

○ 4. ability to earn a weekend pass if he can behave well at mealtimes.

31. The nurse judges that Gary's problematic behavior stems from feelings of resentment toward his mother. Gary's resentment seems to represent an attempt to punish his mother for what he perceives as her lack of concern for him. The *best* thing for the nurse to do with this information is to

○ 1. explain it to the patient but in an indirect manner.

○ 2. assist the patient to discover it gradually for himself.

○ 3. record it on the patient's chart so that the psychiatrist can deal with it.

○ 4. include his mother in therapy sessions so that she can discover it for herself.

32. If Gary and his mother improve their relationship and Gary accomplishes the normal developmental task of identity, which of the following age-related developmental tasks should he be expected to master *next*?

○ 1. A sense of intimacy.

○ 2. A sense of integrity.

○ 3. A sense of autonomy.

○ 4. A sense of productivity.

33. Which of the following terms *best* describes Gary's sense of self-awareness of his attitudes and defense mechanisms as well as his self-understanding of his behavior?

○ 1. Insight.

○ 2. Rapport.

○ 3. Lucidity.

○ 4. Cathexis.

34. During the latter part of Gary's hospitalization, his progress slows, and he seems to be making more enemies than friends. Which of the following evaluations of this situation is probably *most accurate*?

○ 1. The patient probably has too many problems to overcome.

○ 2. The patient probably has been unable to develop trust in the nurse.

○ 3. The patient probably is reacting to the termination of his hospitalization.

○ 4. The patient probably is experiencing only a temporary setback in his overall progress.

## THE PATIENT WITH PROBLEMS WITH EXPRESSION OF ANGER

Mr. Ted Talbot, 24, is admitted to a psychiatric hospital for evaluation after numerous incidents of threatening, angry outbursts and two episodes of hitting a co-worker at the grocery store where he works. Mr. Talbot is very anxious and tells Ms. Turner, the nurse who admits him, "I didn't mean to hit him. He made me so mad I just couldn't help it. I hope I don't hit anyone here."

**35.** Which of the following responses is the *most therapeutic* response for the nurse to make?
○ 1. "You'd better not hit anyone here even if you do get mad."
○ 2. "Tell me more about what happened."
○ 3. "It sounds like you were quite angry. When you feel angry here, you'll need to tell us about it instead of hitting."
○ 4. "I'm sure you didn't mean to hit him and that it won't happen here."

**36.** Ms. Turner knows that providing a safe environment for Mr. Talbot and the other patients is a nursing care priority. Which of the following is the *most important initial* action she should take to ensure a safe environment?
○ 1. Let other patients know that he has a history of hitting others so that they will not provoke him.
○ 2. Put him in a private room and limit his time out of the room to when staff can be with him.
○ 3. Tell him that hitting others is not acceptable behavior and ask him to let a staff member know when he begins feeling angry so they can talk.
○ 4. Obtain an order for a medication to decrease his anxiety.

**37.** Mr. Talbot rushes out of the day room where he has been watching TV with other patients. He is hyperventilating, flushed, and his fists are clenched. He says to Mr. Moss, his primary nurse, "That bastard! He's just like Tom. I almost hit him." Which of the following would be the *best* response for Mr. Moss to make?
○ 1. "You're angry and you did well to leave the situation. Let's walk up and down the hall while you tell me about it."
○ 2. "Even if you're angry, you can't use that language here."
○ 3. "I'm glad you left the situation. Why don't you go to your room and calm down. I'll come in soon to talk."
○ 4. "I can see you're angry. Let me get you some Ativan to help you calm down. Then we'll talk about what happened."

**38.** Which of the following factors in Mr. Talbot's history is *least likely* to contribute to his difficulty in coping with anger?
○ 1. A history of abuse as a child.
○ 2. Frequent drinking episodes.
○ 3. A family history of bipolar disorder.
○ 4. A learning disability.

**39.** In the first group meeting after Mr. Talbot is admitted, Ms. Twill, a 65-year-old patient, sits near the nurse and says loudly, "I'm sitting here because I'm afraid of Ted. He's so big and I heard him talk about hitting people." Which of the following responses would be the *most therapeutic* for the nurse to make?
○ 1. "Everyone is here for different problems, Ms. Twill. You know you don't have to worry. We'll keep you safe."
○ 2. "Ted is new to the group. Since he doesn't know anyone here, let's go around and introduce ourselves."
○ 3. "You don't know Ted yet, Ms. Twill. When you do know him, I'm sure you won't be afraid."
○ 4. "It can be frightening to have new people on the unit. The purpose of this group is for people to get to know each other so we can talk together about things like being afraid."

**40.** After Mr. Talbot tells the group why he is in the hospital, Anna Welch, a 22-year-old woman, says, "My doctor tells me I need to get mad more and not let people tell me what to do. Maybe she thinks I should be more like Ted." In order to respond to Ms. Welch, it is *most important* for the nurse to understand that
○ 1. denial of anger and the inability to be assertive can be as serious a problem as the aggressive expression of anger.
○ 2. it is appropriate for a woman to deny her anger since assertive behavior in women is not culturally acceptable.
○ 3. since patients frequently distort what they are told by physicians, it is unlikely that Ms. Welch has been told what she reports.
○ 4. since she and Mr. Talbot are about the same age, Ms. Welch is trying to help him feel accepted by the group.

**41.** In developing a nursing care plan for Mr. Talbot, the staff decides to take an educational approach. *All* of the following would be steps in the plan *except*
○ 1. Assist the patient to recognize anger.
○ 2. Identify all the important people in the patient's life with whom he is angry.
○ 3. Identify alternative ways to express anger.
○ 4. Practice the expression of anger.

42. In talking about discharge with his nurse, Mr. Talbot says, "It's been easy not to get mad and hit people here because the staff won't let me. It's not the same at work." The *most effective* response for the nurse to make would be
    ○ 1. "We have helped, but you are the one who decided not to hit when you were angry. You can do that at work, too."
    ○ 2. "Lots of people feel this way. It's just worry about leaving the hospital. You've learned so much you won't have any problems at work."
    ○ 3. "You sound worried about going back to work. The things you've learned here can help at work, too. Let's talk about what you learned and how you can use it."
    ○ 4. "It's hard to leave the hospital, I know. But you're better and need to get back to work. You'll be OK, I know."

43. After the group meeting, Ms. Welch tells Ms. Dobb, her primary nurse, "My doctor says I'm really mad inside and I'm passive-aggressive. I don't know what she means. You know I don't get angry. Do you think I'm passive-aggressive?" Which of the following responses would be *most inappropriate* for the nurse to make?
    ○ 1. "Most people get mad sometimes. Can you remember any times when you've felt angry about something?"
    ○ 2. "Since this is something you've discussed with your doctor, I think you need to keep talking to her about it."
    ○ 3. "Do you have any thoughts about what your doctor meant?"
    ○ 4. "I think it is hard for you to recognize when you feel angry, and that means you can't express it very well."

44. Ms. Dobb and the treatment team recommend that Ms. Welch take an assertiveness-training course offered in the hospital. Which of the following behaviors indicates that Ms. Welch is becoming more assertive?
    ○ 1. The patient begins to arrive late for unit activities.
    ○ 2. The patient asks the nurse to call her employer about her insurance.
    ○ 3. The patient tells her roommate that smoke bothers her and asks her not to smoke.
    ○ 4. The patient follows the nurse's advice and asks her doctor about being passive-aggressive.

45. Anger is a complex emotion that triggers both physiological and psychological responses. Which of the following physiological responses does *not* occur when a patient is angry?
    ○ 1. Increased respiratory rate.
    ○ 2. Decreased blood pressure.
    ○ 3. Increased muscle tension.
    ○ 4. Decreased peristalsis.

46. Which of the following psychological responses to anger is *least common* in psychiatric patients?
    ○ 1. Decreased self-esteem.
    ○ 2. Feelings of invulnerability.
    ○ 3. Fear of retaliation.
    ○ 4. Feelings of guilt.

47. Anger is a common human emotion and one nurses often encounter as they care for patients with psychosocial alterations. Which of the following statements is *least accurate* and *least useful* to the nurse caring for patients who express anger?
    ○ 1. Anger can be an adaptive response and should be discussed with the patient.
    ○ 2. Feeling angry may be frightening and cause anxiety in the patient.
    ○ 3. When a patient is angry, it is usually because the nurse has done something wrong.
    ○ 4. Anger is frequently used by patients to keep the nurse from getting too close.

48. Which of the following factors is *most important* for the nurse to consider when assessing the angry patient's potential for violence?
    ○ 1. The time of day and level of activity on the unit.
    ○ 2. The attitude of the staff toward the angry patient.
    ○ 3. The staff-patient ratio.
    ○ 4. The patient's past history of violent behavior.

49. Indirect expression of anger is more common than direct expression. Which of the following patient behaviors is *most likely* to be an indirect expression of anger?
    ○ 1. Responding sarcastically to an invitation to join a unit activity.
    ○ 2. Refusing to take medication.
    ○ 3. Organizing a card game with other patients.
    ○ 4. Shouting at another patient.

## THE PATIENT WITH FAMILY ABUSE AND VIOLENCE

Mrs. Ellen Taws, a 35-year-old married homemaker, is referred to the mental health center because she is depressed.

50. Seeing Mrs. Taws for the first time, the nurse notices bruises on her upper arms and asks about them. After denying any problems, Mrs. Taws

starts to cry and says, "He didn't really mean to hurt me, but I hate the kids to see. I'm so worried about them." During the interview it would be *most important* for the nurse to determine

○ 1. the type and extent of abuse in the family.

○ 2. the potential of immediate danger to the patient and her children.

○ 3. the resources available to the patient.

○ 4. whether the patient wants to be separated from her husband.

**51.** Mrs. Taws describes her husband as a "good man" who works hard and provides well for his family. She does not work outside the home and states that she is proud to be a wife and mother just like her own mother. The family pattern that the patient describes *best* illustrates which characteristic of abusive families?

○ 1. Tight, impermeable boundaries.

○ 2. Imbalanced power ratio.

○ 3. Role stereotyping.

○ 4. Dysfunctional feeling tone.

**52.** The nurse discusses the Taws family in a staff meeting. Which of the following statements made by other staff members is likely to be *most helpful* to the nurse as she develops a treatment plan?

○ 1. "The patient sounds like a lot of women I know who don't want to change. You can try family therapy, if he'll come."

○ 2. "Have you thought about suggesting that she attend the group we have for women in abusive families?"

○ 3. "I think the police should be notified in case he hits her again and she wants to call them."

○ 4. "Have you thought about calling the school nurse to find out what she knows about the family?"

**53.** As the nurse learns more about the Taws family, which of the following characteristics is she *least likely* to find to be true about Mr. Taws?

○ 1. Between episodes of abuse, he has a warm, empathetic relationship with his wife.

○ 2. He grew up in an abusive family.

○ 3. He is a college graduate and has a stable work history.

○ 4. He has not met his own expectations for career achievement.

**54.** Mrs. Taws tells the nurse that her 8-year-old daughter refuses to go to school because she is afraid her mother will not be home when she returns. Which of the following is the *most therapeutic* response for the nurse to make?

○ 1. "She must be feeling insecure right now. Let her stay home with you for a few days to reassure her."

○ 2. "Children often feel responsible for trouble in the family. Have you talked with her about what she is afraid might happen?"

○ 3. "You know she is too young to be home alone after school. If you can't be there, you should find someone else to meet her so she won't be afraid."

○ 4. "She is aware of the trouble in the family and is worried about what might happen. Would you like to have her talk to the child therapist here? I think it would be helpful."

**55.** The nurse finds herself dreading Mrs. Taws' appointments and feels she is not working effectively with her. Which of the following actions would be *most appropriate* for the nurse to take?

○ 1. Request that the case be transferred to another staff member who likes to work with women.

○ 2. Recognize that these are normal feelings in working with women in abusive families.

○ 3. Tell the patient about her feelings and ask if she thinks treatment is helping.

○ 4. Discuss her feelings with her clinical supervisor.

**56.** As the nurse develops a treatment plan for Mrs. Taws, which of the following factors would be *least important* for her to consider?

○ 1. Mr. Taws' refusal to be involved in treatment.

○ 2. The patient's coping skills.

○ 3. The recent promotion of the patient's husband.

○ 4. The birthday party next week for the patient's 5-year-old.

**57.** After months of treatment, Mrs. Taws tells the nurse that she has decided to stop treatment. There has been no abuse during this time and because she is less depressed, she feels better able to cope with the needs of her husband and children. In discussing this decision with Mrs. Taws, it would be *most important* for the nurse to

○ 1. tell the patient that this is a bad decision which she will regret.

○ 2. find out more about the patient's decision.

○ 3. warn the patient that abuse often stops when one partner is in treatment, only to begin again.

○ 4. remind the patient of her duty to protect the children by continuing treatment.

Andrew Dudley, a third grader, is referred to the clinic by the school nurse because he is fearful, anxious, and socially isolated.

**58.** Before meeting Andrew for the first time, it would be *most important* that the nurse

○ 1. plan for appropriate play therapy equipment.

○ 2. obtain as much background information about him as possible from the school.

○ 3. make certain that the school has informed the parents of the visit.

○ 4. discuss the case with the child psychologist.

**59.** During the first visit, Andrew is very quiet and finally says to the nurse, "I don't like this. We don't talk to people we don't know in my family." The nurse's *best* response would be

○ 1. "Well, talking is what we do here. Maybe when you know me better, it will be easier for you."

○ 2. "Talking to someone you don't know isn't easy, I know. Let me tell you about this place and what we do here. Then you can ask me questions about it, if you'd like."

○ 3. "It's hard to be in a new place and to talk to people you don't know. And you probably wonder why you had to come."

○ 4. "Well, if you don't want to talk, I have some things to play with here. Why don't you have a look at them?"

**60.** After meeting with Andrew, the nurse talks with his mother, who says, "It's that school nurse again. She's done nothing but try to make trouble for our family since Andrew went to school. And now you're part of it." Which of the following responses is *least likely* to help the clinic nurse develop a relationship with this family?

○ 1. "The school nurse is concerned about Andrew and is only doing her job. Does this bother you?"

○ 2. "We see a number of children who go to Andrew's school. He isn't the only one, if you're worried about that."

○ 3. "You sound pretty angry with the school nurse. Can you tell me what has happened?"

○ 4. "It sounds like you've had some bad experiences with the school. Let me tell you why Andrew was referred, and then you tell me about your concerns."

**61.** After seeing Andrew several times for evaluation, the clinic nurse decides that treatment is indicated. The nurse meets with Andrew's parents to discuss her recommendations with them. During the visit, Mr. Dudley says, "There's nothing wrong with him. He's just like I was at that age. I know what you're after. You think my wife is hitting him again, don't you?" Mrs. Dudley begins to cry and Mr. Dudley puts his arm around her. Which of the following is the *most therapeutic* response for the nurse to make?

○ 1. "I didn't know that was a problem in your family. You are both upset, but we do need to talk about this."

○ 2. "If she is hitting him, something will have to be done. Have you been hitting your son, Mrs. Dudley?"

○ 3. "I am concerned about Andrew. He is too fearful and anxious. I need to know about anything you think might make him this way, including hitting him."

○ 4. "Neither Andrew nor the school have talked about your hitting him, Mrs. Dudley. Can you tell me about it, please?"

**62.** Mrs. Dudley tells the nurse that the year Andrew was 7 was a very bad time for the family. Mr. Dudley was unemployed and she worked a second job to help. In addition, her mother, who helped with Andrew, died unexpectedly. Twice during the year, she slapped Andrew repeatedly when he refused to obey. Both parents say it has not happened again and that the family is back to normal. In assessing the family, the nurse decides that Andrew is not at risk for abuse. Which of the following observations would *not* support this decision?

○ 1. The caring and supportive relationship between the Dudleys.

○ 2. Andrew has not talked about violence during his visits.

○ 3. The infrequent episodes were limited to a time of intense family stress.

○ 4. The Dudleys' defensive attitude toward the school nurse.

## THE PATIENT WITH A PSYCHOPHYSIOLOGICAL DISORDER

Mr. Eric Jasper, 24, is admitted to the hospital with a diagnosis of chronic ulcerative colitis. He has had frequent bouts of diarrhea, causing him to lose another 10 pounds from his already slight frame, in the last month.

**63.** Since this is Mr. Jasper's fourth admission to the hospital in 9 months, he is a familiar person to the nurse caring for him. Which of the following remarks the nurse could make to Mr. Jasper upon his admission would be *most beneficial* to the patient?

○ 1. "It's nice to see you again, Mr. Jasper. Did you get lonesome for us on the outside?"

○ 2. "I thought we had seen the last of you for a while, Mr. Jasper. What are you doing back?"

○ 3. "It's been 2 months since you were last here, Mr. Jasper. What do you think about being back in the hospital?"

○ 4. "I see you have your old room again, Mr. Jasper. No need to explain things to you, since you are such an old pro."

**64.** Mr. Jasper tells the nurse that he would give anything to be rid of his illness. He sighs and says he often daydreams about being healthy, sometimes imagining himself as showing powers of endurance that would put others to shame. When he thinks of himself in this way, which of the following ego defense mechanisms is Mr. Jasper using?

○ 1. Fantasy.
○ 2. Projection.
○ 3. Repression.
○ 4. Compensation.

**65.** The nurse feels sorry for Mr. Jasper but does not want him to know it. Regardless of precautions she might take to hide her feelings, in which of the following ways would Mr. Jasper *best* be able to detect the nurse's true feelings toward him?

○ 1. By listening carefully to what she says to him.
○ 2. By asking her for a description of her feelings toward him.
○ 3. By observing her facial expressions and nonverbal behavior when she is with him.
○ 4. By reading, with permission, what she has written and concluded about him on his chart.

**66.** The nurse realizes she feels sympathy for Mr. Jasper instead of empathy. Which of the following descriptions *best* defines empathy?

○ 1. To identify with another person's feelings.
○ 2. To have parallel feelings with another person.
○ 3. To feel condolence and agreement with another person.
○ 4. To experience and perceive the feelings of another person.

**67.** Mr. Jasper becomes tense and nauseated when he hears the cart containing meal trays approaching. He knows that eating increases his loose stools and discomfort. Which of the following practices would be *best* for the nursing staff to plan to use to prevent the premeal buildup of tension Mr. Jasper experiences?

○ 1. Reroute the meal cart so that the patient will not be disturbed by it.
○ 2. Order a special early tray for the patient to let him finish eating before the meal cart comes.
○ 3. Turn the patient's television or radio on before meals to mask the noise of the approaching meal cart.
○ 4. Arrange for someone to keep the patient engaged in a relaxing activity or conversation before the meal time.

**68.** Mr. Jasper should be involved in suitable activities in his room while his illness is being treated. For which of the following attributes *in particular* should the activities be chosen?

○ 1. The activities should be conducive to rest and relaxation.
○ 2. The activities should enhance improvement of social skills.
○ 3. The activities should include insight and self-awareness experiences.
○ 4. The activities should involve manual dexterity rather than intellectual processes.

**69.** Certain personality characteristics are often attributed to persons with ulcerative colitis. Based on this theory, which of the following traits should the nurse expect Mr. Jasper to have?

○ 1. Self-reliance.
○ 2. Decisiveness.
○ 3. Perfectionism.
○ 4. Ambitiousness.

**70.** The nurse *correctly* recognizes that she has encountered an obstacle to Mr. Jasper's therapy when the patient's behavior is characterized by his being

○ 1. closed off emotionally from others.
○ 2. highly intelligent and manipulative.
○ 3. prone to become dependent on the therapist.
○ 4. unable to tolerate the therapist's suggestions and guidance.

**71.** The physician recommends that Mr. Jasper have part of his bowel resected and an ileostomy constructed. Later, Mr. Jasper says to the nurse, "That doctor of mine surely likes to play big. I'll bet the more he can cut, the better he likes it." Which of the following replies would be *most therapeutic* for the nurse to make?

○ 1. "You sound upset. We could talk about it, if you'd like."
○ 2. "'...the better he likes it.' What do you mean by that?"
○ 3. "Aren't you being a bit hard on him? He is trying to help you."
○ 4. "Does that remark have something to do with the operation he wants you to have, by any chance?"

**72.** Mr. Jasper becomes increasingly morose and irritable after thinking more about his physician's recommendations. He is rude to his visitors and pushes nurses away when they attempt to give him medications and treatments. Which of the following nursing interventions would be *best* when the patient has a hostile outburst?

○ 1. Offer the patient positive reinforcement each time he cooperates.
○ 2. Encourage the patient to discuss his immediate concerns and feelings.

○3. Continue with the assigned tasks and duties as though nothing has happened.

○4. Encourage the patient to direct his anger at staff members who can handle his angry outbursts.

73. One evening Mr. Jasper uses a stream of profanities directed at the nurse, then abruptly hangs his head and pleads, "Please forgive me. Something just came over me. Why do I say those things?" The nurse should judge that the type of behavior the patient is exhibiting is called

○1. punning.

○2. confabulation.

○3. flight of ideas.

○4. emotional lability.

74. The nursing staff begins teaching Mr. Jasper what to expect following surgery but finds that he does not retain the information and seems indifferent to these efforts. The *most likely* reason Mr. Jasper is not learning is because he lacks

○1. an acceptance of the idea of having surgery.

○2. an interest in obtaining information about his impending surgery.

○3. the intelligence to grasp what he is being taught about the surgery.

○4. confidence in the members of the nursing staff who are teaching him about his surgery.

75. Arrangements are made for a member of the ileostomy club to meet with Mr. Jasper. Which of the following aims illustrates the *chief purpose* for having a representative from the club visit Mr. Jasper preoperatively?

○1. To let the patient know he has resources in the community to help him.

○2. To provide support for the physician's plan of therapy for the patient.

○3. To show the patient support and give realistic information on the ileostomy.

○4. To convince the patient that he will not be disfigured and can lead a full life.

76. If Mr. Jasper's immediate physical problems are solved by successful surgical intervention, which of the following actions will be *least important* to his continued health?

○1. Learning about the effects of his coping strategies on his body.

○2. Having physical examinations regularly.

○3. Adhering faithfully to a rigid dietary regimen.

○4. Participating actively in a social group that he enjoys.

77. Mr. Jasper's family has seen Mr. Jasper through many exacerbations and remissions of his illness. Of the following possible effects of chronic invalidism on the patient's family, the most detrimental to their interrelationships would *most probably* be that the illness may make family members feel

○1. guilty and dominated.

○2. put upon and overworked.

○3. superior and self-sufficient.

○4. sympathetic and concerned.

78. The organs of the body involved in a psychophysiological disease such as the one with which Mr. Jasper suffers are ordinarily under the control of the

○1. central nervous system.

○2. autonomic nervous system.

○3. peripheral nervous system.

○4. reticular activating system.

79. The physical symptoms of a person with overconcern for the body often center on the gastrointestinal tract. The *least likely* reason for this finding is that

○1. cultural rituals are related to the alimentary tract throughout life.

○2. there is a strong emphasis during early childhood on eating and toileting behaviors.

○3. the gastrointestinal tract is a fragile body part and easily susceptible to damage.

○4. the functioning of the digestive and intestinal tracts is readily noted and subject to some amount of manipulation.

80. The *most important* distinction for the nurse to make between a psychophysiological disorder, such as ulcerative colitis, and a neurotic disorder, such as conversion reaction, is that when a psychophysiological disorder is present, the physical ailment may be

○1. consciously selected by the person.

○2. fatal to the person if left untreated.

○3. relieved when the mental conflict is arrested.

○4. handled by the person with a characteristic attitude of indifference.

## THE PATIENT WITH A TERMINAL ILLNESS

Greg Shaw, 13, is admitted to the hospital for the third time. His illness is diagnosed as acute lymphatic leukemia. The liaison psychiatric nurse is asked by the team leader to help the nursing staff work more effectively with this terminally ill child and his family.

81. One of the nurses says to the liaison nurse, "Whenever I go to Greg's room, I feel that I have to smile and act happy even though I want to cry when I see him." Which of the following responses

that the liaison nurse could make would be *best* in this situation?

- ○ 1. "Call me when you feel that way. We can talk it over at the time."
- ○ 2. "Try not to show emotion, such as crying. You will likely upset the patient."
- ○ 3. "Keep smiling. The patient and his parents need all the support they can get."
- ○ 4. "Tell the patient that you feel bad that he is ill. If it seems appropriate, you can cry too."

82. Greg suspects that he will not live. However, others talk about only pleasant matters with him and have a persistently cheerful manner around him. Feelings Greg *most likely* will develop as a result of such behavior are feelings of

- ○ 1. relief.
- ○ 2. isolation.
- ○ 3. hopefulness.
- ○ 4. independence.

83. Most authorities would agree that Greg's parents should be told as much about Greg's disease and prognosis as

- ○ 1. they wish to know.
- ○ 2. the nurse believes they can understand.
- ○ 3. the physician can tell them.
- ○ 4. their clergyman thinks is advisable for them to know.

84. Mrs. Shaw tells the nurse, "How much we wish we had taken that trip to Europe last year. Greg wanted to go but we foolishly put it off. It makes me furious that we didn't go as originally planned!" Which of the following stages of adaptation to dying is Greg's mother *most likely* experiencing?

- ○ 1. Anger.
- ○ 2. Denial.
- ○ 3. Bargaining.
- ○ 4. Depression.

85. Since Greg is increasingly prone to outbursts concerning his treatments, which of the following approaches by the nurses when treatments are to be done would likely be *most helpful* in gaining his cooperation?

- ○ 1. Tell him how the treatment can be expected to help him each time.
- ○ 2. Describe the probable effect on his body that missing each treatment would have.
- ○ 3. Ask him to be a good boy and not make the treatment any harder for himself or the staff.
- ○ 4. Promise to give him a backrub every 2 hours if he does not make a fuss about the treatment.

86. Which of the following behaviors, if displayed by Greg, would indicate *most clearly* his need for emotional support?

- ○ 1. He teases his sister about her new boyfriend.
- ○ 2. He wants to have someone with him at all times.
- ○ 3. He has the nurse wait with his bath while he makes a phone call.
- ○ 4. He complains about the limited number of choices on the dietary list.

87. The liaison nurse suggests that some recreational diversion be planned for Greg. Which of the following guidelines *in particular* should the recreational activities selected for Greg reflect?

- ○ 1. They should be of a nonviolent nature.
- ○ 2. They should stimulate the imagination.
- ○ 3. They should require some physical effort.
- ○ 4. They should be geared to early adolescent interests.

88. The team leader makes no comments about Greg during a nursing report, other than to list tasks and routines completed for Greg. Which of the following kinds of behavior is the nurse *most likely* demonstrating when she emphasizes the technical aspects of caring for a dying patient?

- ○ 1. Tactful behavior.
- ○ 2. Efficient behavior.
- ○ 3. Objective behavior.
- ○ 4. Defensive behavior.

89. The nurse who usually is *most effective* when caring for Greg and when helping his family cope with death is one who demonstrates that she

- ○ 1. has contemplated her own death and mortality.
- ○ 2. attends continuing education classes on death and dying.
- ○ 3. can provide caring and physical care but remain distant emotionally.
- ○ 4. views dying persons as distinct populations of people in need of comfort.

90. Greg's 10-year-old sister asks the nurse, "Can you check my blood? When Greg got the measles so did I. And I think I have this, too." Appropriate actions by the nurse include *all* of the following *except*

- ○ 1. asking Greg's doctor to take a sample of the sister's blood.
- ○ 2. explaining that leukemia is not a communicable disease.
- ○ 3. discussing the sister's concern with her parents.
- ○ 4. telling the sister's parents about a group for siblings of patients with terminal illness.

91. When talking with the nurse, Greg's 15-year-old brother says, "We used to play pretty rough games together. Maybe some of the bruises he got when I tackled him caused this." The *most helpful* response by the nurse would be

○ 1. "Don't feel guilty. You didn't cause Greg's illness."

○ 2. "I can see you're worried about this. Let's talk about how people get leukemia."

○ 3. "Here is some information about leukemia for you to read. You'll see you didn't cause it."

○ 4. "Lots of people worry about things like this. It isn't your fault."

92. The liaison nurse explains to the staff that because Mrs. Shaw's best friend recently died after a brief illness, Mrs. Shaw can be expected to react to the impending loss of her son even more intensely than is usually expected. Which of the following concepts *best* explains this expected grief experience?

○ 1. Losses are cumulative in effect.

○ 2. Losses take time to become resolved.

○ 3. Losses affect one's emotional reserves.

○ 4. Losses involve objects or people that are significant to oneself.

93. After a period of depression and preoccupation with his son's death, Mr. Shaw has started to adjust to the idea of life without Greg. This phenomenon of emotionally reacting to a person's death before it actually occurs is known as

○ 1. neurotic depression.

○ 2. acute grief reaction.

○ 3. pathological mourning.

○ 4. anticipatory mourning.

94. At Greg's age of 13, which of the following psychosocial issues would he normally be expected to be resolving, according to Erik Erikson's theory?

○ 1. A lifetime vocation.

○ 2. A social conscience.

○ 3. A personal and sexual identity.

○ 4. A sense of initiative and industry.

95. Which of the following statements that Greg makes about himself indicates that he has *most probably* come to healthy terms with his death?

○ 1. "Why did I have to get leukemia?"

○ 2. "I don't want to talk about it anymore. I'm going to die anyway."

○ 3. "I would like you to sit with me. I feel as though it's OK now."

○ 4. "I think a new drug will be discovered very soon to cure leukemia."

96. Which of the following philosophies that Greg and his family could adopt would most likely help them cope *best* during the final stages of Greg's illness?

○ 1. To live each day as it comes as fully as possible.

○ 2. To relive the pleasant memories of days gone by.

○ 3. To expect the worst and be grateful when it does not happen.

○ 4. To plan ahead for the remaining good times that will be spent together.

97. Greg's physician and parents contemplate discontinuing the chemotherapy and blood transfusions that are keeping Greg alive and in a state of suffering. They are contemplating the act of

○ 1. homicide.

○ 2. decerebration.

○ 3. active euthanasia.

○ 4. passive euthanasia.

98. Greg dies quietly one morning. Nursing intervention to assist the family at this time should include *all* of the following measures *except*

○ 1. providing an unobtrusive place for the family to gather.

○ 2. encouraging the family members to express their feelings.

○ 3. supporting the defense mechanisms in use by the family members.

○ 4. staying with the family while they make the funeral arrangements.

99. The time of death for Greg was recorded as 5:48 a.m. While there is no universally accepted definition of death, the current trend in the United States is to define death as occurring at the time when there is irreversible cessation of functioning of the person's

○ 1. lungs.

○ 2. brain.

○ 3. heart.

○ 4. kidneys.

100. Which of the following behaviors that Greg's family might show after his death should be considered a part of the *normal* sequence of grief and mourning, as opposed to being a sign of pathological mourning?

○ 1. Mourning for him for as long as 1 year.

○ 2. Acknowledging only positive memories of him.

○ 3. Becoming upset as each death anniversary approaches.

○ 4. Developing symptoms similar to those demonstrated by the deceased.

# CORRECT ANSWERS AND RATIONALES

Numbers appear in parentheses following the rationales. The numbers identify textbooks listed in the references at the end of Part I, where correct answers can be verified.

## *The Patient with Anxiety*

1. 4. Excess elimination of carbon dioxide from the lungs by hyperventilation will cause respiratory alkalosis. $HCO_3^-$ and base excess levels help determine whether nonrespiratory (metabolic) alkalosis or acidosis is present. (5, 9)

2. 1. The best measure to ease symptoms caused by hyperventilation is to have the patient rebreathe into a paper bag. Having the patient put his head between his knees, giving him low concentrations of oxygen, and having him take deep, slow breaths and exhale normally will not alleviate symptoms of hyperventilation. (9)

3. 1. Neurotic anxiety is out of proportion to its cause. Normal anxiety is characterized as lessening with the passage of time, being a rational response to an objective danger, and being easily traceable to a consciously recognized stimulus. (2, 5)

4. 3. The patient with neurotic anxieties experiences feelings of inadequacy and inferiority. Distrust, alienation, and superiority are not associated with neurotic anxiety. (2, 5)

5. 1. The defense mechanism repression operates to banish unacceptable ideas from conscious awareness. Repression occurs automatically and involuntarily. Projection occurs when feelings and wishes from within oneself are attributed to others. Regression denotes a return to more infantile patterns of reacting. Sublimation involves diverting instinctual drives into socially acceptable channels. (2, 12)

6. 3. Using optimistic verbalization avoids the patient's feelings and offers little help when an anxious patient feels uneasy. Being present, demonstrating competence, and respecting how the patient feels are helpful nursing measures when a patient is anxious. (2, 12)

7. 1. Tachycardia is a sympathetic response that usually occurs in the presence of anxiety. Bradycardia, constricted pupils, and excessive salivation describe typical parasympathetic responses. (2, 5, 12)

8. 1. A nurse has feelings also. When the nurse is being adversely affected by the patient's feelings, it is best for her to leave if her anxiety is too high for her to function effectively. She can return to the patient when her anxiety subsides. It is less helpful to be untruthful with the patient, suggest that the subject of conversation be changed, or try to stay despite overwhelming feelings. (2, 12)

9. 2. The neurotic patient tends to be self-centered and needs a range of outside interests to help divert attention from himself. (2, 12)

10. 2. Being unable to make sexual advances for fear of being turned down best illustrates the tendency of the neurotic patient to expect negative reactions from others. No physical complaint or ineffective method is depicted in the situation described in this item. The goal—marital sexual relations—would seem attainable. (2, 12)

11. 3. The use of antianxiety agents may become habit-forming, decrease muscular tension, reduce motivation for change, and have little effect on anxiety of panic proportions. However, the primary reason for some persons preferring not to use them during psychotherapy is that they tend to reduce motivation for change. Psychotherapy is most effective when the patient's motivation for change is high. (11, 12)

12. 3. Using alcohol, or any central nervous system depressant, when taking chlordiazepoxide (Librium) is contraindicated because of the additive effects of the alcohol and drug. (5, 11)

13. 3. The role playing, role reversal, and doubling techniques of psychodrama help the patient see his behavior in a different light and to view it more objectively. He can then practice responding differently to problematic situations, with group support, input, and feedback. (2, 12)

14. 3. The patient with anxiety may be able to learn to recognize when he is feeling anxious, understand the reasons for his anxiety, and be able to describe situations that preceded his feelings of anxiety. However, he is likely to continue to experience neurotic symptoms unless he has also learned to alter his methods of behaving so as to handle his anxiety successfully. (2, 5)

15. 1. Oxazepam (Serax) and hydroxyzine pamoate (Vistaril) are minor tranquilizers. Thiothixene (Navane) and thioridazine hydrochloride (Mellaril) are major tranquilizers. Biperiden hydrochloride (Akineton) and procyclidine hydrochloride (Kemadrin) are used in the treatment of Parkinson's disease. Desipramine hydrochloride (Pertofrane) and protriptyline hydrochloride (Vivactil) are antidepressants. (2, 11)

16. 2. Minor tranquilizers are prescribed when possi-

ble because they cause fewer undesirable side effects than major tranquilizers and barbiturates. (11)

**17.** 3. Some anxiety is necessary to help develop adaptive behavior. Increasing one's alertness to the environment is adaptive behavior. For example, the anxiety associated with taking an examination motivates one to study. (2, 12)

## The Patient with Maladaptive Behavior Patterns

**18.** 4. The best initial course of action when admitting a patient is to observe him in order to get to know him and to establish baseline information. This is part of assessment in the nursing process. It is not recommended that patients be isolated unless there is a very good reason for it. An example would be the very active, combative patient who is dangerous to himself and others. Interventions, such as telling the patient that the staff has authority to subdue him or providing the patient with rules he must follow, threaten the patient and are likely to promote trouble. (2, 5)

**19.** 4. A self-fulfilling prophecy is when the patient acts the way he has been described. It is the tendency to behave according to the views and expectations that significant others have of the individual. Congruency refers to consistency in thinking, feeling, and acting. Double-bind is a type of interaction demanding a response to a message that has contradictory signals. Consensual validation is the process of checking out words and events to ensure a shared meaning. (2, 12)

**20.** 3. The antisocial person needs to be confronted by his behavior in order to learn what is expected of him and how to achieve what is expected. An intervention that indicates the patient needs a better excuse than he is using to avoid a social function encourages the use of excuses and belittles the patient. The patient is unlikely to cooperate when he is told that he should try to make a social event successful. Having the patient use an activity other than the one he has planned avoids dealing with a problem and would not be a first choice of action. (2, 12)

**21.** 1. A norm is a rule of behavior for a group and specifies pressures and rewards for adherence. The individual who does not conform may be labeled a deviant. A more is a norm that specifies behavior of vital importance to the society and embodies basic moral values. A folkway is a cultural norm that specifies behavior regarded by society as having

relatively minor importance. Proscribed behaviors are behaviors that society labels acceptable for certain individuals in that society. (2, 5)

**22.** 1. When the nurse asks the patient described in this item if he understands why others find him repulsive, the patient is likely to feel defensive and defiant. The question is belittling, and a natural tendency is to counterattack the threat to the self-image. Since the person with an antisocial personality is egocentric and unconcerned about his effect on others, he is unlikely to feel ashamed, remorseful, or embarrassed. (5, 12)

**23.** 2. Society tends to stigmatize those who vary from its value system. Therefore, the patient's behavior described in this situation is a source of anxiety because it is alien to the staff's and patients' value systems. (2, 10)

**24.** 1. The patient in this situation is trying to provoke the nurse and wants a reaction from the nurse when he taunts him. Behavior that is reinforced will continue. Behavior that is not reinforced tends to become extinguished. Hence, ignoring the patient's comment is the best course of action. The other responses would tend to reinforce the patient's behavior. (5, 12)

**25.** 2. In the situation described in this item in which the patient enjoys making bomb threats, it would be least helpful to respond to the patient's comment by moralizing, such as by saying that the patient could go to jail for these threats. It would be better to validate and clarify the meaning of the patient's message. Such comments give feedback to the patient and promote self-evaluation. (2, 12)

**26.** 4. When the patient described in this item says he plans to make a bomb threat to the hospital, the results of the patient's action if he carries out his threat are too serious to risk bargaining with the patient. The best course of action, and the one most likely to promote trust, is to tell the patient honestly what must be done about the bomb threat. It is possible that the patient is also asking to be stopped and that he is indirectly pleading for help. (2, 12)

**27.** 1. The most basic and important idea to convey to the patient described in this item is that, as a person, he is accepted although his behavior may not be. (2, 12)

**28.** 2. When the nurses wish to influence the behavior of the patient described in this item in a positive way, the best course of action should be based on treating the patient's behavior more objectively than others have in the past. This represents a staff response to the patient's behavior that counteracts the harmful effects of parental attitudes and, in the case described in this item, the mother's overindulgence of the patient and lack of limit setting. (2, 5)

**29.** 2. The developing child needs limits set on his destructive tendencies in order to learn right from wrong. Being afraid to say "no" provides no limits. Heredity, birth trauma, and poverty are not significant factors in the development of antisocial behavior. (2, 12)

**30.** 1. The best approach in the situation described in this item is to capitalize on the patient's strengths and his responsibilities in a given situation. Patients such as this are skillful at placing the blame or focus on others. The interaction should be present-oriented and have a positive focus. (5, 12)

**31.** 2. Therapy is usually most effective when the patient is helped to understand why he behaves as he does. The therapist's insight is not likely to be accepted by the patient until he understands himself. Explaining the patient's behavior to him is usually not beneficial. Documenting the patient's behavior so that the physician can deal with a problem delegates a nursing responsibility to someone else. Bringing the mother into therapy sessions at this time is likely to focus on someone other than the patient. (2, 12)

**32.** 1. Intimacy is a developmental task of early adulthood. It is mastered after a sense of identity is established, normally during adolescence. A sense of integrity is a developmental task of the elderly. A sense of autonomy is a developmental task of early childhood. A sense of productivity, or generativity, is a developmental task of middle adulthood. (2, 12)

**33.** 1. The term "insight" best describes a patient's self-awareness and self-understanding. Rapport is the manner in which the patient and nurse perceive each other and relate to each other; it is a positive feeling. Lucidity is the state of being intelligible or clear to the understanding of others. Cathexis refers to an emotional investment in a person, object, or idea. (2, 5, 12)

**34.** 3. Various behaviors, including a slowing of progress, may surface during the final phases of the relationship between the patient and nurse. The nurse needs to redirect the patient to the issues of termination and help him deal with the feelings associated with it. (2, 5)

## *The Patient with Problems with Expression of Anger*

**35.** 3. Describing acceptable behavior to the patient focuses on the immediate problem concerning the patient. Asking the patient to explain what hap-

pened is a therapeutic statement likely to elicit assessment data; however, it is less focused on the patient's immediate problem. Threatening statements do not elicit further information and are not therapeutic. Providing false reassurance is not therapeutic. (2, 12)

**36.** 3. The nurse clearly addresses behavioral expectations and provides alternatives for the patient. Isolating the patient and making others responsible for the patient's behavior are inappropriate because they do not include the patient in managing his behavior. Medication may be helpful but does not involve the patient in responsibility for his behavior. (2, 12)

**37.** 1. The nurse acknowledges and labels the patient's emotion and acknowledges the patient's appropriate behavior. Recognizing the patient's physiological arousal, the nurse suggests an activity and stays with the patient. Setting limits on the patient's language does not acknowledge the patient's control. Offering the patient medication suggests that he cannot control his behavior. (2, 12)

**38.** 3. Childhood abuse, alcohol abuse, and learning disabilities are all associated with angry, impulsive behavior. A family history of bipolar disorder predisposes the patient to that illness but is not specifically associated with difficulty in coping with anger. (2, 12)

**39.** 4. This response acknowledges the patient's feelings and helps the group accept a new member. The nurse's response should acknowledge the patient's fear and address the purpose of the group but should not provide false reassurance. (2, 12)

**40.** 1. Both denial of anger with passive, unassertive behavior and the aggressive expression of anger are maladaptive behavior patterns. Gender-based stereotypes of assertive behavior are not conducive to mental health. Options 3 and 4 are unwarranted assumptions based on inadequate data. (2, 12)

**41.** 2. Identifying individuals with whom the patient is angry is not important to the overall plan. Helping the patient recognize anger, identifying alternative ways to express anger, and practicing the expression of anger are all steps in the process of teaching an individual to recognize and respond appropriately to anger. (2, 12)

**42.** 3. The nurse acknowledges the patient's concern and provides an opportunity to review his progress and to prepare for the work situation. The first option is therapeutic but does not review the patient's progress or prepare him for the work situation. The second and fourth options provide false reassurance. (2, 12)

**43.** 2. To refuse to discuss the patient's concern is

inappropriate. It is important to help the patient recognize that anger is a normal emotion and to invite the patient to talk about her concern with the label of passive-aggressive. (2, 12)

**44.** 3. By requesting that her roommate respect her rights, the patient asserts herself. Arriving late is often passive resistance, and asking the nurse to call is dependent behavior. Asking the doctor is more assertive, but the patient relies on the nurse's direction to do so. (2, 12)

**45.** 2. Blood pressure, as well as respiratory rate and muscle tension, increase in anger due to the response of the autonomic nervous system to the secretion of epinephrine. Peristalsis decreases. (2, 9)

**46.** 2. Fear of retaliation, guilt, and decreased self-esteem are common psychological responses to feelings of anger. While anger may provide an initial feeling of strength and invulnerability, this is rarely a sustained response. (2, 12)

**47.** 3. Anger has many sources and functions. If the nurse personalizes the anger, she misses the opportunity to understand its meaning to the patient. Anger is an adaptive response in many situations and serves to energize the individual. To understand the use of anger, the nurse must discuss it with the patient. Anger also causes anxiety and can serve to protect the patient from closeness. (2, 12)

**48.** 4. Violent behavior is more likely to occur when there is a demand for high patient activity, when there is inadequate staffing, and when the staff feels hopeless about a patient. However, the patient's past history of violent behavior is the *most accurate* predictive factor. (2, 12)

**49.** 1. Sarcasm is frequently used to express anger indirectly. Refusing medication and shouting are both more direct expressions of angry, negative feelings. Assuming responsibility for a unit activity is a positive, assertive action. (2, 12)

## The Patient with Family Abuse and Violence

**50.** 2. The immediate safety of the patient and her children is the immediate concern. If there is immediate danger, action must be taken to protect them. The level of abuse in the family, the patient's plans, and the resources available are also important in developing a treatment plan, but are not the most important concerns. (2, 12)

**51.** 3. Impermeable boundaries, imbalanced power ratio, and dysfunctional feeling tone are all common in abusive families. However, the traditional and rigid gender roles described by the patient are examples of role stereotyping. (2, 12)

**52.** 2. Group therapy with a group of women with similar problems may help the patient reduce her isolation and sense of shame. The idea that victims of abuse do not want to change is inaccurate and leads to feelings of hopelessness among professionals. Contacting other people about the patient and family without the patient's consent violates confidentiality. (2, 12)

**53.** 1. Lack of empathy characterizes relationships in abusive families. A history of family violence and low self-esteem are common among abusers. The idea that only poorly educated, poorly employed men are abusive is a myth. (2, 12)

**54.** 4. It is important for the nurse to address the family problem and include the patient in making decisions about her daughter. Allowing the child to remain home and having someone else at home to meet her ignore the basic family problem. To ask the patient to talk to her daughter is appropriate but is not sufficient intervention in this family situation. (2, 12)

**55.** 4. Feelings of frustration and ineffectiveness are not unusual. Discussing such feelings with a clinical supervisor helps the nurse understand and deal with her own feelings. To transfer the patient or to ask her for reassurance will neither help the patient nor facilitate the professional growth of the nurse. (2, 12)

**56.** 4. While any event in a family may contribute to an abusive episode, the birthday party is less important to treatment planning than the husband's promotion, which is potentially a major stressor. His refusal of treatment and the patient's coping skills are both very important in treatment planning. (2, 12)

**57.** 2. The nurse needs more information about the patient's decision before deciding what intervention is most appropriate. Judgmental responses could make it difficult for the patient to return for treatment should she want to do so. (2, 12)

**58.** 3. Parental consent is required in order to see a minor unless it is an emergency. The nurse will assess the use of play therapy as she gets to know the patient. Both school information and consultation with the child psychologist will be useful but are not the first priority. (2, 13)

**59.** 2. Children as well as adult patients need to be oriented to the setting and have a chance to ask questions. The nurse acknowledges the patient's feelings and provides information. Stating that the patient is expected to talk does not encourage him to do so. The nurse could orient a 9-year-old child to the setting before starting play therapy. (2, 12)

**60.** 1. To defend the school nurse puts the patient's mother on the defensive. All the other responses address, either directly or indirectly, the mother's concerns and ask for her view of the situation. This is important in building a relationship with the family. (2, 12)

**61.** 1. The nurse is supportive and nonjudgmental but makes it clear that the alleged abuse must be discussed. Threatening responses will not help build the relationship with the parents, and the nurse must recognize the feelings of the couple. (2, 12)

**62.** 4. A strong defensive reaction by parents to an appropriate concern by a teacher or other professional may indicate family problems. A caring, supportive relationship between family members and infrequent episodes of abuse during a time of intense family stress are not characteristic of abusive, violent families. (2, 12)

## The Patient with a Psychophysiological Disorder

**63.** 3. When the patient described in this item returns to the hospital for the fourth time in 9 months, it is best for the nurse to acknowledge his readmission and give the patient an opportunity to express his feelings. Telling the patient it is nice to see him and asking him if he had become lonesome serves little purpose except as social comments. Telling the patient that the nurse thought she had seen the last of the patient and asking him what he is doing back in the hospital could be interpreted as being rude and challenging. The nurse is making an assumption when she states that the patient will not need to be oriented to the hospital because of previous admissions. (2, 5)

**64.** 1. The defense mechanism being used by the patient in this situation is fantasy. He is daydreaming and making up a mental picture in his mind. Repression is preventing painful thoughts from entering consciousness. Projection is attributing one's own unacceptable traits to others. Compensation covers up a weakness by emphasizing a desirable trait. (2, 12)

**65.** 3. Nonverbal communication, much more than verbal communication, expresses a person's true feelings. Listening to what a person is saying, asking a person to describe how he feels, and reading the chart are forms of verbal communication. (2, 5)

**66.** 4. Empathy is described as the ability to feel as another person feels and to be able to understand and respond to the feelings. Having parallel feelings with another person and feeling condolence and agreement with another person describe sympathy more accurately than empathy. Identifying with another person's feelings is only part of the process of empathizing with another person. (2, 12)

**67.** 4. Using people for therapeutic interventions is usually more helpful than manipulating the environment, as is the case in this item when a patient becomes upset when he hears meal trays approaching. Tension is less likely to develop when a patient is interpersonally involved than when the time element in relation to eating has been altered. (2, 12)

**68.** 1. Activity within physical limits is desirable. However, the emphasis of treatment lies in providing rest and freedom from emotional stress to the extent possible for a patient suffering with a psychophysiological disorder, such as the one described in this item. This goal is best met when activities that promote rest and relaxation are chosen for the patient. The goal is less well met by activities that promote improvement of social skills, insight and self-awareness, and manual rather than intellectual dexterity. (5, 12)

**69.** 3. Persons with ulcerative colitis have a personality described as obsessive-compulsive. Behavior such as perfectionism, conformity, rigidity, being emotionally on guard, and being obstinate is typical. (5, 9)

**70.** 1. Patients with psychophysiological disorders, such as ulcerative colitis, tend to close themselves off emotionally from others and do not reveal their feelings easily. These characteristics are often an obstacle in therapy. These patients may expect the therapist to help them without having to disclose feelings. (2, 5)

**71.** 2. In the situation described in this item, when the patient seems to be questioning his physician's goals, it is best for the nurse to present an open statement by repeating part of what the patient said and ask him what he means by what he said. This technique helps the patient express his feelings. It is less therapeutic to tell the patient that he sounds upset, that he is being hard on his physician, or that his remark apparently has something to do with the surgery he is about to have. (5, 12)

**72.** 2. When the patient described in this item has hostile outbursts, it is best for the nurse to help the patient express his feelings. This serves as a release valve for the patient. Other types of actions by the nurse are less therapeutic than helping him to express himself. (2, 5, 12)

**73.** 4. The patient described in this item directs profanities at the nurse and then is sorry for his behavior. This type of behavior illustrates emotional lability, which is a readily changeable or unstable emotional affect. Punning is using a word when it can have two or more meanings, or a play on words. Confabulation is replacing memory loss by fantasy to hide confusion; it is unconscious behavior. Flight of ideas refers to a rapid succession of verbal expressions that jump from one topic to another and are only superficially related. (2, 5)

**74.** 1. From information given about this patient, it is most likely that he has not accepted the idea of having surgery. Hence, he is not in a state of readiness for learning. Lacking an interest in obtaining information, intelligence to grasp the teaching, and confidence in the nursing staff are unlikely reasons for this patient's failure to grasp what the nurses are teaching, although these factors may sometimes also play a role in influencing learning. (2, 5)

**75.** 3. Preoperative visits and talks with patients who have made successful adjustments to ileostomies are helpful and tend to make the patient less fearful of the operation and its consequences. (5)

**76.** 3. An ileostomy for treatment of ulcerative colitis eliminates the need for a strict dietary regimen. Development of more effective coping skills and more satisfying social relationships are both important to the resolution of psychophysiological disorders. (2, 9)

**77.** 1. When a member of a family has been chronically ill, feelings of guilt and domination tend to cause the greatest amount of intrapsychic conflict in the family's interrelationships. Also, these feelings are least easy to express and communicate openly. Hence, feelings of guilt and domination would tend to have the most negative and destructive effect on interrelationships in terms of behavioral symptomatology. (2, 5)

**78.** 2. The body systems and organs affected by psychophysiological disorders are usually innervated by the autonomic nervous system. In the presence of stress, the autonomic nervous system prepares the gastrointestinal tract for the body's response with hyperemia, hypermotility, and hypersecretion. Lesions in the form of ulcers may result in the lining of the intestine from chronic irritation. (5, 12)

**79.** 3. Overconcern for the body often centers on the gastrointestinal tract for a variety of reasons. For example, cultural rituals are related to the alimentary tract throughout life, there is a strong emphasis during early childhood on eating and toileting, and functioning of the digestive tract is readily noted and subject to some amount of manipulation. An unlikely reason for overconcern with the gastro-

intestinal tract is that it is fragile. It is a sturdy part of the body and is not easily susceptible to damage. (5, 12)

**80.** 2. Psychophysiological disorders, if untreated, may prove fatal. Persons with psychophysiological disorders do not select the physical ailment with which they suffer, find relief from physical symptoms when a mental conflict is arrested, or handle them with an attitude of indifference. (2, 12)

## The Patient with a Terminal Illness

**81.** 4. Patients very often sense a nurse's feelings. Therefore, when the nurse described in this item becomes emotionally upset while caring for the terminally ill child, it is best for the nurse to share her emotions with the child when it seems appropriate. It is also acceptable to cry. Such practices as trying not to show emotion and trying to smile regardless of how one feels are inappropriate responses. It is of little help to the patient or the nurse who is upset if the nurse waits until a later time when she can speak to someone about the situation. (5, 12)

**82.** 2. Children are aware of and show anxieties about death at an earlier age than was once thought, and they recognize false cheerfulness. They tend to experience isolation and loneliness when those around them are trying to hide or mask the truth. They are then left to face the realities of death alone. (2, 5)

**83.** 1. Most authorities recommend that the parents of an ill child, including the child who is terminally ill, should be told as much as *they* wish to know. The nurse determines this by talking with the parents and child. (2, 5)

**84.** 1. The family appears to be experiencing anger in the situation described in this item, much of which stems from feelings of guilt. During the stage of denial, the parents are more likely to deny their child's diagnosis and prognosis. During the stage of bargaining, the parents tend to offer to do certain things in exchange for more time before their child dies. In depression, parents are likely to make few or no comments and appear and act dejected. (2, 5)

**85.** 1. In the situation described in this item, the best course of action when the patient has outbursts concerning his treatments is to tell him how the treatment can be expected to help him. Describing the effect on his body if he misses a treatment is a negative approach and is threatening to the patient.

The patient is likely to feel angry if he is told to be a good boy during treatments. Offering to give the patient a backrub if he does not fuss does not give the patient information to which he is entitled and old enough to understand. (2, 3)

**86.** 2. When a patient wants to have someone with him at all times, he is displaying dependency, and for the patient described in this item, who is 13 years old, the behavior illustrates regression. It would be considered normal for a 13-year-old boy to tease a sister, make the nurse wait while he uses the telephone, and complain about his dietary choices. (2, 5)

**87.** 4. Recreational activities selected for the 13-year-old described in this item should be geared to the interests of an adolescent. Activities that are physical in nature are likely to be too strenuous for a terminally ill child. Activities of a nonviolent nature and those that stimulate the child's imagination are satisfactory, but the first criterion should be that the activity be appropriate for the patient's age level. (2, 5)

**88.** 4. When a nurse caring for a terminally ill patient reports only tasks and routines completed for the patient, the nurse is most probably behaving defensively. It is very likely that she has not come to grips with death and dying. (2, 5)

**89.** 1. It is best to examine one's own feelings about death and dying before caring for the terminally ill patient. Many authorities consider self-examination of one's own finiteness essential before one can successfully meet the needs of the dying patient. (2, 5, 12)

**90.** 1. Having a blood sample taken is an unnecessary, invasive procedure and would not directly address the child's fear. An age-appropriate explanation by the nurse and alerting the parents to the sibling's concern and the resources available to assist siblings with the terminal illness are all appropriate interventions. (2, 10, 13)

**91.** 2. A response that acknowledges the brother's concern and provides him with information is most helpful. Reassurance without addressing the expressed concern and providing information without acknowledging the expressed concern are not as helpful as acknowledgement plus information. (2, 10, 13)

**92.** 1. Losses tend to be cumulative. Old losses are relived or reexperienced with each new loss and add to the intensity of the present grief experience. (5)

**93.** 4. When a person starts to adjust to life without a family member before the patient actually dies, the person is experiencing anticipatory grief or mourning. It is an early "giving up" of the loved one and accomplishes some of the grieving for the loved one before he dies. (2, 5)

**94.** 3. According to Erikson, a child of age 13 is normally seeking to meet his needs for a personal identity. (2, 5)

**95.** 3. When the child described in this term indicates that "it's OK now," he is indicating an acceptance of his impending death and being at peace with the surroundings. If the child says he does not want to talk about his illness, he is probably showing denial, or maybe anger. When the child says he does not want to talk because he is going to die anyway, he reveals bitterness and anger. Thinking that a new drug may be found to cure his illness suggests that the child is probably bargaining or denying his illness. (2, 5)

**96.** 1. It is best when supporting the family of a terminally ill patient to focus on the present, the "here and now." This can be accomplished by living each day at a time to its fullest. Families also want to know what to expect and want someone to listen to them as they experience grief over death. (2, 5, 12)

**97.** 4. The parents described in this item are contemplating passive euthanasia, which is allowing the patient to die without using life-prolonging measures. Active euthanasia is performing an act that would result in the death of the patient. (5)

**98.** 4. The least important intervention measure for a nurse to use when a patient dies is to stay with the family while it makes funeral arrangements. It is more important to intervene with such measures as providing privacy for the family, encouraging family members to express their feelings, and supporting defense mechanisms the family members may be using to ease their sorrow. (2, 12)

**99.** 2. Because of scientific achievements in prolonging life, the definition of death has become more complicated. However, a generally accepted definition states that death is present when an individual has sustained either irreversible cessation of circulatory *and* respiratory functioning *or* irreversible cessation of functions of the brain, including the brain stem. (5, 9)

**100.** 1. The process of resolution of loss by death may take up to 1 year. Such behaviors as acknowledging only positive memories of the deceased, becoming upset with each anniversary of the death, and developing symptoms similar to those demonstrated by the deceased would not be considered normal signs of grief. (12)

## REFERENCES FOR PART I
### The Nursing Care of Patients with Psychosocial Alterations

1. American Psychiatric Association. Diagnostic and Statistical Manual of Mental Disorders III-R. 4th ed. Washington, D.C.: American Psychiatric Association, 1987.
2. Beck DM, Rawlins RP, Williams SR. Mental Health-Psychiatric Nursing: A Holistic Life-Cycle Approach. 2nd ed. St. Louis: CV Mosby, 1988.
3. Brunner LS, Suddarth DS. The Lippincott Manual of Nursing Practice. 3rd ed. Philadelphia: JB Lippincott, 1983.
4. Burgess AW. Psychiatric Nursing in the Hospital and the Community. 4th ed. Englewood Cliffs, NJ: Prentice-Hall, 1985.
5. Haber J, Hoskins PP, Leach AM, Sideleau BV. Comprehensive Psychiatric Nursing. New York: McGraw-Hill, 1987.
6. Ingalls AJ, Salerno MC. Maternal and Child Health Nursing. 6th ed. St. Louis: CV Mosby, 1987.
7. Jorm AF. A Guide to the Understanding of Alzheimer's Disease and Related Disorders. New York: New York University Press, 1987.
8. Lego S. The American Handbook of Psychiatric Nursing. Philadelphia, JB Lippincott, 1984.
9. Luckmann J, Sorensen KC. Medical-Surgical Nursing: A Psychophysiologic Approach. 3rd ed. Philadelphia: WB Saunders, 1987.
10. Mace NL, Rabins PV. The 36-Hour Day: A Guide to Caring for Persons with Alzheimer's Disease, Related Dementing Illnesses and Memory Loss in Later Life. Baltimore: Johns Hopkins University Press, 1981.
11. Rodman MJ, Smith D. Pharmacology and Drug Therapy in Nursing. 3rd ed. Philadelphia: JB Lippincott, 1985.
12. Stuart GW, Sundeen SF. Principles and Practice of Psychiatric Nursing. 3rd ed. St. Louis: CV Mosby, 1987.
13. Whaley LF, Wong DL. Nursing Care of Infants and Children. 3rd ed. St. Louis: CV Mosby, 1987.
14. Wormser GP, Staff RE, Buttone ER. AIDS (Acquired Immune Deficiency Syndrome). Park Ridge, IL: Noyes, 1987.

# PART II

## The Nursing Care of Maternity Patients and Newborns

# *test* 1

*The Pregnant Patient Receiving Prenatal Care*

*The Pregnant Patient in Childbirth Preparation Class*

*The Preconception Patient*

*The Patient with a Spontaneous Abortion*

*Correct Answers and Rationales*

Select the one *best* or *correct* answer and indicate your choice by filling in the circle with a pencil in front of the option you have chosen. If the answer you would prefer is not given, select the one you think is *most appropriate*.

## THE PREGNANT PATIENT RECEIVING PRENATAL CARE

Mrs. Mary Adams schedules an appointment at the prenatal clinic because she has missed two menstrual periods.

**1.** From the initial interview, the nurse learns that Mrs. Adams' last menstrual period began July 13. According to Naegele's rule, Mrs. Adams' estimated date of confinement is
- ○ 1. February 10.
- ○ 2. April 20.
- ○ 3. October 20.
- ○ 4. December 16.

**2.** While the nurse is preparing her for a pelvic examination, Mrs. Adams says, "I am afraid of this examination." Which of the following responses would be *best* for the nurse to make?
- ○ 1. "I will be with you to explain everything the doctor is doing."
- ○ 2. "Nearly all mothers have some fears about this type of examination."
- ○ 3. "Please tell me more about what you mean when you say you are afraid."
- ○ 4. "The examination will not take long. You will be draped to ensure privacy."

**3.** Which of the following nursing measures would help Mrs. Adams relax during insertion of the speculum?
- ○ 1. Having her bear down slightly.
- ○ 2. Helping her take slow chest breaths.
- ○ 3. Having her grasp the nurse's hand snugly.
- ○ 4. Conversing with her to distract her attention.

**4.** The physician determines that Mrs. Adams is approximately 10 weeks gestation. At this time, it is possible to assess *all* of the following signs of pregnancy *except*
- ○ 1. palpation of fetal movements.
- ○ 2. an increase in the size of the uterus.
- ○ 3. a softening of the lower uterine segment (Hegar's sign).
- ○ 4. a bluish color of the vaginal mucous membranes (Chadwick's sign).

**5.** Mr. and Mrs. Adams tell the nurse, "We just can't believe that we are going to have a baby!" Which of the following responses by the nurse would be *best* in this situation?
- ○ 1. "Would you like some pamphlets on the childbirth experience?"
- ○ 2. "These feelings are normally experienced by couples during early pregnancy."
- ○ 3. "You should not have doubts now. The doctor has confirmed that you are pregnant, Mrs. Adams."
- ○ 4. "Would you like me to make an appointment for you at the mental health clinic for counseling on pregnancy?"

**6.** The nurse evaluates the Adamses' expression of surprise at the confirmation of the pregnancy as being an indication of
- ○ 1. normal ambivalence.
- ○ 2. rejection of the pregnancy.
- ○ 3. acceptance of the pregnancy.
- ○ 4. need for further developmental assessment.

**7.** The nurse correctly determines that Mrs. Adams is attempting to verify the reality of her pregnancy when Mrs. Adams states that she has
- ○ 1. always had irregular menstrual cycles.
- ○ 2. noticed that her bra fits a little tighter than usual.
- ○ 3. no difficulty in wearing her most tight-fitting pants.

○ 4. been successful in losing four pounds during the past month.

8. If Mr. Adams experiences *mitleiden* ("suffering along"), the symptom the nurse will *least likely* expect to be identified by Mr. Adams during the first trimester is
○ 1. nausea.
○ 2. weight gain.
○ 3. fetal movement.
○ 4. various types of discomfort.

9. Which of the following statements, if made by Mr. Adams, would the nurse interpret as being *least likely* to express feelings common to expectant fathers during the first trimester?
○ 1. "I don't understand why Mary starts crying for no reason."
○ 2. "I always thought Mary was very healthy, but now she complains about being tired all the time."
○ 3. "I feel really good about all the attention our friends and family are giving Mary since she's been pregnant."
○ 4. "I'm planning to work weekends at another job to make sure we have enough money for any unexpected expenses."

10. Mrs. Adams tells the nurse that she has been vomiting her breakfast nearly every morning. Which of the following nursing measures would *most likely* help Mrs. Adams with early-morning nausea and vomiting?
○ 1. Sip whole milk with breakfast.
○ 2. Drink only liquids for breakfast.
○ 3. Eat some crackers before arising from bed in the morning.
○ 4. Drink a carbonated beverage before arising from bed in the morning.

11. In what way, if any, should Mr. and Mrs. Adams' sexual activity change during pregnancy, if Mrs. Adams remains free of complications?
○ 1. The Adamses should practice coitus interruptus during pregnancy.
○ 2. It is generally agreed that sexual activity need not be altered during pregnancy.
○ 3. It is best to avoid sexual intercourse until Mrs. Adams is at least 16 weeks gestation.
○ 4. Ideally, the Adamses should have sexual intercourse no more often than once a week during pregnancy.

12. Mrs. Adams asks if she may have an occasional alcoholic beverage during her pregnancy. The *best* advice the nurse can provide Mrs. Adams, in relation to alcohol during pregnancy, is for her to
○ 1. limit drinking to beer or wine.
○ 2. abstain from drinking alcoholic beverages.

○ 3. drink no more than 1 ounce of liquor per day.
○ 4. dilute liquor with water or soda before drinking it.

13. Mrs. Adams asks the nurse how much weight would be safe for her to gain during her pregnancy. The nurse *appropriately* teaches Mrs. Adams that in relation to gaining weight during pregnancy, it has been found that
○ 1. a maximum weight gain of about 20 pounds (9 kg) is usually recommended.
○ 2. weight gain has little significance as long as the patient does not feel hungry.
○ 3. a weight gain of approximately 12 pounds (5.5 kg) each trimester is recommended.
○ 4. weight gain varies, but a range of 25 to 30 pounds (11 to 13.6 kg) is usually considered normal.

14. Mrs. Adams is taught the importance of having sufficient protein in her diet. The nurse would evaluate her teaching as being successful if Mrs. Adams includes which of the following foods rich in protein in her diet in addition to meat, fish, and poultry?
○ 1. Beans and nuts.
○ 2. Mushrooms and melons.
○ 3. Spinach and turnip greens.
○ 4. Citrus fruits and tomatoes.

15. The nurse explains to Mrs. Adams that she will need to take supplemental iron during her pregnancy. Mrs. Adams can increase the absorption of the supplemental iron by taking it
○ 1. at bedtime.
○ 2. between meals.
○ 3. at the same time every day.
○ 4. with a good source of vitamin C.

16. In addition to taking supplemental iron, Mrs. Adams is taught to increase her dietary intake of iron. Mrs. Adams would correctly choose which of the following two foods that are *especially* rich in iron content?
○ 1. Beef and pork.
○ 2. Bananas and figs.
○ 3. Carrots and tomatoes.
○ 4. Cottage cheese and yogurt.

17. The nurse determines *correctly* that Mrs. Adams is including foods rich in folic acid (folacin) in her meal planning when Mrs. Adams recalls that each day she eats at least two servings of
○ 1. fresh fruit.
○ 2. dairy products.
○ 3. whole wheat bread.
○ 4. green leafy vegetables.

18. During Mrs. Adams' first prenatal visit in the second trimester, the nurse describes quickening and

asks Mrs. Adams to note the date carefully on which she first feels fetal movement. This information is used *primarily* to help
○ 1. determine fetal well-being.
○ 2. assess the growth of the fetus.
○ 3. document the estimated date of delivery.
○ 4. determine the lie of the fetus in the uterus.

**19.** The nurse would *correctly* evaluate the highlight of the second trimester for Mrs. Adams as being her report that she
○ 1. has experienced quickening.
○ 2. has bought a cradle for the nursery.
○ 3. is now able to wear maternity clothes.
○ 4. is no longer experiencing morning sickness.

**20.** The nurse *correctly* determines that the nursing measure that would *most likely* facilitate Mr. Adams' involvement in the pregnancy during the second trimester is
○ 1. suggesting that Mr. Adams develop a new hobby.
○ 2. helping Mr. Adams identify new acquaintances at work.
○ 3. encouraging Mr. Adams to listen to the fetal heart beat.
○ 4. referring Mr. Adams to an expectant fathers' bowling team.

**21.** Mrs. Adams calls the clinic one day and tells the nurse that she has some vaginal discharge and local itching. Which of the following courses of action is *best* for the nurse to take in this situation?
○ 1. Ask the patient to come to the clinic for an examination.
○ 2. Advise the patient to take a vinegar douche under low pressure.
○ 3. Tell the patient that her symptoms are normal during pregnancy.
○ 4. Explain to the patient that she should avoid sexual intercourse as long as the symptoms persist.

**22.** Mrs. Adams continues to visit the clinic regularly during her pregnancy. During one visit, she asks about the brown discoloration across her nose and cheeks. Which of the following statements by the nurse *most accurately* reflects authoritative opinion concerning such skin discolorations?
○ 1. The discoloration is related to the sex of the fetus.
○ 2. The discoloration is potentially serious and may require treatment.
○ 3. The discoloration will fade if an antihistaminic drug is prescribed.
○ 4. The discoloration usually disappears after delivery and is without clinical significance.

**23.** The nurse will use Leopold maneuvers while ex-

amining Mrs. Adams. In order for Mrs. Adams to be more comfortable and the results to be more accurate, the nurse will plan to prepare Mrs. Adams for Leopold maneuvers by having her
○ 1. empty her bladder.
○ 2. lie on her left side.
○ 3. hyperventilate for a short time.
○ 4. avoid eating immediately before the examination.

**24.** The nurse performs Leopold maneuvers on Mrs. Adams *primarily* in order to
○ 1. turn the fetus in the uterus.
○ 2. ease the fetus into the pelvis.
○ 3. assess the location of the placenta.
○ 4. determine the fetal position in the uterus.

**25.** As Mrs. Adams is lying supine on the examining table, she tells the nurse that she is becoming dizzy. The nurse observes that Mrs. Adams is pale and perspiring freely. The *first* course of action the nurse should take in this situation is to
○ 1. turn the patient onto either side.
○ 2. obtain the patient's blood pressure.
○ 3. assess the patient for vaginal bleeding.
○ 4. lower the patient's head below the level of her feet.

**26.** Mrs. Adams tells the nurse, "I hope I don't get varicose veins during pregnancy. What causes them?" The nurse should explain that varicose veins are usually due to
○ 1. a decrease in normal cardiac output.
○ 2. an increase in maternal blood volume.
○ 3. an interference with venous return from extremities.
○ 4. a constriction in the blood vessel walls in the extremities.

**27.** Mr. Adams asks to listen to the fetal heart. At what gestational age will Mr. Adams *most likely first* be able to hear the fetal heart when using a stethoscope?
○ 1. At approximately 6 weeks.
○ 2. At approximately 12 weeks.
○ 3. At approximately 18 weeks.
○ 4. At approximately 24 weeks.

**28.** Mrs. Adams says she is often constipated. In relation to relieving constipation, the nurse should teach Mrs. Adams that it is *best* to
○ 1. use a glycerine suppository as necessary.
○ 2. drink a glass of hot water in the morning.
○ 3. eat foods that contain a minimum of seasoning.
○ 4. use a mild laxative, such as milk of magnesia, as necessary.

**29.** Mrs. Adams complains of discomfort due to hemorrhoids. Which of the following measures should the nurse recommend that Mrs. Adams use sev-

eral times a day as necessary to relieve the discomfort of hemorrhoids?
- ○1. Lie down with her hips elevated on a pillow.
- ○2. Alternately raise and lower each leg while lying down.
- ○3. Sit with the knees spread and well flexed (tailor sitting).
- ○4. Rest on the hands and knees while rocking the pelvis (pelvic tilt).

**30.** Mrs. Adams tells the nurse that she and her husband wish to drive to visit relatives who live several hundred miles away. Which of the following recommendations concerning traveling by automobile is *best* for the nurse to offer Mrs. Adams?
- ○1. Automobile travel should be avoided during the first half of pregnancy.
- ○2. Automobile travel during pregnancy should be limited to 1- to 2-hour trips.
- ○3. Automobile travel during pregnancy should include intermittent rest periods.
- ○4. Automobile travel is safe, but the pregnant woman should avoid driving the car.

**31.** Mrs. Adams complains of leg cramps. The exercise that helps *most* to relieve leg cramps is to
- ○1. walk until the cramps disappear.
- ○2. alternately flex and extend the legs.
- ○3. push upward on the toes and downward on the knees.
- ○4. lie flat in bed with the legs extended and elevated.

**32.** The nurse should also teach Mrs. Adams that leg cramps can be relieved by adding a small amount of which of the following to milk?
- ○1. Psyllium hydrophilic mucilloid (Metamucil).
- ○2. Unflavored gelatin granules.
- ○3. Sodium bicarbonate (baking soda).
- ○4. Aluminum hydroxide gel (Amphojel).

**33.** When Mrs. Adams complains of heartburn, the nurse teaches her preventive measures. Which of the following measures is *least* recommended in preventing heartburn?
- ○1. Eat smaller and more frequent meals.
- ○2. Remain in an upright position following meals.
- ○3. Drink an adequate amount of fluid (6 to 8 glasses) daily.
- ○4. Take a half-teaspoon of sodium bicarbonate (baking soda) dissolved in a half-cup of water.

**34.** When Mrs. Adams complains of ankle edema, the nurse teaches coping strategies to avoid aggravating her ankle edema. The nurse determines that the teaching has been effective when Mrs. Adams says that she will
- ○1. wear knee-high hose instead of pantyhose.
- ○2. complete at one time all tasks that require standing.
- ○3. reduce her fluid intake.
- ○4. dorsiflex her feet frequently.

**35.** Mrs. Adams telephones the nurse complaining of an intense, "grabbing" pain in the lower abdomen. The nurse *correctly* recommends that Mrs. Adams apply warmth to her lower abdomen when the nurse's assessment indicates that the pain is
- ○1. radiating to the epigastric area.
- ○2. accompanied by nausea and vomiting.
- ○3. located in the right lower quadrant.
- ○4. due to stretching of the round ligament.

**36.** At her next prenatal visit, Mrs. Adams tells the nurse that she is exhausted because she has been unable to sleep at night. The nurse teaches Mrs. Adams several strategies to promote sleep. The nurse determines that Mrs. Adams has *incorrectly* learned the strategies when Mrs. Adams states that she will
- ○1. drink hot chocolate before going to bed.
- ○2. ask her husband to give her a soothing backrub.
- ○3. place pillows at her back and between her legs.
- ○4. practice deep-breathing exercises before she goes to sleep.

**37.** Which of the following feelings would the nurse expect that Mrs. Adams would be *least likely* to experience during the third trimester?
- ○1. Fear of possible miscarriage.
- ○2. Vulnerability to loss, rejection, or insult.
- ○3. Anxiety, tension, or sense of worry about a variety of things.
- ○4. Hesitation to go out unless someone who cares about her accompanies her.

**38.** Which of the following questions asked by Mr. Adams would *not* be a common concern of expectant fathers during the third trimester?
- ○1. "Should I look for a new job?"
- ○2. "Can we afford to have a baby?"
- ○3. "What kind of parents will we be?"
- ○4. "Will I really be able to help Mary in labor?"

**39.** Late in her pregnancy, Mrs. Adams tells the nurse that she is voiding frequently. While assessing Mrs. Adams because of her frequency, the nurse questions her concerning symptoms of pyuria, hematuria, and dysuria. When Mrs. Adams reports no symptoms, the nurse's *next* course of action in this situation should be to
- ○1. weigh the patient.
- ○2. assess the patient for lightening.
- ○3. obtain a urine specimen from the patient.
- ○4. ask the patient if she is aware of fetal movements.

*quickening 16 - 18 weeks*

# THE PREGNANT PATIENT IN CHILDBIRTH PREPARATION CLASS

Sara and Paul Buxkemper are pregnant for the first time. They voice interest in the childbirth preparation classes being offered in the community. They have the support of their physician for a family-centered birth experience.

**40.** At what time during Mrs. Buxkemper's pregnancy should the nurse advise the Buxkempers to begin the childbirth preparation classes?
- ○ 1. As soon as Mrs. Buxkemper experiences quickening.
- ○ 2. After the Buxkempers have read pamphlets on the anatomy and physiology of reproduction that the nurse gives them.
- ○ 3. As soon as possible so that the Buxkempers have sufficient time to learn techniques used during labor and delivery.
- ○ 4. In the late second trimester or early third trimester, by which time the Buxkempers can be expected to be anticipating birth with eagerness.

**41.** The nurse who is teaching the childbirth preparation class explains the purpose of the classes. She *correctly* explains that the *primary* focus of the classes will be on the physiology of labor and delivery, and the preparation for coping with
- ○ 1. discomfort.
- ○ 2. parenthood.
- ○ 3. sibling rivalry.
- ○ 4. sleep deprivation.

**42.** The nurse who teaches the classes explains the sequence of maneuvers the fetus goes through during labor and delivery. When the head presents, the *normal* sequence of maneuvers is
- ○ 1. engagement, external rotation, flexion, and expulsion.
- ○ 2. descent, flexion, external rotation, internal rotation, and extension.
- ○ 3. descent, flexion, internal rotation, extension, and external rotation.
- ○ 4. internal rotation, descent, engagement, expulsion, and external rotation.

**43.** In response to a question about preparation for breast-feeding, the nurse recommends that the mother prepare her nipples during pregnancy by
- ○ 1. wearing a supportive but loose-fitting bra.
- ○ 2. tugging and rolling the nipples between the thumb and forefinger.

- ○ 3. rubbing the nipples with a terrycloth towel when drying them after bathing.
- ○ 4. patting the nipples once a day with a gauze sponge moistened with alcohol.

**44.** As the nurse evaluates all the causes of pain during labor, she *correctly* decides to teach the members of the childbirth preparation class that the *primary* cause of pain during the first stage of labor is due to
- ○ 1. hypoxia of the myometrium.
- ○ 2. cultural response to pain.
- ○ 3. pressure on pelvic structures.
- ○ 4. dilatation and effacement of the cervix.

**45.** In evaluating class member response to the teaching of techniques for coping with discomfort during labor, the nurse determines that Mrs. Buxkemper has *correctly* understood the techniques for coping when she indicates that she has been practicing *all* of the following methods *except*
- ○ 1. effleurage.
- ○ 2. progressive relaxation.
- ○ 3. various chest breathing patterns.
- ○ 4. rapid, deep breathing techniques.

**46.** Mrs. Buxkemper asks the nurse teaching the classes how much blood she is likely to lose during delivery. The nurse's response is based on the knowledge that the *maximum* blood loss considered to be within *normal* limits during delivery and the first few hours after delivery is approximately
- ○ 1. 100 ml.
- ○ 2. 300 ml.
- ○ 3. 500 ml.
- ○ 4. 700 ml.

**47.** The Buxkempers have questions about the amniotic fluid and sac. The nurse teaches *correctly* that they serve *all* the following functions *except*
- ○ 1. helping to dilate the cervix.
- ○ 2. protecting the fetus from injury.
- ○ 3. providing the fetus with immune bodies.
- ○ 4. keeping the fetus at an even temperature.

**48.** The nurse explains *correctly* to the Buxkempers when she teaches that the umbilical cord contains blood vessels, the total number *normally* being
- ○ 1. one vein and one artery.
- ○ 2. two veins and one artery.
- ○ 3. one vein and two arteries.
- ○ 4. two veins and two arteries.

**49.** The nurse teaches that the infant's source of oxygen before birth is through the umbilical cord. The fetal blood vessel in which the oxygen content is *highest* is the

○ 1. aorta.
○ 2. umbilical vein.
○ 3. pulmonary artery.
○ 4. inferior vena cava.

50. Mrs. Buxkemper asks what she can do for back-aches. Which of the following exercises should the nurse teach Mrs. Buxkemper as *most helpful* to relieve backaches during pregnancy?
    ○ 1. Sit-ups.
    ○ 2. Leg lifts.
    ○ 3. Knee bends.
    ○ 4. Pelvic rock.

51. Mrs. Buxkemper asks the nurse what she can do about the varicose veins in her legs. The type of clothing Mrs. Buxkemper should be taught to *avoid* because of her varicosities is
    ○ 1. sandal-type shoes.
    ○ 2. knee-length hosiery.
    ○ 3. a two-way stretch girdle.
    ○ 4. slacks with an elasticized waist.

52. Because of the varicosities in Mrs. Buxkemper's legs, the nurse teaches her to lie down with her feet elevated and a pillow under one hip (to avoid compression of the vena cava) several times a day. The purpose of this procedure is to help
    ○ 1. strengthen the valves in the veins.
    ○ 2. increase the muscle tone of the legs.
    ○ 3. facilitate drainage from the extremities.
    ○ 4. decrease the supply of blood through the arteries.

53. The nurse teaches the expectant mothers in the class to alternately contract and relax the peri-neum (pubococcygeal muscle) several times a day. The *primary* purpose of Kegel exercises is that they help
    ○ 1. prevent vulvar varicosities.
    ○ 2. relieve lower back discomfort.
    ○ 3. strengthen the perineal muscles.
    ○ 4. strengthen the abdominal muscles.

## THE PRECONCEPTION PATIENT

Ms. Sandy Cox, 20, visits a birth-control clinic. She and her boyfriend are planning their wedding and want to plan the spacing of their children. Ms. Cox asks about conception and contraception.

54. The nurse discusses fertilization. Ms. Cox asks, "How long does it take for sperm to reach an ovum?" The nurse's response should be guided by knowledge that, when an ideal situation exists, the *shortest* time it takes for sperm to reach the ovum is approximately
    ○ 1. 1 to 5 minutes.
    ○ 2. 15 to 20 minutes.
    ○ 3. 30 to 35 minutes.
    ○ 4. 60 to 65 minutes.

55. Ms. Cox asks, "Why do people who use natural methods to prevent pregnancy have such a high failure rate?" The nurse should explain that natural methods depend on knowing when ovulation occurs, which is not always easy to determine. Another reason why the actual length of time that fertilization can occur varies and can last as long as 15 days or more is that
    ○ 1. ova are capable of fertilization for up to 24 hours.
    ○ 2. sperm and ova can unite to fertilize with remarkable ease.
    ○ 3. large numbers of ova are discharged from the ovaries occasionally.
    ○ 4. thousands of sperm are deposited in the vagina with each ejaculation.

56. The nurse teaches Ms. Cox that the time during the menstrual cycle when most women ovulate is
    ○ 1. during the menstrual period.
    ○ 2. shortly before the menstrual period.
    ○ 3. about one week following the menstrual period.
    ○ 4. approximately two weeks before the beginning of the menstrual period.

57. Ms. Cox asks how oral contraceptives ("the pill") work. The nurse's response should be based on knowledge that biological preparations used as oral contraceptives prevent pregnancy by
    ○ 1. destroying ova.
    ○ 2. destroying sperm.
    ○ 3. inhibiting ovulation.
    ○ 4. preventing implantation.

58. The nurse assesses Ms. Cox to determine whether she is a candidate for oral contraceptives. If Ms. Cox indicates she has experienced any of the following conditions in the past, the one that would preclude her from using oral contraceptives would be
    ○ 1. dysmenorrhea.
    ○ 2. irregular menses.
    ○ 3. thrombophlebitis.
    ○ 4. pulmonary tuberculosis.

59. If Ms. Cox chooses to use an oral contraceptive and forgets to take her pill one day, she should be instructed to
    ○ 1. wait until menstruation occurs and then start the next series of pills.
    ○ 2. take two pills as soon as she remembers that she missed taking the one pill.

○3. take it as soon as she remembers and take the next pill at the regular time.

○4. take the next pill at the regular time without compensating for the missed pill.

60. Ms. Cox says that her husband-to-be objects to using "rubbers" (condoms). The *major* complaint for using condoms for contraception is that they
○1. irritate the penis.
○2. tear relatively easily.
○3. disrupt the sexual act.
○4. predispose to vaginal infections.

61. Ms. Cox asks, "What do men do if they wish to be sterilized?" The nurse should respond that a commonly used procedure involves clamping or cutting the
○1. epididymis.
○2. seminal vesicles.
○3. ejaculatory duct.
○4. ductus deferens (vas deferens).

62. Ms. Cox asks about douching as a contraceptive method. The nurse should teach her that, as a contraceptive method, a vaginal douche is
○1. unreliable.
○2. satisfactory when a spermicidal solution is used for the douche.
○3. moderately reliable provided the douche is used in conjunction with a spermicidal agent.
○4. fairly reliable provided the douche is used as soon after intercourse as possible, within a minute or two.

63. Ms. Cox inquires about using a diaphragm for contraception. Ms. Cox should be taught that the recommended *minimum* length of time to wait after intercourse before removing the diaphragm is
○1. 1 hour.
○2. 6 hours.
○3. 12 hours.
○4. 24 hours.

64. Ms. Cox is taught the relationship between basal temperatures and fertility. When should a woman who is obtaining her basal temperatures take her temperature?
○1. Every evening before retiring.
○2. Every morning before breakfast.
○3. Every afternoon between three and four o'clock.
○4. Every morning upon awakening and before arising.

65. Ms. Cox and the nurse discuss various sexual myths. Which of the following statements describes a *fact*, rather than a myth, concerning sexuality?
○1. Alcohol acts as a depressant for sex.

○2. Sexual intercourse should be avoided during menstruation.
○3. Masturbation is a sexual dysfunction when used by married persons.
○4. Having an orgasm is a necessary part of a satisfactory sexual experience.

66. The nurse discusses sexual arousal and orgasm with Ms. Cox. The nurse asks Ms. Cox which *primary* anatomic structure in the female is involved in sexual arousal and orgasm. The nurse's teaching will be considered effective if Ms. Cox's answer is the
○1. vagina.
○2. clitoris.
○3. mons pubis.
○4. labia minora.

67. Ms. Cox asks the nurse, "If the time is right for sex, why is foreplay important?" The nurse should base her response on the knowledge that, in addition to arousing the sexual urge, foreplay helps to
○1. relax the vaginal orifice.
○2. increase vaginal secretions.
○3. delay premature clitoral orgasm.
○4. prevent early ejaculation in the male.

68. If Ms. Cox has understood the nurse's discussion of sexual response in the male, Ms. Cox will *correctly* respond that the *primary* anatomic structure in the male involved in sexual arousal and orgasm is the
○1. penis.
○2. testes.
○3. scrotum.
○4. epidiymides.

69. As Ms. Cox is repeating in her own words the knowledge she has gained from the discussion of the sexual response cycle, as described by Masters and Johnson, Ms. Cox will *correctly* include *all* of the following as phases of the sexual response cycle *except* the
○1. nascent phase.
○2. plateau phase.
○3. orgasmic phase.
○4. resolution phase.

70. Ms. Cox asks several questions about becoming pregnant. She says, "How do sperm ever manage to reach the ovum?" The nurse is *correct* when she explains that sperm are propelled in the female primarily by
○1. cilia in the female reproductive tract.
○2. movements of the sperm's tail-like portion.
○3. peristalsis-like contractions in the cervix and uterus.
○4. gravity and the force generated by the process of ejaculation.

71. After learning about fertilization, Ms. Cox asks where it occurs in the body. The nurse responds *correctly* when she explains that the anatomic structure in which fertilization of the ovum *normally* occurs is the
    - ○ 1. ovary.
    - ○ 2. uterus.
    - ○ 3. corpus luteum.
    - ○ 4. fallopian tube.

72. The nurse teaches Ms. Cox that the fertilized ovum implants itself in the uterus. Approximately how many days after conception does the fertilized ovum *normally* implant in the uterine wall?
    - ○ 1. 3 days.
    - ○ 2. 7 days.
    - ○ 3. 11 days.
    - ○ 4. 15 days.

73. In describing the pelvic area changes that occur with pregnancy, the nurse tells Ms. Cox that the uterus receives its blood supply directly from the uterine artery and from the
    - ○ 1. iliac artery.
    - ○ 2. ovarian artery.
    - ○ 3. hypogastric artery.
    - ○ 4. uterosacral artery.

74. The nurse describes the development of the placenta. The nurse teaches *correctly* that the placenta is formed by the fusion of chorionic villi and the
    - ○ 1. decidua vera.
    - ○ 2. chorion laeve.
    - ○ 3. decidua basalis.
    - ○ 4. chorion frondosum.

75. Ms. Cox asks what the placenta does during pregnancy. The nurse explains the specific functions that the placenta performs for the embryo/fetus during pregnancy. The nurse *correctly* determines that Ms. Cox has understood the discussion of placental functions when Ms. Cox identifies the organ that *least likely* performs functions similar to those of the placenta as the
    - ○ 1. brain.
    - ○ 2. lungs.
    - ○ 3. kidney.
    - ○ 4. stomach.

76. The nurse also teaches Ms. Cox that the placenta produces *all* the following hormones *except*
    - ○ 1. aldosterone.
    - ○ 2. progesterone.
    - ○ 3. human placental lactogen.
    - ○ 4. human chorionic gonadotropin.

77. The nurse explains that one of the following hormones stimulates ovulation and the development of the corpus luteum. Which is the correct hormone?
    - ○ 1. Estrogenic hormone (EH).
    - ○ 2. Luteinizing hormone (LH).
    - ○ 3. Adrenocorticotropic hormone (ACTH).
    - ○ 4. Follicle-stimulating hormone (FSH).

78. Ms. Cox says that her sister-in-law is unable to become pregnant. Which of the following conditions will result in a woman's being unable to conceive?
    - ○ 1. Absence of an ovary.
    - ○ 2. A dilated hymenal ring.
    - ○ 3. Occluded fallopian tubes.
    - ○ 4. An obstructed Bartholin's gland duct.

79. Ms. Cox says a friend of hers failed to become pregnant and artificial insemination by her husband was not advised. She asks why this could not be done. The nurse should recognize that artificial insemination is *contraindicated* when the male has
    - ○ 1. hypospadias.
    - ○ 2. undescended testicles.
    - ○ 3. premature ejaculations.
    - ○ 4. difficulty maintaining an erection.

80. It is generally agreed that before beginning to counsel Ms. Cox about sexuality, it is *best* for the nurse *first* to
    - ○ 1. obtain a sexual history from the patient.
    - ○ 2. have the patient undergo a complete physical examination.
    - ○ 3. suggest that the patient's sexual partner attend the counseling sessions.
    - ○ 4. discuss the normal anatomy and physiology of the reproductive system with the patient.

81. Authorities recommend that the nurse can *best* prepare to counsel Ms. Cox concerning sexuality when the nurse *first* has
    - ○ 1. had personal experience with a sexual relationship.
    - ○ 2. reviewed the literature on the subject of human sexuality.
    - ○ 3. worked to understand her own personal attitudes concerning human sexuality.
    - ○ 4. completed an educational program for preparation as a clinical specialist in sexual counseling.

82. About a year later, Ms. Cox-Davis returns to the clinic for a pregnancy test. The hormone used for this test is
    - ○ 1. estrogen hormone.
    - ○ 2. luteinizing hormone.
    - ○ 3. follicle-stimulating hormone.
    - ○ 4. human chorionic gonadotropin hormone.

83. While Ms. Cox-Davis is waiting for the results of her pregnancy test, she asks the nurse several questions concerning pregnancy. She asks the

nurse if it is true that the *primary* cause of maternal deaths in this country is
○ 1. hemorrhage.
○ 2. puerperal infections.
○ 3. hypertensive disorders.
○ 4. hematologic disorders.

**84.** The nurse explains to Ms. Cox-Davis that the infant mortality rate is defined as the number of deaths in infants under
○ 1. 1 year of age per 1,000 live births.
○ 2. 1 month of age per 1,000 live births.
○ 3. 1 year of age per 100,000 live births.
○ 4. 1 month of age per 100,000 live births.

**85.** The nurse tells Ms. Cox-Davis that of the following factors, the *greatest* single factor for decreasing maternal deaths during the past three decades is *most often* credited to
○ 1. improved prenatal care.
○ 2. fetal monitoring during labor.
○ 3. the use of analgesia during delivery.
○ 4. medical supervision of care during the puerperium.

**86.** Ms. Cox-Davis asks the nurse how the sex of the infant is determined. The nurse should base her response on knowledge that the chromosome combination that must exist to produce a male infant is
○ 1. XX.
○ 2. XY.
○ 3. XYY.
○ 4. XXY.

## THE PATIENT WITH A SPONTANEOUS ABORTION

Julie Eagle is admitted to the hospital when she is 12 weeks gestation. She has abdominal cramping and bright-red vaginal spotting. Her cervix is not dilated.

**87.** The type of abortion Ms. Eagle is *most probably* experiencing is called
○ 1. a missed abortion.
○ 2. a threatened abortion.
○ 3. an inevitable abortion.
○ 4. an incomplete abortion.

**88.** Ms. Eagle is discharged when her symptoms subside, although she is still having slight vaginal spotting occasionally. Of *special* importance is that Ms. Eagle be instructed to
○ 1. weigh herself daily.
○ 2. follow a salt-free diet temporarily.

○ 3. save her perineal pads for inspection.
○ 4. have intercourse no more often than once a week.

**89.** Ms. Eagle returns to the hospital for a dilatation and curettage (D&C) when it is determined that she has passed some of the products of conception. At this time, Ms. Eagle is *most probably* experiencing which of the following types of abortion?
○ 1. Missed.
○ 2. Induced.
○ 3. Threatened.
○ 4. Incomplete.

**90.** While Ms. Eagle is being prepared for the D&C, she is given butorphanol tartrate (Stadol), *primarily* to
○ 1. prevent nausea.
○ 2. reduce discomfort.
○ 3. control hemorrhage.
○ 4. promote uterine relaxation.

**91.** Postoperatively, the nurse finds Ms. Eagle crying. Which of the following comments would be *best* for the nurse to make in this situation?
○ 1. "Why are you crying?"
○ 2. "Will a pill help your pain?"
○ 3. "I am sorry you lost your baby."
○ 4. "A baby still was not formed in your uterus."

**92.** In evaluating Ms. Eagle's reaction to the loss of her pregnancy, the nurse would observe Ms. Eagle for expected feelings and perceptions. Which of the following is *least likely* to be considered an expected response to a spontaneous abortion?
○ 1. Guilt.
○ 2. Denial.
○ 3. Euphoria.
○ 4. Alienation.

**93.** Following her assessment of Ms. Eagle, the nurse suggests that Ms. Eagle receive pentazocine hydrochloride (Talwin) *primarily* to
○ 1. inhibit lactation.
○ 2. aid uterine involution.
○ 3. relieve abdominal discomfort.
○ 4. prevent conception for about 6 weeks.

**94.** Ms. Eagle is Rh negative and her husband is Rh positive. Since analysis of her blood indicates that she is unsensitized, she receives human anti-D globulin (RhoGam) before her discharge from the hospital. The purpose of administering RhoGam to Ms. Eagle is to help prevent her from
○ 1. becoming Rh positive.
○ 2. developing Rh sensitivity.
○ 3. developing AB antigens in her blood.
○ 4. becoming pregnant with an Rh-positive fetus.

# CORRECT ANSWERS AND RATIONALES

Numbers appear in parentheses following the rationales. The numbers identify textbooks listed in the references at the end of Part II, where correct answers can be verified.

## The Pregnant Patient Receiving Prenatal Care

**1.** 2. When using Naegele's rule, count back three calendar months from the first day of the last menstrual period. That would be April 13 for the patient described in this item. Then add seven days and one year, which would be April 20 of the following year for this patient. (7)

**2.** 3. When the patient described in this item expresses fear of the examination she is about to have, it is best for the nurse to say something that allows the patient an opportunity to describe her feelings. The nurse can then determine what nursing measure to use to help the patient. It is of no help to a fearful patient when the nurse describes her own role to the patient and when she says nearly all patients have some fears. Telling the patient the examination will not take long or that she will be draped for privacy ignores her fears. (7, 9)

**3.** 1. Having the patient bear down for speculum insertion helps relax the perineum at that time. Techniques of relaxation, such as taking slow chest breaths, are often used during labor and are also useful when a patient feels tense during a pelvic examination. Grasping the nurse's hand could result in more tension. Trying to distract the patient with conversation during an examination is likely to be annoying and therefore is a poor way to help a patient relax. (7)

**4.** 1. By the time a pregnancy has reached its 10th week, the uterus has enlarged to about twice its normal size. Chadwick's sign, which is the bluish coloring of the vaginal mucosa, is noted as early as the 6th week of pregnancy. Hegar's sign, which is a softening of the lower uterine segment, may be noted at 6 to 8 weeks of pregnancy. Fetal movements cannot be palpated until about 18 to 20 weeks of pregnancy. (7, 1)

**5.** 2. The couple described in this item are expressing a *feeling* about having a baby. The nurse is responding to their feeling when she explains that such feelings are normal and experienced by many couples early in pregnancy. Studies have shown that a common reaction to pregnancy is summa-

rized as "someday, but not now." Fathers as well as mothers go through a phase of having to come to terms with the realization of pregnancy when it is confirmed. The physician's confirmation of the pregnancy is something the couple already knows. Offering the couple a pamphlet on pregnancy does not respond to the couple's feelings. There is no indication that the couple described in this item is in need of psychological counseling. (1)

**6.** 1. When the pregnancy is confirmed, the initial reaction is surprise at the reality of conception, regardless of whether the pregnancy was planned or unplanned. Expressions of surprise and wrong timing reflect the predominant feeling of ambivalence common during the first trimester. Acceptance of pregnancy is one of the developmental tasks of pregnancy. Rejection of the pregnancy, especially early in pregnancy, may result in a decision to terminate the pregnancy. (7)

**7.** 2. The only evidence of pregnancy the expectant mother has during the first trimester is amenorrhea and confirmation by the health professional. Thus, she watches her body carefully for evidence of "pregnancy" changes such as waist enlargement, breast development, and weight gain. (7)

**8.** 3. Expectant fathers who experience *mitleiden* ("suffering along") during the first trimester may develop symptoms similar to those of the expectant mother (*i.e.*, nausea, weight gain, and various aches and pains). The sharing of common symptoms may be a means of identifying with the pregnancy for the father. The expectant father will not be able to observe fetal movement until the second trimester. (7)

**9.** 3. During the first trimester, the expectant father commonly feels left out of the pregnancy. He may be confused by the mood swings the expectant mother is experiencing; he may resent the attention given to the expectant mother and the changes in their relationship necessitated by maternal fatigue, and he begins to worry about the expense of having a baby. (7)

**10.** 3. Eating a dry carbohydrate food, such as crackers or toast, before arising from bed in the morning often relieves the early-morning nausea and vomiting that many pregnant women experience. Foods high in fat content and fluids tend to exacerbate the condition for many women. (7)

**11.** 2. It is generally agreed that couples need not change their patterns of sexual activity during pregnancy unless complications arise. Some women find intercourse uncomfortable during late pregnancy, but this discomfort can usually be overcome by using lateral positions, rather than the face-to-face man-on-top position. (7)

**12.** 2. It has not been determined how much alcohol may be consumed during pregnancy without harming the fetus. Therefore, it is recommended that pregnant women should be taught that it is best to abstain from drinking alcoholic beverages during pregnancy. The fear is that alcohol consumed during pregnancy *may* cause birth defects. (7)

**13.** 4. Weight gain during pregnancy varies considerably among pregnant women, but it has been found that a gain of between about 25 and 30 pounds (11 kg and 13.6 kg) is normal and common. The *pattern* of weight gain appears more important than the total amount of weight gained. There is little weight gain during the first trimester of pregnancy, a rapid increase in weight during the second trimester, and a rate that slows somewhat during the third trimester. The normal weight curve during pregnancy is sigmoid. (7)

**14.** 1. Rich sources of protein include meat, fish, poultry, beans, nuts, milk, eggs, cheese, and wheat germ. Such foods as mushrooms, melons, spinach, turnip greens, citrus fruits, and tomatoes are poor sources of protein but good sources of other nutrients. (7)

**15.** 4. Absorption of supplemental iron and nonmeat sources of iron is enhanced by combining them with meat or a good source of vitamin C. The pregnant woman should be taught to take the iron tablets with meals to decrease adverse gastrointestinal symptoms. (7)

**16.** 1. Foods rich in iron content include almost all flesh foods, including shellfish, as well as green vegetables. Eggs also are rich in iron. Poor sources of iron include carrots, tomatoes, bananas, figs, cottage cheese, and yogurt. Milk and milk products are poor sources of iron. (7)

**17.** 4. Green leafy vegetables, such as asparagus, spinach, Brussels sprouts, and broccoli, are rich sources of folic acid. It is important for a well-balanced diet to include whole grains, dairy products, and fresh fruits; however, these foods are rich sources of other nutrients. (7)

**18.** 3. In conjunction with Naegele's rule, the date of quickening is used to help determine the estimated date of delivery. Using the date when quickening is first noted is not an entirely accurate way to estimate the date of delivery, but it is judged that it occurs when the mother is approximately 20 weeks pregnant. (7)

**19.** 1. The highlight of the second trimester for the expectant mother is feeling fetal movement. Quick-

ening provides evidence that her baby is a real person. Perceiving the baby as a person usually increases excitement about the pregnancy, as evidenced by her wearing maternity clothes and making purchases for the nursery. (7)

**20.** 3. The father's involvement in the pregnancy can be facilitated during the second trimester by watching and feeling fetal movements and by hearing the fetal heart beat. Developing new time-consuming interests outside the home may be an indication that the father is not coping positively with the changes precipitated by the pregnancy. (7)

**21.** 1. There is normally an increased vaginal discharge during pregnancy, but local itching is associated with infections, such as those due to *Trichomonas vaginalis* or *Candida albicans*. The best advice to give the patient described in this item is that she should discuss the discharge with a physician. It may be serious and require treatment. Douches are not often prescribed during pregnancy. Intercourse may be contraindicated, depending on the cause of the discharge and the discomfort associated with it. (7)

**22.** 4. The discoloration on the face that often appears during pregnancy is called *chloasma*. It usually disappears after delivery and is without clinical significance. The patient bothered by the appearance of the pigment change may be able to decrease its prominence with the proper use of make-up. No treatment is recommended for chloasma. (7)

**23.** 1. The patient should empty her bladder before the nurse palpates the abdomen while using Leopold maneuvers. This increases the patient's comfort and makes palpation a more accurate procedure. (7)

**24.** 4. Leopold maneuvers are used to determine the position of the fetus in the uterus. After the back of the fetus is located, it becomes easier to assess fetal heart tones, which can best be heard through the fetal back. (7)

**25.** 1. The most common reason for a pregnant woman to feel dizzy, become pale, and perspire freely when she lies in the supine position is that there is pressure on the vena cava. The condition is often referred to as supine hypotension. It is alleviated when the patient turns onto either side. (7)

**26.** 3. The enlarging uterus places pressure on blood vessels carrying blood to and from the lower part of the body, especially the extremities, and predisposes to varicosities. The prevention and management of varicosities include abandoning anything that places constriction on the legs or thighs, such as round garters; lying on the back with the legs extended straight up in the air while resting them against a wall several times a day; and wearing elastic stockings or bandages. (7)

**27.** 3. With the use of a stethoscope, fetal heart tones may be heard after a woman has been pregnant about 17 to 20 weeks. They may be heard as early as the 10th week of pregnancy with a doppler. (7)

**28.** 2. Various measures are helpful in relieving constipation, such as drinking a glass of hot water in the morning, increasing roughage and fluid in the diet, and exercising regularly. It is best not to suggest laxatives or suppositories because the patient may become dependent on them. The patient should use them only when diet, fluid intake, and exercise do not control the problem, and after consulting the nurse again. (7)

**29.** 1. Various measures are helpful in relieving the discomfort of hemorrhoids, such as lying down while the hips are elevated on a pillow, taking sitz baths, and applying witch-hazel compresses to the anal area. Having the woman position herself with the hips elevated facilitates the movement of blood from engorged veins in the rectum toward the central circulation. Tailor sitting and pelvic tilts are most often used to relieve lower backaches. Leg lifts help improve circulation and muscle tone in the legs. (1)

**30.** 3. Traveling by automobile is not contraindicated during pregnancy unless the woman develops complications; in that case, decisions should be made on an individual basis. However, the woman should be advised to take intermittent rest periods of 10 to 15 minutes every 2 hours while traveling and walk about in order to stimulate circulation, which becomes sluggish during long periods of sitting. (7)

**31.** 3. It has been found that pushing up on the toes and down on the knees is an effective measure to relieve leg cramps. Keeping the legs warm and elevating them as much as possible are good preventive measures. (7)

**32.** 4. Large amounts of milk or dicalcium phosphate tend to bring on leg cramps. Cramps are believed to be due to excessive phosphorus absorption. Adding a small amount of aluminum hydroxide gel to milk is suggested because it removes some phosphorus from the intestinal tract so that it is not absorbed in excessive quantities. (7)

**33.** 4. Sodium bicarbonate (baking soda) should be avoided during pregnancy because of the potential for electrolyte imbalance. The patient should be taught to avoid eating fatty foods, and to eat smaller, more frequent meals. Other helpful measures include an adequate fluid intake, wearing loose clothing around the waist, taking small sips of water, milk, or a carbonated beverage, remaining in a sitting position (lying down increases heartburn), and trying to remain relaxed. (1, 7)

**34.** 4. Frequent dorsiflexion of the feet facilitates circulatory fluid return in the lower extremities by stimulating muscle contraction. Other strategies that avoid an increase in ankle edema include avoiding standing or sitting for long periods; avoiding restrictive bands around the legs; and resting with the legs and hips elevated several times a day. (7)

**35.** 4. Round-ligament pain is often intense and is described as a "grabbing" sensation. After it is determined that the pain is not due to a medical complication, using heat or warmth may be suggested to reduce the discomfort. Explaining to the expectant mother the cause of the discomfort usually relieves her anxiety. (7)

**36.** 1. The expectant mother should avoid caffeine products and stimulating activities. A warm, caffeine-free beverage, a soothing backrub, extra pillows to support a side-lying position, and relaxation techniques usually benefit the expectant mother who is experiencing difficulty sleeping. (7)

**37.** 1. The fear of miscarriage is a primary concern of the first trimester for the expectant mother. Third-trimester concerns are those related to increased vulnerability, anxiety and tension about a variety of situations and events, and intensified need for security. (7)

**38.** 1. The concern about financial capabilities is intensified in the third trimester and the expectant father asks whether or not he and his partner can afford a baby and whether or not his job is stable. However, it is not common for the father to ask about finding a new job. Other concerns that resurface during the third trimester are questions about what kind of parents the partners will be and whether or not the father will be able to help his partner during labor. (7)

**39.** 2. Most patients pregnant for the first time and many who have been pregnant before experience lightening 1 or 2 weeks before delivery. This means the fetus descends into the pelvis. The mother can breathe better when this occurs because there is less pressure on the chest cavity. However, the patient often experiences frequency of urination because the head of the fetus compresses the bladder. If the patient has no symptoms of pyuria, hematuria, or dysuria, frequency is most probably caused by lightening, and the patient should be assessed for signs of lightening. Leopold maneuvers often help determine whether the fetus has descended into the pelvis. (7)

## *The Pregnant Patient in Childbirth Preparation Classes*

**40.** 4. Toward the end of pregnancy, especially the third trimester, couples are usually psychologically ready for the termination of the pregnancy and are very receptive to preparation for classes dealing with labor and delivery. The couple should have grown in their relationship by this time and be ready to prepare for the coming birth. (7)

**41.** 1. The primary focus of classes that prepare expectant parents for childbirth is the physiology of childbirth and the techniques and aids that facilitate coping with the discomfort of childbirth. Prenatal education programs often include a variety of classes, each with specific goals. Early pregnancy classes focus on changes, discomforts, danger signs, and nutritional needs during pregnancy. Sibling classes focus on preparation of siblings for attending the birth and acceptance of the newborn. Postpartum classes focus on changes expected during the fourth trimester and preparation for parenthood. (7)

**42.** 3. In order, the maneuvers occurring during labor and delivery when the head of the fetus presents are descent, flexion, internal rotation, extension, and external rotation. These maneuvers occur as the head passes through the mother's bony pelvis. (7)

**43.** 2. Opinions differ on the best preparation of nipples for breast-feeding. Tugging and rolling the nipples between the thumb and forefinger is thought to be beneficial in distributing natural lubrication from Montgomery's tubercles, stimulating blood flow to the breast, and developing a protective layer of skin over the nipples (all goals of nipple preparation). Recommendations that the nipples be rubbed gently with a rough towel, such as a terrycloth towel, when being dried after bathing to help toughen them, remove protective lubrication and should be avoided. Such agents as alcohol are believed to predispose to cracked nipples because they may remove normal oils on the nipples. Some authorities recommend massaging the nipples with a cream. (7)

**44.** 4. The primary source of pain in the first stage of labor is the stretching and dilating of the cervix. Perception of pain determined by cultural patterning affects the discomfort of labor. During the sec-

ond stage of labor, discomfort is caused by myometrial cell hypoxia, distention of the vagina and perineum, and pressure on the adjacent structures. (7)

**45.** 4. Hyperventilation results in maternal respiratory alkalosis, with the consequence of reduced placental oxygen exchange for the fetus. Thus, rapid breathing in labor is no longer advocated. Techniques that decrease discomfort during labor are progressive relaxation, effleurage (except during the transition phase of labor), and a variety of chest-breathing patterns. (7)

**46.** 3. In a normal delivery and the first 24 hours after delivery, a total blood loss not exceeding approximately 500 ml is generally considered normal. (7)

**47.** 3. Amniotic fluid does not provide the fetus with immune bodies but it does help dilate the cervix, protect the fetus from injury, and keep the fetus at an even temperature. (7)

**48.** 3. The umbilical cord normally consists of two arteries and one vein. Oxygen and other nutrients are carried to the fetal circulation by the one umbilical vein. The oxygen-poor blood is pumped back to the placenta by the fetal heart through two umbilical arteries. A single umbilical artery is sometimes associated with congenital anomalies. (7)

**49.** 2. Oxygenated blood flows through the umbilical vein to the fetus; blood leaving the fetus to return to the placenta travels through the umbilical arteries. (7)

**50.** 4. The pelvic rock, or pelvic tilt, which seems to help strengthen back muscles, has been found to help many women who have backaches during pregnancy. The exercise is done as follows: while standing with hands on hips, alternately "tuck" the buttocks under and then relax. The exercise may be done standing, sitting, lying, or on hands and knees. (7)

**51.** 2. The patient with varicosities should be taught to avoid wearing knee-length hosiery because it inhibits circulatory functioning in the legs. There is no reason for a patient with varicosities in the legs to avoid wearing sandal-type shoes, a stretch girdle, and slacks with an elasticized waist. (7)

**52.** 3. Elevating the legs enhances venous return from the legs and decreases venous stasis to relieve varicosities. This positioning does not strengthen vessel valves, increase muscle tone, or decrease the supply of blood through the arteries. (7)

**53.** 3. Alternately contracting and relaxing the perineum (that is, the pubococcygeal muscle) is frequently referred to as Kegel exercises. They help strengthen the perineal muscles, tone the vagina, prevent hemorrhoids, and control stress incontinence. (7)

## The Preconception Patient

**54.** 1. It takes only 1 to 5 minutes for sperm to reach the ovum under ideal conditions. This is an important point to make with a person seeking help in relation to contraception. Many people believe that the time interval is much longer and that they can take steps to prevent conception after intercourse, which is usually too late. (7)

**55.** 1. Determining the exact length of fertility in the female each month is difficult, partly because ova can be fertilized for about 24 hours after ovulation. Since ovulation is difficult to detect, the couple may need to abstain from sexual intercourse for several consecutive days. The beginning of the period during which fertilization can occur is determined by subtracting 18 days from the length of the shortest cycle recorded in a 6-month period; the end of the period is determined by subtracting 11 days from the end of the longest recorded cycle. Sperm and ova do unite easily, but this does not increase the difficulty of determining fertility; nor does the fact that large numbers of sperm are deposited in the vagina with each ejaculation. Typically, one ovum is discharged each month. Occasionally, two may be discharged, and if both are fertilized the mother will have twins. (7)

**56.** 4. Ovulation occurs approximately 2 weeks before menstruation begins. Stated another way, menstruation occurs approximately 2 weeks after ovulation. (7)

**57.** 3. Oral contraceptives consist most commonly of estrogen and a synthetic progestational agent. They inhibit ovulation by suppressing follicle-stimulating hormone (FSH) and luteinizing hormone (LH). No ova are discharged from the ovaries when ovulation is inhibited, and therefore conception cannot occur. (7)

**58.** 3. It is recommended that women with a history of thrombophlebitis, embolic diseases, liver impairment, cardiovascular accident, and malignancies of the reproductive system, including the breasts, not use oral contraceptives. Most authorities also recommend that women with hypertension, migraine headaches, diabetes mellitus, gall bladder disease, sickle-cell anemia, cystic breast disease, and vaginal bleeding of unknown causes not use oral contraceptives. Women who are not yet 4 weeks postpartum, those who have recently aborted, and

those over 35 years of age are not generally advised to use oral contraceptives. (7)

**59.** 3. When a woman forgets to take a contraceptive pill, it is recommended that she take it as soon as she remembers and to take the next pill at the regular time. (7)

**60.** 3. A common complaint about using condoms is that applying them disrupts the sexual act. They break relatively infrequently when properly used, they are not reported to irritate the penis (although lubrication may be needed to reduce vaginal irritation), and they do not predispose to vaginal infection. (7)

**61.** 4. A relatively common surgical procedure for male sterilization is a vasectomy, in which the ductus deferens (vas deferens) is cut or clamped. (7)

**62.** 1. Vaginal douching is an unreliable method of contraception. Because sperm enter the cervix within seconds after ejaculation, the douche is highly unlikely to be used in time and may even facilitate conception by pushing sperm farther up the birth canal. Spermicidal agents are minimally effective when used alone, and a douche would wash away the agent, reducing its effectiveness even more. A douche should be reserved for cleansing the vagina or for vaginal infections, when a medicated solution may be appropriate. (7)

**63.** 2. A diaphragm should be left in place at least 6 hours after intercourse. If it is removed earlier, sperm may still be alive and may migrate to the fallopian tube to cause conception. (7)

**64.** 4. The patient determining her basal temperature should take her temperature every morning upon awakening and before arising. At this time, her temperature is least likely to be influenced by other factors. There is a slight drop in body temperature before ovulation in some but not all women. A rise in temperature is noted at ovulation. A woman cannot determine exactly when ovulation occurs until it has actually happened. (7)

**65.** 1. It is a myth that alcohol acts as a sexual stimulant. Alcohol is a central nervous system depressant and acts accordingly on libido and the sexual drive. Masturbation is not a dysfunction, having intercourse during menstruation is not harmful, and having an orgasm is not necessary for a satisfactory sexual experience. (4)

**66.** 2. The clitoris is composed of erectile tissue and is especially sensitive to foreplay and movements of the shaft of the penis against its surface. (1, 7)

**67.** 2. Sexual arousal (foreplay, excitement) helps increase vaginal secretions, which help prepare the vagina for penile penetration and increase comfort during sexual intercourse by lubricating the vagina. (1)

**68.** 1. The glans penis is very sensitive to sexual arousal. During orgasm, rhythmic muscle contractions occur in the penis. Other pelvic anatomic structures are affected by the vasocongestion and myotonia that occur during the excitement and plateau phases of the sexual response cycle. (1, 7)

**69.** 1. The four phases used by Masters and Johnson to describe the physiology of the sexual response cycle are the excitement, plateau, orgasmic, and resolution phases. (1, 7)

**70.** 2. The sperm's tail propels it along the female reproductive tract. Muscular action in the uterus *may* help move sperm toward the fallopian tube, but there are no peristalsis-like contractions in the cervix and uterus. (1, 7)

**71.** 4. Fertilization normally occurs in the fallopian tubes. If the fertilized ovum does not move into the uterus, the condition is known as a tubal pregnancy. A tubal pregnancy is one type of ectopic pregnancy. (7)

**72.** 2. The fertilized ovum remains in the fallopian tube about 3 days and in the uterus about 4 days until it implants itself in the uterine wall. (7)

**73.** 2. The uterus receives its blood supply from the uterine and the ovarian arteries. The ovarian artery is a branch of the aorta. It enters the broad ligament and supplies the ovary with blood, while its main stem makes its way to the upper margin of the uterus. (7)

**74.** 3. The chorionic villi and decidua basalis fuse to become the placenta. The decidua vera is also a layer of the decidua, but neither it nor the decidua capsularis is in direct contact with the ovum. The chorionic frondosum is the part of the chorionic villi that fuses with the decidua basalis. The chorionic laeve is the part of the chorionic villi that does not fuse with the decidua basalis; it degenerates and finally almost disappears. (7)

**75.** 1. During pregnancy, the placenta performs the same functions in the embryo/fetus as the lungs, kidney, and stomach (respiration, elimination, and nutrition). The placenta does not perform functions normally performed by the brain. (1, 7)

**76.** 1. Aldosterone is produced by the adrenal cortex and stimulates the maternal kidney tubules to reabsorb sodium and water. Human placental lactogen (HPL), human chorionic gonadotropin (HCG), and progesterone are three of the hormones produced by the placenta during pregnancy. (7)

**77.** 2. The anterior lobe of the pituitary gland releases gonadotropins. There are two principal gonado-

tropins: the luteinizing hormone (LH), which affects ovulation and the development of the corpus luteum, and the follicle-stimulating hormone (FSH), which stimulates development of the follicle. Estrogen, among other things, brings about a thickening of the endometrium. Adrenocorticotropic hormone (ACTH) affects the body's response to stress. (7)

**78.** 3. Occluded or obstructed fallopian tubes make it impossible for a woman to conceive because the sperm cannot reach the ovum. Such conditions as absence of an ovary, a dilated hymenal ring, or an obstructed Bartholin's duct gland do not result in infertility. (7)

**79.** 2. A man with cryptorchidism, or undescended testicles, is sterile. Therefore, he is not a candidate for artificial insemination. (7)

**80.** 1. When acting as a sexuality counselor, the nurse should begin by obtaining a sexual history from the patient. Obtaining the history is an example of assessment in the nursing process. Only after the nurse has collected necessary information can she analyze the data, plan appropriate care for the patient, put the plan into effect, and then evaluate the plan. (7)

**81.** 3. Nurses who do sexual counseling should first have a good understanding of their own personal attitudes about sex. Such activities as having had a sexual relationship, reviewing the literature, and completing requirements to be a sexual counselor may also help, but they do not replace good self-understanding. (7)

**82.** 4. Human chorionic gonadotropin is the hormone used in the pregnancy test. Estrogen stimulates uterine development during pregnancy. Luteinizing hormone stimulates ovulation. Follicle-stimulating hormone is involved in follicle maturation during the menstrual cycle. (7)

**83.** 3. The three most common causes of maternal mortality in the United States are, in order of frequency, hypertensive disorders, puerperal infections, and hemorrhage. Until recently, hemorrhage was the primary cause of maternal death, and a decrease in this cause of death is the largest single factor responsible for a decrease in maternal mortality in the last three decades. (7)

**84.** 1. The infant mortality rate is defined as the number of deaths in infants under 1 year of age per 1,000 live births. The neonatal death rate is the number of deaths in infants under 1 month of age per 1,000 live births. (7)

**85.** 1. Many factors are credited with decreasing maternal mortality, but improved antepartal care is a major one. Other factors include improved medical management, improved educational programs for health professionals, and the work of public health agencies and community health nurses. (7)

**86.** 2. Female sex cells normally contain two X chromosomes, and the male cell one X chromosome and one Y chromosome. The mature ovum always has the X type, but the spermatozoon may be either X or Y. If a male X chromosome combines with the ovum, the infant will be a female (XX). If a male Y chromosome combines with the ovum, the result is a male infant (XY). (7)

## *The Patient with a Spontaneous Abortion*

**87.** 2. A threatened abortion is one in which there is vaginal bleeding or spotting. The cervix is not dilated and abdominal cramping may be present. An inevitable abortion is characterized by more bleeding and cramping than a threatened abortion; the cervix is dilating, and termination of the pregnancy cannot be prevented. An incomplete abortion is one in which some but not all the products of conception have been expelled; usually the placenta remains. A missed abortion is one in which the fetus is dead but has not been expelled from the uterus. (7)

**88.** 3. The patient threatening to abort may be sent home if only slight bleeding or spotting is present and she is free of abdominal pain. However, she should be taught to save her perineal pads and tissue or clots she passes for inspection so that it can be determined if she is expelling any products of conception. She should refrain from having sexual intercourse, because coitus is likely to increase bleeding and cramping. A light or regular diet is satisfactory. The patient need not weigh herself daily. (7)

**89.** 4. In an incomplete abortion, part of the products of conception are retained. In a missed abortion, the fetus dies *in utero* but is not expelled. A threatened abortion results when bleeding and cramping occur but the cervix remains closed and no products of conception have been expelled. An induced abortion is an elective termination of pregnancy. (7)

**90.** 2. Butorphanol tartrate (Stadol) exerts an analgesic effect. It does not prevent nausea, relax the uterus, or control hemorrhage. (7)

**91.** 3. When a patient aborts spontaneously, she can be expected to be suffering from grief that may last months. When offering the patient support, a simple statement such as, "I'm sorry you lost your baby" is appropriate. The nurse should stay with the patient and allow her to express her feelings. Asking why the mother is crying suggests that the nurse sees no need for the patient's sorrow. Offering the patient an analgesic and saying that the aborted fetus was not a formed baby offer the mother no support. (7)

**92.** 3. Euphoria or cheerfulness may signal pathologic mourning. The expected responses or feelings of expectant mothers who experience spontaneous abortion or ectopic pregnancy are feelings of assault to self-concept, guilt, anger, and/or alienation. Shock, denial, or disbelief immediately after the loss is common. (1)

**93.** 3. Pentazocine hydrochloride (Talwin) is an analgesic and does not provide contraceptive protection, inhibit lactation, or promote uterine involution. (2)

**94.** 2. Rh sensitization can be prevented by human anti-D globulin, which clears the maternal circulation of Rh-positive fetal cells and prevents sensitization. (7)

# test 2

The Teenaged Patient with Pregnancy-Induced
Hypertension (PIH)

The Pregnant Patient with Third-Trimester
Bleeding

The Pregnant Patient with Premature Labor

The Pregnant Patient with Diabetes Mellitus

The Patient with an Ectopic Pregnancy

The Pregnant Patient with a Hydatidiform Mole

Correct Answers and Rationales

Select the one *best* or *correct* answer and indicate your choice by filling in the circle with a pencil in front of the option you have chosen. If the answer you would prefer is not given, select the one you think is *most appropriate*.

## THE TEENAGED PATIENT WITH PREGNANCY-INDUCED HYPERTENSION (PIH)

Ms. Cecilia Flores, 17, is unmarried and pregnant. She has been receiving prenatal care at a clinic and has early signs of pregnancy-induced hypertension (PIH).

1. Which of the following information available to the nurse in Ms. Flores' chart, would the nurse determine as being the *least likely* risk factor for PIH?
   ○ 1. Age.
   ○ 2. Primigravid status.
   ○ 3. Family history of PIH.
   ○ 4. High socioeconomic level.

2. The nurse determines that Ms. Flores is experiencing a *typical* symptom of preeclampsia when she complains of
   ○ 1. abdominal cramping.
   ○ 2. swelling of the fingers.
   ○ 3. increased urinary output.
   ○ 4. intermittent bloody spotting.

3. A symptom Ms. Flores is also *most likely* to describe that is typical of preeclampsia is
   ○ 1. sleeplessness.
   ○ 2. a sudden excessive weight gain.
   ○ 3. bleeding of the oral mucous membranes.
   ○ 4. intermittent tightening of the uterus.

4. The sign that is *typical* of preeclampsia and that Ms. Flores's health practitioners are *most likely* to note is
   ○ 1. mental confusion.
   ○ 2. a slow, bounding pulse.
   ○ 3. elevated blood pressure.
   ○ 4. elevated blood urea nitrogen (BUN).

5. Which of the following criteria would the nurse determine as being the *best* description of the blood pressure changes that Ms. Flores would experience at this time?
   ○ 1. A systolic blood pressure value of at least 140 mm Hg.
   ○ 2. A diastolic blood pressure value in excess of 90 mm Hg.
   ○ 3. An increase in systolic or diastolic blood pressure of at least 20 mm Hg.
   ○ 4. An increase above baseline of at least 30 mm Hg in systolic pressure and 15 mm Hg in diastolic pressure.

6. The supervision of Ms. Flores' preeclampsia will continue while she remains at home. The nurse should be prepared to teach her home therapy, which is *most likely* to consist *primarily* of
   ○ 1. diet therapy.
   ○ 2. rest therapy.
   ○ 3. drug therapy.
   ○ 4. physical therapy.

7. Ms. Flores' preeclampsia is *least likely* to affect her fetus by causing
   ○ 1. stillbirth.
   ○ 2. prematurity.
   ○ 3. congenital anomalies.
   ○ 4. intrauterine growth retardation.

8. To monitor fetal status during home therapy, the nurse asks Ms. Flores to keep a record of fetal movement patterns. The nurse would determine that the teaching-learning process has been *successful* when Ms. Flores makes which of the following statements?
   ○ 1. "I will count the number of times the baby moves in 30 minutes three times a day."
   ○ 2. "I will count the number of times the baby moves in 30 minutes after lunch each day."
   ○ 3. "I will count the number of times the baby moves in 30 minutes every morning before I get up."

**101**

○ 4. "I will count the number of times the baby moves in 30 minutes each night just before bedtime."

9. Ms. Flores reports that each time she counts fetal movements, the fetus is moving 6 to 12 times. The nurse decides *correctly* that this report
○ 1. is reassuring.
○ 2. requires follow-up assessment.
○ 3. is characteristic of acute fetal distress.
○ 4. should be called to the physician's attention.

10. The nurse counsels Ms. Flores about her diet. Although the exact cause is not known, preeclampsia has been noted to be more prevalent among women whose diets are low in
○ 1. fats.
○ 2. proteins.
○ 3. carbohydrates.
○ 4. vitamins and minerals.

11. If Ms. Flores is taking a typical supplemental mineral and vitamin preparation, for which of the following food nutrients is she *unlikely* to require an increased dietary intake as well?
○ 1. Iron.
○ 2. Protein.
○ 3. Calcium.
○ 4. Vitamin D.

12. To help Ms. Flores avoid a folic acid (folacin) deficiency, the nurse recommends a diet with adequate folic acid content. Of the following types of foods, the one *richest* in folic acid is
○ 1. poultry.
○ 2. fresh fruit.
○ 3. dairy products.
○ 4. green leafy vegetables.

13. Ms. Flores prepares her own meals at home. She says, "I love vegetables and cook up lots of them almost every day." The nurse should teach Ms. Flores to *avoid* overcooking vegetables because this practice readily destroys vitamin
○ 1. A.
○ 2. C.
○ 3. E.
○ 4. K.

14. At the nurse's request, Ms. Flores records her typical daily menu as follows:

Breakfast: two pieces of toast and coffee
Lunch: bean burrito and a cola drink
Dinner: beef and bean taco salad in a flour tortilla shell.

Which of the following supplements to the above menu would *best* provide the necessary nutrients for Ms. Flores for one day?
○ 1. One glass of milk with each meal, one egg, one serving of green beans, one orange, and one apple.
○ 2. One milkshake, one serving of meat, one banana, and two slices of bread with two pats of butter.
○ 3. One glass of milk with each meal and one at bedtime, one dish of custard, one serving of liver, one apple, and one banana.
○ 4. One glass of milk with each meal, two eggs, two slices of bread with two pats of butter, one apple, and one serving of carrots.

15. Ms. Flores tells the nurse that she uses a little mineral oil for occasional constipation. The nurse should teach Ms. Flores to *avoid* taking mineral oil because it tends to interfere with the normal
○ 1. production of bile.
○ 2. secretion of gastric juices.
○ 3. relaxation of stomach sphincters.
○ 4. absorption of fat-soluble vitamins.

16. Ms. Flores complains of flatulence. Which of the following suggestions should the nurse recommend to her to help overcome flatulence during her pregnancy?
○ 1. Decrease the number of meals each day.
○ 2. Avoid eating gas-producing foods.
○ 3. Drink carbonated beverages several times a day.
○ 4. Drink a little bicarbonate of soda in water as necessary.

17. Ms. Flores asks why she has heartburn. The nurse should teach that heartburn is due to
○ 1. an increase in peristaltic action.
○ 2. a displacement of the stomach by the uterus.
○ 3. an increase in the secretion of hydrochloric acid.
○ 4. a backflow of stomach contents into the esophagus.

18. Ms. Flores calls the nurse at the clinic one morning and says she has had a headache for two days. She says she is nauseated and does not want to take aspirin. She asks the nurse to recommend something for her. Of the following responses, which would be *best* for the nurse to make?
○ 1. "Take one of the new buffered aspirin. It isn't as likely to upset your stomach."
○ 2. "I think the doctor needs to see you today. Could you come to the clinic this morning?"
○ 3. "We can't prescribe on the phone. I will make an appointment for you to see the doctor."
○ 4. "I'll have your doctor phone a prescription for you to your pharmacy. You can pick it up later today."

19. The nurse asks Ms. Flores how often the baby has moved today. Ms. Flores replies that she hasn't

counted the baby's movements today, but that she counted a total of 6 times that the baby moved yesterday. The nurse is *correct* in evaluating that the fetus

○ 1. requires follow-up evaluation.

○ 2. is showing signs of central nervous system maturation.

○ 3. could be experiencing an increase in deep sleep periods.

○ 4. is moving an adequate number of times in a 12-hour period.

**20.** Which of the following clinical manifestations, if present in Ms. Flores, would the nurse determine is *least likely* to indicate that Ms. Flores' preeclampsia is progressing toward severe preeclampsia?

○ 1. Oliguria.

○ 2. Elevated hematocrit.

○ 3. Proteinuria greater than 5 g in 24 hours.

○ 4. Weight gain of less than 1 pound in 1 week.

**21.** Ms. Flores is admitted to the hospital because her preeclampsia worsens. Which room would be *most appropriate* for this patient if the following choices are available?

○ 1. A room that is brightly lighted and close to the nurses' station.

○ 2. A room in the labor suite where the patient can be transferred quickly for delivery.

○ 3. A room where the patient will have quiet and where personnel can observe her frequently.

○ 4. A room on a surgical unit where the patient can be transferred quickly to the operating room for an emergency cesarean.

**22.** Of the following equipment, the *least important* to keep in Ms. Flores' room and readily available is

○ 1. restraints.

○ 2. a padded tongue blade.

○ 3. equipment for aspirating mucus.

○ 4. a catheterization tray with an indwelling catheter.

**23.** An infusion of 5% dextrose in Ringer's solution is started on Ms. Flores. Of the following signs, which assessment finding should the nurse report *promptly,* if it is present?

○ 1. Proteinuria.

○ 2. Flushed skin.

○ 3. Moist rales in the lung fields.

○ 4. A urinary output that exceeds her fluid intake.

**24.** Ms. Flores' hourly urine output is monitored. Of the following actions, which should the nurse take when she notes that for 2 consecutive hours, Ms. Flores' output was between 15 and 17 ml?

○ 1. Notify the physician of the observation.

○ 2. Continue with the present regimen of care.

○ 3. Obtain an order to insert an indwelling catheter.

○ 4. Encourage the patient to take more fluids by mouth.

**25.** Ms. Flores is to receive magnesium sulfate intravenously. Before administering the magnesium sulfate, it is important for the nurse *first* to obtain the

○ 1. fetal heart rate.

○ 2. maternal pulse rate.

○ 3. maternal temperature.

○ 4. maternal respiratory rate.

**26.** While Ms. Flores receives magnesium sulfate, the drug the nurse should have ready as an antidote for magnesium sulfate is

○ 1. calcium gluconate.

○ 2. diazepam (Valium).

○ 3. levallorphan (Lorfan).

○ 4. nalorphine hydrochloride (Nalline).

**27.** While magnesium sulfate is being administered to Ms. Flores, the nurse should assess her regularly for hypermagnesemia. An important sign of magnesium toxicity is

○ 1. hyperactivity.

○ 2. rapid pulse rate.

○ 3. tingling of the fingers.

○ 4. decreased deep tendon reflexes.

**28.** Based on her knowledge of the pathophysiology of pregnancy-induced hypertension and the physiologic changes of pregnancy, the nurse determines that the *best* position for Ms. Flores to assume is the

○ 1. supine position.

○ 2. semi-Fowler's position.

○ 3. left lateral position.

○ 4. Trendelenburg position.

**29.** If Ms. Flores complains of the following symptoms, which should suggest to the nurse that Ms. Flores may be about to have a convulsion?

○ 1. Fetal movements.

○ 2. A severe headache.

○ 3. Feeling very warm.

○ 4. Inability to void.

**30.** If Ms. Flores has signs of an impending convulsion, the nurse's *first* course of action should be to

○ 1. start the patient on oxygen therapy.

○ 2. place the patient in wrist and ankle restraints.

○ 3. increase the flow rate of the patient's intravenous infusion.

○ 4. insert a padded mouth gag between the patient's upper and lower teeth.

**31.** If Ms. Flores develops eclampsia, which of the following would the nurse determine is *not* a phase of an eclamptic convulsion?

○ 1. Coma phase.
○ 2. Tonic phase.
○ 3. Clonic phase.
○ 4. Resolution phase.

**32.** If eclampsia develops, the nurse will anticipate *correctly* that the cure for Ms. Flores' pregnancy-induced hypertension will be
○ 1. strict bedrest.
○ 2. delivery of the fetus.
○ 3. sedation with diazepam (Valium).
○ 4. administration of hydralazine (Apresoline).

**33.** In planning for Ms. Flores' labor, the two *primary* goals of her care should be to
○ 1. lessen edema and reduce blood pressure.
○ 2. prevent convulsions and deliver the baby safely.
○ 3. increase urinary output and limit kidney damage.
○ 4. sedate the patient and decrease reflex excitability.

**34.** The two problems *most commonly* seen among pregnant teenagers, such as Ms. Flores, are pregnancy-induced hypertension and
○ 1. hypoglycemia.
○ 2. gestational diabetes.
○ 3. excessive weight gain.
○ 4. iron-deficiency anemia.

**35.** Ms. Flores tells the nurse about the father of her infant. If the relationship between Ms. Flores and the father of her baby is *typical,* the father is *most likely* to be
○ 1. an older man who has taken advantage of her.
○ 2. a younger boy with whom she has engaged in sexual experimentation.
○ 3. one of many with whom she has had a series of casual relationships.
○ 4. a member of her peer group with whom she has had a relationship over a period of time.

## THE PREGNANT PATIENT WITH THIRD-TRIMESTER BLEEDING

Ms. Sheryl Guichard is approximately 32 weeks gestation. She is admitted to the hospital because she is bleeding vaginally. This is her second pregnancy.

**36.** Ms. Guichard asks if she has an ectopic pregnancy. The nurse should explain by basing her response on knowledge that if implantation occurs in one of the fallopian tubes, the time during pregnancy when the tube will generally rupture is during the

○ 1. first 3 months.
○ 2. 4th or 5th month.
○ 3. 6th or 7th month.
○ 4. 8th or 9th month.

**37.** After helping Ms. Guichard into bed upon admission, the nurse's *most appropriate* action would be to
○ 1. perform a vaginal examination.
○ 2. give the patient a cleansing enema.
○ 3. shave the patient's abdomen and perineal area.
○ 4. check the fetal heart rate and the mother's blood pressure.

**38.** A differential diagnosis between placenta previa and abruptio placenta is made at the time of Ms. Guichard's admission. Of the following symptoms, the one that is *most typical* of abruptio placenta is
○ 1. lack of pain.
○ 2. a rigid abdomen.
○ 3. lack of uterine contractions.
○ 4. early rupture of the membranes.

**39.** In using the medical record to facilitate the differentiation of Ms. Guichard's diagnosis, the nurse would assess the medical record for contributing factors of placenta previa and abruptio placenta. Which of the following would the nurse evaluate as being the *least likely* contributing factor of abruptio placenta?
○ 1. Cigarette smoking.
○ 2. Maternal hypertension.
○ 3. Increased maternal age or parity.
○ 4. A previous low transverse cesarean delivery.

**40.** Ms. Guichard asks the nurse what the difference between abruptio placenta and placenta previa is. The nurse will evaluate the differences between abruptio placenta and placenta previa and base her response on the knowledge that the implantation of the abruptio placenta is
○ 1. normal.
○ 2. abnormal.
○ 3. outside the uterus.
○ 4. in the lower uterine segment.

**41.** If Ms. Guichard has abruptio placenta, a complication she may develop is hypofibrinogenemia. A *typical* late sign of this complication is
○ 1. headaches.
○ 2. a tendency to bleed.
○ 3. an elevated blood pressure.
○ 4. a tendency to form excessive scar tissue.

**42.** If Ms. Guichard has placenta previa, the *most likely* symptom she will present is
○ 1. painless bleeding.
○ 2. a boardlike abdomen.
○ 3. intermittent pain with spotting.
○ 4. a dull pain in the lower abdomen.

**43.** The nurse prepares Ms. Guichard for ultrasonography. Part of her preparation should include explaining to Ms. Guichard that the procedure
- ○ 1. is painless.
- ○ 2. uses a contrast dye.
- ○ 3. takes at least 2 hours.
- ○ 4. requires a topical anesthesia.

**44.** The nurse determines that Ms. Guichard has *correctly* understood the pretest teaching for the ultrasound procedure when Ms. Guichard indicates that she has
- ○ 1. shaved her abdomen without assistance.
- ○ 2. expelled a large bowel movement before admission.
- ○ 3. emptied her bladder immediately before the procedure.
- ○ 4. ingested 1.5 quarts of water about 2 hours before the procedure.

**45.** It is determined that Ms. Guichard has a partial placenta previa. In explaining the diagnosis to Ms. Guichard, the nurse would differentiate the implantation of the partial placenta previa from the low or complete placenta previa implantation by explaining that the partial placenta previa implantation site
- ○ 1. is near the internal os.
- ○ 2. covers the entire internal os.
- ○ 3. is over a portion of the internal os.
- ○ 4. lies within 5 cm of the internal os.

**46.** The nurse explains that the bleeding Ms. Guichard is experiencing results from
- ○ 1. premature labor.
- ○ 2. a heavy bloody show.
- ○ 3. the birth of a macrosomic fetus.
- ○ 4. exposure of maternal blood sinuses.

**47.** After 3 days of bed rest in the hospital, Ms. Guichard is discharged and told to remain in bed until the onset of labor. Ms. Guichard's husband works and she has a 2-year-old child. After assessing that Ms. Guichard needs assistance at home, which of the following courses of action would be *most appropriate* for the nurse to take?
- ○ 1. Explore with the patient the kinds of assistance available to her.
- ○ 2. Suggest that the patient's mother come to stay until after the baby is born.
- ○ 3. Suggest that the patient's husband take a leave of absence from work until the baby is born.
- ○ 4. Tell the patient that bed rest seems difficult under the circumstances but that she should rest as much as possible.

**48.** If the nurse gives the following going-home instructions to Ms. Guichard, which is in *error*?
- ○ 1. Eat a low-calorie diet.
- ○ 2. Avoid sexual intercourse.
- ○ 3. Come to the hospital if her membranes rupture.
- ○ 4. Call the physician if fetal movements decrease.

**49.** The nurse is notified that Ms. Guichard is being readmitted to the hospital to have a cesarean section. Ms. Guichard is now 34 weeks gestation and is having bright-red vaginal bleeding. Upon her admission, the nursing measure to which the nurse should give *highest* priority is to
- ○ 1. shave the patient's abdomen.
- ○ 2. evaluate the status of the fetus.
- ○ 3. start an intravenous infusion on the patient.
- ○ 4. insert an indwelling catheter into the patient's bladder.

**50.** The nurse *correctly* evaluates that Ms. Guichard is being prepared for a cesarean delivery at this time because
- ○ 1. the fetus is now mature.
- ○ 2. profuse bleeding is occurring.
- ○ 3. the patient is becoming anemic.
- ○ 4. the patient is unable to maintain bed rest.

**51.** After the birth, the nurse will assess Ms. Guichard for expression of feelings usually experienced by mothers who give birth prematurely. The feeling *least likely* expected from Ms. Guichard is
- ○ 1. fear.
- ○ 2. failure.
- ○ 3. depression.
- ○ 4. attachment.

## THE PREGNANT PATIENT WITH PREMATURE LABOR

Ms. Tanya Hall, who has previously delivered two nonviable fetuses, is now at approximately 28 weeks gestation. She is admitted to a perinatal center with contractions occurring every 3 to 4 minutes. Her contractions are of moderate intensity.

**52.** Ms. Hall is a candidate for ritodrine (Yutopar) therapy. The use of this agent would ordinarily be *contraindicated* if Ms. Hall
- ○ 1. has intact membranes.
- ○ 2. is experiencing marked fatigue.
- ○ 3. is more than 28 weeks gestation.
- ○ 4. has a cervical dilatation of 5 cm or more.

**53.** The *primary* reason ritodrine (Yutopar) is prescribed for Ms. Hall is that the agent's desired effect is to help inhibit
- ○ 1. bleeding.
- ○ 2. uterine contractions.

○ 3. placental insufficiency.
·○ 4. prostaglandin production.

54. If Ms. Hall is experiencing an adverse effect to the use of ritodrine (Yutopar), she will *very likely* have
○ 1. hypotension.
○ 2. seizure activity.
○ 3. itchy skin.
○ 4. jitteriness.

55. An increase in the blood plasma volume is sometimes associated with ritodrine (Yutopar) therapy. If Ms. Hall experiences this condition, a laboratory finding that will help confirm it is
○ 1. a decrease in the patient's hemoglobin level.
○ 2. the presence of protein in the patient's urine.
○ 3. a decrease in the patient's blood glucose level.
○ 4. the presence of mucus in the patient's vaginal secretions.

56. Ms. Hall's labor contractions are being monitored with a tokodynamometer (external monitor). The optimal placement of the tokodynamometer disc is
○ 1. directly over the fundus.
○ 2. over the body of the fetus.
○ 3. over the circumference of the patient's abdomen.
○ 4. at the site of discomfort during a contraction.

57. When the monitor is applied to Ms. Hall, she tells the nurse she is afraid to move because of the monitor. Which of the following responses would be *most appropriate* for the nurse to make to Ms. Hall?
○ 1. "Don't worry. Your monitor is applied very securely."
○ 2. "Lying on your back is the best position. You won't need to move."
○ 3. "You may lie in any position that is comfortable, except on your back."
○ 4. "It is best to lie quietly on your left side. However, you may flex and extend your legs freely."

58. When the monitor has been in place on Ms. Hall for about 2 hours, the nurse notes that the pattern of contractions recorded by the monitor has changed from a regular wave pattern to an almost flat pattern. Which of the following actions should the nurse take *first*?
○ 1. Notify the physician.
○ 2. Administer oxygen to the patient.
○ 3. Turn the patient onto her left side.
○ 4. Adjust the placement of the tokodynamometer.

59. The doppler (ultrasound) method is used to monitor the fetal heart rate. The transducer is *best* located on Ms. Hall's abdomen
○ 1. near her umbilicus.

○ 2. approximately 2″ above the symphysis pubis.
○ 3. over the area where the fetal heart tones are best heard.
○ 4. approximately midway between the mother's umbilicus and symphysis pubis.

60. The *major* advantage of monitoring the fetal heart rate electronically, compared with obtaining the rate with a fetoscope, is that an electronic monitor
○ 1. takes much less nursing time to use.
○ 2. causes less discomfort to the mother.
○ 3. provides a continuous recording of the fetal heart rate.
○ 4. records the intensity of the uterine contractions simultaneously.

61. If Ms. Hall's fetal heart rate is within the *normal* range, it will be
○ 1. 80 to 120 beats per minute.
○ 2. 100 to 140 beats per minute.
○ 3. 120 to 160 beats per minute.
○ 4. 140 to 180 beats per minute.

62. Ms. Hall is discharged after her contractions are effectively suppressed. She returns later in the third trimester of her pregnancy in questionable labor and is scheduled for an amniocentesis. The nurse should anticipate that preparation for the amniocentesis should *most certainly* include
○ 1. shaving the patient's abdomen.
○ 2. having the patient empty her bladder.
○ 3. giving the patient a cleansing enema.
○ 4. withholding fluids and food for 4 hours.

63. An ultrasound is performed on Ms. Hall before the amniocentesis. In explaining the purpose of the ultrasound to Ms. Hall, the nurse *correctly* evaluates that the *least likely* purpose of the ultrasound at this time is to
○ 1. locate the placenta.
○ 2. measure the biparietal diameter.
○ 3. show where to insert the needle.
○ 4. identify a pool of amniotic fluid.

64. Ms. Hall asks the nurse about the significance of the tests that are performed. The nurse's explanation concerning the L/S (lecithin/sphingomyelin) ratio should be based on the knowledge that these substances are the major components of surfactant, which functions in the infant to
○ 1. regulate the heart rate.
○ 2. prevent coagulation defects.
○ 3. stimulate the respiratory center.
○ 4. maintain the expansion of the lungs.

65. Another test performed on Ms. Hall's amniotic fluid is the "shake" test. This test, which evaluates the stability of foam after amniotic fluid and ethyl

alcohol are combined, helps *primarily* to determine the maturity of the fetus'
- ○ 1. biliary system.
- ○ 2. urinary system.
- ○ 3. vascular system.
- ○ 4. pulmonary system.

**66.** The nurse *correctly* explains to Ms. Hall that the concentration of creatinine in amniotic fluid is an indirect measure of the ability of the fetus to adapt to extrauterine life because creatinine
- ○ 1. increases as the liver matures and secretes it.
- ○ 2. decreases as the fetus swallows and metabolizes it.
- ○ 3. increases as the fetal kidneys mature and excrete it.
- ○ 4. decreases as the size of the fetus increases and absorbs it.

**67.** The nurse should teach Ms. Hall that if the following symptoms occur after the amniocentesis, the one she should report *promptly* is
- ○ 1. nausea.
- ○ 2. vaginal bleeding.
- ○ 3. urinary frequency.
- ○ 4. irregular, painless uterine tightness.

## THE PREGNANT PATIENT WITH DIABETES MELLITUS

Ms. Emma Jackson is a Class B, insulin-dependent diabetic and is receiving prenatal care in a high-risk obstetric clinic.

**68.** When obtaining Ms. Jackson's health history, the nurse learns that Ms. Jackson frequently eats clay. One danger in her practice of pica (eating nonfood items) is that Ms. Jackson is *most likely* to
- ○ 1. predispose her infant to congenital anomalies.
- ○ 2. develop allergies to foods that are essential to her health.
- ○ 3. cause her infant to have a dislike for many nutritious foods.
- ○ 4. crowd foods out of her diet that are important to her health.

**69.** Which of the following predictions in relation to Ms. Jackson's need for insulin during pregnancy is *most accurate*? Ms. Jackson's need for insulin during pregnancy
- ○ 1. will increase.
- ○ 2. will decrease.
- ○ 3. will remain essentially the same as it was before she became pregnant.

- ○ 4. cannot be predicted and will have to be calculated on an individual basis.

**70.** Based on her understanding of the effect of diabetes mellitus on pregnancy, the nurse will assess Ms. Jackson for complications of pregnancy that occur with diabetes. The *least likely* complication the nurse would expect to notice in Ms. Jackson is
- ○ 1. infection.
- ○ 2. ketoacidosis.
- ○ 3. oligohydramnios.
- ○ 4. pregnancy-induced hypertension.

**71.** The nurse prepares to teach Ms. Jackson how to monitor glucose control and insulin dosage at home. The nurse would base her teaching on knowledge that the *most accurate* method of assessment is
- ○ 1. urine testing.
- ○ 2. blood glucose testing.
- ○ 3. 50 g 1-hour screen.
- ○ 4. 3-hour glucose tolerance testing.

**72.** The nurse teaches Ms. Jackson about symptoms of hypoglycemia and hyperglycemia. The nurse evaluates that Ms. Jackson *correctly* understands the teaching when she tells the nurse that which of the following is a manifestation of hypoglycemia?
- ○ 1. Polyuria.
- ○ 2. Tiredness.
- ○ 3. Drowsiness.
- ○ 4. Nervousness.

**73.** At 37 weeks gestation, Ms. Jackson tells the nurse that she has had to decrease her dosage of insulin markedly to prevent hypoglycemia. The nurse is *correct* in determining that the *most likely* reason for Ms. Jackson's symptom is that her
- ○ 1. placenta is failing.
- ○ 2. diabetes is out of control.
- ○ 3. diet should include more calories.
- ○ 4. fetus is compressing the umbilical cord.

**74.** Ms. Jackson is admitted to the hospital for evaluation. She receives an intravenous solution of 5% dextrose and regular insulin. The nurse is given discretion to increase or decrease insulin dosages as necessary. If at 10 a.m. Ms. Jackson's blood glucose level is 80 mg/100 ml of blood and at 11 a.m. it is 90 mg/100 ml, the *best* course of action for the nurse to take at this time is to
- ○ 1. increase the insulin dosage immediately.
- ○ 2. decrease the insulin dosage promptly.
- ○ 3. allow the insulin dosage to remain unchanged for the time being.
- ○ 4. obtain another reading of the patient's blood glucose level before bedtime and then adjust the insulin dosage as necessary.

**75.** Ms. Jackson is evaluated for induction of labor. Which of the following cervical conditions is the *least likely* to be favorable for induction?
○ 1. Soft.
○ 2. Posterior.
○ 3. 75% effaced.
○ 4. 3 cm dilated.

## THE PATIENT WITH AN ECTOPIC PREGNANCY

Ms. Jenny Koh is admitted to a hospital. It is suspected that she is pregnant with gestation occurring outside the uterus.

**76.** Upon Ms. Koh's admission, information that is *particularly* important for the nurse to obtain from Ms. Koh because she is suspected of having an ectopic pregnancy is to determine
○ 1. when the patient last had sexual intercourse.
○ 2. whether the patient has been pregnant previously.
○ 3. whether the patient is taking birth control pills.
○ 4. when the patient started her last normal menstrual period.

**77.** Sonography confirms that Ms. Koh has an ectopic pregnancy. In which anatomic structure do *most* implantations of fertilized ova occur when there is an ectopic pregnancy?
○ 1. In an ovary.
○ 2. In the cervix.
○ 3. In a fallopian tube.
○ 4. In the peritoneal cavity.

**78.** Ms. Koh has a tubal rupture. The symptom that caused Ms. Koh to seek health care is *most likely* to have been
○ 1. sharp abdominal pain.
○ 2. uncontrollable vomiting.
○ 3. severe vaginal bleeding.
○ 4. marked abdominal distention.

**79.** Ms. Koh is scheduled for emergency surgery. The nurse preparing her should be *especially* careful to include regular monitoring of Ms. Koh's blood pressure and
○ 1. pulse rate.
○ 2. uterine cramping.
○ 3. vaginal discharge.
○ 4. pupillary reflexes.

**80.** When the nurse reads Ms. Koh's past health history, she finds that a condition that *most likely* predisposed Ms. Koh to having an ectopic pregnancy is a history of having had

○ 1. infectious hepatitis.
○ 2. an incompetent cervix.
○ 3. late onset of menarche.
○ 4. pelvic inflammatory disease.

**81.** The nurse provides discharge teaching about self-care at home and adverse manifestations to report to the physician. To evaluate Ms. Koh's understanding of the discharge teaching about adverse manifestations, the manifestation the nurse would *least likely* expect Ms. Koh to report would be
○ 1. pain.
○ 2. edema.
○ 3. fever.
○ 4. bleeding.

## THE PREGNANT PATIENT WITH A HYDATIDIFORM MOLE

Ms. Edith Lewis is thought to be beginning her 4th month of pregnancy based on uterine size and has had "morning sickness" during the first 3 months. She calls her physician's office nurse to report that her morning sickness has reached the point that she has not been able to "keep anything down for 3 days."

**82.** When the nurse receives the call, of the following suggestions, it would be *best* for her to recommend that Ms. Lewis
○ 1. take sips of carbonated beverages.
○ 2. come to the physician's office that day.
○ 3. consider obtaining psychological counseling.
○ 4. eat saltine crackers before arising in the morning.

**83.** Because Ms. Lewis has been unable to retain food, her body has been using reserve fat tissues. Consequently, which of the following substances not normally found in the urine can the nurse anticipate will be present when Ms. Lewis' urine is examined?
○ 1. Protein.
○ 2. Albumin.
○ 3. Glucose.
○ 4. Acetone.

**84.** If Ms. Lewis' excessive vomiting continues, she is *most likely* to have a deficit in her body of the electrolyte
○ 1. calcium.
○ 2. potassium.
○ 3. bicarbonate.
○ 4. organic acid.

**85.** The hormone that is *most probably* implicated

and playing a role in nausea and vomiting of pregnancy is

○ 1. estrogen.

○ 2. progesterone.

○ 3. human chorionic gonadotropin.

○ 4. human chorionic somatotropin.

**86.** Ms. Lewis is admitted to the hospital. If the nurse observes that Ms. Lewis has the following symptoms, which would be *least indicative* of dehydration?

○ 1. Lassitude.

○ 2. Scanty urine.

○ 3. Puffiness about her eyelids.

○ 4. Oral temperature of 99.5° F. (37.5° C.).

**87.** Ms. Lewis receives intravenous therapy. Thiamine (vitamin B$_1$) is added to Ms. Lewis' intravenous solution because thiamine helps

○ 1. control vomiting.

○ 2. metabolize carbohydrates.

○ 3. improve kidney filtration.

○ 4. correct acid-base imbalance.

**88.** Ms. Lewis receives intravenous fluids that are to be administered continuously over a period of time. It is generally recommended that the intravenous tubing on Ms. Lewis' setup be changed at least every

○ 1. 24 hours.

○ 2. 36 hours.

○ 3. 48 hours.

○ 4. 72 hours.

**89.** Ms. Lewis is suspected of having a hydatidiform mole. Which of the following symptoms is *most likely* to make it necessary for Ms. Lewis to be examined for the presence of a hydatidiform mole?

○ 1. Seizure activity.

○ 2. Periods of amnesia.

○ 3. A rapidly enlarging uterus.

○ 4. Painful uterine contractions.

**90.** Sonography confirms the presence of a hydatidiform mole and Ms. Lewis' uterus is emptied by dilatation and curettage. The nurse should teach Ms. Lewis that it is important to have regular checkups following the removal of the mole because Ms. Lewis' clinical picture may be complicated by

○ 1. severe anemia.

○ 2. the presence of choriocarcinoma.

○ 3. invasion of the mole into the ovaries.

○ 4. the presence of polyps in the fallopian tubes.

# CORRECT ANSWERS AND RATIONALES

Numbers appear in parentheses following the rationales. The numbers identify textbooks listed in the references at the end of Part II, where correct answers can be verified.

## The Teenaged Patient with Pregnancy-Induced Hypertension (PIH)

**1.** 4. Pregnancy-induced hypertension (PIH) is seen more often in primigravidas, teenagers from a low socioeconomic class, older primigravidas (over 35 years of age), women with a family history of PIH, and women with additional complications such as multiple gestation, diabetes mellitus, Rh incompatibility, and hydatidiform mole. (7)

**2.** 2. Preeclampsia is characterized by weight gain in excess of that expected based on caloric intake. The gain is due to water retention and results in symptoms of edema. The patient is most likely to note swelling of her fingers. Other classical signs of preeclampsia include proteinuria and elevated blood pressure. Epigastric pain is a late symptom of the disease. (7)

**3.** 2. A very common sign of preeclampsia that the patient usually describes is a sudden excessive weight gain due to the accumulation of water in tissues that manifests itself in edema. Finger and facial edema can be noted. Urinary output decreases. Such symptoms as sleeplessness, nervousness, anorexia, bleeding of the oral mucosa, and intermittent tightening of the uterus are not associated with preeclampsia. (7)

**4.** 3. The three most common signs and symptoms of preeclampsia are elevated blood pressure, edema, and proteinuria. (7)

**5.** 4. The *best* description of the blood pressure changes occurring in PIH and upon which the diagnosis of PIH is based is an increase of 30 mm Hg or more in systolic pressure and 15 mm Hg or more in diastolic pressure. A blood pressure value between $^{120}/_{80}$ and $^{140}/_{90}$ is usually considered the general range of blood pressure in mild preeclampsia. Both systolic and diastolic pressures increase in PIH. (7)

**6.** 2. The preeclamptic patient whose symptoms are mild is often treated at home. Of prime importance is that the patient restrict her activities, and bed rest during most of the day is recommended. Drug therapy is not used, with the exception of a sedative if indicated. The diet should be well balanced. Phys-

ical therapy plays no part in the care of the patient with preeclampsia. (7)

**7.** 3. Congenital anomalies are not associated with hypertensive disease. Such conditions as stillbirth, prematurity, and a low birth weight in relation to gestational age are associated with preeclampsia. (7)

**8.** 1. A common method of fetal status assessment requires the mother to count the number of times the fetus moves in a 30-minute time period three times per day. In addition, the expectant mother is instructed to note the strength of the movements. She may be taught to assess the movements in the early morning, mid-afternoon, and late evening. (7)

**9.** 1. A report of at least five or six fetal movements during each counting period is reassuring rather than a sign of acute fetal distress, and does not require follow-up assessment or notification of the physician. (7)

**10.** 2. Preeclampsia is most often noted among women with a low socioeconomic status. Their diets are characteristically low in protein and high in carbohydrates and salt. The incidence of the disease is also high in young primigravida women and in women with multiple pregnancies. Counseling patients who have factors predisposing to preeclampsia should include teaching the importance of a diet that contains adequate proteins. (1)

**11.** 4. The fetus needs iron, protein, and calcium for proper growth, and the mother should have increased amounts of these nutrients in her diet to supply the fetus. It has not been demonstrated that increased amounts of vitamin D are indicated, because the amount the mother normally ingests is adequate for both her needs and those of the fetus. Most vitamin D is obtained from milk fortified with the vitamin. Some vitamin D can be produced by the body from sunlight, but this source is unreliable because of air pollution and the inconsistency with which most people obtain sunlight on the skin. (7)

**12.** 4. Folic acid is crucial during pregnancy because it is required for rapid cell division. Rich sources of folic acid include plant foods and especially green leafy vegetables, liver, wheat germ, orange juice, and cooked legumes. Such foods as fresh fruit, dairy products, and poultry are not considered good sources of folic acid. (7)

**13.** 2. Heat destroys certain nutrients in food but especially water-soluble vitamins, such as vitamin C, thiamine, and folacin. Therefore, it is best to cook vegetables in the shortest time and with the least amount of water possible. It is preferable to eat raw fruits and vegetables when possible to avoid the destruction of vitamin C. (7)

**14.** 1. An adolescent's daily requirements from the basic four food groups are approximately as follows:

Milk—four or more glasses

Meat—two or more servings

Vegetables and fruit—four or more servings

Bread and cereal—four or more servings

The diet of the patient described in this item has no milk, three servings of protein, one serving of vegetables, and four servings of bread. Therefore, she needs four cups of milk and three servings of fruit and vegetables. (7)

**15.** 4. Mineral oil, especially when taken near mealtime, interferes with the proper absorption of fat-soluble vitamins from the gastrointestinal tract. This could lead to a reduction in the production of vitamin K, a fat-soluble vitamin, and predispose the infant to hemorrhagic disease. If dietary measures and an adequate to above-average fluid intake do not prevent constipation and a laxative is indicated, it is better to use a stool softener or a mild laxative such as milk of magnesia. Harsh laxatives are contraindicated. (1, 7)

**16.** 2. Flatulence is an annoying and fairly common discomfort of pregnancy. Suggestions to help overcome it include eating smaller but more frequent meals, chewing food well, and avoiding gas-producing foods, such as carbonated beverages. Bicarbonate of soda should be avoided during pregnancy because of the potential for electrolyte imbalance. (1, 7)

**17.** 4. Heartburn is caused by stomach contents that enter the distal end of the esophagus. This results in a burning sensation usually referred to as heartburn. (7)

**18.** 2. When a patient with preeclampsia complains of a headache for 2 days, as the patient described in this item did, it is best to have a physician examine the patient as soon as possible. Continuous headache is a symptom of preeclampsia, and immediate care is recommended. (7)

**19.** 1. Fewer than 10 fetal movements in a 12-hour period is not reassuring and requires physician notification for follow-up assessment. (7)

**20.** 4. Due to edema, weight gain in pregnancy-induced hypertension (PIH) is more than 1 pound (0.5 kg) per week. Signs of severe preeclampsia are blood pressure of $^{160}/_{110}$ mm Hg or greater on two different occasions at least 6 hours apart, oliguria, proteinuria of 5 g or greater in 24 hours, and such changes in laboratory values as elevated hemato-crit, BUN, serum creatinine, and plasma uric acid. (7)

**21.** 3. The patient with preeclampsia may develop eclampsia, which is characterized by convulsions. To decrease the likelihood of convulsions and their dangers, it would be best to place this patient in a room that is quiet (in order to decrease stimuli that could trigger a convulsion) and convenient for frequent observations by nursing personnel. (7)

**22.** 1. Because a patient with preeclampsia may have a seizure (convulsion), certain equipment must be ready should seizure activity start. Such equipment includes a padded tongue blade, equipment for aspirating mucus, equipment to administer oxygen, a catheterization tray with an indwelling catheter, and equipment for the administration of emergency drugs. Water retention is an important aspect of preeclampsia; therefore, it may become necessary to use an indwelling catheter for the most accurate determination of urinary output. Respiration may become depressed, requiring the aspiration of mucus and the administration of oxygen. A padded tongue blade is used to prevent the patient from injuring her mouth if seizure activity occurs. It is least important to have restraints at the patient's bedside. Their use is not recommended, even during a seizure. (7)

**23.** 3. When a patient is receiving an intravenous infusion, the nurse should report promptly if moist rales are heard in the lung fields. These indicate fluid overload and pulmonary edema. Proteinuria can be expected in the patient with preeclampsia. A urinary output greater than fluid intake is desirable because the preeclamptic patient typically retains excess fluids. Flushed skin is probably unrelated to preeclampsia. (7)

**24.** 1. The patient with preeclampsia tends to produce scanty amounts of urine due to impaired kidney functioning. Therapy may be needed when the hourly urine output is less than 20 to 30 ml. The nurse should notify the physician of her observation in this situation. (7)

**25.** 4. Magnesium sulfate is a central nervous system depressant often used as an anticonvulsant. Because of its actions on the central nervous system, it may depress respiration to a dangerously low and even life-threatening level. Magnesium sulfate should not be administered without consulting the physician if the patient's respiratory rate is below 12 to 14/minute. (7)

**26.** 1. The antidote for magnesium sulfate is calcium, which is commonly administered as calcium gluconate. It should be readily available when magnesium sulfate is being used. (7)

**27.** 4. Typical signs of an above-normal blood level of magnesium include decreased deep tendon reflexes, lethargy progressing to coma with increasing toxicity, and impaired respiration. The nurse should check the patellar, biceps, and radial reflexes regularly when a patient is receiving magnesium sulfate. Hyperactivity and tingling of the fingers are common with hypocalcemia. A rapid pulse rate is common with hypomagnesemia. (7)

**28.** 3. To prevent potential fetal injury due to alteration of placental tissue perfusion, the best maternal position is the left lateral position. If the mother insists on the supine position, supine hypotension can be avoided by elevating the head of the bed and placing a rolled towel under her right hip. (1)

**29.** 2. A typical symptom that often warns of an impending convulsion is a severe headache. Such symptoms as feeling warm, being unable to void, and feeling fetal movements are not precursors of an eclamptic convulsion. (7)

**30.** 4. The patient who shows signs of an impending convulsion should be cared for in such a way that she is protected from injury during the convulsion. A padded mouth gag should be placed between her upper and lower teeth to prevent injury in the mouth and to help keep the airway open. The bed rails are padded to prevent injury in case the patient strikes them. *Gentle* restraint, best done with the nurse's hands, may be necessary during a convulsion, but restraining the patient's arms and legs is not advised. Increasing the patient's intravenous infusion and administering oxygen are not recommended. (7)

**31.** 4. Resolution is not one of the phases of an eclamptic seizure. The first, second, and third phases of the convulsion are, respectively, the tonic, clonic, and coma phases. (7)

**32.** 2. The only known cure for pregnancy-induced hypertension (PIH) is delivery of the fetus. Early diagnosis and careful management are used to control PIH. Medical treatment for severe preeclampsia often includes bed rest, a high-protein (moderate sodium) diet, restoration of fluid and electrolyte balance, sedation, and administration of antihypertensives. Medical treatment for eclampsia includes steps to control convulsions, correct hypoxia and acidosis, lower blood pressure, and stabilize the mother for delivery of the fetus. (7)

**33.** 2. Highest priorities during the labor and delivery of a patient who has preeclampsia are to prevent convulsions and to deliver the infant safely. Efforts to decrease edema, reduce blood pressure, increase urinary output, limit kidney damage, and keep the patient comfortable are desirable, but these aspects of care are not as important as preventing convulsions and delivering an infant safely. (7)

**34.** 4. Pregnant teenagers have iron-deficiency anemia more frequently than other pregnant women. (7)

**35.** 4. Although pregnancy may occur in various relationships, the father of a baby whose mother is an unmarried adolescent is usually a member of the mother's peer group. Usually, she has had a relationship with him over a period of time. (7)

## The Pregnant Patient with Third-Trimester Bleeding

**36.** 1. An ectopic pregnancy ordinarily occurs early in pregnancy, during the first 3 months. Vaginal bleeding may occur and be described as spotting, but bleeding also occurs within the peritoneal cavity when a woman has an ectopic pregnancy. Tubal gestation occurs in about 95% of instances. (1)

**37.** 4. When a patient is admitted with bleeding in the third trimester of pregnancy, the nurse should first check the fetal heart rate and the mother's blood pressure. A vaginal examination and an enema are contraindicated for this patient. There is no need to prepare the patient for delivery because she is not in labor. (7)

**38.** 2. The most typical sign when the placenta separates prematurely is a rigid abdomen. Pain is common. The amnion does not ordinarily rupture, nor are uterine contractions likely to be present. (7)

**39.** 4. A previous low transverse (low cervical uterine incision) cesarean delivery is associated with increased risk for placenta previa. Excessive uterine pressure (hydramnios or multiple gestation), sudden release of uterine pressure (amniotomy), maternal hypertension, trauma, increased maternal age and parity, and maternal habits of daily living, such as cigarette smoking and alcohol ingestion, are associated with abruptio placenta. (7)

**40.** 1. The implantation of an abruptio placenta is normal. By definition, an abruptio placenta is the premature separation of a normally implanted placenta. (7)

**41.** 2. Hypofibrinogenemia is a coagulation defect that predisposes the patient to excessive bleeding. It is caused when thromboplastin from the uterus and placenta enters the bloodstream. This causes small fibrin clots and uses fibrinogen, which results in blood that clots poorly. (7)

**42.** 1. Placenta previa is present when the placenta has attached itself in the lower segment of the uterus. It may partially or completely cover the cervical os.

The most characteristic sign of placenta previa is painless bleeding during the last trimester of pregnancy. (7)

**43.** 1. The patient in this item should be taught that ultrasonography is painless and will help determine the location of the placenta. Ultrasound is most commonly used for diagnostic purposes in obstetrics, although it is used to help diagnose a variety of conditions involving the brain, aorta, pancreas, urinary system, biliary system, thyroid, and eyes. No topical anesthesia or contrast dye is used for the examination. The examination requires an average of 20 to 30 minutes. (7)

**44.** 4. Preparatory procedures for ultrasound are ingesting 1 to 1.5 quarts of water about 2 hours before the ultrasound is performed. A full bladder is necessary to assess the vagina and cervix in relation to the bladder. Assessing the cervix is especially important when vaginal bleeding due to placenta previa is suspected. The abdomen is prepared for the procedure by spreading mineral oil or a transmission gel over it. An empty rectum is not required for the ultrasound. (7)

**45.** 3. The site of implantation of the partial placenta previa is over a portion of the internal cervical os, but the internal os is not covered entirely as it is with a complete placenta previa. A low placental implantation site is near the internal os. (7)

**46.** 4. Bleeding precipitated by placenta previa results from exposure of maternal blood sinuses when placental villi are torn from the uterine wall as the lower uterine segment contracts and dilates in the later weeks of pregnancy. Bleeding in placenta previa is not initiated because of the birth of a macrosomic fetus, heavy bloody show, or preterm labor. (7)

**47.** 1. When a patient requires help at home because she must remain in bed, it is best for the nurse first to explore the kinds of assistance available to the patient. The patient's order for bed rest should not be changed to one of getting as much rest as possible. It is usually unrealistic to expect a husband who works to stay with the patient. The nurse must first determine whether the patient's mother is in a position to help the patient. This item illustrates how the nurse uses the nursing process. *First*, she assesses by gathering information. Then she continues by analyzing her findings, planning a course of action, implementing care, and finally evaluating care. (7)

**48.** 1. No information is given about the patient described in this situation to indicate that a low-calorie diet is necessary. A regular diet would be more appropriate. However, the patient with pla-

centa previa should avoid sexual intercourse because of the danger of starting vaginal bleeding. She should return to the hospital if her membranes rupture and should notify the physician if fetal movements decrease. (7)

**49.** 3. When a patient with placenta previa who is having bright-red vaginal bleeding is admitted and will have a cesarean section, the nurse should place highest priority on starting an intravenous infusion to correct/prevent hypovolemia. No doubt this patient will require an indwelling catheter and will have her abdomen shaved in preparation for the cesarean section. The fetal status should also be evaluated. But these measures are less urgent for this patient than starting an intravenous infusion upon her admission. (7)

**50.** 2. A cesarean section delivery for placenta previa is performed prior to 37 weeks gestation when frequent, recurrent, or profuse bleeding occurs or the well-being of the fetus is threatened. Otherwise, delivery is postponed until approximately 37 weeks to allow for fetal maturity. (7)

**51.** 4. Feelings of attachment are often postponed until the infant's health improves. Parents are often overwhelmed by feelings of fear, loss, sadness, and failure. (1)

### The Pregnant Patient with Premature Labor

**52.** 4. Pharmaceutical agents to suppress labor are ordinarily contraindicated when the patient has a cervical dilatation of 5 cm or more and when the patient's membranes have ruptured. The drug may be used beyond the 28th week of pregnancy. The patient's fatigue, described in this item, should be investigated but would not necessarily contraindicate the use of ritodrine (Yutopar). (7)

**53.** 2. The desired effect of ritodrine (Yutopar) therapy is to inhibit uterine contractions. The drug acts primarily on the $\beta_2$ receptors in smooth muscles to help control activity of the uterine muscles. Certain drugs have been used to control prostaglandin production in order to inhibit premature labor, but ritodrine is not one of them. (7)

**54.** 4. Common adverse effects to ritodrine (Yutopar) therapy include jitteriness, apprehension, and tremors, but not seizure activity such as a convulsion. Hypotension, itchy skin, and a skin rash are not reported as adverse effects to ritodrine therapy. (7)

**55.** 1. When blood plasma volume increases, a type of blood dilution occurs that causes a decrease in hemoglobin and hematocrit levels. Hyperglycemia is associated with ritodrine (Yutopar) therapy, not hypoglycemia. Proteinuria is not associated with ritodrine therapy and increased blood plasma volume. Mucus is normally present in vaginal secretions. (7)

56. 1. As the uterus contracts, the abdominal wall rises and, when external monitoring is used, presses against the transducer. This movement is transmitted into an electrical current, which is then recorded. For best results, the tokodynamometer should be placed where uterine displacement during contractions is greatest. (7)

57. 3. Although the patient's activity is limited when using a monitor because she cannot get out of bed, she may and should be encouraged to change positions in bed. The patient should be assured that she may move about in bed and assume any position of comfort, except the supine position, while she is being monitored. Lying flat on the back during labor causes pressure on major abdominal vessels, and as a result decreases blood supply to the fetus. Telling a patient not to worry is not helpful. (1, 7)

58. 4. A transducer may have slipped out of place if a regular wave pattern noted for several hours becomes almost flat. This may occur when, for example, the patient moves about in bed. The first course of action in this situation would be for the nurse to adjust the placement of the tokodynamometer. (1, 7)

59. 3. When the fetal heart rate is being monitored, the best placement of the doppler is over the area where the best sharp fetal heart tones are heard. The heart tones are less likely to be heard as well when the doppler is placed elsewhere on the abdomen. (7)

60. 3. A major advantage of monitoring the fetal heart rate electronically is that it provides for a continuous recording of the fetal heart rate, during as well as between contractions. Using a fetoscope allows only a sampling of readings, and the method is not as accurate in determining variables in the fetal heart rate. Neither manual nor electronic monitoring is uncomfortable for the mother. Electronic monitoring may require less nursing time, but this is not considered a major advantage for using electronic monitoring. The type of monitoring described in this item does not determine the intensity of uterine contractions. (7)

61. 3. The fetal heartbeat is normally between 120 and 160 beats per minute. (7)

62. 2. To help avoid the danger of puncturing a full bladder, the patient should be *sure* to void before an amniocentesis. Giving the patient a cleansing enema, shaving her abdomen, and withholding fluids and food prior to the amniocentesis are ordinarily not indicated. (7)

63. 2. Before amniocentesis, an ultrasound is valuable in localizing the placenta to avoid puncturing it with the needle, locating a pool of amniotic fluid, and showing the physician where and how deep to insert the needle. Assessing the gestational age by measuring the biparietal diameter is not a prerequisite to performing an amniocentesis. (7)

64. 4. Surfactant helps eliminate the stickiness of alveolar tissues in the lungs. This allows for lung expansion. Insufficient amounts of surfactant predisposes to respiratory distress in the newborn. (7)

65. 4. The "shake" test, as described in this item, helps determine the maturity of the fetal pulmonary system. The more stable the foam, the more mature the fetus' pulmonary system is. The test may be used in combination with the L/S ratio, described in the previous item. (7)

66. 3. The concentration of creatinine in amniotic fluid increases with maturity of the fetal kidneys. Maturity of the kidneys increases their ability to excrete creatinine. (7)

67. 2. Following an amniocentesis, the woman should promptly report vaginal bleeding, rupture of the membranes, or a decrease or increase in fetal movements. Painless uterine tightness is most probably due to Braxton-Hicks contractions. (7)

## The Pregnant Patient with Diabetes Mellitus

68. 4. Pica, which is the ingestion of nonfood items, tends to crowd out nutritious foods from the diet. Pica may also interfere with the proper utilization of nutrients and, in some instances, may cause an intestinal obstruction. Pica is sometimes noted to be culturally acquired. The cause of the practice is not clearly understood. (7)

69. 1. The placenta produces human placental lactogen (HPL), also called human chorionic somatomamotropin (HCS). This hormone (and to a lesser degree, estrogen and progesterone) is an insulin antagonist. As a result, the woman with diabetes who is insulin dependent will need more insulin during pregnancy. (7)

70. 3. The expectant diabetic mother has a higher risk for complications, such as hydramnios, pregnancy-induced hypertension (PIH), ketoacidosis, dystocia, and infections, than the expectant non-diabetic mother. (7)

71. 2. The most accurate method for home monitoring

of glucose control and insulin dose is blood glucose testing. In pregnancy, the renal threshold for glucose is lower, resulting in the presence of glucose in the urine at lower blood glucose levels than is usual for the nonpregnant adult. The 50 g 1-hour test is used to screen pregnant women for gestational diabetes. The 3-hour glucose tolerance test is used to diagnose diabetes. (7)

**72.** 4. Nervousness is an early sign of hypoglycemia. Polyuria, tiredness, and drowsiness are manifestations of hyperglycemia. (7)

**73.** 1. When a pregnant diabetic reports that her dosage of insulin has to be decreased markedly to avoid hypoglycemia, the nurse should suspect that the patient's placenta is failing and the fetus could be in serious jeopardy due to placental insufficiency. In particular, the small blood vessels in the body are affected by diabetes, including those in the placenta. The patient with placental insufficiency may require the induction of labor to reduce fetal risk. (7)

**74.** 3. In general, it is desirable to maintain a blood glucose level between 60 mg/100 ml and 100 to 110 mg/100 ml. For the patient described in this item whose blood glucose level is 90 mg/100 ml of blood, action is not required now because the blood glucose level is within normal range. However, the nurse should check the blood glucose level in another hour and not wait until bedtime. The nurse should be alert to the patient's need for an increased amount of insulin because the patient is receiving dextrose intravenously and presumably is about to eat a noon meal. (7)

**75.** 2. A cervix favorable for successful induction is anterior, soft, more than 50% effaced, and at least 3 cm dilated. (7)

## The Patient with an Ectopic Pregnancy

**76.** 4. It may be important to obtain information from a patient suspected of having an ectopic pregnancy concerning when she last had sexual intercourse, whether she is taking birth control pills, and whether she has been pregnant previously. However, it is of *particular* importance to determine when the patient started her last normal menstrual period. Such information helps establish an accurate diagnosis. Usually, the patient with an ectopic pregnancy will have missed a menstrual period or two and knows she is pregnant. Some patients may not know whether they are pregnant, especially if their menstrual cycles are irregular. (7)

**77.** 3. An ectopic pregnancy is defined as any gestation that is located outside the uterus. The word "ectopic" comes from a Greek word meaning displaced. Approximately 95% of ectopic pregnancies occur in a fallopian tube. (7)

**78.** 1. The most typical symptom when a patient has an ectopic pregnancy and the tube has ruptured is severe abdominal pain. It is knifelike in quality and in a lower quadrant of the abdomen. There is ordinarily slight vaginal bleeding, more often described as spotting. Vomiting and abdominal distention are not associated with an ectopic pregnancy in which the tube has ruptured. (7)

**79.** 1. When the fallopian tube of a patient with an ectopic pregnancy ruptures, the patient presents an emergency situation because of extensive bleeding into the peritoneal cavity. Shock will develop if precautionary measures are not taken. The nurse readying such a patient for surgery should be especially careful to include monitoring of the patient's blood pressure and pulse rate for signs of impending shock. The nurse should be prepared also to administer blood or plasma expanders as necessary through an intravenous line that should already be in place. (7)

**80.** 4. Anything that causes a narrowing or some constriction in the fallopian tubes so that a fertilized ovum cannot be properly transported to the uterus for implantation predisposes to an ectopic pregnancy. Pelvic inflammatory disease is most often the cause of constricted or narrow tubes. Developmental defects may also cause a constriction or narrowing of the fallopian tubes. (7)

**81.** 2. The expected symptoms that the patient would report are pain, bleeding, and/or temperature elevation. (7)

## The Pregnant Patient with a Hydatidiform Mole

**82.** 2. When a woman entering her 4th month of pregnancy has had "morning sickness" but now has been vomiting for 3 days, as described in this item, it would be best that the patient come to the physician's office that day. Early-morning nausea often occurs during the first trimester. Vomiting that persists into the second trimester should be investigated because the vomiting may be serious and its causes need to be assessed. (7)

**83.** 4. Combustion cannot be completed when fat is burned in the body in the absence of carbohydrate. Improper fat metabolism results in acetone and diacetic acid in the urine from the starvation the patient described in this item is experiencing. (7)

**84.** 2. Gastrointestinal secretion losses from vomiting, as well as from diarrhea and excessive perspiration, will result in a potassium deficit (hypokalemia) if precautionary measures are not taken. (7)

**85.** 3. Human chorionic gonadotropin, a placental hormone that peaks in the first trimester of pregnancy and levels off at about the 12th week of pregnancy, has been theorized to be the major hormone that contributes to nausea and vomiting during pregnancy. (7)

**86.** 3. Puffiness about the eyelids is a sign of water retention. Common signs of dehydration include scanty urine, lassitude, and temperature elevation. (7)

**87.** 2. Thiamine is converted to a coenzyme that plays an important part in carbohydrate metabolism. It has an important role in providing nutrients for all cells in the body. Thiamine has not been found to be effective in controlling vomiting, improving kidney filtration, or correcting an acid-base imbalance. (7)

**88.** 3. It is generally recommended that the tubing be changed every 48 hours to decrease the likelihood of infection. Changing the tubing every 24 hours has been common practice, but the Centers for Disease Control now says that 48 hours is a safe interval. (9)

**89.** 3. A characteristic symptom when a patient has a hydatidiform mole is a rapidly enlarging abdomen of a size greater than would be expected for the length of time the patient thinks she has been pregnant. Trophoblastic tissue rapidly proliferates, so the uterus grows out of proportion to a pregnancy of comparable length. The patient may also have vaginal bleeding that may become profuse. Vomiting and signs of preeclampsia may also be present. (7)

**90.** 2. A patient who has had a hydatidiform mole removed should have regular checkups to rule out the presence of choriocarcinoma, which may complicate the patient's clinical picture. The patient's human chorionic gonadotropin (HCG) levels are monitored to rule out choriocarcinoma. (7)

# test 3

Select the one *best* or *correct* answer and indicate your choice by filling in the circle with a pencil in front of the option you have chosen. If the answer you would prefer is not given, select the one you think is *most appropriate*.

## THE PRIMIGRAVID PATIENT IN LABOR

Mrs. Ellen Miller, 22, is pregnant for the first time. She is 40 weeks gestation and is admitted to the hospital in the first stage of labor.

1. Mrs. Miller's uterine contractions are about 10 minutes apart. At this time, Mrs. Miller's emotions can be expected to be
   - ○ 1. serious.
   - ○ 2. irritable.
   - ○ 3. happy.
   - ○ 4. panicky.

2. Mrs. Miller asks how long she will be in labor. *All of* the following factors will influence the length of her labor *except*
   - ○ 1. size of the placenta.
   - ○ 2. mental attitude of the mother.
   - ○ 3. position of the fetus *in utero*.
   - ○ 4. power of the uterine contractions.

3. Mrs. Miller is ordered to have a cleansing enema p.r.n. Under which of the following conditions would an enema be *contraindicated*?
   - ○ 1. The patient is in early labor.
   - ○ 2. The patient has vaginal bleeding.
   - ○ 3. The patient's membranes have ruptured.
   - ○ 4. The fetal head is estimated to be at station zero.

4. The nurse performs a nitrazine test to determine whether Mrs. Miller's membranes have ruptured. The nurse is justified in determining that the membranes have *most probably* ruptured if the color on the nitrazine paper is
   - ○ 1. blue.
   - ○ 2. olive.
   - ○ 3. orange.
   - ○ 4. yellow.

5. Mrs. Miller says, "The doctor says the baby is at 'plus one.' What does that mean?" The nurse *correctly* explains that the point to which the baby has descended during labor is described as a station; when the station is "plus one," the part of the baby to be born first is located
   - ○ 1. 1 cm above the ischial spines.
   - ○ 2. 1 cm below the ischial spines.
   - ○ 3. 1 fingerbreadth above the ischial spines.
   - ○ 4. 1 fingerbreadth below the ischial spines.

6. Mr. Miller coaches Mrs. Miller to help her with breathing and relaxation techniques, as they were taught in childbirth preparation classes. When Mrs. Miller reaches the transition phase of labor, she screams out, "I can't have this baby!" The technique that Mr. Miller should use to help his wife at this time is to
   - ○ 1. leave the room until his wife gains control.
   - ○ 2. ask the nurse to give his wife the prescribed analgesia.
   - ○ 3. tell his wife that she is doing well and it will soon be over.
   - ○ 4. talk to his wife while using direct eye contact and breathe with her.

7. Mrs. Miller has a low subarachnoid (saddle) block in preparation for delivery. After Mrs. Miller receives this regional anesthesia, it is *most certainly* important for the nurse to monitor Mrs. Miller's
   - ○ 1. blood pressure.
   - ○ 2. urinary output.
   - ○ 3. level of anesthesia.
   - ○ 4. level of consciousness.

8. Newborn Baby Miller is assessed by using the Apgar rating system. If his score is 8, the nurse can safely determine that this newborn's physical condition is

○ 1. good.
○ 2. fair.
○ 3. poor.
○ 4. critical.

9. The nurse prepares prescribed oxytocin, which she is to add to Mrs. Miller's intravenous infusion when the placenta has been delivered. The nurse determines *correctly* that the placenta has separated and is about to be delivered when the
○ 1. abdominal wall relaxes noticeably.
○ 2. cord lengthens outside of the vagina.
○ 3. patient complains of pain in her back.
○ 4. uterus falls below the level of the symphysis pubis.

10. While Mrs. Miller holds and looks at her newborn baby, the nurse observes that Mrs. Miller is crying. The *best* interpretation of the mother's behavior is that
○ 1. the patient is disappointed in the baby's sex.
○ 2. the patient is grieving the loss of her pregnancy.
○ 3. crying is a common, normal response following delivery.
○ 4. a mother-newborn bonding problem is most likely present.

11. While Mrs. Miller holds her newborn soon after delivery, she asks the nurse when she can start breast-feeding her baby. Based on knowledge of infant alertness, it is *best* for the nurse to reply by saying
○ 1. "You may begin to nurse your baby right now if you like."
○ 2. "You may nurse your baby in about 2 hours after the baby is bathed."
○ 3. "You may nurse your baby in about 8 hours after the baby has had some rest."
○ 4. "You may nurse your baby after he has had water to assess his gastrointestinal tract."

## THE INTRAPARTAL PATIENT WITH SINGLE-ROOM MATERNITY CARE

Mrs. Dorothy Nickols is admitted to a hospital that provides single-room maternity care. Mrs. Nickols is in labor and will be delivering her third child.

12. Mr. and Mrs. Nickols decided to use the single-room maternity care when Mrs. Nickols was about 6 months pregnant. The popularity of units that provide family-centered care instead of traditional care is due to provision of care that
○ 1. promotes unity of the family.
○ 2. allows the father to deliver the infant.

○ 3. reduces the risks of postpartum complications.
○ 4. permits the parents to practice techniques of prepared childbirth.

13. Mr. and Mrs. Nickols learned active relaxation techniques as part of the psychoprophylaxis method of childbirth preparation. A characteristic of active relaxation is that it includes
○ 1. using techniques of relaxation of uninvolved body muscles during uterine contractions.
○ 2. accepting a supreme power that can help relieve the discomfort of uterine contractions.
○ 3. considering the discomfort of uterine contractions to be more psychological than physical.
○ 4. assuming a state of mind that is open to suggestion from an attendant during uncomfortable uterine contractions.

14. Mrs. Nickols, who is in early labor, asks the nurse if she has to stay in bed. Which of the following replies that the nurse could make reflects the *most common* practice concerning ambulating during early labor?
○ 1. "It is best to stay in bed to help prevent the cord from prolapsing."
○ 2. "You may walk about but let me know immediately when your membranes rupture."
○ 3. "It is best to stay in bed and lie on your left side so that your baby receives a good supply of oxygen."
○ 4. "You may walk to the bathroom but it is best for you to stay in bed at other times so that I can observe your contractions accurately."

15. Mrs. Nickols is progressing but still in the first stage of labor. She is happy and appears relaxed, although she is aware of labor contractions. At this time, Mr. Nickols can be of *most* assistance by
○ 1. keeping a record of the patient's urinary output.
○ 2. playing a game of cards that the patient and he enjoy.
○ 3. helping the patient focus on an object in the room during contractions.
○ 4. suggesting that the patient start slow chest breathing during contractions.

16. When Mrs. Nickols returns to bed, she is encouraged to assume a position of comfort but preferably not to lie on her back for long periods of time. The supine position is likely to predispose her to
○ 1. nausea.
○ 2. dyspnea.
○ 3. backache.
○ 4. hypotension.

17. Mrs. Nickols uses effleurage to help herself "keep on top" of her contractions. Effleurage means a type of massage that consists of

○ 1. deep kneading of muscular tissues.

○ 2. secure grasping of muscular tissues.

○ 3. light stroking on the skin's surface.

○ 4. punctuated tapping on the skin's surface.

18. The effectiveness of skin massage to control discomfort, as Mrs. Nickols is using, is often explained by the gate control theory. According to this theory of pain, where in the body is the gating mechanism located?

○ 1. In the spinal cord.

○ 2. In reticular fibers.

○ 3. In the cerebral cortex.

○ 4. In cutaneous nerve fibers.

19. According to the gate control theory of pain, a *closed* gate means that the person should experience

○ 1. no pain.

○ 2. dull pain.

○ 3. light pain.

○ 4. reduced pain.

20. At the beginning of Mrs. Nickols' labor, a moderate increase in the amount of bloody vaginal discharge (show) should be interpreted by the nurse as an indication of

○ 1. progressive fetal descent.

○ 2. increased cervical dilatation.

○ 3. rupture of the fetal membranes.

○ 4. premature separation of the placenta.

21. Mrs. Nickols is using personalized concentration points or ideas to promote muscular relaxation during labor. These points or ideas serve as a

○ 1. projection for pain.

○ 2. distraction from pain.

○ 3. rationalization for pain.

○ 4. counter-irritant for pain.

22. The nurse should plan to check Mrs. Nickols' blood pressure *between* contractions *primarily* because

○ 1. the blood pressure normally increases during a contraction.

○ 2. the blood pressure is normally erratic during a contraction.

○ 3. a patient is unable to cooperate sufficiently with the procedure during a contraction.

○ 4. the procedure interferes with techniques the patient has been been taught to use during a contraction.

23. Mrs. Nickols is to have only fluids during labor. The *primary* reason for observing this practice is that during labor

○ 1. solid foods tend to cause nausea.

○ 2. the digestive process is normally slow.

○ 3. the patient's appetite can be expected to be poor.

○ 4. the body has a sufficient store of nutrients to make eating unnecessary.

24. The nurse assesses Mrs. Nickols and determines that her cervix is dilated 6 cm. Her contractions are becoming stronger and closer together. The nurse can expect that it is *most probable* that Mrs. Nickols' mental attitude will now reflect feelings of

○ 1. depression.

○ 2. excitement.

○ 3. seriousness.

○ 4. irritability.

25. Mrs. Nickols is beginning to have considerable discomfort during contractions. While observing techniques learned in childbirth preparation classes, Mr. Nickols suggests that Mrs. Nickols change from slow chest breathing to a type of breathing during the peak of contractions that is *best* described as

○ 1. deep chest breathing.

○ 2. pursed lip breathing.

○ 3. rapid panting breathing.

○ 4. shallow chest breathing.

26. The nurse should judge that Mrs. Nickols is *most probably* hyperventilating during labor when she complains of

○ 1. feeling warm.

○ 2. feeling dizzy.

○ 3. having a headache.

○ 4. being short of breath.

27. Which of the following actions should the nurse take to help Mrs. Nickols overcome the effects of hyperventilation?

○ 1. Have the patient breathe into a paper bag.

○ 2. Have the patient take several whiffs of oxygen.

○ 3. Have the patient breathe rapidly and shallowly.

○ 4. Have the patient breathe with forceful expirations.

28. Which of the following acid-base imbalances is Mrs. Nickols likely to experience when she hyperventilates excessively?

○ 1. Metabolic acidosis.

○ 2. Metabolic alkalosis.

○ 3. Respiratory acidosis.

○ 4. Respiratory alkalosis.

29. Mrs. Nickols is not completely dilated, but she has a strong urge to push. The *best* course of action for the nurse to take at this time is to

○ 1. position the patient for pushing.

○ 2. give the patient a prescribed sedative.

○ 3. suggest that the patient use a pant-blow pattern of breathing.

○ 4. let the patient push but tell her to push as lightly as possible.

**30.** If Mrs. Nickols develops back labor and the fetal head is presenting, what position is the fetus *most likely* assuming in the uterus?
- 1. The occipitodiagonal position.
- 2. The occipitoanterior position.
- 3. The occipitoposterior position.
- 4. The occipitotransverse position.

**31.** The nurse should anticipate that if Mrs. Nickols has back labor, an expected consequence is that she will *very likely*
- 1. require an episiotomy.
- 2. have a precipitate delivery.
- 3. experience marked discomfort.
- 4. be at risk for postpartum hemorrhage.

**32.** While Mrs. Nickols is in the transition phase of labor, she is *most* in need of nursing care that includes providing her with
- 1. fluids.
- 2. extra warmth.
- 3. distractions from pain.
- 4. encouragement and support.

**33.** Mrs. Nickols vomits, and her arms and legs begin to shake while she is in the transition phase of labor. She cries out, "I can't take it! I can't take it!" Which of the following actions is *most appropriate* for the nurse to take at this time?
- 1. Teach Mrs. Nickols a new breathing pattern.
- 2. Remind Mrs. Nickols that she must stay in control.
- 3. Suggest that Mr. Nickols breathe with Mrs. Nickols.
- 4. Provide rest for Mrs. Nickols until the peak of each contraction.

**34.** After assessing Mrs. Nickols, the nurse determines that she is beginning the second stage of labor. Of the following situations the nurse finds, the one that *best* confirms her judgment is that Mrs. Nickols'
- 1. show is bloody.
- 2. membranes rupture.
- 3. contractions are very strong.
- 4. cervix is completely dilated.

**35.** Mrs. Nickols elects to deliver in the side-lying position. The nurse should help position Mrs. Nickols so that she is lying on her
- 1. left side with her right knee flexed.
- 2. left side with her right knee extended.
- 3. right side with her left knee flexed.
- 4. right side with her left knee extended.

**36.** Mrs. Nickols delivers a girl. After Mrs. Nickols has eye-to-eye contact with her newborn, it can be expected that Mrs. Nickols will *most probably* next
- 1. kiss the infant.
- 2. fold the infant in her arms.
- 3. examine the infant for deformities.
- 4. touch the infant with her fingertips.

**37.** Mr. and Mrs. Nickols are heard to make the comments given below shortly after the infant is born. Which comment should the nurse interpret as a possible sign of eventual parent-infant bonding problems?
- 1. "She is so cute."
- 2. "I wish she were a boy."
- 3. "She looks just like you."
- 4. "I want to nickname her Sugar Bear."

**38.** Approximately 10 minutes after delivery, Mrs. Nickols experiences a chill. Which of the following actions is *most appropriate* for the nurse to take?
- 1. Administer an analgesic.
- 2. Obtain the patient's temperature.
- 3. Cover the patient with additional blankets.
- 4. Notify the physician of the patient's condition.

**39.** The Nickolses' oldest child wants to see his new sister's eyes. Which of the following methods is the *easiest* way to get the infant to open her eyes?
- 1. Place the infant in an upright position.
- 2. Place the infant under an overhead light.
- 3. Pull down the lower eyelid with the thumb.
- 4. Separate the eyelids with the thumb and forefinger.

## THE INTRAPARTAL PATIENT WITH RISK FACTORS

**40.** Ms. Li Nguyen is a 39-year-old primigravida admitted in labor. She asks how long her labor will last. The nurse should base her response on knowledge that the *average* length of time a woman pregnant for the first time is in labor is approximately
- 1. 4 hours.
- 2. 12 hours.
- 3. 20 hours.
- 4. 28 hours.

**41.** Ms. Nguyen has rheumatic heart disease. The nursing management of Ms. Nguyen during pregnancy should *most certainly* include helping her find ways to reduce physical activity when she
- 1. is irritable.
- 2. complains of anorexia.
- 3. has dyspnea upon exertion.
- 4. demonstrates an elevated hemoglobin value.

**42.** The nurse assesses Ms. Nguyen upon admission to the labor suite. Which of the following questions that the nurse asks Ms. Nguyen should have *first* priority?
- 1. "Are you feeling life?"

○ 2. "When did you last eat?"

○ 3. "How frequent are your labor contractions?"

○ 4. "Will you breast-feed or bottle-feed your infant?"

**43.** Ms. Nguyen has not attended childbirth preparation classes during her pregnancy. After admission procedures are completed, the nurse demonstrates some breathing and relaxation techniques. Ms. Nguyen listens politely to the instructions but says, "I was told that I would be having epidural anesthesia. Will I need to use those techniques?" The nurse's *best* response to Ms. Nguyen would be

○ 1. "You may need to use breathing and relaxation techniques in case your anesthesia does not take effect."

○ 2. "Breathing and relaxation techniques may help you during labor before you receive your anesthesia."

○ 3. "Breathing and relaxation techniques will help you after you deliver when you could use them to advantage."

○ 4. "You will still have discomfort during delivery, when you could then use breathing and relaxation techniques."

**44.** The recommended position for Ms. Nguyen during administration of the epidural anesthetic agent is the

○ 1. sitting position.

○ 2. side-lying position.

○ 3. knee-chest position.

○ 4. supine position with knees flexed.

**45.** Fifteen minutes after injection of the anesthetic agent, Ms. Nguyen's blood pressure drops to 92/64. Based on this observation, which of the following actions is *least effective* for the nurse to take?

○ 1. Administer oxygen by mask.

○ 2. Elevate the head of the bed.

○ 3. Displace the uterus to the right.

○ 4. Increase the intravenous infusion rate.

**46.** When Ms. Nguyen's cervix is fully dilated, the nurse should plan to instruct Ms. Nguyen to push when

○ 1. the patient feels the urge to push.

○ 2. the patient feels the onset of a contraction.

○ 3. the nurse observes a bulging of the perineum.

○ 4. the nurse palpates the onset of a contraction.

**47.** Ms. Nguyen's newborn has Down syndrome. This syndrome is caused by

○ 1. a congenital anomaly.

○ 2. a chromosomal defect.

○ 3. a maternal metabolic disorder.

○ 4. improper development of the fetal thymus gland.

**48.** The nurse assesses Baby Nguyen after birth. A physical finding the nurse *most likely* observes is that Baby Nguyen has

○ 1. flared nares.

○ 2. bulging fontanels.

○ 3. a protruding tongue.

○ 4. an absence of the rooting reflex.

**49.** The nurse begins preparation to counsel Ms. Nguyen concerning her infant with Down syndrome. Which of the following statements about Down syndrome *lacks* scientific support?

○ 1. Down syndrome is ordinarily easy to diagnose at the time of birth.

○ 2. Persons with Down syndrome are especially susceptible to infections.

○ 3. Treatment for curing Down syndrome has met with little success to date.

○ 4. Down syndrome occurs more frequently in babies born of mothers who are intellectually limited.

**50.** If the following findings are noted on Ms. Nguyen's record, which predisposed her *most* to having an infant with Down syndrome?

○ 1. Being 39 years old.

○ 2. Having cerebral palsy.

○ 3. Having a history of hypertension.

○ 4. Having rubella (German measles) while pregnant.

Ms. Alice O'Malley, 22, is a Class B, insulin-dependent diabetic who is being induced at 39 weeks gestation for suspected placental insufficiency. An oxytocic agent is administered via intravenous infusion.

**51.** The nurse is given the discretion to increase the rate of the infusion every 15 minutes as indicated. The nursing measure that is *essential* while caring for Ms. O'Malley during induction is to

○ 1. remain with the patient continuously.

○ 2. keep the patient awake during induction.

○ 3. change the patient's position every half hour.

○ 4. stop the oxytocic infusion as soon as the patient's contractions are 5 to 6 minutes apart.

**52.** When Ms. O'Malley's membranes are ruptured, the nurse notes that the amniotic fluid is meconium-stained. The *most likely* reason for the presence of meconium in the amniotic fluid is that the fetus is

○ 1. experiencing hypoxia.

○ 2. in the breech position.

○ 3. congenitally malformed.

○ 4. large for gestational age.

**53.** If the fetal head is still quite high in the pelvis

when Ms. O'Malley's membranes are ruptured, the *most important* action for the nurse to take is to

○ 1. auscultate the fetal heart rate.

○ 2. position the patient on her left side.

○ 3. be prepared for a precipitate delivery.

○ 4. determine the patient's blood pressure.

54. If Ms. O'Malley's cord prolapses, initial and *immediate* nursing measures should be directed toward helping

○ 1. relieve pressure on the cord.

○ 2. expedite delivery of the infant.

○ 3. replace the cord into its normal position.

○ 4. give the mother oxygen therapy.

55. While Ms. O'Malley is receiving the infusion of oxytocin, she has a strong contraction that lasts about 90 seconds. Of the following courses of action, the one the nurse should take *first* is to

○ 1. stop the infusion.

○ 2. notify the physician.

○ 3. start oxygen therapy.

○ 4. turn the patient onto her left side.

56. To prevent meconium aspiration at the time of birth, Baby O'Malley's care should include

○ 1. intubating the infant as soon as it is delivered.

○ 2. administering oxygen to the infant as soon after delivery as possible.

○ 3. suctioning the infant's nasopharynx as soon as the head is delivered.

○ 4. administering an agent to dilate the bronchi promptly after the infant's delivery.

Ms. Leta Pachelli, who is pregnant for the fifth time and has had four normal deliveries, is admitted to the hospital in active labor. Her condition and that of the fetus have been good since admission.

57. Ms. Pachelli calls out, "Nurse, the baby is coming." When the nurse responds to Ms. Pachelli's call, the *first* course of action the nurse should take is to

○ 1. inspect the perineum.

○ 2. time the contractions.

○ 3. auscultate the fetal heart rate.

○ 4. rush the patient to the delivery room.

58. It appears that delivery of Ms. Pachelli's baby is imminent and the nurse has no help immediately available to her. Of the following actions, which is *most appropriate* for the nurse to take *first*?

○ 1. Have the patient pant to delay the delivery.

○ 2. Administer a prescribed analgesic to the patient.

○ 3. Prepare a clean area upon which to deliver the baby.

○ 4. Prepare to administer intravenous fluids to the patient.

59. Which of the following statements is *most likely* to assist Ms. Pachelli to remain calm and cooperative during the delivery?

○ 1. "The baby is coming. Just relax and everything will be fine."

○ 2. "Even though the baby is coming, the doctor will be here very soon."

○ 3. "The baby is coming. I will explain what is happening and tell you what to do as we go along."

○ 4. "There is no need for concern. Many babies are born safely without the assistance of a doctor."

60. When should the nurse plan to deliver Ms. Pachelli's baby's head?

○ 1. Between contractions.

○ 2. At the end of a contraction.

○ 3. At the peak of a contraction.

○ 4. At the beginning of a contraction.

61. As soon as Baby Pachelli's head is delivered, the nurse should *next*

○ 1. tell the mother to avoid strenuous pushing.

○ 2. feel around the infant's neck for the umbilical cord.

○ 3. apply gentle traction on the infant's anterior shoulder.

○ 4. place gentle pressure with one hand on the mother's lower abdomen.

62. Assuming sterile equipment is available, what, if anything, should the nurse do in relation to the umbilical cord after Ms. Pachelli's baby is born?

○ 1. Cut it.

○ 2. Clamp it.

○ 3. Leave it untouched.

○ 4. Wrap it in normal saline.

63. In relation to the delivery of Ms. Pachelli's placenta, which of the following actions is *most appropriate* for the nurse to take?

○ 1. Have the patient bear down.

○ 2. Massage the fundus for a few minutes.

○ 3. Wait for signs of placental separation before taking any action.

○ 4. Pull gently on the cord until the placenta begins to appear at the vaginal orifice.

64. If some membrane remains just inside the vagina after Ms. Pachelli's placenta delivers, it is *best* for the nurse to handle this membrane by

○ 1. cutting the trailing membrane away from the placenta.

○ 2. teasing the trailing membrane out of the vagina with a gentle motion.

○ 3. massaging the uterus lightly until the trailing membrane is expelled.

○ 4. clamping the trailing membrane carefully at a point as near the placenta as possible.

**65.** Of the following complications, the one Ms. Pachelli or her infant is *least likely* to develop as a result of a precipitate delivery is
- ○ 1. a ruptured uterus.
- ○ 2. trauma to the baby's head.
- ○ 3. excessive postpartal bleeding.
- ○ 4. lacerations of the maternal soft tissues.

**66.** Ms. Pachelli has a history of smoking one to two packs of cigarettes daily. Which of the following observations of her infant will reflect effects of smoking during pregnancy?
- ○ 1. The infant's pulse rate is above average.
- ○ 2. The infant's hemoglobin is below average.
- ○ 3. The infant's birth weight is below average.
- ○ 4. The infant's respiratory rate is above average.

**67.** If the following factors are present in Ms. Pachelli's health history, which should have alerted the nurse to the possibility of Ms. Pachelli's having a rapid labor and delivery?
- ○ 1. The patient has had four previous pregnancies.
- ○ 2. The patient attended prepared childbirth classes.
- ○ 3. The patient had a 12-hour labor with her previous pregnancy.
- ○ 4. The patient had signs of hypertension earlier in this pregnancy.

Ms. Patty Quinn, who is pregnant for the second time, is admitted to the hospital in labor. She is pregnant with twins.

**68.** Ms. Quinn is in active labor. She is observed to have contractions no more often than two or three times in a 10-minute period. The discomfort during contractions that Ms. Quinn is *most likely* to experience is best described as being
- ○ 1. mild.
- ○ 2. severe.
- ○ 3. gnawing.
- ○ 4. continuous.

**69.** When getting ready for the delivery of Ms. Quinn's twins, the *least important* measure for the nurse to take while preparing for a safe delivery is to have which of the following ready?
- ○ 1. A double set of cord care equipment.
- ○ 2. A double set of oxygen therapy equipment.
- ○ 3. Two persons skilled in resuscitation techniques.
- ○ 4. A double set of local anesthetic block equipment.

**70.** Ms. Quinn delivers a boy and a girl. The twins are described as dizygotic twins. Dizygotic twins are the result of the fertilization of

- ○ 1. two ova with one sperm.
- ○ 2. two ova with two sperm.
- ○ 3. one ovum with one sperm.
- ○ 4. one ovum with two sperm.

**71.** Of the following complications, the one to which Ms. Quinn is *especially* susceptible is
- ○ 1. thrombophlebitis.
- ○ 2. puerperal infection.
- ○ 3. rupture of the uterus.
- ○ 4. postpartum hemorrhage.

**72.** Ms. Quinn's twins require additional hospitalization after Ms. Quinn is discharged. Unless plans are made to prevent it, a problem likely to arise later relates to
- ○ 1. resentment for having had twins.
- ○ 2. jealousy later in life between the twins.
- ○ 3. bonding between the newborns and parents.
- ○ 4. lack of interest in the eventual care and nurture of the twins.

Ms. Debbie Raab is admitted to the hospital's delivery suite in active labor. She is almost 2 weeks postterm.

**73.** Ms. Raab, now in the second stage of labor, pushes with a contraction. If she uses the following techniques, which is in *error*?
- ○ 1. The patient is in a semi-Fowler's position.
- ○ 2. The patient flexes her thighs sharply onto her abdomen.
- ○ 3. The patient exerts downward pressure as though she is about to have a bowel movement.
- ○ 4. The patient holds her breath during several bearing-down efforts for the length of each contraction.

**74.** Ms. Raab has a bilateral pudendal block for anesthesia before her delivery. The nurse can expect that the pudendal block will normally relieve Ms. Raab's discomfort *primarily* in the
- ○ 1. back.
- ○ 2. uterus.
- ○ 3. cervix.
- ○ 4. perineum.

**75.** The physician performs an episiotomy on Ms. Raab, the *primary* reason being to
- ○ 1. relieve pressure on the rectum.
- ○ 2. shorten the second stage of labor.
- ○ 3. facilitate the third stage of labor.
- ○ 4. provide room for flexion of the infant's head in the pelvis.

**76.** After delivery, it would be *best* for the nurse to remove Ms. Raab's legs from the stirrups and lower them together slowly in order to help prevent Ms. Raab's having

1. leg cramps; rapid extension of muscle tissue predisposes to cramping.
2. shortness of breath; sudden release of intraabdominal pressure affects chest capacity.
3. chilling sensations; changes in body temperature result from sudden muscular exertion.
4. nerve damage; rapid extension of nerves in the popliteal space predisposes to nerve tissue damage.

77. If the nurse uses deep suctioning of Baby Raab's nasopharynx, there is danger of
    1. injuring tender mucous membranes.
    2. abolishing the infant's normal efforts to clear mucus.
    3. stimulating the vagus nerve.
    4. removing too much carbon dioxide.

78. The nurse evaluates Baby Raab's condition. The nurse assesses the newborn's heart rate, respiratory effort, muscle tone, and reflex irritability while using the Apgar scoring chart. The nurse should *next* evaluate the newborn's
    1. eyes.
    2. color.
    3. suck reflex.
    4. urethral patency.

79. Baby Raab has an Apgar score of 7 at 1 minute and 9 at 5 minutes. Based on these scores, the nurse *accurately* determines Baby Raab's condition to be
    1. fair.
    2. poor.
    3. good.
    4. critical.

80. If Baby Raab's Apgar score indicates that he is in fair condition, the nurse should first clear his airway. The nursing measure of *highest* priority indicated *next* for Baby Raab is to
    1. supply the neonate with warmth.
    2. give the neonate oxygen therapy.
    3. assist with intubating the neonate.
    4. perform cardiac massage on the neonate.

Mrs. Lydia Sanchez is pregnant for the first time. There is a question about whether her pelvis is adequate for vaginal delivery. Mrs. Sanchez has started labor contractions.

81. If the following findings are noted in Mrs. Sanchez, which is important to report because it strongly suggests that there is a disproportion between the size of the fetus and the birth canal?
    1. The patient's cervix is 90% effaced.
    2. The patient's cervix is dilated 3 cm.
    3. The patient's membranes remain intact.
    4. The fetal head has not engaged.

82. Pelvic measurements are obtained on Mrs. Sanchez. A pair of waterproof gloves are required when the measurement to be obtained is the
    1. true conjugate.
    2. biischial diameter.
    3. diagonal conjugate.
    4. obstetric conjugate.

83. The pelvic measurement that is *most* important when determining whether Mrs. Sanchez's pelvis is adequate for a vaginal delivery is the
    1. true conjugate.
    2. biischial diameter.
    3. diagonal conjugate.
    4. transverse diameter.

84. Based on magnetic resonance imaging (MRI) studies, Mrs. Sanchez's physician elects to perform a cesarean section. When the nurse takes the consent form (permit) to the Sanchezes for signing, Mr. Sanchez says, "I'll sign it. I always take care of our business affairs." Which of the following responses would be *most appropriate* for the nurse to make in this situation?
    1. "Is that all right with you, Mrs. Sanchez?"
    2. "All right, Mr. Sanchez. You may sign right here."
    3. "Thank you, Mr. Sanchez, but Mrs. Sanchez must also sign her consent form."
    4. "Just a minute. I will have to ask the doctor if that is satisfactory with him."

85. Mrs. Sanchez is prepared for a cesarean delivery. If Mrs. Sanchez's preoperative orders include the following types of preparation, which should the nurse question before carrying it out?
    1. Shaving the patient's abdomen.
    2. Giving the patient a narcotic drug.
    3. Giving the patient atropine sulfate.
    4. Inserting an indwelling catheter into the patient's bladder.

86. Mr. Sanchez is asked if he would like to be with his wife during the cesarean delivery. Research studies regarding the father's presence during a cesarean delivery indicate that there is
    1. no evidence of harm.
    2. no evidence of benefit.
    3. an increase in postpartum infection rates.
    4. an increase in lawsuits with charges of malpractice.

87. Mr. and Mrs. Sanchez select general anesthesia for the cesarean delivery. The nurse should plan to observe Mrs. Sanchez for adverse effects of general anesthesia, which generally include *all* of the following *except*

○ 1. a delay in the production of breast milk.

○ 2. a delay in the onset of spontaneous respiration in the newborn.

○ 3. an increased likelihood of uterine atony and excessive bleeding.

○ 4. a greater risk for maternal vomiting and aspiration than when general anesthesia is not used.

**88.** To be prepared for possible problems when caring for Baby Sanchez, the nurse should be guided by knowledge that, compared to babies born vaginally, babies born by cesarean section tend to have an increased incidence of

○ 1. cold stress.

○ 2. convulsions.

○ 3. umbilical cord infections.

○ 4. respiratory distress syndrome.

**89.** Before Mrs. Sanchez's newborn is removed from the operating room and taken to the newborn nursery, which of the following measures is of *utmost importance* for the nurse to complete?

○ 1. Being sure the surgical sponge count is correct.

○ 2. Fingerprinting the mother and footprinting the baby.

○ 3. Instilling prophylactic drops/ointment in the baby's eyes.

○ 4. Keeping the baby with the mother until she is awake from anesthesia and able to see her baby.

**90.** While caring for Mrs. Sanchez after the cesarean delivery, the nurse should anticipate that Mrs. Sanchez is likely to experience *all* of the following emotions *except*

○ 1. relief.

○ 2. frustration.

○ 3. indifference.

○ 4. disappointment.

# CORRECT ANSWERS AND RATIONALES

Numbers appear in parentheses following the rationales. The numbers identify textbooks listed in the references at the end of Part II, where correct answers can be verified.

## *The Primigravid Patient in Labor*

1. 3. In the first stage of labor when complications are absent and while contractions are still not strong, about 10 to 15 minutes apart, the patient is usually not very uncomfortable. She is excited that the big day has finally arrived, and she can be expected to be happy and eager. As labor progresses, the patient becomes serious and ready to get down to "work." As transition approaches, she is likely to become irritable, tired, and sometimes panicky. (7)

2. 1. The size of the placenta is the factor least likely to influence the length of labor. Such factors as the position of the fetus and the mother's attitude have been found to influence the length of labor. Fetal malpositions may prolong labor. Ambulation of the mother and a side-lying position when not out of bed decrease the length of labor. A major influence on the length of the first stage of labor is the power of labor (frequency, intensity, and duration of the uterine contractions). (7)

3. 2. There is some controversy concerning whether an enema is beneficial during labor. When an enema is ordered to be given at the nurse's discretion, the nurse should *avoid* giving an enema if vaginal bleeding is present, labor is progressing rapidly, imminent delivery is noted, or the presenting part of the fetus is not engaged. An enema would also not be given if the patient has had a bowel movement or diarrhea very recently. If the membranes are ruptured, an enema *may* be given but it should be expelled into a bedpan. (7)

4. 1. The nitrazine test helps determine the acidity of a fluid. The membranes have no doubt ruptured if the acidity of the fluid is above 6.5, and the nitrazine test paper then becomes blue-green, blue-gray, or deep blue in color. If the pH of the fluid is below about 6.0, the fluid is most likely vaginal secretions, and the color of the nitrazine test paper will be olive, olive-yellow, or olive-green. (7)

5. 2. The ischial spines are used as landmarks to determine the descent of the presenting part. When the station is plus one, the presenting part is 1 cm below the ischial spines. When the station is minus one, the presenting part is 1 cm above the ischial spines. (7)

6. 4. The transition stage of labor requires reinforcement of techniques learned during childbirth preparation classes. It is best when the husband described in this item speaks to his wife while using direct eye contact and breathes with her when she loses control during the transition stage. This often helps the mother regain control. The mother should be encouraged to focus on one contraction at a time at this point in labor. (7)

7. 1. One complication of regional anesthesia is hypotension. It may develop because the anesthetic acts as a sympathetic blocker. The nurse should monitor blood pressure, pulse, respiration, and fetal heart rate every 5 minutes until delivery and should report any drop in blood pressure immediately. To overcome hypotension, the administration of intravenous fluids to the patient is usually increased. The person administering the anesthesia is responsible for monitoring the level of anesthesia. The patient will normally be conscious while under the influence of this type of anesthesia. (7)

8. 1. The Apgar rating system rates a newborn on the basis of his or her heart rate, respiratory effort, muscle tone, reflex irritability, and color. The infant is given a score between 0 to 10. The higher the score, the better is the newborn's condition. The newborn described in this item has an Apgar score of 8 and is rated in good condition. A score between 4 and 6 indicates the newborn's condition is fair. A score between 0 and 3 indicates the newborn's condition is extremely poor. (7)

9. 2. The most reliable sign that the placenta has detached from the uterine wall is observing the cord lengthen outside the vagina. The drug oxytocin is administered to promote uterine contractions and thereby control bleeding. (7)

10. 3. The birth of a baby is a very emotional experience. An expression of happiness with tears is not an abnormal reaction. (7)

11. 1. Very soon after birth, a newborn is active and alert. The American Academy of Pediatrics recommends beginning breast-feeding as soon after delivery as possible. A baby that will be breast-fed should not be given water or formula by bottle at this time. Many institutions provide sterile water for the initial feeding at 1 to 6 hours after birth to assess for esophageal atresia. A breast-fed baby may nurse before or after the initial sterile water feeding. (7)

## *The Intrapartal Patient with Single-Room Maternity Care*

**12.** 1. One reason why birthing centers or single-room maternity units that offer parents an alternative to a traditional delivery are gaining popularity is that they are administered in a manner that promotes family unity while still offering physical safety and care for the mother and her newborn. Policies vary widely, although ordinarily the father does not actually deliver the baby but may be allowed to move the newborn upon its birth to the mother's abdomen. Family-centered centers or units do not necessarily reduce the risk of postpartum complications, although women at risk usually are informed and participate in the decision-making process. Parents may use techniques they learned in prepared childbirth classes in traditional hospital settings, just as they may in the family-centered centers or units. (1, 7)

**13.** 1. Many childbirth educators use a variety of techniques and methods to prepare parents for childbirth, and active relaxation is one such technique. Active relaxation is concerned primarily with teaching relaxation of uninvolved muscle groups while contracting a specific group, and teaching chest breathing techniques to lift the diaphragm off the contracting uterus. Hypnosis is a technique in which the person assumes a state of mind that makes him or her open to suggestions from an attendant. (1)

**14.** 2. Most authorities suggest that a woman in an early stage of labor be allowed to walk if she wishes. This practice is *not* used if complications are present. Birthing centers or single-room maternity units allow women considerable latitude without a great deal of supervision at this time in labor. But it is wise for the nurse to check the patient for possible prolapse of the cord when the membranes rupture, especially if she has been ambulating. (7)

**15.** 2. It is best to use techniques of breathing and concentration when the woman in labor needs them. While she is still fairly comfortable and in early labor, distraction activities such as reading, cards, or games are recommended. No information given in this situation indicates that it is necessary to keep an accurate record of urinary output for this patient, although the nurse should be aware of whether or not the patient is voiding. (7)

**16.** 4. It is generally recommended that patients in labor assume a comfortable position in bed. However, the prolonged use of the supine position is not recommended because it tends to predispose the mother to hypotension. (7)

**17.** 3. Effleurage is light stroking of the skin. It is a French word that means grazing, or touching lightly in passing. Some describe effleurage as a "feather touch." (7)

**18.** 1. The gating mechanism is in the spinal cord, perhaps in the substantia gelatinosa, according to the gate control theory of pain. (7)

**19.** 1. A closed gate means that a person should have no pain because pain impulses cannot be transmitted to the brain. An open gate results in the opposite effect. (7)

**20.** 2. Show normally occurs when cervical dilatation increases. Fetal descent is unrelated to show. Rupture of the fetal membranes will result in the escape of amniotic fluid. Premature separation of the placenta is accompanied by bleeding, which is frequently concealed. (7)

**21.** 2. Personalized concentration points or ideas serve as a distraction from pain. They do not act as a projection, rationalization, or counter-irritant for pain. (7)

**22.** 1. Blood pressure normally increases during a contraction, which is why it is best to take a patient's blood pressure between uterine contractions. (7)

**23.** 2. The digestive process is normally slow during labor, and as a result solid foods are generally withheld. Nausea and vomiting are not unusual late in the first stage of labor, even when food is omitted. (7)

**24.** 3. As a woman progresses into the first stage of labor and her contractions become stronger and closer together, she typically becomes less talkative and more serious. She tends to turn her thoughts inward as she now begins to concentrate on the work at hand. (1, 7)

**25.** 4. The psychoprophylaxis method of childbirth suggests using slow chest breathing until it becomes ineffective during labor contractions. The patient is taught to use shallow chest breathing during the peak of a contraction. When transition nears, a pant-blow pattern of breathing is used. (7)

**26.** 2. When a patient is hyperventilating during labor, she is eliminating more carbon dioxide than usual. The result is that she very often complains of feeling dizzy and light-headed. Feeling warm or having headaches or shortness of breath is not associated with hyperventilation. (1, 7)

**27.** 1. The symptoms of hyperventilation are due to excess carbon dioxide elimination from the body. Hence, rebreathing into a paper bag is beneficial because it increases the intake of carbon dioxide during respirations. Taking whiffs of oxygen, breathing rapidly and shallowly, and breathing with

The Nursing Care of Maternity Patients and Newborns

forceful expirations are likely to aggravate the situation. (7)

**28.** 4. The carbon dioxide insufficiency that occurs during hyperventilation will lead to respiratory alkalosis. (7)

**29.** 3. Pushing during labor when the urge is present but the cervix is still not completely dilated is likely to produce swelling of the cervix and make labor and delivery more difficult. The psychoprophylaxis method of childbirth suggests that at such times, the mother should be encouraged to use a pant-blow (blow-blow) pattern of breathing to help overcome the urge to push. Using a sedative is not recommended, nor is it helpful to tell the patient to push but to do so as lightly as possible. (7)

**30.** 3. When a woman has back labor, the fetus is most probably in an occipitoposterior position. This means the fetal head presses against the mother's sacrum, which causes marked discomfort during contractions. Transverse and anterior occiput positions do not cause pressure on the mother's sacrum. No position of the fetus is described as being occipitodiagonal. (7)

**31.** 3. It is estimated that about 25% of women in labor have back labor. The woman with back labor will experience marked discomfort, more so than when the fetal vertex is in the anterior position. Back labor does not necessarily predispose to a precipitate delivery or postpartum hemorrhaging. The woman with back labor does not *require* an episiotomy, although the physician may elect to do one. (7)

**32.** 4. During the transition phase of labor, the mother most needs encouragement and support. It is a difficult and painful time when contractions are especially strong. During this phase, the woman usually finds it very difficult to keep herself in control. Everything else seems secondary to the mother as she strives to progress into the second stage of labor and delivery. (7)

**33.** 3. The psychoprophylaxis method of childbirth encourages a woman in strong labor to deal with one contraction at a time. It is often helpful when her coach (in the situation described in this item, the husband) breathes with her when the patient appears to be losing control. If the patient rests until the contraction peaks, she might not be able to "get on top" of the contraction. It is unreasonable to expect a patient in the transition phase of labor to learn new techniques of breathing. (7)

**34.** 4. The second stage of labor begins with the complete dilation of the cervix and ends with the delivery of the infant. The membranes often rupture when the patient enters the second stage of labor,

but they may also rupture earlier, in some instances even before labor begins. Show normally is bloody during the first stage of labor, especially when the patient reaches the transition phase. Contractions are very strong during the second stage of labor, but they are also very strong during the transition phase in the first stage of labor. (7)

**35.** 1. The left lateral position is preferred when a patient decides to deliver while lying on her side. The right knee, which should be flexed, is supported by the nurse or the labor coach. Lying on the left side results in less interference with maternal and fetal circulation and greater uterine efficiency. (7)

**36.** 4. The process of bonding between a mother and her newborn ordinarily follows a pattern, starting with eye-to-eye contact. The mother then tends to touch the infant with her fingertips. Next, she is likely to massage the infant, usually with the palm of a hand, and proceed to examine the infant. (7)

**37.** 2. Expressions of disappointment over the sex of a newborn may lead to problems with parent-infant bonding in the future. Behavior that is hostile or very low-key (passive) about the infant may also lead to eventual bonding problems. (7)

**38.** 3. A chill shortly after delivery is not uncommon. There is no need to call the physician. An analgesic is not indicated for a chill. It takes time for the temperature to change following a chill. (7)

**39.** 1. The most effective position in which to place the infant so that he will open his eyes is the upright position. Rocking may also cause the eyes to open. (7)

## The Intrapartal Patient with Risk Factors

**40.** 2. The average length of time a primigravida is in labor is approximately 12 hours. The first stage of labor lasts about 11 hours; the second stage averages about 1 hour, and the last stage averages 1 to 5 minutes. (7)

**41.** 3. A woman who has a heart disease concurrent with pregnancy needs close supervision so that she puts no undue stress on her heart. Signs of heart failure may occur insidiously, and therefore the nurse should be alert to signs typical of the condition. Increased dyspnea with exertion is used most often to indicate that the patient most certainly should decrease her physical activity. A rapid pulse rate, palpitations, and a cough are additional signs that suggest the patient may be experiencing heart failure. (7)

**42.** 3. When admitting a patient to the labor suite of a

hospital, certain information about the patient is important to obtain promptly in order to plan care. The information should most certainly include the frequency, intensity, and duration of labor contractions; when labor started; and whether the membranes have ruptured. From this information, the nurse obtains a quick overview of the woman's status and proceeds accordingly with nursing care, including validating information. It is important to know such information as whether the patient feels life, when she last ate, and how she plans to feed her infant. But knowledge of this type is less influential in making initial plans for the patient's care. (7)

**43.** 2. Regional anesthesia, such as a lumbar epidural block, is ordinarily not administered until the patient is in an active phase of labor and has cervical dilatation of about 4 to 5 cm. Therefore, before regional anesthesia is given, the patient may well benefit if she knows how to use breathing and relaxation techniques. Responses to the patient that indicate the patient can use breathing and relaxation techniques after delivery, that discomfort during delivery will still be present, and that the anesthesia may not take effect are less accurate. (7)

**44.** 2. Lumbar epidural anesthesia is administered with the patient in a side-lying position. After anesthesia is introduced, the head of the bed may be elevated slightly to prevent the level of anesthesia from ascending above the desired level. (7)

**45.** 2. A drop in the mother's blood pressure may occur after a lumbar epidural anesthetic is introduced. Measures to combat hypotension and its effects include expanding vascular volume, increasing oxygen concentration of inspired air, and removing pressure of the gravid uterus from the great vessels. (7)

**46.** 4. Lumbar epidural anesthesia eliminates the urge to bear down. The nurse must tell the patient when the contraction begins and determines this by palpating for a contraction. The perineum will not bulge until the fetus is being pushed against it. (7)

**47.** 2. Down syndrome is due to a chromosomal defect. There is trisomy of chromosome 21, which results in a total chromosomal count of 47 instead of the normal 46. Translocation of chromosomes and having a different number of chromosomes within cells of one person also lead to the disorder, but occur very rarely.(7)

**48.** 3. Typical physical findings on a newborn with Down syndrome include slanting eyes set closely together, a protruding tongue, a flat nose, short thick hands, and simian creases on palmar surfaces.

Such findings as bulging fontanels, flared nares, and an absence of the rooting reflex are not associated with Down syndrome. (7)

**49.** 4. Down syndrome is not associated with the mother's intellectual level. The condition is ordinarily easy to diagnose at birth; children with the condition are very susceptible to infections and an infection is a usual cause of death. There has been little or no success in attempts to cure the disease. (7)

**50.** 1. The incidence of Down syndrome increases with the age of the mother. The pregnant woman who contracts rubella, especially during the first 16 weeks of pregnancy, is likely to deliver a baby with various anomalies, but Down syndrome is not associated with rubella. (7)

**51.** 1. The induction of labor with an oxytocic agent carries risks. It is *essential* that a nurse remain with the patient at all times to monitor uterine contractions and the fetal heart rate. Even if the patient is being monitored with electronic equipment, which is common, the nurse should monitor the patient also. It is not safe to rely on the patient to report when contractions begin. Usual protocol is to increase the administration of the oxytocic agent, according to agency policy, until a regular pattern of contractions begins. Then, the infusion should be held at that rate or decreased. The infusion should be stopped and the physician notified if contractions are occurring less than 2 minutes apart, last longer than 60 seconds, or the fetal heart rate becomes abnormal. (7)

**52.** 1. A typical sign of fetal distress due to an inadequate transfer of oxygen to the fetus is meconium-stained amniotic fluid. The woman described in this situation has presented symptoms of placental insufficiency, and therefore the fetus is at risk for hypoxia. (7)

**53.** 1. The nurse should auscultate the fetal heart rate when the membranes are ruptured and the head of the fetus is high in the pelvis. As amniotic fluid rushes out, the cord may prolapse. A drop in the heart rate suggests fetal distress which may be caused by pressure of the head on the umbilical cord. (7)

**54.** 1. The first step for the nurse to take when a cord prolapses is to use measures that relieve pressure on the cord. An infant's condition can be compromised seriously when pressure on the cord does not allow blood to reach the infant. Immediate measures include lowering the mother's head by using the Trendelenburg position or knee-chest position so that the presenting part of the infant will move away from the pelvis, and moving the presenting part off the cord by applying pressure through the vagina with a sterile gloved hand. (1, 7)

**55.** 1. If a patient receiving an oxytocic agent to induce labor has a contraction lasting longer than 60 seconds, the nurse should *first stop* the infusion. She should then place the patient on her left side to help promote maternal and fetal circulation, start oxygen therapy via mask at 6 to 8 liters/minute, and notify the physician. (7)

**56.** 3. The aspiration of meconium is best prevented by suctioning the infant's nasopharyngeal area immediately after the head is delivered but before the chest is delivered. As long as the chest is compressed in the vagina, the infant cannot inhale and aspirate meconium in the upper respiratory tract. The aspiration of meconium blocks the flow of air to the alveoli, which leads to respiratory complications that could threaten the infant's life. (1, 7)

**57.** 1. The nurse should first inspect the perineum when the mother says she feels the baby is about to be born. The nurse should observe for crowning. It is vital in the situation described in this item to validate the patient's symptoms. If the mother is not ready to deliver, the nurse might then use such measures as timing the contractions and auscultating the fetal heart rate. (7)

**58.** 3. The nurse should immediately prepare a clean area for delivery of the baby when birth is imminent and no additional help is available. Trying to delay the birth is contraindicated. Therefore, the nurse must make the best preparations possible in the limited amount of time she has available. (7)

**59.** 3. When a nurse assumes responsibility during a precipitate delivery, explaining what is happening as the birth moves along and how the mother can assist is likely to help the mother remain calm and cooperative. The cliché "Everything is fine" is of little value and may arouse suspicion in the mother. Saying the physician will arrive soon may not be an accurate statement and is not very reassuring if the mother is concerned about the delivery. Telling the mother that many babies are born without benefit of a physician is nonsupportive of the mother. (7)

**60.** 1. It is best to deliver the head between contractions to prevent the head from emerging suddenly with subsequent damage to the perineum and possible cerebral damage to the infant. (7)

**61.** 2. As soon as the baby's head is delivered, it is important to check the infant's neck for the umbilical cord. If the cord encircles the neck, it should be pulled down *gently* and slipped over the infant's head, if possible. This is done to avoid cutting off the infant's oxygen supply, which may occur while the infant's shoulder presses on the cord during deliv-

ery, cutting off the infant's blood supply. If a loop of the cord around the neck cannot be removed, the cord is clamped and cut and the infant is delivered quickly to prevent asphyxiation. (7)

**62.** 2. Most authorities recommend clamping the cord about a minute after the baby is born, provided sterile equipment is available. There is no hurry to cut the cord, and in the situation described in this item it would be better to wait to cut the cord at a more convenient time. Using sterile technique and equipment is essential. (7)

**63.** 3. The best course of action is to wait for a sign of placental separation. Pulling on the cord before the placenta is detached may cause an eversion of the uterus. After separation occurs, the patient can be asked to bear down. After delivery of the placenta, the fundus may be massaged. (7)

**64.** 2. It is not uncommon to note that some membrane may trail after the birth of the placenta. The recommended procedure is to tease the membrane from the vagina with gentle up, down, and out motions. The trailings should not be cut or clamped. The uterus should be massaged after all parts of the placenta are delivered. Uterine contractions will not help the vagina contract and expel trailings of the placenta. (8)

**65.** 1. Birthing moves very rapidly when a precipitate delivery occurs. As a result, maternal tissue often tears, cerebral trauma to the infant may occur, and excessive postpartum bleeding may be present. Excessive bleeding is usually due to lacerations and often to having exhausted uterine musculature. The uterus is unlikely to rupture. (7)

**66.** 3. Babies born of mothers who smoke have lower-than-average birth weights. (7)

**67.** 1. Some of the factors that predispose to a rapid labor and delivery and the possibility of an emergency delivery include a history of multiparity, delivering an unanticipated premature infant, and a history of rapid labors in the past. Patients who must travel a long distance when in labor are also at risk for emergency deliveries. (7)

**68.** 1. During active labor when contractions occur only a few times within a 10-minute period, the patient is most likely to describe her discomfort as mild, or even painless. This type of labor is sometimes called hypotonic labor. It is exhausting because it prolongs the length of labor. (7)

**69.** 4. When preparing for the birth of twins, the nurse should be sure to have a double set of equipment available for two newborns. Twins are generally smaller than singlets and are at greater risk for various complications. Therefore, two persons skilled in resuscitation techniques should be available, as well as two sets of equipment for oxygen therapy and two resuscitators. Because there will be two infants, the nurse should also have two sets for cord care, identification, bassinets, clothing, and the like. However, two sets of anesthesia equipment are not needed for the mother who is about to deliver twins. (7)

**70.** 2. Dizygotic, or fraternal, twins develop from two ova and two sperm. They may be of the same sex, but their chances of resembling each other are no greater than that of any brother and sister. Identical, or monozygotic, twins develop from a single ovum and a single sperm. (7)

**71.** 4. Any complication is possible following delivery, but the woman who has delivered twins is especially likely to have uterine atony, which is the primary cause of postpartum hemorrhage. The uterus has been distended to a larger degree than normal by the presence of a multiple birth and this predisposes to uterine atony and postpartum hemorrhage. (7)

**72.** 3. When newborns must remain in the hospital after the mother is discharged, a problem in relation to parent-infant bonding is likely. To prevent it, a plan should be worked out for a reasonable method for the parents to visit their newborns and to handle and care for them as much as possible. Rivalry with siblings at home may also become a problem. Less likely to occur are feelings of resentment for having had twins, jealousy later in life between twins, and lack of interest in the care and nurture of newborns after their release from a hospital. (7)

**73.** 4. The patient should use exhale breathing while pushing to avoid the adverse physiologic effects of the Valsalva maneuver, which occurs with prolonged breath-holding during pushing. The technique for exhale breathing includes inhaling several deep breaths, then holding the breath for 5 to 6 seconds, and, finally, exhaling slowly every 5 to 6 seconds through pursed lips while continuing to hold the breath. Then another breath is taken and the process repeated. The Valsalva maneuver can also be avoided by exhaling continuously while pushing. The semi-Fowler's position enhances the effectiveness of abdominal muscle efforts during pushing. (7)

**74.** 4. A bilateral pudendal block is used for vaginal deliveries to relieve pain primarily in the perineum and vagina. It does not relieve discomfort in the uterus, cervix, or back. Pudendal-block anesthesia is adequate for an episiotomy and its repair and for most low-forceps deliveries when there are no complications. (7)

**75.** 2. An episiotomy serves several purposes. It shortens the second stage of labor, substitutes a clean surgical incision for a tear, and decreases undue stretching of muscles in the perineum. Flexion occurs early in the descent of the infant's head into the pelvis and will not be facilitated by an episiotomy. An episiotomy helps prevent a tear into the anal area but does not necessarily relieve pressure on the rectum during delivery. The third stage of labor is affected by an episiotomy. (7)

**76.** 1. Slowly removing the mother's legs from the stirrups helps prevent cramping. Also, lowering the legs increases blood flow to the extremities; if the legs are moved rapidly, the sudden demand for blood may cause fainting sensations. (7)

**77.** 3. Deep suctioning of the nasopharynx immediately after birth carries the danger of stimulating the vagus nerve, which causes a slow heartbeat. If the suctioning is carried out carelessly, mucous membranes can be injured. Suctioning does not abolish the infant's efforts to clear mucus. Oversuctioning may remove too much oxygen, which can cause respiratory distress. (7)

**78.** 2. The Apgar scoring chart evaluates a newborn on the basis of his or her color, heart rate, respiratory effort, muscle tone, and reflex irritability. (7)

**79.** 3. An Apgar score of 7 to 10 indicates the infant's condition is good. A score of 0 to 3 denotes very poor, or critical, condition. A score of 4 to 6 means the baby is in fair condition. (7)

**80.** 2. An infant judged to be in fair condition at birth has an Apgar score of between 4 and 6. The infant first should have his or her airway cleared. The next highest priority is to administer oxygen therapy to the infant. Cardiac massage is used only if the infant's heart stops beating. The infant needs warmth, but establishing satisfactory respirations has higher priority. (7)

**81.** 4. A disproportion between the size of the fetus and the birth canal is called cephalopelvic disproportion. It is usually caused when the woman has a contracted pelvis. When the head of the fetus fails to engage in the pelvis after "trial labor," cephalopelvic disproportion is very likely present. (7)

**82.** 3. Obtaining the diagonal conjugate requires the use of gloves because it involves vaginal penetration. The true conjugate (conjugata vera) is determined by subtracting 1.5 to 2 cm from the diagonal conjugate. The obstetric conjugate is equivalent to the true conjugate. The biischial diameter determines the transverse diameter of the pelvic outlet, which is the distance between the ischial tuberosities. It is measured with a pelvimeter. (7)

**83.** 1. The most important pelvic measurement is the

true conjugate (obstetric conjugate) when judging whether a woman's pelvis will allow for a normal vaginal delivery. (7)

**84.** 3. Preparation for a cesarean section is similar to preparation for any abdominal surgery. The patient must give the consent. Another person may not sign for the patient unless the patient is unable to sign for herself, in which case only certain designated persons may do so legally. (7)

**85.** 2. Preparing a patient for a cesarean delivery is similar in many ways to preparing other patients for abdominal surgery. For example, an indwelling catheter ensures that the urinary bladder will remain empty during surgery, atropine sulfate is used to help dry respiratory secretions, and the abdomen is shaved. However, the nurse should question an order for a narcotic drug before a cesarean delivery because of the depressing effects it is likely to have on the infant. The preoperative care of a patient having a cesarean delivery also includes monitoring the fetus's heart tones. (7)

**86.** 1. Studies have shown that there is no evidence of harm from a father's presence during a cesarean delivery. The father can offer support to the extent possible and, if the mother has general anesthesia, the father is present to help with parental-infant bonding at delivery. (7)

**87.** 1. The postoperative care of a patient who has general anesthesia for a cesarean section includes being prepared for a possible delay in the onset of spontaneous respirations in the infant, an increased likelihood of uterine atony, and a greater risk of maternal vomiting and aspiration than when

general anesthesia is not used. A general anesthetic does not influence milk production. (7)

**88.** 4. Respiratory distress syndrome is more common among babies born by cesarean section than among babies born vaginally. Such conditions as convulsions, cold stress, and umbilical-cord infections are not more greatly associated with cesarean births than with vaginal births. (7)

**89.** 2. Before an infant born by cesarean delivery and its mother are separated in the operating room, it is important that the mother has been fingerprinted and the infant has been footprinted. This measure is necessary for legal and safety reasons to avoid possible errors in identification. It is better if the mother awakens from anesthesia before the infant is removed to the nursery to promote maternal-infant bonding, but this is often impractical when the mother has had general anesthesia. Prophylactic eyedrops must be placed in a newborn's eyes—this is a legal requirement—but this need not be done in the operating room as long as it is done within 1 hour, 2 hours at most, after delivery. Having an accurate sponge count is unrelated to when the infant and mother are separated after a cesarean delivery. (7)

**90.** 3. In studies, women who had cesarean deliveries reported being frustrated, angry, disappointed, and having feelings of loss and grief. Some women felt relieved, even happy, especially if they had a complicated labor or if the timing of the cesarean delivery was elective. Indifference was not expressed as a result of having a cesarean delivery. (7)

# *test* 4

*The Postpartal Patient with a Vaginal Birth*
*The Postpartal Patient Who Breast-Feeds*
*The Postpartal Patient Who Bottle-Feeds*
*The Postpartal Patient with a Cesarean Birth*
*The Postpartal Patient with Risk Factors*
*Correct Answers and Rationales*

Select the one *best* or *correct* answer and indicate your choice by filling in the circle with a pencil in front of the option you have chosen. If the answer you would prefer is not given, select the one you think is *most appropriate*.

## THE POSTPARTAL PATIENT WITH A VAGINAL BIRTH

Ms. Kathleen Thames has delivered her first baby in a hospital that uses mother-baby nursing care (mother and baby are cared for in the mother's room by the same nurse).

1. The *primary* goal of the mother-baby method of care is to
   - ○ 1. allow for easier supervision of the baby.
   - ○ 2. decrease the risk of cross-infection among infants.
   - ○ 3. eliminate the necessity of having a routine for mother and baby.
   - ○ 4. provide opportunities for developing a positive relationship between mother and baby.
2. Baby Thames is breast-fed immediately after birth and then falls asleep. Ms. Thames asks the nurse when she should next breast-feed her infant. The nurse should base her response on knowledge concerning a newborn's activity periods and therefore should tell Ms. Thames to
   - ○ 1. wake the newborn in an hour to offer a feeding.
   - ○ 2. plan to feed the newborn in about 2 to 4 hours.
   - ○ 3. plan to feed the newborn again in about 8 hours.
   - ○ 4. plan *not* to feed the newborn again until the next day.
3. To instill a medication properly into Baby Thames' eyes, where in the eye should the medication be placed?
   - ○ 1. On the cornea.
   - ○ 2. At the inner canthus.
   - ○ 3. At the outer canthus.
   - ○ 4. In the lower conjunctival sac.

4. Which of the following biologic preparations is *inappropriate* as a prophylactic agent for ophthalmia neonatorum?
   - ○ 1. Gentian violet.
   - ○ 2. Penicillin drops.
   - ○ 3. Silver nitrate 1%.
   - ○ 4. Erythromycin (Ilotycin) ointment.
5. Baby Thames is ordered to have an intramuscular injection of phytonadione (AquaMEPHYTON). Which of the following muscles is *most often* recommended as the *best* to use?
   - ○ 1. The deltoid muscle.
   - ○ 2. The gluteus medius muscle.
   - ○ 3. The gluteus maximus muscle.
   - ○ 4. The vastus lateralis muscle.
6. When the nurse accidentally bumps the bassinet, Baby Thames throws out his arms, hands open, and begins to cry. The reflex Baby Thames is demonstrating is called the
   - ○ 1. Moro reflex.
   - ○ 2. rooting reflex.
   - ○ 3. grasping reflex.
   - ○ 4. tonic neck reflex.
7. The nurse assesses Ms. Thames' feelings during the recovery period. In response to the nurse's question about how she is feeling, Ms. Thames replies that she is tired, sore, and hungry. Ms. Thames then begins to discuss her birth experience. Based on the assessment data, the nurse will *correctly* place Ms. Thames in which of the following phases of postpartal psychological adaptation?
   - ○ 1. Giving-up.
   - ○ 2. Taking-in.
   - ○ 3. Letting-go.
   - ○ 4. Taking-hold.
8. As the nurse plans nursing interventions for Ms.

**133**

Thames for the first 24 hours, the nurse will anticipate that Ms. Thames' primary concern will *most
likely* be focused on her
○ 1. baby.
○ 2. husband.
○ 3. own comfort.
○ 4. mothering skills.

9. In preparing for modification of Ms. Thames' plan
of care to include continued postpartal psychological adaptation, the nurse would anticipate that
the *optimal* phase for providing the teaching-
learning experience for infant care skills and personal hygiene skills will be when Ms. Thames is in
which of the following postpartal psychological
adaptation phases?
○ 1. Taking-in.
○ 2. Letting-go.
○ 3. Taking-hold.
○ 4. Letting-down.

10. About 4 hours after delivery, Ms. Thames says she
has to urinate. The *best* course of action for the
nurse to take in this situation is to
○ 1. catheterize the patient.
○ 2. offer the patient a bedpan.
○ 3. check the patient's bladder for distention.
○ 4. assist the patient to walk to the bathroom.

11. Ms. Thames' bladder is noted to be distended.
When Ms. Thames tries to void, she has difficulty
starting urination. Ms. Thames' problem with
voiding is *most probably* due to having
○ 1. delivered a term infant.
○ 2. an infection in the bladder.
○ 3. pressure of the uterus on the bladder.
○ 4. edema in the area of the lower urinary organs.

12. Ms. Thames is unable to urinate and the nurse
prepares to catheterize her. Resistance to the
catheter is felt on catheter insertion. Which of the
following courses of action would be *most appropriate* for the nurse to take?
○ 1. Remove the catheter and wait about an hour
before trying again.
○ 2. Pull the catheter back about a half-inch before
trying to move it inward again.
○ 3. Allow the labia to fall into place and then gently
move the catheter inward again.
○ 4. Ask the patient to bear down gently as if to
void and slowly advance the catheter 2 to 3
inches.

13. Twelve hours after delivery, at what height would
the nurse expect to find Ms. Thames' uterine
fundus, if involution is normal?
○ 1. Slightly above the level of the umbilicus.
○ 2. Midway between the umbilicus and the symphysis pubis.

○ 3. Barely palpable above the upper margin of the
symphysis pubis.
○ 4. No specific height due to individual variation
among patients.

14. When the nurse checks Ms. Thames' fundus about
24 hours after delivery, she notes that it is to the
right of the midline. Which of the following conditions is the *most likely* cause for this finding?
○ 1. Constipation.
○ 2. Uterine atony.
○ 3. Urinary retention.
○ 4. Retention of blood clots.

15. Ms. Thames is to take her first shower since delivery. The nurse should stay nearby while Ms.
Thames showers *primarily* because she is most
likely to
○ 1. chill.
○ 2. faint.
○ 3. vomit.
○ 4. hemorrhage.

16. On Ms. Thames' 2nd postpartal day, the nurse
notes a large ecchymotic area to the right of
the perineum. Which of the following nursing
measures would be *most appropriate* in this situation?
○ 1. Apply an ice bag to the perineum.
○ 2. Continue with the patient's usual care.
○ 3. Increase the number of sitz baths from three to
six each day.
○ 4. Consult the physician about whether he wishes
to evacuate the hematoma.

17. The nurse observes that Ms. Thames is assuming
more of her own care and beginning to initiate
care for her infant as well. The phase of maternal
behavior that Ms. Thames is *most clearly* demonstrating is the
○ 1. let-down phase.
○ 2. taking-in phase.
○ 3. letting-go phase.
○ 4. taking-hold phase.

18. Ms. Thames wishes to start postpartum exercises.
Which of the following exercises should the nurse
teach her to use beginning on her 1st postpartum
day?
○ 1. While in a sitting position, lie back and then
return to a sitting position.
○ 2. While in a prone position, do push-ups by using
the arms to lift the upper body.
○ 3. While in a supine position with the knees
flexed, inhale deeply while allowing the abdomen to expand and then exhale while contracting the abdominal muscles.
○ 4. While in a supine position with the knees
flexed, bring the chin onto the chest wall while

inhaling, and reach for the knees by lifting the head and shoulders while exhaling.

**19.** If Ms. Thames experiences afterpains, a position in bed she could assume to help relieve them is the
- ○ 1. prone position.
- ○ 2. Sims' position.
- ○ 3. knee-chest position.
- ○ 4. mid-Fowler's position.

**20.** Of the following exercises, which is *best* for Ms. Thames to use the first few days after delivery?
- ○ 1. Leg lifts.
- ○ 2. Side-leg raises.
- ○ 3. Partial sit-ups.
- ○ 4. Perineal contractions (Kegel's exercises).

**21.** If progress is normal, on Ms. Thames' 2nd postpartal day the nurse should anticipate that her lochia will be
- ○ 1. pink.
- ○ 2. white.
- ○ 3. bright red.
- ○ 4. dark yellow.

**22.** Ms. Thames tells the nurse she has "cramps" every time she breast-feeds her newborn. The nurse's *best* course of action in this situation is to
- ○ 1. offer the patient a prescribed analgesic.
- ○ 2. advise the patient to nurse her infant less frequently.
- ○ 3. suggest to the patient that she ambulate more frequently.
- ○ 4. recommend to the patient that she take a prescribed laxative.

**23.** The nurse should explain to Ms. Thames that the "cramps" are uterine contractions caused by
- ○ 1. blood loss during delivery.
- ○ 2. retention of small placental tags.
- ○ 3. excessive stretching of the uterus.
- ○ 4. release of oxytocin during nursing.

**24.** Ms. Thames says that her baby spits up after feeding and asks why he does. The nurse should base her response on knowledge that regurgitation is believed to be due to an infant's normally having
- ○ 1. an immature cardiac sphincter.
- ○ 2. a small stomach in relation to his total size.
- ○ 3. slower peristaltic action than an older child.
- ○ 4. a proportionately longer gastrointestinal tract than an older child.

**25.** Ms. Thames asks the nurse, "How do I know that my baby is spitting up and not vomiting?" The nurse should teach Ms. Thames that, in contrast to regurgitated material, vomited material is characterized by
- ○ 1. being variable in amount.
- ○ 2. having a curdled appearance.

- ○ 3. appearing brownish in color.
- ○ 4. usually occurring before a feeding.

**26.** Ms. Thames asks, "Can my baby see?" Which of the following responses is *most accurate* concerning a newborn's eyesight?
- ○ 1. "Yes, but your baby can see but only moving figures."
- ○ 2. "Yes, your baby can see but only within a limited range."
- ○ 3. "No, your baby cannot see but he can distinguish light from dark."
- ○ 4. "No, your baby cannot see now but will be able to when he is about a week old."

**27.** The nurse teaches Ms. Thames to provide visual stimulation for her baby, which is *best* accomplished when Ms. Thames
- ○ 1. provides eye-to-eye contact with the infant.
- ○ 2. holds the infant so that he can look outdoors.
- ○ 3. wiggles her fingers in front of the infant's eyes.
- ○ 4. moves a brightly colored rattle in front of the infant's eyes.

**28.** Ms. Thames seems embarrassed when the nurse finds her talking to her newborn. In this situation, it is *best* for the nurse to base her response on knowledge that a newborn
- ○ 1. prefers high-pitched speech with tonal variations.
- ○ 2. responds to low-pitched speech with sameness of tone.
- ○ 3. likes communication that uses cooing sounds rather than words.
- ○ 4. cannot hear well enough to be aware of speech until he is about 4 weeks old.

**29.** Ms. Thames asks the nurse how often she may hold her baby without "spoiling him." Which of the following suggestions would be *best* for the nurse to offer Ms. Thames?
- ○ 1. "Hold him only when he is fussy. Then you will not spoil him."
- ○ 2. "Hold him as much as you like. Holding him will not spoil him."
- ○ 3. "Hold him only when he is being fed. Then you will not spoil him."
- ○ 4. "Hold him occasionally. But use an infant seat as much as possible to prevent spoiling him."

**30.** The night nurse finds Ms. Thames drenched in perspiration. The nurse should explain to Ms. Thames that the condition
- ○ 1. is uncommon but related to her milk coming in.
- ○ 2. is common and due to a temporary increase in sweat-gland activity.
- ○ 3. will be called to her physician's attention because excessive perspiration in the early puerperium is unusual.

○ 4. is often an early sign of infection and her physician will most likely order an antibiotic for her in the morning.

**31.** On the evening before she is to be discharged, Ms. Thames begins to cry because she worries about being able to care for her baby. Of the following interpretations, it would be *most appropriate* for the nurse to evaluate Ms. Thames as experiencing the

○ 1. taking-in phase of childbearing and exhibiting typical signs of sleep deprivation.

○ 2. postpartal blues phase of childbearing and possibly needing psychological counseling.

○ 3. letting-down phase of childbearing and needing help to take responsibility for caring for her newborn.

○ 4. taking-hold phase of childbearing and reacting to her feelings of inadequacy in relation to the care of her newborn.

**32.** Ms. Thames asks the nurse what method of contraception she should use until she has her 6-week checkup. The nurse should teach that one recommended choice is the condom, to be used by her husband in conjunction with

○ 1. a diaphragm.

○ 2. a spermicide.

○ 3. a vaginal douche.

○ 4. the rhythm method.

**33.** As part of discharge teaching, the nurse instructs Ms. Thames about the care of her newborn's umbilical cord area. Teaching should include having Ms. Thames care for the area by

○ 1. washing the umbilical cord area with soap and water.

○ 2. applying petrolatum jelly to the umbilical cord area.

○ 3. cleaning the umbilical cord area with hydrogen peroxide.

○ 4. swabbing the umbilical cord area with a pledget moistened with alcohol.

**34.** Ms. Thames asks the nurse, "What can I do so that my baby will not suck his thumb?" The nurse should explain that one way to minimize or eliminate thumb-sucking is to

○ 1. give the baby a pacifier.

○ 2. bandage the thumb the baby sucks.

○ 3. increase the amount of the baby's feedings.

○ 4. give the baby water each time he starts to suck his thumb.

**35.** When the baby is 1 month old, Ms. Thames stops by the hospital to show her primary nurse how the baby has grown. Ms. Thames tells the nurse that at first the baby's crying really bothered her, but that it doesn't bother her so much any more. Ms.

Thames says she now realizes her baby needs a fussy period each evening to work through frustrations. Based on these data, the nurse would determine that Ms. Thames is moving in which of the following directions in terms of her postpartal psychological adaptation?

○ 1. Backward to the taking-in phase.

○ 2. Forward to the letting-go phase.

○ 3. Continuously within the taking-hold phase.

○ 4. Between the taking-in and letting-go phases.

## THE POSTPARTAL PATIENT WHO BREAST-FEEDS

Ms. Andrea Underwood decides when she is 6 months pregnant to breast-feed her baby. She discusses this with a nurse in her physician's office during pregnancy and later after delivery.

**36.** Ms. Underwood says, "I'm worried that I won't be able to nurse my baby because my breasts are so small." Which of the following statements offers the nurse the *best* guide when she responds to Ms. Underwood's statement?

○ 1. Breast size does not influence the ability to nurse a baby.

○ 2. Women with small breasts tend to produce less milk than women with large breasts.

○ 3. The woman's belief in her ability to nurse is less important than the size of her breasts.

○ 4. The baby is able to grasp the nipples more easily when the breasts are small than when they are large.

**37.** Ms. Underwood asks what she can do to prepare for nursing the baby. The nurse should teach her that it would be *best* to

○ 1. apply alcohol to her nipples daily to toughen them for nursing.

○ 2. do nothing special since the breasts prepare themselves for nursing.

○ 3. keep her breasts clean by washing them daily with warm water.

○ 4. wash her breasts three times a day and follow that with a lanolin massage.

**38.** The nurse notes that Ms. Underwood has inverted nipples. Which of the following courses of action is *most appropriate* to teach Ms. Underwood during pregnancy?

○ 1. Wear a brassiere that is cut open at the nipples.

○ 2. Brush the nipples lightly daily with a terry-cloth towel.

○ 3. Do nothing until late in pregnancy; the nipples usually correct themselves without treatment.

○ 4. Push the areolar tissues away from the nipples; then grasp the nipples to tease them out of the tissues.

**39.** During her 7th month of pregnancy, Ms. Underwood calls the nurse because she notes fluid leaking from her nipples. The nurse should explain to her that

○ 1. this is colostrum and indicates her breasts are being readied for nursing.

○ 2. her milk has come in early and she should pump her breasts until the baby is born.

○ 3. she should come to the office because her physician will most likely prescribe a medication for this.

○ 4. she should limit her salt intake because most likely she is retaining fluids, which results in the discharge.

**40.** Ms. Underwood delivers a normal baby. The nurse teaches Ms. Underwood that she should *not* take medications while she is lactating unless the physician prescribes them. The rationale for this advice is that many drugs

○ 1. have been found to suppress milk production.

○ 2. have been found to depress the baby's appetite.

○ 3. are excreted in breast milk and will affect the baby.

○ 4. interfere with the milk-ejection reflex and predispose to breast engorgement.

**41.** If a medication is prescribed for Ms. Underwood, the nurse should teach her that, in relation to the time she nurses her baby, it is *best* to take the medication

○ 1. during a feeding.

○ 2. midway between feedings.

○ 3. immediately after a feeding.

○ 4. immediately before a feeding.

**42.** When counseling Ms. Underwood about her diet during lactation, the nurse should stress that, of the following food constituents, the one *especially* important for the lactating mother to have in larger amounts than the nonlactating mother is

○ 1. fats.

○ 2. protein.

○ 3. calories.

○ 4. vitamin K.

**43.** Ms. Underwood asks the nurse if she needs to adjust her intake of fluids. In relation to fluid intake during lactation, the nurse should explain that

○ 1. satisfying a normal appetite for fluid intake is appropriate.

○ 2. an increase in fluid intake is recommended to foster the production of milk.

○ 3. a decrease in fluid intake is recommended to avoid diluting the quality of the milk.

○ 4. a definite answer has not been established concerning fluid intake during lactation.

**44.** The nurse should teach Ms. Underwood that, of the following actions, the one that *best* stimulates the baby to open his mouth and grasp the nipple is to

○ 1. pull down on the infant's chin.

○ 2. squeeze the infant's cheek gently.

○ 3. place the nipple into the infant's mouth.

○ 4. brush the infant's lips lightly with the nipple.

**45.** Ms. Underwood asks the nurse about bubbling her baby. The nurse's response should be guided by knowledge that

○ 1. babies eat more if they are bubbled frequently.

○ 2. babies fed on demand rarely need to be bubbled.

○ 3. proper techniques of nursing eliminate the need for bubbling.

○ 4. breast-fed babies usually do not swallow as much air as bottle-fed babies.

**46.** Ms. Underwood tells the nurse that her nipples are sore from the baby's nursing. Which of the following measures would be *least likely* to alleviate the soreness?

○ 1. Nursing more frequently.

○ 2. Avoiding engorgement of the breasts.

○ 3. Changing nursing positions with nursing.

○ 4. Wearing a breast binder between nursings.

**47.** Ms. Underwood tells the nurse that her baby has trouble grasping the nipples. Upon assessment, the nurse notes that Ms. Underwood's breasts are engorged. Of the following measures, the one that is *least likely* to help relieve engorgement of the breasts is to

○ 1. take a hot shower before nursing the baby.

○ 2. massage the breasts before nursing the baby.

○ 3. express a little milk before nursing the baby.

○ 4. rub the nipples gently with lanolin before nursing the baby.

**48.** The nurse explains to Ms. Underwood that the *best* way to prevent breast engorgement is to

○ 1. increase her activities.

○ 2. wear a supportive brassiere.

○ 3. empty both breasts regularly.

○ 4. decrease fluid intake temporarily.

**49.** The nurse teaches Ms. Underwood how to express milk manually. The proper method for manual expression includes using the thumb and forefinger to

○ 1. alternately compress and release the nipple.

○ 2. compress and release the breast at the edge of the areola.

○ 3. slide forward from the edge of the areola toward the end of the nipple.

○ 4. roll the nipple between the fingers while exerting a gentle pull on the nipple.

50. Ms. Underwood asks the nurse how she will stop producing milk when she wishes to wean the baby. The nurse's response should be based on knowledge that the

○ 1. milk supply will diminish as the baby nurses less.

○ 2. physician usually orders a medication to suppress lactation.

○ 3. wearing of a tight breast binder usually is effective to suppress lactation.

○ 4. milk supply normally diminishes at approximately 4 to 6 months after delivery.

51. Ms. Underwood asks to be referred to someone to answer breast-feeding questions after discharge. Which of the following organizations would be *best* able to give Ms. Underwood information about breast feeding?

○ 1. The LaLeche League.

○ 2. The American Red Cross.

○ 3. The International Childbirth Education Association.

○ 4. The American Society for Psychoprophylaxis in Obstetrics.

52. Ms. Underwood says she is aware of the letdown sensation in her breasts and asks what causes it. The nurse should teach that the letdown sensation causes milk to move through milk ducts to sinuses and this movement is stimulated by a hormone called

○ 1. estrogen.

○ 2. oxytocin.

○ 3. prolactin.

○ 4. parathormone.

## THE POSTPARTAL PATIENT WHO BOTTLE-FEEDS

The nurse discusses formula preparation with a group of postpartal mothers at the pediatric clinic.

53. Ms. Vanslyke is using a commercial, premodified milk for her baby's formula. The nurse teaches *correctly* that commercial, premodified milks are diluted to have approximately the same number of calories per ounce as human milk, which normally is about

○ 1. 10 calories.

○ 2. 20 calories.

○ 3. 30 calories.

○ 4. 40 calories.

54. As a *general* rule, approximately how many calories each day per pound of body weight are required by newborns in order to maintain normal growth and development?

○ 1. 20 to 24 calories.

○ 2. 30 to 35 calories.

○ 3. 40 to 45 calories.

○ 4. 50 to 55 calories.

55. Ms. Washington expresses concern about the number of calories her baby is receiving. The nurse should explain that the factor having the *most* influence on determining the number of calories the infant requires is the

○ 1. sex of the baby.

○ 2. baby's birth weight.

○ 3. comparison of her baby's serial weights.

○ 4. type of feeding the baby receives (breast or formula).

56. Ms. Xhu lives in a community where tap water meets public health requirements for safety. How should Ms. Xhu be taught to prepare her baby's bottles before filling them with formula?

○ 1. Boil the bottles for a minimum of 10 minutes.

○ 2. Wash the bottles in soapy water and then rinse them well.

○ 3. Place the bottles in a warm oven (225° F.) for a minimum of 20 minutes.

○ 4. Soak the bottles in a vinegar solution for about a half-hour and then rinse them well.

57. After Ms. Xhu is taught how to prepare bottles for formula, Ms. Ybarra asks, "Is that the only way it can be done?" The nurse explains that there is an alternative. If Ms. Ybarra has the following kitchen appliances, which should the nurse recommend she use?

○ 1. A dishwasher.

○ 2. A toaster oven.

○ 3. A microwave oven.

○ 4. A slow-cooker pot.

58. Ms. Anderson uses the terminal method of sterilization when preparing formula. She uses clean equipment and formula. She then sterilizes filled, loosely capped bottles and places them in a tightly covered boiling-water bath. The *minimum* number of minutes *most* authorities recommend that bottles of formula be kept in the boiling-water bath when using terminal sterilization is

○ 1. 15 minutes.

○ 2. 25 minutes.

○ 3. 35 minutes.

○ 4. 45 minutes.

**59.** Ms. Zamora lives in a one-room cabin in a migrant workers' village. The nurse recommends that Ms. Zamora use powdered formula and prepare each bottle of formula as it is needed. The nurse *most probably* makes this recommendation to Ms. Zamora when she learns that Ms. Zamora's home is *without* access to

○ 1. an oven.

○ 2. a telephone.

○ 3. a refrigerator.

○ 4. a safe water supply.

**60.** When teaching the mothers how to care for the nipple after bottle-feeding their infants, the nurse explains that it is *best* to

○ 1. scrub the nipple in warm soapy water.

○ 2. wash the nipple under hot running water.

○ 3. boil the nipple for a short time before handling it.

○ 4. soak the nipple in a mild disinfectant before washing it.

## THE POSTPARTAL PATIENT WITH A CESAREAN BIRTH

Ms. Mary Zak delivered a term female infant by cesarean section due to cephalopelvic disproportion. This is her first birth.

**61.** The nurse assesses Ms. Zak's feelings about having a cesarean birth instead of a vaginal birth. The nurse would anticipate that the feeling *least likely* to be expressed by Ms. Zak will be

○ 1. anger.

○ 2. fatigue.

○ 3. disappointment.

○ 4. enhancement of self-esteem.

**62.** In an attempt to help Ms. Zak view her cesarean delivery as a birthing experience rather than a surgical experience, the nurse would focus intervention efforts on reinforcing the basic purpose for the use of cesarean birth. Cesarean birth would *least likely* be used as an intervention for

○ 1. fetal distress.

○ 2. maternal fatigue.

○ 3. fetal well-being.

○ 4. maternal distress.

**63.** Ms. Zak is to have a clear liquid diet as tolerated following her cesarean section. Under which of the following circumstances would serving Ms. Zak's diet be *contraindicated*?

○ 1. The patient has no bowel sounds.

○ 2. The patient has abdominal distention.

○ 3. The patient has marked discomfort in the operative area.

○ 4. The patient has had no bowel movement since she had surgery.

**64.** Ms. Zak complains of "gas pains" postoperatively. Of the following measures, it would be *best* for the nurse to

○ 1. offer the patient ice chips.

○ 2. keep the patient on bed rest.

○ 3. serve the patient orange juice.

○ 4. increase the patient's activities.

**65.** Ms. Zak should turn, cough, and deep-breathe regularly following her cesarean birth, *primarily* to help prevent

○ 1. pleurisy.

○ 2. adhesions.

○ 3. subinvolution.

○ 4. respiratory congestion.

**66.** After determining that Ms. Zak's fundus is firm and in the midline, the nurse ambulates Ms. Zak for the first time after delivery. A moderate amount of lochia gushes from Ms. Zak's vagina. Of the following courses of action, it would be *best* for the nurse to

○ 1. put the patient to bed and notify the physician.

○ 2. place the patient in bed in the Trendelenburg position promptly.

○ 3. help the patient lie down in bed and massage her fundus until firm.

○ 4. continue to ambulate the patient and explain that the gush is caused by pooling of discharge in the vagina.

**67.** The nurse has determined that Ms. Zak is in the taking-in phase of postpartal psychological adaptation. As the nurse anticipates Ms. Zak's need during the taking-in phase, the nursing intervention that the nurse would *least likely* expect to provide would be

○ 1. providing nourishing food and snacks.

○ 2. facilitating uninterrupted periods of rest.

○ 3. discussing the birthing experience with Ms. Zak.

○ 4. asking for a return demonstration of infant care skills.

**68.** When Ms. Zak is changing her baby's diaper, she questions the nurse about some red-tinged drainage from the baby's vagina. Of the following responses, which would be the *most appropriate* for the nurse to make?

○ 1. "It is of no concern because it is such a small amount."

○ 2. "The cause of vaginal bleeding in newborns is unknown. I'll report it to your physician."

○ 3. "Sometimes baby girls have a small amount of

vaginal bleeding due to hormones received from the mother."

○ 4. "Vaginal bleeding in newborns is caused by a temporary bleeding problem. I'll check to see whether your baby has received a medication for it."

69. A week after she is discharged, Ms. Zak calls the maternity unit and says that she is afraid she is losing her milk because the baby has been nursing every 4 hours and now is crying to be fed every 2 hours. Which of the following statements is the *most likely* reason for the baby's need for more frequent feedings?
   ○ 1. The baby is not digesting the breast milk properly.
   ○ 2. The mother is having a temporary decrease in her milk supply.
   ○ 3. The mother is most likely not allowing the baby enough time to suck with each feeding.
   ○ 4. The baby is in a temporary growth spurt and requires more frequent feedings for the time being.

## THE POSTPARTAL PATIENT WITH RISK FACTORS

Ms. Jennifer Brown delivered her second infant prematurely and the infant died. Ms. Brown is Rh negative and the infant Rh positive.

70. Ms. Brown asks to see the the baby soon after his death. Which of the following statements offers the nurse the *best* guide for answering Ms. Brown's request?
   ○ 1. The mother should be allowed to view the body but only if the fetus is physically normal.
   ○ 2. The mother should be allowed to view the body because this has been found to help complete the grieving process.
   ○ 3. The mother should not be allowed to view the body because seeing the baby may precipitate postpartum depression.
   ○ 4. The mother should not be allowed to view the body because it is the nurse's responsibility to protect her from unnecessary trauma.

71. Ms. Brown asks how she should tell her 4-year-old son about the baby's death. Of the following responses, which is *most appropriate* for the nurse to make?
   ○ 1. "Tell him God took the baby to heaven."

○ 2. "Explain to him that death is a long sleep."
○ 3. "I think he is too young to understand what happened."
○ 4. "He may be lonely at first. Tell me how you think he will feel."

72. Ms. Brown is a candidate for RhoGAM. The nurse should anticipate that the *best* time for Ms. Brown to receive the immunoglobulin
   ○ 1. was during labor.
   ○ 2. at her 6-week postpartal checkup.
   ○ 3. immediately after delivery of the placenta.
   ○ 4. within 3 days after the birth of her infant.

73. The nurse should question the physician's order *unless* the route by which the Rh immunoglobulin (RhoGAM) is to be administered to Ms. Brown is the
   ○ 1. oral route.
   ○ 2. intravenous route.
   ○ 3. subcutaneous route.
   ○ 4. intramuscular route.

74. Two days after Ms. Brown receives the Rh immunoglobulin, the decision is made to do either a Kleihauer-Betke test or an indirect Coombs test on her blood. The *primary* purpose for doing one of these tests is to determine whether Ms. Brown has
   ○ 1. developed an ABO incompatibility.
   ○ 2. experienced prior Rh sensitization.
   ○ 3. had a transfusion reaction sometime in the past.
   ○ 4. received an adequate amount of the Rh immunoglobulin.

Ms. Pattie Crawford is admitted to have her tenth baby. She is an insulin-dependent class A diabetic.

75. Ms. Crawford's children are all living and include one set of twins and one set of triplets. At this time, what gravida is Ms. Crawford?
   ○ 1. Gravida 5.
   ○ 2. Gravida 7.
   ○ 3. Gravida 9.
   ○ 4. Gravida 11.

76. Ms. Crawford delivers a normal infant. Which of the following postpartum complications is Ms. Crawford *more likely* to have than a woman who has delivered only one or two babies?
   ○ 1. Uterine atony.
   ○ 2. Vaginal hematoma.
   ○ 3. Puerperal infection.
   ○ 4. Urinary tract infection.

77. During the first 24 hours after delivery, the nurse can expect that Ms. Crawford's insulin require-

ments, when compared with requirements during pregnancy, are *most likely* to be

- ○ 1. markedly decreased.
- ○ 2. markedly increased.
- ○ 3. the same as during pregnancy.
- ○ 4. so varied that adjustments need to be made on an individual basis.

**78.** The nurse notes that Ms. Crawford's fundus is "boggy." Which of the following actions would be *most appropriate* for the nurse to take?

- ○ 1. Notify the physician.
- ○ 2. Massage the patient's fundus.
- ○ 3. Elevate the foot of the patient's bed.
- ○ 4. Express clots from the patient's uterus.

**79.** Later, when the nurse is assessing Ms. Crawford, she observes that Ms. Crawford's fundus has risen above the umbilicus and is displaced to the right. In this situation, the *best* course of action for the nurse to take is to

- ○ 1. assist the patient to void.
- ○ 2. massage the patient's fundus.
- ○ 3. place an abdominal binder on the patient's abdomen.
- ○ 4. help the patient into a mid-Fowler's position in bed.

Ms. Mary Moore is a 32-year-old primipara who delivered a 3,600-g infant vaginally with the aid of low-forceps application and a midline episiotomy

**80.** In preparing to develop a plan of care for Ms. Moore, the nurse would review Ms. Moore's prenatal and birthing records. Which of the following information, if present in the records, would *most likely* alert the nurse to anticipate that Ms. Moore could be at risk for infection?

- ○ 1. Vaginal laceration.
- ○ 2. Leukocytosis of 15,000/mm$^3$.
- ○ 3. Blood loss of 500 ml at delivery.
- ○ 4. Moniliasis during the third trimester.

**81.** In order to plan the assessments of Ms. Moore for signs of infection, the nurse analyzes interventions that have resulted in the decrease in maternal morbidity and mortality. The nurse determines that the intervention that has *least likely* resulted in decreased maternal morbidity and mortality rates is

- ○ 1. aseptic technique.
- ○ 2. antibiotic therapy.
- ○ 3. increase in surgical intervention.
- ○ 4. reduction of debilitative disease.

**82.** The routine nursing assessment of Ms. Moore's episiotomy would be *least likely* to include assessment for

- ○ 1. pallor.
- ○ 2. edema.
- ○ 3. discharge.
- ○ 4. approximation.

**83.** As part of the preparation for assessing Ms. Moore's perineum and anus, the nurse should decide that the *best* position for Ms. Moore to be placed in for the assessment would be

- ○ 1. Sims' position.
- ○ 2. Fowler's position.
- ○ 3. the prone position.
- ○ 4. the supine position.

**84.** Nursing assessment reveals that Ms. Moore has a temperature of 100.6° F. and 100.8° F., respectively, on her 2nd and 3rd postpartal days. The nurse *correctly* interprets the temperature elevation to be

- ○ 1. precipitated by breast engorgement.
- ○ 2. a potential sign of postpartal infection.
- ○ 3. normal postpartal adjustment to being N.P.O. during labor.
- ○ 4. the result of intensified postpartal diaphoresis and diuresis.

**85.** Ms. Moore is diagnosed as having a puerpural infection. In analyzing factors that contributed to the development of the infection, the nurse decides that the *most likely* contributor to the infection was

- ○ 1. maternal age (over 30).
- ○ 2. vaginal manipulation and trauma.
- ○ 3. normal vaginal flora present in pregnancy.
- ○ 4. presence of bacteria in the hospital environment.

**86.** Ms. Moore begins antibiotic therapy consisting of ampicillin sodium (Polycillin) intravenously and kanamycin sulfate (Kantrex) intramuscularly. Ms. Moore says she has no drug allergies. The nurse reviews the adverse effects of ampicillin and kanamycin to plan for the assessment of potential adverse reactions. Based on a review of the medications, the nurse would be *least likely* to assess Ms. Moore for

- ○ 1. a rash.
- ○ 2. dizziness.
- ○ 3. increased bleeding.
- ○ 4. difficulty breathing.

Ms. Nelda Newsom, 39, is a grand multipara who weighed 305 pounds at her last prenatal visit. Ms. Newsom was delivered by cesarean section for fetal distress.

**87.** After reviewing Ms. Newsom's prenatal and delivery records, the nurse determines that Ms.

Newsom is at risk for development of thromboembolic disease. Of the following data, which was *least likely* to be interpreted by the nurse as a factor predisposing to thromboembolic disease?

○ 1. Obesity.
○ 2. Maternal age.
○ 3. Maternal gravida.
○ 4. Anesthesia and surgery.

**88.** Since Ms. Newsom is considered at risk for thromboembolic disease, the nurse plans to assess her for signs and symptoms of the disease. The nurse decides that the nursing assessment *most likely* to identify a symptom of thromboembolic disease would be

○ 1. Homan's sign.
○ 2. Chandelier sign.
○ 3. deep tendon reflexes.
○ 4. costovertebral angle tenderness.

**89.** Ms. Newsom's physician orders heparin (Panheprin) therapy prophylactically. Ms. Newsom asks the nurse why she needs the medicine. The nurse reviews the desired effect of heparin and *correctly* responds that Ms. Newsom is receiving the medication to

○ 1. make her blood thinner.
○ 2. hasten discharge of lochia.
○ 3. promote uterine involution.
○ 4. prevent blood-clot formation.

**90.** Nursing assessment to evaluate the effectiveness of the heparin (Panheprin) therapy and the prevention of side effects would *least likely* include assessment of

○ 1. lochia alba.
○ 2. the intravenous site.
○ 3. calf tenderness.
○ 4. peripheral pulses.

Opal Overton is a gravida 2 who delivered twins vaginally a few hours ago.

**91.** The nurse who is recovering Ms. Overton should assess her for symptoms of early postpartum hemorrhage. Which of the following data used by

the nurse to determine Ms. Overton's predisposition for hemorrhage would *most likely* support the nurse's anticipation of early postpartal hemorrhage?

○ 1. Oligohydramnios.
○ 2. Multiple gestation.
○ 3. A 12-hour labor.
○ 4. Birth of a 3,600-g infant.

**92.** The nurse evaluates Ms. Overton for clinical manifestations of the *primary* cause of early postpartum hemorrhage. Of the following symptoms, which is the *primary* cause of early postpartum hemorrhage?

○ 1. Uterine atony.
○ 2. Vulvar hematoma.
○ 3. Vaginal lacerations.
○ 4. Retained placental fragments.

**93.** The nurse evaluates the plan of care for Ms. Overton. Which of the following nursing interventions would the nurse be *least likely* to use in assessing Ms. Overton for early postpartum hemorrhage?

○ 1. Assessment of uterine tone.
○ 2. Assessment of lochia amount.
○ 3. Assessment of bladder fullness.
○ 4. Assessment of vulvar discomfort.

**94.** If Ms. Overton develops early postpartal hemorrhage, the nurse would be prepared to perform which of the following interventions *first*?

○ 1. Uterine massage.
○ 2. Intravenous infusion.
○ 3. Foley catheter insertion.
○ 4. Notification of the physician.

**95.** Ms. Overton's fundus remains firm and her lochia is rubra and moderate in amount during the first 24 hours after delivery. Based on the uterine and lochia assessment data, the nurse is *correct* in deciding that Ms. Overton

○ 1. is at risk for late postpartum hemorrhage.
○ 2. remains at risk for early postpartum hemorrhage.
○ 3. is no longer at risk for early postpartum hemorrhage.
○ 4. needs to be assessed for 24 hours more for hemorrhage risk.

# CORRECT ANSWERS AND RATIONALES

Numbers appear in parentheses following the rationales. The numbers identify textbooks listed in the references at the end of Part II, where correct answers can be verified.

## *The Postpartal Patient with a Vaginal Birth*

**1.** 4. The mother-baby method of care has been developed primarily to provide convenient and frequent opportunities for developing a positive relationship between the mother and her infant. (7)

**2.** 2. The newborn is awake and alert for about the first 30 minutes after delivery, when he may be fed. Then, he usually falls asleep for about 2 to 4 hours, when he awakens and can be fed again. Typically, the newborn will not awaken to eat while he is in a sleep phase. (7)

**3.** 4. A medication placed in the eye is best instilled into the lower conjunctival sac. Much of the medication is likely to be lost if placed in the inner or outer canthus. The medication may irritate and damage the cornea if placed on it. (7)

**4.** 1. Gentian violet is not used as a prophylactic agent for ophthalmia neonatorum. Such agents as penicillin drops, silver nitrate 1%, and erythromycin (Ilotycin) ointment are appropriate. (7)

**5.** 4. The vastus lateralis muscle is most frequently recommended for intramuscular injections in the newborn. The muscle affords the best tissue and the least likelihood of injuring other structures. The gluteus muscles are not recommended because of the danger of injuring the sciatic nerve. The deltoid muscle is too small in a newborn for administering medications intramuscularly. (7)

**6.** 1. The Moro, or startle, reflex is present when the infant responds to stimuli by extending the arms, hands open, and then by moving the arms in an embracing motion. The Moro reflex should be present at birth but disappears when the infant reaches about 3 months of age. The grasping reflex is present when the infant grasps an object placed in his hand. The rooting reflex is present when the infant turns his head and opens his mouth after being stimulated on the cheek. This reflex is also called the sucking reflex. The tonic neck reflex is demonstrated when the infant, while lying on his back, turns his head to one side. (7)

**7.** 2. The mother is in the taking-in phase during the first hours and up to 2 to 3 days immediately following birth. During this time food and sleep are a major focus for her. In addition, she works through her birth experience to sort out reality from fantasy and clarify any misunderstandings. The taking-hold phase is the second phase of postpartal psychological adaptation, and the letting-go phase is the final phase of postpartal psychological adaptation. (3, 7)

**8.** 3. During the taking-in phase of maternal postpartum adjustment, the mother's primary concern is with her own needs. The taking-in phase usually lasts for the first 2 to 3 days after birth. (3, 7)

**9.** 3. The taking-hold phase begins after completion of the taking-in phase and lasts about 10 days. During the taking-hold phase of postpartal psychological adaptation, the mother is concerned with her need to resume control of all facets of her life in a competent manner. Thus, at this time she is ready to learn self-care and infant care skills. The letting-go phase is the final phase of postpartal psychological adaptation. (3)

**10.** 4. Usually, the patient is able to begin ambulating sufficiently to walk to the bathroom, with the nurse's assistance, between about 4 and 8 hours after delivery. It is usually unnecessary to use the bedpan. Catheterization should be used only as the *last* resort if a patient is unable to void after delivery. (7)

**11.** 4. Edema is ordinarily present in the area of the lower urinary organs following delivery. This condition often makes it difficult to start voiding. Hyperemia of the bladder mucosa is also noted to be present. The combination of hyperemia and edema predisposes to a decrease in the sensation to void, overdistention of the bladder, and incomplete emptying of the bladder. Nursing care of the postpartum patient should include careful monitoring of the urinary bladder to help prevent retention and its associated problems. (7)

**12.** 4. The catheter may have caused a temporary spasm at the internal sphincter resulting in resistance. It is recommended that the patient be asked to bear down gently as if to void to promote sphincter relaxation. This technique usually helps overcome a temporary spasm. If the catheter is removed entirely, a new sterile catheter must be obtained and a second attempt made to introduce it. Pulling the catheter out a bit and allowing the labia to fall into place are contraindicated because of the danger of introducing organisms that could cause a urinary tract infection. (9)

**13.** 1. It can be expected that the height of the patient's uterus will be felt slightly above the umbilicus. This is normal approximately 12 hours after delivery. Unless complications occur, this mother could expect normal progress of involution. Immediately after delivery, however, the top of the uterus will normally be midway between the umbilicus and the symphysis pubis. It descends at the rate of approximately one fingerbreadth each day. It will be barely palpable above the upper margin of the symphysis pubis approximately 7 to 10 days after delivery. Although there is individual variation, these are the common normal ranges. (7)

**14.** 3. A full bladder is likely to push the uterus to the right of the midline. When the bladder is empty, the uterus normally lies approximately in the midline. Other causes for a uterus observed to be on one side include having the mother lying or sleeping on the side or having a relaxation of the uterus; the latter instance may cause bleeding. (7)

**15.** 2. Patients sometimes feel faint owing to the sudden change in blood circulation in the body when ambulating for the first time after delivery. Primarily for this reason, the nurse should stay nearby while the patient takes her first shower after delivery. (1, 7)

**16.** 2. No special treatment is indicated when an ecchymotic area is observed. Ice is effective immediately to reduce bleeding or swelling but not on the 2nd postpartal day. Heat would be more appropriate, but three sitz baths daily would appear to be adequate. (7)

**17.** 4. Maternal behavior has been observed to pass through distinct phases after the birth of an infant. The first phase is the taking-in phase, when the mother is consumed primarily with her own dependency needs. The second phase is the taking-hold phase when the mother is concerned with taking care of her own needs and with initiating her first motherly (caretaker) tasks with her infant. The third phase, letting go, is present when the mother begins to realize the separateness of her life and that of her infant and that she is no longer childless. She adjusts to her life and takes responsibility for the care of her child. Another phase is the let-down phase, often called the postpartal or "baby" blues, when feelings of depression and irritability are typical. (7)

**18.** 3. When delivery has been uncomplicated, postpartum exercises may begin on the 1st postpartum day with exercises to strengthen the abdominal muscles. This is done by inhaling deeply while allowing the abdomen to expand and exhaling while contracting the abdominal muscles. Such exercises as reaching for the knees, push-ups, and sit-ups are ordinarily too strenuous to use as early as the 1st postpartum day but may be worked up to later in the postpartum period. (7)

**19.** 1. A position in bed that may help relieve the afterpains is lying on the abdomen. A pillow placed under the abdomen to apply additional pressure may increase comfort and/or relief. (7)

**20.** 4. For the first few days after delivery, the recommended exercise is perineal contractions. The exercise stimulates muscle tone in the area of the perineum and around the urinary meatus and vaginal orifice. Such exercises as leg lifts, head raising, and partial sit-ups are generally too strenuous for the first few days postpartum. (1)

**21.** 3. The vaginal discharge that normally occurs for approximately 3 days after delivery is called rubra because it contains mostly blood and is bright red. The discharge then becomes more serous and watery and is called serosa. About the 10th day after delivery, the discharge becomes thinner, scanty, and almost without color; it is called alba. (7)

**22.** 1. Multiparas, more frequently than primiparas, tend to experience cramps when they breast-feed their newborns. This is because breast-feeding causes oxytocin to be released, which causes uterine muscles to contract. The uterine muscles tend to be more tonically contracted after delivery in primiparas. An analgesic is most commonly offered to provide relief from the discomfort. (7)

**23.** 4. Breast-feeding stimulates the secretion of oxytocin, which causes the uterine muscles to contract. These contractions account for the discomfort associated with afterpains. They are not related to blood loss. Afterpains tend to be more common when small placental tags have been retained, when the uterus has been excessively stretched, and with increasing parity. (7)

**24.** 1. Regurgitation in the newborn is thought to be due to the infant's having an immature cardiac sphincter. The spitting represents an overflow of the stomach and is probably due to feeding the infant too fast or too much. (1, 7)

**25.** 2. Vomited material has been digested and looks very much like curdled milk. It has a sour odor. Vomiting usually occurs between feedings and empties the stomach of its content. In contrast, infants regurgitate undigested material that does not have a sour odor during or immediately after a feeding. The amount of material is not a safe guide in distinguishing vomiting from regurgitation. (6)

**26.** 2. The newborn has immature oculomotor coordination, an inability to accommodate for distance, and poorly developed eyes, visual nerves, and brain. However, the normal newborn has eyesight and can see with clarity within a distance of about 9 to 12 inches (22 to 30 cm). (7)

**27.** 1. Newborns like to look at eyes, and providing eye-to-eye contact between parents and their infant is a good way to provide visual stimulation. The parents' eyes are circular, move from side to side, and become larger and smaller, and newborns have been observed to fix on them. It has been demonstrated that in general newborns prefer circular objects of darkness against a white background. (7)

**28.** 1. Speaking to infants is very important, and the nurse should encourage mothers to do so. Some authorities believe it is the most important aspect of sensory stimulation in a newborn. Newborns respond best when speech has variations in tone and is associated with a high-pitched voice. Words should be spoken slowly. Cooing can be used but a newborn responds to words, and they should be used too as a stimulus to language development later in life. A newborn can hear all sounds greater than about 55 decibels. (7)

**29.** 2. Tactile stimulation of the newborn is important and should be encouraged. Holding and patting infants helps them develop trust. (7)

**30.** 2. Excessive perspiration is common during the puerperium. As described in this item, it is an unlikely sign of infection. It is temporary and does not ordinarily require any treatment other than to keep the patient comfortable. (7)

**31.** 4. A new mother often has concerns about her ability to care for her infant properly during the taking-hold phase of childbearing. During this phase, the mother is working toward independence and autonomy, and she wants to be able to perform well. She needs emotional support, advice on how to manage, reassurance, and reinforcement of appropriate behavior. Postpartal blues are characterized by irritability and generally occur later in the puerperium. Psychological counseling is rarely necessary. The let-down phase is sometimes used to describe the postpartal blues. (7)

**32.** 2. A spermicide is often recommended for contraception after delivery until the patient has her 6-week checkup, after which another type may be used. Also, the husband can use a condom, and some authorities recommend that both a condom and a spermicide be used. The rhythm method is unsafe because the patient is unlikely to be able to determine when she ovulates until her menstrual cycle returns. Neither a vaginal douche nor a diaphragm are recommended. (7)

**33.** 4. It is best to clean the newborn's umbilical cord area with a pledget moistened with alcohol. The alcohol promotes drying and helps decrease the incidence of infection. Sometimes, an antibiotic ointment may be used instead of alcohol. Such agents as hydrogen peroxide, petrolatum jelly, and soap and water have not been found to be as effective as using alcohol or an antibiotic ointment. (7)

**34.** 1. Infants suck fingers for comfort and security. If the primary caretaker objects to thumb sucking, a pacifier can be offered. Giving the infant a blanket may also be used if a pacifier is objectionable to the mother. Thumb sucking is considered harmless unless used to an extreme. If an infant sucks a finger a great deal into late infancy, dental malformation may occur. Increasing feedings, offering water, and bandaging the thumb are not advised. (7)

**35.** 2. The mother described in this situation is progressing forward into the letting-go phase. This phase is initiated as the third phase of postpartal psychological adaptation and continues throughout life. This phase is characterized by the mother's acceptance that the infant is a separate individual rather than an extension of herself; the mother recognizes the infant's/child's need for increased independence at various stages of growth and development. (3)

## *The Postpartal Patient Who Breast-Feeds*

**36.** 1. Various hormones play a role in lactation. Prolactin, a pituitary hormone, has a central role. A variety of factors influence milk supply, such as the infant's suckling, emptying of the breasts, and the mother's diet, exercise, rest, and level of contentment. The size of the breasts is not important as long as there is glandular tissue to secrete the milk. The fat in breast tissue plays no role in milk production. (7)

**37.** 3. The best preparation for breast-feeding is washing the breasts daily with warm water. The expectant mother should avoid soap because of its drying effect. Retracted nipples may be prepared by stretching or rolling or by using nipple cups. Exposing the nipples to sunlight when possible during the last trimester may help decrease soreness when first nursing. Using alcohol and massaging several times a day are not recommended. (1, 7)

**38.** 4. The areolar tissues can be pushed in and away from the nipples. Then the nipples can be grasped and pulled out gently. Using a Woolwich breast shield, which pushes the nipples through openings in the shield, is also effective to help overcome inverted nipples. (7)

**39.** 1. During the last trimester of pregnancy, a woman may notice that she is leaking a fluid from her nipples. This is colostrum, a precursor of milk. It is recommended that the mother keep the nipples clean so that colostrum does not dry and form a crust on the nipples, a condition that would predispose to sore and cracked nipples. (7)

**40.** 3. Medications can be secreted in the milk and then influence the baby. Except for prescribed drugs, medications are not recommended for lactating mothers. (7)

**41.** 3. Taking a drug after nursing will help minimize the infant's exposure to the drug because drugs are most highly concentrated in the body soon after they are taken. (7)

**42.** 3. One of the most important factors for the lactating mother to include in her diet is calories. An inadequate calorie intake can reduce milk volume, but milk quality should not be affected. (7)

**43.** 2. An increase in fluid intake is recommended during lactation to foster milk production and to replace the fluids that the baby consumes with nursing. Inadequate fluid intake may decrease milk volume. Eight to ten glasses of fluid (water, juice, milk, soup) a day are recommended. (7)

**44.** 4. Lightly brushing the infant's lips with the nipple causes the infant to open his mouth and begin sucking. Such techniques as pulling down on the infant's chin, squeezing his cheek, or placing the nipple directly into the infant's mouth force his mouth open or force him to take the nipple. The infant should be taught to open his mouth and grasp the nipple on his own; he should not be forced to nurse. (7)

**45.** 4. While it is true that breast-fed babies do not swallow as much air as bottle-fed babies, breast-fed babies still should be bubbled in the middle and at the end of each feeding. (7)

**46.** 4. Wearing a breast binder will not alleviate the discomfort of sore nipples. Suggestions to help avoid sore nipples include changing position with each nursing so that different areas of the nipples have the greatest stress from nursing, avoiding engorgement of the breasts, which makes it difficult for the infant to grasp the nipple, nursing more frequently so that a ravenous infant is not vigorously sucking during the beginning of nursings, and feeding the infant on demand so that he is not overly hungry, which causes him to suck vigorously. Exposing the nipples to light is recommended as necessary. Some authorities have also recommended using warm tea bags, which contain tannic acid, as compresses to help healing. (7)

**47.** 4. A variety of measures may be tried to relieve engorgement of the breasts, such as massaging the breasts before nursing to help bring the milk down to the sinuses where the infant can obtain it and expressing a little milk before nursing the infant. Taking a hot shower or applying hot packs to the breasts are techniques that have been found helpful to improve the milk flow. Using an oxytocic nasal spray has also been used because it acts to promote the letdown reflex in the breasts. Applying lanolin to the nipples will not relieve engorgement. (7)

**48.** 3. It is better to prevent engorgement if possible. The best technique is to empty the breasts regularly and frequently with nursings. It has been found that engorgement is less likely to occur when the mother and infant are together, as in single-room maternity care, because nursing can occur conveniently to meet the infant's and mother's needs. Increasing activity and wearing a supportive brassiere will not prevent engorgement. Decreasing fluid intake is not advised. (7)

**49.** 2. The best technique to express milk from the breast is to alternately compress and release the breast at the edge of the areola. The thumb is positioned on top and two fingers on the bottom of the breast at the edge of the areola. The mother pushes in toward her chest and then squeezes her thumb and fingers together while pulling forward on the areola without sliding her fingers or thumb on her skin. Manipulating the nipples may injure them. (7)

**50.** 1. The milk supply diminishes normally as the baby nurses less. The gradual method of weaning by eliminating one feeding at a time over several weeks is the *best* recommendation. Lactation suppression by medication is most effective when it is started as soon after delivery as maternal vital signs are stable. Mechanical methods of lactation suppression (a breast binder) are most effective when used as soon after delivery as possible. The milk supply remains beyond 4 to 6 months after delivery if the breasts are emptied regularly. (7)

**51.** 1. The LaLeche League was formed to assist mothers who wish to learn the art of breast-feeding. The American Red Cross, the Childbirth Education Association, and the American Society for Psychoprophylaxis in Obstetrics *may* give advice, but teaching and helping the nursing mother is not their primary function. (7)

**52.** 2. Oxytocin is believed to be responsible for bringing on the letdown sensation when milk is carried to the nipples. Prolactin stimulates milk production. Parathormone acts principally to regulate calcium concentration in body fluids. Estrogen influences development of secondary sex characteristics in the woman and controls menstruation. (7)

## The Postpartal Patient Who Bottle-Feeds

**53.** 2. Mother's milk normally contains about 20 calories per ounce. (7)

**54.** 4. As a general rule, most newborns require about 50 to 55 calories each day per pound of body weight, or about 117 calories per kilogram of weight. (7)

**55.** 3. When an infant shows weight gain at a steady rate and an amount of gain that can be normally expected for his age, the infant can be judged to be receiving sufficient calories. The sex of the infant results in only a slight variation in terms of caloric needs. The infant's birth weight and whether he is breast- or bottle-fed are not used to determine his caloric needs. (7)

**56.** 2. When the tap water a mother is using is safe, authorities no longer recommend boiling bottles before filling them with formula. As long as cleanliness is observed while preparing formula, it is safe to wash the bottles in hot, soapy water and then rinse them well before filling them with formula. (7)

**57.** 1. It is considered safe to prepare nursing bottles in a dishwasher. (7)

**58.** 2. To ensure sterilization, most authorities recommend keeping bottles of formula in a boiling-water bath for at least 25 minutes in terminal sterilization. The bottles of formula are then stored in a refrigerator. (7)

**59.** 3. When formula cannot be refrigerated, it is best to recommend that a mother use powdered formula and mix it with water one bottle at a time when needed. The lack of a safe water supply is not necessarily a factor in the situation described in this item; formula can be made with a questionable water supply by boiling the water first, which the patient described in this item should be taught to do before reconstituting the powdered formula, or by using the terminal method of sterilization. The lack of a telephone or oven is of no significance in this situation. (7)

**60.** 1. A nipple should be washed in warm, soapy water as soon as possible after use to prevent remaining formula from coagulating and drying in the nipple. A nipple brush should be used, and water should be forced through the nipple holes. The nipple should be rinsed thoroughly. Boiling unclean equipment is not recommended because organisms can lodge in waste materials on the article. Rinsing the nipple under hot water will tend to coagulate the remaining milk and will make cleaning more difficult. A disinfectant is unnecessary. (7)

## The Postpartal Patient with a Cesarean Birth

**61.** 4. Feelings typically identified by women experiencing an emergency cesarean birth are fear, discouragement, disappointment, frustration, anger, mutilation, and loss of self-esteem. (1)

**62.** 2. The basic purpose for performing a cesarean delivery is to preserve the life or health of the mother or fetus and is based on evidence of maternal or fetal distress. Thus, fetal or maternal distress and fetal well-being are purposes for performing cesarean delivery. Maternal fatigue without evidence of maternal and/or fetal distress is not a purpose of cesarean delivery. (1)

**63.** 1. A patient's postoperative diet should be withheld if the nurse does not hear bowel sounds. She makes this assessment when auscultating the patient's abdomen. Loss of peristalsis may be due to manipulation of the abdominal contents and to the general anesthesia, or the patient may have paralytic ileus. (1)

**64.** 4. The accumulation of gas in the intestinal tract following abdominal surgery is best relieved by increasing the patient's activities with such measures as changing her position frequently, ambulating her to the extent possible, and avoiding offering her items that may increase distention. Orange juice and cold liquids are examples of items that predispose to distention. A rectal tube may also be used. A gastric or intestinal tube is sometimes used when other measures to relieve distention fail. (7)

**65.** 4. Turning, coughing, and deep-breathing are used postoperatively to help prevent respiratory congestion. These activities are not associated with the prevention of such conditions as pleurisy, adhesions, and subinvolution. (7)

**66.** 4. It can be expected that the lochia will increase when the patient is first ambulated. Lochia tends to pool in the uterus and vagina when the patient is recumbent and flows out when she arises. If bright-red bleeding continues, the patient should be put to bed. Massaging the fundus is not indicated because the lochia is normal. (7)

**67.** 4. During the taking-in phase, the mother has dependency needs such as the need for rest, nourishment, and opportunities to relive her birthing experience. She will be ready to demonstrate infant care skills during the taking-hold phase, when she is concerned about resuming control of her life. (3)

**68.** 3. It is believed that the hormone estrogen causes slight vaginal bleeding in the newborn girl. The condition disappears spontaneously; there is no need for concern, and no treatment is indicated. (7)

**69.** 4. Newborns normally increase the number of breast-feedings during periods of rapid growth. Periods of rapid growth (growth spurts) are expected at 10 to 14 days, 5 to 6 weeks, 2.5 to 3 months, and 4.5 to 6 months of age. Following each growth spurt, the infants usually settle into a regular pattern. (7)

## The Postpartal Patient with Risk Factors

**70.** 2. If the mother wishes to view the body, it is her right to do so. Viewing the body has been found to help the grieving process. (1)

**71.** 4. In the situation described in this item, it is best for the nurse first to learn something about the child and then to allow the mother to express how she thinks her son may feel. Offering opinions and giving advice are not recommended; it is better to explore various courses of action and leave the final decision to the mother. If a youngster is told God took a loved one or that the loved one is asleep, the child may be afraid of God or afraid to go to sleep. (3)

**72.** 4. Candidates for Rh immunoglobulin therapy are women who are unsensitized and Rh negative. The immunoglobulin is of no value after sensitization has occurred. It is recommended that Rh immunoglobulin be administered within 3 days after delivery. Some authorities advocate an antepartal dose when the patient is between about 28 and 32 weeks pregnant and then another dose early in the postpartal period. (7)

**73.** 4. Rh immunoglobulin (RhoGAM) is administered intramuscularly. (7)

**74.** 4. The primary reason for doing a follow-up about 2 days after a patient has received Rh immunoglobulin is to determine whether an adequate amount of the immunoglobulin has been administered to the patient. The Kleihauer-Betke test determines whether fetal cells are still present. The indirect Coombs test determines whether excess antibodies are present. (7)

**75.** 2. Gravida means a pregnant woman. The patient described in this situation has five children delivered singly, including her present one, which account for five pregnancies; the twins and triplets account for two pregnancies. This patient's gravida is 7. (7)

**76.** 1. A mother who has delivered ten babies, as described in this item, is more likely to have uterine atony following delivery than the woman who has delivered only one or two babies. Such conditions as vaginal hematoma and puerperal and urinary tract infections are not necessarily related to the number of pregnancies a woman has. (7)

**77.** 1. For about 24 hours after delivery, a diabetic woman's insulin requirements are most likely to be markedly decreased, maybe even to the point of requiring no insulin. The work of labor and delivery decreases insulin requirements (exercise decreases the amount of insulin required by a diabetic). The placenta, which has been allowing glucose but not insulin to cross to the fetus, has been removed and no longer disrupts the mother's usual glucose/insulin balance. (7)

**78.** 2. The most frequent cause of a "boggy" fundus shortly after delivery is relaxation of uterine muscles. The nurse's first course of action would be to massage the fundus. If the fundus does not become firm with this action, it may then be necessary to call the physician. Elevating the foot of the bed and attempting to express clots from the uterus will not firm a relaxed uterus. (7)

**79.** 1. The postpartal fundus rises in the abdomen and displaces to the right side when the patient's bladder is distended. When this occurs, the patient should be encouraged to void. (7)

**80.** 1. Localized infections may occur in the puerperium at laceration, episiotomy, or abdominal incision sites. During pregnancy and the puerperium, the white blood cell count may be slightly elevated, and moniliasis may occur frequently during pregnancy. (7)

**81.** 3. Maternal morbidity and mortality have decreased due to the use of antibiotic therapy, aseptic technique, fewer traumatic operative deliveries, increased understanding of labor dystocia, improved (not increased) surgical intervention, and reduction of malnutrition and debilitative disease in the population. (7)

**82.** 1. The nurse could use the REEDA (*R*edness, *E*dema, *E*cchymosis, *D*ischarge, and *A*pproximation) method to assess the episiotomy for signs of infection. (7)

**83.** 1. The best position for assessing the episiotomy is the Sims' position, with the top leg over the bottom leg. The nurse lifts the top buttock and exposes the perineum and anus for assessment. (7)

**84.** 2. A temperature of 100.4° F. on any two of the first ten postpartal days, excluding the first 24 hours, is associated with postpartal reproductive tract infection. (7)

**85.** 2. Vaginal examination during labor results in deposits of pathogens in the cervix and later invasion of the decidua by the pathogens. Vaginal trauma, such as vaginal lacerations, increase the risk of infection. (7)

**86.** 3. The adverse effects of ampicillin sodium (Polycillin) and kanamycin sulfate (Kantrex) include skin rashes, anaphylaxis, ototoxicity (hearing loss and disequilibrium), renal toxicity, and neuromuscular blockade. Increased bleeding is not an adverse effect. (2)

**87.** 3. Factors predisposing to thromboembolic disease include maternal obesity, increased maternal age, high parity, anesthesia and surgery (possible vessel trauma and venous stasis due to prolonged immobility), history of thrombosis, maternal anemia, hypothermia, heart disease, and lactation suppression with estrogen. (7)

**88.** 1. Homan's sign is used in assessing for deep leg vein thromboembolic disease. The sign may or may not be positive, but usually results in tenderness or pain due to calf pressure as the foot is dorsiflexed. Costovertebral angle tenderness (Chandelier sign) is used to assess for potential urinary tract infection. Deep tendon reflexes are assessed for central nervous system irritability in pregnancy-induced hypertension. (7)

**89.** 4. Heparin (Panheprin) therapy is ordered to prevent clot formation. A side effect of heparin therapy in the puerperium is an increase in lochia flow. (7)

**90.** 1. Lochia alba is a creamy to yellow vaginal discharge that occurs during the final healing process of the uterus as it returns to its prepregnant state. Nursing assessment for the effectiveness and side effects of heparin (Panheprin) therapy includes assessment for symptoms of deep leg vein thromboembolic disease and hemorrhage. (7)

**91.** 2. Risk factors predisposing to early postpartal hemorrhage include overdistention of the uterus (hydramnios, macrosomic infant, multiple gestation), grandmultiparity, anesthetic agents (Halothane), trauma (midforceps, intrauterine manipulation), prolonged or very rapid labor, oxytocin therapy, uterine infection, maternal malnutrition, pregnancy-induced hypertension, or history of hemorrhage. (7)

**92.** 1. Uterine atony is the primary cause of early postpartum hemorrhage. The second leading cause is lacerations of the birth canal. Retained placental fragments is the primary cause of late postpartum hemorrhage. (1, 7)

**93.** 4. Vulvar discomfort could be due to an episiotomy or a vulvar hematoma. However, since the primary cause of early postpartum hemorrhage is uterine atony, nursing assessment to detect early postpartum hemorrhage would include assessments for uterine atony, such as uterine tone, bladder fullness, and amount of lochia discharged. (7)

**94.** 1. Uterine massage to prevent excessive blood loss due to uterine atony is the first intervention for early postpartum hemorrhage. While one nurse massages the uterus, another nurse should notify the physician and prepare to implement the physician's orders. These may include starting an intravenous infusion and administering medications to stimulate uterine contractions. (1)

**95.** 3. Early postpartum hemorrhage is defined as a blood loss of more than 500 ml in the first 24 hours after delivery. Unless this patient's blood loss was excessive at the time of delivery, a moderate amount of blood loss during the first 24 hours after birth would not constitute hemorrhage. Late postpartum hemorrhage occurs after the first 24 hours and is most often caused by retained placental fragments. (7)

# *test* 5

Select the one *best* or *correct* answer and indicate your choice by filling in the circle with a pencil in front of the option you have chosen. If the answer you would prefer is not given, select the one you think is *most appropriate*.

## THE NEONATAL PATIENT

Baby DeBusk is admitted to the nursery. His Apgar scores were 8 and 9 at 1 and 5 minutes after birth, respectively. His gestational age is estimated at 39 weeks.

1. The nurse notes that for almost an hour after birth, Baby DeBusk was awake and alert and startled and cried easily. Respirations rose to 70 per minute and his heart rate on two occasions was 180 beats per minute. Baby DeBusk then slept quietly for about 2 hours, awakened with a start, cried and extended and flexed all four extremities. Baby DeBusk choked, gagged, and regurgitated some mucus. Of the following actions, which would be *best* for the nurse to take?
   - ○ 1. Call the physician; the neonate appears to have hypoglycemia.
   - ○ 2. Change the neonate's position and aspirate mucus as necessary; the signs the neonate presents are normal.
   - ○ 3. Place the neonate in an incubator; these signs suggest that he needs humidity and well-oxygenated air to breathe.
   - ○ 4. Wrap the neonate carefully in a blanket and offer formula; he appears hungry and needs to be protected from injuring himself.

2. The nurse observes Baby DeBusk gagging on mucus and becoming cyanotic during the first feeding. Of the following measures, the *first* one the nurse should take is to
   - ○ 1. start mouth-to-mouth breathing.
   - ○ 2. administer a little 100% oxygen.
   - ○ 3. raise the neonate's head and pat him on the back.
   - ○ 4. clear the neonate's airway with gravity or suction.

3. The nurse is able to retract Baby DeBusk's foreskin only slightly beyond the urethral opening without using force. In this situation, before cleansing the penis, it would be *best* for the nurse to
   - ○ 1. retract the foreskin as far as it will move back with ease.
   - ○ 2. use gentle but steady force to retract the foreskin gradually farther each day.
   - ○ 3. allow the foreskin to remain in place but prepare to use a bulb syringe to help with cleansing.
   - ○ 4. allow the foreskin to remain in place but report the situation to the physician for possible corrective measures.

4. Ms. DeBusk plans to place her baby for adoption but asks to hold and feed Baby DeBusk while she is hospitalized. Of the following responses, which is the *most appropriate* for the nurse to make?
   - ○ 1. "All right, Ms. DeBusk. We'll bring the baby to you for his next feeding."
   - ○ 2. "We'll ask your physician if she thinks that is a good idea. She knows you better than we do."
   - ○ 3. "It is not a good idea to hold and feed the baby. It will be that much harder to give him up to other parents."
   - ○ 4. "We will ask your social worker the next time she visits. Policies concerning your request vary among agencies."

5. Baby DeBusk weighs 8 pounds, 1 ounce (3.7 kg) at birth; at 3 days of age, he weighs 7 pounds, 12 ounces (3.5 kg). In view of Baby DeBusk's weight change, the nurse *appropriately* determines that Baby DeBusk should be
   - ○ 1. fed as he demands since his weight loss is within normal limits.
   - ○ 2. given more than average amounts of fluid to prevent further dehydration.
   - ○ 3. switched to a different formula since the current one appears to be inadequate.
   - ○ 4. given additional feedings since his weight loss indicates inadequate intake.

6. The nurse notes that Baby DeBusk's skin appears jaundiced. When assessing the infant's skin for jaundice, the *best* technique is to

**151**

○ 1. blanch the skin on the forehead.
○ 2. blanch the skin on the buttocks.
○ 3. observe the skin in natural daylight.
○ 4. observe the skin when the infant cries.

## PHYSICAL ASSESSMENT OF THE NEONATAL PATIENT

A nurse is performing a complete physical assessment on Baby Jones, who is approximately 24 hours old. The infant was delivered vaginally.

**7.** At what time in relation to feedings would it be *best* to assess Baby Jones' physical condition?
○ 1. Midway between her feedings.
○ 2. Immediately after she has a feeding.
○ 3. The time of her feeding is unimportant.
○ 4. Immediately before she is to have a feeding.

**8.** The nurse notes a swelling on Baby Jones' scalp and determines that the baby has caput succedaneum. Which of the following criteria differentiates cephalhematoma from a caput succedaneum?
○ 1. The area of involvement.
○ 2. The size of the swelling.
○ 3. The kind of trauma at delivery.
○ 4. The period of time required for absorption.

**9.** Baby Jones was born at term and weighed 7 pounds, 8 ounces (3,400 g) at birth. Which of the following statements is *most accurate* in relation to the neonate's birth weight?
○ 1. The neonate's birth weight is large for her gestational age (LGA).
○ 2. The neonate's birth weight is small for her gestational age (SGA).
○ 3. The neonate's birth weight is appropriate for her gestational age (AGA).
○ 4. The neonate's birth weight cannot be assessed accurately without more information.

**10.** The nurse measures the circumference of the head and chest. If Baby Jones is normal, it would be *typical* to find that when the two measurements are compared, the head will be
○ 1. the same size as the chest.
○ 2. 2 cm larger than the chest.
○ 3. 2 cm smaller than the chest.
○ 4. 4 cm larger than the chest.

**11.** The nurse finds that Baby Jones' head is asymmetrical because of molding. When Baby Jones' parents ask about it, the nurse should explain that the effects of molding will *most likely* disappear when the neonate's age is about

○ 1. 2 to 3 days.
○ 2. 1 to 2 weeks.
○ 3. 5 to 6 weeks.
○ 4. 3 to 4 months.

**12.** Baby Jones' anterior fontanel is normal if it is shaped like a
○ 1. circle.
○ 2. square.
○ 3. diamond.
○ 4. triangle.

**13.** An effective way for the nurse to evaluate the patency of Baby Jones' nostrils is to
○ 1. insert a catheter through each nostril.
○ 2. cover the mouth and auscultate the chest on each side.
○ 3. observe for ciliary movements within each of the nostrils.
○ 4. occlude one nostril at a time and observe for respiratory effort.

**14.** Which of the following findings, if noted by the nurse while assessing Baby Jones' chest, should be reported *promptly* for further investigation?
○ 1. A heart murmur.
○ 2. An expiratory grunt.
○ 3. Bronchial breath sounds.
○ 4. Fine crackles at the end of deep inspiration.

**15.** The nurse assesses Baby Jones' tonic neck reflex. Which of the following statements *best* describes movement when the tonic neck reflex is normal and when the baby is on her back?
○ 1. The neonate is able to touch her chin on the acromial process of either shoulder.
○ 2. The neonate resists pull on her arms and does not move her chin beyond the point of her elbows.
○ 3. The neonate turns her head to her left side, extends her left extremities, and flexes her right extremities.
○ 4. The neonate turns her head to her left side, extends all her extremities, and flexes then promptly relaxes them.

**16.** The parents are concerned about marks on Baby Jones' cheeks from the use of forceps during delivery. The nurse should teach the parents that *most typically* such bruises require
○ 1. no special type of treatment.
○ 2. cleansing with an antiseptic daily until healed.
○ 3. applying an antibiotic ointment daily until healed.
○ 4. covering the area with a sterile dressing until healed.

**17.** Ms. Jones expresses concern when she notes that her baby's eyes are crossed. The nurse should explain that strabismus in a newborn is considered to be

○ 1. normal; the eyes drift until the newborn can see.

○ 2. normal; there is lack of eye-muscle coordination in newborns.

○ 3. abnormal; the eye muscles are of unequal strength and will probably need surgical intervention to correct.

○ 4. abnormal; the condition is common in prematurely born neonates, but full-term neonates ordinarily can focus their eyes well.

18. If Baby Jones is typical of *most* newborns, the color of her eyes will be

○ 1. blue or gray.

○ 2. gray or black.

○ 3. blue or brown.

○ 4. brown or black.

19. The nurse notes a white cheeselike substance in Baby Jones' body creases. This substance is called

○ 1. milia.

○ 2. lanugo.

○ 3. smegma.

○ 4. vernix caseosa.

20. When the nurse notes the white cheeselike substance on Baby Jones' skin, the nurse's *best* course of action is to

○ 1. remove it with oil.

○ 2. notify the physician.

○ 3. allow it to remain on the skin.

○ 4. brush it off the skin with a dry cotton ball.

21. The nurse inspects Baby Jones' palms. Which of the following findings in relation to creases is *most often* associated with chromosomal abnormalities?

○ 1. Many creases across the palm.

○ 2. Absence of creases on the palm.

○ 3. A single crease across the palm.

○ 4. Two large creases across the palm.

22. Which of the following organs is the nurse *least likely* to be able to palpate during her examination of Baby Jones?

○ 1. The liver.

○ 2. The spleen.

○ 3. The kidneys.

○ 4. The thyroid gland.

23. The bottoms of Baby Jones' feet are examined. Which of the following statements about creases would be *typical* of a newborn who is at term?

○ 1. There are no creases on the bottom of the feet.

○ 2. There are creases in the area under the heels only.

○ 3. There are creases spread over the entire bottoms of the feet.

○ 4. There are creases in the area forward of the transverse arch only.

24. Which of the following observations in relation to

Baby Jones' cord should be reported to the physician promptly?

○ 1. The cord clamp has been removed.

○ 2. The cord stump is bluish and dry.

○ 3. The cord stump has three blood vessels.

○ 4. The base of the cord stump is moist and pink.

25. Ms. Jones asks when the "soft spots" close. The nurse should teach her that Baby Jones' anterior fontanel will normally close when she reaches the age of approximately

○ 1. 2 to 3 months.

○ 2. 6 to 8 months.

○ 3. 12 to 18 months.

○ 4. 20 to 24 months.

26. The nurse should teach Ms. Jones that Baby Jones' posterior fontanel will normally close when the baby reaches the age of approximately

○ 1. 2 to 3 weeks.

○ 2. 2 to 3 months.

○ 3. 6 to 8 months.

○ 4. 12 to 18 months.

27. The nurse notes that Baby Jones' hands and feet have changed from a pink to a bluish color during the examination. Appropriate action for the nurse to take in relation to this finding is to

○ 1. wrap the neonate warmly.

○ 2. massage the neonate's extremities.

○ 3. administer oxygen to the neonate promptly.

○ 4. report the change to the physician promptly.

28. Baby Jones receives an injection of vitamin K. This is *usually* administered to newborns because

○ 1. newborns have no intestinal bacteria.

○ 2. newborns are susceptible to avitaminosis.

○ 3. hemolysis of the fetal red blood cells destroys vitamin K.

○ 4. the newborn's liver is incapable of producing sufficient vitamin K.

29. The nurse notes that Baby Jones has a higher red blood cell count than normally noted in children and adults. This relatively high level in the newborn is due *primarily* to the fetus' having a

○ 1. need for more red blood cells for adequate oxygenation.

○ 2. less mature system to destroy mature red blood cells adequately.

○ 3. greater abundance of red bone marrow to manufacture red blood cells.

○ 4. need to remove wastes from internal organs not yet functioning to capacity.

30. What is the approximate range of hemoglobin in a normal newborn at birth?

○ 1. 5 to 10 g/100 ml of blood.

○ 2. 10 to 15 g/100 ml of blood.

○ 3. 15 to 20 g/100 ml of blood.

○ 4. 20 to 25 g/100 ml of blood.

31. *All* of the following observations are normal in Baby Jones at this age *except*
    ○ 1. dark stools.
    ○ 2. peeling skin.
    ○ 3. a high-pitched cry.
    ○ 4. irregular respirations.

32. The nurse notes small, shiny white spots on Baby Jones' gums and hard palate. When the nurse observes this finding, it is *best* for her to
    ○ 1. place Baby Jones in isolation.
    ○ 2. notify the physician promptly.
    ○ 3. send a specimen obtained by swabbing the spots to the laboratory.
    ○ 4. consider them to be Epstein's pearls, which have no clinical significance.

33. If the nurse notes the following findings while assessing Baby Jones' eyes, which should she refer to the physician for evaluation?
    ○ 1. An absence of tears.
    ○ 2. An opacity of the lenses.
    ○ 3. Constriction of the pupils in response to a bright light directed onto them.
    ○ 4. The presence of a red circle on the pupils when an ophthalmoscope's light is directed onto them.

34. When the nurse stimulates the soles of Baby Jones' feet, the infant fans her toes and dorsiflexes her feet, indicating a positive Babinski reflex. From this finding, the nurse is *correct* in determining that Baby Jones is demonstrating
    ○ 1. immaturity of muscle coordination.
    ○ 2. immaturity of the central nervous system.
    ○ 3. a possible defect in the lower spinal cord.
    ○ 4. a possible injury to nerves that innervate the feet.

35. While Baby Jones lies on her back, the nurse flexes the infant's hips and knees at right angles and then abducts the legs until the sides of the knees touch the examining table. If the nurse feels or hears a clicking sound when she carries out this maneuver, Baby Jones is demonstrating Ortolani sign. The nurse's findings should be reported promptly because this sign is *typical* if the neonate has
    ○ 1. a fracture of the femur.
    ○ 2. legs of an unequal length.
    ○ 3. a congenital dislocation of the hip.
    ○ 4. a lateral deviation of the spine (scoliosis).

36. When the soles of Baby Jones' feet are observed, they appear flat. Ms. Jones asks if there is anything she should do about her infant's feet. The nurse should base her response on knowledge that the neonate

○ 1. can be expected to have feet that appear flat for several years.
○ 2. should be seen by a pediatrician for further evaluation of her feet.
○ 3. is likely to injure her feet if she is encouraged to walk at an early age.
○ 4. will develop the longitudinal arch in her feet if she wears corrective shoes when she starts to walk.

37. The nurse should expect to find that, of the following senses, the one that is probably *most highly* developed in Baby Jones is her sense of
    ○ 1. taste.
    ○ 2. smell.
    ○ 3. touch.
    ○ 4. hearing.

## THE POST-TERM NEONATAL PATIENT

Baby Kennedy is a post-term infant with an Apgar score of 7 and 9 at 1 and 5 minutes after birth, respectively.

38. When assessing Baby Kennedy, the nurse can expect to observe which of the following physical characteristics?
    ○ 1. Oily skin.
    ○ 2. A long, thin body.
    ○ 3. Very little scalp hair.
    ○ 4. An abundance of vernix caseosa.

39. When Baby Kennedy is 2 hours old, the nurse notes an increased respiratory rate and tremors of his hands and feet. These signs are *most likely* to be the result of the neonate's having
    ○ 1. hypothermia.
    ○ 2. hypocalcemia.
    ○ 3. hypoglycemia.
    ○ 4. respiratory distress syndrome.

40. Because of his postmaturity, Baby Kennedy is predisposed to problems with
    ○ 1. digesting fats.
    ○ 2. nursing at the breast.
    ○ 3. establishing parental bonding.
    ○ 4. maintaining a normal temperature.

41. A nurse reports that she thinks Baby Kennedy may have thrush when she notes that he has
    ○ 1. frequent hiccups.
    ○ 2. jaundiced sclera.
    ○ 3. a red rash on the abdomen.
    ○ 4. white patches in the mouth.

**42.** It is determined that Baby Kennedy has thrush. To help determine the source of Baby Kennedy's infection, steps will *no doubt* be taken to request a laboratory examination of Ms. Kennedy's
○ 1. blood.
○ 2. sputum.
○ 3. breast milk.
○ 4. vaginal exudate.

**43.** Baby Kennedy is circumcised. The *most common* protection used to cover the penis following a circumcision using the Yellen or Gomco clamp is a sterile dressing embedded with
○ 1. petrolatum.
○ 2. talcum powder.
○ 3. an antibiotic ointment.
○ 4. benzalkonium chloride (Zephiran).

**44.** The nurse observes a small amount of bright-red bleeding from Baby Kennedy's circumcision site. Of the following actions, which is the *most appropriate* for the nurse to take *first?*
○ 1. Notify the physician immediately.
○ 2. Do nothing because a small amount of bleeding is usual.
○ 3. Secure the diaper to cause pressure on the bleeding area.
○ 4. Apply gentle pressure to the area with a sterile gauze pad.

**45.** The nurse should teach Ms. Kennedy to cleanse the circumcision site with
○ 1. mild soap.
○ 2. warm water.
○ 3. hexachlorophene (pHisoHex).
○ 4. benzalkonium chloride (Zephiran).

## THE NEONATAL PATIENT WITH RISK FACTORS

Baby Ellis is delivered by cesarean section and is classified as a preterm, appropriate-for-gestational-age infant. The cesarean delivery was performed for placenta previa.

**46.** Based on her knowledge of care of the newborn immediately after delivery, the nurse should be prepared to help *first* with which of the following activities as soon as Baby Ellis is removed from the uterus?
○ 1. Stimulate the neonate to cry.
○ 2. Administer oxygen to the neonate.
○ 3. Place the neonate in a resuscitator.
○ 4. Aspirate mucus from the neonate's mouth.

**47.** Baby Ellis is to be given oxygen via a mask attached to a hand-operated bag. While administering oxygen, it is *best* to position Baby Ellis on her
○ 1. side with her neck slightly flexed.
○ 2. back with her head turned slightly to the side.
○ 3. abdomen with her head slightly turned to the side.
○ 4. back with her neck slightly extended (sniffing position).

**48.** Of the following observations, the one that indicates *best* that the oxygen is being administered properly is when the nurse notes that with each compression of the bag, Baby Ellis'
○ 1. chest rises.
○ 2. abdomen rises.
○ 3. heart rate increases slightly.
○ 4. efforts to breathe on her own offer resistance.

**49.** External heart massage becomes necessary for Baby Ellis. Which of the following techniques for giving heart massage is *in error?*
○ 1. Cardiac massage is alternated with ventilation.
○ 2. The midsternum is compressed with the heel of the hand.
○ 3. The heart is compressed approximately 100 to 120 times per minute.
○ 4. The downward displacement of the chest wall is no more than $3/4''$.

**50.** After respirations and heartbeat are established, Baby Ellis is placed in an oxygen hood. Which of the following actions is *unnecessary* when administering oxygen by the hood method?
○ 1. Humidifying the air.
○ 2. Covering the neonate's eyes.
○ 3. Deflecting the oxygen from the neonate's head.
○ 4. Measuring the oxygen concentration in the hood.

**51.** Baby Ellis is transferred to a neonatal center for high- risk infants to receive intensive care. Which of the following actions is *least likely* to be helpful to the parents in relation to their baby's care and condition at this time?
○ 1. Suggesting that the parents call or visit the neonatal center.
○ 2. Accompanying the parents to see and touch the neonate before transport.
○ 3. Assisting the parents to participate in as much of the neonate's care as possible.
○ 4. Reporting the positive aspects of the neonate's condition rather than the negative aspects.

**52.** Which of the following factors *most* increases Baby Ellis' risk for having respiratory distress syndrome (hyaline membrane disease)?
○ 1. The mother's having placenta previa.

○ 2. The neonate's being born before term.

○ 3. The mother's being delivered by cesarean section.

○ 4. The neonate's having sluggish respiratory activity after delivery.

**53.** Baby Ellis is likely to develop respiratory distress syndrome (hyaline membrane disease), which is caused by an alteration in the body's excretion of

○ 1. ptyalin.

○ 2. surfactant.

○ 3. vasopressin.

○ 4. aldosterone.

**54.** If Baby Ellis develops respiratory distress syndrome, it is likely that she will have expiratory grunting. It is believed that this type of breathing *most likely* occurs because the neonate

○ 1. has aspirated some meconium.

○ 2. has a partial collapse of the trachea.

○ 3. is attempting to increase intra-alveolar pressure in the lungs.

○ 4. is attempting to develop negative pressure in the pleural spaces.

**55.** Baby Ellis receives oxygen therapy. Efforts are made to help prevent Baby Ellis from developing retinopathy of prematurity. It has been demonstrated that this condition is *most likely* to develop when a preterm infant's care has included the indiscriminate use of

○ 1. oxygen.

○ 2. vitamin K.

○ 3. blood transfusions.

○ 4. respiratory stimulants.

**56.** If Baby Ellis develops retinopathy of prematurity, the child will *most likely* be

○ 1. deaf.

○ 2. mute.

○ 3. blind.

○ 4. mentally retarded.

**57.** The nurse *best* determines the adequacy of Baby Ellis' oxygen therapy by

○ 1. observing the neonate for cyanosis.

○ 2. monitoring the neonate's pulse rate.

○ 3. observing the neonate's arterial blood gas levels.

○ 4. monitoring the amount of oxygen the neonate receives.

**58.** Baby Ellis is to have continuous positive airway pressure therapy through nasal prongs. If the following nursing orders appear on the infant's care plan, which should the nurse question before implementing it?

○ 1. Change nasal prongs p.r.n.

○ 2. Keep infant on her left side.

○ 3. Provide mouth and nasal care p.r.n.

○ 4. Empty condensation in the delivery tube p.r.n.

**59.** Cold stress is to be avoided for Baby Ellis. Of the following measures, the one that will help *most* to prevent cold stress is being sure that Baby Ellis

○ 1. is dry at all times.

○ 2. does not receive unwarmed oxygen.

○ 3. does not touch the sides of the incubator.

○ 4. is located in the nursery away from an outside wall.

**60.** The *primary* purpose for humidifying the oxygen before Baby Ellis receives it is to help

○ 1. promote dilitation of the bronchioles.

○ 2. decrease bacterial growth in the delivery tube.

○ 3. prevent drying of the respiratory mucous membranes.

○ 4. enhance blood circulation in the respiratory system.

**61.** Baby Ellis is fed by gavage. After inserting the catheter but before introducing nourishment, the nurse's *best* course of action is to

○ 1. clamp the catheter momentarily.

○ 2. place the free end of the catheter under water.

○ 3. aspirate stomach contents through the catheter.

○ 4. instill about 5 ml of sterile water into the catheter.

**62.** Before introducing the catheter for gavaging Baby Ellis, the nurse should lubricate the catheter with

○ 1. mineral oil.

○ 2. sterile water.

○ 3. petrolatum jelly.

○ 4. a water-soluble jelly.

**63.** Following gavage, Baby Ellis should have her head slightly elevated and be positioned on her

○ 1. back.

○ 2. abdomen.

○ 3. left side.

○ 4. right side.

**64.** Ms. Ellis asks the nurse if her baby can have breast milk. The nurse's *best* response to Ms. Ellis' question is

○ 1. "No. Your baby requires a special high-calorie formula."

○ 2. "Yes, but not until your baby can suck and swallow better."

○ 3. "No. It is not recommended that breast milk be given by gavage."

○ 4. "Yes. I will show you how to pump your breasts and store your milk."

**65.** Which of the following emotions is Ms. Ellis *most likely* to experience *first* because her baby was born before term?

○ 1. Fear.

○ 2. Guilt.

○ 3. Anger.
○ 4. Dependency.

66. Ms. Ellis is afraid her 2-year-old daughter will be jealous of the new baby when she comes home and asks for help. Which of the following suggestions would be *most appropriate* for the nurse to make?
    ○ 1. Suggest that Ms. Ellis divide her time equally between the two children.
    ○ 2. Suggest that Ms. Ellis ignore signs of jealousy to diminish the behavior.
    ○ 3. Suggest that Ms. Ellis let her daughter hold the baby once or twice every day.
    ○ 4. Suggest that Ms. Ellis give undivided attention to her older daughter several times each day.

Ms. Laura Fullingham, a gravida 2, has learned that her fetus may be affected by hemolytic disease. She is hospitalized for further assessment.

67. If Baby Fullingham has hemolytic disease, then the combination of the parents' blood Rh findings that *most often* leads to the disease is when the blood of
    ○ 1. both parents is Rh positive.
    ○ 2. both parents is Rh negative.
    ○ 3. the mother is Rh positive and the father is Rh negative.
    ○ 4. the mother is Rh negative and the father is Rh positive.

68. Ms. Fullingham had no problem with Rh sensitization during her first pregnancy *primarily* because
    ○ 1. the first baby is usually Rh negative.
    ○ 2. most women today are immunized against the Rh factor.
    ○ 3. antibodies are not ordinarily formed until there is exposure to an antigen.
    ○ 4. the mother's blood is able to neutralize antibodies formed in the first pregnancy.

69. The *most likely* reason for Ms. Fullingham's sensitization to the Rh factor is that she
    ○ 1. has an excess of immunoglobulins.
    ○ 2. had an Rh-positive infant the first time she was pregnant.
    ○ 3. had an Rh-negative infant the first time she was pregnant.
    ○ 4. has an overabundance of hemagglutination-inhibition antibodies.

70. Which of the following effects of hemolysis due to Rh sensitization is *least likely* to be present in Baby Fullingham at the time of delivery?

○ 1. Edema.
○ 2. Anemia.
○ 3. Jaundice.
○ 4. Heart failure.

71. Antibody titers were done on Ms. Fullingham during pregnancy to monitor the severity of Rh sensitivity. What specimen is used to determine the antibody titer?
    ○ 1. Fetal blood.
    ○ 2. Amniotic fluid.
    ○ 3. Maternal urine.
    ○ 4. Maternal blood.

72. An amniocentesis is to be done on Ms. Fullingham. Before the amniocentesis is performed, it is *most important* for the nurse to obtain
    ○ 1. the heart rate of the fetus.
    ○ 2. the mother's body temperature.
    ○ 3. a urine specimen from the mother.
    ○ 4. a blood specimen from the mother.

73. A specimen of amniotic fluid is obtained and is to be examined for bilirubin density. The type of container in which the nurse should place the specimen is a
    ○ 1. dark container.
    ○ 2. warmed container.
    ○ 3. chilled container.
    ○ 4. transparent container.

74. A direct Coombs test is done on the cord blood to detect the presence of
    ○ 1. fetal red cells in the maternal serum.
    ○ 2. maternal red cells in the fetal circulation.
    ○ 3. antibodies coating the baby's red blood cells.
    ○ 4. antigens coating the mother's red blood cells.

75. Ms. Fullingham's fetus is found to be severely affected by hemolytic disease and an intrauterine transfusion is planned. The *primary* reason for an intrauterine transfusion is to
    ○ 1. remove excess bilirubin.
    ○ 2. replace destroyed red blood cells.
    ○ 3. dilute maternal antibody concentration.
    ○ 4. serve as a focus for maternal antibodies.

76. Labor is induced for Ms. Fullingham at 32 weeks gestation and an exchange transfusion is planned immediately after delivery. When this procedure is performed, which of the following actions is *legally* considered a nursing responsibility?
    ○ 1. Cross-matching the blood.
    ○ 2. Having the equipment ready.
    ○ 3. Obtaining an informed consent.
    ○ 4. Obtaining serial red blood counts.

77. Baby Fullingham is given an exchange transfusion to
    ○ 1. replenish the body's white blood cells.
    ○ 2. restore the blood's antigen-antibody balance.

3. lower the blood's concentration of bilirubin.

4. replace Rh-negative blood with Rh-positive blood.

78. The nurse can anticipate that the vein that will *most likely* be used to give Baby Fullingham the exchange transfusion is the

1. jugular vein.

2. femoral vein.

3. temporal vein.

4. umbilical vein.

79. Infection is a potential complication of Baby Fullingham's exchange transfusion. Which of the following signs is *least* reliable when the nurse assesses Baby Fullingham for signs of infection?

1. Lethargy.

2. A poor sucking reflex.

3. An elevated temperature.

4. An above-average respiratory rate.

80. Intravenous albumin is ordered for Baby Fullingham. How will albumin help reduce the infant's blood bilirubin level?

1. Bilirubin production is prevented by maintaining high levels of blood albumin.

2. Bilirubin binds to albumin and is transported to the liver for eventual excretion.

3. Albumin combines with enzymes and couples with bilirubin, which can then be excreted.

4. Albumin acts as a catalyst to convert bilirubin to biliverdin, which can then be excreted.

81. Which organ in Baby Fullingham's body is *most* subject to damage when hemolytic disease remains uncontrolled?

1. The liver.

2. The brain.

3. The spleen.

4. The kidneys.

82. Which of the following precautions should the nurse observe when Baby Fullingham is to receive phototherapy?

1. The neonate's eyes should be patched.

2. The neonate's scalp should be covered.

3. The neonate's feedings should be withheld.

4. The neonate's therapy should be discontinued if a rash develops.

83. Baby Fullingham's condition deteriorates, and death appears imminent. The parents are Roman Catholic, and a priest of the church is not available to baptize the baby. Which of the following statements *most accurately* reflects the tenets of the Roman Catholic Church concerning who may properly baptize an infant?

1. One of the parents.

2. A person who had been baptized.

3. A Roman Catholic.

4. Anyone, regardless of religious beliefs.

Baby Gonzales is an infant of a Class B insulin-dependent diabetic mother.

84. Baby Gonzales' blood glucose level is monitored and is found to be low when the infant is about 2 hours old. This finding is *most likely* due to

1. a reaction to the stresses of labor and the period of increased activity following delivery.

2. an interruption in the source of maternal glucose and a continued high production of insulin by the baby.

3. a physical response of the body that normally occurs during transition from intrauterine to extrauterine life.

4. an increase in the production of urine that occurs when the kidneys are ridding the body of excess glucose.

85. A characteristic behavioral sign Baby Gonzales is *most likely* to exhibit when his blood glucose level is low is

1. sneezing.

2. jitteriness.

3. eagerness to eat.

4. difficulty breathing.

86. The nurse can anticipate that when Baby Gonzales has a low blood sugar level, he is *most likely* to be given

1. sterile water orally.

2. breast or formula feedings.

3. regular insulin subcutaneously.

4. balanced electrolyte solution intravenously.

87. A complication for which the nurse should carefully observe Baby Gonzales is

1. anemia.

2. hypertension.

3. hemolytic disease.

4. respiratory distress syndrome.

88. Ms. Gonzales says to the nurse, "I have diabetes but my husband does not. Will our new baby have diabetes too?" In terms of risk, the nurse should base her response on knowledge that the child has

1. an increased risk of developing diabetes.

2. practically no risk of developing diabetes when one parent is free of the disease.

3. a high risk of developing diabetes when the parent having the disease is the mother.

4. more of a risk of developing diabetes than children born subsequently to a diabetic mother.

Ms. Julie Hansard, who does not have a physician, is admitted to the hospital in early labor. She delivers a 6-pound, 4-ounce (2,835 g) baby after an uneventful 8-hour labor. Ms. Hansard told the nurse on admission that she has been using heroin for the past 2 years.

**89.** When the nurse learns that Ms. Hansard has been using heroin, which of the following actions should she take?
  ○ 1. Inform the police; using heroin is illegal.
  ○ 2. Inform the head nurse; she is responsible for taking next steps.
  ○ 3. Inform no one; the information the nurse learns is confidential.
  ○ 4. Inform the physician who is called to deliver Ms. Hansard; heroin addiction affects care.

**90.** Ms. Hansard has no access to heroin. In the immediate postpartal period, the symptoms she will *most likely* demonstrate are
  ○ 1. nausea and tremors.
  ○ 2. fatigue and drowsiness.
  ○ 3. euphoria and hyperactivity.
  ○ 4. depression and a desire to be alone.

**91.** Approximately when after birth can the nurse anticipate that Baby Hansard will demonstrate symptoms of heroin withdrawal?
  ○ 1. Within the 1st day.
  ○ 2. During the 3rd day.
  ○ 3. During the 5th day.
  ○ 4. During the 7th day.

**92.** Ms. Hansard should be taught that the effects of heroin addiction may continue in Baby Hansard for as long as
  ○ 1. 1 month.
  ○ 2. 3 months.
  ○ 3. 6 months.
  ○ 4. 1 year or more.

**93.** Which of the following signs related to crying will Baby Hansard *most likely* demonstrate when having symptoms of heroin withdrawal?
  ○ 1. No cry.
  ○ 2. A weak cry.
  ○ 3. A shrill cry.
  ○ 4. A hoarse cry.

**94.** Which of the following medications to help sedate Baby Hansard can the nurse anticipate will *most likely* be used during the period of withdrawal from heroin?
  ○ 1. Levallorphan (Lorfan).
  ○ 2. Nalorphine hydrochloride (Nalline).
  ○ 3. Meperidine hydrochloride (Demerol).

  ○ 4. Chlorpromazine hydrochloride (Thorazine).

**95.** The gastrointestinal problem Baby Hansard is *most likely* to present due to heroin withdrawal is
  ○ 1. colic.
  ○ 2. vomiting.
  ○ 3. constipation.
  ○ 4. paralytic ileus.

**96.** The nurse should teach Ms. Hansard that her *best* course of action to help comfort her infant when he is irritable is to
  ○ 1. offer the infant a pacifier.
  ○ 2. give the infant extra formula.
  ○ 3. let the infant cry out his irritableness.
  ○ 4. place the infant on his abdomen in a cool room.

**97.** Ms. Hansard tells the nurse, "I'm glad my baby can be cured of the heroin addiction he got from me." Which of the following responses would be *most accurate* for the nurse to make in this situation?
  ○ 1. "Yes. Your infant can be cured of his heroin addiction because he has acquired no psychological dependency on the drug."
  ○ 2. "Yes. Your infant can be cured of his heroin addiction because the heroin he received from you during pregnancy has minimal addictive qualities."
  ○ 3. "Not exactly. It will be extremely difficult for your infant to be cured of his heroin addiction because he received it during his entire fetal period."
  ○ 4. "Yes and no. Your infant can be cured of his heroin addiction but only if he has psychological counseling as soon as he is old enough to profit from it."

**98.** Baby Hansard was at risk for fetal malformation because of his mother's drug abuse during pregnancy. The *most important* determinant of the effects of drug-induced malformations of the fetus is the
  ○ 1. amount of the drug the mother took.
  ○ 2. length of time the mother took the drug.
  ○ 3. amount of sensitivity the mother has for the drug.
  ○ 4. stage of embryonic development when the drug was taken.

# CORRECT ANSWERS AND RATIONALES

Numbers appear in parentheses following the rationales. The numbers identify textbooks listed in the references at the end of Part II, where correct answers can be verified.

## The Neonatal Patient

1. 2. The baby's signs described in this item are normal for his age. He appears to be regurgitating and choking on mucus, which is also common during the second period of reactivity. The recommended procedure in this situation is to change the baby's position and aspirate mucus as necessary. (7)

2. 4. If a newborn gags on mucus and becomes cyanotic while having his first feeding, the infant's airway is most probably not open. The nurse should clear the infant's airway with gravity (by lowering the infant's head) and/or suction. (7)

3. 1. It is not recommended that efforts be used to move the foreskin back in a newborn any farther than it will retract with ease. Adhesions between the prepuce and the glans penis are common in the newborn. Current opinion is to wait until the separation occurs normally as the boy grows. By the age of 3, in most cases the foreskin is easy to retract. *The foreskin should never be forcibly retracted.* (7)

4. 1. In the past, it was often thought best for the mother not to see an infant she was giving up for adoption. It is now general procedure to allow the mother to see the baby if she wishes, because authorities agree that the mother has that right. Also, the mother will probably experience grief when she gives up her infant for adoption. Seeing and holding the infant allows the grief process to begin. (7)

5. 1. Newborns tend to lose about 5% to 15% of their birth weight during the first few days after birth. This is very likely due to minimal nutritional intake, since the breasts are still not secreting milk, and to the loss of extracellular fluid. The weight loss of the infant described in this item falls within a normal range, and therefore nothing needs to be done at this time. (7)

6. 1. It is an important nursing responsibility to assess for jaundice in the newborn. The best technique is to blanch the skin over a bony area, such as the forehead or chest, by applying pressure to the area and observing the area before the color in the skin returns. Until blood returns to the area after removing pressure, the yellow color of jaundice is relatively easy to see. (7)

## Physical Assessment of the Neonatal Patient

7. 1. It is best to examine a baby approximately midway between feedings. The hungry baby is often irritable, making examination difficult. Manipulation after eating may cause the baby to regurgitate or vomit, and the infant is also less responsive soon after eating. (5)

8. 1. Caput succedaneum is caused by pressure on the head during labor. It is an edematous area that occurs over the place where the scalp was encircled by the cervix. Cephalhematoma is caused by blood between the bone and the periosteum. Because the bleeding is under the periosteum, it cannot cross a suture line, whereas a caput can. Hence, the area of involvement best differentiates the two. (7)

9. 3. The normal full-term newborn weighs between 6 and 9 pounds (2,700 g and 3,500 g). (7)

10. 2. At birth, the circumference of a newborn's head is approximately 2 cm larger than the circumference of the chest. The average normal circumference of a newborn's head is 33 to 35 cm (13″ to 14″). The average normal circumference of the newborn's chest is 31 to 35 cm (12.5″ to 14″). If the head has molding, it should be measured again after molding has been corrected for an accurate measurement. (7)

11. 1. During vaginal delivery, the cranial bones tend to override when the head accommodates to the size of the birth canal. The phenomenon is called molding, and its effects will subside within a few days after delivery without any special attention. The head appears elongated from molding. (7)

12. 3. The anterior fontanel is normally shaped like a diamond. It is about 2 to 3 cm wide and 3 to 4 cm long. The measurements may be somewhat smaller from the effects of molding. The posterior fontanel is small and shaped like a triangle. (7)

13. 4. The best way to evaluate patency of the baby's nostrils is to occlude one nostril at a time and observe respirations while doing so. An infant initially breathes through his nose and only later learns to breathe through his mouth. Therefore, it is not necessary to cover the mouth while occluding the nostril. (5)

14. 2. An expiratory grunt is significant and should be reported promptly when noted during the assessment of a newborn. A heart murmur is not unusual during the newborn period, although it should be reported. Bronchial breath sounds are normally

heard over most of the chest wall. They often sound harsh and loud because the stethoscope is a very short distance from the interior chest cavity. It is not uncommon to hear fine crackles at the end of deep inspiration when auscultating a newborn's chest. They are probably caused by unabsorbed amniotic fluid. (7)

15. 3. The tonic neck reflex, also often called the fencing position, is present when the infant turns her head to her left side, extends her left extremities, and flexes her right extremities. This reflex disappears in a matter of months, after the newborn's nervous system has had time to mature more. (7)

16. 1. Bruises or marks that result from the use of forceps during delivery require no treatment. The bruises will disappear in a few days. If the skin has been broken by the forceps, special care may be required. (7)

17. 2. Convergent strabismus is common during infancy, until about 6 months of age, because of poor oculomotor coordination. (7)

18. 1. Babies have blue or slate-gray eyes at birth. The baby's eyes will have their permanent color after about 3 months of age. (7)

19. 4. The white cheeselike substance in the newborn's body creases is called vernix caseosa. Milia are small white nodules on the skin, usually caused by plugged sebaceous glands or hair follicles. Lanugo is the fine downy hair found over the newborn's body, except for the palms of the hands and the soles of the feet. Smegma is a cheesy substance found under the prepuce of the penis and around the clitoris and the labia minora. (7)

20. 3. Unless vernix caseosa is stained with meconium or blood, it should be left on the skin because it serves as a protective coating. It disappears within about 24 hours after birth. (1)

21. 3. A single crease across the palm (simian crease) is most often associated with chromosomal abnormalities, notably Down syndrome. (7)

22. 4. In the newborn, the liver, spleen, and kidneys are palpable, but the thyroid gland is normally not palpable. (7)

23. 3. Creases normally are spread over the entire bottoms of the feet in a full-term baby. (7)

24. 4. The physician should be notified if the base of the cord is moist and pink to red in color. The findings are often a sign of an infection at the base of the cord stump. Normal findings include a cord stump that is bluish and dry and a cord stump that had three blood vessels. The cord clamp is ordinarily removed when the umbilical stump is dry. (7)

25. 3. Normally, the anterior fontanel closes between about 12 and 18 months. Premature closure

(craniostenosis or premature synostosis) prevents proper growth and expansion of the brain, resulting in mental retardation. Premature closure of the fontanel is ordinarily treated surgically. (7)

26. 2. Normally, the posterior fontanel closes when the infant is about 2 to 3 months old. (7)

27. 1. When the nurse notes that the color of the newborn's hands and feet change from a pink to a bluish color during a physical examination, she should first wrap the infant warmly. This change in coloring is normal and is caused by the fact that the infant is most probably cold. This change in color is called acrocyanosis. (7)

28. 1. Bacteria that inhabit the large intestine synthesize vitamin K, which is then absorbed. Vitamin K is often given to newborns because they lack bacteria in the intestines. An absence of vitamin K often results in a bleeding tendency. (7)

29. 1. During fetal life, the infant has a great need for oxygen. To help satisfy its need for oxygen, the infant's hemoglobin has a greater affinity for oxygen and more red blood cells than does a child or an adult. Hemoglobin and hematocrit values are correspondingly higher than they are later in life. (7)

30. 3. The normal range of hemoglobin in the normal newborn is between 15 and 20 g/100 ml of blood. After birth, the hemoglobin value gradually decreases. (7)

31. 3. A persistent and high-pitched or shrill cry is not typical of a newborn. A shrill cry is typical of an infant experiencing heroin withdrawal, increased intracranial pressure, or hypoglycemia. The newborn normally has dark stools, irregular respirations, and peeling skin. (7)

32. 4. Epstein's pearls are small shiny spots (cysts) often found on a newborn's gums and hard palate. They have no clinical significance and disappear without treatment within a few weeks. (7)

33. 2. An opacity of a newborn's lenses should be referred to a physician promptly for further evaluation. Lens opacity may indicate the presence of congenital cataracts. An absence of tears is common because the newborn's lacrimal glands are not yet functioning. The presence of a red circle on the pupils when an ophthalmoscope's light is directed onto them is a normal finding. This finding is often called the red reflex and indicates the light is shining onto the retina. The newborn's pupils normally constrict when a bright light is focused onto them. The finding implies that light perception and visual acuity are present, as they should be after birth. (7)

34. 2. A positive Babinski reflex in a newborn is normal. It demonstrates the immaturity of the central nervous system in corticospinal pathways. An in-

fant's muscle coordination is immature, but the Babinski reflex does not help determine this immaturity. A positive Babinski reflex in an adult indicates disease. (7)

**35.** 3. Ortolani sign indicates the infant most probably has a dislocated hip. Ortolani test consists of flexing the infant's knees and hips at right angles and bringing the sides of the knees down to the surface of the examining table. A characteristic click can be felt or heard when Ortolani sign is present. The length of an infant's legs is determined by measuring the distance from the anterior superior iliac spine to the medial malleolus. Scoliosis is a condition most often found in adolescent girls. A fractured clavicle occurs occasionally during delivery, but a fractured femur would be a most unusual finding in a newborn. (7)

**36.** 1. The soles of an infant's feet have pads of fat tissue that give the feet the appearance of being flat because the longitudinal arch is obscured. This is a normal condition and gradually disappears so that by the time the child is about 3 years of age, the feet appear normal. Flat feet (pes planus) is a deformity of the feet caused by a lowering of the longitudinal arch when the bones in the feet are not positioned properly relative to each other. This condition can rarely, if ever, be determined accurately during infancy. (7)

**37.** 3. It is believed that the sense of touch is most highly developed at birth. It is probably for this reason that newborns respond well to being touched. (7)

### The Post-term Neonatal Patient

**38.** 2. Post-term, or postmature, infants are born after pregnancy has reached full term. Typical physical characteristics of the post-term infant include having a long, thin body, abundant scalp hair, absence of vernix caseosa, skin that is dry, thin, and cracked, long nails, and an absence of lanugo. At birth, these infants tend to look as though they are 1 to 3 weeks old. (1)

**39.** 3. Post-term infants often suffer from hypoglycemia. An increased respiratory rate and tremors of the hands and feet are typical when the blood glucose level is below normal. Hypothermia results in a low body temperature. Hypocalcemia is characterized by irritability, twitching, and convulsions, although hand tremors may also be present. Apnea and an expiratory grunt are the prime manifestations of respiratory distress. (7)

**40.** 4. Post-term infants tend to have little subcutaneous fat, which predisposes them to cold stress and problems maintaining a normal temperature. They require extra warmth. Problems related to nursing at breast, digesting fats, and establishing parental bonding are not associated with postmaturity. (7)

**41.** 4. Thrush is an infection caused by *Candida albicans*. The characteristic sign of the infection is the appearance of white patches in the mouth and on the tongue. (7)

**42.** 4. *Candida albicans*, which causes thrush, also causes monilial vaginitis. An infant born of a mother with monilial vaginitis may acquire the infection while passing through the birth canal. Laboratory examination of exudate from lesions in the mother's vagina will reveal whether she has a *Candida albicans* infection. The infection occurs more frequently in pregnant women than in nonpregnant women. The source of infection in the mother is unknown but may be the result of a decrease in vaginal pH, which allows for an overgrowth of the yeast infection. (7)

**43.** 1. Authorities who recommend using a dressing on a circumcision most often recommend one imbedded with petrolatum. Powder is not indicated because of its drying and caking effects. On occasion, a physician may order an antibiotic ointment, such as polymyxin B-bacitracin-neomycin (Neosporin). (7)

**44.** 4. If bleeding occurs following a circumcision, most authorities recommend that the nurse first apply gentle pressure on the area with sterile gauze. Bleeding is not common, but when it occurs it requires attention. Applying pressure with the diaper does not allow the nurse to observe whether bleeding has stopped. It is necessary to notify the physician when bleeding cannot be stopped with conservative measures. (7)

**45.** 2. The most often recommended procedure is to cleanse a circumcision with warm water each time the diaper is changed. Other methods of care may become necessary only if complications develop. (7)

### The Neonatal Patient with Risk Factors

**46.** 4. The first step to take when an infant is delivered by cesarean section is to aspirate mucus from the infant's mouth. If this is not done, the infant will aspirate mucus when it begins to breathe. After this step is taken, the infant may be stimulated to cry, given oxygen, or placed in a resuscitator if the infant's condition warrants such measures. (7)

**47.** 4. When being giving oxygen by mask with a hand-operated bag, an infant should be placed on the back with the neck slightly extended, in the sniffing or neutral position. This position provides the most room for lung expansion and places the upper respiratory tract in the best position for receiving oxygen. A small rolled towel under the infant's shoulders helps extend the neck properly. Overextension of the neck will block the airway. (7)

**48.** 1. Oxygen is being administered properly when it reaches the lungs. When this occurs, the chest rises with each contraction of the hand-operated bag. (7)

**49.** 2. An infant's sternum should be compressed with two fingers, not the hand, in CPR. It is appropriate to alternate cardiac massage with ventilation, to compress the heart at a rate of about 100 to 120 times a minute, and to displace the chest wall $1/2''$ to $3/4''$ (1.0 to 1.5 cm). (1)

**50.** 2. There is no need to cover the infant's eyes when administering oxygen via the hood. The air in a hood should be humidified, the oxygen should be deflected from the infant's head, and the oxygen concentration in the hood should be monitored. (7)

**51.** 4. When an infant must be placed in an intensive care center for preterm babies, the parents should be kept informed of the infant's condition, even when the news is negative. It is appropriate to help the parents develop a relationship with the infant by encouraging them to call or visit the center, allowing them to see and touch the baby before he or she is transferred, and allowing them to participate in the infant's care to the extent possible. (7)

**52.** 2. Respiratory distress syndrome (RDS), also known as hyaline membrane disease (HMD), is a developmental condition that primarily attacks infants born before term. There has been a question about whether cesarean section predisposes infants to RDS, but in uncomplicated full-term cesarean deliveries there appears to be little if any correlation. The fact that the infant described in this item needed respiratory assistance at birth is not the likely cause of RDS but may be a sign that the infant has it. (7)

**53.** 2. When surfactant is present in decreased amounts, the alveoli in the lungs do not expand properly and respiratory distress syndrome (RDS) occurs. The condition prevents proper aeration, resulting in a poor exchange of oxygen and carbon dioxide in the lungs. (7)

**54.** 3. An infant's expiratory grunt is similar to an adult's pursed-lip breathing, except the infant is breathing in this manner involuntarily and the adult is doing so voluntarily. Both types of breathing increase intra-alveolar pressure, making it easier

for the body to empty air in the lungs and enhance carbon dioxide elimination. (7)

**55.** 1. The indiscriminate use of oxygen in high concentrations causes retinopathy of prematurity (ROP). Blindness is likely to result. (7)

**56.** 3. The infant with retinopathy of prematurity is most likely to be blind. (7)

**57.** 3. The best way to determine the adequacy of oxygen therapy is to observe the infant's arterial blood gas findings that describe oxygen and carbon dioxide tensions. Cyanosis can be used to validate laboratory findings but using it without laboratory examination is not sufficiently reliable to evaluate oxygen therapy, nor does the pulse rate serve as a good index. The oxygen should be monitored carefully; only the amount necessary for physiological requirements should be administered. (7)

**58.** 2. The nurse should question a nursing order that states an infant receiving continuous positive airway pressure therapy should be kept on the left side. It is appropriate during continuous positive airway pressure therapy to change the nasal prongs, empty condensation in the delivery tube, and provide mouth and nasal care as indicated. (7)

**59.** 2. A great deal of heat can be lost quickly by convection. If oxygen is not warmed before it is administered to an infant, the infant is likely to suffer from cold stress. It is also helpful to keep the infant dry, but this is not as critical as ensuring that oxygen is warmed before it is administered. Touching the incubator and locating the incubator away from an outside wall are unlikely to prevent cold stress in most instances. (7)

**60.** 3. Oxygen should be humidified before administration to help prevent drying the mucous membranes in the respiratory tract. Drying of mucosa impedes the normal functioning of cilia in the respiratory tract and predisposes to irritation of the mucous membranes. (7)

**61.** 3. After the nurse inserts a catheter for gavaging an infant, she should next check to determine that the catheter is in the stomach before instilling nourishment. The best way is to aspirate stomach contents. Another method is to inject a few milliliters of air into the catheter while auscultating over the stomach with a stethoscope to listen for the sound of the air entering the stomach. In the past, it was common to place the catheter under water; if the appearance of bubbles at regular intervals coordinated with respirations, the nurse judged that the catheter was in the airway. This latter procedure is no longer recommended. (7)

**62.** 2. The catheter to be used for gavaging an infant should be lubricated with sterile water before introducing it. Oil-based lubricants could inadvertently enter the lungs and lead to serious complications. A water-soluble jelly is not recommended. (7)

**63.** 4. Following a gavage, an infant should be placed in the right side-lying position with the head slightly elevated. This positioning facilitates digestion and helps decrease regurgitation. (1)

**64.** 4. Many centers that care for high-risk infants recommend that the mother pump her breasts, store the milk, and bring it to the center so the infant can be fed with it, even if the infant needs to be gavaged. (7)

**65.** 2. Giving birth to a premature infant is most often associated with feelings of guilt by the parents. They tend to ask what they might have done to cause it, or not have done that could have prevented it. (7)

**66.** 4. The most appropriate guideline is to suggest that the mother give some undivided time each day to the 2-year-old child who may feel jealous of a new baby. Dividing time equally between children may not be feasible. Ignoring behavior typical of jealousy will not help meet the youngster's needs. Allowing the older child to hold the baby occasionally is unlikely to help overcome jealousy and may result in the child's hurting the baby. (7)

**67.** 4. When there are Rh problems, most often the mother is Rh negative and the father is Rh positive. About 10% to 15% of marriages in this country have the potential for Rh problems. (7)

**68.** 3. The problem of Rh sensitivity arises when the mother's blood develops antibodies when fetal red blood cells enter the maternal circulation. In cases of Rh sensitivity, this usually does not occur until the first pregnancy; hence, hemolytic disease of the newborn is rare when a mother is having her first baby. A mismatched blood transfusion in the past could also result in hemolytic disease because the transfusion would have had the same effects on the mother. (7)

**69.** 2. The most common cause of Rh sensitization is delivery of an Rh-positive baby, although transfusion with improperly matched blood can also cause the condition. Concentration of immunoglobulins is unrelated to Rh sensitization. Hemagglutination-inhibition tests determine susceptibility or immunity to the rubella virus. (7)

**70.** 3. Jaundice is not present at birth because the mother's liver breaks down the bilirubin and excretes it. Anemia due to the destruction of red blood cells by antibodies may occur as the severity of hemolytic disease of the newborn increases. Heart failure occurs as the heart decompensates because of the severe anemia. The edema results

from the heart failure. The severe form of this condition is called hydrops fetalis. (7)

**71.** 4. Because the antibodies appear in the mother's blood, the specimen required for antibody titer is maternal blood. (7)

**72.** 1. Before performing an amniocentesis, it is important for the nurse to obtain baseline data so that she can compare it with findings during and after the amniocentesis. This procedure helps determine whether complications are present. It is especially important to obtain the fetal heart rate. The mother should be assessed for evidence of uterine contractions and ruptured membranes. (7)

**73.** 1. The optical density of the amniotic fluid is evaluated for bilirubin level with a spectrophotometer. The higher the optical density, the more bilirubin is present in the fluid, indicating that fetal red blood cells are being destroyed. From these findings, the severity of the disease in the fetus can be estimated. Because light destroys bilirubin, a specimen being studied to determine the bilirubin level should be placed in a dark container. (7)

**74.** 3. A direct Coombs test is done on cord blood to detect antibodies coating the baby's red blood cells. (1, 7)

**75.** 2. The fetus severely affected by hemolytic disease is transfused because the severe anemia with which the fetus suffers can produce grave results. The transfusion is done to replace destroyed red blood cells. The mother handles excess bilirubin that results from destroyed blood cells in her own liver. It is not until after delivery that the infant must handle the bilirubin, and the newborn does it poorly, especially if born prematurely, due to liver immaturity. When bilirubin reaches an above-average level in the newborn, the infant will then be jaundiced. (7)

**76.** 2. Preparing necessary equipment for the procedure of an exchange transfusion is a nursing responsibility. Cross-matching the blood, obtaining blood counts, and obtaining an informed consent are not the nurse's legal responsibilities, although she may assist with these procedures. (7)

**77.** 3. The aim of care for this infant is to reduce the blood concentration of bilirubin, in addition to relieving the infant's anemia. (7)

**78.** 4. The vein most commonly used for an exchange transfusion is the umbilical vein. The catheter is placed in the vein and into the body. The umbilical vein is large and easily accessible. An exchange transfusion can be done by cutdown into the jugular or femoral artery, but these sites are not as common as the umbilical vein. (7)

**79.** 3. A premature infant like the one in this item has

an unstable temperature-regulating mechanism, so an elevated temperature is not necessarily a good guide for determining the presence of infection in this case. In fact, the temperature is frequently subnormal in a premature infant with an infection. Such signs as lethargy, a poor sucking reflex, and changes in respirations are better guides to assess this infant for infection. (7)

**80.** 2. The albumin provides binding sites for the bilirubin. This is important because it is the free or unbound bilirubin that causes problems, such as kernicterus, in the infant. (7)

**81.** 2. The organ most subject to damage when uncontrolled hemolytic disease is present is the brain. The bilirubin crosses the blood-brain barrier and damages the cells of the CNS. This condition is called kernicterus. (7)

**82.** 1. Phototherapy is often used in the presence of jaundice. The infant's eyes should be patched while the infant is under the light to prevent eye damage. The scalp is not covered. Some agencies cover the genitalia, especially in a boy infant, because the effects of exposure to phototherapy on the genitalia are unknown. The stools tend to become loose and green and the urine may be green, due to excretion of decomposed bilirubin. A body rash is common and usually disappears spontaneously. (7)

**83.** 4. Tenets of the Roman Catholic Church hold that it would be acceptable for anyone, regardless of his or her religious beliefs, to baptize an infant. Local practice may vary. (1)

**84.** 2. Glucose crosses the placenta but insulin does not. Hence, a high blood sugar in the mother will cause a high blood sugar in the fetus. This causes the fetal pancreas to produce more insulin. At birth, the infant loses its source of glucose from the mother but has a continued high production of insulin, which often results in a drop in blood glucose levels. (7)

**85.** 2. A low blood glucose level in the newborn is likely to cause the infant to be jittery, to have a high-pitched or weak cry and tremors, and to refuse food. (7)

**86.** 2. It is usual to give a newborn with hypoglycemia a breast- or bottle-feeding. Administering intravenous glucose may be prescribed by some physicians, especially if the hypoglycemia is severe. Giving the infant sterile water or a balanced electrolyte solution intravenously will not help overcome hypoglycemia. Giving insulin will aggravate the condition. (7)

**87.** 4. Infants born of diabetic women suffer from respiratory distress syndrome about seven times more often than infants born of nondiabetic women. The infant described in this item should be observed closely for such signs as an expiratory grunt, nasal flaring, rapid respirations, and sternal and subcostal breathing, which are typical of respiratory distress syndrome. (7)

**88.** 1. The genetics involved in diabetes mellitus is not clearly understood, but a familial tendency appears to be present. It is best to tell parents that when either or both parents have the disease, their children have an increased risk of developing the disease. The severity of the disease the child may develop depends on several factors, but it seems that the more severe the disease of the parent(s), the greater the chance their children will develop the disease. (1)

**89.** 4. It is important first of all to tell the physician of the patient's use of heroin; this knowledge will influence the care of the mother and her baby. The information is used only in relation to the patient's care. With the patient's consent, the information may be shared with other community health agencies that become involved with the patient's long-term care. (7)

**90.** 1. Common symptoms associated with heroin withdrawal include nausea, tremors, cramps, diaphoresis, and yawning. (7, 9)

**91.** 1. The newborn can be expected to demonstrate symptoms of heroin withdrawal within the first 24 to 48 hours after birth. (7)

**92.** 4. The mother should be taught that the symptoms of heroin addiction may be present in her infant for as long as 1 year. At times, symptoms may persist for more than a year. (1, 7)

**93.** 3. An infant suffering from heroin withdrawal has a characteristic shrill or high-pitched cry. (7)

**94.** 4. Chlorpromazine hydrochloride (Thorazine) is the drug of choice for helping sedate an infant born with heroin addiction. It acts as a tranquilizer and helps control agitation and tension. Phenobarbital, diazepam (Valium), or paregoric may also be used. Nalorphine hydrochloride (Nalline) and levallorphan (Lorfan) are narcotic antagonists but do not help control the symptoms of withdrawal. Meperidine hydrochloride (Demerol) is a narcotic and depressant that would be inappropriate for this infant. (7)

**95.** 2. The newborn experiencing withdrawal from heroin has gastrointestinal problems similar to those of an adult who is withdrawing from heroin. The infant is likely to have vomiting, diarrhea, regurgitation, and anorexia. Because of these gastrointestinal problems, the newborn withdrawing from heroin needs to be monitored carefully to prevent dehydration. (7)

**96.** 1. A newborn with signs of heroin withdrawal is irritable, often restless, difficult to console, and in need of much sucking activity. It is often helpful to offer the infant a pacifier and to cuddle and rock him. The infant's environment should be kept at a low stimulation level. Offering the infant extra nourishment is not advised because overfeeding tends to increase problems with vomiting, regurgitation, and diarrhea. (1)

**97.** 1. Newborns with a drug addiction acquired from their mothers during pregnancy can be cured, because the infant has no psychological dependency on the drug. However, he does require care for the physical signs of addiction as long as they remain. (1)

**98.** 4. The amount of drug a pregnant woman uses, the length of time she uses it while pregnant, the amount of sensitivity she has for the drug, and the stage of embryonic development when the woman used the drug *may* influence the fetus. However, the most important determinant in terms of influencing the fetus is the stage of embryonic development when the drug was used. (7)

## REFERENCES FOR PART II
### The Nursing Care of Maternity Patients and Newborns

1. Bobak IM, Jensen MD. Essentials of Maternity Nursing: The Nurse and the Childbearing Family. 2nd ed. St. Louis: CV Mosby, 1987.
2. Clark JB, Queener SF, Karb VB. Pharmacological Basis of Nursing Practice. St. Louis: CV Mosby, 1986.
3. Haber J, Hoskins PP, Leach AM, Sideleau, BF. Comprehensive Psychiatric Nursing. New York: McGraw-Hill, 1987.
4. Haas K, Haas A. Understanding Sexuality. St. Louis: Times Mirror/Mosby, 1987.
5. Jones DA, Lepley MK, Baker BA. Health Assessment Across the Life Span. New York: McGraw-Hill, 1984.
6. Marlow DR, Redding BA. Textbook of Pediatric Nursing. 6th ed. Philadelphia: WB Saunders, 1988.
7. Olds SB, London ML, Ladewig PA. Maternal-Newborn Nursing. 3rd ed. Menlo Park: Addison-Wesley, 1988.
8. Oxorn H. Oxorn-Foote Human Labor and Birth. 5th ed. Norwalk: Appleton-Century-Crofts, 1986.
9. Potter PA, Perry AG. Fundamentals of Nursing: Concepts, Process, and Practice. St. Louis: CV Mosby, 1985.
10. Schuster CS, Ashburn SS. The Process of Human Development: A Holistic Life-Span Approach. 2nd ed. Boston: Little, Brown, 1986.

# PART III

## The Nursing Care
## of Children

# test 1

*Health Promotion of the Infant and Family*

*Health Promotion of the Toddler and Family*

*Health Promotion of the Preschooler and Family*

*Health Promotion of the School-Aged Child and Family*

*Health Promotion of the Adolescent and Family*

*Meetings to Discuss Common Childhood and Adolescent Health Problems*

*Correct Answers and Rationales*

Select the one *best* or *correct* answer and indicate your choice by filling in the circle with a pencil in front of the option you have chosen. If the answer you would prefer is not given, select the one you think is *most appropriate.*

## HEALTH PROMOTION OF THE INFANT AND FAMILY

A nurse works in a children's clinic and helps with care for well and ill children of various ages.

1. Ms. Lee brings her 4-month-old infant, Timmy, to the clinic. He appears well. Ms. Lee asks the nurse when she should wean Timmy from breast-feedings and have him use a cup. The nurse should explain that Timmy will show readiness to be weaned when he is
   - 1. taking solid foods well.
   - 2. sleeping through the night.
   - 3. shortening his nursing time.
   - 4. eating on a regular schedule.

2. Ms. Lee says that Timmy's physician recommends certain solid foods, but Timmy refuses to eat them after his breast-feedings. The nurse should suggest that Ms. Lee feed Timmy by
   - 1. offering him dessert followed by his vegetables and meat.
   - 2. giving him breast milk as long as he refuses to eat solid foods.
   - 3. mixing pureed food with cow's milk and feeding it to him through a large-hole nipple.
   - 4. giving him a few minutes of breast nursing and then feeding him his solid foods.

3. Which of the following abilities would be considered *unusual* for an infant of Timmy's age (4 months)?
   - 1. Sitting up without support.
   - 2. Responding to pleasure with smiles.
   - 3. Grasping a rattle when it is offered to him.
   - 4. Turning himself from either side to his back.

4. The nurse plans to administer the Denver Developmental Screening Test (DDST) to 5-month-old Sandra Plitka. The nurse should explain to Sandra's mother that the test measures the child's
   - 1. intelligence quotient.
   - 2. emotional development.
   - 3. social and physical abilities.
   - 4. predisposition to genetic and allergic illnesses.

5. The nurse discusses immunization for Sandra with Ms. Plitka. In addition to immunizing for diphtheria, pertussis, and tetanus (DPT), authorities recommend that during the first 6 months of life, children should also be immunized against
   - 1. mumps.
   - 2. measles.
   - 3. tuberculosis.
   - 4. poliomyelitis.

6. Ms. Plitka asks the nurse, "What about a smallpox vaccination for Sandra?" The nurse should explain that the current recommendation concerning smallpox immunization is that vaccination for this disease
   - 1. should no longer be given.
   - 2. should be postponed until the child is about 2 years old.
   - 3. can safely be delayed until the child starts school.
   - 4. should be postponed until the child is an adolescent.

7. The nurse discusses Sandra's motor skill development with Ms. Plitka. The nurse explains to Ms. Plitka that at about 7 months of age Sandra will *most likely* be able to
   - 1. walk with support.
   - 2. feed herself with a spoon.
   - 3. stand holding onto furniture.
   - 4. sit alone using her hands for support.

8. Ms. Grange brings 1-month-old Ben to the clinic. Which of the following developmental achievements is *normal* for Ben?

○ 1. He smiles and laughs aloud.
○ 2. He rolls from his back to his side.
○ 3. He holds a rattle for a brief period of time.
○ 4. He turns his head from side to side when lying on his abdomen.

9. Two-month-old Casey Crane is brought to the clinic for his first immunization against diphtheria, pertussis, and tetanus (DPT). What route should the nurse use to administer the vaccine?
○ 1. Oral.
○ 2. Intramuscular.
○ 3. Subcutaneous.
○ 4. Intradermal.

10. The nurse should teach Casey's mother about the normal reaction an infant may experience approximately 12 to 24 hours after a diphtheria, pertussis, and tetanus (DPT) immunization. One of these reactions could be
○ 1. lethargy.
○ 2. mild fever.
○ 3. diarrhea.
○ 4. nasal congestion.

11. Ms. Ortiga brings Paula to the clinic. Paula is observed by the nurse to be competent in the following developmental skills: she holds her head erect when in a sitting position, she stares at an object placed in her hand and takes it to her mouth, she coos and gurgles when talked to, and she sustains part of her own weight when held in a standing position. The nurse is correct when she assesses Paula's age to be approximately
○ 1. 2 months.
○ 2. 4 months.
○ 3. 6 months.
○ 4. 8 months.

12. Ms. Ortiga says, "The soft spot near the front of Paula's head is still big. When will it close?" The nurse's response should be guided by knowledge that most often the anterior fontanel closes when the infant's age is between about
○ 1. 2 to 4 months.
○ 2. 4 to 8 months.
○ 3. 8 to 12 months.
○ 4. 12 to 18 months.

13. The nurse explains to Ms. Ortiga the danger of the infant's choking when propping a bottle of formula or fruit juice at bedtime. The nurse also explains that propping a bottle at bedtime when Paula is old enough to handle the bottle safely is *not* recommended *primarily* because the practice predisposes the infant to
○ 1. obesity.
○ 2. dental caries.
○ 3. an abnormally prolonged attachment to a bottle.

○ 4. an abnormally prolonged use of nighttime feedings.

14. Ms. Droege thinks 9-month-old George is developing slowly. When the nurse evaluates the infant's development, she should base her judgments on knowledge that *all* of the following developmental tasks are typical of a normal 9-month-old infant *except*
○ 1. creeping and crawling.
○ 2. beginning to use specific imitative verbal expressions.
○ 3. putting his arm through a sleeve while being dressed.
○ 4. holding his nursing bottle with good hand-mouth coordination.

15. Ms. Droege says it is difficult to add new foods to George's diet. "He spits everything out of his mouth," she says. The nurse is referring to the *most often* recommended way to begin infants on new foods when she suggests that Ms. Droege
○ 1. mix new foods with formula.
○ 2. mix new foods with more familiar foods.
○ 3. offer new foods on a one-at-a-time basis.
○ 4. offer new foods after formula has been offered.

## HEALTH PROMOTION OF THE TODDLER AND FAMILY

16. Ms. Hampton is recently divorced and is seeking employment. She brings her 18-month-old daughter, Dolly, to the clinic because the child eats "ashes, crayons, paper—almost anything she can get into her mouth." Based on knowledge of Dolly's behavior, the nurse should *first* determine if Dolly is
○ 1. cutting large teeth.
○ 2. experiencing a growth spurt.
○ 3. experiencing a change in the home environment.
○ 4. eating a soft, low-roughage diet.

17. The nurse assesses Dolly's physical development. Which of the following tasks is *most typical* of a normally developed 18-month-old child?
○ 1. Copying a circle.
○ 2. Pulling toys.
○ 3. Playing tag with other children.
○ 4. Building a tower of eight blocks.

18. Ms. Baker brings her normally developed 3-year-old son Hal to the clinic for a checkup before enrolling him in nursery school. The nurse would expect Hal to be *least skilled* in
○ 1. riding a tricycle.
○ 2. tying shoelaces.

○ 3. stringing large beads.

○ 4. using blunt scissors.

19. Which of the following people would *most likely* be Hal's "significant others"?

○ 1. Peers.

○ 2. Parents.

○ 3. Siblings.

○ 4. Neighbors.

20. Twenty-four-month-old Christopher Creighton is brought to the clinic by his mother because "he keeps pulling at his ear." Christopher is unco-operative when the nurse tries to look in his ears. Which of the following courses of action would be *best* for the nurse to try *first*?

○ 1. Ask another nurse to assist.

○ 2. Allow the parent to assist.

○ 3. Wait until the child calms down.

○ 4. Restrain the child's arms.

21. Ear drops are prescribed for Christopher. They are to be instilled twice a day. When teaching Mrs. Creighton to instill the drops, the nurse should tell her to pull Christopher's ear lobe

○ 1. up and forward.

○ 2. up and backward.

○ 3. down and forward.

○ 4. down and backward.

22. Before Mrs. Creighton leaves, she tells the nurse that she is having problems toilet-training Chris-topher. Toilet-training in toddlers *most com-monly* fails because the

○ 1. rewards are too limited.

○ 2. training equipment is inappropriate.

○ 3. parents ignore "accidents" that occur during training.

○ 4. child is not developmentally ready to be trained.

23. Niki Cole, 2½ years old, is brought to the clinic by her father. He explains that Niki is afraid of the dark and says "no" to everything she is asked to do. The nurse is aware that the negativism demon-strated by toddlers, like Niki, is frequently an ex-pression of

○ 1. a quest for autonomy.

○ 2. hyperactivity.

○ 3. separation anxiety.

○ 4. sibling rivalry.

24. The nurse is aware that Niki's fear of darkness can be explained by Piaget's theory of intellectual or cognitive development. What concept in the pre-conceptual phase of cognitive development ex-plains Niki's fear of darkness?

○ 1. Reversibility.

○ 2. Animism.

○ 3. Conservation of matter.

○ 4. Object permanence.

25. Mr. Cole reports that Niki often falls while running. This can partially be explained by the fact that a preschooler's vision is

○ 1. myopic.

○ 2. hyperopic.

○ 3. presbyopic.

○ 4. amblyopic.

26. Mrs. Puzak brings 3-year-old Carol to the clinic because she is concerned about Carol's nutritional status. Mrs. Puzak tells the nurse that for the last week Carol has refused to eat anything except animal crackers and peanut-butter-and-jelly sandwiches. Which of the following would be *most appropriate* for the nurse to suggest?

○ 1. "Give Carol extra time to play outside if she eats what the family eats at mealtime."

○ 2. "Consult a physician, because Carol's behavior will cause nutritional deficiency."

○ 3. "Don't be overly concerned about Carol's be-havior. Food fads usually last a short time."

○ 4. "Insist that Carol eat small portions of the fam-ily's meal in order to maintain adequate nutri-tion."

27. The nurse assesses Carol's teeth during the physi-cal exam. Using knowledge of dental health for the toddler, it would be appropriate for the nurse to teach Mrs. Puzak to

○ 1. have Carol brush her teeth after every meal and at bedtime.

○ 2. brush Carol's teeth with a small toothbrush with soft natural bristles.

○ 3. floss Carol's teeth using unwaxed dental floss.

○ 4. add a fluoride supplement to Carol's milk three times daily.

28. Mrs. Puzak asks the nurse for advice about disci-plining Carol. Based on knowledge of the *best approach* toward discipline with a 3-year-old, the nurse should suggest that Mrs. Puzak use

○ 1. structured interactions.

○ 2. spanking.

○ 3. reasoning.

○ 4. scolding.

29. Which of the following pain assessment tech-niques would be *least effective* for the nurse to use when caring for toddlers?

○ 1. Ask them about their pain.

○ 2. Observe them for restlessness.

○ 3. Watch their faces for grimaces.

○ 4. Listen for pain clues in their cries.

30. In discussing the behavior of people with her friends, a clinic nurse discovers that she is less judgmental than her friends. The nurse is *most likely* to be less judgmental because she

○ 1. gave up her values in an attempt to accept people as they are.

2. understands the origin of her own values.
3. consciously overlooks other people's values that are contrary to hers.
4. works gradually to change the detrimental values of others.

## HEALTH PROMOTION OF THE PRESCHOOLER AND FAMILY

Mrs. Zeeb has brought her 4-year-old son Charles to the pediatrician's office for an annual checkup.

31. Mrs. Zeeb is concerned that Charles may be hyperactive. She describes him as always "in motion." He is constantly bruising himself or dropping or spilling something. Which nursing intervention would be *most* appropriate?
    1. Determine if there have been any changes at home.
    2. Explain that this is not unusual behavior.
    3. Explore the possibility that the child is being abused.
    4. Suggest that the child be seen by a pediatric neurologist.

32. Mrs. Zeeb asks the nurse to recommend activities that would help Charles channel his energy. Which of the following activities should the nurse recommend?
    1. Participating in parallel play.
    2. Playing a game like "Simon Says."
    3. Riding a bicycle.
    4. Stringing large beads.

33. Mrs. Zeeb tells the nurse that Charles creates quite a scene every night at bedtime and asks what she can do to make bedtime a little more pleasant. The nurse should suggest that Mrs. Zeeb
    1. allow him to stay up one or two nights a week.
    2. establish a set bedtime and include a predictable routine.
    3. let him play tag with his father just before bedtime.
    4. tell him he can have a cookie if he goes to bed without a fuss.

34. Mrs. Zeeb asks the nurse about dental care for Charles. She explains that Charles does not appear to have any problems, and she helps him brush his teeth daily. However, she has noticed that the neighbors take their 4- and 5-year-old children to the dentist and wonders if she should do the same. Which response from the nurse would be *most* appropriate?

    1. "Since you help him brush his teeth daily, he does not need to visit a dentist."
    2. "You should have begun taking him to the dentist last year, but it is not too late."
    3. "He does not need to see a dentist until he is ready to start school."
    4. "A dental checkup is a good idea, even if he doesn't have any noticeable problems."

35. Mrs. Zeeb says that she will be glad when Charles can brush his teeth without her help. She asks the nurse at what age Charles will be able to do this. The nurse should respond
    1. 3 years.
    2. 5 years.
    3. 6 years.
    4. 7 years.

36. Mrs. Zeeb tells the nurse that Charles does not seem to know the difference between right and wrong. She explains that he knows he should not push other children, but the only reason he can give for not pushing them is that he avoids trouble. Mrs. Zeeb is describing typical behavior of a child who has reached which level of moral development as described by Kohlberg?
    1. Autonomous.
    2. Conventional.
    3. Preconventional.
    4. Principles.

37. Mrs. Zeeb tells the nurse that Charles seems to have developed very strange eating habits. Often he will not finish his meals, and for days he may only eat one food. Mrs. Zeeb says she would like to develop a plan that would "help correct" Charles's eating habits. In developing such a plan, the nurse and Mrs. Zeeb should consider
    1. determining a food reward for him, if he finishes his meals.
    2. allowing him to make some decisions about the foods he eats.
    3. requiring him to eat the foods served at mealtimes.
    4. telling him that he cannot play with his friends unless he finishes his meals.

38. Since both she and her husband are nearsighted, Mrs. Zeeb is concerned that Charles may be nearsighted. She says that he likes looking at his picture books and knows most of the alphabet. What assessment technique should the nurse use to evaluate Charles's visual acuity?
    1. The cover and cross-over test.
    2. Allen picture cards.
    3. Snellen alphabet chart.
    4. Ishihara plates.

39. After having a blood sample drawn, Charles insists

that the site be covered with a Band-Aid. When his mother tries to remove the Band-Aid before they leave the nurse's office, Charles screams that all his blood will come out if the Band-Aid is removed. This behavior indicates

- ○ 1. a normal fear of injury.
- ○ 2. a normal fear of compromised body integrity.
- ○ 3. an abnormal fear of compromised body integrity.
- ○ 4. an abnormal fear of loss of control.

40. Preschool-aged children like Charles may believe that injections are punishment for misdeeds. Which nursing intervention would help prepare a preschool-aged child for an injection?
- ○ 1. Have an older child explain that shots do not hurt big boys.
- ○ 2. Suggest diversionary activities such as singing.
- ○ 3. Give him a play syringe, alcohol sponge, and Band-Aid so the child can give a doll play injections.
- ○ 4. Give him a pounding board so that he can express his fear.

Several employees at a silk flower shop have preschool-aged children. While talking at lunch one day about their children, the employees decide it would be helpful to have an "informational" meeting with a pediatric nurse. An employee arranges for a community pediatric nurse specialist to meet with them.

41. A woman at the meeting says her 5-year-old son seems prone to minor accidents like skinning his knees and elbows and falling off his scooter. In order to analyze the situation, the nurse needs more information. The nurse should base further assessment on the knowledge that childhood accidents are more likely to occur when the family
- ○ 1. consists of only one child.
- ○ 2. has limited formal education.
- ○ 3. is experiencing changes.
- ○ 4. has a high economic status.

42. Several other parents are interested in accident prevention and ask how to teach 4-year-olds about safety. The nurse knows that one of the *most* effective strategies that parents can use to teach 4-year-olds about safety is to
- ○ 1. show them potential dangers to avoid.
- ○ 2. tell them they are bad when they do something dangerous.
- ○ 3. provide good examples of safe behavior.
- ○ 4. show them pictures of children who have been involved in accidents.

43. A woman in the group explains that her 5-year-old daughter has had multiple ear infections and asks how preschool-aged children perceive illness. The nurse should explain that they generally regard it as
- ○ 1. a necessary part of life.
- ○ 2. a test of self-worth.
- ○ 3. punishment for wrongdoing.
- ○ 4. the will of God.

44. A father in the group says that while at the pediatrician's office he saw a brochure about something called the Denver Developmental Screening Test. He asks if his 5-year-old son should have this test. Before answering the question, the nurse would need additional information about the
- ○ 1. father's understanding of the test.
- ○ 2. reason for the visit to the pediatrician.
- ○ 3. child's developmental level.
- ○ 4. child's performance in kindergarten.

## HEALTH PROMOTION OF THE SCHOOL-AGED CHILD AND FAMILY

Nine-year-old Kellie is brought to the pediatrician's office for a camp physical. She has no history of significant health problems.

45. When the nurse asks Kellie and her mother about Kellie's best friend, the nurse is assessing Kellie's
- ○ 1. language development.
- ○ 2. motor development.
- ○ 3. neurological development.
- ○ 4. social development.

46. Kellie proudly tells the nurse that she is completely responsible for brushing and flossing her teeth. When responding to this information, the nurse should realize that Kellie
- ○ 1. is too young to be given this responsibility.
- ○ 2. is most likely quite capable of this responsibility.
- ○ 3. should have assumed this responsibility much sooner.
- ○ 4. is probably just exaggerating her responsibility.

47. Kellie's mother tells the nurse that Kellie is continually telling riddles and jokes to the point of driving the family crazy. The nurse explains that this is a sign of
- ○ 1. inadequate parental attention.
- ○ 2. mastery of language ambiguities.
- ○ 3. inappropriate peer influence.
- ○ 4. watching too much television.

48. Kellie's mother tells the nurse that Kellie is begin-

ning to identify behaviors that please others as "good" behaviors. Kellie's behavior is characteristic of which of Kohlberg's levels of moral development?

○ 1. Preconventional morality.
○ 2. Conventional morality.
○ 3. Postconventional morality.
○ 4. Autonomous morality.

49. Kellie's mother asks the nurse about Kellie's apparent need for between-meal snacks, especially after school. The nurse discusses Kellie's nutritional needs with her mother and develops a nutritional plan with her. In developing this plan, the nurse should recognize that Kellie

○ 1. does not need to eat between meals.
○ 2. should eat the snacks her mother prepares.
○ 3. should help prepare her own snacks.
○ 4. will instinctively select nutritionally sound foods.

50. Kellie's mother is concerned about Kellie's compulsion for collecting things. The nurse explains that this behavior is related to the cognitive ability to perform

○ 1. concrete operations.
○ 2. formal operations.
○ 3. coordination of secondary schemas.
○ 4. tertiary circular reactions.

51. When Kellie's height and weight are compared with standard growth charts, she is found to be in the 85th percentile for height and in the 45th percentile for weight. These findings indicate that Kellie is

○ 1. of normal height and weight.
○ 2. overweight for her height.
○ 3. underweight for her height.
○ 4. taller than average.

52. According to Erikson's framework of psychosocial development, play as a vehicle of development can help the school-aged child develop a sense of

○ 1. initiative.
○ 2. industry.
○ 3. identity.
○ 4. intimacy.

53. The parents of a 6-year-old child tell the nurse that they are concerned about the child's tonsils. On inspection, the tonsils are very large, but are not reddened or inflamed. The nurse explains that these findings *most likely* indicate

○ 1. the need for tonsillectomy.
○ 2. acute tonsillitis.
○ 3. a normal increase in lymphoid tissue.
○ 4. an abnormal growth of lymphoid tissue.

54. The school nurse is planning a series of safety and accident prevention classes for a group of third

graders. What preventive measure does the nurse stress during the first class, knowing the leading cause of accidental injury and death in this age group?

○ 1. The use of flame-retardant clothing.
○ 2. The use of life preservers.
○ 3. The use of protective eyewear.
○ 4. The use of auto seat belts.

55. The immunizations recommended for children between the ages of 4 and 6 years prior to entering school are

○ 1. diphtheria, tetanus, pertussis, and polio.
○ 2. measles, mumps, rubella, and polio.
○ 3. polio, smallpox, measles, and pertussis.
○ 4. tetanus, diphtheria, mumps, and smallpox.

56. The mother of a 10-year-old boy is concerned about the fact that her son is overweight. When developing a plan of care with the mother, the nurse encourages her to

○ 1. limit his between-meal snacks.
○ 2. prohibit him from playing outside if he eats sweets.
○ 3. include the child in meal planning and preparation.
○ 4. limit his caloric intake to 1,200 calories daily.

## HEALTH PROMOTION OF THE ADOLESCENT AND FAMILY

Ms. Mannheim is the school nurse at Jackson High School. Many of the students come to talk with her about a variety of concerns.

57. When interacting with adolescents, the nurse considers their phase of cognitive development. According to Piaget, this phase of development is characterized by the ability to

○ 1. assimilate and accommodate.
○ 2. deal with abstract possibilities.
○ 3. manipulate concrete materials.
○ 4. solve problems of conservation.

58. Mary, 16, comes to see Ms. Mannheim because of dysmenorrhea. Mary explains that she has cramps, backache, and nausea with her periods. Ms. Mannheim considers that the basis for these symptoms is *most likely*

○ 1. pathological.
○ 2. physiological.
○ 3. psychogenic.
○ 4. psychosomatic.

59. Relief of dysmenorrhea at this time in her life is

important for Mary because it will help her develop

○ 1. positive peer relations.
○ 2. positive self-identity.
○ 3. a sense of autonomy.
○ 4. a sense of control.

60. Mary tells Ms. Mannheim that she would like to use tampons during her period. An appropriate nursing intervention would be to
○ 1. assess her understanding of her anatomy.
○ 2. determine if she is sexually active.
○ 3. provide her with information about toxic shock syndrome.
○ 4. refer her to a specialist in adolescent gynecology.

61. Ms. Mannheim is invited to attend a meeting of the Parent-Teacher Association. Several parents express frustration with the amount of time their adolescents spend in front of the mirror and the length of time it takes them to get dressed to leave the house. Ms. Mannheim explains that this behavior is
○ 1. an indication of an abnormal concern with self.
○ 2. a method of procrastination commonly seen in teenagers.
○ 3. a method of testing their parents' limit-setting.
○ 4. a result of rapid body change and developing self-concept.

62. One mother asks Ms. Mannheim if her 16-year-old daughter still needs immunizations. Ms. Mannheim would *correctly* explain that
○ 1. children more than 7 years old do not need immunizations.
○ 2. adolescents should routinely receive measles vaccination at age 16.
○ 3. the last immunization is a tetanus booster at age 16.
○ 4. adolescents and adults should have a tetanus-diphtheria booster every 10 years.

63. Several high-school seniors are referred to Ms. Mannheim because of suspected alcohol misuse. When assessing the situation, it would be *most* important for Ms. Mannheim to determine
○ 1. if they know the legal drinking age.
○ 2. the type of alcohol they usually drink.
○ 3. the reasons they choose to use alcohol.
○ 4. when and with whom they use alcohol.

64. Several parents are concerned about the type and large quantities of food teenagers eat and their refusal to eat foods served at family meals. It would be *most appropriate* for Ms. Mannheim to help the parents develop a plan to
○ 1. evaluate the adolescent's nutritional intake carefully.

○ 2. inform the adolescent about the adverse effects of fad diets and fast foods.
○ 3. give the adolescent responsibility for grocery-shopping for a month.
○ 4. incorporate the adolescent's preferences into meal planning.

65. One of the seniors justifies his actions by saying, "Everyone does it, so it's all right." This is an example of which level of moral reasoning, as defined by Kohlberg?
○ 1. Preconventional level.
○ 2. Conventional level.
○ 3. Postconventional level.
○ 4. Autonomous level.

66. As part of annual health screening, Ms. Mannheim visits the 8th-grade physical education classes. She asks each student to bend forward at the waist with the back parallel to the floor and the hands together at midline. The purpose of this is to observe for signs of
○ 1. slipped epiphysis.
○ 2. congenital hip dislocation.
○ 3. idiopathic scoliosis.
○ 4. physical dexterity.

## MEETINGS TO DISCUSS COMMON CHILDHOOD AND ADOLESCENT HEALTH PROBLEMS

The parents of children attending an elementary school and a high school invite the school nurse to attend some of their Parent-Teacher Association meetings to discuss common health problems related to their youngsters.

67. One parent asks about head lice (pediculosis capitis). Which of the following symptoms is *most* common when a child has been infested with head lice?
○ 1. Itching of the scalp.
○ 2. Scaling of the scalp.
○ 3. Serous weeping on the scalp surface.
○ 4. Pinpoint hemorrhagic spots on the scalp surface.

68. A parent asks, "Can I get head lice too?" The nurse indicates that adults can also be infested with head lice, but she should explain that infestation with pediculosis is more common among school children than among adults *primarily* because
○ 1. an immunity to pediculosis usually is established by adulthood.

2. children of school age tend to be more neglectful of frequent handwashing.

3. pediculosis is most often spread by close contact with infested children in the classroom.

4. the skin of adults is more capable of resisting the invasion of lice than the skin of children.

**69.** One parent asks what causes ringworm of the scalp (tinea capitis). The organism responsible for causing ringworm of the scalp is classified as a

1. virus.

2. fungus.

3. bacillus.

4. protozoan.

**70.** One mother says that her physician ordered griseofulvin (Grisactin) to treat her son's ringworm of the scalp. "He said it is very important to take the medication exactly as ordered for several weeks. Why is that so important?" she asks. The nurse should base her response on knowledge that

1. a sensitivity to the drug may occur if it is not taken over a period of time.

2. fewer side effects occur as the body slowly adjusts to a new substance over a period of time.

3. fewer allergic reactions occur if the drug is maintained at the same level over a period of time.

4. the growth of the causative organism into new cells is prevented when the drug is used over a period of time.

**71.** "How did my children get pinworms?" a mother asks. The nurse should respond by explaining that pinworms are spread *most commonly* by contaminated

1. food.

2. hands.

3. animals.

4. toilet seats.

**72.** A parent says his family will be traveling abroad, and asks why the drinking water there must be boiled. In addition to various types of dysentery, contaminated drinking water is *most often* responsible for the transmission of

1. typhus.

2. brucellosis.

3. poliomyelitis.

4. typhoid fever.

**73.** A mother says one of her children has chicken pox and asks about his care. The nurse should explain that the care of a child with chicken pox is directed *primarily* toward the prevention of

1. anemia and dehydration.

2. anorexia and malnutrition.

3. infection at the site of lesions.

4. infection in the respiratory system.

**74.** A mother says to the nurse, "My sister-in-law's children have chicken pox and she feels helpless because she doesn't know how to relieve the itching." Which of the following home regimens should the nurse suggest to relieve itching areas in children with chicken pox?

1. Applying generous amounts of fine baby powder.

2. Applying a paste made with baking soda and water.

3. Applying terry-cloth towels moistened in warm water.

4. Applying cool compresses moistened with a weak salt solution.

**75.** A mother says that a physician described her youngster as having 20/60 vision. She asks the nurse what 20/60 means. The nurse should base her response on knowledge that the child

1. has lost approximately one-third of his visual acuity.

2. is seeing at 60 feet what he should be seeing at 20 feet.

3. is seeing at 20 feet what he should be seeing at 60 feet.

4. has visual acuity approximately three times better than the average child.

**76.** A parent says her youngster has hemophilia and she worries whenever the child has a bump or cut. The nurse explains that after cleaning the area, the wound should be cared for by applying

1. gentle pressure.

2. warm, moist compresses.

3. a tourniquet above the injured area.

4. dressings moistened with witch hazel.

**77.** Which of the following over-the-counter medications should the mother be taught to *avoid* giving her child with hemophilia?

1. Acetylsalicylic acid (Aspirin).

2. Magnesium hydroxide (Milk of Magnesia).

3. Acetaminophen (Tylenol).

4. Multiple vitamin capsules.

**78.** The parents ask the school nurse how they can best prepare their children for entering school. Of the following courses of action, it would be *best* for the nurse to recommend that the parents

1. have an older sibling tell their children about school.

2. orient their children to the school's physical environment.

3. offer to stay with their children for the first few days of school.

4. discuss school with their children if they ask questions about it.

**79.** The nurse should explain that the *most common* cause for the unhappiness some children experience when first entering school is their

○ 1. feeling of insecurity.
○ 2. inability to pay attention.
○ 3. emotional maladjustment.
○ 4. poor language development.

**80.** Food requirements for school children are discussed. When compared with the food requirements of preschoolers and adolescents, the food requirements of children between about 6 and 12 years of age are not as great because they have a lower

○ 1. growth rate.
○ 2. metabolic rate.
○ 3. level of activity.
○ 4. hormonal secretion rate.

**81.** When the eating habits of children in middle childhood (ages 6 through 12) are discussed, the nurse is guided by knowledge that eating habits of children during this period are *most* influenced by

○ 1. food preferences of their peers.
○ 2. the smell and appearance of food offered them.
○ 3. the atmosphere and examples provided by parents at mealtimes.
○ 4. parents encouraging their children to eat foods that are good for them.

**82.** Adolescent behavior is discussed with the parents. According to Erikson, of the following developmental tasks, the central problem of adolescence is establishing a sense of

○ 1. identity.
○ 2. industry.
○ 3. intimacy.
○ 4. initiative.

**83.** Which of the following statements would be *best* for the nurse to use when she describes findings in relation to the onset of adolescence in boys and girls?

○ 1. "Girls and boys experience the onset of adolescence at approximately the same age."
○ 2. "Boys experience the onset of adolescence approximately 1 to 2 years earlier than girls."
○ 3. "Girls experience the onset of adolescence approximately 1 to 2 years earlier than boys."
○ 4. "Findings do not support a sexual relationship concerning the onset of adolescence."

**84.** In order to illustrate adolescent behavior, the nurse uses a common statement one could expect from an adolescent. Which of the following statements would be *most typical* of a normal adolescent in the United States?

○ 1. "I can hardly wait to grow up."
○ 2. "I know who I am and where I want to go in life."

○ 3. "I usually prefer being with my parents rather than being alone in my room."
○ 4. "I like my friends and I don't mind their choice of clothes and hairdo. But I want to be different."

**85.** One parent says, "I certainly wish I knew how to cut down on conflicts between my teenaged son and myself." The nurse responds to the parent's comment by using a proverb in her explanation. Which of the following proverbs reflects an attitude toward child-rearing that *most often* leads to conflicts between parents and teenagers?

○ 1. "Do as I say, not as I do."
○ 2. "A stitch in time saves nine."
○ 3. "Spare the rod and spoil the child."
○ 4. "Nature is more important than nurture."

**86.** Several parents express concern about problems acne creates in their children and ask the nurse how a teenager with acne should cleanse the affected areas. Of the following courses of action, it would be *best* for the nurse to recommend that teenagers with acne cleanse their skin with

○ 1. witch hazel.
○ 2. soap and water.
○ 3. hydrogen peroxide.
○ 4. lotions and creams.

**87.** A parent in the group says that his neighbor's 15-year-old youngster has mononucleosis and asks the nurse what precautions should be used to prevent its spread. Which of the following responses would *most accurately* reflect present opinion concerning the spread of mononucleosis?

○ 1. No particular precautionary measures are advised.
○ 2. The youngster's eating utensils should be boiled before being reused.
○ 3. The youngster's linens should be washed separately in hot, soapy water.
○ 4. A mask should be used when giving the youngster direct personal care.

**88.** Another parent asks how she would know if her youngster developed mononucleosis. The nurse should explain that in addition to fatigue, the symptom *most typical* of mononucleosis is

○ 1. liver tenderness.
○ 2. enlarged lymph glands.
○ 3. persistent nonproductive cough.
○ 4. generalized skin rash resembling a blush.

**89.** The subject of venereal diseases and their control is discussed at one meeting. The nurse *correctly* explains that community health measures designed to control the incidence of venereal diseases are *most often* directed toward

○ 1. mass screening for venereal diseases.

○ 2. locating the sources of venereal diseases.

○ 3. treating persons who have or are suspected of having venereal diseases.

○ 4. isolating persons who have or are suspected of having venereal diseases.

**90.** A parent asks why it is recommended that adolescent girls not be given "measles vaccine." The *most important* reason why girls after the age of puberty are usually *not* given rubella vaccine is that

○ 1. risks to the fetus are high if the girl is pregnant.

○ 2. chances of contracting the disease are much lower after puberty than before.

○ 3. dangers associated with a strong reaction to the vaccine are increased after puberty.

○ 4. changes occurring within the immunologic system may affect the rhythm of the menstrual cycle.

# CORRECT ANSWERS AND RATIONALES

Numbers appear in parentheses following the rationales. The numbers identify textbooks listed in the references at the end of Part III, where correct answers can be verified.

## Health Promotion of the Infant and Family

1. 3. Readiness for weaning is an individual matter but is usually present when an infant begins to shorten his nursing time. He will be showing independence and will then be ready to take a cup and learn a new skill. The child ready for weaning may also demonstrate that he is able to take solid foods well, sleep through the night, and eat on a regular schedule, but these behaviors are not necessarily evidence of readiness for weaning. (7, 21)

2. 4. Starting an infant on solid foods is a new experience for him and requires new skills. It is typical for the infant to spit out foods because he has not learned how to swallow them. Also, he is hungry and is accustomed to having milk to satisfy his hunger. It is generally recommended that the infant be given at least some milk first and then offered solids. If his hunger has been satisfied by taking all the milk, he will be uninterested in learning to accept solid foods. In starting solid foods with an infant, it has not been found satisfactory to offer dessert before vegetables and meat, to mix pureed foods with cow's milk, or to continue with breast milk only, while delaying offering solid foods. (7, 21)

3. 1. A 4-month-old infant is not able to sit without support, but will normally display such behaviors as responding with smiles, grasping a rattle, and turning from either side to his back. It is normal to expect a child of 7 or 8 months to be able to sit without support. (7, 21)

4. 3. The Denver Developmental Screening Test measures a child's social and physical abilities. It is not designed to measure intelligence and emotional development, nor does it measure predisposition to illnesses. (7, 21)

5. 4. The United States Public Health Service and the American Academy of Pediatrics have developed recommended guidelines for immunization of children. A series of three injections of diphtheria, pertussis, and tetanus (DPT) vaccine is recommended during the 1st year of life. Poliomyelitis protection is administered twice during the 1st year unless the disease is prevalent in the area where the child lives, in which case another dose may be given.

Measles, mumps, and rubella vaccine administration is recommended when the child is 15 months old. Administering these vaccines early in the child's life may interfere with the adequate development of immunity because of the presence of maternal antibodies in the youngster. Immunity for tuberculosis is not done; skin testing for tuberculosis may be done if the disease is prevalent in the area where the child lives. (7, 21)

6. 1. Routine vaccination for smallpox is no longer recommended. The dangers and incidence of complications following vaccination have been determined to be greater than the possibility of contracting the disease. The disease is considered to be eradicated because no cases of smallpox have been reported since 1977. (11, 21)

7. 4. By 7 months of age an infant can sit alone, leaning forward on his hands for support. The ability to sit follows progressive head control and straightening of the back. By 8 months of age, an infant should be able to sit well unsupported. At about 10 months of age, an infant can step with one foot and crawl well. At 11 months, an infant can walk while holding onto furniture and by 12 months, an infant can walk with one hand held. Around 18 months, an infant can feed himself successfully with a spoon. (15, 21)

8. 4. A 1-month-old infant is able to lift his head and turn it from side to side when in the prone position. He has been able to do this since birth if he was full term and no abnormalities or complications were present. Smiling and laughing aloud are expected behaviors for a 2- to 3-month-old infant. Holding a rattle for a brief time and rolling from the back to the side are characteristic behaviors of a 4-month-old infant. (7, 21)

9. 2. The diphtheria, pertussis, and tetanus (DPT) vaccine is given by injection deep into the largest muscle available. The best muscle to use in a 2-month-old infant is the vastus lateralis. This muscle is located in the anteriolateral portion of the upper thigh. The intramuscular route is used to reduce the inflammatory reaction to DPT vaccine. (15, 21)

10. 2. Mild fever 12 to 24 hours after the administration of a diphtheria, pertussis, and tetanus (DPT) vaccine is common in an infant. The infant's mother should be taught to use acetaminophen (Tylenol) for the fever. A fever above 102° F. (39° C.) rectally should be reported to the physician. An infant with a fever tends to be restless, rather than lethargic. Diarrhea and nasal congestion are not associated with the administration of the DPT vaccine. (15, 21)

**11.** 2. Typical behaviors of an infant of about 4 months of age include holding his head erect when sitting, staring at an object placed in his hand, taking the object to his mouth, cooing and gurgling, and sustaining part of his own weight when in a standing position. (7, 21)

**12.** 4. The most common time for the anterior fontanel to close is between 12 and 18 months of age. The small posterior fontanel usually closes by the end of the 2nd month. (7, 11)

**13.** 2. Many mothers prop a bottle of formula or fruit juice at bedtime for their infants after the infants are old enough to handle a bottle safely. The infant then awakens periodically to take more formula or fruit juice, constantly bathing recently erupted teeth with the high-carbohydrate liquid. The practice has been noted to predispose the infant to dental caries, which may eventually require considerable dental work. The practice of propping the bottle does not necessarily lead to obesity or an abnormally prolonged use of a bottle or of nighttime feedings. (7, 21)

**14.** 3. Normally, a 9-month-old infant will not be able to put his arm through a sleeve while being dressed but will be able to carry out such activities as creeping, crawling, holding his nursing bottle, and using imitated verbal expressions. He will be approximately 2 years old before he can put an arm through a sleeve. (7, 21)

**15.** 3. Infants should be offered new foods on a one-at-a-time basis. This provides the infant with an opportunity to become familiar with a variety of food tastes and textures gradually. Also, allergies or adverse reactions to a specific food can be detected when new foods are introduced one at a time. Mixing new foods with formula or other familiar foods would make it impossible to detect allergic or other unfavorable reactions satisfactorily. This practice may also cause the infant to refuse foods with which he is already familiar and likes. If a new food is offered after the infant's appetite is satisfied with formula, he is not likely to eat the new food. (15, 21)

## Health Promotion of the Toddler and Family

**16.** 3. It is important to determine if the child is experiencing a change in the home environment. This could cause anxiety that the child is relieving through oral gratification. Eating non-food substances is called pica. Nutritional deficiencies, especially an iron deficiency, were thought to cause pica, but research has not substantiated this theory. Unlikely causes of pica include teething, experiencing a growth spurt, and eating a diet low in roughage. (15, 21)

**17.** 2. Pulling toys is a typical task of a normally developed 18-month-old child. Copying a circle and building a tower of eight or more blocks are typical behaviors of a 3-year-old child. Playing tag with other children requires cooperative play and the ability to follow rules. This behavior develops at about 5 years of age. (15, 21)

**18.** 2. Tying shoelaces is not expected of a 3-year-old child because it requires fine motor skills that are underdeveloped until the end of the preschool years. A 3-year-old can ride a tricycle, string large beads, and use blunt scissors with one hand. (15, 21)

**19.** 2. The most significant people for a child between 1 and 3 years of age are the child's parents. Siblings are the next most significant people. Peers and neighbors become more important when a child begins school. (15, 21)

**20.** 2. Parents can be asked to assist when their child is unable to cooperate during a procedure. Lack of cooperation is due to fright and the child will feel more secure with a parent present. Other methods may be necessary, but obtaining a parent's assistance is the recommended first course of action. (15, 21)

**21.** 4. The ear lobe should be pulled down and backward because the auditory canals are almost straight in a child. In an adult, the ear lobe is pulled up and backward because the auditory canals are directed inward, forward, and down. (15, 21)

**22.** 4. The most common reason that toilet-training in toddlers fails is that they are not developmentally ready for training. Even with appropriate rewards and proper equipment, the child who is not ready for training will not be able to learn voluntary control. "Accidents" that occur during training should be ignored. They are usually caused by the child's incomplete sphincter control, together with absorption in play until it is too late to get to the potty chair. (7, 21)

**23.** 1. According to Erikson, the developmental task of toddlerhood is acquiring a sense of autonomy while overcoming a sense of doubt and shame. Characteristics of negativism and ritualism are typical of behaviors in this quest for autonomy. In an attempt to achieve autonomy, the toddler often does the opposite of that requested. Hyperactivity, separation anxiety, and sibling rivalry are behaviors that may be demonstrated by the toddler, but they do not explain a toddler's negativism. (15, 21)

**24.** 2. The concept of animism, in which the child attributes lifelike qualities to inanimate objects, is a peculiarity of preconceptual thought. The preconceptual phase of cognitive development, which is a part of the preoperational stage, lasts from ages 2 to 4 years, according to Piaget's theory. Children in the concrete operational stage of Piaget's theory (school age) comprehend the concept of reversibility (an act can be undone by performing an opposite act). Reversibility allows mental action to replace physical action. School-age children also understand the concept of conservation (things are the same even when their form and shape change). Object permanence, a milestone of the sensorimotor period of Piaget's theory, is demonstrated at 6 to 9 months of age when the infant reaches for a hidden object. (15, 21)

**25.** 2. Until 7 years of age, children are normally hyperopic or farsighted. However, because of accommodative ability, these children usually see objects at close range. Myopia or nearsightedness is the ability to see objects at close range but not at a distance. Presbyopia is a vision defect that occurs in persons more than 40 years of age. The lens becomes less elastic and near objects are blurred. Amblyopia or "lazy eye" is reduced visual acuity in one eye despite appropriate optical correction. (10, 21)

**26.** 3. Food preferences and appetite are sporadic during the toddler years. A child may enjoy one food for several days in a row and suddenly refuse to eat it again for days. Attempts to alter such food fads are met with resentment and obstinacy. It is best to accept such extremes and offer small portions of other foods. Offering extra time to play outside and insisting that the child eat small portions of the family's meal are not appropriate nutritional strategies. Consulting a physician is unnecessary because food fads are normal and usually temporary. (15, 21)

**27.** 3. Parents should clean and floss the toddler's teeth. Toddlers do not have the cognitive or motor skills needed for effective cleaning. The parent should brush the toddler's teeth after every meal and at bedtime, using a small toothbrush with soft, rounded nylon bristles that are short and uniform in length. Nylon bristles dry more rapidly and retain their shape better than natural bristles. A fluoride supplement is needed only if the child ingests minimal amounts of tap water. Routine fluoride supplements are not recommended. If the water is fluoridated, the child should get enough fluoride by ingesting frozen concentrated juices, powdered drinks, gelatin, or other foods. (15, 21)

**28.** 1. Structuring interactions with 3-year-old children helps minimize unacceptable behavior. This approach involves setting clear and reasonable rules and calling attention to unacceptable behavior as soon as it occurs. Physical punishment (spanking) does cause a dramatic decrease in a behavior but has serious negative effects. However, slapping a child's hand is effective when the child refuses to listen to verbal commands. Reasoning is more appropriate for older children, especially when moral issues are involved. Reasoning combined with scolding many times takes the form of shame or criticism. Unfortunately, children take such remarks seriously, believing that they are "bad." (15, 21)

**29.** 1. Toddlers usually express pain through such behaviors as restlessness, facial grimaces, irritability, and crying. It is not particularly helpful to ask toddlers about pain: they may not understand or may be unable to describe the experience. They are less able to verbalize and communicate the location of pain. (15, 21)

**30.** 2. Behavior is learned. Understanding one's own behavior enables a person to be less judgmental about the behavior of other people. The nurse should not be expected to give up her values and learn to accept other people's values as her own, nor should she purposefully overlook values contrary to her own. Nurses may work toward changing values that have been found detrimental to wellness, but an ethical and moral concept is at stake. If change is indicated, it is better to present the person with alternatives and consequences and let him decide whether to change. (7, 15)

## Health Promotion of the Preschooler and Family

**31.** 2. Preschool-aged children have been described as powerhouses of gross motor activity who seem to have endless energy. A limitation of their motor ability is that in moving as quickly as they do, they are not always able to judge distances, nor are they able to estimate the amount of strength and balance needed for activities. As a result, they have frequent mishaps. (14, 20)

**32.** 2. A game such as "Simon Says," which requires the preschooler to use a variety of motor skills, can help channel activity and meet developmental needs. Parallel play and stringing large beads are appropriate for a younger child. While the preschooler can ride a tricycle well, riding a bicycle requires more skill in balance than a 4-year-old is likely to have. (14)

**33.** 2. It is not uncommon for bedtime to be a problem with preschoolers. Recommendations for reducing conflicts at bedtime include establishing a set bedtime, having a dependable routine such as story reading, and conveying the expectation that the child will comply. Excitement just prior to bedtime and the misuse of food should be avoided. (8, 14)

**34.** 4. Routine dental exams should begin when a child is young, before any obvious problems develop. Dental caries can occur before a child is 2 years old. Teeth should be brushed after meals and at bedtime. Reprimanding the mother for not taking the child to the dentist is not helpful. (14)

**35.** 3. Children under the age of 6 years do not have the manual dexterity needed for tooth-brushing. Parents should supplement tooth-brushing efforts of preschool-aged children. (14)

**36.** 3. The preconventional level of Kohlberg's stages of moral development is typical of the preschool-aged child. Stage 1 behaviors of the preconventional level have a punishment- obedience orientation. Conventional morality pertains to children 7 to 12 years of age. Autonomous and principles are not stages of moral development as described by Kohlberg. (8, 20)

**37.** 2. Allowing a child to make some decisions about the foods eaten and not insisting that the child finish his meals can avoid power struggles. Refusing to finish meals and to eat all types of foods is normal behavior for a preschool-aged child. It is important to avoid tension at mealtime and to avoid confrontations about food, which can become a weapon, a bribe, or a pacifier. (8)

**38.** 2. Allen picture cards are used to test visual acuity in children who are not proficient with the alphabet. The Snellen alphabet chart is commonly used with children over 8 or 9 years of age. Ishihara plates are used to test for color-blindness. The cover and cross-over test is used to rule out strabismus. (8)

**39.** 2. The preschool-aged child does not have an accurate concept of skin integrity and can view medical and surgical treatments as a hostile invasion that can destroy or damage his body. The preschooler does not understand that he will not exsanguinate from an injection site. The other fears are unrelated to this behavior. (14)

**40.** 3. Allowing the preschool-aged child to give play injections can help him prepare for an injection. Giving play injections after the experience and using a pounding board after the experience help the child feel in control again. Preschool- aged children know that injections hurt. Diversionary activities are appropriate during an injection. (14, 20)

**41.** 3. Family changes and stressors, such as moving, having company, taking vacations, or adding new members, can distract parental attention and contribute to accidents. Only children tend to receive more attention than children with brothers and sisters. The environment of lower socioeconomic families is more conducive to childhood accidents. (8)

**42.** 3. Young children tend to imitate what they see, and parents teach by example whether intentionally or not. Parents should know where their children play and should discuss safety with them. Even though children may know safety measures, they may forget them while playing with friends. A child should not be labeled "bad" or "good" based on behavior, since it is the behavior that is undesirable. As children mature, parental interventions aimed at preventing accidents progress from protection to education. (6, 14)

**43.** 3. Preschool-aged children may view illness as punishment for their fantasies. Preschool-aged children do not have the cognitive ability to separate their fantasies from reality and may expect to be punished for their "evil thoughts." The other options require a higher level of cognition than the preschooler possesses. (14, 20)

**44.** 1. The father's knowledge and understanding of the test must be assessed, as must the reason for asking the question. The Denver Developmental Screening Test is used to evaluate development in children from 1 month to 6 years of age. Gathering information about the other options is premature. (6, 8)

## Health Promotion of the School-Aged Child and Family

**45.** 4. During the school-aged years, the child learns to socialize with children his own age. The "best friend" stage, which occurs around the age of 9 or 10 years, is very important in providing a foundation for self-esteem and later relationships. (14, 20)

**46.** 2. Children are capable of mastering the skills required for flossing when they reach age 9. By age 9 or 10, many children are able to assume responsibility for their personal hygiene. (8)

**47.** 2. School-aged children delight in riddles and jokes. Mastery of the ambiguities of language and of sentence structure allows the school-aged child to manipulate words, and riddles and jokes are a method of practicing this skill. (8, 14)

**48.** 2. Behaviors characteristic of Kohlberg's conventional level of moral development (level 2) are those related to expectations of others and the desire to conform to social expectations. In stage 3 of the conventional level of moral reasoning, good behaviors are seen as those that are approved by others. The other two levels of moral development are preconventional (level 2) and postconventional (level 3). Preconventional morality pertains to children 0 to 7 years of age, while postconventional morality pertains to adolescents and adults. (8, 20)

**49.** 3. Snacks are necessary for school-aged children and they should help prepare their own snacks. School-aged children are in a stage of cognitive development in which they can learn to categorize or classify, and they can also learn cause and effect. By preparing their own snacks, school-aged children can learn the basics of nutrition (for example, what carbohydrates are and what happens when they are eaten). (8, 14)

**50.** 1. The school-aged child (age 7 to 11) who has achieved the cognitive abilities required to master concrete operations often collects various objects when learning to manipulate and classify these objects. Coordination of secondary schemas and tertiary circular reactions are part of the sensorimotor phase of cognitive development (0 to 2 years of age). Formal operations do not emerge until a later age (11 to 15 years of age). (8, 20)

**51.** 3. The values of height and weight percentiles are usually similar for an individual child. Marked discrepancies identify overweight or underweight children. Measurements between the 5th and 95th percentile are considered normal. (20)

**52.** 2. According to Erikson, industry versus inferiority is the theme of psychosocial development during middle and late childhood. The challenge is the mastery of skills to create and complete projects, and this is often done through play. Sense of initiative is the theme of the preschool child. Sense of identity is the theme of early adolescence, and sense of intimacy and solidarity is the theme for late adolescence and young adulthood. (8, 20)

**53.** 3. Lymphoid tissue develops rapidly in relative size until the child is 10 to 11 years old. Lymphatic hyperplasia in the form of enlarged tonsils is normal until the child is 6 or 7 years old, after which the tissue slowly atrophies. Enlarged tonsils are not surgically removed unless they become abscessed or compromise physiological functioning. (8, 14)

**54.** 4. Motor-vehicle accidents are the most common cause of accidental injury and death in children between the ages of 6 and 12 years. Measures that prevent accidents involving motor vehicles, bicycles, or motorized bikes should be emphasized. Other major causes of accidental injury and death

in children between the ages of 6 and 12 years are drowning, burns, and firearms. Accidents among children 0 to 1 year of age involve falls, poisoning, and burns. (7, 8, 14, 17)

**55.** 1. Boosters of diphtheria, tetanus, and pertussis (DPT) and oral polio vaccine (OPV) are the immunizations recommended for children between the ages of 4 and 6 years prior to entering school. The recommended age for measles, mumps, and rubella (MMR) immunization is 15 months. Smallpox vaccinations are no longer routinely given to children. (8)

**56.** 3. Children aged 9 to 10 years can assume increasing responsibility for their health, and helping in meal preparation is an opportunity to learn about nutrition. The food intake of the school-aged child cannot be continually monitored by parents due to the child's expanding world. Physical activity should be encouraged, not restricted. A school-aged child requires approximately 2,400 calories per day. (8)

## Health Promotion of the Adolescent and Family

**57.** 2. The ability to deal with abstract possibilities develops in adolescents, but not all adolescents develop this ability. Assimilation and accommodation are characteristics of the sensorimotor development of infants. Problems of conservation are part of concrete operations learned by children between 4 and 7 years of age. (8, 14)

**58.** 2. The basis for these symptoms is most likely physiological. There are two types of dysmenorrhea, primary and secondary. Primary is the most common type and is believed to be caused by an increased level of prostaglandins. This increased level produces uterine hyperactivity and contractions. Approximately 80% of females who take prostaglandin-inhibitors, such as ibuprofen (Motrin), experience relief of symptoms. (20)

**59.** 2. Relieving dysmenorrhea in adolescence is crucial for the development of positive self-identity, of which positive body image and sexual identity are parts. Menstruation should not be viewed as painful and debilitating. Sense of autonomy, according to Erikson, is the developmental task of toddlers and, if successfully mastered, leads to a sense of self-control. (7, 20)

**60.** 3. Ninety-five percent of cases of toxic shock syndrome occur during menses, and a relationship between tampon use and development of toxic shock syndrome has been found. Most adolescent females can use tampons if they are changed frequently. (8)

**61.** 4. Adolescence is a time of integrating physical changes into the self-concept, and most teenagers spend a great deal of time worrying about their personal appearance. This is normal adolescent behavior. (8, 14)

**62.** 4. Recommended immunization for adolescents and adults is combined tetanus toxoid and diphtheria toxoid every 10 years. Measles vaccination should not be routinely given to adolescent females because of the possible effects on a fetus, if the girl were pregnant. (8, 14)

**63.** 3. Information about why adolescents choose to use alcohol or other drugs can be used to determine whether they are becoming responsible users or problem users. Alcohol may be used out of simple curiosity or as a method to escape life. (14)

**64.** 4. It is important to prevent food intake from becoming the center of an independence-dependence struggle. Nursing responsibilities include helping parents realize that adolescents require a high calorie intake and need to make individual decisions. Adolescents are subject to peer pressure, which often supercedes family pressure. Responsibility for grocery shopping for a month may encourage independence but does not ensure nutritional status. (8, 20)

**65.** 2. Stage 3 behaviors of Kohlberg's conventional level of moral reasoning focus on the approval of others. Moral dilemmas are solved by the group standard with an emphasis on conformity. Adolescents usually function at this level of moral development. Children from 0 to 2 years function at the preconventional level; adolescents and adults function at the postconventional level. (8, 14)

**66.** 3. When bending forward, a person who has idiopathic scoliosis has an obvious rib hump. The two sides of the back at the hips, ribs, and/or shoulders are not level. Slipped epiphysis is characterized by continuous or intermittent hip pain, and the leg tends to externally rotate. Congenital hip dislocation is an abnormality of the hip joint at birth and the most reliable test at birth is the Ortolani test. (14, 20)

## Meetings to Discuss Common Childhood and Adolescent Health Problems

**67.** 1. The most common characteristic of head lice (pediculosis capitis) is severe itching. Itching is also present when lice infest other parts of the body. Scratch marks can almost always be found when lice are present. Head lice is the most common form of lice infestation. (6, 21)

**68.** 3. Lice are spread by personal contact, infested articles of clothing and bed and bathroom linens, and combs and brushes. Lice are more common among school-aged children than among adults because of the close contact in school and the common practice of sharing possessions. Children may be more neglectful of handwashing than adults, but hands do not commonly spread lice. Adults do not have an immunity to lice, nor is their skin resistant to lice. Repeated infestations of lice can occur at any age. (6, 21)

**69.** 2. Ringworm of the scalp is caused by a fungus. The fungus is grouped under the name of dermatophytes. (6, 21)

**70.** 4. Griseofulvin (Grisactin) is an antifungal agent. The drug does not kill the fungus. It acts by binding to the keratin that will be deposited in the skin, hair, and nails as they grow. This keratin is then resistant to the fungus. But as the keratin is shed, as it normally is, the fungus then enters new uninfected cells unless drug therapy continues. Therefore, prolonged therapy lasting from weeks to months is ordinarily required. The long-term administration does not prevent sensitivity or allergic reactions. Generally, the longer a medication is used, the more likely it is that side effects will develop. (7, 21)

**71.** 2. The adult pinworm emerges from the rectum and colon at night onto the perianal area to lay its eggs. Itching and scratching occur, and the infected child will then transfer eggs from his hands and reinfect himself or infect others. Nightclothes and bed linens can also be sources of the infection. The eggs can also be transmitted by dust in the home. It is possible for pinworms to be spread through food and water supplies, but these are rare sources of infection with pinworms. (6, 7)

**72.** 4. Water is usually the culprit for spreading typhoid fever. Typhus is spread through insect bites. Brucellosis (undulant fever) is spread by cow's milk. Poliomyelitis is most probably spread through respiratory secretions. (11, 21)

**73.** 3. The care of a child with chicken pox is concerned primarily with preventing infection in the lesions. The lesions cause severe itching, and organisms are ordinarily introduced into the lesions by scratching them. (7, 21)

**74.** 2. A paste of baking soda and water is often helpful in relieving itching associated with chicken pox. Calamine lotion can be used also. Using baby powder, moist terry-cloth towels, and cool compresses is unlikely to relieve itching. (7, 21)

**75.** 3. A child with 20/60 vision is seeing at 20 feet what he should be seeing at 60 feet. 20/200 is considered the boundary of legal blindness. (6, 15)

**76.** 1. Hemophilia, an inherited bleeding disorder, causes excessive bleeding. A bump, bruise, or cut can cause serious bleeding. After the injured area is cleansed, gentle pressure should be applied over the area to allow clot formation to help stop the bleeding. In addition, the area should be immobilized and elevated. Cold applications are often used to promote vasoconstriction to help control the bleeding. Warmth and moisture are not helpful in promoting coagulation. A tourniquet should not be used because of the high risk of tissue hypoxia and resulting necrosis. (7, 21)

**77.** 1. Acetylsalicylic acid (aspirin) inhibits platelet aggregation, prolongs bleeding time, and inhibits prothrombin synthesis. It is therefore contraindicated for a child with hemophilia. Acetaminophen (Tylenol) is the recommended alternative for analgesic and antipyretic purposes. Magnesium hydroxide (Milk of Magnesia) and multiple vitamin capsules have no effect on bleeding and are not contraindicated for patients with hemophilia. (6, 21)

**78.** 2. To help prepare a child for entering school, it is generally recommended that the child be taken to the school so that he may become oriented to its physical environment. Older siblings are likely to criticize the younger child, and staying with the child for a few days is generally not advised. The child may not ask questions because of his fears, and therefore preparation probably cannot be accomplished well through discussions. (7, 21)

**79.** 1. The child entering school is moving into a new environment. He has experienced security at home and can predict how he influences others in his family. The unhappiness is a normal response to the loss of security with resulting feelings of insecurity. It has been found that usually a stronger-than-usual bond exists between the child and other members of the family, especially parents, in the child who has a school phobia. Such factors as inability to pay attention, emotional maladjustment, and poor language development suggest psychosocial disturbances and should not be playing a role among normal children who seem unhappy about entering school. (7, 21)

**80.** 1. Children between 6 and 12 years of age have a slower growth rate than younger children and adolescents. Their food requirements are comparatively smaller as a result. (15, 21)

**81.** 3. Children are most likely to be influenced by examples and the atmosphere provided by parents, although at times they may be influenced by their peers. It has been found that coaxing and badgering children to eat is most likely to aggravate the situation when eating habits are poor. (7, 15)

**82.** 1. According to Erikson's theory, the central problem confronting adolescents is establishing a sense of identity. The core problem of young adulthood is concerned with intimacy. School-aged children, between about 6 and 13 years of age, are concerned with industry, and preschool children with initiative. (6, 21)

**83.** 3. Girls experience the onset of adolescence approximately 1 to 2 years earlier than boys. The reason for this is not understood. (7, 21)

**84.** 1. The typical statement of a normal adolescent in the United States reflects a desire to grow up and become an adult. Most children of this age are in the process of discovering themselves and do not know where they wish to go in life. Teenagers prefer being with peers or being alone to being with parents. These youngsters do not want to be different and strive to be like their peers. (11, 21)

**85.** 1. A proverb that illustrates a very likely cause for many problems between teenagers and their parents is, "Do as I say, not as I do." Teenagers are generally quick to note when parents "preach" one thing and do something else. (21)

**86.** 2. Acne is a disorder of the pilosebaceous follicles (hair follicles and sebaceous gland complex). During adolescence, the secretions of the sebaceous glands increase with alterations of the follicular lining so that the ducts of the sebaceous glands become occluded with accumulated sebum. Bacteria in the follicle then causes an infection. Frequent washing of affected areas with soap and water is recommended to act as a mild peeling agent and reduce secondary infection. Witch hazel is an astringent that can be used *after* cleansing the skin thoroughly. Lotions and creams aggravate the condition by adding more oily substances to the already oily skin. Hydrogen peroxide is a poor cleansing agent for skin that has acne. (7, 21)

**87.** 1. The cause of infectious mononucleosis is thought to be the Epstein-Barr virus. No precautionary measures are recommended for patients with mononucleosis. The virus is believed to be spread only by direct intimate contact. (11, 21)

**88.** 2. Mononucleosis usually has an insidious onset with fatigue and the inability to maintain usual activity levels as the most common symptoms. The lymph nodes are typically enlarged, particularly in the abdomen, and the spleen also may be enlarged. Fever and a sore throat often accompany mononucleosis. (11, 21)

**89.** 2. Public health measures used for the control of

venereal diseases are most often directed toward locating the sources of the infections. When a person is diagnosed as having a venereal disease, an important responsibility is to identify all the person's sexual contacts and urge them to have treatment. Although venereal diseases are prevalent, mass screening is impractical. Isolating persons after they have therapy is unnecessary. Treatment is important, but for effective control all contacts should also be treated. Sex education has been found to be important also when working toward the control of venereal diseases. (7, 21)

**90.** 1. When rubella vaccine is used, the person develops a mild form of the disease, stimulating the body to develop an immunity. When pregnant women receive rubella vaccine early in pregnancy, the fetus may be deformed and/or aborted. Some authorities recommend withholding immunization for rubella after puberty because if the woman is pregnant, and she may not always know she is, the fetus is placed in jeopardy. (7)

# test 2

*The Patient with Tonsillitis*

*The Patient with Chronic Otitis Media*

*The Patient with Aspiration of a Foreign Body*

*The Patient with Bronchial Asthma*

*The Patient with Cystic Fibrosis and Bronchopneumonia*

*The Patient with Sudden Infant Death Syndrome*

*The Patient Requiring Cardiopulmonary Resuscitation*

*Correct Answers and Rationales*

Select the one *best* or *correct* answer and indicate your choice by filling in the circle with a pencil in front of the option you have chosen. If the answer you would prefer is not given, select the one you think is *most appropriate*.

## THE PATIENT WITH TONSILLITIS

Four-year-old Jason Higgens has been admitted to the pediatric unit for a tonsillectomy and adenoidectomy. His parents plan to stay with him as much as possible. Jason's growth and development are normal.

1. Jason asks the nurse if it will hurt to have his tonsils and adenoids out. Which of the following responses would be *best* for the nurse to make?
   ○ 1. "It will not hurt because you will be asleep."
   ○ 2. "It will not hurt because you're a big boy."
   ○ 3. "It will hurt because of the incisions in the throat."
   ○ 4. "It will hurt, but we have medicine to help you feel better."

2. Preoperatively, the nurse discusses with Jason and his parents the plan of care that will be implemented when Jason returns to his room from the recovery room. Which of the following interventions should the nurse emphasize?
   ○ 1. The patient should cough frequently.
   ○ 2. The patient can have aspirin for pain, as needed.
   ○ 3. The patient should restrict his talking.
   ○ 4. The patient can have sips of clear liquids when awake.

3. Jason falls asleep the night before surgery and breathes loudly through his mouth. The nurse recognizes that this is probably due to
   ○ 1. very dry room air.
   ○ 2. poorly developed jaw muscles.
   ○ 3. enlarged tonsils and adenoids.
   ○ 4. large amounts of nasal drainage.

4. After surgery and a brief stay in the recovery room, Jason returns to his room. In which position should the nurse place Jason to prevent aspiration?
   ○ 1. Supine or Trendelenburg.
   ○ 2. Side-lying or supine.
   ○ 3. Side-lying or prone.
   ○ 4. Prone or Trendelenburg.

5. Jason has finally awakened and Mrs. Higgens asks the nurse for something for Jason to eat or drink. Which of the following is best for Jason *initially*?
   ○ 1. A yellow Popsicle.
   ○ 2. Vanilla ice cream.
   ○ 3. Red Kool-Aid.
   ○ 4. Chocolate pudding.

6. The nurse monitors Jason frequently for signs and symptoms of hemorrhage. Which of the following would be an *early* indication of hemorrhage?
   ○ 1. Drooling of bright-red secretions.
   ○ 2. A pulse rate of 95 beats per minute.
   ○ 3. 25 ml of dark-brown emesis.
   ○ 4. Infrequent swallowing.

7. Which response to hospitalization and trauma of surgery would be *most typical* for a preschool-aged child such as Jason?
   ○ 1. Anger.
   ○ 2. Irritability.
   ○ 3. Self-consciousness.
   ○ 4. Depression.

8. The nurse concludes that Mr. and Mrs. Higgens understand Jason's discharge instructions when they state that medical attention should be sought for which of the following occurrences?
   ○ 1. Low-grade fever.
   ○ 2. Signs of bleeding.
   ○ 3. Slight ear pain.
   ○ 4. Objectionable mouth odor.

**187**

## THE PATIENT WITH CHRONIC OTITIS MEDIA

Fifteen-month-old Susie Platzer is admitted to the pediatric day surgery unit for a bilateral tympanostomy tube insertion. In the past 7 months, Susie has had multiple middle ear infections that have not responded to antibiotic therapy.

9. Otitis media occurs more frequently in infants and young children than in older children and adults. This is because of the unique anatomic features of the infant's/young child's
   - ○ 1. nasopharynx.
   - ○ 2. eustachian tubes.
   - ○ 3. external ear canals.
   - ○ 4. tympanic membranes.

10. Which of the following signs and symptoms are *most characteristic* of acute otitis media?
   - ○ 1. Rhinorrhea, fever, and bulging tympanic membrane.
   - ○ 2. Cough, irritability, and inverted tympanic membrane.
   - ○ 3. Pulling at the ears, earache, and gray tympanic membrane.
   - ○ 4. Vomiting, diarrhea, and yellow tympanic membrane.

11. Which of the following primary assessment techniques would be used to diagnose otitis media?
   - ○ 1. Percussion.
   - ○ 2. Auscultation.
   - ○ 3. Palpation.
   - ○ 4. Inspection.

12. The doctor prescribed sodium ampicillin (Omnipen) for Susie several times when she had acute otitis media. The *primary* purpose of the medication was to
   - ○ 1. shrink swollen tissues in the eustachian tube.
   - ○ 2. treat the probable organism, *H. influenza.*
   - ○ 3. reduce the severe pain.
   - ○ 4. reduce the fever.

13. When Susie completed a course of antibiotic therapy, Susie's parents were instructed to bring her to the office for a recheck. The purpose of the recheck was to
   - ○ 1. determine if the ear infection had affected her hearing.
   - ○ 2. make certain she had taken all of the antibiotic.
   - ○ 3. document that the infection was completely cleared.
   - ○ 4. obtain a prescription for another course of antibiotics.

14. When the nurse attempts to put an identification bracelet on Susie's arm and to help her into a hospital gown, Susie becomes frightened. Which of the following approaches would it be *best* for the nurse to try *first?*
   - ○ 1. Encourage the child's mother to help.
   - ○ 2. Ask another nurse to help.
   - ○ 3. Wait until the child calms down.
   - ○ 4. Use restraints during the procedure.

15. Tympanostomy tubes are inserted while Susie is under general anesthesia. These tubes are inserted to
   - ○ 1. distribute antibiotic solution into the middle ear.
   - ○ 2. shrink the mucosal lining of the middle ear.
   - ○ 3. increase pressure in the middle ear.
   - ○ 4. allow ventilation of the middle ear.

16. A goal of postoperative nursing care is to facilitate drainage from the right ear. Which of the following interventions would be *most likely* to accomplish this goal?
   - ○ 1. Apply external heat to the right ear.
   - ○ 2. Have the child lie on the right side.
   - ○ 3. Apply a gauze pressure dressing to the right ear.
   - ○ 4. Apply cold compresses to the left ear.

17. Two interventions included in Susie's postoperative nursing care plan are to apply external heat or cool compresses, and to avoid chewing by offering liquid or soft foods. Which nursing diagnosis do these interventions address?
   - ○ 1. Hyperthermia related to infectious process.
   - ○ 2. Impairment of skin integrity related to ear drainage: Potential.
   - ○ 3. Alteration in comfort: Pain related to the inflammatory process.
   - ○ 4. Knowledge deficit related to unfamiliarity with the situation.

18. Prior to Susie's discharge from the day surgery center, Susie's parents ask, "What will happen to the tubes in her ears?" Which of the following responses would be *most accurate* for the nurse to make?
   - ○ 1. "The tubes will dissolve in approximately 6 months."
   - ○ 2. "The tubes will probably fall out in about 6 months."
   - ○ 3. "The tubes will remain permanently in place."
   - ○ 4. "The tubes will be removed in approximately 6 months."

19. Ear drops are ordered for Susie at home. The nurse teaches Susie's parents to instill them. Which of the following statements would indicate that Susie's father has understood the teaching?
   - ○ 1. "I'll gently pull the ear lobe up and forward."

○ 2. "I'll gently pull the ear lobe up and backward."

○ 3. "I'll gently pull the ear lobe down and forward."

○ 4. "I'll gently pull the ear lobe down and backward."

**20.** Which of the following techniques is *best* for the nurse to use in evaluating Susie's parents' ability to administer ear drops correctly?

○ 1. Observe the parents instilling drops in the patient's ear.

○ 2. Listen to the parents as they describe the procedure.

○ 3. Ask the parents to list the steps in the procedure.

○ 4. Have each parent critique the other's performance of the procedure.

**21.** An often-recommended practice to help prevent recurrence of otitis media in a youngster such as Susie is to

○ 1. cleanse the ears thoroughly and often.

○ 2. use continuous, small-dose antibiotic therapy.

○ 3. use ear drops regularly to prevent accumulation of ear wax (cerumen).

○ 4. hold a child upright for formula feedings.

## THE PATIENT WITH ASPIRATION OF A FOREIGN BODY

Mr. and Mrs. Jacobs bring their 2-year-old daughter Jane to the emergency department because she has a cough, is short of breath, and has a fever. They tell the nurse that about a week ago Ellen choked on a peanut. They thought that she had coughed it out and had forgotten about the incident until she began to cough and became short of breath. Mrs. Jacobs asks the nurse if Jane's cough, shortness of breath, and fever could be related to aspiration of the peanut.

**22.** The nurse answers, "Yes," and explains that a potential complication that children who aspirate peanuts may develop is

○ 1. pseudomembranous bronchitis.

○ 2. acute bronchitis.

○ 3. vegetal bronchitis.

○ 4. chronic bronchitis.

**23.** Mrs. Jacobs tells the nurse that her pediatrician said that peanuts are "one of the worst things a child can aspirate" and asks why this is true. The nurse explains that this is true because peanuts

○ 1. swell when wet.

○ 2. contain a fixed oil.

○ 3. decompose when wet.

○ 4. contain calcium.

**24.** The nurse plans to discuss with Jane's parents other foods that are easily aspirated. Which of the following foods are *most* likely to be aspirated?

○ 1. Mashed potatoes and bread.

○ 2. Juice and noodles.

○ 3. Round candy and hot dogs.

○ 4. Milk and pudding.

**25.** Jane is admitted to the pediatric unit and a bronchoscopy is scheduled. Her parents attempt to decrease Jane's fear of the hospital by asking for some toys for her. Which of the following toys are safe and appropriate for 2-year-old Jane?

○ 1. A large pink balloon.

○ 2. A rag doll with bright button eyes.

○ 3. Eight large colored plastic blocks.

○ 4. A red beaded necklace.

**26.** Jane begins to fuss and cry when her parents attempt to leave the hospital for an hour. As the nurse tries to take Jane out of the safety crib to console her, Jane pushes her away. What state of separation anxiety does Jane's behavior indicate?

○ 1. Protest.

○ 2. Despair.

○ 3. Denial.

○ 4. Detachment.

**27.** In order to help Jane's parents best manage her separation anxiety, the nurse would suggest that they

○ 1. leave while she is sleeping.

○ 2. bring her favorite toys from home.

○ 3. tell her they are leaving and at what hour they will return.

○ 4. make their visits shorter.

**28.** The bronchoscopy is performed and Jane tolerates the procedure well. Which of the following parameters would be *most important* for the nurse to assess after Jane returns to her room?

○ 1. Cardiac rate and rhythm.

○ 2. Respiratory rate and quality.

○ 3. Sputum quantity and color.

○ 4. Pulse pressure and deficit.

**29.** Before Jane is discharged, the nurse teaches Mr. and Mrs. Jacobs the three signs that indicate a child is *truly* choking and needs immediate life-saving. The nurse knows that the Jacobs understand the teaching when they identify the three signs as the following: The child cannot speak,

○ 1. turns blue, and vomits.

○ 2. turns red, and collapses.

○ 3. turns blue, and gags.

○ 4. turns blue, and collapses.

**30.** Mrs. Jacobs asks the nurse how long it is before brain death occurs if a child's airway is completely obstructed. The nurse is *correct* when she responds

○ 1. "1 to 3 minutes."
○ 2. "4 to 6 minutes."
○ 3. "7 to 10 minutes."
○ 4. "More than 10 minutes."

## THE PATIENT WITH BRONCHIAL ASTHMA

Six-year-old Jordan Farmer, who has bronchial asthma, is brought to the hospital's emergency room by his mother. He is having an acute asthmatic attack.

31. During the asthmatic episode, Jordan has difficulty breathing and attempts to take in more air by breathing deeply. The nurse recognizes that this compensatory mechanism frequently results in the acid-base imbalance of
○ 1. metabolic acidosis.
○ 2. metabolic alkalosis.
○ 3. respiratory acidosis.
○ 4. respiratory alkalosis.

32. Which of the following manifestations is *most closely* related to Jordan's probable acid-base imbalance?
○ 1. His breath sounds are greatly diminished.
○ 2. He complains of a tingling sensation in his fingertips.
○ 3. His heart rate is 68 beats per minute.
○ 4. He has had no need to urinate for several hours.

33. During Jordan's acute attack of bronchial asthma, his breathing is *most likely* to be characterized by
○ 1. periods of apnea.
○ 2. crowing on inspiration.
○ 3. wheezing on expiration.
○ 4. abdominal muscle retractions.

34. The standard dosage of epinephrine (Adrenalin) 1:1,000 in the treatment of asthma is 0.01 ml per kilogram of body weight. Jordan weighs 45 pounds. Which amount of epinephrine will most likely be ordered for him?
○ 1. 0.15 ml.
○ 2. 0.20 ml.
○ 3. 0.30 ml.
○ 4. 0.45 ml.

35. Fifteen minutes after administering a dose of epinephrine (Adrenalin), the nurse assesses Jordan for evidence that the medication has produced the desired therapeutic effect. Indications that Jordan is responding to the epinephrine include
○ 1. a decrease in wheezing.

○ 2. tachycardia.
○ 3. a rise of 0.2° in temperature.
○ 4. paroxysms of sneezing.

36. The nurse is justified in judging that Jordan is having a *typical* side effect from epinephrine (Adrenalin) when she observes that Jordan is
○ 1. having tremors.
○ 2. feeling sleepy.
○ 3. developing a skin rash.
○ 4. experiencing nasal congestion.

37. Jordan fails to respond to the epinephrine (Adrenalin), and aminophylline (Aminophyllin) is administered intravenously. During the infusion, the nurse plans to monitor Jordan for
○ 1. a decrease in level of consciousness.
○ 2. shaking chills.
○ 3. circumoral erythema.
○ 4. vital-sign changes.

38. In addition to medication administration, other measures to alleviate Jordan's asthmatic episode may include
○ 1. postural drainage.
○ 2. fluid restriction.
○ 3. prone positioning.
○ 4. oxygen administration.

39. Episodes of asthma may be triggered by various mechanisms, including allergy to certain foods. If Jordan's asthma attack were triggered by a certain food, which of the following is *most likely* to be responsible?
○ 1. Whitefish.
○ 2. Tossed salad.
○ 3. Hamburger patty.
○ 4. Hot-fudge sundae.

40. Mrs. Farmer expressed concern that Jordan's 6-month-old baby brother, Myron, may also have food allergies. When discussing feeding techniques for Myron, the nurse suggests that Mrs. Farmer
○ 1. avoid giving him commercially prepared infant food.
○ 2. limit his fruit juice intake to apple juice.
○ 3. introduce new foods to him one at a time.
○ 4. discontinue formula feedings when he begins to eat baby foods.

41. Mrs. Farmer asks about the measures she can take at home to decrease the frequency of Jordan's asthmatic episodes. Which of the nurse's suggestions would be appropriate?
○ 1. Cover his mattress with a sheepskin pad.
○ 2. Use an aerosol spray disinfectant in his bedroom.
○ 3. Dust and vacuum the entire house frequently.
○ 4. Have him sleep with his bedroom window open.

42. Jordan is about to be discharged from the hospital. During discharge teaching, the nurse would instruct Mrs. Farmer to protect Jordan from
    ○ 1. extreme environmental temperatures.
    ○ 2. chest mobility exercises.
    ○ 3. the knowledge that he has asthma.
    ○ 4. synthetic material in clothing.

43. Jordan's mother tells the nurse that Jordan wishes to have a pet. Of the following pets, the one that would be *most appropriate* for Jordan is a
    ○ 1. cat.
    ○ 2. fish.
    ○ 3. gerbil.
    ○ 4. canary.

44. Cromolyn sodium (Aarane) is prescribed for Jordan to use at home. How should he and his mother be taught to administer the drug?
    ○ 1. The drug should be inhaled.
    ○ 2. The drug should be swallowed.
    ○ 3. The drug should be placed under the tongue.
    ○ 4. The drug should be given rectally by suppository.

45. The nurse discusses the use of cromolyn sodium (Aarane) with Mrs. Farmer. The nurse should teach the mother that the medication will be of no use to Jordan if it is administered when Jordan is
    ○ 1. about to eat a meal.
    ○ 2. having an asthmatic attack.
    ○ 3. being readied for sleep at night.
    ○ 4. about to engage in strenuous exercise.

46. Which of Mrs. Farmer's statements *best* reflects the family's positive adjustment to Jordan's disorder?
    ○ 1. "We give Jordan what he wants because he has an asthma attack if we don't."
    ○ 2. "We keep him away from other children so he won't be exposed to colds."
    ○ 3. "Although Jordan's disease is serious, we try to not let it be the focus of our family."
    ○ 4. "I'm afraid that when Jordan gets older, I won't be able to supervise what he does."

47. Mrs. Farmer tells the nurse that Jordan wants to participate in sports and asks the nurse to suggest activities appropriate for him. The nurse's response is based on the knowledge that
    ○ 1. physical activities are inappropriate for the asthmatic child.
    ○ 2. asthmatic children should be excluded from team sports.
    ○ 3. vigorous physical exercise frequently precipitates an asthmatic episode.
    ○ 4. most asthmatic children can participate in sports if the asthma is controlled.

## THE PATIENT WITH CYSTIC FIBROSIS AND BRONCHOPNEUMONIA
12|93

Three-year-old Debby Skiff is admitted to the hospital because of bronchopneumonia. She has cystic fibrosis.

48. A sputum specimen for culture is collected from Debby, the *primary* reason being to learn
    ○ 1. whether the child's cystic fibrosis is under control.
    ○ 2. the organism responsible for the child's pneumonia.
    ○ 3. whether old blood is present in the child's tracheobronchial tree.
    ○ 4. which portion of the child's lungs is affected by the pneumonia.

49. Debby is to receive penicillin three times in every 24-hour period. If the following choices are available, which schedule for administering the medication is *best?*
    ○ 1. Noon, 4 p.m., and 8 p.m.
    ○ 2. 9 a.m., 2 p.m., and 7 p.m.
    ○ 3. 10 a.m., 4 p.m., and 10 p.m.
    ○ 4. 8 a.m., 4 p.m., and midnight.

50. Debby is to have postural (bronchial) drainage. It is *best* for the nurse to plan to carry out postural drainage shortly
    ○ 1. after meals.
    ○ 2. before meals.
    ○ 3. after rest periods.
    ○ 4. before rest periods.

51. Before evaluating the effects of postural drainage, the nurse should understand that the *primary* reason for Debby's having this type of therapy is to help
    ○ 1. dilate the bronchioles.
    ○ 2. promote better use of the diaphragm.
    ○ 3. improve circulation in the chest cavity.
    ○ 4. clean the lungs of mucopurulent material.

52. Debby is placed in a mist tent. The *primary* reason for using this tent for Debby is that it helps
    ○ 1. lower the child's temperature.
    ○ 2. provide the child with clean air.
    ○ 3. reduce the viscosity of the child's respiratory secretions.
    ○ 4. provide a means for administering inhalant medications to the child.

53. The nurse can expect Debby to have stools that are *typically*
    ○ 1. bulky and foul in odor.
    ○ 2. watery and sweet in odor.
    ○ 3. dry and have the odor of ammonia.
    ○ 4. dark in color and have almost no odor.

**54.** When several unmet needs are present, the body will direct extra energies toward meeting those needs that are most necessary for sustaining life. If Debby demonstrates the following behaviors, which can be explained on the basis of the previous statement?

○ 1. The patient cries to be near her mother.

○ 2. The patient tries hard to eat her meals.

○ 3. The patient has a rapid respiratory rate.

○ 4. The patient is uncooperative when her intravenous therapy is started.

**55.** The nurse plans recreational therapy for Debby. Which of the following toys would provide Debby with the *most* support while she is ill?

○ 1. A jigsaw puzzle.

○ 2. Her favorite doll.

○ 3. A fuzzy stuffed animal.

○ 4. Scissors, paper, and paste.

**56.** Because of Debby's health, Mr. and Mrs. Skiff do not look forward to the approaching summer weather. The reason that hot weather is hazardous for Debby is that, characteristically, a child with cystic fibrosis has

○ 1. no sweat glands.

○ 2. little skin pigment to prevent sunburn.

○ 3. a poorly functioning temperature control center.

○ 4. an abnormally high salt loss through perspiration.

**57.** The nurse judges that Mr. and Mrs. Skiff understand the nature of cystic fibrosis *correctly* when they tell her that Debby's disease is characterized *primarily* by

○ 1. an abnormality in the glands of the body that secrete mucus.

○ 2. the formation of fibrous cysts in various organs of the body.

○ 3. the failure of pancreatic ducts to develop properly.

○ 4. an abnormal interaction between the body's antigens and antibodies.

**58.** The Skiffs go on to explain *correctly* that cystic fibrosis affects many organs in Debby's body, but *not* her

○ 1. lungs.

○ 2. kidneys.

○ 3. pancreas.

○ 4. salivary glands.

**59.** Which of the following instructions should the nurse include when she teaches Debby's parents how to care for Debby at home?

○ 1. Restrict the child's activities in order not to tire her.

○ 2. Carry out breathing exercises and postural drainage for the child at home.

○ 3. Give the child cough suppressants at bedtime to allow for restful sleep.

○ 4. Regulate the child's medication dosage according to daily urine tests for bilirubin and acetone.

**60.** Debby's parents ask the nurse how Debby's disease is transmitted from them. Which of the following statements is *false* concerning cystic fibrosis, which is an autosomal recessive mendelian disorder?

○ 1. A carrier of the disease is free of symptoms of the disease.

○ 2. Two persons with the disease will bear children with the disease.

○ 3. Two persons who are carriers of the disease cannot produce children with the disease.

○ 4. A person with the disease and an unaffected person will bear children free of the disease.

**61.** The nurse refers Debby's parents to the local chapter of the National Cystic Fibrosis Foundation. The Foundation has been *especially* helpful for parents with children who have cystic fibrosis by assisting the parents with

○ 1. finding tutors to educate children with cystic fibrosis at home.

○ 2. offering genetic counseling to the parents of children with cystic fibrosis.

○ 3. meeting with other parents of children with cystic fibrosis for mutual support.

○ 4. giving financial help to purchase medications for children with cystic fibrosis.

**62.** When planning Debby's long-term care, the nurse should take into account that Debby's prognosis can *best* be described as being

○ 1. good; she is likely to experience permanent regression of the disease as she grows older.

○ 2. fair; she can look forward to a full life as an adult provided she has good health care during childhood.

○ 3. unfavorable; she is unlikely to survive past early adulthood.

○ 4. unpredictable; her prognosis depends on an extremely large number of variables.


## THE PATIENT WITH SUDDEN INFANT DEATH SYNDROME

Mr. and Mrs. Lopez have just brought their 3-month-old infant son, Nigel, into the emergency room. He is not breathing and a tentative diagnosis of Sudden Infant Death Syndrome (SIDS) is made.

**63.** What would be the *best* action for the nurse to take in regard to the parents?

○ 1. Offer to telephone their pastor.

○ 2. Tell them that the doctor will talk with them soon.

○ 3. Ask another patient to sit with them.

○ 4. Accompany them to a private area and stay with them.

**64.** The emergency room nurse takes a brief history of events occurring before and after the parents found Nigel. Which of the following questions would be *most* appropriate for the nurse to ask the parents?

○ 1. "Was Nigel wrapped in a blanket?"

○ 2. "Was Nigel's older brother jealous of him?"

○ 3. "At what time did you find Nigel?"

○ 4. "When had you last checked Nigel?"

**65.** Mr. and Mrs. Lopez have been told that Nigel has died. Which of the following interventions should the nurse include in the plan to assist the parents in their grieving process?

○ 1. Reassure them that his death is not their fault.

○ 2. Provide an opportunity for them to see him.

○ 3. Ask them if they would like to call their pastor.

○ 4. Give them a package containing his clothing.

**66.** Before Mr. and Mrs. Lopez leave the hospital, the nurse evaluates their understanding of the cause of Nigel's death. The parents should know that the etiology of SIDS is

○ 1. unknown.

○ 2. apnea.

○ 3. infection.

○ 4. cardiac dysrhythmias.

**67.** Given the crisis associated with the loss of a child from SIDS, the nurse arranges for a community health nurse to visit Mr. and Mrs. Lopez at home. When should the nurse visit the parents?

○ 1. A few days after the funeral.

○ 2. Two weeks after the funeral.

○ 3. As soon as the parents are ready to talk.

○ 4. As soon after the infant's death as possible.

**68.** The nurse develops nursing goals for the visits to Mr. and Mrs. Lopez. The *primary* goal for the second visit is to help them

○ 1. express their feelings.

○ 2. gain an understanding of the disease.

○ 3. assess the impact of the infant's death on his siblings.

○ 4. deal with issues such as having other children.

## THE PATIENT REQUIRING CARDIOPULMONARY RESUSCITATION

The nurse prepares to discharge 5-year-old Robin Loomis from the one-day surgery unit, where she had a cyst removed from her leg. The nurse leaves the room to get supplies and when she returns finds that Robin is not breathing.

**69.** Which of the following nursing measures is the *priority* action?

○ 1. Clear the airway.

○ 2. Begin mouth-to-mouth resuscitation.

○ 3. Initiate oxygen therapy.

○ 4. Start chest compressions.

**70.** Continuing the cardiopulmonary resuscitation (CPR) assessment, the nurse palpates for a pulse. Which of the following sites is *best* for checking the pulse during CPR in a 5-year-old child?

○ 1. Femoral.

○ 2. Carotid.

○ 3. Radial.

○ 4. Brachial.

**71.** What is the recommended rescue breathing rate during CPR for 5-year-old Robin?

○ 1. 10 breaths/minute.

○ 2. 12 breaths/minute.

○ 3. 15 breaths/minute.

○ 4. 30 breaths/minute.

**72.** Robin is pulseless. The nurse begins chest compressions. Since effective chest compressions depend on proper technique, the nurse should apply pressure

○ 1. on the lower sternum with the heel of one hand.

○ 2. midway on the sternum with the tips of two fingers.

○ 3. over the apex of the heart with the heel of one hand.

○ 4. on the upper sternum with the heel of both hands.

**73.** What is the recommended rate of external chest compression for Robin?

○ 1. 50 to 70 compressions/minute.

○ 2. 60 to 80 compressions/minute.

○ 3. 70 to 80 compressions/minute.

○ 4. 80 to 100 compressions/minute.

**74.** When providing chest compressions, the nurse should compress the chest to a depth of

○ 1. 1″ to 1.5″.

○ 2. 1.5″ to 2″.

○ 3. 2″ to 2.5″.

○ 4. 2.5″ to 3″.

**75.** Which of the following signs would indicate that the cardiopulmonary resuscitation was effective for Robin?

○ 1. The appearance of mottling.

○ 2. Dilatation of pupils.

○ 3. Palpable peripheral pulses.

○ 4. Cool, dry skin.

**76.** A 10-month-old child is choking and the nurse attempts to clear the airway. What should the nurse do *next* after opening the infant's mouth?
  ○ 1. Use blind finger sweeps.
  ○ 2. Deliver four back blows.
  ○ 3. Apply four subdiaphragmatic abdominal thrusts.
  ○ 4. Attempt to visualize the object.

**77.** In which of the following positions should the nurse place an infant in order to deliver back blows?
  ○ 1. Face up, with the head lower than the trunk.
  ○ 2. Face down, with the head lower than the trunk.
  ○ 3. Face to the side, with the head lower than the trunk.
  ○ 4. Face up, with the head supported above the trunk.

**78.** What is the appropriate technique for delivering back blows to an infant?

  ○ 1. Slowly with the palm of the hand.
  ○ 2. Slowly with the heel of the hand.
  ○ 3. Rapidly with the palm of the hand.
  ○ 4. Rapidly with the heel of the hand.

**79.** Suddenly the infant begins to cry. What is the nurse's *most* appropriate action?
  ○ 1. Deliver four chest thrusts.
  ○ 2. Deliver four back blows.
  ○ 3. Finger-sweep the mouth.
  ○ 4. Observe the infant closely.

**80.** If the nurse had to perform mouth-to-mouth breathing for the infant, the nurse should tilt the infant's head back slightly in order to
  ○ 1. prevent airway obstruction.
  ○ 2. minimize gastric distention.
  ○ 3. prevent excessive pressure on the neck.
  ○ 4. inhibit extensor posturing.

# CORRECT ANSWERS AND RATIONALES

Numbers appear in parentheses following the rationales. The numbers identify textbooks listed in the references at the end of Part III, where correct answers can be verified.

## *The Patient with Tonsillitis*

1. 4. Preschool children are fearful of physical injury to themselves. Truthful but simple explanations will minimize distorted fears and reduce anxiety. A detailed explanation may be beyond their understanding and add to their fears. (7)

2. 4. Once the child is alert, he may have sips of clear liquids. Eating enhances the blood supply to the throat, which promotes rapid healing. Coughing is discouraged because it promotes bleeding. Aspirin is contraindicated because it causes bleeding. Talking is not restricted. (14)

3. 3. Tonsillectomy and adenoidectomy are indicated in children who have severe chronic upper airway obstruction leading to alveolar hypoventilation, difficulty swallowing, or extreme discomfort in breathing. Enlargement of the adenoids blocks the space behind the posterior nares. Because it is difficult for air to pass from the nose to the mouth, the child breathes through the mouth. Dry room air does not necessarily make a child breathe through the mouth. Poorly developed jaw muscles and large amounts of nasal drainage could cause mouth breathing, but are not problems necessarily associated with enlarged tonsils and adenoids. (21)

4. 3. Placing the child in a prone (on the abdomen) position or in a side position facilitates drainage of secretions and helps prevent aspiration. Trendelenburg position is contraindicated because it decreases effective lung volumes. The supine position is contraindicated due to the risk of aspiration. (21)

5. 1. The nurse must consider both the color and consistency of foods and fluids given initially. Red or brown-colored foods and fluids should be avoided so that if vomiting occurs, fresh or old blood can be distinguished from the ingested liquids. Ice cream and pudding are not offered until clear liquids are retained. (21)

6. 1. Drooling of bright-red blood indicates hemorrhage. Children tend to avoid swallowing after surgery because of the discomfort. Therefore, they drool. It is not unusual for the secretions to be slightly blood-tinged due to the small amount of oozing after surgery. A pulse rate of 95 beats per minute is within normal limits for a 4-year-old. A small amount of dark-brown blood is often present in postoperative emesis because of the surgical procedure. (21)

7. 1. Preschool children often become angry with their parents because they cannot understand why their parents allow physicians and nurses to hurt them. Irritability is a response more characteristic of infants. Self-consciousness and depression are most characteristic of school-aged children. (21)

8. 2. Any bleeding warrants medical attention. Hemorrhage may occur 5 to 10 days after a tonsillectomy when tissue is sloughed as a result of the healing process. Low-grade fever, slight ear pain, and objectionable mouth odor commonly occur for a few days after surgery. (21)

## *The Patient with Chronic Otitis Media*

9. 2. The eustachian tubes of infants and young children are short and lie in a relatively horizontal position. This anatomic position favors the development of otitis media because it is easy for materials from the nasopharynx to enter the tubes. Bacteria may be present in the nasopharynx, but the structure of this region does not affect middle-ear function. The external ear canal leads to the tympanic membrane, and when this membrane is intact bacteria are prevented from entering the middle ear. The tympanic membrane changes appearance with an ear infection, but the structure of this membrane does not predispose infants and young children to ear infections. (20, 21)

10. 1. A bulging, bright-red tympanic membrane (because of increased middle-ear pressure) usually indicates otitis media. Other characteristic findings are rhinorrhea, fever, cough, irritability, pulling at the ears, earache, and vomiting and diarrhea. A reddened, nonbulging tympanic membrane may indicate otitis media if the membrane has ruptured. A gray or yellow tympanic membrane may indicate infection, but the most conclusive indication of otitis media is a red and bulging tympanic membrane. (20, 21)

11. 4. The otoscope is the device used to inspect the tympanic membrane. Using the otoscope, the nurse examines the tympanic membrane for color, bulging, landmarks, mobility, and the presence of light reflex. Percussion is the striking or tapping of the body surface to learn the condition of the parts beneath the resultant sound. Auscultation involves

evaluation of body sounds. Palpation is the use of touch to detect bodily characteristics. (21)

**12.** 2. Sodium ampicillin (Omnipen) is a synthetic penicillin effective against *H. influenza*, pneumococci, and streptococci. These organisms most frequently cause acute otitis media. Oral decongestants, such as pseudoephedrine hydrochloride (Sudafed), may be prescribed to relieve eustachian tube obstruction due to inflammation. A topical analgesic, in the form of otic drops, may be given to relieve an earache. Acetaminophen (Tylenol) may be given for a fever. (8, 21)

**13.** 3. Because ear infections are sometimes difficult to treat, it is important to determine if the antibiotics have resolved the infection. If the patient is not rechecked, it will be difficult to determine if another infection is a continuation of a previous infection or a separate infection. Studies may be done to determine if an infection has impaired the child's hearing, but they are not done after each course of antibiotics. A visit to the physician's office cannot validate that all the medication was taken. If the infection is resolved with one course of antibiotics, another course will not be prescribed. (8)

**14.** 1. Strangers and separation from the parent are extremely stressful for the toddler. Toddlers manifest anxiety by protest, physical resistance, and regression. Often the parent's presence and involvement in the care decreases the child's anxiety and helps prepare the child for surgery. Asking another nurse (a stranger) and using restraints may be required, but these approaches should not be used unless necessary because they will heighten the child's fears. In a strange environment, it is unrealistic to expect the toddler to change behavior. Postponing the actions may only increase the child's anxiety. (21)

**15.** 4. Tympanostomy tubes allow ventilation of the middle ear and facilitate drainage of fluid by maintaining the patency of the eustachian tube. The pressure-equalizing tubes do not distribute medication into the ear. Decongestants may be used to shrink mucous membranes and increase eustachian tube function. (21)

**16.** 2. Positioning the child on the affected right side will promote drainage from the middle ear via gravity. The application of heat may facilitate drainage of exudate from the ear, but only if the child is lying on the affected side. The application of an ice bag may help reduce pressure and edema. A gauze dressing is not applied after surgery, though a loose wick may be inserted in the external canal to absorb drainage. (21)

**17.** 3. The application of external heat or cool compresses and the avoidance of chewing address the management of pain or discomfort. Approaches for the nursing diagnosis "potential for impaired skin integrity" include keeping the skin around the ear clean and dry, cleansing with hydrogen peroxide, and protecting the skin with a protective coating. Interventions for the diagnosis of hyperthermia include removing bedclothes and extra clothing, reducing environmental temperature, and encouraging fluids. Knowledge deficit interventions include educating parents about follow-up care, avoiding activities that allow water to enter the ears, and teaching preventive practices. (21)

**18.** 2. The tympanostomy tubes remain in place for approximately 6 months. The tiny, white, spool-shaped tubes are made of a polyurethane material that does not change in structure or composition while in the ear. The tubes are spontaneously ejected from the ear. Parents should be told about their appearance so they can observe them if they fall out. (21)

**19.** 4. For children 3 years old and younger, the external auditory canal is straightened by gently pulling the ear lobe down and backward. For the older child and adult, the ear lobe is gently pulled up and backward. (21)

**20.** 1. Return demonstrations are the best way of evaluating a person's ability to perform a skill. This technique enables the teacher to observe not only the sequencing of the steps of the procedure, but also the learner's ability in performing the skill. (21)

**21.** 4. Sitting or holding a child upright for formula feedings helps prevent the pooling of formula in the pharyngeal area. Formula is a good medium for bacterial growth. When the vacuum in the middle ear opens into the pharyngeal cavity, formula along with bacteria is drawn into the middle ear. Cleansing the ears will not reduce the incidence of otitis media because the pathogenic bacteria are in the nasopharynx. Continuous, small doses of antibiotics are used only in cases of recurrent otitis media. (21)

## The Patient with Aspiration of a Foreign Body

**22.** 3. A child who aspirates a peanut into the bronchus is at risk for vegetal bronchitis, which is characterized by cough, dyspnea, and fever. The child may have choked immediately after the incident, but complications do not develop until later. Pseudomembranous bronchitis is characterized by violent cough and dyspnea, in which casts of bronchial tubes are expectorated. It is not associated with aspiration of peanuts. Acute bronchitis, which is caused by inflammation of one or more bronchi, is not associated with the aspiration of peanuts. Chronic bronchitis probably does not exist as a clinical entity in children. (7)

**23.** 1. Peanuts swell and become soft when moistened with bronchial secretions, which makes them difficult to remove. Because peanuts contain a fixed oil, they can cause lipoid pneumonia, but this is not the factor that makes them so dangerous when aspirated. Peanuts do begin to decompose when wet, and they do contain calcium, but neither of these factors makes them dangerous when aspirated. (7)

**24.** 3. Spherical or cylindrical objects are more likely to be aspirated and plug the airway than any other shaped objects. The size, shape, and consistency of foods are important determinants of obstruction. (21)

**25.** 3. The eight large plastic blocks have neither small removable parts nor sharp or rough edges and promote appropriate developmental skills of a toddler. Balloons are hazardous; they can burst and can be aspirated. The button eyes of the rag doll and the beads of the necklace are potentially removable parts that can be swallowed or aspirated. (7)

**26.** 1. Young children have specific reactions to separation and hospitalization. In the protest stage, the toddler physically and verbally attacks anyone who attempts to provide care. In the despair stage, the toddler becomes withdrawn and obviously depressed. Denial or detachment occurs if the toddler's stay in the hospital without the parent is prolonged. The toddler "settles in" to hospital life and denies the parents' existence. (7)

**27.** 2. Bringing a child's favorite toys, security blanket, or familiar objects from home can make the transition from home to hospital less stressful. Leaving without telling the toddler may impair the child's trust in the parents. Parents should tell the toddler when they are leaving and when they will return, not by time but in relation to the child's activities; 2-year-olds have a very limited sense of time. Short visits do not satisfy the toddler's overwhelming need for comfort. (7)

**28.** 2. After a bronchoscopy, the patient should be observed for signs and symptoms of respiratory distress. Laryngeal edema may occur and cause airway obstruction. Signs and symptoms of respiratory distress include tachypnea, increased stridor and retractions, and tachycardia. The sputum may be bloody after bronchoscopy. A change in pulse pressure is not associated with bronchoscopy, but rather with intracranial pressure and shock. Pulse

deficit is associated with some dysrhythmias. Cardiac rate and rhythm are important to assess but are not the most important parameters to assess because tachycardia may be present normally after the procedure. (14)

**29.** 4. The three signs that indicate a child is *truly* choking and requires immediate life-saving interventions are: the child cannot speak, turns blue (becomes cyanotic), and collapses. These are symptoms of airway obstruction. (21)

**30.** 2. Brain death will begin to occur within 4 to 6 minutes if oxygen is not restored. Complete obstruction of the upper airway results in anoxia to vital organ systems. (7)

## The Patient with Bronchial Asthma

**31.** 4. Children experiencing mild asthmatic episodes often hyperventilate to move more air, causing increased exhalation of carbon dioxide. This reduces the plasma $PCO_2$, carbonic acid, and hydrogen ion concentration, leaving a base bicarbonate excess. These imbalances constitute respiratory alkalosis. (21)

**32.** 2. In respiratory alkalosis, the alkalinity of the body fluids results in a decrease in the ionization of calcium. Low levels of circulating ionized calcium increase the excitability of nerve and muscle tissue. This is manifested by paresthesia (numbness and tingling) of the digits, upper lip, and ear lobes. In mild asthma with respiratory alkalosis, the breath sounds are typically loud with expiratory wheezing. The pulse rate is elevated, and urinary production is increased because of the increased renal circulation. (18, 21)

**33.** 3. During an acute asthma attack, the bronchi and bronchioles narrow and become obstructed. This causes dyspnea. Because the obstruction of the flow of air is more marked during expiration, air tends to be trapped in the lungs, and the child must use great effort to rid the lungs of air. This produces a characteristic wheeze on expiration. Accessory muscles of the chest wall are used predominantly to assist with breathing. (7, 21)

**34.** 2. Forty-five pounds equals about 20 kilograms (2.2 pounds/kg). 20 kg × 0.01 ml/kg = .20 ml of epinephrine. (15)

**35.** 1. Epinephrine relaxes bronchial muscle and reduces congestion and edema in the pulmonary system, resulting in decreased wheezing. Tachycardia is a side effect of epinephrine. Minor temperature alterations and sneezing are unrelated to the desired improvement in pulmonary status. (15)

**36.** 1. Common side effects of epinephrine include tremors or trembling, anxiety or nervousness, nausea and vomiting, headache, palpitations, tachycardia, and dyspnea. (6, 7)

**37.** 4. Early signs of possible aminophylline (Aminophyllin) toxicity include hypotension, dysrhythmias, and seizures. Assessment for these manifestations should be made frequently. (4, 16)

**38.** 4. Oxygen administration is one of the most important therapies in the treatment of asthma. Supplemental oxygen decreases the cardiopulmonary work required to supply adequate amounts of oxygen to the body tissues. Chest physiotherapy is contraindicated in the acute phases of asthma because it often worsens the situation. Fluids should be offered liberally to help thin bronchial secretions. A high-Fowler's position promotes chest expansion and diaphragmatic descent. (5)

**39.** 4. Asthma is a disease in which the airways react to certain external and internal stimuli including allergens, infections, exercise, and emotions. Food allergens most frequently associated with asthma include wheat, egg white, dairy products, citrus fruits, corn, and chocolate. (15)

**40.** 3. When introducing solid foods to infants, only one new food should be added at a time so that if an allergic reaction occurs, the food allergen can be easily identified. In the absence of evidence of allergy, all foods are appropriate except mixed foods. Mixed foods should be avoided to facilitate allergen identification. Infant formula is a major source of nutrition for the 1st year, and should not be eliminated when solids are introduced. (15)

**41.** 3. Inhaled irritants and allergens are a common trigger for asthmatic episodes. Frequent dusting and vacuuming decrease the amount of inhaled allergens available to the asthmatic child. Wool fibers (from the sheepskin), aerosols, and open windows are all potential sources for respiratory irritants. (21)

**42.** 1. Parents should be taught that extremes of weather, such as excessively cold temperatures, may precipitate an asthmatic episode because of the effect on the airways. A child with asthma should do chest mobility exercises to strengthen respiratory muscles. Children with asthma need to be taught about the disease so they can become active participants in their care. Children with asthma should wear clothing made of synthetic material and cotton, not real fur or wools, because they are potential respiratory irritants. (11, 21)

**43.** 2. Having pets is discouraged when trying to allergy-proof a home for a child with bronchial asthma, unless the pets are kept outside. Pets with hair or feathers are especially likely to bring on attacks of asthma. A fish would be a satisfactory pet for the child described in this item, but the mother should be taught to prevent the fish tank from harboring mold. (15, 21)

**44.** 1. Cromolyn sodium (Aarane) is administered by inhalation in its powdered form. (21)

**45.** 2. Cromolyn sodium (Aarane) is used as a prophylactic agent (that is, to help prevent bronchial asthmatic attacks). The drug is not an anti-inflammatory, bronchodilator, or antihistamine agent. Therefore, cromolyn sodium is of no use to a patient who is having an asthmatic attack. The drug acts to inhibit the release of histamine and acts locally to prevent the release of mediator substances from mast (connective tissue) cells following exposure to allergens. (7, 21)

**46.** 3. The family is constantly involved in day-to-day living with the asthmatic child. Developing a positive family life requires placing the illness in its proper prospective. Some parents have a tendency to overprotect the child with a chronic illness. This overprotectiveness may cause a child to have an exaggerated feeling of importance or later, as an adolescent, to rebel against the overprotectiveness. Children with asthma need to be treated as normally as possible within the scope of the illness. (21)

**47.** 4. In 1984, the American Academy of Pediatrics stated that physical activities are beneficial to asthmatic children. The majority of these children can engage in school and sports activities with minimal difficulty, if the asthma is kept in check. (21)

## The Patient with Cystic Fibrosis and Bronchopneumonia

**48.** 2. The primary reason for culturing a sputum specimen when the patient has bronchopneumonia is to determine the organism causing the infection in the respiratory tract. Blood may be found in the sputum, but this will be determined by using methods other than a culture. Sputum cultures do not help determine whether a child's cystic fibrosis is under control or what portion of the child's lungs is affected by pneumonia. (15, 21)

**49.** 4. It is important to give antibiotics spaced at equal intervals over a 24-hour period to help maintain therapeutic levels of the medication in the bloodstream. Therefore, if a medication is to be given three times in each 24-hour period, good times to give the drug are at 8 a.m., 4 p.m., and midnight. A patient should be awakened to keep such a schedule. (7)

**50.** 2. It is generally recommended that postural drainage be used before eating to avoid the possibility of vomiting or regurgitating food. Rest periods do not play as important a role in scheduling postural drainage. (7, 21)

**51.** 4. Postural drainage uses the force of gravity to accomplish its primary goal, which is to clear the lungs and respiratory passages of mucopurulent material. Inhalant or systemic medications are used to dilate bronchioles. Developing better use of the diaphragm is best accomplished with breathing exercises. Improving the circulation in the chest cavity is not a goal of postural drainage. (7, 21)

**52.** 3. The primary reason for using a mist tent for a child with cystic fibrosis is that the humid air helps liquefy and decrease the viscosity of respiratory secretions. This, in turn, helps the patient raise these secretions and expectorate them. (7, 21)

**53.** 1. Poor digestion and absorption of foods, especially of fats, result in frequent bowel movements with stools that are bulky and very foul-smelling in a child with cystic fibrosis. The stools also contain abnormally large quantities of fat, which is called steatorrhea. (7, 21)

**54.** 3. Oxygen is essential for life. When a respiratory disease is present, the body will place first priority on obtaining oxygen by increasing the respiratory rate. Behaviors such as the child crying to be near her mother, trying to eat, and being uncooperative during therapy reflect efforts to meet such needs as affection, escaping from something fearful, and gaining self-esteem. But these needs are not as essential for maintaining life as the need for oxygen and are ordinarily met only after essentials for maintaining life have been met first. A hierarchy of needs as described in this rationale was first developed by Abraham Maslow. His theory is used extensively by nurses in planning and implementing nursing care. (7, 21)

**55.** 2. A child's favorite doll would be a good choice of toys for a 3-year-old girl. The doll provides support and is a familiar toy. In view of lung pathology, a fuzzy stuffed animal is not advised. Scissors, paper, and paste are not appropriate for a 3-year-old unless the child is supervised. A jigsaw puzzle is not particularly appropriate for an ill 3-year-old child. (7, 21)

**56.** 4. A characteristic of cystic fibrosis is that excess amounts of salt are lost through perspiration. During warm weather or whenever the child perspires more than usual, salt supplements are almost always necessary. Having no sweat glands, little skin pigment, and a poorly functioning temperature control center are conditions unrelated to cystic fibrosis. (7, 21)

**57.** 1. Cystic fibrosis is characterized by a dysfunction in mucus-producing exocrine glands in the body. The mucus secretions are very thick and sticky, rather than thin and slippery. The mucus obstructs various passages in the body, especially in the bronchi, bronchioles, and pancreatic ducts. Obstruction with plugs of mucus in the pancreatic ducts prevents pancreatic digestive enzymes from reaching the small intestine, resulting in poor digestion and absorption of various food nutrients. (7, 11)

**58.** 2. The organs most often attacked by cystic fibrosis are the pancreas, lungs, liver, and salivary glands. The kidneys are not involved unless complications arise that would affect their functioning. (7, 21)

**59.** 2. The best course of action for the home care of a child with cystic fibrosis is to carry out breathing exercises and postural drainage. Although the child should not exert herself to the point of fatigue, in general children with cystic fibrosis should be encouraged to do as much as they can. This practice helps improve respiratory functioning and improves the child's psychological outlook. A cough suppressant is contraindicated because it is important to expectorate secretions from the respiratory passages. Medication dosage will not be altered for the child with cystic fibrosis on the results of urine tests for bilirubin and acetone. (7, 21)

**60.** 3. The manner in which cystic fibrosis is transmitted from parents to their children is the same as for sickle-cell disease, which is also an autosomal recessive mendelian disorder. Affected children inherit the defective gene from both parents; therefore, the chances are that it will occur in one of four of their children. Cystic fibrosis does not cause a woman to become sterile, but 95% of men with cystic fibrosis are sterile. (7, 21)

**61.** 3. If parents of children with cystic fibrosis are unfamiliar with the work of the National Cystic Fibrosis Foundation, the nurse should refer the parents to the Foundation. An important function of the Foundation is to put parents of children with cystic fibrosis in touch with each other. Parents are often able to offer each other support and help. In some instances, the Foundation has given parents financial assistance for equipment required for the home care of children with cystic fibrosis, but not for medications. The Foundation does not obtain tutors for the children or provide genetic counseling for the parents. (7, 21)

**62.** 3. Although some people with cystic fibrosis have survived beyond young adulthood, most do not. The prognosis for the disease remains unfavorable, even with good health care. (7, 21)

## The Patient with Sudden Infant Death Syndrome

**63.** 4. The most important nursing intervention is to reach out to the anxious parents and to stay with them while the infant is being evaluated. (14)

**64.** 3. A sensitive approach to the parents can help minimize their guilt and prevent later emotional disturbances. Questions that imply parental neglect, wrongdoing, or abuse should not be asked. (21)

**65.** 2. Parents should have the opportunity to say their final farewell to their infant. This last contact helps them focus on the reality of death. Reassuring them that they are not at fault does not focus on the reality of death. The presence of their pastor may be helpful, but enabling them to see their son is more important. For some parents, clothes may be too painful a reminder of their child's death, and they may not wish to take them home. (7)

**66.** 1. One of the main techniques used in crisis intervention in the hospital includes helping parents to begin to gain an intellectual understanding of SIDS. Numerous theories have been proposed, but no specific cause of SIDS has been identified. Evidence suggests that infants with SIDS had chronic hypoxia, possibly from prolonged periodic apnea. (7)

**67.** 4. The nurse visits as soon after the death as possible. The parents need expert counseling to deal not only with the death of their child, but also with a tragedy that is extremely sudden, unexpected, and unexplained. (21)

**68.** 1. The goal of the second visit is to help the parents express their feelings. Gaining an understanding of the disease is a goal of the first visit. Although it is important to assess the impact of SIDS on siblings, this is not the primary goal for the second visit, although plans must be flexible. Parents are unable to deal with decisions such as having other children during the second visit; this should be discussed later. (21)

## The Patient Requiring Cardiopulmonary Resuscitation

**69.** 1. When breathlessness is determined, the priority nursing action is to clear the patient's airway. This action alone may re-establish spontaneous respiration. If the patient does not begin breathing, mouth-to-mouth resuscitation is begun. Oxygen therapy would not be initiated at this time. Chest compressions are begun only after the patient is determined to be pulseless. (21)

**70.** 2. Checking the carotid artery pulse during CPR in a child provides information about perfusion of the brain. The brachial pulse is checked in an infant because the infant's short and often fat neck makes it difficult to palpate the carotid pulse. The femoral and radial arteries might indicate perfusion to the peripheral body sites, but the critical need is for adequate circulation to the brain. (21)

**71.** 3. The rescue breathing rate is one every 4 seconds or 15 times per minute in a child. Rescue breaths should be delivered slowly. The appropriate volume of a rescue breath is the volume that makes the chest rise and fall. (21)

**72.** 1. The chest is compressed with the heel of *one* hand positioned on the lower sternum, two finger-breadths above the sternal notch. Fingertips are used to compress the sternum in infants, and the heel of *two* hands is used in adult cardiopulmonary resuscitation. (21)

**73.** 4. Chest compressions are delivered at a rate of 80 to 100 times per minute for a 5-year-old child. This rate approximates the resting minimum pulse, which allows for adequate brain perfusion. A rate less than 80 does not provide adequate brain perfusion for the 5-year-old child. (21)

**74.** 1. In a 5-year-old child, the chest is compressed to a depth of 1″ to 1.5″. This depth forces blood out of the heart into the vital organs (lungs and brain). Deeper compressions could damage the liver, lungs, or other underlying structures. Less deep compression would not provide adequate circulation to the vital organs. (21)

**75.** 3. Signs of recovery from cardiopulmonary arrest include palpable peripheral pulses, the disappearance of mottling and cyanosis, the return of pupils to normal size, and warm, dry skin. To determine if the victim of cardiopulmonary arrest has resumed spontaneous breathing and circulation, chest compressions must be stopped for 5 seconds at about the end of the 1st minute and every few minutes thereafter. (21)

**76.** 4. After opening the infant's mouth, the nurse attempts to visualize and remove the object. The nurse attempts to remove only a visible object; blind finger sweeps are not used in infants and children because the foreign body may be pushed back into the airway. If the foreign body cannot be visualized, mechanical force is used in an attempt to dislodge the object. Back blows and chest thrusts are used. Subdiaphragmatic abdominal thrusts are not used for infants of 1 year of age or less because of potential injury to abdominal organs. (21)

**77.** 2. The infant is placed face down, straddled over the nurse's arm with the head lower than the trunk and the head supported. This position, together with the back blows, facilitates the dislodgement and removal of a foreign object and minimizes aspiration if vomiting occurs. (21)

**78.** 4. Back blows are delivered rapidly and forcefully with the heel of the hand between the infant's shoulder blades. Slowly delivered back blows are less likely to dislodge the object. Using the heel of the hand enables more force to be applied, increasing the possibility of loosening the object. (21)

**79.** 4. Crying indicates that the airway obstruction has been relieved and the infant needs close observation. Delivering chest thrusts or back blows could jeopardize a patent airway. Blind finger sweeps are contraindicated in infants. (21)

**80.** 1. Tilting the head slightly prevents the tongue from obstructing the airway. Gastric distention interferes with diaphragmatic excursion, which occurs when breaths are delivered too rapidly. Excessive pressure on the neck does not directly affect an obstructed airway. Extensor posturing indicates brain damage and is not related to airway obstruction. (21)

# test 3

The Patient with a Ventricular Septal Defect

The Patient with Tetralogy of Fallot

The Patient with Down Syndrome

The Patient with Rheumatic Fever

The Patient with Sickle-Cell Anemia

The Patient with Iron-Deficiency Anemia

The Patient with Hemophilia and Acquired
  Immune Deficiency Syndrome

The Patient with Leukemia

Correct Answers and Rationales

Select the one *best* or *correct* answer and indicate your choice by filling in the circle with a pencil in front of the option you have chosen. If the answer you would prefer is not given, select the one you think is *most appropriate*.

## THE PATIENT WITH A VENTRICULAR SEPTAL DEFECT

Matt Stone was born with a ventricular septal defect (VSD) that was never corrected. Matt, now 4 years old, is admitted for cardiac catheterization.

1. When admitting Matt, the nurse should recall that a ventricular septal defect
   ○ 1. is a cyanotic heart defect.
   ○ 2. is rarely associated with other defects.
   ○ 3. may or may not require surgical repair.
   ○ 4. is frequently associated with brain damage.

2. Given the altered hemodynamics of ventricular septal defect, a consequence that may develop is
   ○ 1. increased pulmonary vascular resistance.
   ○ 2. decreased arterial perfusion of the lower extremities.
   ○ 3. enlargement of the third and fourth ventricles in the brain.
   ○ 4. left ventricular hypertrophy.

3. In planning Matt's care, the nurse considers his stage of development. Since 4-year-old Matt seems to be developing normally, he is most likely resolving Erikson's stage of
   ○ 1. autonomy vs. shame and doubt.
   ○ 2. identity vs. identity diffusion.
   ○ 3. initiative vs. guilt.
   ○ 4. industry vs. inferiority.

4. Matt is scheduled for a cardiac catheterization tomorrow. The nurse's plan of care for Matt should be based on the knowledge that cardiac catheterization for children usually involves the use of
   ○ 1. ultra-high-frequency sound waves.
   ○ 2. a right-sided approach.
   ○ 3. a cutdown procedure.
   ○ 4. general anesthesia.

5. The nurse considers Matt's need for psychological preparation for the cardiac catheterization. The nurse should base interventions on the fact that
   ○ 1. overpreparing a preschooler decreases his level of anxiety considerably.
   ○ 2. preschoolers are cognitively unable to understand the procedure.
   ○ 3. little psychological preparation can be given to preschoolers.
   ○ 4. preparation is a joint responsibility of the physician, parents, and nurse.

6. The catheterization is performed and Matt is returned to his room with a pressure dressing in place. Matt has an intravenous infusion and is slightly drowsy. The nurse would give *highest priority* to which of the following post-procedure assessments?
   ○ 1. Vital signs every 4 hours.
   ○ 2. Pulse checks above the catheterization site.
   ○ 3. Temperature checks of the right leg.
   ○ 4. Comparison of color in right and left legs.

7. The cardiac catheterization confirmed the diagnosis of a small membranous ventricular septal defect. Matt is to be discharged tomorrow. When preparing Matt's parents for his discharge, the nurse should tell them that
   ○ 1. his activities should be limited for 3 weeks.
   ○ 2. he should take sponge baths until the stitches are removed.
   ○ 3. he will need antibiotics before any dental work is done.
   ○ 4. the stitches will be removed in 2 weeks.

**203**

## THE PATIENT WITH TETRALOGY OF FALLOT

Five-year-old Allison Kolling is admitted to the hospital for heart surgery to repair tetralogy of Fallot. The nurse observes that Allison is cyanotic at admission.

**8.** What is the underlying cause of Allison's cyanosis?
- ○ 1. The aorta is constricted.
- ○ 2. There is stenosis of the mitral valve.
- ○ 3. There is stenosis of the pulmonary artery.
- ○ 4. The aorta receives blood directly from the vena cava.

**9.** Allison undergoes an electrocardiogram. The *primary* reason for performing this procedure is to determine the
- ○ 1. electrical activity in heart muscle.
- ○ 2. pressure of the blood in the heart.
- ○ 3. amount of blood entering the heart.
- ○ 4. various sounds made by each heartbeat.

**10.** A cardiac catheterization is ordered for Allison. Allison asks the nurse if the procedure will hurt. Which of the following statements offers the nurse the *best* guide for responding to Allison's query?
- ○ 1. Some pressure may be felt when the catheter is introduced into the vein.
- ○ 2. Momentary sharp pain will usually occur when the catheter enters the heart.
- ○ 3. It is unusual for a 5-year-old to be aware of discomfort or pain during the procedure.
- ○ 4. It is a painless procedure, although a tingling sensation is often noted in the extremities.

**11.** Allison experiences attacks of dyspnea. During Allison's attacks, the nurse makes a typical observation when she notes that Allison positions herself in a
- ○ 1. squatting position.
- ○ 2. Trendelenburg position.
- ○ 3. semi-sitting position.
- ○ 4. left side-lying position.

**12.** Allison is taught coughing and deep-breathing exercises before corrective heart surgery. Of the following teaching-learning principles for the nurse to take into account when teaching Allison, which should assume *first* priority?
- ○ 1. Building the teaching on the patient's present level of knowledge.
- ○ 2. Arranging the order of information to be taught to the patient in a logical sequence.
- ○ 3. Arranging to use actual equipment for demonstrations that will be used when teaching the patient.
- ○ 4. Presenting the information to be taught to the patient in order from the simplest to the most complex.

**13.** On her 2nd postoperative day, Allison suddenly stops breathing, and peripheral pulses are absent. Of the following measures, the one the nurse should take *first* is to
- ○ 1. clear the patient's airway.
- ○ 2. begin mouth-to-mouth resuscitation.
- ○ 3. start the patient on oxygen therapy.
- ○ 4. start external cardiac compressions.

**14.** Two nurses administer cardiopulmonary resuscitation (CPR) to Allison. The number of rescue breaths that should be administered per minute by the nurse giving artificial ventilation is
- ○ 1. 12.
- ○ 2. 15.
- ○ 3. 18.
- ○ 4. 20.

**15.** The number of cardiac compressions the second nurse should deliver each minute to Allison when administering cardiopulmonary resuscitation (CPR) should be approximately
- ○ 1. 60 to 70.
- ○ 2. 70 to 80.
- ○ 3. 80 to 100.
- ○ 4. 100 to 120.

**16.** Which of the following techniques should the nurse use for applying pressure on the heart when she is performing cardiopulmonary resuscitation on Allison?
- ○ 1. Apply pressure midway on the sternum with the heel of one hand.
- ○ 2. Apply pressure midway on the sternum with the tips of two fingers.
- ○ 3. Apply pressure over the apex of the heart with the heel of one hand.
- ○ 4. Apply pressure over the apex of the heart with the tips of two fingers.

**17.** If Allison's sternum is depressed too deeply and too vigorously during cardiopulmonary resuscitation (CPR), there is danger of
- ○ 1. injuring the patient's liver.
- ○ 2. rupturing the patient's heart.
- ○ 3. tearing the patient's diaphragm.
- ○ 4. distending the patient's stomach.

**18.** Over which of the following arteries is it recommended that the nurse palpate for evidence of a pulse while administering cardiopulmonary resuscitation (CPR) to five-year-old Allison?
- ○ 1. The radial artery.
- ○ 2. The femoral artery.
- ○ 3. The carotid artery.
- ○ 4. The dorsalis pedis artery.

**19.** Allison's parents express concern when they note

that Allison wants to be held more frequently than usual postoperatively. The term that *best* describes this behavioral response to stress is
- ○ 1. repression.
- ○ 2. depression.
- ○ 3. regression.
- ○ 4. rationalization.

20. Ms. Kolling asks the nurse why Allison has clubbed fingers. The nurse should base her response on knowledge that the clubbing of Allison's fingers is due to
- ○ 1. polycythemia.
- ○ 2. peripheral hypoxemia.
- ○ 3. delayed physical growth.
- ○ 4. destruction of bone marrow.

21. The nurse should anticipate that the *most likely* fear Allison's parents will have when they plan to take Allison home is fear of
- ○ 1. allowing the child to lead a normal active life.
- ○ 2. persuading the child of the need for extra rest.
- ○ 3. having the child develop postoperative complications.
- ○ 4. having the child's siblings treat her as a handicapped person.

22. Allison's 3-year-old sister has become quiet and shy and demonstrates more than the usual amount of sexual curiosity, according to her mother. According to Erikson's description of the central psychosocial problem of the preschooler, Allison's sister is demonstrating an attempt to resolve a conflict between
- ○ 1. trust and mistrust.
- ○ 2. initiative and guilt.
- ○ 3. industry and inferiority.
- ○ 4. autonomy and shame or doubt.

## THE PATIENT WITH DOWN SYNDROME

A community health nurse has visited the Stevens' home regularly to help with the personal care of their severely retarded daughter, Patty, age 10. Patty's mother has a back ailment of recent origin that has prevented her from assuming responsibility for Patty's care.

23. Patty is mentally retarded because of Down syndrome. *Most* mental retardation in this country results from
- ○ 1. unknown causes.
- ○ 2. hydrocephalus.
- ○ 3. phenylketonuria.
- ○ 4. Down syndrome.

24. Patty's disability was apparent at birth, and she was slow to develop. Which of the following behaviors is *least* characteristic of a delay in early development common to mentally retarded children?
- ○ 1. Not using expressive language.
- ○ 2. Not responding to verbal commands.
- ○ 3. Starting to walk at 20 months of age.
- ○ 4. Being able to sit up at 6 months of age.

25. Patty has undergone extensive testing. Which of the following information is *least likely* to be determined through the use of psychological testing?
- ○ 1. The presence and extent of organic brain damage.
- ○ 2. A differential diagnosis and profiles of symptoms.
- ○ 3. The patient's response to drug and other therapies.
- ○ 4. A differential diagnosis from other forms of psychopathology.

26. Patty has an intelligence quotient (IQ) of approximately 40. The kind of environment and interdisciplinary program from which Patty is likely to profit *most* would *best* be described as
- ○ 1. custodial.
- ○ 2. educational.
- ○ 3. habit training.
- ○ 4. sheltered workshop.

27. By which of the following means can the intelligence quotient of a mentally handicapped child like Patty *most likely* be raised?
- ○ 1. By serving her hearty, nutritious meals.
- ○ 2. By giving her vasodilating medications as prescribed.
- ○ 3. By letting her play with children more able than herself.
- ○ 4. By providing her with stimulating, non-threatening life experiences.

28. Patty has no major physical defects. When the nurse instructs her parents about physical problems most commonly associated with Down syndrome, she should teach the parents to be *especially* observant of Patty's
- ○ 1. weight.
- ○ 2. pulse rate.
- ○ 3. respirations.
- ○ 4. blood pressure.

29. The *basic* aim of the nurse working with Patty's parents is to increase their sense of
- ○ 1. liking for the child.
- ○ 2. responsibility for their child's welfare.
- ○ 3. understanding of their child's disability.
- ○ 4. confidence in their abilities to care for their child.

30. Mrs. Stevens' childbearing days are over, but she inquires about genetic counseling for her younger sister. The *primary* role of the genetic team working with a family is to
    ○ 1. provide the parents with the facts about their birth defect risks.
    ○ 2. report to the parents on the chromosome analysis of the amniotic cells.
    ○ 3. prepare the parents psychologically for the birth of a defective child.
    ○ 4. prescribe birth control or abortion measures for parents to take as needed.

31. The nurse mentions to Mrs. Stevens that a group meeting for the mothers of retarded children is to be held soon. "Not retarded!" blazes Mrs. Stevens. "Exceptional." To respond to this outburst by the mother, which of the following possible replies by the nurse would be *best?*
    ○ 1. "Why do you prefer the term 'exceptional?'"
    ○ 2. "I'm sorry if I offended you by my thoughtless remark."
    ○ 3. "No matter what it's called, the condition is still the same, isn't it?"
    ○ 4. "I'd like to hear more of your thoughts and feelings on that, if I may."

32. In relation to teaching goals, Mrs. Stevens' desire for Patty to be able to dress herself would *best* be written in a nursing care plan as
    ○ 1. a single attainable goal.
    ○ 2. a goal that may be postponed.
    ○ 3. a series of small, short-term goals.
    ○ 4. a part of the overall larger goal of optimal functioning.

33. Sometimes Patty seems deliberately to do things that cause her mother to become displeased and upset, such as taking off her clothes. Which of the following reasons probably *best* explains why Patty tends to act this way?
    ○ 1. To annoy her mother.
    ○ 2. To get attention from her mother.
    ○ 3. To express anger with her mother.
    ○ 4. To relieve her boredom with herself.

34. The community health nurse observes the Stevens family at mealtime. She notes that Patty is messy and eats noisily. Which of the following approaches that the nurse could recommend to decrease the undesirable eating habits would provide the *most positive* reinforcement for Patty's desirable table manners?
    ○ 1. Praising her when she chews quietly.
    ○ 2. Scolding her when she smacks her lips.
    ○ 3. Ignoring her when she plays with her food.
    ○ 4. Making her leave the table when she spills her milk.

## THE PATIENT WITH RHEUMATIC FEVER

Seven-year-old Cathy Scoby visits a physician's office with her mother. Cathy is sent to the hospital for admission. The medical diagnosis is rheumatic fever.

35. The nurse obtains a nursing history from Cathy's mother after Cathy is admitted to the hospital. It is *most likely* that the nurse will learn that Cathy was recently ill with
    ○ 1. mumps.
    ○ 2. measles.
    ○ 3. viral flu.
    ○ 4. a sore throat.

36. The health-illness continuum is used to assist the nurse in determining Cathy's needs for nursing care. The continuum helps illustrate that
    ○ 1. the human body has the ability to adapt within a rather wide range.
    ○ 2. there is a point at which a patient is beyond help.
    ○ 3. there are certain well-defined points at which a patient should be considered well or ill.
    ○ 4. the human body handles illness in relation to its ability to regenerate diseased tissues.

37. Maslow's theory concerning a hierarchy of needs is also used to plan Cathy's nursing care. The theory holds that, after physiological needs are met, the need having *highest priority* is that for
    ○ 1. security.
    ○ 2. affection.
    ○ 3. self-respect.
    ○ 4. self-fulfillment.

38. Which of the following nursing diagnoses is *most appropriate* for the nurse to make for Cathy?
    ○ 1. Alteration in comfort.
    ○ 2. Impaired fluid volume.
    ○ 3. Unsatisfactory dietary habits.
    ○ 4. Dysfunction in the respiratory processes.

39. Of the following laboratory blood findings, which would help *most* to confirm that Cathy very likely has rheumatic fever?
    ○ 1. A high leukocyte count.
    ○ 2. A low hemoglobin count.
    ○ 3. An elevated antibody level.
    ○ 4. A sensitivity of the causative organisms to penicillin.

40. Procaine penicillin (Crysticillin) is prescribed for Cathy. This drug acts *primarily* on microorganisms by
    ○ 1. destroying them.
    ○ 2. inhibiting their growth.
    ○ 3. neutralizing their toxins.

○ 4. decreasing their pathogenicity.

41. Activity is sharply restricted during the acute phase of Cathy's illness. In order to evaluate the effectiveness of bed rest, the nurse must recognize that activity restriction is used for Cathy *primarily* to help
   ○ 1. prevent injury to tender joints.
   ○ 2. reduce the workload on the heart.
   ○ 3. promote full benefit of drug therapy.
   ○ 4. minimize the severity of the disease's inflammatory process.

42. During the acute phase of Cathy's illness, it would be *least desirable* to interest Cathy in which of the following diversional activities?
   ○ 1. Reading a book.
   ○ 2. Playing with a doll.
   ○ 3. Listening to the radio.
   ○ 4. Playing checkers with a roommate.

43. It is determined that Cathy has carditis as a result of having rheumatic fever. Which of the following physical findings is *most* indicative of Cathy's having carditis?
   ○ 1. A heart murmur.
   ○ 2. Low blood pressure.
   ○ 3. An irregular pulse rate.
   ○ 4. Pain over the anterior chest wall.

44. When it is determined that Cathy has carditis, she is given digoxin (Lanoxin). The *primary* reason for giving this drug to Cathy is that it helps
   ○ 1. relax the walls of the heart's arteries.
   ○ 2. improve the strength of the heartbeat.
   ○ 3. prevent irregularities in ventricular contractions.
   ○ 4. eliminate dissociation of ventricular and atrial rhythms.

45. The physician prescribes digoxin (Lanoxin), 0.15 mg, p.o. daily for Cathy. The digoxin is available in liquid form with 0.05 mg/ml. How much of the medication should the nurse administer with each dose?
   ○ 1. 0.2 ml.
   ○ 2. 0.5 ml.
   ○ 3. 3.0 ml.
   ○ 4. 5.0 ml.

46. Cathy's nursing care plan indicates that her pulse should be obtained several times during the night without waking her. The *primary* reason for obtaining a sleeping pulse rate is to ensure that Cathy's pulse rate is free of influence from
   ○ 1. having had a morning dosage of digitalis.
   ○ 2. carrying out normal activity during waking hours.
   ○ 3. being in a warmer environment during the day than at night.

○ 4. having various nurses obtaining the pulse rate during day/evening hours.

47. Cathy is to receive 5 grains of acetylsalicylic acid (aspirin) every 4 hours. The metric equivalent of 5 grains is
   ○ 1. 0.032 g.
   ○ 2. 0.32 g.
   ○ 3. 3.2 g.
   ○ 4. 32 g.

48. Which of the following signs or symptoms should lead the nurse to suspect that Cathy is experiencing early salicylate toxicity?
   ○ 1. Pain in the chest.
   ○ 2. Pink-colored urine.
   ○ 3. A slow pulse rate.
   ○ 4. Ringing in the ears.

49. Which of the following measures is likely to be *most effective* in minimizing the joint pain Cathy is experiencing?
   ○ 1. Massaging the affected joints.
   ○ 2. Applying ice to the affected joints.
   ○ 3. Limiting movement of the affected joints.
   ○ 4. Putting the affected joints through range-of-motion.

50. Which of the following nursing measures is also likely to help alleviate Cathy's joint pains?
   ○ 1. Changing the patient's position in bed frequently.
   ○ 2. Applying gentle traction to the patient's affected joints.
   ○ 3. Supporting the patient's body in proper alignment with rolled pillows.
   ○ 4. Using a bed cradle to remove the weight of bed linens on the patient's joints.

51. Which of the following eating utensils is *contraindicated* if Cathy develops chorealike movements?
   ○ 1. A fork.
   ○ 2. A spoon.
   ○ 3. A plastic cup.
   ○ 4. A drinking tube.

52. The nurse discusses long-term care for Cathy with her parents. The nurse should teach them that a necessary part of Cathy's long-term care is that she receive
   ○ 1. physical therapy.
   ○ 2. antibiotic therapy.
   ○ 3. psychological therapy.
   ○ 4. anti-inflammatory therapy.

53. The nurse discusses Cathy's illness and its predisposing factors at a nursing team conference. Which of the following statements *best* describes research findings in relation to factors that predispose to rheumatic fever?

○ 1. Rheumatic fever is more common among girls than boys.

○ 2. Rheumatic fever is most common among Caucasians.

○ 3. Rheumatic fever is most common in families of low socioeconomic status.

○ 4. Rheumatic fever strikes without regard to socioeconomic status, race, or age.

# THE PATIENT WITH SICKLE-CELL ANEMIA

Jenny Otley, 1 year of age, is admitted to the hospital suffering from sickle-cell crisis.

54. When preparing for Jenny's admission, the nurse should anticipate and prepare for therapy that is *most likely* to include the use of
    ○ 1. parenteral iron therapy.
    ○ 2. an exchange transfusion.
    ○ 3. intravenous fluid therapy.
    ○ 4. a fast-acting anticoagulant.

55. The local tissue damage Jenny is likely to show at admission is due to
    ○ 1. a general inflammatory response due to an autoimmune reaction complicated by hypoxia.
    ○ 2. air hunger and resultant respiratory alkalosis due to deoxygenated red blood cells.
    ○ 3. cell damage with signs of ischemia and necrosis due to the obstruction of circulation.
    ○ 4. hypersensitivity of the central nervous system due to high serum bilirubin levels and adrenocortical imbalance.

56. The nurse notes that Jenny prefers lying on her side with her knees sharply flexed. Jenny's positioning should cause the nurse to assess Jenny further for evidence of
    ○ 1. nausea.
    ○ 2. a backache.
    ○ 3. abdominal pain.
    ○ 4. emotional regression to early infancy.

57. The crisis subsides and Jenny is to be discharged. The nurse should teach Mr. and Mrs. Otley to seek prompt health care if Jenny develops
    ○ 1. headaches and nausea.
    ○ 2. fatigue and lassitude.
    ○ 3. a skin rash and itching.
    ○ 4. a sore throat and fever.

58. Mr. and Mrs. Otley are planning a vacation. Which of the following geographic areas would be *contraindicated* for Jenny?

○ 1. Desert areas.
○ 2. Oceanside areas.
○ 3. Large urban areas.
○ 4. Mountainous areas.

59. Mrs. Otley says she does not understand how Jenny could be so healthy and normal at birth and then develop symptoms of sickle-cell disease. Which of the following statements *best* explains why Jenny was symptom-free at birth and shortly thereafter?
    ○ 1. The placenta bars passage of the hemoglobin S from the mother to the fetus.
    ○ 2. The red bone marrow does not begin to produce hemoglobin S until several months after birth.
    ○ 3. Antibodies transmitted from the mother to the fetus provide the newborn with temporary immunity.
    ○ 4. The newborn has a high concentration of fetal hemoglobin in the blood for a period of time after birth.

60. It has been determined that Mr. and Mrs. Otley are both carriers of the sickle-cell trait. They ask about the chances of sickle-cell disease occurring in their children. The nurse should respond to their question based on knowledge that the gene responsible for sickle-cell disease is autosomal recessive and the percentage of the Otleys' children subject to having the *disease* is
    ○ 1. 25%.
    ○ 2. 50%.
    ○ 3. 75%.
    ○ 4. 100%.

61. Jenny is black, and it is known that sickle-cell disease has a high incidence among American blacks. In which other ethnic group is there also a significant incidence of the disease?
    ○ 1. Greek-Americans.
    ○ 2. German-Americans.
    ○ 3. Oriental-Americans.
    ○ 4. Spanish-Americans.

# THE PATIENT WITH IRON-DEFICIENCY ANEMIA

Alexander Gray, age 11 months, is seen in an outpatient pediatric clinic. Alexander is very pale, and his mother explains that he drinks more than a quart of cow's milk daily, eats few solids, and sleeps excessively. A diagnosis of iron-deficiency anemia is made.

**62.** Mrs. Gray asks the nurse what she could have done to prevent the iron-deficiency anemia. The nurse bases the response on knowledge that solid foods should be introduced into the diet of an infant at

○ 1. 1 to 2 months of age.

○ 2. 5 to 6 months of age.

○ 3. 8 to 10 months of age.

○ 4. 10 to 12 months of age.

**63.** Alexander's current diet needs to be modified. The nurse should base Alexander's diet on which of the following modifications?

○ 1. Equal intake of iron-rich solids and milk.

○ 2. Increased intake of iron-rich solids and de-____ ____take.

____ ____e intake of iron-rich solids.

____ ____e of iron-rich solids and mainte-____ ____t milk intake.

____ Mrs. Gray about iron-rich foods

____ *priate* for 11-month-old Alex-____ ____lection of which of the follow-____ ____that she has understood the

____ eals, meats, and green vege-

____ k, and yellow vegetables.

____ ____nd mixed vegetables.

____ ____ruits, milk, and red meats.

**65.** Mrs. Gray asks the nurse about the relationship between iron-deficiency anemia and infection. The nurse should explain that

○ 1. little is known about iron-deficiency anemia and its relationship to infection in children.

○ 2. children with iron-deficiency anemia are more susceptible to infection than are other children.

○ 3. children with iron-deficiency anemia are less susceptible to infection than are other children.

○ 4. children with iron-deficiency anemia are no more susceptible to infection than are other children.

# THE PATIENT WITH HEMOPHILIA AND ACQUIRED IMMUNE DEFICIENCY SYNDROME

Neonate Greg Aldridge is suspected of having hemophilia A (classic hemophilia) because he experienced prolonged bleeding following circumcision.

**66.** Greg's physician has ordered several laboratory tests to help diagnose the bleeding disorder. Which test result would most likely be *abnormal* if Greg has hemophilia?

○ 1. Bleeding time.

○ 2. Tourniquet test.

○ 3. Clot retraction test.

○ 4. Partial thromboplastin time.

**67.** Which datum from Greg's family history supports a diagnosis of hemophilia?

○ 1. He has an older brother and sister who are healthy.

○ 2. The ethnic background of his family is Italian and German.

○ 3. His maternal grandfather had prolonged bleeding after surgery.

○ 4. His paternal grandmother died from chronic lymphocytic leukemia.

**68.** A diagnosis of hemophilia A is confirmed. As Greg enters the second half of infancy, the nurse should teach his parents to

○ 1. give him one-half of a children's aspirin if he has a fever above 101° F.

○ 2. sew thick padding into the elbows and knees of his clothing.

○ 3. check his urine for occult blood every day.

○ 4. expect the eruption of his primary teeth to produce moderate to severe bleeding.

**69.** The nurse plans to teach Greg's parents to recognize hemarthrosis. An *early* sign of hemarthrosis is

○ 1. reluctance to move a body part.

○ 2. a cool, pale, clammy extremity.

○ 3. petechiae formation around a joint.

○ 4. instability of a long bone on passive movement.

**70.** Greg's mother tells the nurse that when Greg reaches school age, she is going to teach him at home. She does not want to send him to school because the teacher will not look after him as well as she would. Greg's mother's comments represent what common parental reaction to a child's chronic illness?

○ 1. Overprotection.

○ 2. Devotion.

○ 3. Mistrust.

○ 4. Insecurity.

**71.** Greg experiences a bleeding episode in his elbow, and his parents bring him to the emergency department. A lyophilized concentrate of Factor VIII is administered intravenously. In addition to monitoring the infusion, the nurse initiates measures that minimize bleeding in the affected area. Which of the following interventions would be appropriate?

○ 1. Apply constant pressure to the elbow.

○ 2. Keep the elbow below the level of the heart.

3. Place a warm, moist pack on the elbow.
4. Immobilize and elevate the elbow.

72. Because of the risks associated with the administration of Factor VIII concentrate, the nurse would teach Greg's family to recognize and report
    1. yellowing of the skin.
    2. horizontal ridges on the nails.
    3. abdominal distention.
    4. paroxysmal, nonproductive coughing.

73. Greg's mother tells the nurse she is afraid to allow Greg to be very active because he could injure himself and bleed. The nurse explains that physical fitness is very important for children with hemophilia and that an ideal activity for them is
    1. snow skiing.
    2. swimming.
    3. football.
    4. gymnastics.

74. Greg and his parents have coped successfully with hemophilia and Greg just celebrated his 3rd birthday. However, he has been treated for pneumonitis three times in the last three months and on physical examination his liver and spleen are found to be enlarged. What screening test is likely to be ordered for Greg?
    1. Serum glutamic-pyruvic transaminase (SGPT).
    2. Creatinine phosphokinase (CPK).
    3. Enzyme-linked immunosorbent assay (ELISA).
    4. Hemagglutination inhibition test (HAI).

75. Laboratory tests confirm the diagnosis of acquired immune deficiency syndrome (AIDS). What is the *most likely* route of transmission of AIDS in Greg's situation?
    1. The causative virus contaminated some of the Factor VIII replacement he received during bleeding episodes.
    2. He had casual contact with a child who tested positive for human immunodeficiency virus (HIV).
    3. A needle used to obtain a sample of his blood transmitted the virus to him.
    4. He ate food prepared by a cook who tested positive for human immunodeficiency virus (HIV).

76. Infection is an ongoing problem for the individual with AIDS. The nurse teaches Greg's family signs and symptoms of infection. For which of the following signs and symptoms should they be *especially* alert?
    1. Erythema around the infected area.
    2. Fever.
    3. Tenderness of the infected area.
    4. Warmth of the infected area.

77. The nurse teaches Greg's parents to avoid the spread of AIDS by
    1. washing his clothing and linens separately in hot water.
    2. cleaning his bedroom and bathroom daily with disinfectant.
    3. having him use disposable plates, cups, and silverware at all times.
    4. using plastic or latex gloves when helping him control external bleeding.

# THE PATIENT WITH LEUKEMIA

Scott Warren, an acutely ill 10-year-old, is hospitalized with an upper respiratory infection and right otitis media. He is pale and lethargic. When Scott was 7, it was determined that he had leukemia. After a long initial regimen of care, Scott has had a remission, during which he has been symptom-free and his parents have become optimistic about his prognosis.

78. Which of the following statements *best* describes Scott's leukemia?
    1. His disease is infectious in nature and characterized by increased white blood cell production.
    2. His disease is neoplastic in nature and characterized by a proliferation of immature white blood cells.
    3. His disease is inflammatory in nature and characterized by solid tumor formation in the lymph nodes.
    4. His disease is allergic in nature and characterized by an increased number of circulating antibodies in his bloodstream.

79. Which of the following statements *best* describes a condition that made Scott especially prone to infections?
    1. The child's play activities were too strenuous in view of his illness.
    2. The child's vitamin C intake had been inadequate over a period of time.
    3. The child's red blood cells were inadequate for carrying oxygen for tissue nourishment.
    4. The child's white blood cells were incapable of handling an infectious process.

80. Laboratory findings show that Scott is anemic, which has *most probably* resulted from blood loss and
    1. an inadequate intake of iron in the diet.
    2. a decrease in the production of red blood cells.

○ 3. an increase in destruction of red blood cells by lymphocytes.

○ 4. a progressive replacement of the bone marrow with scar tissue.

81. The nurse notes that Scott has petechiae, that his gums, lips, and nose bleed easily, and that there are bruises on various parts of his body. Which of the following laboratory findings would be *typical* when these symptoms appear?

○ 1. Low platelet count.

○ 2. Low serum calcium level.

○ 3. Faulty thrombin production.

○ 4. Insufficient fibrinogen concentration.

82. Which of the following measures should be kept at a *minimum*, when possible, because Scott is prone to bruise and bleed easily?

○ 1. Giving the patient a stool softener.

○ 2. Changing the patient's position in bed.

○ 3. Offering the patient food at frequent intervals.

○ 4. Administering drugs to the patient intramuscularly.

83. Which of the following measures would be *contraindicated* when the nurse gives Scott oral hygiene?

○ 1. Applying petrolatum jelly to the lips.

○ 2. Cleaning the teeth with a toothbrush.

○ 3. Swabbing the mouth with moistened cotton swabs.

○ 4. Rinsing the mouth with a nonirritating mouthwash.

84. Which of the following items is likely to be *most* effective for promoting hemostasis over a lesion when the nurse observes that an area in Scott's mouth is bleeding?

○ 1. Chewing gum.

○ 2. A cotton ball.

○ 3. A gauze sponge.

○ 4. A dry tea bag.

85. Which of the following beverages is Scott likely to tolerate *best* when he feels nauseated?

○ 1. Milk.

○ 2. Weak tea.

○ 3. Plain water.

○ 4. A carbonated beverage.

86. The nurse should question the order if the drug prescribed for Scott to help control discomfort is

○ 1. acetaminophen (Tylenol).

○ 2. acetophenetidin (phenacetin).

○ 3. acetylsalicylic acid (aspirin).

○ 4. propoxyphene hydrochloride (Darvon).

87. Scott is scheduled for a bone marrow aspiration. Over which of the following bone sites should the nurse prepare Scott's skin for entry of the needle?

○ 1. The radius.

○ 2. The sternum.

○ 3. A cervical vertebra.

○ 4. The posterior iliac crest.

88. Scott is also scheduled for a lumbar puncture. The rationale for this procedure is to

○ 1. relieve undue pressure in the central nervous system.

○ 2. inject drugs that will help control an infection in the central nervous system.

○ 3. determine whether the central nervous system has been invaded by the disease.

○ 4. identify organisms that may be causing an infection in the central nervous system.

89. Mercaptopurine (Purinethol), 75 mg daily, is prescribed for Scott. Mercaptopurine is marketed in 50-mg tablets for oral administration. How many tablets should the nurse give Scott each day?

○ 1. Half of one tablet.

○ 2. One and a half tablets.

○ 3. Two tablets.

○ 4. Two and a half tablets.

90. Which of the following signs and symptoms, if present in Scott, should suggest to the nurse that toxicity to mercaptopurine (Purinethol) is occurring?

○ 1. Nausea, vomiting, and diarrhea.

○ 2. Skin rash, constipation, and polyuria.

○ 3. Dry mouth, blurred vision, and headache.

○ 4. Drowsiness, malaise, and low blood pressure.

91. Methotrexate (Amethopterin) is ordered for Scott also. The nurse should question the order before preparing to help administer the drug if an order has *not* also been written for

○ 1. having the patient in a state of fasting.

○ 2. obtaining a white blood cell count on the patient.

○ 3. an x-ray examination of the patient's spinal canal.

○ 4. collecting a specimen from the patient for urinalysis.

92. Methotrexate (Amethopterin) is given to Scott by injecting it into his spinal canal. This type of drug administration is called

○ 1. subdural.

○ 2. intrathecal.

○ 3. intraosseous.

○ 4. intra-arterial.

93. Mercaptopurine (Purinethol) and methotrexate (Amethopterin) are classified as antimetabolites. Antimetabolites function in the body to

○ 1. selectively destroy malignant cells, thereby slowing tumor growth.

○ 2. create a hormonal imbalance within the body that acts to suppress tumor growth.

**211**

3. damage deoxyribonucleic acid (DNA) within cell nuclei, which in turn disrupts cell growth and division.

4. imitate nutrients essential for malignant cell growth, thus preventing those cells from using natural nutrients.

94. Allopurinol (Zyloprim) is ordered for Scott. Which of the following nursing measures should be observed while Scott is taking allopurinol?

1. Encouraging a high fluid intake.
2. Omitting carbonated fluids.
3. Giving foods high in potassium.
4. Limiting foods high in natural sugar.

95. When Scott fails to respond to therapy, as he did in the past, his parents are told of his imminent death. Which of the following statements offers the nurse the *best* guide as she makes plans to assist Scott's parents?

1. Knowing for years that the prognosis was poor helps prepare relatives for the death of children.
2. Relatives are especially grieved when a remission in a disease process was thought to be a good sign of cure.
3. Trust in health personnel who wish to help relatives in grief is most often destroyed by a death that is considered untimely.
4. It is more difficult for relatives to accept the death of a 10-year-old than the death of a younger child whose family membership has been short.

96. The nurses caring for Scott and his family describe how they wish to offer the Warrens the best care. Authorities generally agree that in order to help others deal with death, the nurse *first* must have

1. experienced the death of a loved one herself.
2. worked out her own personal philosophy of life and death.

3. taken a course that considered how to deal with death and grieving.
4. developed a belief of her own that accepts a supreme being and a life hereafter.

97. Which of the following courses of action would be *most appropriate* for the nurse when she is planning to meet Scott's emotional needs during his last days of life?

1. Restrict Scott's visitors to his parents so as not to overtax him.
2. Answer Scott's questions about his illness and imminent death honestly.
3. Concentrate nursing efforts on meeting Scott's physical needs in order to help him think of things other than himself.
4. Encourage Scott to play quietly with his roommate in order to replace thoughts of sadness with thoughts of pleasurable things.

98. After Scott's death, his mother asks the nurse, "What if we had brought Scott in when he first complained of an earache? Would he have lived if we had brought him to the hospital sooner?" Which of the following statements offers the nurse the *best* guide for responding to Mrs. Warren's questions?

1. The nurse should explain that everything possible was done for the child.
2. The nurse should provide comfort by saying that the child is no longer suffering with an incurable illness.
3. The nurse should explain that the child's physician is in the best position to explain what happened.
4. The nurse should describe how infections are often the result of leukemia rather than a cause of it.

# CORRECT ANSWERS AND RATIONALES

Numbers appear in parentheses following the rationales. The numbers identify textbooks listed in the references at the end of Part III, where correct answers can be verified.

## The Patient with a Ventricular Septal Defect

1. 3. A ventricular septal defect is an acyanotic heart defect; oxygenated blood is shunted from the left ventricle to the right ventricle through the defect because of the pressure gradient. Although frequently associated with other defects such as pulmonary stenosis and coarctation of the aorta, ventricular septal defect is not associated with brain damage. Eighty percent of children with a small ventricular septal defect will experience spontaneous closure of the defect. (21)

2. 1. Increased pulmonary vascular resistance may develop because of the higher pressure within the left ventricle and because the systemic circulation offers more resistance than the pulmonary circulation. Blood is shunted through the defect from the left ventricle to the right ventricle into the pulmonary artery. This increased blood volume can eventually result in increased pulmonary vascular resistance. (21)

3. 3. Erikson maintains that the chief psychosocial task of the preschool period is acquiring a sense of initiative. The child's activities center around energetic learning and seeking accomplishment and satisfaction in these activities. The conflict of guilt arises when the child oversteps the limits of his abilities and behaves or acts inappropriately. Autonomy vs. shame and doubt is the psychosocial task of toddlers. Identity vs. identity diffusion is the task of early adolescents, and industry vs. inferiority is the task of school-aged children. (21)

4. 2. In children, cardiac catheterization usually involves a right-sided approach because septal defects permit entry into the left side of the heart. The catheter is usually inserted into the femoral vein via a percutaneous puncture; a cutdown procedure is rarely used. The catheterization is usually performed under local anesthesia with sedation. Echocardiography involves the use of ultra-high-frequency sound waves. (20, 21)

5. 4. Preparation is the joint responsibility of the physician, parents, and nurse. Overpreparing a preschooler can *increase* his anxiety level, rather than decrease it. Preschoolers are cognitively ready to understand information that is individualized to their level. Little psychological preparation can be given to infants and toddlers. (21)

6. 4. The involved and uninvolved extremities should be compared in terms of color, temperature, pedal pulses, and capillary filling time. Vital signs, including blood pressure, are checked as often as every 15 minutes after the procedure to detect dysrhythmias and hypotension. Pulses, especially *below* the catheterization site, are checked for equality and symmetry. Fluids should be encouraged following the procedure. The dye used during the catheterization causes an osmotic diuresis. (21)

7. 3. Antibiotics are suggested for children with heart defects before any dental work is done to reduce the incidence of bacterial endocarditis. Activities are not restricted. Stitches are not necessary with a percutaneous approach. The pressure dressing will be removed before the child is discharged, making it possible to shower or bathe as usual. (8)

## The Patient With Tetralogy of Fallot

8. 3. The congenital defects present in a child with tetralogy of Fallot are (1) a stenosis of the pulmonary artery, (2) an interventricular septal defect, and (3) a deviation of the aorta. The fourth defect (tetralogy means a series of four) is hypertrophy of the right ventricle, which occurs as an adaptive mechanism to help overcome the effects of the three congenital defects. When pulmonary stenosis is severe, the patient will be cyanotic because blood is unable to reach the lungs satisfactorily for oxygenation. The pulmonary stenosis tends to worsen in the older infant or child. (7, 21)

9. 1. An electrocardiogram (ECG) records the electrical impulses in heart muscle and provides a graphic tracing of the pattern of the impulses and their sequence and magnitude. An ECG does not provide information about the pressure of the blood in the heart. A cardiac catheterization is used to measure the pressure in the chambers of the heart and major vessels and to measure the amount of blood entering the heart. Auscultation with a stethoscope is required to detect the various sounds made with each heartbeat. A phonocardiogram provides a graphic representation of heart sounds. (7, 21)

10. 1. The best guide for a nurse to follow when a child asks if cardiac catheterization is painful is to explain that the patient will experience some pres-

sure when the catheter is introduced. The child's trust will be quickly lost if the nurse is untruthful. Most children are sedated and feel little during the procedure. (7, 21)

**11.** 1. Flexing the legs reduces the venous flow of blood from the lower extremities. This reduces the volume of blood being shunted through the interventricular septal defect and the overriding aorta in the child with tetralogy of Fallot. The result is that the blood then entering the systemic circulation has a better content of oxygen and dyspnea is reduced. Flexing the legs also increases the vascular resistance and the pressure in the left ventricle. An infant will often assume a knee-chest position in a crib, or the mother learns to put him over her shoulder while holding him in a knee-chest position to relieve dyspnea. (11, 21)

**12.** 1. Before planning any teaching program for a child or an adult, the nurse's first step is to assess the patient to determine what he already knows. Even a 5-year-old child has some understanding of a condition he has had since birth. The child's interest will soon be lost if material with which he is familiar is repeated. Such techniques as placing information in a logical sequence, presenting the material in a progression from simple to complex, and using actual equipment for demonstrations are recommended, but should be used after obtaining baseline information about what the child already knows. (11, 21)

**13.** 1. When a person stops breathing and has no pulse, the nurse should prepare to administer cardiopulmonary resuscitation (CPR). The first course of action is to clear the patient's airway. Other measures such as administering oxygen, starting artificial ventilation, or beginning cardiac compressions will be futile if the airway is not patent so that oxygen can be delivered to the pulmonary system. (7, 21)

**14.** 2. The recommended rate per minute for administering artificial ventilation during cardiopulmonary resuscitation (CPR) is: for infants, 20 rescue breaths per minute; for children, 15 rescue breaths per minute; for adults, 12 rescue breaths per minute. (15, 21)

**15.** 3. Chest compressions are delivered at a rate of 80 to 100 times per minute for a 5-year-old child. This rate approximates the resting minimum pulse, which allows for adequate brain perfusion. A rate less than 80 does not provide adequate brain perfusion for the 5-year-old child. (21)

**16.** 1. The sternum should be compressed when pressure is applied to massage the heart during cardiopulmonary resuscitation (CPR). In a child, the pres-

sure should be applied about midway on the sternum with the heel of one hand. The tips of the fingers are used for an infant. Two hands are used, one on top of the other with fingers interlaced, for an adult. (6, 7)

**17.** 1. The greatest danger when the sternum is depressed too deeply and vigorously during cardiopulmonary resuscitation (CPR) is injury to the liver and possibly also fracture of the patient's ribs. Tearing the diaphragm, rupturing the heart, and causing gastric distention are not ordinarily complications of CPR. (7)

**18.** 3. The carotid artery should be used to palpate for evidence of a pulse rate in children, adolescents, and adults during cardiopulmonary resuscitation (CPR). The carotid artery is large, centrally located, and ordinarily easily accessible. The brachial artery, which courses along the inner aspect of the upper arm, should be used when CPR is administered to infants because the short neck of an infant makes palpating the carotid artery difficult. (7, 21)

**19.** 3. Regression is defined as the act of moving backward. In psychology, the term is used to describe a person who reverts to an earlier stage of behavior or emotion. Depression is characterized by feelings of sadness, gloom, and low spirits. Repression is a defense mechanism by which an unacceptable or painful experience is put out of the conscious mind. Rationalization is characterized by the person's making explanations and excuses for behavior. (6, 7)

**20.** 2. A patient with persistent hypoxia will eventually experience tissue changes in the body because of the low oxygen content of the blood (hypoxemia). Clubbing of the fingers is one common finding. It is believed to be due to tissue fibrosis and hypertrophy from the hypoxemia and to an increase in capillaries in the area, which occurs as the body attempts to improve blood supplies. This same phenomenon is noted in adults with chronic obstructive pulmonary disease (COPD) and occurs for the same reason as it does in the child with tetralogy of Fallot, as described in this situation. The child may be small for her age, but clubbing does not result from slow physical growth. Clubbing of the fingers is also associated with polycythemia, but polycythemia is not a component of tetralogy of Fallot. Destruction of bone marrow is not related to a cyanotic heart malformation. Instead, bone marrow is actively producing erythrocytes to compensate for the chronic hypoxia. (21)

**21.** 1. Most parents find it especially difficult to allow a child who has been unable to be normally active before corrective heart surgery to lead a normal and active life after surgery. These parents are less likely to be apprehensive about persuading the child for the need for rest, having the child develop postoperative complications, and having the child's siblings treat the child as a handicapped person. (7, 21)

**22.** 2. The central psychosocial task for the preschool child is to develop a sense of initiative vs. guilt, according to Erikson's theory. Any environmental change may affect a child. In this situation, the sister is very likely feeling less attention from her mother and is attempting to resolve the conflict with her behavior. (7, 21)

## *The Patient with Down Syndrome*

**23.** 1. The cause of mental retardation in most children in the United States is unknown. The causes are not precisely understood, but are believed to include genetic factors, social factors, and physiologic factors. (6, 21)

**24.** 4. Being able to sit up at 6 months of age is a typical developmental skill of a normal infant and could be expected to be delayed in a mentally retarded infant. Mentally retarded children tend not to use expressive language and not to respond to verbal commands at an age level that would be appropriate for their biological age. Walking, which normally occurs at or relatively soon after 1 year of age, is almost always delayed in the mentally retarded youngster. (7, 21)

**25.** 3. Psychological tests are used primarily to measure intelligence and personality. They are not used to determine a patient's response to drugs and other therapies. (7, 21)

**26.** 3. With recent advances in the care of the mentally retarded, it has been found that persons with an IQ between about 35 and 50 are trainable. They can be taught to take care of their hygienic needs, use acceptable social manners, and manage speech and other simple means of communication. Patients with an IQ between about 50 and 75 are educable. Custodial care is required for the severely and profoundly retarded; these persons have an IQ below about 35. (7, 21)

**27.** 4. Nonthreatening experiences that are stimulating and interesting to the child have been observed to help raise an IQ. Such practices as serving nutritious meals, administering vasodilating drugs, and letting the youngster play with more able children than herself have not been demonstrated to increase intelligence. (7, 21)

**28.** 3. It is especially important to observe the nature of the child's respirations because children with Down syndrome are prone to develop respiratory infections. (7, 21)

**29.** 4. The parents must continue to work daily with their retarded child when the nurse is not there. Instructions and counseling are directed toward increasing their ability to care for the child confidently. A sense of liking for, responsibility for, and understanding of the child tends to grow as the former goal is accomplished. (7, 21)

**30.** 1. The primary aim of genetic counseling is to inform couples of birth defect risks. Reporting to couples about chromosome analysis of the amniotic cells and preparing a couple psychologically for the birth of a defective child are secondary and vary among facilities. A decision about birth control methods should be left to the couple. (7, 21)

**31.** 4. To respond to a mother who becomes angry when a nurse calls her child retarded instead of exceptional, the nurse should give the mother a chance to explore her feelings on the subject because the mother is upset. Trying to use logic, defending the comment, or apologizing cannot be expected to be effective in handling the situation described in this item. Asking "why" questions may cause the mother to become defensive and does not encourage exploration of feelings. (7, 21)

**32.** 3. Goals set for a mentally retarded child should be simple and attainable. It is best to break skills, such as dressing oneself, into many small parts and have the child repeat each part with slowly advancing variations. Hence, a series of small, short-term goals would be the most appropriate. (7, 21)

**33.** 2. The most likely explanation when the mentally retarded child described in this item tends deliberately to do things that displease her mother is that the child is seeking attention from her mother. Often, the need to get attention is greater than the fear of being punished and worth the mother's displeasure with the child. (19)

**34.** 1. Very often, the best reinforcement for desired behavior in children is reward, or praise, as described in this item. Such techniques as scolding the child, ignoring her, or making her leave the table when she misbehaves do not serve the purpose of reinforcing desired behavior. (7, 21)

## *The Patient With Rheumatic Fever*

**35.** 4. Rheumatic fever is an inflammatory collagen disease that typically follows an infection by Group A beta-hemolytic streptococci. The infection ordinarily occurs in the throat. Rheumatic fever generally follows the infection with streptococci in approximately 2 weeks. It is believed that the disease involves an autoimmune or allergic response to the organism. The name "rheumatic fever" was given to the disease because of the joint involvement and the fever during the acute stage. Mumps, measles, and viral influenza are caused by viruses and do not predispose to rheumatic fever. (7, 21)

**36.** 1. The health-illness continuum is based on the concept that there is no one point at which health or illness occurs. Both are relative, and there is considerable range and latitude in what might be called illness or wellness. The continuum can be used for planning all patient care, including care for the acutely ill child described in this item. (7)

**37.** 1. Maslow built his theory on the knowledge that needs motivate behavior. These needs fall into a characteristic order. The most demanding needs are physiological needs for maintaining life. The remaining needs according to Maslow's theory are (in order of priority) needs for security and survival, affection and love, self-respect, self-fulfillment, and self-actualization. (7)

**38.** 1. A nursing diagnosis should state a health problem derived from existing evidence about the patient and from sound nursing knowledge. The health problem should be amenable to nursing care and should serve as a basis for planning and carrying out patient-centered nursing care. A typical health problem that a child with rheumatic fever has is painful joints, and therefore an appropriate nursing diagnosis for the child described in this item is an alteration in comfort. Promoting comfort is a nursing responsibility and serves as a basis for planning and carrying out nursing care. Patients may have more than one nursing diagnosis, but based on the information given about the patient described in this item, it is less likely for the child to have impaired fluid volume, a dysfunction in the respiratory processes, or unsatisfactory dietary habits. (7, 21)

**39.** 3. It is not known exactly why rheumatic fever follows a streptococcal infection, but it is theorized that there is an antigen-antibody response in the body to an M protein that is noted to be present in certain strains of streptococci. The antibodies developed by the body attack certain tissues, such as in the heart and joints. Antibody levels are found to be elevated or rising through the use of antistreptolysin O (ASO) titer. This blood finding is the most reliable evidence indicating that the patient has had a streptococcal infection. The antibody levels are likely to be elevated for weeks after a child develops rheumatic fever. (7, 21)

**40.** 1. The penicillins are bactericidal for many organisms (that is, they destroy microorganisms). They inhibit the proper synthesis of bacterial cell walls. For children with rheumatic fever, penicillin is used to destroy streptococcal organisms. (7, 21)

**41.** 2. Every effort is made to reduce the work of the heart during the acute phase of rheumatic fever when the heart is suffering with an inflammatory condition. Bed rest with very limited activity is recommended to help attain the goal of preventing heart failure. Rheumatic fever is among the leading causes of heart failure and death in youngsters between 5 and 15 years of age. (7, 21)

**42.** 4. School-age children enjoy board games, and they are very intense about following rules. Their play can often become very emotional. Obtaining rest is of utmost importance during the acute stage of rheumatic fever. Therefore, playing a game with another child will most probably be too strenuous for the youngster described in this item, especially when the game involves competition for winning, such as checkers. Such diversional activities as reading a book, playing with a doll, and listening to a radio are satisfactory. (7, 21)

**43.** 1. The connective tissue of the heart of a patient with rheumatic fever is inflamed, and signs of carditis indicate inflammation severe enough to compromise heart function. The most common signs of carditis include heart murmurs, tachycardia during rest, cardiac enlargement, and changes in the electrical conductivity of the heart. Heart murmurs are present in about 75% of all patients during the first week of carditis and in 85% of patients by the third week. Low blood pressure, an irregular pulse rate, and pain over the anterior chest wall are not related to the inflammatory process of rheumatic fever. (7, 21)

**44.** 2. Digitalis preparations, such as digoxin (Lanoxin), act to improve and strengthen the heartbeat. They increase cardiac output by increasing the strength of the heart's contractions and decrease the heart rate. Digitalis is not used to relax artery walls, prevent irregularities in ventricular contractions, or eliminate dissociation of ventricular and atrial rhythms. (7, 11)

**45.** 3. The following method describes how the correct amount of medication is determined when 0.15 mg of a drug is prescribed for each dose and the preparation on hand contains 0.05 mg/ml:

$$0.15 \text{ mg} : x \text{ ml} :: 0.05 \text{ mg} : 1 \text{ ml}$$
$$0.05x = 0.15$$
$$x = \frac{0.15}{0.05} = 3 \text{ ml}$$

The correct dosage will be contained in 3 ml of the drug in solution. (13)

**46.** 2. An above-average pulse rate that is out of proportion to the amount of fever the patient has is an early sign of cardiac failure in a patient with rheumatic fever. The sleeping pulse is used to determine whether mild tachycardia is present during sleep or whether it is the result of normal daytime activity. (7, 21)

**47.** 2. Five grains of a drug are equivalent to 0.32 g or 0.3 g. (13)

**48.** 4. Signs and symptoms of early salicylate toxicity include tinnitus (ringing in the ears), disturbances in hearing and vision, and dizziness. Salicylate toxicity may cause nausea, vomiting, diarrhea, and bleeding from mucous membranes when salicylates are used over a period of time. Such symptoms as chest pain, pink-colored urine, and a slow pulse rate (bradycardia) are not associated with salicylate toxicity. (11, 16)

**49.** 3. The joints of a patient with rheumatic fever, usually the knees, ankles, elbows, and wrists, are painful, swollen, red, and hot to the touch. Pain is ordinarily minimized when movement of the affected joints is limited. Exercise should not be used, as it usually is for patients with other forms of arthritis. Despite joint involvement in a patient with rheumatic fever, permanent deformities do not occur. Massaging the joints and applying ice to them are unlikely to relieve pain. (7, 21)

**50.** 4. For a child with arthritis associated with rheumatic fever, the joints are generally so tender that even the weight of bed linens can increase the pain. Using a bed cradle is recommended to help remove the weight of the linens on painful joints. Supporting the body in good alignment and changing the patient's position are recommended, but these nursing measures are not likely to relieve pain. Applying traction to the joints is not recommended. Traction is usually used to relieve muscle spasms, and these are not associated with rheumatic fever. (7, 21)

**51.** 1. The safety of a child with chorealike movements is of prime importance. Feeding the child may be difficult. The use of a fork should be avoided because of the danger of injury to the mouth and face with the tines of the fork. (11)

**52.** 2. A person who has had rheumatic fever is likely to develop the illness again after a future streptococcal infection. Therefore, it is advised that a child who has had rheumatic fever receive antibiotic prophylaxis for at least 5 years and sometimes for an even longer period after the acute attack to prevent recurrence of the disease. (7, 11)

**53.** 3. It has been observed that rheumatic fever occurs most often among those in lower socio-economic groups, in which streptococcal infections spread among people living in crowded conditions. Its incidence is not affected by race, sex, or ethnicity, and adults as well as children contract the disease. (7, 15)

## The Patient With Sickle-Cell Anemia

**54.** 3. A major therapeutic consideration during a sickle-cell crisis is increasing the transport and availability of oxygen to the body's tissues. Methods of doing this include administering a high volume of intravenous fluid and electrolytes to help compensate for the acidosis resulting from hypoxemia associated with sickle-cell crisis. The fluids also help overcome the dehydration with which the patient usually suffers. Rest and analgesics are commonly used during therapy for sickle-cell crisis. Anticoagulants have been suggested, but they are not included in the general treatment of crisis. Exchange transfusions are used only in highly specific situations. Iron therapy is contraindicated for this condition. (7, 21)

**55.** 3. Characteristic sickle cells tend to "log jam" in capillaries. This results in poor circulation to local tissues, causing ischemia and necrosis. The basic defect in sickle-cell disease is an abnormality in the structure of the red blood cells. Erythrocytes are sickle-shaped, rough in texture, and rigid, and because of this morphology they obstruct normal blood flow through capillaries. (7, 21)

**56.** 3. Because of the infant's self-positioning on her side with her knees sharply flexed, the nurse should assess further for evidence of abdominal pain. Such positioning has been noted by health personnel to indicate the presence of abdominal pain in most instances. Regression is common in acutely ill hospitalized children but insufficient data are given in this item to confirm regression to early infancy. Nausea usually causes an infant to refuse nourishment. A backache would most probably cause an infant to lie on her back to relieve discomfort. (21)

**57.** 4. Children with sickle-cell disease are prone to develop infections as a result of the necrosis of areas within the body and a generalized less-than-optimal health status. The child is often anorexic, gains weight slowly, and has malaise and irritability. Specific signs of infection are a sore throat and fever. Fatigue, lassitude, headaches, and nausea could be prodromal signs of an infection, but these symptoms could also be signs of other illnesses.

More information should be gathered in such instances. A skin rash and itching has a low probability of indicating an infection; more likely, it is due to an unrelated contact dermatitis. The exception would be varicella (chicken pox), and therefore an assessment should include questions about recent contacts with an infected person. An infection in children with sickle-cell anemia often brings on a crisis and should therefore be treated promptly. (7, 21)

**58.** 4. Sickling is more likely to occur where oxygen levels are low. Mountainous areas and flying in non-pressurized planes are contraindicated for those with sickle-cell disease. An oceanside area would be satisfactory; so would desert and urban areas, unless they are in mountainous places. (21)

**59.** 4. Sickle-cell disease is an inherited disease that is present at birth. However, 60% to 80% of a newborn's hemoglobin is fetal hemoglobin, which has a structure different from hemoglobin S and A. Sickling with symptoms generally occurs about 4 months after birth. Some hemoglobin S is produced by the fetus near term. The fetus produces all its own hemoglobin from the earliest production in the first trimester. Passive immunity from antibodies from the mother is not related to sickle-cell disease, but this transmission of antibodies is important in protecting the infant from various infections during early infancy. (7, 21)

**60.** 1. Sickle-cell disease is an autosomal recessive mendelian disorder. Therefore, if both parents have the trait, there is a one in four chance that a child will have the disease. There is a one in two chance that a child will have the trait. (6, 15)

**61.** 4. Sickle-cell disease is prevalent among blacks. Approximately 8% of blacks have sickle-cell trait and about 1 out of 600 black infants born in this country has the disease. Spanish-Americans also have a high incidence of sickle-cell disease. Caucasians rarely have the disease, but those who do are most often of Mediterranean descent. (10)

## The Patient with Iron-Deficiency Anemia

**62.** 2. Solids should be introduced when an infant is approximately 5 to 6 months of age. Full-term infants use up their prenatal iron stores within 4 to 6 months after birth. Cow's milk contains insufficient iron. Introducing solids before the age of 5 to 6 months could increase the likelihood of food allergies, which would increase the risk of gastric irritation. (21)

**63.** 2. Intake of iron-rich solids needs to be increased and intake of milk needs to be decreased to one quart per day. It is impossible to obtain the needed iron from milk alone, but the milk contains essential minerals and vitamins. Decreasing milk intake will increase hunger for and tolerance of solids. Nearly exclusive intake of iron-rich solids can cause constipation and inadequate absorption of essential nutrients. (21)

**64.** 1. Relatively large amounts of iron are contained in eggs, iron-fortified cereals, meats, and green vegetables. Fruits, non-fortified cereals, milk, yellow vegetables, and juices contain less iron than eggs, iron-fortified cereals, meats, and green vegetables. (21)

**65.** 2. Children with iron-deficiency anemia are more susceptible to infection because of marked decreases in bone marrow functioning with microcytosis. (21)

## The Patient with Hemophilia and Acquired Immune Deficiency Syndrome

**66.** 4. The partial thromboplastin time (PTT) measures the activity of thromboplastin, which is dependent on intrinsic clotting factors. In hemophilia, the intrinsic clotting Factor VIII, called antihemophilic factor, is deficient, resulting in a prolonged PTT. Bleeding time, tourniquet test, and clot retraction test measure platelet function, vasoconstriction, and capillary fragility. These are unaffected in the individual with hemophilia. (21)

**67.** 3. Hemophilia A is a genetically transmitted disorder. It is an X-linked recessive disorder characterized by a deficiency of plasma Factor VIII. A hemophiliac male and a normal female have normal male children and female children who carry the hemophilia trait. The carrier females pass the abnormal gene to half their sons. Ethnic background and familial leukemia are unrelated to the development of hemophilia. (21)

**68.** 2. As the hemophilic child begins to acquire motor skills, the risk of bleeding increases because of falls and bumps. Such injuries can be minimized by padding vulnerable joints. Aspirin is contraindicated because of its anti-platelet properties. Since genitourinary bleeding is not a typical problem in the young hemophiliac, urine testing is not indicated. Tooth eruption does not normally cause bleeding episodes in hemophiliac children. (21)

**69.** 1. Bleeding into the joints in the hemophiliac child leads to pain and tenderness, resulting in restricted movement. If the bleeding continues, the area becomes hot, swollen, and immobile. Petechial bleeding is not a problem in hemophilia. (17)

**70.** 1. Overprotection is a parental reaction to chronic illness. Its characteristics include sacrifice of self and family for the child, failure to recognize the child's capabilities and sense of responsibility, restrictions on play and peer friendship, and a lack of confidence in other peoples' capabilities. (21)

**71.** 4. When a bleeding episode occurs, the affected area should be immobilized and elevated to slow blood flow to the area and to promote hemostasis. Pressure should be applied to the area for 10 to 15 minutes to promote clot formation. Cold packs promote vasoconstriction; warm packs promote vasodilation and bleeding. (21)

**72.** 1. Because Factor VIII concentrate is derived from large pools of human plasma, the risk of hepatitis is always present. Clinical manifestations of hepatitis include jaundice of the skin, mucous membranes, and sclera. (21)

**73.** 2. Swimming is an ideal activity for the hemophiliac child. Noncontact sports and physical activities that do not place excessive strain on joints are appropriate for the child with hemophilia. Such activities strengthen the muscles surrounding joints and help control bleeding in these areas. Noncontact sports also enhance general mental and physical well-being. (21)

**74.** 3. Hepatosplenomegaly and interstitial pneumonitis, together with failure to thrive and diffuse lymphadenopathy, are clinical manifestations of acquired immune deficiency syndrome (AIDS) in children. When these manifestations are present in a high-risk child, an enzyme-linked immunosorbent assay (ELISA) is performed to screen for the presence of the AIDS virus. (15)

**75.** 1. The AIDS virus is spread by direct contact with blood or blood products and by sexual contact. Children with hemophilia are especially at risk for AIDS infection because of the factor concentrates they receive. These concentrates are derived from great quantities of pooled plasma, exposing recipients to thousands of blood donors. There is no evidence that casual contact between infected and uninfected persons transmits the responsible virus. The sterile, disposable needles used in all hospitals and clinics to perform venipunctures are not a source of AIDS transmission. (21)

**76.** 2. Fever is a cardinal manifestation of infection in those with AIDS. Because the major physiological alteration in patients with AIDS is generalized dysfunction of the immune system, typical indicators of the body's response to infection, such as erythe-

ma, warmth, and/or tenderness of an area, may be absent. (21)

**77.** 4. AIDS is spread by direct contact with blood or blood products and by sexual contact. Gloves must be worn when handling the blood or articles contaminated with the blood of the individual with AIDS. (21)

## The Patient With Leukemia

**78.** 2. Leukemia is a neoplastic disorder of blood-forming tissues in the body that is characterized by a proliferation of immature white blood cells. Leukemia is not an infectious, inflammatory, or allergic disease. (7, 21)

**79.** 4. Normal white blood cells are decreased (that is, they fail to mature); hence, a child with leukemia is subject to infection. Infection is secondary to granulocytopenia. The major morbidity and mortality factor associated with leukemia is infection due to the presence of granulocytopenia. (7, 21)

**80.** 2. The production of red blood cells, as well as of blood platelets, is prevented when leukemic cells replace normal bone marrow. This pathologic process results in poor red-blood-cell development and, eventually, in anemia. (7, 21)

**81.** 1. Megakaryocytes, from which platelets derive, are decreased when leukemia is present. Platelet counts are low (thrombocytopenia) and the patient is subject to easy bruising and bleeding. Bruising and bleeding in a child with leukemia are not related to a low serum calcium level, faulty thrombin production, or insufficient fibrinogen concentration. (7, 21)

**82.** 4. All treatments should be performed gently in the care of a leukemic child prone to bruising and bleeding. When there is a choice, injections should be avoided or limited. Such measures as using a stool softener, changing the patient's position in bed, and offering the patient food at frequent intervals are indicated and need not be curtailed because of proneness to bleeding in the patient with leukemia. (7, 21)

**83.** 2. The mucous membranes of the mouth are easily damaged and are often ulcerated in the person with leukemia. It is better to give oral hygiene without using a toothbrush, because a toothbrush can easily damage sensitive oral mucosa. Applying petrolatum jelly to the lips, swabbing the mouth with moistened cotton swabs, and rinsing the mouth with a nonirritating mouthwash are appropriate measures when caring for the mouth of a child with leukemia. (6, 21)

**84.** 4. A dry tea bag, placed on the bleeding area, can be used effectively to control bleeding from lesions on the oral mucosa. Tannic acid in the tea apparently helps control the bleeding. (21)

**85.** 4. Carbonated beverages are ordinarily best tolerated when a patient feels nauseated. Many find cola drinks especially easy to tolerate, but noncola beverages are also recommended. (21)

**86.** 3. Acetylsalicylic acid (aspirin) lengthens the bleeding time by interfering with proper blood clotting. This drug is contraindicated in patients who have a tendency to bleed, such as a patient with leukemia. Nonnarcotic drugs other than aspirin may be prescribed to control pain. Narcotic analgesics may be required when pain is severe. (16, 21)

**87.** 4. Although bone marrow specimens may be obtained from various sites, the most commonly used site in children is the posterior iliac crest. The area is close to the body's surface and removed from vital organs. Also, the area is large, so specimens can be obtained easily. The sternum is rarely used in children because it is fragile and very near vital organs. For infants, the proximal tibia and the posterior iliac crest are used. (11, 21)

**88.** 3. A lumbar puncture is performed on a patient with leukemia to determine whether the central nervous system has been invaded by the disease. An antineoplastic agent such as the antimetabolite methotrexate may be injected intrathecally, but antineoplastic agents are not given to control infection. A lumbar puncture is not used to relieve undue pressure or to identify organisms in the central nervous system in a patient with leukemia. (11, 21)

**89.** 2. The number of tablets each containing 50 mg of a drug to be used when the patient is to receive 75 mg of the drug for each dosage is determined by using ratios as follows:

$$1 \text{ tablet}: 50 \text{ mg} :: x \text{ tablets}: 75 \text{ mg}$$
$$50x = 75$$
$$x = {}^{75}/_{50} = 1\tfrac{1}{2} \text{ tablets}$$

**90.** 1. Toxic doses of mercaptopurine (Purinethol) are most likely to produce anorexia, nausea, vomiting, and diarrhea. This drug also tends to cause bone marrow depression, and observations of the blood count then are especially important. Some of the other signs described in this item may be present but are not characteristic of toxicity to this drug. (16)

**91.** 2. Methotrexate (Amethopterin) may be used alone or in combination with other antineoplastic drugs. The drug is not highly toxic in low doses but may cause severe leukopenia at higher doses. It is customary and recommended that blood tests be done prior to therapy so that there is a baseline from which to study the effects of the drug on white blood cell levels. (16)

**92.** 2. The drug is administered intrathecally when injected into the spinal canal. This route is also called the intraspinal route, and the technique is the same as that for a lumbar puncture. The space between the dura mater and the arachnoid is the subdural area. A drug is placed in bone tissue when the intraosseous route is used and into an artery when the intra-arterial route is used. (11, 21)

**93.** 4. Antimetabolites have chemical structures resembling those of substances used normally for cell growth and metabolism. These drugs keep cancer cells from using natural nutrients in metabolic processes and therefore interfere with the cellular growth and development of cancer cells. (16)

**94.** 1. The destruction of malignant cells during periods of chemotherapy produces large amounts of uric acid. The kidneys may not be able to eliminate the uric acid, and tubular obstruction from the crystals could result in renal failure and uremia. Allopurinol (Zyloprim) interrupts the process of purine degradation to reduce the uric acid. The patient should be encouraged to increase fluid intake to further assist in eliminating uric acid. Allopurinol is often used also for patients with gout. (16)

**95.** 2. The patient's parents usually feel optimistic when a child with leukemia is in remission. It has been found that parents are more grieved when optimism is followed by defeat, and the nurse should recognize this when she plans various ways to help the parents of a dying child. It is not necessarily true that knowing for years when a prognosis is poor helps prepare relatives for a child's death, that trust in health personnel is destroyed when a death is untimely, or that it is more difficult for relatives to accept the death of a child who has been with a family for longer periods than a younger child. (21)

**96.** 2. The nurse caring for terminally ill patients is better prepared to do so when she has worked out her own philosophy of death. Although other experiences, such as having lost a loved one to death, taking classes in the care of the dying patient and in grieving, and developing her own belief in a supreme being and a life hereafter may be helpful in assisting the nurse in her thinking about death, of prime importance are her own feelings about life and death. (7, 21)

**97.** 2. Most patients, even children, are aware when their death appears imminent. The best policy is to answer the patient's questions honestly. When this is done, the patient tends to feel less isolated and alone. Such actions as restricting visitors, concentrating on efforts to make the patient think of something other than death, and encouraging the patient to replace thoughts of sadness with thoughts of pleasurable things are not recommended and tend to increase the dying person's fears, isolation, and feelings of loss of control. (7, 21)

**98.** 4. Just as with the patient, it is best to answer relatives honestly when they ask questions about their loved one's condition. For the situation described in this item, the nurse answers the parents' question honestly when she explains that infections are often the result of leukemia rather than a cause of it. It is less satisfactory to tell the parents that everything possible has been done for their child, that the child is no longer suffering from his illness, and that the physician is in the best position to answer their questions. (7, 21)

# test 4

*The Patient with Cleft Lip and Palate*
*The Patient with Tracheoesophageal Fistula*
*The Patient with Imperforate Anus*
*The Patient with Pyloric Stenosis*
*The Patient with Intussusception*
*The Patient with Inguinal Hernia*
*The Patient with Hirschsprung's Disease*
***Correct Answers and Rationales***

Select the one *best* or *correct* answer and indicate your choice by filling in the circle with a pencil in front of the option you have chosen. If the answer you would prefer is not given, select the one you think is *most appropriate*.

## THE PATIENT WITH CLEFT LIP AND PALATE

Tommy Taylor is born with a cleft lip and palate. He is transferred from the hospital's newborn nursery to a pediatric unit for care.

**1.** Tommy's parents are shocked when they see Tommy for the first time. Which of the following nursing actions would *most* help the parents accept Tommy's anomaly?
- ○ 1. Bring the infant to them more often.
- ○ 2. Tell them that surgery will correct the defect.
- ○ 3. Show them pictures of babies before and after surgery.
- ○ 4. Allow them to complete their grieving process before seeing the infant again.

**2.** Which of the following factors is of *primary* concern in caring for Tommy preoperatively?
- ○ 1. Preventing an infection in the infant's mouth.
- ○ 2. Using techniques to minimize the infant's crying.
- ○ 3. Altering the usual methods for feeding the infant.
- ○ 4. Preventing the infant from putting his fingers in his mouth.

**3.** Which of the following nursing measures is *most likely* to help Tommy retain his feedings?
- ○ 1. Bubble him at frequent intervals.
- ○ 2. Feed him small amounts at a time.
- ○ 3. Place the nipple on the back of his tongue.
- ○ 4. Hold him in a lying position while feeding him.

**4.** Tommy has surgery to repair his cleft lip. The nurse observes Tommy having difficulty breathing postoperatively. Which of the following nursing measures would be *most helpful* in bringing relief?
- ○ 1. Raising the infant's head.
- ○ 2. Turning the infant onto his abdomen.
- ○ 3. Inserting an airway into the infant's mouth.
- ○ 4. Placing downward pressure on the infant's chin.

**5.** The *most frequently* recommended method for feeding an infant following the surgical repair of a cleft lip is to use
- ○ 1. gastric gavage.
- ○ 2. intravenous fluids.
- ○ 3. a rubber-tipped medicine dropper.
- ○ 4. a bottle with a large-holed nipple.

**6.** To keep Tommy's surgical suture line clean and free of debris, the nurse should remove formula and drainage with cotton-tipped applicators moistened with
- ○ 1. mineral oil.
- ○ 2. distilled water.
- ○ 3. a mild antiseptic solution.
- ○ 4. half-strength hydrogen peroxide.

**7.** Tommy's grandmother asks what type of toy would be appropriate for Tommy while he is hospitalized. The nurse should suggest that the grandmother bring
- ○ 1. several small plastic toys.
- ○ 2. a large cuddly stuffed animal.
- ○ 3. a brightly colored mobile to hang over the infant's crib.
- ○ 4. a cassette tape recording of traditional children's stories.

**8.** Before Tommy's discharge from the hospital, Tommy's mother is taught to seek health care if the child develops an upper respiratory infection because Tommy is prone to develop which complication?
- ○ 1. Pneumonia.
- ○ 2. Dehydration.
- ○ 3. Otitis media.
- ○ 4. Laryngotracheobronchitis.

**223**

9. Tommy's parents ask the nurse when it is likely that Tommy's cleft palate will be repaired. The nurse should base her response on knowledge that the time when the first repair of a cleft palate is *usually* done is
   - ○ 1. prior to the eruption of teeth.
   - ○ 2. after the child learns to sit alone.
   - ○ 3. prior to the development of speech.
   - ○ 4. after the child learns to drink from a cup.

10. Tommy is eventually admitted to the hospital for repair of his palate. Which of the following eating utensils would be *most appropriate* for Tommy on the second day after the surgery?
    - ○ 1. A cup.
    - ○ 2. A drinking tube.
    - ○ 3. An Asepto syringe.
    - ○ 4. A large-holed nipple.

11. Which of the following types of restraints would be *best* for the nurse to use for Tommy immediately postoperatively after the repair of his cleft palate?
    - ○ 1. A safety jacket.
    - ○ 2. Elbow restraints.
    - ○ 3. Arm and leg restraints.
    - ○ 4. Arm and body restraints.

12. Which of the following positions would be *best* for Tommy when the nurse irrigates his mouth after the repair of his cleft palate?
    - ○ 1. On the back with the head turned to the side.
    - ○ 2. In a low Fowler's position with the head straight.
    - ○ 3. In a sitting position with the head tilted forward.
    - ○ 4. On the abdomen with the head over the side of the bed.

13. Mrs. Taylor is encouraged to stay with Tommy as much as possible for the first few days after his surgery. Which of the following activities carried out by the mother would offer the *most* support to Tommy during this time?
    - ○ 1. Holding and cuddling the child.
    - ○ 2. Helping the child play with some of his toys.
    - ○ 3. Reading some of the child's favorite stories to him.
    - ○ 4. Staying at the child's bedside and holding his hand.

14. Which of the following problems is *most common* among children, such as Tommy, who have had cleft palate repairs?
    - ○ 1. A speech defect.
    - ○ 2. Nutritional inadequacies.
    - ○ 3. Difficulty in developing a healthy self-image.
    - ○ 4. Difficulty in developing an independent personality.

# THE PATIENT WITH A TRACHEOESOPHAGEAL FISTULA

Several hours after Joseph Michael is born, it is noted that he has a tracheoesophageal fistula (TEF).

15. Mr. and Mrs. Michael express feelings of guilt about Joseph's anomaly. Which of the following approaches would be *best* for the nurse to use to support the parents?
    - ○ 1. Help the parents accept their feelings as being normal.
    - ○ 2. Explain that the parents did nothing to cause the infant's defect.
    - ○ 3. Encourage the parents to concentrate on long-term plans for the infant.
    - ○ 4. Have the parents visit their infant as often as possible during his hospitalization.

16. Joseph is admitted to the pediatric surgical unit. In her initial assessment of Joseph, the nurse can expect to observe which *typical* sign of a tracheoesophageal fistula (TEF)?
    - ○ 1. Continuous drooling.
    - ○ 2. Diaphragmatic breathing.
    - ○ 3. A slow response to stimuli.
    - ○ 4. The passage of large amounts of frothy meconium.

17. The nurse caring for Joseph reports that the infant responds to her initial feeding attempts with behavior characteristic of TEF. She states that she has not been able to feed him because the
    - ○ 1. infant's sucking attempts were too poorly coordinated to be effective.
    - ○ 2. infant's rooting and sucking reflexes were too poor to give him formula.
    - ○ 3. infant coughed after several swallows, choked, and became cyanotic.
    - ○ 4. infant took about 10 ml of formula, fell asleep, and could not be stimulated to take more formula.

18. Joseph is found to have a blind upper pouch and a fistula into the trachea from the lower pouch of the esophagus. Aspiration of material into Joseph's lungs occurs *primarily* from the
    - ○ 1. inability to expectorate mucus.
    - ○ 2. overflow of secretions from the upper pouch.
    - ○ 3. reflux of gastric secretions into the bronchi.
    - ○ 4. obstruction of the fistula leading into the trachea.

19. A gastrostomy is created for Joseph, the *primary* reason being to
    - ○ 1. reduce reflux of gastric contents into the infant's trachea.

○ 2. prevent aspiration of mucus and saliva swallowed by the infant.

○ 3. prevent abdominal distention with excessive air taken with the infant's oral feedings.

○ 4. enable the infant to adjust to gastrostomy feeding before having corrective surgery.

**20.** Before corrective surgery, Joseph is placed on his back in a crib with his head and shoulders elevated. The reasons for positioning Joseph in this manner are to reduce the reflux of gastric secretions into the trachea through the fistula and to

○ 1. reduce the cardiac workload, which has been increased by the anomaly.

○ 2. alleviate the pressure of the distended abdominal contents on the diaphragm.

○ 3. enhance pooling of the secretions in the bottom of the upper esophageal pouch.

○ 4. allow air to escape from the fistula into the trachea to reduce gastric distention.

**21.** Which of the following signs should indicate to the nurse that Joseph needs tracheal suctioning?

○ 1. A brassy cough.

○ 2. ‛Substernal retractions.

○ 3. A decrease in activity.

○ 4. An increased respiratory rate.

**22.** Joseph is placed in a heated isolette with high humidity. The *major* reason for maintaining high humidity in Joseph's environment is to help

○ 1. lower his metabolic rate.

○ 2. replace some of his fluid losses.

○ 3. decrease the likelihood of infection.

○ 4. decrease the viscosity of his respiratory secretions.

**23.** Joseph has gastrostomy feedings following surgery to correct the TEF. A pressure clamp is on the gastrostomy tube, and a syringe barrel is used to instill formula into the tube. While Joseph is being fed, which of the following techniques helps *most* to prevent air from entering the stomach after the syringe barrel is attached to the gastrostomy tube?

○ 1. Open the clamp after pouring all the infant's formula into the syringe barrel.

○ 2. Open the clamp before pouring all the infant's formula into the syringe barrel.

○ 3. Open the clamp and continuously pour the infant's formula down the side of the syringe barrel.

○ 4. Open the clamp and allow a small portion of the infant's formula to enter the stomach before pouring additional formula into the syringe barrel.

**24.** Which of the following nursing measures will help *most* to meet Joseph's psychological needs while

his formula is given to him through the gastrostomy tube?

○ 1. Holding the infant.

○ 2. Talking to the infant.

○ 3. Giving the infant a pacifier.

○ 4. Lightly stroking the infant's abdomen.

**25.** After feeding Joseph through the gastrostomy tube, the nurse cradles the infant in her arms and rocks him for about 15 minutes, the *primary* purpose being to help

○ 1. promote relaxation.

○ 2. prevent regurgitation of formula.

○ 3. relieve pressure on the surgical repair.

○ 4. associate eating with a pleasurable experience.

**26.** When Joseph begins oral feedings, his nursing care plan should be based on the principle that

○ 1. an infant adjusts to oral feedings better when small, frequent feedings are offered.

○ 2. a well-followed feeding schedule helps the infant accept oral feedings more readily.

○ 3. oral feedings following intubation are best accepted when offered by the same nurse repeatedly or by the infant's mother.

○ 4. oral feedings following intubation are best planned in conjunction with observations of the infant's behavior.

**27.** When preparing for Joseph's discharge from the hospital, the nurse teaches Mrs. Michael about her son's need for long-term health care because Joseph has a high probability of developing

○ 1. speech problems.

○ 2. an esophageal stricture.

○ 3. delay in psychosocial development.

○ 4. recurrent mild diarrhea with dehydration.

**28.** Which of the following conditions, if it occurred in Mrs. Michael's pregnancy with Joseph, would have provided a clue that Joseph might have an anomaly of the gastrointestinal tract?

○ 1. Meconium in the amniotic fluid.

○ 2. Low implantation of the placenta.

○ 3. Increased amount of amniotic fluid.

○ 4. Premature separation of the placenta.

## THE PATIENT WITH IMPERFORATE ANUS

The nurse assesses newborn Darren Smith. Newborn assessment reveals an imperforate anal membrane, and a diagnosis of imperforate anus is made.

**29.** Given the diagnosis of imperforate anus, the nurse would expect further newborn assessment to reveal

○ 1. an absence of meconium stool.
○ 2. abdominal distention.
○ 3. ribbon-like stools.
○ 4. herniation of abdominal viscera.

30. The doctor explains the diagnosis to Mr. and Mrs. Smith and suggests that Darren be scheduled for radiographic examination. Mrs. Smith asks about the purpose of this examination. The nurse should base the response on knowledge that the examination determines the distance between the anal dimple and the
○ 1. perineum.
○ 2. closed end of the rectum.
○ 3. scrotum.
○ 4. rectovesical pouch.

31. Darren's mother asks the nurse about the incidence of imperforate anus. The nurse should explain that imperforate anus occurs once in every
○ 1. 2,000 live births.
○ 2. 3,000 live births.
○ 3. 5,000 live births.
○ 4. 8,000 live births.

32. The nurse monitors Darren's urine output for the presence of meconium. Passage of meconium in the urine would indicate the presence of what type of fistula?
○ 1. Vesicocervical.
○ 2. Vesicovaginal.
○ 3. Rectourinary.
○ 4. Rectovaginal.

33. Mr. Smith observes that Darren's big toe dorsiflexes and his other toes fan when the nurse gently strokes the sole of his foot. When Mr. Smith asks about this response, the nurse should explain that this is
○ 1. an abnormal tonic foot sign.
○ 2. a normal plantar reflex.
○ 3. a normal Galant reflex.
○ 4. a normal Babinski reflex.

34. Mrs. Smith says the doctor told her that Darren has anal membrane atresia and that it is a "low" anorectal anomaly. She asks the nurse what "low" means. The nurse bases her response on the knowledge that this classification indicates that the rectum
○ 1. is at or below the level of the puborectalis muscle.
○ 2. has descended normally through the puborectalis muscle.
○ 3. is above the level of the abdominus rectus muscle.
○ 4. is at or below the level of the abdominus rectus muscle.

35. Given the diagnosis of anal membrane atresia,

which of the following surgical procedures would the nurse expect Darren to undergo?
○ 1. Transplantation of the anus dorsally.
○ 2. Dilatation of the cloaca.
○ 3. Incision of the membrane.
○ 4. Creation of a temporary colostomy.

36. Before surgery, Darren is to receive an intramuscular injection of an antibiotic. Which of the following needles should the nurse select?
○ 1. 19G, 1½″.
○ 2. 20G, 1″.
○ 3. 22G, 2″.
○ 4. 25G, ⅝″.

37. Based on the knowledge of the preferred intramuscular injection site in infants, what muscle would the nurse select for injection?
○ 1. Deltoid.
○ 2. Dorsogluteal.
○ 3. Ventrogluteal.
○ 4. Vastus lateralis.

38. The surgery is successfully completed, and Darren is returned to his crib with only an intravenous infusion. Mrs. Smith asks whether Darren will have normal bowel function. The nurse should base her answer on the fact that children who have corrective surgery as infants for low anorectal anomalies
○ 1. may or may not be continent.
○ 2. generally achieve social continence.
○ 3. are rarely continent.
○ 4. are generally continent.

39. A postoperative nursing goal is to prevent tension on the perineum. In order to achieve this goal, the nurse should *avoid* placing Darren on his
○ 1. abdomen with his legs pulled up under him.
○ 2. back with his legs suspended at a 90° angle.
○ 3. left side with his hips elevated.
○ 4. right side with his hips elevated.

40. Mr. Smith asks the nurse how newborns like Darren respond to painful stimuli. The *best* response for the nurse to make would be that newborns generally cry loudly and
○ 1. the crying does not cease with distraction.
○ 2. try to roll away.
○ 3. move the whole body.
○ 4. withdraw the affected part.

41. Darren's anorectal malformation and subsequent surgery are stressors for Mr. and Mrs. Smith. A nursing goal is to facilitate parental/infant bonding. Which of the following interventions would *most likely* achieve this goal?
○ 1. Explain that they can visit Darren anytime.
○ 2. Encourage them to hold Darren.

○ 3. Ask them to help monitor the intravenous infusion.

○ 4. Help them plan for Darren's discharge.

## THE PATIENT WITH PYLORIC STENOSIS

Four-week-old Jeremy Moore is admitted to the hospital with a history of vomiting. Mrs. Moore explains that initially Jeremy seemed to have a problem with regurgitation. He then developed nonprojectile vomiting that occurred during and after feedings. The vomiting became more forceful until "one time he vomited across the room."

**42.** Which of the following serum electrolyte values would *most likely* occur with Jeremy's persistent vomiting?

○ 1. $K^+$ 3.2 mEq/L; $Cl^-$ 92 mEq/L; $Na^+$ 120 mEq/L.

○ 2. $K^+$ 3.4 mEq/L; $Cl^-$ 120 mEq/L; $Na^+$ 140 mEq/L.

○ 3. $K^+$ 3.5 mEq/L; $Cl^-$ 90 mEq/L; $Na^+$ 145 mEq/L.

○ 4. $K^+$ 5.5 mEq/L; $Cl^-$ 110 mEq/L; $Na^+$ 130 mEq/L.

**43.** For which of the following acid-base imbalances should the nurse monitor Jeremy *most closely?*

○ 1. Respiratory alkalosis.

○ 2. Respiratory acidosis.

○ 3. Metabolic alkalosis.

○ 4. Metabolic acidosis.

**44.** A tentative diagnosis of hypertrophic pyloric stenosis is made. Given this diagnosis, the nurse would anticipate that Jeremy's vomitus would contain gastric contents,

○ 1. bile, and streaks of blood.

○ 2. mucus, and bile.

○ 3. mucus, and streaks of blood.

○ 4. bile, and gross blood.

**45.** Jeremy's skin is inelastic and his upper abdomen is distended. In order to feel the pyloric tumor most easily, the nurse should palpate the epigastrium just to the right of the umbilicus

○ 1. just before the patient vomits.

○ 2. while the patient is eating.

○ 3. while the patient is lying on the left side.

○ 4. just after the patient eats.

**46.** A diagnosis of hypertrophic pyloric stenosis is confirmed. Mrs. Moore asks the nurse about the occurrence of this problem. The nurse should explain that hypertrophic pyloric stenosis is

○ 1. equally common in male and female infants.

○ 2. five times more common in female than in male infants.

○ 3. five times more common in male than in female infants.

○ 4. ten times more common in male than in female infants.

**47.** When the diagnosis of hypertrophic pyloric stenosis cannot be made on the basis of clinical findings, the nurse could anticipate preparing the patient for a barium study of the upper gastrointestinal tract or

○ 1. a cytology of the gastric mucosa.

○ 2. a gastric analysis.

○ 3. an ultrasound scan.

○ 4. an endoscopy.

**48.** Results of a barium study of the upper gastrointestinal tract in a patient with pyloric stenosis would most likely indicate an elongated, thread-like pyloric channel. This finding is known as a positive

○ 1. olive sign.

○ 2. string sign.

○ 3. pearl sign.

○ 4. stenotic sign.

**49.** Before scheduling Jeremy for surgery, the physician wants to rehydrate him and orders the administration of parenteral fluids and electrolytes. Monitoring which of the following parameters would provide the nurse with the *least accurate* information about Jeremy's hydrational status?

○ 1. Urine specific gravity.

○ 2. Skin color.

○ 3. Urine output.

○ 4. Daily weight.

**50.** Which of the following should the nurse write on Jeremy's care plan as an expected patient outcome related to the nursing diagnosis of fluid volume deficit due to vomiting?

○ 1. The patient's abdomen is undistended.

○ 2. The patient exhibits no manifestations of dehydration.

○ 3. The patient does not vomit.

○ 4. The patient breathes easily without dyspnea.

**51.** For which of the following problems is Jeremy at risk secondary to a decrease in circulating fluid volume?

○ 1. Diabetes insipidus.

○ 2. Acute renal failure.

○ 3. Paralytic ileus.

○ 4. Adrenal insufficiency.

**52.** Jeremy undergoes a pyloromyotomy and returns to his room in stable condition. While standing by his crib, Mrs. Moore says, "Perhaps if I had brought Jeremy to the hospital sooner, he would not have needed surgery." What would be the nurse's *best* response?

○ 1. "Surgery is the most effective treatment for pyloric stenosis."

○ 2. "Try not to worry; your son will be fine."

○ 3. "Do you feel that this problem reflects your mothering skills?"

○ 4. "You think that earlier hospitalization could have avoided surgery?"

**53.** The surgical operation most often performed to treat pyloric stenosis is called the

○ 1. Holt-Oram procedure.

○ 2. Fredet-Ramstedt procedure.

○ 3. Taussig-Bing procedure.

○ 4. Olive-Waterston procedure.

**54.** Mrs. Moore asks when Jeremy will be able to take liquids by mouth. The nurse would base her response on the knowledge that if Jeremy does not vomit, he most likely would be taking feedings of clear liquids containing glucose and electrolytes

○ 1. 6 hours after surgery.

○ 2. 24 hours after surgery.

○ 3. 36 hours after surgery.

○ 4. 48 hours after surgery.

**55.** Jeremy's parents want to be involved in his care postoperatively, and the nurse teaches them proper feeding techniques. The nurse would know that they understood the teaching if after feeding Jeremy, they position him in his crib with his head elevated and on the

○ 1. left side.

○ 2. abdomen.

○ 3. right side.

○ 4. back.

**56.** Jeremy does not seem to be satisfied with the first few feedings of formula. Based on a correct interpretation of the cause of this dissatisfaction, the nurse would

○ 1. encourage the infant's parents to hold him.

○ 2. hang a mobile over the infant's crib.

○ 3. feed the infant more often.

○ 4. give the infant a pacifier.

**57.** Jeremy's hospitalization and surgery are stressful events for Mr. and Mrs. Moore. Which of the following would the nurse *correctly* interpret as a *positive* indication of parental coping?

○ 1. They tell the nurse they have to get away for a while.

○ 2. They discuss the infant's care realistically.

○ 3. They discuss the infant's care superficially.

○ 4. They fear that they will disturb the infant.

## THE PATIENT WITH INTUSSUSCEPTION

Four-month-old Amy Javitz is a healthy, thriving infant who suddenly had episodes of acute abdominal pain. She is admitted to the hospital with a diagnosis of intussusception.

**58.** Which term describes the basic problem associated with intussusception?

○ 1. Infection.

○ 2. Inflammation.

○ 3. Obstruction.

○ 4. Perforation.

**59.** When the nurse interviews Mrs. Javitz, she describes Amy's behavior prior to admission. Mrs. Javitz is *most likely* to describe Amy as crying

○ 1. constantly and extending the legs.

○ 2. intermittently and drawing the knees to the chest.

○ 3. shrilly when ingesting food.

○ 4. intermittently when positioned on the left side.

**60.** Of the questions the nurse could ask Mrs. Javitz during Amy's admission history, which would be *least* likely to result in pertinent diagnostic data?

○ 1. "What did Amy's last stool look like?"

○ 2. "When was Amy last immunized?"

○ 3. "What has Amy had to drink in the last 24 hours?"

○ 4. "When did you notice that Amy wasn't feeling well?"

**61.** Prior to palpating Amy's abdomen, the nurse lightly strokes it. The nurse uses this technique to

○ 1. assess abdominal tenderness.

○ 2. relax the abdominal musculature.

○ 3. stimulate peristalsis.

○ 4. assess abdominal distention.

**62.** Because nonsurgical intervention was unsuccessful, Amy underwent surgery to reduce the invagination. Amy returns to her room with a nasogastric tube in place. She is allowed nothing by mouth and is receiving intravenous fluids. Which of the following parameters would be used to calculate the amount of intravenous fluid and electrolyte solution to be infused over the next 24 hours?

○ 1. Body weight.

○ 2. Urine output.

○ 3. Body weight and gastric output.

○ 4. Body weight and urine output.

**63.** The nasogastric tube is no longer freely removing gastric secretions. Which troubleshooting technique should the nurse use to determine the position of the tube?

○ 1. Aspirate gastric contents with a syringe.

○ 2. Irrigate the tube with distilled water.

○ 3. Increase the level of suction.

○ 4. Rotate the tube.

**64.** When fluids by mouth are appropriate for Amy, the physician will *most likely* initiate feeding with which of the following solutions?
○ 1. Cereal-thickened formula.
○ 2. Full-strength formula.
○ 3. Half-strength formula.
○ 4. Glucose water.

**65.** Amy is at risk postoperatively for developing an ileus. Which observation would the nurse *not* include in an assessment for this complication?
○ 1. Measurement of urine specific gravity.
○ 2. Assessment of bowel sounds.
○ 3. Documentation of the first stool.
○ 4. Measurement of gastric output.

**66.** Which of the following phases is *most characteristic* of the newborn and infant period with respect to growth and development?
○ 1. Dependent on having needs met.
○ 2. Achieving impulse control.
○ 3. Demonstrating autonomy.
○ 4. Exploring the environment.

**67.** When Amy resumes taking oral feedings after surgery, her parents comment that she seems to be sucking on her pacifier more since surgery. Which explanation of this behavior is *most accurate*?
○ 1. Amy's sucking provides an outlet for emotional tension.
○ 2. Amy's sucking indicates she is ready to take solid foods.
○ 3. Amy's sucking indicates she is thirsty.
○ 4. Amy's sucking is an attempt to get attention from her parents.

## THE PATIENT WITH INGUINAL HERNIA

Mrs. Perez brings her 7-month-old son Roberto to the clinic because she has noticed a swelling in his right groin. The swelling varies in size. It disappears when Roberto rests, but appears when he cries. A tentative diagnosis of inguinal hernia is made.

**68.** The nurse examines Roberto. Which of the following assessment findings should concern the nurse *most?*
○ 1. The inguinal swelling is reddened and Roberto's abdomen is distended.
○ 2. Roberto is irritable and a thickened spermatic cord can be palpated on his right side.
○ 3. The inguinal swelling can be reduced and Roberto has a stool in his diaper.

○ 4. Roberto's diaper is wet with urine and his abdomen is nontender.

**69.** Roberto is admitted to the pediatric unit. He is given a warm bath and meperidine hydrochloride (Demerol) to help him relax before the physician attempts to reduce the hernia. The physician reduces the hernia nonoperatively and schedules Roberto for a herniorrhaphy in 2 days. Mrs. Perez asks the nurse why the surgery is not performed now. The nurse should explain that delaying surgery
○ 1. ensures proper preoperative preparation.
○ 2. ensures that the patient will be n.p.o. 24 hours before surgery.
○ 3. allows the edema and inflammation in the area to subside.
○ 4. allows the patient to wear a truss for 24 hours.

**70.** Mrs. Perez is concerned about her son's surgery. She asks the nurse if 7-month-old Roberto would have been scheduled for surgery even if the hernia had been asymptomatic. The nurse answers, "Yes." Which of the following statements offers the *best* explanation concerning why Roberto's repair would be done at this time?
○ 1. From a physiological viewpoint, an infant will tolerate surgery better than an older child.
○ 2. The experience of surgery is less frightening for an infant than it is for an older child.
○ 3. There is less danger of complications when surgery is an elective procedure rather than an emergency procedure.
○ 4. There is a preference for doing surgery near the genital organs before a child becomes conscious of his sexual identity.

**71.** Mrs. Perez does not understand the cause of the hernia and is concerned that she has somehow caused it. The nurse reassures Mrs. Perez that she has done nothing to cause the hernia. Her response is based on the knowledge that an inguinal hernia is caused by the incomplete closure of the inguinal ring or
○ 1. recanalization of the embryologic gut.
○ 2. a congenital weakness.
○ 3. an open umbilical ring.
○ 4. severe hyperperistalsis.

**72.** Roberto is scheduled for a herniorrhaphy tomorrow. The nurse's goal should be to prepare Roberto and his mother psychologically for the surgery. What would be the *best* method of preparing Roberto psychologically for surgery?
○ 1. Explain pre- and postoperative procedures to his mother.
○ 2. Have his mother stay with him.

○ 3. Make sure he has his own blanket.

○ 4. Allow him to play with sterile dressings.

73. Roberto underwent an inguinal herniorrhaphy and has been back in his room on the pediatric unit for several hours. Mrs. Perez says the surgeon told her that Roberto can go home today and asks the nurse when he will be able to leave. The nurse should tell her that before the surgeon will discharge him, Roberto must be completely recovered from the anesthesia and

○ 1. resume his normal activity.

○ 2. have a bowel movement.

○ 3. have a systolic blood pressure of 90.

○ 4. retain an oral feeding.

74. The nurse prepares Mrs. Perez for Roberto's discharge. Based on knowledge of the postoperative complication that Roberto is *most likely* to develop, the nurse should tell Mrs. Perez to

○ 1. change his diaper as soon as it is soiled.

○ 2. have him wear an abdominal binder.

○ 3. cover the incision with a dry sterile dressing.

○ 4. keep his hands away from the incision.

75. Mrs. Perez asks the nurse what to do about bathing Roberto. The nurse should tell Mrs. Perez to give Roberto

○ 1. daily sponge baths for 2 weeks.

○ 2. full tub baths twice a day.

○ 3. daily sponge baths for 1 week.

○ 4. full tub baths every day.

76. Peter Barnes, age 15, had an inguinal hernia repaired earlier today and is getting ready to go home. The nurse instructs him about the resumption of physical activities. Which of the following statements would indicate that Peter has understood the instructions?

○ 1. "I can ride my bike next week."

○ 2. "I have to skip physical education classes for 2 weeks."

○ 3. "I can start wrestling again in 3 weeks."

○ 4. "I will postpone my weight-lifting class for 6 weeks."

## THE PATIENT WITH HIRSCHSPRUNG'S DISEASE

Seven-month-old Ken Carter is admitted to the hospital with a tentative diagnosis of Hirschsprung's disease.

77. Which parental statement obtained during the nursing history *most accurately* describes infants with this disorder?

○ 1. "Our baby has occasional episodes of diarrhea."

○ 2. "Our baby wants to nurse all the time."

○ 3. "Our baby sometimes has trouble sleeping."

○ 4. "Our baby has a really flat tummy."

78. In preparing Ken's hospital room, the nurse selects toys for him. Which of the following toys is most appropriate for 7-month-old Ken?

○ 1. Large colorful alphabet blocks.

○ 2. Several balloons on a string.

○ 3. Crayons and drawing paper.

○ 4. A mobile to hang above the crib.

79. During the physical assessment, the nurse would be *most* likely to note that Ken

○ 1. exhibits a prominent venous network over his thighs and calves.

○ 2. weighs less than expected for his height and age.

○ 3. has clubbing and cyanosis of his fingers and toes.

○ 4. demonstrates hyperactive deep tendon reflexes.

80. The nurse assesses Ken's growth and development. Which behavior would the nurse consider *unusual*?

○ 1. He grasps a raisin neatly between his index finger and the base of his thumb.

○ 2. He raises his chest and upper abdomen off the bed with his hands.

○ 3. He imitates sounds that the nurse makes to him.

○ 4. He cries loudly in protest when his mother leaves the room.

81. Ken is scheduled for a barium enema to confirm the diagnosis. A primary concern following this procedure is evacuation of barium from the colon. What intervention should the nurse use to identify this evacuation?

○ 1. Test the pH of the stool.

○ 2. Observe the color of the stool.

○ 3. Palpate the left lower abdomen.

○ 4. Auscultate for bowel sounds.

82. Diagnostic evaluation confirms the diagnosis of Hirschsprung's disease, and a colostomy is planned. When *initially* discussing the diagnosis and treatment with Ken's parents, it would be *most* appropriate for the nurse to

○ 1. assess the adequacy of their coping skills.

○ 2. reassure them that he will be fine.

○ 3. encourage them to ask questions.

○ 4. use printed materials.

83. Mrs. Carter asks the nurse to explain the basic problem involved in Hirschsprung's disease. The nurse's response is based on her knowledge that the primary defect in Hirschsprung's disease is

○ 1. atrophy of the junction between the small and large intestine.
○ 2. lack of internal anal sphincter muscle contraction.
○ 3. atresia of the lower portion of the rectosigmoid colon.
○ 4. absence of nerve innervation in the distal colon.

84. Ken is to have a temporary colostomy created. Prior to this surgery, he is to take oral neomycin sulfate for 3 days. The *major* purpose of this medication is to
○ 1. inhibit intestinal nitrogen formation.
○ 2. suppress intestinal bacteria.
○ 3. prevent urinary tract infection.
○ 4. promote stool evacuation from the colon.

85. The appropriate pediatric dosage of neomycin sulfate is 10.3 mg/kg q 4 hours. Ken weighs 5 kg. Which of the following dosages *most closely* approximates a safe daily dose for him?
○ 1. 50 mg per day.
○ 2. 100 mg per day.
○ 3. 300 mg per day.
○ 4. 500 mg per day.

86. The nurse anticipates that 24 to 48 hours before surgery, Ken's preoperative preparation will *most likely* include
○ 1. administration of a Fleet's enema.
○ 2. insertion of a gastrostomy tube.
○ 3. restriction of oral intake to clear liquids.
○ 4. preparation of the perineum with povidone-iodine (Betadine).

87. Which of Mrs. Carter's statements about Ken's colostomy indicates that she needs further teaching?
○ 1. "We will take care of the colostomy until Ken is old enough to do it."
○ 2. "The colostomy will give the intestine time to shrink to its normal size."
○ 3. "The colostomy may include two separate abdominal openings."
○ 4. "Right after the procedure is done, the stoma will appear big and red."

88. The surgery is performed, and Ken's postoperative recovery is uneventful. The nurse prepares Mr. and Mrs. Carter for Ken's discharge. Which of the following instructions should the nurse give them?
○ 1. Position Ken so that there is no pressure on the stoma site.
○ 2. Allow the diaper to absorb the colostomy drainage.
○ 3. Give Ken plenty of liquids to drink.
○ 4. Expect the stoma to become dusky red within 2 weeks.

89. While at home, Ken has begun to eat table foods and Mrs. Carter is concerned about the foods he should eat while he has the colostomy. The nurse explains that Ken should *avoid* eating
○ 1. ground beef.
○ 2. ripe bananas.
○ 3. ice cream.
○ 4. green beans.

90. Ken is now 15 months old and has been readmitted to the hospital for colostomy closure. The surgery is over, and Ken is returned to the unit with an intravenous line in place. The infusion set delivers 1 ml per 60 drops. A total of 250 ml over the next 3 hours has been ordered. How many drops per minute should the infusion deliver?
○ 1. 14 drops per minute.
○ 2. 21 drops per minute.
○ 3. 60 drops per minute.
○ 4. 83 drops per minute.

91. Ken is going to be discharged within a day or two. In anticipation of concerns that Mr. and Mrs. Carter may have about the effects of Ken's surgery on his development and care at home, the nurse tells them that
○ 1. abdominal distention is to be expected.
○ 2. toilet training may be difficult.
○ 3. dairy products should be avoided.
○ 4. vitamin supplements will be needed until Ken reaches adolescence.

# CORRECT ANSWERS AND RATIONALES

Numbers appear in parentheses following the rationales. The numbers identify textbooks listed in the references at the end of Part III, where correct answers can be verified.

## *The Patient with Cleft Lip and Palate*

**1.** 3. Pre- and postoperative pictures of babies with cleft palates and lips provide a clear and concrete image of expectations of corrective surgery described by health personnel. Providing these pictures is specific to the parents' behavior, because the parents reflect societal values that emphasize the infant's facial appearance and responsive expressiveness. The bonding process also reflects this emphasis. Bringing the infant described in this item to his parents more often may be beneficial but would not help the parents accept the infant's anomaly and expectations from surgery. Allowing the completion of the grieving process prior to another interaction between the infant and parents could result in a separation that could last months. (6, 21)

**2.** 3. It is important for the newborn to have foods and fluids prior to corrective surgery for a cleft lip. Methods for feeding will need to be adjusted to fit his needs. Commonly, a rubber-tipped syringe or medicine dropper is used to feed the infant described in this item. Infection in the mouth is uncommon, and minimizing crying is of no particular help. There is no special need to keep the infant's fingers out of his mouth preoperatively and that may upset him even further. Also, being able to put his fingers in his mouth may provide comfort for the infant. (6, 21)

**3.** 1. An infant with a cleft palate and lip swallows large amounts of air when he is being fed and therefore should be bubbled frequently. The defect in the soft palate allows air to be drawn into the pharynx with each swallow of formula. The stomach will become distended with air, and regurgitation, possibly with aspiration, is likely if the infant is not bubbled frequently. Feeding the infant frequently would not prevent swallowing large amounts of air. A nipple is likely to cause the infant to gag and predisposes him to aspiration. Holding the infant in a lying position during feedings can also produce aspiration and regurgitation of formula. (6, 21)

**4.** 4. Following the repair of a cleft lip, the infant must become accustomed to nasal breathing. However, if the infant is having difficulty breathing, it would be best to open his mouth by placing downward pressure on his chin. This helps relieve distress. In some instances, an airway is used postoperatively, but when it is not in place it is best to try pressure on the chin first. Raising the infant's head and turning the infant onto his abdomen are likely to aggravate the situation. (6, 21)

**5.** 3. A rubber-tipped medicine dropper has been found to be a very satisfactory method for feeding an infant who has had surgical repair of a cleft lip. Gastric gavage is ordinarily not used unless complications develop. Intravenous fluids will not supply complete nutrition for the infant. A large-holed nipple may cause the child to aspirate because formula enters the mouth too rapidly. Feeding methods for the infant described in this item should produce the least tension possible on the sutures to promote effective healing of the cleft lip repair. (6, 21)

**6.** 4. Half-strength hydrogen peroxide is recommended for cleansing the suture line following the repair of a cleft lip. The bubbling action of the hydrogen peroxide is effective for removing debris. Normal saline may be the preferred solution in some agencies. (6, 21)

**7.** 3. Toys and play activities enable the child to learn about the world around him. The lack of motor and manipulative development in the young infant limits him to sensory learning that involves his eyes, ears, and touch. Thus, a mobile is most appropriate for him because the changes in the hanging moving objects interest him. Stuffed animals would be more appropriate for a child who has developed manipulative skills, later in his first year. The cassette tape recording provides some variation in the auditory environment, but stories would be more appropriate for the child who has developed language. Small plastic toys can be dangerous for infants and young children because they tend to put these toys in their mouths. This would be especially unsuitable for a child with a recently repaired cleft lip and with a cleft palate. (6, 21)

**8.** 3. Inadequate drainage through the eustachian tubes often causes otitis media when a child with a cleft palate develops an upper respiratory infection. Recurrent otitis media and the accumulation of serous drainage in the middle ear prevent normal movement of the tympanic membrane and a resulting hearing deficit. If nutrition is maintained and overall health is good, the child with a cleft palate should have no more respiratory infections than his peers of the same age. Although eating is a problem for these children, their intake is not reduced enough to predispose them to dehydration unless another condition predisposing to dehydration occurs. (21)

**9.** 3. Optimal time for the surgical repair of a cleft palate depends on many factors, but it is best when it can be done before speech development and before the child learns faulty speech habits. Such factors as when teeth erupt, when the child can sit alone, and when the child learns to drink from a cup are not ordinarily used to determine the time for palate repair. (6, 21)

**10.** 1. A cup is the preferred utensil for eating after the repair of a cleft palate. At the age when repair is done, the child is ordinarily able to drink from a cup, and using it avoids having to place a utensil in the mouth, where surgery has just been completed. (6, 21)

**11.** 2. Recommended restraints for a child who has had palate surgery would be elbow restraints. They minimize the limitation placed on the child but still prevent him from injuring the repair with his fingers and hands. A safety jacket, arm and leg restraints, and arm and body restraints restrict the child unnecessarily and would probably frustrate him immeasurably. (6, 21)

**12.** 3. A sitting position (that is, with the trunk of the body upright and the head tilted forward) is recommended when the mouth of a child who has had palate surgery is being irrigated. This position is best because the child is least likely to choke and aspirate fluid during the irrigation. (7, 21)

**13.** 1. The mother of a child who has had palate surgery should be encouraged to hold and cuddle him, thus offering him necessary emotional support. Such activities as helping the child play with toys, reading stories to him, and staying with him are not contraindicated but do not offer as much emotional support as holding and cuddling him. (6, 21)

**14.** 1. A speech defect is common following the repair of a cleft palate, and many children require speech therapy following surgery. Such conditions as nutritional inadequacies and difficulty in developing a healthy self-image and an independent personality are uncommon if a child receives adequate care and support. (6, 21)

### The Patient With a Tracheoesophageal Fistula

**15.** 1. The parents of children born with defects often have feelings of guilt and ask what they might have done to cause the condition or how they might have avoided it. It is important to allow parents to express their feelings and to accept these feelings as normal reactions. Encouraging the parents to begin long-term planning and having them visit the infant as often as possible are generally of little help when a nurse is offering emotional support to distraught parents, and it may appear to the parents as though they are being talked out of their feelings. Explaining that the parents are not at fault would not be appropriate until they have dealt with their feelings of guilt. (6, 21)

**16.** 1. An atresia of the esophagus prevents the passage of swallowed mucus and saliva into the stomach. After fluid has accumulated in the pouch, it flows from the mouth and the infant then drools continuously. The lack of swallowed amniotic fluid prevents the accumulation of normal meconium; lack of stool results. Responsiveness of the infant to stimuli would depend on the overall condition of the infant and is not considered a classic sign of a tracheoesophageal fistula (TEF). Diaphragmatic breathing is not associated with TEF. (6, 21)

**17.** 3. The infant with TEF swallows normally, but the fluids quickly fill the blind pouch. He then coughs, chokes, and becomes cyanotic while the fluid returns through the nose and mouth. Poor rooting and sucking reflexes are typical of infants who have neurologic dysfunctions; these reflexes may also be depressed by medication given to the mother during labor. Falling asleep after taking little formula is characteristic of an infant who becomes exhausted with the exertion of feeding and is often caused by a cardiac anomaly. (6, 21)

**18.** 2. Gastric secretions reflux into the trachea and bronchi through the fistula in the infant with TEF. Although fluid can be aspirated as mucus and saliva from the mouth and nose and from secretions overflowing from the blind pouch, most of the fluid comes from the stomach. Swallowing will not result in fluid moving into the lower pouch. The fistula has no connection with the upper esophagus and mouth in most instances of TEF. (6, 21)

**19.** 1. A gastrostomy created for an infant with TEF allows air that enters the stomach through the fistula from the trachea to escape. Excess air increases the reflux of stomach contents into the trachea. Oral feedings are contraindicated until corrective surgery has repaired the fistula. Mucus and saliva cannot enter the stomach in an infant with TEF because the upper portion of the esophagus ends in a blind pouch. (6, 21)

**20.** 3. Gravity encourages the flow of secretions with pooling in the bottom of the upper pouch when an infant with TEF is placed on his back with his head and shoulders elevated. More effective removal of secretions will then result when a catheter is positioned in this pool of secretions. Each breathing cycle forces some air into the stomach, which prevents the upward passage of air into the trachea. Although abdominal distention would eventually result from air entering the stomach, this is a much later manifestation of TEF. There is generally no additional cardiac workload and little possibility of cardiac failure unless other anomalies complicate TEF. (6, 21)

**21.** 2. Laryngospasms result from the overflow of secretions into the larynx in an infant with TEF. The obstruction to inspiration stimulates the strong contraction of accessory muscles of the thorax to assist the diaphragm in breathing. This produces substernal retractions. A brassy cough is related to a relatively constant laryngeal narrowing, usually due to edema. A decrease in activity and an increased respiratory rate are usually due to hypoxia. This is a relatively long-term and constant phenomenon in infants with TEF. The laryngospasms with TEF clear quickly when secretions are removed from the oropharynx area. (6, 21)

**22.** 4. High humidity in inspired air increases the humidity in the air passages and makes the secretions less viscid. Ciliary action can then bring the secretions to the larger bronchi, where they cause coughing and expectoration. The heat rather than the humidity influences the rate of metabolism. Fluid loss can be reduced by the high humidity, but the humidity cannot replace fluid already lost. The high humidity is likely to increase the possibility of infection because it fosters the growth of microorganisms. (6, 21)

**23.** 1. The best way to prevent air from entering the stomach when feeding an infant through a gastrostomy tube is to open the clamp *after* all the formula has been placed in the syringe barrel. Other techniques will allow air to enter the stomach through the gastrostomy tube. (6, 21)

**24.** 3. Giving the infant a pacifier while feeding him through a gastrostomy tube allows normal sucking activity. Talking or singing to him would not be contraindicated but would not best meet the infant's psychological needs at this time. It is difficult to feed an infant by tube while holding him. Therefore, it would be better to hold him before and after feeding him. Stroking his abdomen may not be contraindicated but does not satisfy the child's need to suck. (6, 21)

**25.** 4. Helping meet the psychological needs of an infant being fed through a gastrostomy tube can be accomplished when the infant is rocked after feed-

ing him. He will soon learn to associate eating with a pleasurable experience. Holding and rocking an infant can well accomplish certain other goals, but these are not primary goals in caring for the infant described in this item. (6, 21)

**26.** 4. It is best to follow a care plan based on the principle that oral feedings started after an infant has been fed through a gastrostomy tube are best planned in conjunction with observations of the infant's needs and behavior. When the infant's needs and behavior are overlooked, care plans are likely to be unsatisfactory and are more likely to meet the nurse's needs rather than those of the patient. (6, 21)

**27.** 2. Dilatation at the anastomosis site is needed over the first years of childhood in approximately half the children who have had corrective surgery for TEF. Speech problems are likely if other malformations or abnormalities are present to produce them. The larynx and structures for speech are not affected by TEF. Dysphagia and strictures may decrease food intake and poor weight gain may be noted, but diarrhea and dehydration are not associated with TEF repair. Delayed psychosocial development is possible with long hospitalization and separation from the parents during TEF treatment. However, encouraging parental involvement in children's facilities greatly reduces this possibility. (6, 21)

**28.** 3. Maternal hydramnios occurs with infants that have a congenital obstruction of the gastrointestinal tract, such as occurs in the presence of a TEF. The fetus normally swallows amniotic fluid and absorbs the fluid from the gastrointestinal tract. Excretion then occurs through the kidneys and placenta. The majority of fluid absorption occurs in the colon. This course of events cannot occur when the fetus has a gastrointestinal obstruction. Meconium in the amniotic fluid, low implantation of the placenta, and premature separation of the placenta could occur but are more specifically associated with fetal hypoxia. Meconium in the amniotic fluid is a manifestation of fetal hypoxia. Blood loss from a low-lying placenta and premature separation of the placenta could result in fetal hypoxia by decreasing the oxygen available to the fetus. (6, 21)

## The Patient with Imperforate Anus

**29.** 1. The absence of meconium stool is consistent with a diagnosis of imperforate anus. Abdominal distention is a later sign of imperforate anus. Ribbonlike stools are associated with anal stenosis;

herniation of abdominal viscera is not associated with anorectal malformations. (7, 21)

**30.** 2. The purpose of the radiographic examination is to ascertain the distance between the anal dimple and the closed end of the rectum. (7, 21)

**31.** 3. Imperforate anus occurs once in approximately every 5,000 live births, making it one of the more common congenital malformations. (7, 21)

**32.** 3. The passage of meconium in the urine is diagnostic of a rectourinary fistula. The rectum and bladder are connected. A vesicocervical fistula communicates the bladder and cervical canal. In a vesicovaginal fistula, the bladder and vagina communicate. Similarly, in a rectovaginal fistula the rectum and vagina are connected. (7, 21)

**33.** 4. A normal Babinski reflex consists of extension of the big toe and fanning of the other toes. While normal in infants, this response is abnormal after about 1 year of age or when locomotion begins. The tonic foot sign does not exist. Plantar reflex is elicited by scratching the sole of the foot near the lateral aspect, from heel to toe. A normal Galant reflex is initiated by stroking an infant's back alongside the spine. The hips move toward the stimulated side. (7, 21)

**34.** 2. In a low anorectal anomaly, the rectum has descended normally through the puborectalis muscle. In an intermediate anomaly, the rectum is at or below the level of the puborectalis muscle; in a high anomaly, the rectum ends above the puborectalis muscle. (7, 21)

**35.** 3. When anal membrane atresia is present, the membrane is surgically incised or perforated. Transplantation of the anus dorsally is done if the patient has a true low rectovaginal fistula. The cloaca is an embryonic structure involved in most anorectal malformations. A colostomy is the treatment of choice for infants with the high types of imperforate anus (more than 1.5 cm between the anal dimple and the blind end of the colon). (7, 21)

**36.** 4. A 25G to 27G needle ½″ to 1″ long is appropriate for administering an intramuscular injection to an infant. (7, 21)

**37.** 4. The vastus lateralis muscle of the thigh is preferred for administering intramuscular injections to infants because there is less danger of injuring nerves, blood vessels, or bony structures. The deltoid muscle is used for intramuscular injections only when other areas are unavailable. The dorsogluteal site is contraindicated for use in children who have not been walking for at least a year. The ventrogluteal site is relatively free of major nerves and blood vessels, but the vastus lateralis remains the preferred intramuscular injection site in infants. (21)

**38.** 4. Children who have corrective surgery as infants for low anorectal anomalies are generally continent. Fecal continence can be expected after successful correction of anal membrane atresia. Children with high anomalies may or may not achieve continence. (7, 21)

**39.** 1. When placed on their abdomens, neonates pull their legs up under them, which puts tension on the perineum. Therefore, postoperative neonates should be positioned either supine with the legs suspended at a 90° angle or on either side with the hips elevated. (7, 21)

**40.** 3. The newborn responds to pain with total body movement associated with brief, loud crying that ceases with distraction. After 6 months of age, infants react to pain with intense physical resistance and try to escape by rolling away. A toddler reacts by withdrawing the affected part. (7, 21)

**41.** 2. Encouraging the parents to hold the neonate promotes parental/infant bonding. Explaining that the parents can visit anytime will promote bonding only if they do visit the infant, talk to him and hold him. Asking the parents to help monitor the intravenous infusion may be anxiety-producing. Helping the parents plan for the child's discharge involves them in the child's care, but holding and comforting the child are more likely to promote parental/infant bonding. (7, 21)

## *The Patient with Pyloric Stenosis*

**42.** 1. Serum electrolyte values in a patient with persistent vomiting reflect hypokalemia (normal 3.9 to 5.9 mEq/L), hypochloremia (normal 97 to 110 mEq/L), and hyponatremia (normal 134 to 146 mEq/L). (7, 21)

**43.** 3. Metabolic alkalosis occurs because of the excessive loss of potassium, hydrogen, and chloride in the vomitus. Chloride loss results in a compensatory increase in the number of bicarbonate ions. The bicarbonate side of the carbonic acid-base bicarbonate is increased and the pH becomes more alkaline. Metabolic acidosis results from severe diarrhea and starvation. Respiratory acidosis is caused by conditions that result in the excessive retention of $PaCO_2$ (for example, chronic obstructive pulmonary disease and central nervous system dysfunction). Respiratory alkalosis is caused by conditions that result in loss of $PaCO_2$ (such as hyperventilation and gram-negative bacteremia). (7, 21)

**44.** 3. The vomitus of a patient with hypertrophic pyloric stenosis contains gastric contents, mucus, and streaks of blood. The vomitus does not contain bile because the pyloric constriction is proximal to the ampulla of Vater. (7, 21)

**45.** 2. The pyloric tumor is most easily palpated when the abdominal muscles are relaxed during a feeding or immediately after vomiting. (7, 21)

**46.** 3. Hypertrophic pyloric stenosis is five times more common in male than in female infants. (7, 21)

**47.** 3. An upper gastrointestinal radiographic study or an ultrasound scan is used to confirm the diagnosis of pyloric stenosis if the history and physical signs are inconclusive. Cytologic study of the gastrointestinal tract is done to diagnose benign and malignant diseases of the gastrointestinal tract. Gastric analysis is performed to determine the amount or absence of digestive juices. Endoscopy is used to visualize internal body structures. (7, 21)

**48.** 2. A barium study of the upper gastrointestinal tract in pyloric stenosis reveals a fine, elongated stringlike pyloric canal. (7, 21)

**49.** 2. Skin color reflects hemodynamic status. Urine specific gravity, intake and output, and daily weight provide information about hydrational status. (7, 21)

**50.** 2. An expected patient outcome relative to the nursing diagnosis of fluid volume deficit due to vomiting is that the patient exhibits no evidence of dehydration such as weight loss or decreased skin turgor. (21)

**51.** 2. Acute renal failure can occur secondary to a decrease in circulating fluid volume because of renal hypoperfusion. Paralytic ileus, adrenal insufficiency, and diabetes insipidus can result in fluid volume deficit but do not occur secondary to a decrease in circulating fluid volume. (7, 21)

**52.** 4. Restating a patient's response provides the opportunity for clarification and validation. Surgery *is* the most effective treatment for pyloric stenosis, but this response does not give the child's mother an opportunity to express her feelings. The nurse should avoid giving premature reassurance and should give the mother an opportunity to express her concerns. (21)

**53.** 2. Fredet and Ramstedt were the two surgeons who standardized the surgical procedure for repairing the pyloric sphincter. Holt-Oram syndrome is a hereditary heart disease associated with skeletal malformation. The Taussig-Bing syndrome is a rare congenital malformation of the heart characterized by transposition of the great vessels and a ventricular septal defect straddled by a large pulmonary artery. There is no such procedure as Olive-Waterston. (21)

**54.** 1. Clear liquids containing glucose and electrolytes are usually prescribed 4 to 6 hours after surgery. If vomiting does not occur, formula or breast milk can be gradually substituted for clear liquids until the infant is taking normal feedings, usually 48 hours postoperatively. The postoperative feeding of the postpyloromyotomy patient is generally a slow resumption in amount and concentration. (7, 21)

**55.** 3. Positioning the infant on the right side with the head elevated facilitates passage of food through the pyloric sphincter into the intestine. Furthermore, this position minimizes aspiration, if the infant should vomit. (7, 21)

**56.** 4. Giving the infant a pacifier would help meet his non-nutritive sucking needs and ensure oral gratification. Encouraging his parents to hold him and hanging a mobile over the crib will not meet this need. The postpyloromyotomy infant does not need to be fed more frequently. (7, 21)

**57.** 2. The fact that the parents can verbalize the infant's care realistically indicates they are working through their fears and concerns. Without further data, the fact that the parents "have to get away" could be interpreted as ineffective coping. Superficial discussion of the infant's care does not indicate positive coping, nor does fear of disturbing the infant. (7, 21)

## The Patient with Intussusception

**58.** 3. Intussusception is an invagination or telescoping of one portion of the intestine into another. This telescoping causes an obstruction, usually at the ileocecal valve. Intestinal inflammation, hemorrhage, perforation, and peritonitis will occur if the condition is untreated. (21)

**59.** 2. The infant with intussusception experiences acute episodes of colic-like abdominal pain. Typically, the infant screams and draws the knees to the chest. In between these episodes of acute abdominal pain, the infant appears comfortable and normal. The ingestion of food does not precipitate episodes of pain. Pain that occurs when the infant is positioned on the left side is not associated with intussusception. (21)

**60.** 2. Questions about an infant's immunization status are routinely asked during the admission history. However, this question will not elicit diagnostic data relative to intussusception. Diagnostic data associated with an early diagnosis of intussusception include intermittent abdominal pain, vomiting, and the passage of currant-jelly stools. (8)

**61.** 2. Lightly stroking the abdomen relaxes the abdominal musculature so the nurse can proceed with abdominal palpation. Abdominal tenderness and distention are determined by light palpation. It is not desirable to stimulate peristalsis. (20)

**62.** 3. The volume of parenteral fluids needed is based on fluid requirements determined according to body weight and, in this situation, gastric output. If these fluids are not replaced with an appropriate intravenous solution, serious fluid and electrolyte imbalances could develop. Urine output is monitored but is not used to calculate maintenance and replacement needs. (21)

**63.** 1. To check the position of the tube, the nurse should aspirate gastric contents or inject a small amount of air while listening with a stethoscope over the epigastric area. The tube is irrigated with normal saline and only after the position of the tube is confirmed. The suction level should not be increased since an increased level could damage the mucosa. Rotating the tube could irritate or traumatize the nasal mucosa. (8)

**64.** 4. When a child is ready to take fluids by mouth postoperatively, clear liquids are given initially. If clear liquids are tolerated, the osmolarity and amount of oral feeding are gradually increased. This means advancing to half-strength, then full-strength formula while increasing the amount given with each feeding. (21)

**65.** 1. A postoperative ileus is a functional obstruction of the bowel. Assessment of bowel sounds, a record of the first stool, and the amount of gastric output provide information about the return of gastric function. The measurement of urine specific gravity provides information about the infant's fluid and electrolyte status. (8)

**66.** 1. Both newborns and infants depend on the adult for satisfaction of basic needs. Achieving impulse control is characteristic of the early school-age period. Demonstrating autonomy and exploring the environment characterize development of the toddler. (21)

**67.** 1. Sucking provides the infant with a sense of security and comfort. It also is an outlet for releasing tension. The infant should not be discouraged from sucking on the pacifier. Fussiness and irritability after feeding may indicate that the infant's appetite is not satisfied. Sucking is not manipulative in the sense that the infant is seeking parental attention. (20)

## The Patient with Inguinal Hernia

**68.** 1. A hernia that cannot be reduced, together with abdominal distention, area tenderness, and redness

indicate an incarcerated hernia. An incarcerated hernia can lead to strangulation, necrosis, and gangrene of the bowel. Other findings associated with strangulation include irritability, anorexia, and difficulty in defecation. A palpable thickened spermatic cord on the affected side is diagnostic of inguinal hernia. (7, 21)

**69.** 3. If nonoperative reduction is successful, delaying surgery 2 to 3 days allows the edema and inflammation in the inguinal area to subside. Preoperative preparation is minimal and the infant is fed until a few hours before surgery to prevent dehydration. Trusses do not prevent incarceration, and there is no reason to use a truss preoperatively. (7, 21)

**70.** 3. The repair of an inguinal hernia is ordinarily done promptly after diagnosis in healthy infants and children. If surgery is delayed, there is a possibility of a partial obstruction when a loop of the bowel protrudes into the inguinal canal. Serious progression with complete obstruction and perhaps strangulation of the bowel requires emergency surgery to prevent gangrene, which could be fatal. The infant does not have a physiological or psychological advantage over children of older ages. Although performing surgery on areas near the genitals prior to the preschool years is recommended, the *best* reason for doing surgery on the child with an inguinal hernia is to avoid having to perform emergency surgery. (7, 21)

**71.** 2. An inguinal hernia is caused by a congenital weakness or an incomplete closure of the inguinal ring. A portion of the intestine prolapses through the inguinal ring. Failure of the embryologic gut to recanalize results in intestinal atresia or stenosis. An open umbilical ring causes an umbilical hernia. Hyperperistalsis due to gastroenteritis may cause intussusception. (7, 17)

**72.** 2. The *best* method of preparing a 7-month-old child for surgery psychologically is to have the primary caretaker stay with the child. In the second 6 months of life, infants develop separation anxiety. Teaching the mother what to expect may decrease her anxiety; this is important because infants sense anxiety and distress in parents. Taking a favorite toy or blanket to the operating room provides additional security for the child. Actual play and acting out life experiences are appropriate for preschool-aged children. (7, 11, 14)

**73.** 4. Before discharge, the infant must be completely recovered from the anesthesia and take and retain an oral feeding. A normal systolic blood pressure for a 7-month-old is approximately 116. (7, 21)

**74.** 1. Changing the diaper as soon as it becomes soiled helps prevent wound infection. This is the complication most likely to occur following repair of an inguinal hernia in an infant because of possible contamination of the wound with urine and feces. Because the surgical wound is unlikely to dehisce, an abdominal binder is unnecessary. Infants who are not toilet-trained may or may not have the incision covered with a dressing. A topical spray that protects the wound may be applied. (7)

**75.** 3. The incision should be kept as clean and dry as possible. Therefore, daily sponge baths are given for about a week postoperatively. (7)

**76.** 3. Activities such as bicycle-riding, physical education classes, weight-lifting, and wrestling are contraindicated for about 3 weeks. (7, 21)

## The Patient with Hirschsprung's Disease

**77.** 1. Infants with Hirschsprung's disease have episodes of diarrhea when liquid portions of the stool leak around the semi-obstructed colon. These infants demonstrate failure to thrive, constipation, and abdominal distention, and also typically appear unhappy and are poor feeders. (21)

**78.** 1. Infants 5 to 8 months old begin to acquire the motor skills necessary to pick up objects and transfer them from one hand to the other. These infants enjoy holding toys in each hand and banging them together. Appropriate toys are larger than the infant's mouth, bright, sturdy, and easy to manipulate. Balloons can be broken or deflated and aspirated, and string can cause strangulation. Crayons are neither safe nor appropriate for a child this age. A mobile does not stimulate motor development. (15)

**79.** 2. Infants with Hirschsprung's disease typically demonstrate failure to thrive with poor weight gain. This is due to the malabsorption of nutrients secondary to the pathophysiology of the disorder. Prominent thigh and calf veins, clubbing and cyanosis of fingers and toes, and hyperactive deep tendon reflexes are not associated with Hirschsprung's disease. (21)

**80.** 1. Infants 6 to 8 months of age grasp objects between the index and middle fingers and the base of the thumb. A neat pincer grasp usually develops around 10 months of age. At 6 months of age, the infant can partially lift his weight on his hands, enjoys imitating sounds, and is developing separation anxiety. (21)

**81.** 2. Barium causes white or clay-colored stools. The passage of white or clay-colored stools after a bar-

ium enema indicates that the barium is being expelled. (12)

**82.** 3. By encouraging parents to ask questions during information-sharing sessions, the nurse can clarify misconceptions and determine their understanding of information. Assessing the adequacy of the parent's coping skills is important, but it is secondary to encouraging them to express their concerns. The questions they ask and their interaction with the nurse may provide clues about the adequacy of their coping skills. False reassurance should never to given to parents. Written materials are appropriate for augmenting the nurse's verbal communication but also are secondary to encouraging questions. (21)

**83.** 4. The primary defect in Hirschsprung's disease is an absence of autonomic parasympathetic ganglion cells in the distal portion of the colon. (21)

**84.** 2. Neomycin sulfate, an aminoglycoside antibiotic, is given prior to gastrointestinal surgery to suppress intestinal bacteria. Neomycin is poorly absorbed by the gastrointestinal tract, which makes it effective in sterilizing the intestine. This minimizes the incidence of postoperative infection. (4)

**85.** 3. The dose is calculated by multiplying 10.3 mg × 5 kg = 51.5 mg. In computing a daily dosage, the dose is multiplied by the number of times it will be given per day (51.5 mg × 6 = 308 mg per day). (4)

**86.** 3. Dietary intake 24 to 48 hours before intestinal surgery is limited to clear liquids. A clear liquid diet meets the child's fluid needs and avoids the formation of fecal material in the intestine. Repeated saline enemas are given to empty the bowel, and a nasogastric tube may be inserted for gastric decompression. The perineal area is not prepared because it is not involved in the surgery. (17)

**87.** 1. The goal of surgery is to remove the aganglionic bowel and to improve functioning of the internal sphincter. A temporary loop or double-barreled colostomy is usually created to rest the bowel. This enables the normal distal bowel to regain its original tone and size. Final corrective surgery is done when the child is 6 to 12 months old and/or weighs about 10 kg. Thus, the colostomy will likely be reversed before the child will be old enough to care for it himself. A normal, newly created stoma is swollen and erythematous. (15)

**88.** 3. Because of decreased fluid reabsorption from the colon, the child with a colostomy benefits from a liberal fluid intake. There is no reason to avoid normal pressure on the stoma; it has a good blood supply and no nerve endings. An appliance should be fitted for stool collection to help prevent skin breakdown. The stoma should always be reddish-pink and moist. A dusky-colored stoma may indicate impaired circulation to the area. (15)

**89.** 4. A low-residue diet is usually prescribed postoperatively. Such a diet causes less bulky stools and facilitates their passage. High-fiber foods such as raw or whole cooked vegetables are avoided because they increase the bulk of the stool. (21)

**90.** 4. The drop rate is determined as follows:

$$\frac{250 \text{ ml fluid}}{3 \text{ hours}} = 83.3 \text{ ml fluid delivered per hour}$$

$$\frac{83 \text{ ml (approximately)} \times 60 \text{ drops/ml}}{60 \text{ minutes}} = \frac{4,980}{60}$$

$$= 83 \text{ drops}$$

The amount of fluid to be infused each minute is 83 drops. (12)

**91.** 2. Toilet-training the child who has undergone surgery for Hirschsprung's disease is commonly more difficult than in the normal child. This is due to the trauma to the area and the psychological associations involved. Parents should be informed that toilet-training may be prolonged and that patience and a relaxed approach will facilitate the child's efforts. Distention is an early sign of infection. Dietary restrictions or vitamin supplements are usually not required. (15)

# test 5

- *The Patient with Diarrhea/Gastroenteritis*
- *The Patient with Appendicitis*
- *The Patient with Ingestion of Toxic Substances*
- *The Patient with Celiac Disease*
- *The Patient with Phenylketonuria*
- *The Patient with Colic*
- *The Patient with Obesity*
- *The Patient with Cow's Milk Sensitivity*
- *Correct Answers and Rationales*

Select the one *best* or *correct* answer and indicate your choice by filling in the circle with a pencil in front of the option you have chosen. If the answer you would prefer is not given, select the one you think is *most appropriate.*

## THE PATIENT WITH DIARRHEA/GASTROENTERITIS

Six-month-old Brad Hunt is admitted to the hospital because he is ill with severe diarrhea.

1. Brad's diarrhea is *best* defined on the basis of his stools'
   - ○ 1. color.
   - ○ 2. amount.
   - ○ 3. frequency.
   - ○ 4. consistency.
2. The nurse readies a room for Brad's admission. The nurse should *most certainly* have supplies and equipment ready for
   - ○ 1. transfusing the infant with whole blood.
   - ○ 2. obtaining rectal temperatures on the infant.
   - ○ 3. adding humidity to the air in the infant's room.
   - ○ 4. carrying out isolation techniques when caring for the infant.
3. The nurse assesses Brad when he is admitted. She should anticipate that in addition to dehydration, Brad is *most likely* also experiencing
   - ○ 1. urinary retention.
   - ○ 2. hyperactive reflexes.
   - ○ 3. pulmonary congestion.
   - ○ 4. electrolyte imbalances.
4. An intravenous infusion is to be administered through a vein on Brad's scalp. The nurse should prepare Brad's parents for the procedure by explaining that
   - ○ 1. a portion of hair will be removed from the infant's scalp.
   - ○ 2. a sedative will be given to the infant to help keep him quiet.
   - ○ 3. visiting the infant should be delayed until the infusion has been completed.
   - ○ 4. holding the infant will be contraindicated while the infusion is being administered.
5. Compared with a 6-year-old youngster, the percentage of water Brad's body normally contains is
   - ○ 1. less.
   - ○ 2. more.
   - ○ 3. approximately the same.
   - ○ 4. variable.
6. No oral fluids and food are to be given to Brad. He is irritable and cranky. Which of the following nursing measures will help *most* to comfort the infant?
   - ○ 1. Offering him a pacifier.
   - ○ 2. Placing a mobile above his crib.
   - ○ 3. Sitting at his cribside while talking to him.
   - ○ 4. Placing him near other infants sharing the same room.
7. Because the usual course of events associated with diarrhea is no doubt occurring in Brad's intestinal tract, the nurse should recognize that Brad is *especially* susceptible to skin breakdown because his stools contain above-average amounts of
   - ○ 1. bile.
   - ○ 2. acids.
   - ○ 3. bacteria.
   - ○ 4. potassium.
8. Brad needs special care to prevent skin irritation. In addition to the effects of the stool on the skin, which of the following practices is believed to contribute *most* to the breakdown of an infant's skin?
   - ○ 1. Cleansing the area with soap that is inadequately rinsed away.
   - ○ 2. Using disposable diapers to which the infant eventually develops a sensitivity.
   - ○ 3. Dusting the area with powder so often that the

241

skin becomes dry and subject to easy breakdown.

○ 4. Applying an ointment so generously that the skin becomes soft and subject to easy breakdown.

9. A heat lamp is used when Brad's skin appears irritated. Which of the following explanations *best* describes why the application of dry heat is effective for skin irritation?

○ 1. Heat acts as a local anesthetic to damaged tissues.

○ 2. Heat relaxes the infant, which helps him remain on his abdomen.

○ 3. Heat increases the blood supply to damaged tissues to promote healing.

○ 4. Heat constricts blood vessels in damaged tissues to decrease the swelling.

10. The *minimum* number of inches the heat lamp should be placed away from Brad's skin is

○ 1. 8".

○ 2. 10".

○ 3. 18".

○ 4. 24".

Two-year-old Blake Williams is admitted to the hospital with gastroenteritis. His mother states that he vomited seven or eight times in the past 24 hours and has large green liquid stools. Mr. and Mrs. Williams have two other children, an 11-month-old son and a 4½-year-old daughter.

11. Mrs. Williams says she cannot stay with Blake because of the other two children at home. Which response would be *best* for the nurse to make?

○ 1. "You really should stay. Blake is a very sick child."

○ 2. "I understand. You may visit anytime or call to see how he is doing."

○ 3. "It really isn't necessary to stay with Blake because we are here to care for him."

○ 4. "Is it possible for you to get someone to stay with your children? Blake needs you because he seems very afraid of us."

12. Enteric precautions are used with Blake. Which of the following precautions is *unnecessary* for the nurse to observe in this situation?

○ 1. Placing the patient in a private room.

○ 2. Wearing a gown when giving the patient nursing care.

○ 3. Wearing a mask when giving the patient nursing care.

○ 4. Wearing gloves when changing the patient's soiled diapers.

13. Blake is suffering from moderate (10%) dehydration. Which of the following signs is characteristic of this degree of dehydration?

○ 1. Vomiting.

○ 2. Increased perspiration.

○ 3. Absence of tear formation.

○ 4. A decrease in the specific gravity of urine.

14. Because Blake's diarrhea is severe, which of the following electrolytes is he *most probably* losing in excessive amounts?

○ 1. Calcium.

○ 2. Phosphate.

○ 3. Potassium.

○ 4. Magnesium.

15. The physician orders that Blake receive 500 ml of intravenous fluids every 8 hours. The drop factor on the equipment used for Blake is 60 drops per ml. How many drops of fluid should be infused each minute?

○ 1. 10 drops.

○ 2. 25 drops.

○ 3. 42 drops.

○ 4. 63 drops.

16. Because Blake is to receive 500 ml of fluid every 8 hours, how many ml of intravenous fluid will Blake receive every 24 hours?

○ 1. 1,000 ml.

○ 2. 1,500 ml.

○ 3. 2,000 ml.

○ 4. 2,500 ml.

17. The nurse determines that Blake is experiencing discomfort and has swelling in the region where the intravenous needle is inserted. These findings *usually* mean that the

○ 1. needle has come out of the vein.

○ 2. intravenous site has been used too long.

○ 3. patient is allergic to the metal in the needle.

○ 4. rate of fluid administration is too rapid for the size of the vein.

18. Because of problems with Blake's intravenous infusion, the decision is made to use a surgical cutdown procedure to insert a small catheter into one of Blake's veins. The location on Blake's body that the nurse should prepare for the surgical cutdown and site of entry is on the inner surface of either

○ 1. elbow.

○ 2. forearm near the wrist.

○ 3. leg just below the knee.

○ 4. leg in front of the medial malleolus.

19. After Blake's intravenous fluids have been infusing for several hours, the nurse suspects that Blake may have circulatory overload when she

○ 1. finds the child's blood pressure has dropped.

   2. notes that the child's respirations are slow but deep.

   3. hears moist rales when auscultating over the child's chest wall.

   4. observes that the child's urinary output has decreased markedly.

20. A culture shows that Blake's diarrhea is due to *Salmonella bacillus*. Which of the following statements *best* describes the course of *Salmonella* enteritis?

   1. Some persons become chronic carriers of the causative organism and remain infectious for long periods of time.

   2. After the acute stage of the disease is past, it is rare that the causative organism continues to be shed from the body.

   3. The causative organism may live in the body indefinitely, but it becomes so attenuated in time that it is of no danger to anyone.

   4. For persons excreting the causative organism as long as 2 to 3 months after contracting salmonella, an antitoxin has been found helpful to destroy the organism.

21. The nurse attempts to determine the possible source of Blake's infection with *Salmonella*. The *most unlikely* source of *Salmonella* in the home is

   1. fresh eggs.

   2. kitty litter.

   3. a pet turtle.

   4. tropical fish.

22. Mrs. Williams tells the community health nurse that Blake answers "No!" to everything and is difficult to manage. The nurse should explain that the *most probable* explanation for his behavior is that Blake is

   1. exhibiting beginning leadership qualities.

   2. demonstrating an inherited personality trait.

   3. beginning to assert himself as an individual.

   4. showing a typical 2-year-old's lack of interest in everything.

23. Blake's mother says that when Blake cannot have his way, he often throws his arms and legs about, screams, and cries. She says, "I don't know what to do when he acts like that." The community health nurse should explain that when Blake exhibits such behavior, it is *most probably* best for the mother to

   1. ignore the behavior.

   2. let the child have his way occasionally.

   3. give the child part of what he is demanding.

   4. tell the child that she is disappointed in his behavior.

24. If Blake's parents report that Blake is exhibiting the following behaviors since he has been hospitalized, the one that is *least typical* of regressive behavior is

   1. refusing to drink from his cup.

   2. sleeping 10 to 12 hours each day.

   3. crying when a stranger approaches him.

   4. soiling his diapers more often than he did.

25. Of the following courses of action, which is the *best* one for the community health nurse to suggest that Blake's parents take when Blake demonstrates regressive behavior?

   1. Punishing the child's unacceptable behavior.

   2. Accepting the child's behavior as a coping mechanism.

   3. Comparing the child's behavior with that of his older sister.

   4. Explaining to the child that it is now time for him to grow up.

26. The community health nurse observes Blake at play in the same room as his older sister. The play of a normal 2-year-old is *most often* described as being

   1. parallel.

   2. associative.

   3. cooperative.

   4. distributive.

27. Mr. and Mrs. Williams say they are exasperated because Nancy, their 4½-year-old child, frequently tattles on her younger brothers. Which of the following statements offers the *best* explanation for Nancy's behavior?

   1. The child is probably seeking to maintain status.

   2. The child is probably demonstrating readiness for school.

   3. The child is probably expressing a developing personality trait.

   4. The child is probably trying to demonstrate feelings of motherliness.

28. Mr. and Mrs. Williams tell the community health nurse that their first-born child died at age 4 of a "terrible cancer." Which of the following neoplasms in children remains *most* ominous in terms of cure rates?

   1. Lymphoma.

   2. Wilms' tumor.

   3. Neuroblastoma.

   4. Soft-tissue sarcoma.

## THE PATIENT WITH APPENDICITIS

Clark Nunez, age 14, is brought to the emergency department because of right lower quadrant pain. The tentative diagnosis is acute appendicitis.

29. When assessing Clark, the nurse would be alert for signs and symptoms of appendicitis. A clinical finding consistent with appendicitis is
    ○ 1. costovertebral angle tenderness.
    ○ 2. bradycardia.
    ○ 3. an oral temperature of 100° F.
    ○ 4. gross hematuria.

30. While in the emergency department, Clark complains of severe abdominal pain. The *most appropriate* action the nurse could take to help manage the pain is to get an order for
    ○ 1. a heating pad.
    ○ 2. a laxative.
    ○ 3. an ice bag.
    ○ 4. an intravenous narcotic.

31. After assessing Clark's abdomen, the nurse documents the findings. Which notation represents a deviation from normal that could indicate appendicitis?
    ○ 1. The abdomen appears slightly rounded.
    ○ 2. Bowel sounds are heard twice in 2 minutes.
    ○ 3. Tympany is heard in all four quadrants.
    ○ 4. No masses are felt.

32. Which of Clark's signs and symptoms does the nurse *correctly* judge to be *unrelated* to the sympathetic effects caused by the abdominal pain?
    ○ 1. Tachycardia.
    ○ 2. Chills.
    ○ 3. Rapid breathing.
    ○ 4. Dilated pupils.

33. A diagnosis of appendicitis is made. Clark is scheduled for an emergency appendectomy and is to be transferred directly from the emergency room to the operating room. While waiting to be transferred, Clark makes all the following statements. Which statement does the nurse consider to be *most significant*?
    ○ 1. "It suddenly doesn't hurt at all."
    ○ 2. "The pain is around my navel."
    ○ 3. "I feel like I'm going to throw up."
    ○ 4. "It hurts when you press on my stomach."

34. During surgery, Clark was found to have a ruptured appendix. Postoperatively, Clark is to receive gentamicin sulfate (Garamycin) for 10 days. The nurse recognizes that one indication of potential gentamicin toxicity is
    ○ 1. dizziness.
    ○ 2. anorexia.
    ○ 3. hirsutism.
    ○ 4. constipation.

35. Clark returns from surgery alert and oriented. He is receiving parenteral fluids and has a nasogastric tube that is to be attached to continuous suction. Which of the following nursing measures is appropriate for Clark in the *early* postoperative period?
    ○ 1. Irrigate the nasogastric tube every hour.
    ○ 2. Test all stools for occult blood.
    ○ 3. Remove the nasogastric tube when he is fully alert.
    ○ 4. Encourage him to urinate frequently.

36. The nurse recognizes that the *most beneficial* position for Clark in the early postoperative period is
    ○ 1. semi-Fowler's.
    ○ 2. supine.
    ○ 3. left Sims'.
    ○ 4. prone.

37. Which of the following nursing interventions would *most likely* be beneficial *initially* in helping Clark's parents deal with his hospitalization?
    ○ 1. Reassure them that Clark will be fine.
    ○ 2. Assess their current level of knowledge before providing information.
    ○ 3. Encourage them to participate in his physical care.
    ○ 4. Avoid interacting with them if they appear angry or hostile.

38. Which of Clark's statements reflects a typical concern of adolescents after surgery?
    ○ 1. "I hope I won't have problems from this surgery when I'm older."
    ○ 2. "I'm glad that no one can see my scar."
    ○ 3. "I don't want my appendectomy to keep me from playing football."
    ○ 4. "I wish my scar were located where all my friends could see it."

39. While in the hospital, Clark is likely to be *most anxious* about
    ○ 1. having an erection when the nurse assesses his incision.
    ○ 2. being separated from his parents and siblings.
    ○ 3. missing school and having to make up his lessons.
    ○ 4. experiencing potentially painful procedures.

40. Which of Clark's actions does the nurse judge to be a healthy coping behavior?
    ○ 1. He insists on wearing a shirt and gym shorts rather than pajamas.
    ○ 2. He avoids interacting with the adolescents on the unit.
    ○ 3. He refuses to fill out the menu, allowing the nurse to do so.
    ○ 4. He discontinues his intravenous infusion because he is afraid that his blood will leak out.

41. Which approach is likely to be *most effective* in communicating with Clark during his hospitalization?
    ○ 1. Give him only essential information.
    ○ 2. Offer advice and opinions frequently.

○ 3. Use diagrams when explaining procedures.
○ 4. Use adolescent slang terms.

**42.** Clark asks the nurse, "What causes appendicitis?" The nurse bases her response on the fact that there seems to be a relationship between the development of appendicitis and
○ 1. diet.
○ 2. exercise.
○ 3. fluid intake.
○ 4. personality type.

## THE PATIENT WITH INGESTION OF TOXIC SUBSTANCES

A nurse works in the children's unit of a hospital's emergency room.

**43.** The nurse checks the drug supplies in the emergency room. She notes that syrup of ipecac is readily available. This drug is used *primarily* to
○ 1. induce vomiting.
○ 2. promote diuresis.
○ 3. relieve seizure activity.
○ 4. stimulate rapid intestinal elimination.

**44.** Barry Scherer is brought to the emergency room after he has ingested an undetermined amount of drain cleaner. The nurse plans *typical* initial care for Barry when she prepares to assist with
○ 1. administering an emetic.
○ 2. performing a tracheostomy.
○ 3. performing gastric lavage.
○ 4. administering cardiopulmonary resuscitation.

**45.** After the acute stage following the ingestion of drain cleaner, the *most likely* complication Barry will develop is esophageal
○ 1. ulcers.
○ 2. varices.
○ 3. strictures.
○ 4. diverticuli.

**46.** Pearl Adam's mother brings Pearl to the emergency room after the child has taken "some white pills." If Pearl presents one of the following signs, which should lead the nurse to judge that the "pills" Pearl took were *most probably* aspirin?
○ 1. A nosebleed.
○ 2. Seizure activity.
○ 3. Projectile vomiting.
○ 4. Deep, rapid respirations.

**47.** Dean Byrne has drunk kerosene. The complication Dean is *most likely* to experience is
○ 1. uremia.

○ 2. hepatitis.
○ 3. meningitis.
○ 4. pneumonitis.

**48.** Carl Jefferson is brought to the emergency room because of unexplained vomiting. After a health history is obtained and laboratory studies are completed, Carl is found to have lead poisoning. Which of the following treatments should the nurse anticipate will *most probably* be used for Carl?
○ 1. Detoxification with chelating agents.
○ 2. Exchange transfusions with whole blood.
○ 3. Radiation therapy with low-voltage x-rays.
○ 4. Gastric lavages with fluids high in electrolyte content.

**49.** Which of the following complications is Carl *most likely* to develop if lead poisoning goes untreated for a long time?
○ 1. Cirrhosis of the liver.
○ 2. Retarded growth rate.
○ 3. Neurologic changes.
○ 4. Pathologic fractures.

**50.** Of the following measures, the one that has been found to be the *most effective* in preventing lead poisoning in patients such as Carl is to
○ 1. condemn old housing developments.
○ 2. educate the public concerning common sources of lead.
○ 3. educate the public concerning the importance of good nutrition.
○ 4. inoculate children who live in areas where lead poisoning is common.

**51.** Lois Penny, who is being cared for in the emergency room following an accident, demonstrates fear of being exposed for the physical examination. In which of the following age groups is fear of exposure *most typical?*
○ 1. Toddlerhood (ages 1 to 3 years).
○ 2. Preschool age (ages 4 to 5 years).
○ 3. School age (ages 6 to 12 years).
○ 4. Adolescence (ages 13 to 15 years).

**52.** After Lois is cared for, Mrs. Penny asks the nurse, "What is the best way for me to protect my infant son when he is with me in the car?" Which of the following diagrams (see figures on the next page) illustrates how *best* to apply a car's seat belt to protect an infant while traveling?
○ 1. Baby should be lying on car seat with seat belt around it. Better to have infant facing driver.
○ 2. Infant seat is sitting flat on car seat with infant facing driver. Seat belt around infant seat.
○ 3. Infant seat facing forward with seat belt around infant and seat.
○ 4. Infant seat facing backwards with face of infant toward back of car with seat belt in place.

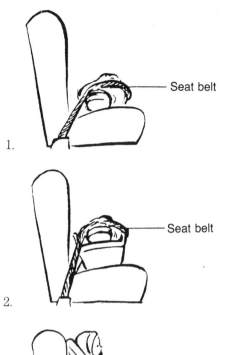

Baby should be lying on car seat with seat belt around it. Better to have infant facing driver.

1.

Infant seat is sitting flat on car seat with infant facing driver. Seat belt around infant seat.

2.

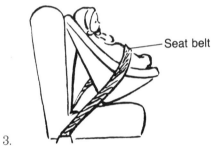

Infant seat facing forward with seat belt around infant and seat.

3.

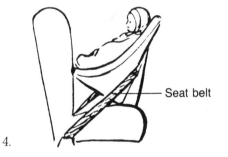

Infant seat facing backwards with face of infant toward back of car with seat belt in place.

4.

**53.** When Rose Benito arrives in the emergency room with aspirin poisoning, the nurse should be prepared to assist with the administration of
○ 1. oxygen.
○ 2. an emetic.
○ 3. a diuretic.
○ 4. a sedative.

**54.** The nurse plans to help familiarize parents with typical behavioral traits of children who are accident-prone. Which of the following characteristics is *most typical* of an accident-prone child?
○ 1. The child is passive and quiet.
○ 2. The child is quick to mimic his elders.

○ 3. The child is not easily frustrated and angered.
○ 4. The child has a normal attention span for his age.

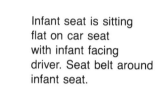

### THE PATIENT WITH CELIAC DISEASE

Matt Johnson, age 18 months, has celiac disease.

**55.** Matt's nurse should expect that because Matt has celiac disease, his stools are *most likely* to be

○ 1. especially dark in color.
○ 2. abnormally small in amount.
○ 3. unusually hard in consistency.
○ 4. particularly offensive in odor.

56. During assessment, a physical finding the nurse is *most likely* to observe is that Matt has
    ○ 1. an enlarged liver.
    ○ 2. a protuberant abdomen.
    ○ 3. tender inguinal lymph nodes.
    ○ 4. edema in the lower extremities.

57. Celiac disease is also referred to as gluten enteropathy. Matt's diet should *not* include foods containing gluten, such as
    ○ 1. wheat, oats, rye, and barley.
    ○ 2. milk, yogurt, cheese, and butter.
    ○ 3. rice, corn, sorghum, and soybeans.
    ○ 4. peanuts, almonds, pecans, and walnuts.

58. For how long is it likely that Matt will need to remain on a special diet?
    ○ 1. For the rest of his life.
    ○ 2. Until the disease is well controlled.
    ○ 3. Until approximately puberty.
    ○ 4. For the period required to desensitize him to offending foods.

59. Matt wears reusable diapers at night. His mother asks what safety precautions she should take with his wet, soiled diapers. Which of the following statements should guide the nurse when she responds to Mrs. Johnson's question?
    ○ 1. The diapers should be boiled after they are washed.
    ○ 2. The diapers should be soaked in an antiseptic solution before they are washed.
    ○ 3. It would be best to use disposable diapers until the diarrhea is under control.
    ○ 4. No special precautions are necessary in the care of this infant's diapers.

## THE PATIENT WITH PHENYLKETONURIA

*avoid milk*

Two-year-old Chrissy Little has phenylketonuria (PKU). Chrissy's mother brings her to a physician's office for a routine checkup.

60. Which of the following conditions would *most likely* have resulted if Chrissy had remained untreated for PKU?
    ○ 1. Heart failure.
    ○ 2. Hepatic coma.
    ○ 3. Renal shutdown.
    ○ 4. Mental retardation.

61. According to Chrissy's health record, when she was 10 days old she was screened for PKU by a community health nurse, using a urine test. When a 10% ferric chloride solution is placed on an infant's diaper that is wet with urine, the test is assessed as positive for PKU if the nurse notes that the ferric chloride and urine combine to produce
    ○ 1. a foul odor.
    ○ 2. a green color.
    ○ 3. a foaming effect.
    ○ 4. precipitate matter.

62. Chrissy was not screened for PKU in the hospital when she was born. If a screening test for PKU is performed on a newborn during the first few days of life, a *false-negative* result may occur that is *most frequently* due to the infant's
    ○ 1. inadequate fluid intake.
    ○ 2. decreased vitamin K level.
    ○ 3. insufficient protein intake.
    ○ 4. increased bilirubin blood level.

63. When comparing the physical characteristics of a well child with those of Chrissy, the nurse can expect that the child with PKU *typically* has
    ○ 1. a shorter stature.
    ○ 2. a larger abdomen.
    ○ 3. a larger head size.
    ○ 4. lighter skin pigmentation.

64. Mrs. Little asks the nurse to explain how PKU is transmitted. The nurse should base her response on knowledge that the disease is transmitted by
    ○ 1. a translocation of a gene.
    ○ 2. a nondisjunction of a gene.
    ○ 3. an autosomal recessive gene.
    ○ 4. a homozygous dominant gene.

65. Chrissy is given Lofenalac, one of several products on the market used to provide an adequate daily protein intake to a child with PKU. Lofenalac and other similar products help attain the goal of diet therapy for Chrissy, which is to keep low blood levels of the constituent
    ○ 1. tyrosine.
    ○ 2. galactose.
    ○ 3. tryptophan.
    ○ 4. phenylalanine.

66. Which of the following foods should be *omitted* from Chrissy's diet?
    ○ 1. Squash.
    ○ 2. Tapioca.
    ○ 3. Cheese.
    ○ 4. Bananas.

67. Several teaching sessions have been documented in Chrissy's health record. Yet Mrs. Little asks the nurse again what caused Chrissy's PKU. Which of

the following explanations offers the *best* reason for the mother's asking repeatedly for information she has already received?

○ 1. Parents of chronically ill children often want very detailed explanations about the causes of and treatments for their children's diseases.

○ 2. Parents of chronically ill children often require long periods of time to work through a grieving process for their children's lack of health.

○ 3. Parents of chronically ill children often try to test a health worker's knowledge about the causes of and treatments for their children's diseases.

○ 4. Parents of chronically ill children often deal with their guilt about possibly causing the children's ill health with hostility and challenging questions about their children's diseases.

## THE PATIENT WITH COLIC

Two-week-old Amy Strunk is brought to the health clinic by her parents. They state that she has been crying almost constantly since birth and brings her knees up to her abdomen frequently. Colic is suspected.

**68.** Which of the following findings would be consistent with a diagnosis of colic?

○ 1. Failure to gain weight.
○ 2. Expulsion of flatus.
○ 3. Soft abdomen.
○ 4. Frequent vomiting.

**69.** While obtaining information about Amy's problem, the nurse asks Amy's parents to describe her bowel movements. Which of the following descriptions would the nurse expect if Amy does have colic?

○ 1. Soft yellow stools.
○ 2. Frequent watery stools.
○ 3. Ribbon-like stools.
○ 4. Mucus-like stools.

**70.** A diagnosis of colic is made. Mrs. Strunk tells the nurse that the diagnosis upsets her because she knows that Amy will continue to have colicky pain. Which of the following responses would be *most appropriate* for the nurse to make?

○ 1. "I know that Amy's crying upsets you, but she needs your undivided attention for the next few months."

○ 2. "It can be very difficult to listen to your baby cry so often, so try to arrange some free time."

○ 3. "It is distressing to see her in pain, but at least she does not have an intestinal obstruction."

○ 4. "It will be a rough 3 months, but she will outgrow it by then."

**71.** Because many of the problems associated with colic seem to be associated with feeding, the nurse develops a teaching plan for Mrs. Strunk after assessing the feeding process. Which of the observations that the nurse makes while Mrs. Strunk is feeding Amy would indicate that she understood the teaching?

○ 1. She holds Amy supine while feeding her.
○ 2. She burps Amy with her sitting on her lap.
○ 3. She places Amy prone after the feeding.
○ 4. She burps Amy during and after the feeding.

**72.** Mrs. Strunk tells the nurse that it is difficult to get Amy comfortable when she sleeps. The nurse should suggest that Mrs. Strunk lay Amy on her

○ 1. back.
○ 2. abdomen.
○ 3. right side.
○ 4. left side.

## THE PATIENT WITH OBESITY

Sam Heinrich, age 17, comes to the clinic for a pre-college physical exam. Based on Sam's appearance, the nurse judges him to be overweight.

**73.** Which of the following is the *most common* method used to determine the extent of obesity?

○ 1. Height and weight growth charts.
○ 2. Skinfold thickness measurement.
○ 3. Hydrometry.
○ 4. Comparison with other family members.

**74.** The *most prevalent* complication of adolescent obesity is its association with

○ 1. adult obesity.
○ 2. orthopedic problems.
○ 3. narcolepsy.
○ 4. psychosocial problems.

**75.** Sam tells the nurse that he is concerned about being obese and wants to lose weight. He asks the nurse what technique might be most effective. The nurse answers that the treatment modality shown to be the *most effective* for adolescents involves

○ 1. taking appetite-suppressant drugs such as antihistamines and/or amphetamines.

○ 2. following a strict dietary regimen.

○ 3. surgical intervention, either gastric bypass or gastric partitioning.

○ 4. participation in a weight-reduction program with other obese adolescents.

Mrs. Disch gave birth to her first child, Jill, 4 months ago and brings her to the clinic for a routine checkup. Mrs. Disch reports that Jill is taking five 8-ounce bottles of formula every day. The nurse realizes that this is an excessive amount of formula.

**76.** What information supports a diagnosis of obesity for Jill?
- ○ 1. She wears clothing in size 9 to 12 months.
- ○ 2. She has a double chin, fat arms and hands, and rolls of fat in the thigh area.
- ○ 3. She weighs 13¼ pounds (50th percentile) and is 23½″ long (25th percentile).
- ○ 4. She has not yet rolled over, either prone to supine or supine to prone.

**77.** In order to help decrease Jill's total caloric intake, the nurse recommends that Mrs. Disch
- ○ 1. decrease the number of feedings to three bottles per day.
- ○ 2. change Jill's feeding from formula to skim milk.
- ○ 3. add a small amount of rice cereal to the formula so Jill will be more satisfied.
- ○ 4. prepare each bottle with 5 ounces of correctly diluted formula and 3 ounces of water.

**78.** While the nurse is talking with her about ways to decrease Jill's caloric intake, Mrs. Disch asks when she should introduce solid foods into Jill's diet. The nurse answers, "At 5 to 6 months of age." The answer is based on the fact that *before* this time, the infant's
- ○ 1. tongue thrusts forward in the mouth.
- ○ 2. ability to push food away deliberately is highly developed.
- ○ 3. gastrointestinal tract blocks absorption of macromolecules.
- ○ 4. sense of taste is not well developed.

**79.** What anticipatory guidance does the nurse give Mrs. Disch regarding the method of introducing solid foods into Jill's diet?
- ○ 1. Decrease the amount of formula to about 900 ml (30 ounces) per day when Jill is regularly taking solid foods.
- ○ 2. Encourage custards, milk puddings, and yogurt when Jill is 18 months old.
- ○ 3. Choose commercially prepared baby foods because they tend to be more nutritious than home-prepared foods.
- ○ 4. Feed Jill solid foods when she is hungriest so that she will not take as much formula.

**80.** At the next clinic visit, Mrs. Disch explains that she and her husband plan to have more children and want to prevent overnourishing them. The nurse teaches Mrs. Disch about ways to prevent overnourishment of infants. Which of the following statements indicates that Mrs. Disch has understood the teaching?
- ○ 1. "I will give the baby a daily supplemental bottle of sterile water."
- ○ 2. "I will establish a regulated feeding schedule for the baby."
- ○ 3. "I will give the baby commercially prepared formula."
- ○ 4. "I will watch for clues that indicate the baby is full."

## THE PATIENT WITH COW'S MILK SENSITIVITY

Mr. and Mrs. Eller bring their 1-month-old daughter Katie to the clinic because she has had diarrhea, has been vomiting, and cries excessively. Based on her history, a tentative diagnosis of cow's milk sensitivity is made.

**81.** Mr. Eller says he has heard of cow's milk sensitivity but knows almost nothing about it. The nurse would explain that it is
- ○ 1. an adverse reaction to cow's milk protein.
- ○ 2. an uncommon nutritional allergy.
- ○ 3. a hereditary disorder of carbohydrate metabolism.
- ○ 4. usually a life-long allergy.

**82.** Mrs. Eller asks the nurse what the medical plan is for Katie. The nurse explains that an evaluation will be done to differentiate cow's milk sensitivity from lactose intolerance. Mrs. Eller asks what lactose intolerance is. The nurse's answer is based on the fact that lactose intolerance is characterized by
- ○ 1. an allergic reaction to lactose.
- ○ 2. a deficiency in the enzyme lactase.
- ○ 3. the breakdown of lactose into lactase.
- ○ 4. the inability to digest lactase.

**83.** Katie undergoes a series of tests to differentiate cow's milk sensitivity from lactose intolerance. Which of the following diagnostic test results confirms the diagnosis of lactose intolerance?
- ○ 1. A blood glucose of 20 mg/dl or less.
- ○ 2. A stool pH of 7.5.
- ○ 3. Positive hydrogen breath test.
- ○ 4. Galactosuria.

**84.** If Katie were lactose-intolerant, what dairy products could Mrs. Eller add to Katie's diet after she was 1 year old?
- ○ 1. Pudding and cream soup.
- ○ 2. Ice cream and cream soup.

○ 3. Yogurt and cheese.
○ 4. Cream soup and buttermilk.

**85.** Lactose intolerance is ruled out and the diagnosis of cow's milk sensitivity is confirmed. The decision is made to put Katie on a diet that does not contain cow's milk. The nurse develops a teaching plan for Mr. and Mrs. Eller about substitute formula. A fact that forms the basis for the teaching plan is that the *initial* milk substitute given is

○ 1. goat's milk.
○ 2. hydrolyzed protein.
○ 3. soy protein.
○ 4. meat-based formula.

**86.** The appropriate formula is prescribed for Katie. Which of the following suggestions should the nurse make to Mr. and Mrs. Eller about purchasing the formula?

○ 1. Buy a month's supply at a time.
○ 2. Buy several brands of the same substitute.
○ 3. Buy only a few containers initially.
○ 4. Buy the same brand consistently.

**87.** Mrs. Eller asks the nurse how to manage Katie's diet during the next year. The nurse should tell her to

○ 1. add pureed squash to Katie's diet when she is 8 months old.
○ 2. avoid giving Katie milk products until she is 10 months old.
○ 3. avoid giving Katie wheat crackers until she is 6 months old.
○ 4. add eggs to Katie's diet when she is 6 months old.

**88.** Jimmy Eller, Katie's 10-month-old brother, is recovering from a severe bout of acute gastroenteritis. He has had no loose stools for 2 days and has been tolerating Pedialyte well. This morning Mrs. Eller started him on half-strength Similac, the formula he was taking before his illness. Subsequently, he has had two diarrheal stools. The *most likely* reason for the recurrent diarrhea is that

○ 1. the gastroenteritis has recurred.
○ 2. he has developed a milk allergy.
○ 3. he cannot tolerate the fat in cow's milk.
○ 4. the brush border of the intestine has been injured.

**89.** Mrs. Eller telephones the clinic nurse and explains what has happened since she brought Jimmy to the clinic 3 days ago. She wants to make sure that Jimmy receives adequate nutrition and asks what she should do. Based on knowledge of the underlying problem, the nurse should tell her to

○ 1. bring him to the hospital for intravenous infusion therapy.
○ 2. feed him Pedialyte until he has no more diarrhea.
○ 3. give him soy-based formula until he can tolerate his regular diet.
○ 4. give him half-strength milk to which a lactase enzyme product has been added.

**90.** Mrs. Eller tells the nurse that she and her husband plan to have other children. Given that Katie had cow's milk intolerance, Mrs. Eller is concerned about how to feed the newborn and asks the nurse for suggestions. The nurse should tell her that the *most practical* approach is to

○ 1. alternate breast-feeding with feeding of soy-based formula.
○ 2. feed the infant a soy-based formula exclusively.
○ 3. breast-feed exclusively while increasing her own fluid intake.
○ 4. alternate breast-feeding with feedings of goat's milk.

# CORRECT ANSWERS AND RATIONALES

Numbers appear in parentheses following the rationales. The numbers identify textbooks listed in the references at the end of Part III, where correct answers can be verified.

## The Patient with Diarrhea/ Gastroenteritis

1. 4. Diarrhea is best defined on the basis of the stools' consistency, which is ordinarily liquid in nature. The color of diarrheal stools is usually greenish, but the color of stools is also affected by food and fluid intake. The amount of stool varies according to estimates made by various people and therefore is not a safe criterion on which to define diarrhea. The frequency of stools varies also, although usually stools occur more frequently than normal when diarrhea is present. (6, 21)

2. 4. An infant with diarrhea should be isolated from others by using isolation techniques until it is determined that the diarrhea is noninfectious. The use of a rectal thermometer is contraindicated in a patient with diarrhea because of the danger of injuring rectal mucosa, which is already tender and swollen. The thermometer may also stimulate peristalsis, causing more diarrhea. Obtaining the infant's temperature by using an axillary determination is recommended. It would be unusual for an infant with diarrhea to require a blood transfusion or humid air in his room. (6, 21)

3. 4. The pathologic processes that produce dehydration with diarrhea also cause electrolyte and acid-base imbalances. Urinary retention is unlikely, but the infant may void less frequently than usual because of a decrease in the volume of urine production. Pulmonary congestion is unlikely because a dehydrated patient suffers from hypovolemia. Hypervolemia is likely to cause pulmonary congestion. Hyperactive reflexes are not typical findings in the presence of diarrhea. (6, 21)

4. 1. Parents are quick to notice changes in their infant's physical appearance. The removal of the infant's hair may be very upsetting to them if they are not told why it will be done. Hair is removed on the scalp at the site of needle insertion for intravenous therapy for better visualization and to provide a smooth surface on which to attach tape to secure the needle. Some parents appreciate receiving the removed hair as a keepsake. Sedatives are ordinarily not prescribed prior to the administration of an intravenous infusion. Visiting the infant and holding him while he receives an infusion are not contraindicated and are usually encouraged to help comfort an ill infant. (21)

5. 2. A newborn's body is approximately 75% to 80% water. The infant approaches adult levels after about 2 years of age. By adulthood, the percentage of body water is between about 50% and 60%. In the elderly person, the percentage of body water drops to approximately 45%. (6, 21)

6. 1. An irritable infant receiving nothing by mouth, like the infant described in this item, is usually best comforted when given a pacifier to satisfy his sucking needs. Such activities as placing a mobile over an infant's crib, speaking to the infant, and placing the infant with others (unless the infant has an infectious disease) may not necessarily be contraindicated, but they will not offer the comfort that a pacifier will. (21)

7. 2. During the course of diarrhea, the intestinal mucosa becomes edematous and inflamed with the result that nutrients are poorly absorbed. Undigested carbohydrate in the intestinal tract leads to bacteria growth and fermentation, which produces lactic and acetic acid. The highly acid stool predisposes the infant to skin breakdown on the buttocks. (6, 21)

8. 1. Many authorities believe that of the practices given in this item, the one that contributes most to skin breakdown is cleansing the area with soap that is inadequately rinsed away. This same theory holds for adults whose skin often breaks down when diarrhea is present. (6, 21)

9. 3. A heat lamp provides heat to the exposed area. Because it stimulates vasodilatation, heat increases the blood supply to damaged tissue and enhances healing. Cold tends to act as a local anesthetic and initially causes vasoconstriction. Heat may be relaxing, but this is not the primary reason for using the heat lamp over an area of irritated skin. (6, 21)

10. 3. A heat lamp should be placed at least 18″ from the skin's surface and the heat treatment should last no more than about 20 minutes. A 25-watt bulb is recommended. The bulb should be protected to help prevent burns from handling the equipment. An active infant or child may require restraining during the treatment, or the nurse may choose to hold the infant or child while administering the treatment. (6, 21)

11. 2. The mother's decision described in this item is that she cannot stay with her hospitalized child because of other responsibilities. In this situation, the nurse's best course of action is to support the

mother, and this is best done when the nurse indicates that she understands and that the mother can visit or call as she is able. Indicating to the mother that she should stay with her ill child is being critical of the mother and seems insensitive. Commenting that the child will be cared for suggests the mother is not necessary. The nurse seems to be telling the mother how to solve her dilemma without sufficient knowledge to warrant the statement when she indicates that the child is being well cared for without her. (21)

**12.** 3. A mask is unnecessary when enteric precautions are used because the organisms are in the stool and are not transmitted through air droplets. A private room is used for a child on enteric precautions. A gown is worn when the nurse is in direct contact with the patient, and gloves are necessary when the nurse is in contact with the patient's stools. (6, 12)

**13.** 3. The absence of tears is typically found when moderate dehydration is observed. Other typical findings associated with moderate dehydration include a dry mouth, sunken eyes, poor skin turgor, and an increased pulse rate. Perspiration would be decreased with dehydration because the body is attempting to conserve fluids. The specific gravity of urine increases with decreased output in the presence of dehydration. (6, 21)

**14.** 3. The stool and intestinal juices contain potassium, which is lost in excessive amounts when diarrhea is present. (6, 21)

**15.** 4. The number of drops the patient should receive each minute is determined as follows:

$$\frac{500 \text{ ml}}{8 \text{ hr}} = 63 \text{ ml approximately to be infused each hour}$$

$$\frac{63 \text{ ml} \times 60 \text{ (drop factor)}}{60 \text{ min}} = \frac{3,780}{60} = 63 \text{ drops/min}$$

The number of drops to be infused each minute is about 63 drops. (12, 13)

**16.** 2. If the patient is to receive 500 ml of fluid every 8 hours, in every 24 hours he should receive 1,500 ml.

$$\frac{24}{8} = 3$$
$$3 \times 500 = 1500 \text{ ml}$$

(12,13)

**17.** 1. The needle has most probably come out of the vein when a patient with an intravenous infusion has pain and swelling in the area of needle insertion. The swelling occurs as the fluid infuses into subcutaneous tissues. Other typical signs of infiltration include skin pallor in the area of needle insertion and coldness of the skin in the area. An inflammation is likely to have occurred if the intravenous site has been used too long. Because an inert metal is used for manufacturing intravenous needles, the possibility of an allergic reaction is remote. If the fluid is administered too rapidly for the size of the vein, fluid would most probably leak around the needle at the area of assembly onto the tubing. (12, 21)

**18.** 4. Most often, when a cutdown is used to start an intravenous infusion, the saphenous vein is chosen at a site on the inner aspect of the ankle near the medial malleolus. The internal saphenous vein courses down the lower leg to the foot and passes anteriorly at the medial malleolus, which is the prominence on the inner aspect of the ankle. (21)

**19.** 3. Typical signs of circulatory overload include the following: moist rales when auscultating over the chest wall; a rise in blood pressure; engorged neck veins; a wide variation between fluid intake and output, with a higher intake than output; shortness of breath; an increased respiratory rate; dyspnea; and cyanosis. (6, 10)

**20.** 1. Some persons become chronic carriers of the causative organism and remain infectious for long periods of time after having *Salmonella* enteritis. The organism continues to be shed from the body. No antitoxin is available to treat or prevent salmonellae infections. (21)

**21.** 4. *Salmonella bacilli* are not spread by tropical fish. Fowl and their eggs are common sources, as are pet turtles and kittens. (6, 21)

**22.** 3. The behavior of the toddler described in this item is typical for his age as he attempts to assert himself as an individual. The negativism reflects the developmental task of establishing autonomy. The child is attempting to exert control over his environment and himself. It is too early to assess leadership qualities when a child is only 2 years old. Negativism does not show disinterest, nor does it demonstrate an inherited personality characteristic. (6, 21)

**23.** 1. Toddlers are busy developing a sense of autonomy. This requires an opportunity to make decisions and express individuality. Temper tantrums occur relatively frequently among toddlers and are considered normal behavior as toddlers search for autonomy. Ignoring the outbursts is most probably best. However, the mother should be taught that during a temper tantrum, she should intervene if the child is likely to injure himself. Allowing the child to have his way, giving him part of what he wants, and expressing disappointment in his behavior are likely to add to the problems associated with temper tantrums. (6, 21)

**24.** 2. Regressive behavior is behavior that reverts to actions typical of an earlier age. Regressive behaviors for a 2-year-old would include refusing to drink from a cup, crying when a stranger approaches, and soiling his diapers more often than he did at home. Sleeping 10 to 12 hours a day is normal behavior for a toddler. (6, 21)

**25.** 2. Regression is a method of coping and represents a retreat to an earlier pattern of behavior that typically occurred prior to current stresses and discomforts. It is best for the child's parents and nurses to accept the regressive behavior of a child for what it represents: a coping mechanism in the face of stress. Acceptance of the child helps increase his feelings of worth and self-esteem, which will in turn increase his ability to cope with stress. Punishing him and comparing his behavior with that of an older sibling tend to reinforce the behavior he is using. Shaming a child is detrimental and causes the child to feel self-doubt. (6, 27)

**26.** 1. A normal 2-year-old is deeply absorbed in his own self. He tends to play among others, but the play is characteristically parallel (that is, the child plays independently of others). During associative play, children play together but without any organization. Cooperative play is organized play among children. Associative and cooperative play is typically observed in children older than the toddler age. Play is not described as being distributive. (6, 21)

**27.** 1. Sibling rivalry is fairly common, and a preschooler often attempts to maintain status and develop initiative in the situation. In order to maintain status, he may show resentment and anger by such behavior as tattling. Parents are often advised to pay more attention to the child to help him maintain status in the family. (6, 21)

**28.** 3. Neuroblastoma presents the gravest prognosis among children, and the survival rate has changed very little in the past two decades. Metastasis usually occurs before a diagnosis is made. This type of neoplasm has not responded well to any type of therapy. Lymphomas have been contained with current forms of therapy. Wilms' tumor carries a high recovery rate. Many soft-tissue sarcomas have been well contained and even cured with continued aggressive therapy. (21)

## The Patient with Appendicitis

**29.** 3. The most common manifestations of appendicitis are right lower quadrant pain, localized tenderness, and a fever of 99° to 102° F. Other signs of inflammation may be present, including increased pulse and respiratory rates. Costovertebral angle tenderness and hematuria are associated with urologic problems. (21)

**30.** 3. An ice bag may help relieve pain. A heating pad is contraindicated because heat may increase circulation to the appendix and lead to rupture. Laxatives are contraindicated because they stimulate bowel motility and can exacerbate abdominal pain. Narcotics may mask symptoms and are not given until a diagnosis is made. (21)

**31.** 2. Manifestations of appendicitis include decreased or absent bowel sounds. Normally, bowel sounds are heard every 10 to 30 seconds. The contour of the male adolescent abdomen is normally flat to slightly rounded. Tympany is typically heard over most of the abdomen. Masses should be absent. (21)

**32.** 2. Chills are a normal response of the body's immune system to infection and are not a response of the sympathetic nervous system to pain. Tachycardia, increased respiratory rate, and dilated pupils are sympathetic effects. (17)

**33.** 1. A sudden relief from pain in the patient with appendicitis may indicate that the appendix has ruptured. This relieves the pressure within the appendix, but spreads the infection to the peritoneal cavity. Periumbilical pain, vomiting, and abdominal tenderness are common manifestations of appendicitis. (21)

**34.** 1. Gentamicin sulfate (Garamycin) is a broad spectrum aminoglycoside antibiotic that can cause nephrotoxicity and ototoxicity. Manifestations of ototoxicity include auditory dysfunctions and vestibular disturbances such as dizziness. Anorexia, hirsutism, and constipation are not side effects of this antibiotic. (16, 20)

**35.** 4. After an appendectomy, the patient should be encouraged to void frequently to prevent bladder distention, which could cause strain on the incision. There is no reason to irrigate the nasogastric tube unless it ceases to function and there is no reason to test the stools for occult blood. The nasogastric tube remains in place until peristalsis returns. (15)

**36.** 1. After an appendectomy for a ruptured appendix, the semi-Fowler's or a right side-lying position helps localize the infection. These positions promote drainage from the peritoneal cavity and decrease the incidence of subdiaphragmatic abscess. (21)

**37.** 2. Before giving information, it is important to assess the learner's current level of knowledge. When dealing with parents of an ill child, the nurse considers their emotions and the intensity of the situa-

**38.** 3. Typically, the adolescent is concerned about the immediate state of his body and its functioning. He needs to know if any changes, such as illness, trauma, or surgery, will alter his lifestyle or interfere with his quest for physical perfection. (15)

**39.** 1. Fears of the adolescent include body changes and emerging sexual urges. The young adolescent is typically concerned about the inability to control these changes and feelings and about embarrassing himself because of them. The typical adolescent is more concerned about being separated from his peer group than from his family and schoolwork and is not unrealistically worried about experiencing pain. (15)

**40.** 1. Adolescents struggle for independence and identity. Typical concerns are peer acceptance, body changes, and sexuality. The adolescent needs to feel in control of the situation and to conform with his peers. Control and conformity are often manifested in appearance, including clothing, and this carries over into the hospital experience. The adolescent feels best about himself when he is able to look and act as he normally does. The adolescent usually understands scientific principles and does not have unrealistic fears of bodily harm. (15)

**41.** 3. Adolescents can comprehend scientific rationale and complexity. They appreciate detailed description and explanations using charts, diagrams, and models. The adolescent dislikes lectures and unsolicited advice and opinions. The use of jargon is a way to establish the identity of the peer group, and adult use of adolescent jargon may be viewed as false or dishonest. (15)

**42.** 1. The exact cause of appendicitis is unknown, but obstruction of the lumen of the appendix is the principal factor. There is increasing evidence that people who eat more fiber have a lower incidence of appendicitis than those who have a low fiber intake. Dietary fiber contributes to the softness and bulk of the stool, decreasing the potential for obstruction. (21)

## The Patient with Ingestion of Toxic Substances

**43.** 1. Syrup of ipecac is an emetic that exerts its action by direct stimulation of the vomiting center and by producing irritating effects on the stomach mucosa. It is given with one to two glasses of water or fruit juice. If the patient does not vomit within about 20 minutes after taking syrup of ipecac, a second dose may be administered. Syrup of ipecac should be removed from the stomach by gavage if emesis does not occur, because it is cardiotoxic and is likely to produce various dysrhythmias. Most authorities recommend that syrup of ipecac be available in the home for emergency use, but it should be kept out of reach of children in the home. (6, 16, 21)

**44.** 2. Drain cleaner almost always contains lye. The mouth, pharynx, and esophagus are burned from the caustic effects of the lye. The nurse should be prepared to assist with a tracheostomy, which may be necessary because of swelling around the area of the larynx. Gastric lavage and emetics are contraindicated because they may cause perforations in the necrotic mucosa. Cardiopulmonary resuscitation is not indicated because lye does not poison by interfering with cardiopulmonary functioning. (6, 21)

**45.** 3. As the burn from lye ingestion heals, scar tissue is most likely to cause esophageal strictures. Ulcers, varices, and diverticuli following lye ingestion do not ordinarily occur. (21)

**46.** 4. The salicylate ion in aspirin stimulates the respiratory center. As a result, an early sign of aspirin poisoning is deep, rapid respirations. Hyperventilation is the most impressive sign of salicylate poisoning. Other signs, such as vomiting and seizure activity, may occur later, when the overdose is large. (6, 21)

**47.** 4. Chemical pneumonitis is the most common complication following the ingestion of hydrocarbons, such as kerosene. The pneumonitis is due to irritation from the hydrocarbon that has been aspirated into the lungs. (6, 21)

**48.** 1. Treatment of a child with lead poisoning is aimed toward mobilizing lead from body tissues, especially from brain tissues. The metal ions damage nervous system cells. Chelating agents are used that tie up the metal ions in the blood and tissues before they enter cells. The lead is then excreted from the body through the kidneys. The most common chelating agent used today is calcium disodium edetate (EDTA). Such therapy as exchange transfusions, radiation therapy, and gastric lavages are ineffective for treating the patient with lead poisoning. (6, 21)

**49.** 3. The most serious and irreversible consequence of lead poisoning is mental retardation due to neurologic changes. It can be expected to occur if lead poisoning is long-standing and goes untreated. Lead poisoning also affects the hematologic and renal systems. (6, 21)

**50.** 2. Public education about the sources of lead that could cause poisoning has been found to be the most effective measure to prevent lead poisoning. Condemning old housing developments has been ineffective because lead paint still exists in other dwellings. Education about good nutrition is not an effective preventive measure. There is no agent for inoculating children against lead poisoning. (6, 21)

**51.** 3. It has been observed that school-aged children are most fearful of being exposed due to increasing body awareness. Children of other ages have concerns about body image but are not unduly modest about exposure. Because of the child's reluctance to undress, the nurse should use every precaution to ensure that the child is properly draped during a physical examination. (6, 21)

**52.** 4. In a front-end impact, the infant seat will be held securely by the seat belt and the child's head will be protected by the back of the infant seat and the back of the car seat when the infant seat faces backwards (with the infant's face toward the back of the car). The seat belt is secured around the infant seat. Other positions offer less satisfactory positioning of an infant seat in the car. The infant seat may be tipped forward and the child's head and neck will be unprotected. If the infant seat is flat on the car seat, the seat belt is in an awkward position and the infant can slip out of both the seat and the belt. (21)

**53.** 2. The emergency treatment of a child who has taken an overdose of aspirin is to induce vomiting. An emetic, such as syrup of ipecac, is almost always given. Vomiting will stop absorption of the drug by removing it from the stomach. Vomiting is not contraindicated when the patient has had an overdose of aspirin because the drug causes no damage to tissues in the mouth, pharynx, and esophagus. (6, 21)

**54.** 2. Many childhood accidents are believed due to a child's mimicking his elders without realizing the dangers associated with such behavior. For example, a child who observes his parents taking medications is likely to ingest medications not intended for him. The accident-prone child tends to be highly active, curious, daring, and aggressive. He is unable to wait for the things he wants and has a short attention span for his age. (6, 21)

### The Patient with Celiac Disease

**55.** 4. The stools of a youngster with celiac disease are characteristically offensive in odor, pale in color, large (bulky) in amount, and soft (loose) in consistency. The presence of excessive flatus is common and there may be bouts of diarrhea. (6, 21)

**56.** 2. The intestines of children with celiac disease fill with accumulated undigested food and flatus with the result that the abdomen characteristically protrudes. Celiac disease is not ordinarily complicated with poor liver functioning that may cause the liver to enlarge, or with edema in the extremities. Tender inguinal lymph nodes are often associated with an infection, and celiac disease is not an infectious disease. (6, 21)

**57.** 1. Damage to intestinal mucosa, which occurs in celiac disease, is caused by gliadin. Gliadin is a part of the protein found in wheat, rye, barley, and oats. Foods containing these grains must be eliminated entirely from the diet of children with celiac disease and of adults with gluten-induced enteropathy (celiac sprue). (6, 21)

**58.** 1. Celiac disease is believed to be inherited. This lifelong disease is most probably due to an inborn error of metabolism or an immunologic error. A child will not outgrow the disease. With good health care, the severity of the disease can be limited. (6, 21)

**59.** 4. When a child has celiac disease, special precautions, such as boiling or soaking his diapers in antiseptic, are unnecessary. The disease is not infectious. If reusable diapers are used, they should be well rinsed following washing in soap or detergent to minimize skin irritation. (6, 21)

### The Patient with Phenylketonuria

**60.** 4. Mental retardation is a common result when children with phenylketonuria (PKU) remain untreated. Abnormal myelination of neural tissue appears to cause mental retardation. Seizure activity occurs in about one-fourth of children with untreated PKU. (6, 21)

**61.** 2. The ferric chloride solution combined with urine containing phenylpyruvic acid produces a green color. Children with PKU have been observed to have a peculiar body odor and the urine has a musty odor. (21)

**62.** 3. The result of testing a newborn for PKU is likely to be negative, even if the infant has the condition, because the infant is still not receiving either formula or breast milk, both of which are high in phenylalanine content. This insufficient intake of protein causes a false-negative result in a screening test because the blood level of phenylalanine is not yet elevated. (6, 21)

**63.** 4. A buildup of phenylalanine in the blood inhibits the proper production of the pigment melanin from tyrosine. As a result, the characteristic skin coloring of a child with PKU is light. The child is also likely to have blue eyes and light hair. Short stature, enlarged abdomen, and large head size are not associated with PKU. (6, 21)

**64.** 3. PKU is due to an inborn error of metabolism. It is an autosomal recessive disorder that makes the conversion of phenylalanine to tyrosine impossible. (6, 21)

**65.** 4. PKU is a disease in which amino acid metabolism is abnormal. Phenylalanine is an amino acid in many foods. When the hepatic enzyme phenylalanine hydroxylase is missing, phenylalanine is not converted to tyrosine. Dietary treatment is directed toward keeping the phenylalanine blood level within a safe range, about 5 to 9 mg/dl in infants and children. Higher levels of phenylalanine in the blood are likely to result in brain damage. (6, 21)

**66.** 3. Natural protein foods contain relatively large amounts of phenylalanine. Animal proteins, such as milk and cheese, are omitted from the diet of a child with PKU. The diet may include fruits and vegetables, which are low in protein and phenylalanine. For example, such fruits and vegetables as squash and bananas are allowed; so, also, is tapioca. The only treatment for PKU is dietary. (6, 21)

**67.** 2. Parents typically grieve about the loss of health in their children afflicted with a chronic disease. Many times, they repeat questions, as though they are trying to deny what is really happening. This type of behavior is important as the parents attempt to integrate the experience and their feelings within their own self-image. Asking for detailed explanations, testing the competence of health workers, and expressing hostility toward health workers may explain the parents' behavior, but explaining the behavior described in this item as a part of the grieving process seems most plausible. (6, 21)

## The Patient with Colic

**68.** 2. Infants with colic have paroxysmal abdominal pain or cramping caused by the production and accumulation of gas. This causes pain and abdominal distention. They may expel flatus or eructate, but do not vomit. Despite this pain, infants tolerate the formula well, gain weight, and thrive. (7, 11, 21)

**69.** 1. Infants with colic have normal stools, and normal stools for an infant are soft and yellow. Abnormal stools may indicate bowel obstruction or infection. (11)

**70.** 2. The nurse needs to provide the parents with support. Parents are stressed and need to be en-

couraged to get out of the house and arrange for some free time. Comparing colic to other problems is inappropriate; parents have the right to be upset. Although colic usually disappears spontaneously by the time the child is 3 months old, guarantees should not be made. (21)

**71.** 4. Infants with colic should be burped frequently during and after the feeding. Much of the discomfort of colic appears to be associated with the presence of air in the stomach and intestines. Infants with colic should be held fairly upright while being fed, to facilitate air rising. Infants with colic should be burped using the shoulder position and should be placed in an infant seat after feedings. (7, 11, 21)

**72.** 2. Infants with colic seem to sleep more comfortably on their abdomen than on their backs or sides. (7, 11, 21)

## The Patient with Obesity

**73.** 2. Measuring skinfold thickness with special skinfold calipers is the most common method used to assess obesity. The skinfold thickness test, which determines the amount of subcutaneous fat, more accurately determines obesity than does a growth chart. Hydrometry, a method that estimates body fat from measurement of total body water, is a more sophisticated technique. Comparing body size with other family members may shed light on the etiology of obesity, but not on the degree of obesity. (21)

**74.** 1. The most prevalent complication of adolescent obesity is its persistence into adulthood. Obese adolescents are at risk for becoming obese adults: the odds are 28 to 1 that an obese adolescent will become a normal-weight adult. Narcolepsy is the most serious physical effect of severe adolescent obesity, and obese children have an increased incidence of orthopedic problems. Psychosocial problems are the most destructive complications associated with adolescent obesity. (7, 17, 21)

**75.** 4. Weight loss treatment modalities that include peer involvement have been the most successful with obese adolescents. This is because developmentally, peer support is critical to adolescents, especially in an all-encompassing problem such as obesity. Use of drugs may lead to habituation. A strict dietary regimen does not allow the adolescent to make choices. Surgical intervention is a drastic method of weight control and should be used only for morbid obesity. (7, 21)

**76.** 2. The obese infant appears fat, with rolls of fat and flabby skin areas. Height-weight tables are used to compare a child's measurements with norms. A difference between height and weight of one standard deviation is acceptable. An infant in the 95th percentile for weight and the 60th percentile for height is obese. Not having rolled over is not a developmental delay, although obesity may cause a delay in the development of motor skills. Clothing size is an arbitrary measurement of a child's size. (7)

77. 4. Preparing each bottle with 5 ounces of correctly diluted formula and 3 ounces of water provides the infant with the same amount of sucking time and simultaneously reduces the caloric intake. If a baby is accustomed to sucking five bottles per day, reducing the feedings to three bottles will not provide adequate sucking time. Skim milk is never recommended for babies because it does not provide essential fatty acids for growth and development in the first year or two. Furthermore, skim cow's milk provides excessive protein, which elevates the renal solute load and water demands. Cereal should never be mixed in formula and given in a bottle because it does not allow the infant to learn to eat from a spoon. (21)

78. 1. Solid foods are introduced when an infant is physiologically ready, usually between the ages of 5 and 6 months. Before this age, an infant has a strong sucking reflex and the tongue thrusts forward, pushing food out of the mouth. The infant is unable to push food away deliberately, and early introduction of solid food can be perceived as forced feeding. Before the age of 5 or 6 months, the gastrointestinal tract is unable to block macromolecules from absorption, which can lead to food-protein allergy. A newborn's sense of taste is well developed, but this developmental factor is unrelated to the introduction of solids into the diet. (7)

79. 1. Decreasing the amount of formula to 900 ml (30 ounces) per day helps prevent excessive caloric intake. Desserts such as custards, milk puddings and yogurt are introduced in the later part of the first year. Commercially prepared foods have no nutritional advantages over those prepared at home. Spoon-feeding a baby when he is hungriest can lead to frustration because the hunger cannot be satisfied quickly enough. This leads to a panicky baby and distraught parents. (7, 21)

80. 4. Infants generally do not overeat unless urged to do so. Parents should watch for clues that indicate the baby is full. For example, when full, an infant stops sucking and pushes the nipple out of the mouth. Giving an infant an *occasional* supplemental bottle of sterile water provides stimulation and fluid without additional calories. This technique is encouraged after excessive weight gain is noted

during the first few months of life. A demand schedule, rather than a regulated schedule, allows the infant to regulate intake according to individual needs. Bottle-feeding may lead to excessive caloric intake. (7)

## The Patient with Cow's Milk Sensitivity

81. 1. Cow's milk sensitivity is an adverse local and systemic gastrointestinal reaction to cow's milk protein. This is the most common nutritional allergy in infants. Galactosemia is a hereditary disorder of carbohydrate metabolism. Almost all sensitive children can tolerate cow's milk by 2 years of age. (7, 21)

82. 2. Lactose intolerance is caused by a lack of the digestive enzyme lactase. This enzyme, found in intestinal juice, is necessary for the digestion of lactose, the primary carbohydrate in cow's milk. (7, 20)

83. 1. A lactose tolerance test is used to confirm the diagnosis of lactose intolerance. A blood glucose level of 20 mg/dl or less confirms the diagnosis. The fecal pH in lactose intolerance is less than 6 (very acidic). A positive hydrogen breath test is associated with, but does not confirm, the diagnosis of lactose intolerance. Hydrogen gas is produced in the intestinal tract of a child who does not digest lactose completely. The air that the child exhales is tested and gas chromatography is used to analyze the level of the hydrogen gas. Galactosuria, or galactose in the urine, indicates galactosemia, a hereditary disorder of carbohydrate metabolism. (7, 21)

84. 3. Lactose-intolerant individuals are usually able to tolerate dairy products in which lactose has been fermented, such as yogurt, cheese, and buttermilk. Pudding, ice cream, and cream soup contain unfermented lactose. (21)

85. 3. Soy protein is the initial milk substitute. Goat's milk is not used because of cross-reactions with cow's milk. If soy protein is not tolerated, hydrolyzed protein and meat-based formulas may be used. (7, 21, 23)

86. 3. One milk substitute may not be acceptable to a particular infant, so parents are encouraged to buy only a few containers instead of a case until the infant's response is determined. Once an accepted substitute has been identified, they can buy a case and should buy that product consistently. (7)

87. 1. Pureed squash and other hypoallergenic foods can be introduced at the appropriate age. Milk products should be avoided until the child is about

1 year old. Eggs, wheat, and other hyperallergenic foods are also avoided until the child is 1 year old. (7, 21)

**88.** 4. During severe cases of diarrhea, the brush border of the intestine, which produces lactase, is sloughed. In such instances, the child is temporarily unable to digest lactose, the primary carbohydrate in cow's milk. It is unlikely that the infection has recurred 2 days after the symptoms disappeared. Milk allergy usually occurs within the first 3 months of life after ingestion of cow's milk. (8, 21)

**89.** 3. A lactose-free diet, such as soy-based formula, is indicated for a few weeks, until the brush border of the intestine rejuvenates. Milk, which contains lactose, should be avoided. Intravenous fluids are not indicated at this time. Pedialyte will not meet the child's nutritional needs. (8)

**90.** 3. Breast-feeding exclusively for the first few months and eliminating cow's and goat's milk from the infant's diet is the most practical approach to preventing cow's milk sensitivity. Increasing fluid intake increases the mother's milk production. Mothers with allergies or a family history of allergies should avoid all milk products while breast-feeding. (7, 21)

# test 6

**The Patient with Cryptorchidism**

**The Patient with Hydrocele**

**The Patient with Hypospadias**

**The Patient with a Urinary Tract Infection**

**The Patient with Acute/Chronic Glomerulonephritis**

**The Patient with Nephrotic Syndrome**

**The Patient with Acute/Chronic Renal Failure**

**The Patient with Wilms' Tumor**

**Correct Answers and Rationales**

Select the one *best* or *correct* answer and indicate your choice by filling in the circle with a pencil in front of the option you have chosen. If the answer you would prefer is not given, select the one you think is *most appropriate*.

## THE PATIENT WITH CRYPTORCHIDISM

One-month-old Michael Vandarm is brought to the clinic by his father for a checkup. Mr. Vandarm explains that he is very concerned because the right side of his son's scrotum seems incompletely developed.

1. Mr. Vandarm says he is afraid that his son's testicle has not descended and asks when it should descend. The nurse should base her answer on the knowledge that an undescended testicle should descend into the scrotal sac by the age of
   - ○ 1. 24 hours.
   - ○ 2. 6 weeks.
   - ○ 3. 6 months.
   - ○ 4. 18 months.
2. When preparing to palpate Michael's testes, the nurse notices that he has been circumcised. While palpating the testes, the nurse should remember that testes ascend and are often nonpalpable after
   - ○ 1. every feeding.
   - ○ 2. circumcision.
   - ○ 3. exposure to cold.
   - ○ 4. defecation.
3. While the nurse is examining Michael, Mr. Vandarm seems extremely anxious and says that he never expected anything like this to happen. What would be the *best response* for the nurse to make?
   - ○ 1. "Would you like to talk with a parent of a child who has the same problem?"
   - ○ 2. "It must be difficult to have an infant with a problem."
   - ○ 3. "Try not to worry; the testes will more than likely descend spontaneously."

   - ○ 4. "Please tell me more about how you're feeling about the situation."
4. A tentative diagnosis of undescended right testis (cryptorchidism) is made. Mr. Vandarm asks the nurse how an undescended testis compares with one that has descended. The nurse should base her answer on the fact that an undescended testis is
   - ○ 1. generally larger than one that has descended.
   - ○ 2. unlikely to produce sperm normally.
   - ○ 3. unlikely to develop a malignancy after puberty.
   - ○ 4. more prone to develop epididymitis in adolescence.
5. Several other conditions are associated with undescended testes. Therefore, in addition to hydrocele, the nurse should also assess Michael for
   - ○ 1. inguinal hernia and urinary tract anomalies.
   - ○ 2. esophageal fistula and tracheal anomalies.
   - ○ 3. meningomyelocele and spinal tract anomalies.
   - ○ 4. gastroschisis and cardiac anomalies.
6. Several weeks pass and Michael's right testis has still not descended. The physician explains that the testis is below the inguinal ring and suggests that further treatment be postponed until Michael is at least a year old. Mr. Vandarm says he heard about hormone shots that might help Michael. Which of the following hormones is given to stimulate descent of the testis?
   - ○ 1. Growth hormone (GH).
   - ○ 2. Adrenocorticotropic hormone (ACTH).
   - ○ 3. Thyroid hormone.
   - ○ 4. Human chorionic gonadotrophic hormone (HCG).
7. When Michael is 3 years old, he is scheduled for surgical repair (orchiopexy) of his undescended right testicle. Which of the following information would be *critical* for the nurse to give Michael preoperatively?

**259**

○ 1. His penis will not be involved in the surgery.
○ 2. His penis will be involved in the surgery.
○ 3. His scrotum, not his penis, will be involved in the surgery.
○ 4. He will not be able to see any evidence of the surgery.

8. Michael returns from surgery with traction applied to the testis. In the early postoperative period, the nurse should ensure that this traction is
○ 1. removed after 12 hours.
○ 2. maintained consistently.
○ 3. increased gradually.
○ 4. decreased gradually.

9. Michael's parents take turns staying with him so that one of them is with him all the time. They want to participate in his care as much as possible. Which of the following goals should be emphasized *most* in the nurse's teaching?
○ 1. Relieve postoperative discomfort.
○ 2. Prevent contamination at the surgical site.
○ 3. Protect healthy skin surfaces.
○ 4. Promote a positive self-image.

10. The nurse explains the impact of cryptorchidism on Michael's long-term health care needs. Which of the following statements by his mother would indicate that she has understood the nurse's teaching?
○ 1. "Michael will need to have his hormone level checked every 6 months until he is 10 years old."
○ 2. "Michael's testes should be examined periodically for lumps."
○ 3. "Michael will need plastic surgery to repair scrotal scarring when he is 14 years old."
○ 4. "Michael's scrotum should be examined monthly for an accumulation of fluid."

## THE PATIENT WITH HYDROCELE

11. Two-week-old Kiroki Paav is at the clinic for evaluation of a hydrocele that was noted on newborn assessment. A hydrocele is *best* described as an accumulation of fluid in the
○ 1. epididymis and ductus deferens due to a patent seminal vesicle.
○ 2. testicle and peritoneal cavity due to a patent processus vaginalis.
○ 3. scrotum due to an obliterated processus vaginalis.
○ 4. tunica vaginalis of the testicle or along the spermatic cord due to a patent processus vaginalis.

12. Mrs. Paav tells the nurse that when she first saw Kiroki she thought he had a hernia. She asks the nurse what differentiates a hydrocele from a hernia. The nurse explains that
○ 1. both hydroceles and hernias can be reduced.
○ 2. a distended hydrocele can be transilluminated.
○ 3. a hydrocele is bilateral, a hernia unilateral.
○ 4. the scrotum is much larger with a hernia than with a hydrocele.

13. When the hydrocele was found, the physician explained the medical treatment to Mr. and Mrs. Paav. When the nurse tells the Paavs that Kiroki's scrotum is smaller now than it was 2 weeks ago, which response by Mrs. Paav indicates that she understood the teaching?
○ 1. "More time is needed for the fluid to be reabsorbed."
○ 2. "Surgery is needed to remove the fluid and tissue."
○ 3. "I will massage the groin more often to help move the fluid into the abdomen."
○ 4. "Elevating the scrotum will promote gravity drainage."

14. Twelve months later, Kiroki undergoes surgery to correct the hydrocele. The surgery is successful, but immediately after surgery the nurse notices that his scrotum is swollen and bruised. The nurse *correctly* interprets these postoperative findings as
○ 1. normal, requiring no medical intervention.
○ 2. abnormal, requiring further surgery.
○ 3. normal, but requiring medical intervention.
○ 4. abnormal, indicating hemorrhage and damaged testes.

15. As the nurse is applying an ice bag to Kiroki's scrotum, Mrs. Paav says that she worries about other problems that Kiroki may develop. She asks the nurse about other conditions that may accompany hydrocele. The nurse explains that hydrocele may be associated with
○ 1. bowel obstruction.
○ 2. sterility.
○ 3. an endocrine deficiency.
○ 4. inguinal hernia.

## THE PATIENT WITH HYPOSPADIAS

16. Mr. and Mrs. Erika bring their 12-month-old son Andrei to the clinic for evaluation of hypospadias, with associated congenital chordee.

Which of the following statements *best* describes hypospadias?

○ 1. The bladder is turned out and the urethral orifices are visible.

○ 2. The urethra opens on the ventral surface of the penis.

○ 3. A band of fibrous tissue pulls the penis ventrally in an arc.

○ 4. The urethra opens on the dorsal surface of the penis.

**17.** The hypospadias and chordee were noted at birth, and Andrei's parents were advised not to have Andrei circumcised. What was the rationale for this advice?

○ 1. The poorly developed penile vasculature makes the surgical procedure too risky.

○ 2. The associated chordee is very difficult to remove during circumcision.

○ 3. The meatus can become stenosed, leading to symptoms of urinary obstruction.

○ 4. The foreskin is used to repair the deformity surgically.

**18.** Twelve-month-old Andrei is scheduled for surgery that will correct the hypospadias and chordee. This is a preferred time for surgical repair because

○ 1. Andrei is too young to have developed castration anxiety.

○ 2. Andrei will experience less pain at this age.

○ 3. repair is easier before Andrei is toilet-trained.

○ 4. the reconstructed tissue will grow with Andrei.

**19.** The hypospadias and chordee were repaired and Andrei tolerated the procedure well. Andrei is returned to his room on the pediatric unit; he has an intravenous infusion and both a urethral and a suprapubic catheter in place. While assessing Andrei, the nurse tells Mrs. Erika that the *primary* purpose of the suprapubic catheter is to provide

○ 1. an entry port for bladder irrigation.

○ 2. accurate measurement of urinary output.

○ 3. an alternate urinary elimination route.

○ 4. an opportunity to observe the color of the urine.

**20.** As the nurse is assessing Andrei, Mrs. Erika says that she was told preoperatively that Andrei would have a urethral catheter. The nurse knows that Mrs. Erika understood the teaching when she explains that the *major* purpose of the urethral catheter is to

○ 1. prevent bladder spasms.

○ 2. maintain patency of the reconstructed urethra.

○ 3. immobilize the reconstructed urethra completely.

○ 4. ensure accurate measurement of urine.

**21.** Before examining the surgical site, the nurse prepares Mr. and Mrs. Erika for its appearance. She explains that since this is the first of two surgeries, the penis will appear swollen and

○ 1. somewhat misshapen.

○ 2. dusky blue.

○ 3. almost physically perfect.

○ 4. very pale.

**22.** A nursing goal for Andrei is to minimize postoperative pain. In addition to administering an analgesic, which of the following nursing measures would *most likely* achieve this goal?

○ 1. Allowing him to play with other children.

○ 2. Making sure he has adequate rest.

○ 3. Giving him age-appropriate toys.

○ 4. Having his parents comfort him.

**23.** Considering Andrei's age, stage of development, and operative procedure, which of the following postoperative interventions should the nurse emphasize with Mr. and Mrs. Erika?

○ 1. Hold and comfort Andrei as much as possible.

○ 2. Prevent Andrei from disrupting the catheters.

○ 3. Encourage Andrei to play with his favorite toys.

○ 4. Allow Andrei to become familiar with the catheters.

**24.** Mr. and Mrs. Erika tell the nurse that they want to participate in Andrei's care. The nurse encourages their participation and teaches them infection control measures. What is the *most effective* infection control measure the nurse could teach them?

○ 1. Wear a mask.

○ 2. Wash their hands.

○ 3. Wear a cover gown.

○ 4. Wear gloves.

**25.** The nurse reviews Andrei's urinalysis results. Which of the following values should the nurse report to the physician?

○ 1. Specific gravity 1.020.

○ 2. 10 red blood cells per high-powered field.

○ 3. Urinary pH 5.8.

○ 4. 25 white blood cells per high-powered field.

## THE PATIENT WITH URINARY TRACT INFECTION

Three-year-old Beth Nichols is brought to the children's clinic by her father because she has a fever and is very irritable. Beth's health history indicates that she has had a urinary tract infection (UTI) within the past year.

**26.** Because UTIs are fairly common in preschool-aged girls, the nurse asks Beth's father whether Beth has recently had

○ 1. an increased appetite.
○ 2. a skin rash.
○ 3. abdominal pain.
○ 4. back pain.

27. The nurse obtains a clean-voided urine specimen from Beth. The specimen is positive for bacteriuria because the bacterial count is more than
○ 1. 100 colonies/ml.
○ 2. 1,000 colonies/ml.
○ 3. 10,000 colonies/ml.
○ 4. 100,000 colonies/ml.

28. Another characteristic of urine in the presence of bacteria is
○ 1. the presence of protein.
○ 2. a pH of 3.
○ 3. dark amber color.
○ 4. a specific gravity of 1.005.

29. After the diagnosis of urinary tract infection has been confirmed, the nurse should tell Beth's father to
○ 1. decrease her oral fluid intake.
○ 2. give her warm bubble baths.
○ 3. encourage her to void frequently.
○ 4. wash her perineum with soap after she voids and defecates.

30. Co-trimoxazole (Bactrim) is prescribed for Beth, and her father is given a prescription for a 10-day supply. Which of the following information should the nurse give Beth's father?
○ 1. Beth may discontinue the antibiotic when her symptoms disappear completely.
○ 2. The medication will turn Beth's urine reddish-orange.
○ 3. He should bring a clean-voided urine specimen from Beth to the clinic in 3 days.
○ 4. If Beth is reluctant to take the antibiotic, he may mix it with her food.

31. Two days later, Beth's father telephones the clinic nurse. He explains, "Things at home have changed quite a bit since Beth's urinary tract infection was diagnosed. She often ignores our frequent reminders to urinate. She refuses to take the antibiotic unless we promise to buy her gifts, and we are reluctant to discipline her because she is sick." The nurse would base her response on the knowledge that
○ 1. this is normal behavior for a 3-year-old.
○ 2. Beth's psychosocial development has been altered.
○ 3. daily routines should be altered while Beth is ill.
○ 4. the parents should ignore Beth's behavior.

32. Two weeks after being diagnosed, Beth is seen at

the clinic to determine if the urinary tract infection has been eradicated. The *most* significant evaluation datum is that
○ 1. the abdominal pain has disappeared.
○ 2. the urine culture is negative for bacteria.
○ 3. Beth completed 10 days of antibiotic treatment.
○ 4. Beth has become less irritable.

## THE PATIENT WITH ACUTE/CHRONIC GLOMERULONEPHRITIS

Acutely ill Mike Moreno, a 17-year-old high-school basketball player, is admitted to the hospital. He has acute glomerulonephritis. Edema with swelling of the ankles is present.

33. While the nurse is obtaining Mike's health history, Mike says he has voided "very little" during the previous 24 hours. The nurse understands that the production of scanty amounts of urine is called
○ 1. anuria.
○ 2. dysuria.
○ 3. enuresis.
○ 4. oliguria.

34. While the nurse obtains Mike's health history, she is *most likely* to find that Mike has recently had an infection caused by microorganisms classified as
○ 1. pneumococci.
○ 2. meningococci.
○ 3. streptococci.
○ 4. influenza viruses.

35. During the interview when Mike's health history is obtained, Mike describes having "wet dreams" several times during the previous couple of weeks. When analyzing the significance of wet dreams, the nurse should consider the phenomenon to be
○ 1. a symptom of a sexual disorder.
○ 2. a normal occurrence at the patient's age.
○ 3. an early symptom of acute glomerulonephritis.
○ 4. a positive sign that the patient is producing live sperm.

36. The nurse assesses Mike's physical growth. Of the following statements, which offers the *best* guideline for the nurse to analyze her findings?
○ 1. The rate of growth varies among individuals.
○ 2. Various parts of the body grow at about the same rate.
○ 3. Growth does not normally follow a continuous pattern.

○ 4. There is no particular order in which normal growth occurs.

37. While admitting Mike to the hospital, the nurse notes that the patient is wearing a roller bandage on his knee. Mike explains that he put the bandage on earlier in the day. He says he sprained his knee playing basketball before becoming ill. If the nurse makes the following observations, which should prompt her to change the bandage?
   ○ 1. The patient's toes appear swollen.
   ○ 2. The patient's knee is slightly flexed.
   ○ 3. The bandage is made of elastic material.
   ○ 4. The bandage has been applied using a figure-of-eight turn.

38. Mike's mouth is dry and his lips are encrusted with mucus (sordes). It is *best* for the nurse to cleanse the patient's mouth with
   ○ 1. a jelly-type toothpaste.
   ○ 2. a mild white vinegar solution.
   ○ 3. undiluted antiseptic mouthwash.
   ○ 4. half-strength hydrogen peroxide.

39. Mike's fluid intake is to be restricted to 1,000 ml in each 24-hour period. Which of the following fluids would it be *best* for the nurse to offer the patient while helping to prevent excessive thirst?
   ○ 1. Ice chips.
   ○ 2. Tap water.
   ○ 3. Ginger ale.
   ○ 4. Hot bouillon.

40. Mike complains about the food served in the hospital and says he would like any of the four foods listed below. Which should the nurse explain is *contraindicated* for him?
   ○ 1. A ham sandwich.
   ○ 2. An ice-cream sundae.
   ○ 3. A piece of apple pie.
   ○ 4. A waffle with maple syrup.

41. If all of the following diversional activities are available and not contraindicated for Mike, the one the nurse is *most likely* to observe him enjoy *most* during convalescence is
   ○ 1. watching television with a classmate.
   ○ 2. playing a game of chess with his father.
   ○ 3. explaining the rules of basketball to a 12-year-old patient.
   ○ 4. having his mother read a mystery novel to him.

42. A high-school teacher visits Mike and tells the nurse, "I never worry about Mike. He always lands on his feet and seems to know where he is going." This description of Mike's personality is characteristic of a teenager who, according to the psychologist Erik Erikson,
   ○ 1. has a sense of self-identity.
   ○ 2. is of above-average intelligence.
   ○ 3. has a poor relationship with his parents.

○ 4. is emotionally independent of his family at an earlier age than is typical.

43. The nurse can expect that if Mike demonstrates the following developmental characteristics, the one that is *least typical* of his age is being
   ○ 1. moody.
   ○ 2. submissive.
   ○ 3. concerned with personal appearance.
   ○ 4. interested in members of the opposite sex.

Mike's condition worsens on the second morning of the hospitalization. His blood pressure is elevated and he has not voided since 7 p.m. the previous evening.

44. Which of the following would be the *most* appropriate *initial* nursing action?
   ○ 1. Encourage the patient to eat a low-sodium breakfast.
   ○ 2. Help the patient ambulate.
   ○ 3. Encourage the patient to drink more water.
   ○ 4. Assess the patient's neurologic status.

45. Mike's nursing care plan should include *all* of the following actions *except*
   ○ 1. checking the patient's urinary pH daily.
   ○ 2. weighing the patient daily.
   ○ 3. recording the patient's intake and output daily.
   ○ 4. checking the patient's vital signs every 4 hours.

46. When developing Mike's discharge plan, the nurse should assign *lowest* priority to teaching him about
   ○ 1. avoiding fatigue.
   ○ 2. participating in sports.
   ○ 3. restricting dietary protein.
   ○ 4. preventing respiratory infections.

47. Gary Smith, age 15, was diagnosed at 1 year of age as having sickle-cell disease. He is admitted to the hospital with a chief complaint of "losing weight and feeling tired and irritable for about a month." Gary's physician has confirmed the diagnosis of chronic glomerulonephritis. A nursing care plan for Gary should include *all* of the following nursing actions *except*
   ○ 1. teaching measures to prevent infection.
   ○ 2. recording intake and output.
   ○ 3. restricting ambulation.
   ○ 4. monitoring vital signs routinely.

48. Based on knowledge of its pathophysiology, the nurse knows that chronic glomerulonephritis (CGN)
   ○ 1. includes a variety of different disease processes.

○ 2. is symptomatic until kidney destruction occurs.

○ 3. is usually preceded by several attacks of acute glomerular disease.

○ 4. is heralded by renal tubular acidosis.

## THE PATIENT WITH NEPHROTIC SYNDROME

Three-year-old Neil Preston, who has nephrotic syndrome, is hospitalized for observation. He is edematous. At present, he is free of infection.

49. At admission, the nurse notes a *typical* finding in relation to Neil's vital signs when she observes that Neil's
○ 1. pulse rate is slow.
○ 2. respiratory rate is slow.
○ 3. body temperature is elevated.
○ 4. blood pressure is within normal range.

50. According to laboratory findings, Neil is demonstrating a *common* sign of nephrotic syndrome that reflects its pathology, which is that the body
○ 1. excretes protein in the urine.
○ 2. retains red blood cells in the bloodstream.
○ 3. excretes urine of an abnormally low specific gravity.
○ 4. retains unusually large amounts of albumin in the bloodstream.

51. When the nurse obtains Neil's history his mother says that Neil had been "breathing hard and his urine looked foamy." Another clinical manifestation of nephrotic syndrome is an increase in
○ 1. urination.
○ 2. weight.
○ 3. appetite.
○ 4. constipation.

52. Given the insidious onset of nephrotic syndrome, the most common *initial* reaction in parents is
○ 1. anger.
○ 2. guilt.
○ 3. denial.
○ 4. rage.

53. When the nurse obtains a nursing history from Mrs. Preston concerning Neil, it is *particularly* important for the nurse to obtain information concerning Neil's
○ 1. elimination pattern.
○ 2. rest and sleep habits.
○ 3. food likes and dislikes.
○ 4. favorite playtime activities.

54. Based on knowledge of the therapeutic management of nephrotic syndrome, the nurse would anticipate that Neil's treatment will include
○ 1. surgical excision of the diseased glomeruli.
○ 2. fluid intake greater than 500 ml/kg of body weight per day.
○ 3. sodium restriction during periods of massive edema.
○ 4. administration of the somatotropic hormone (STH).

55. Which of the following nursing orders is *least likely* to appear on the care plan that the nurse prepares for Neil after his admission to the hospital?
○ 1. Weigh daily.
○ 2. Fluids as desired.
○ 3. Observe strict bed rest.
○ 4. Record intake and output.

56. Of the following nursing measures to help reduce edema in Neil's eyelids, it would be *best* for the nurse to
○ 1. elevate the head of the patient's bed.
○ 2. irrigate the patient's eyes with warm normal saline.
○ 3. limit the patient's television-watching to short periods of time.
○ 4. apply cool compresses to the patient's eyes several times a day.

57. The drug *most likely* to be used for Neil because of its effectiveness in reducing the mortality rate of children with nephrotic syndrome is
○ 1. streptomycin.
○ 2. prednisone (Deltra).
○ 3. epinephrine (Adrenalin).
○ 4. ascorbic acid (vitamin C).

58. Cyclophosphamide (Cytoxan) is also to be used for Neil. The nurse should be aware that a disadvantage of this drug is that one *common* side effect is
○ 1. sodium retention.
○ 2. loss of muscular coordination.
○ 3. a decreased white blood cell count.
○ 4. an interference with the normal growth rate.

59. Which of the following nursing actions would be *most* helpful in evaluating Neil's fluid balance?
○ 1. Measuring urinary output.
○ 2. Measuring abdominal girth.
○ 3. Assessing urine specific gravity.
○ 4. Obtaining a daily weight.

60. Neil responds well to treatment and is going home soon in remission. The nurse develops a plan to prepare Neil's family for his discharge. As a means of attaining this goal, the nurse should teach Neil's parents to

○ 1. test Neil's urine for pH daily.

○ 2. prevent Neil's contact with infected playmates.

○ 3. notify the physician if Neil's urine output increases.

○ 4. administer Neil's pain medication routinely.

## THE PATIENT WITH ACUTE/ CHRONIC RENAL FAILURE

Mara Ross, age 14, has been hospitalized with acute renal failure (ARF). Two weeks ago she had a Tenckhoff catheter inserted for peritoneal dialysis (PD).

**61.** When Mara asks about the advantages of peritoneal dialysis compared with hemodialysis, the nurse should explain that peritoneal dialysis involves

○ 1. less protein loss.

○ 2. more rapid fluid removal.

○ 3. less chance of infection.

○ 4. fewer dietary restrictions.

**62.** As Mara's nurse performs the daily catheter exit site care, an important step would be to

○ 1. examine the site for signs of infection.

○ 2. hold the catheter taut while cleansing the skin.

○ 3. change the dressing when the peritoneal space is empty.

○ 4. apply an occlusive dressing after cleansing the site.

**63.** Mara's nurse plans discharge teaching for Mara and her family. In regard to diet teaching, the nurse should emphasize that Mara should restrict her intake of

○ 1. iron-rich foods.

○ 2. calories.

○ 3. fluids.

○ 4. phosphorus.

**64.** The nurse wants to emphasize to Mara's parents the importance of maintaining Mara's positive self-concept. An indicator of positive self-concept would be

○ 1. eating and drinking restricted foods.

○ 2. taking medications and participating in dressing changes.

○ 3. withdrawing from friends and after-school activities.

○ 4. complaining about headaches, sore throat, and nausea.

**65.** When evaluating Mara's fluid status, the nurse observes that Mara's most recent drain was 500 ml less than the amount instilled. The nurse also notes that Mara complains of abdominal fullness and distention after draining, and that her weight is 0.5 kg more than it was 8 hours ago. Which of the following findings would be the *best* clinical indicator that recovery of dialysate was incomplete?

○ 1. The patient's weight increased 0.5 kg within 8 hours.

○ 2. The patient's activity increased during the last 8 hours.

○ 3. The patient's abdomen appears distended.

○ 4. The patient feels abdominal fullness.

**66.** Before Mara's discharge from the hospital, the nurse plans to discuss psychosocial aspects of going home with a Tenckhoff catheter in place. A topic of *high* priority for the nurse to discuss with Mara would be the

○ 1. effect of having an abdominal catheter on self-concept.

○ 2. importance of relying on parents to do the peritoneal dialysis.

○ 3. advantages of limiting social activities for a few months.

○ 4. advisability of not disclosing information about peritoneal dialysis to people outside the family.

Five-year-old Billy Askhoff has chronic renal failure following vesicoureteral reflux. He has been on intermittent peritoneal dialysis at home for the past year.

**67.** During a routine home visit, the public health nurse assesses the Tenckhoff catheter exit site. Which of the following findings indicates infection at the catheter exit site?

○ 1. Granulation tissue.

○ 2. Tissue swelling.

○ 3. Dialysate leakage.

○ 4. Rebound tenderness.

**68.** The public health nurse reviews the signs and symptoms of peritonitis with Billy's mother. Identification of which of the following findings indicates that Mrs. Askhoff has understood the teaching?

○ 1. Cloudy dialysate drainage returns.

○ 2. A weight gain of 3 pounds in 3 days.

○ 3. Shortness of breath.

○ 4. Distended abdomen.

**69.** If peritonitis were suspected, which of the following nursing interventions would be *most* appropriate?

○ 1. Discontinue the peritoneal dialysis until peritoneal cultures are negative for bacteria.
○ 2. Check the dialysate drains for occult blood.
○ 3. Have the patient increase his intake of clear
liquids until the infection resolves.
○ 4. Notify the physician.

**70.** The public health nurse assesses Billy for edema.
Which of the following findings is associated with
edema?
○ 1. Lower than normal blood pressure.
○ 2. Absence of pulmonary rales.
○ 3. Pallor.
○ 4. Increased dialysis outflow.

**71.** Mrs. Askhoff tells the public health nurse that she
worries about Billy dying: "I haven't been able to
eat or sleep and have lost 10 pounds over the past
month." She has not discussed her concerns with
anyone but her husband. The public health nurse
attributes Mrs. Askhoff's problem to
○ 1. lack of trust.
○ 2. anxiety.
○ 3. inadequate communication skills.
○ 4. overprotectiveness.

**72.** During the public health nurse's next visit, Mrs.
Askhoff tells the nurse that for the past 2 days, it
has taken 30 minutes to fill the peritoneal space
with dialysate and another 30 minutes to drain the
dialysate at the end of a run. These data indicate
which of the following situations?
○ 1. The inflow and drain times are normal.
○ 2. The inflow and drain times are more than twice
normal.
○ 3. The inflow time is normal, but the drain time is
slower than normal.
○ 4. The inflow time is slower than normal, but the
drain time is normal.

**73.** The public health nurse discusses factors that can
affect inflow and drain times with Mrs. Askhoff.
Kinked or blocked tubing can prolong both these
times. Which of the following factors decreases
drain time?
○ 1. Tensing the abdominal muscles.
○ 2. Inflammation of the peritoneal tissue.
○ 3. Catheter exit site infection.
○ 4. Warming the dialysate.

**74.** Which of the following interventions would be
appropriate if inflow and drain times increase?
○ 1. Increase the amount of dialysate infused for
each dwell.
○ 2. Assess the patient for constipation.
○ 3. Incorporate the increased inflow and drain
times into the dialysis schedule.
○ 4. Monitor the patient for shoulder pain during
inflow and drain times.

## THE PATIENT WITH WILMS' TUMOR

Henry Causey, age 3, is admitted to the hospital because Wilms' tumor is suspected. His mother says, "He
has no energy and has just about quit eating."

**75.** When assessing Henry, the nurse could expect to
find which of the following signs?
○ 1. Hypotension.
○ 2. Petechiae.
○ 3. Pallor.
○ 4. Hypothermia.

**76.** Which of the following examining techniques
should the nurse *avoid* when physically examining Henry?
○ 1. Testing his reflex activity.
○ 2. Placing him in an upright position.
○ 3. Palpating his abdomen.
○ 4. Measuring his chest circumference.

**77.** Which of the following diagnostic tests would be
*least* helpful in confirming a diagnosis of Wilms'
tumor?
○ 1. A chest x-ray.
○ 2. Intravenous pyelogram.
○ 3. Ultrasonography.
○ 4. Computerized tomography.

**78.** A diagnosis of Wilms' tumor is confirmed and
Henry is scheduled for a nephrectomy tomorrow morning. In planning preoperative care for
Henry, the nurse would identify which of the following nursing actions as having the *lowest* priority?
○ 1. Monitoring the patient's vital signs frequently.
○ 2. Bathing the patient carefully.
○ 3. Teaching the patient's parents about the staging of Wilms' tumor.
○ 4. Providing the patient's family with emotional
support.

**79.** During surgery, the malignant tumor is classified
as stage II. Based on a knowledge of staging, the
nurse knows that the tumor
○ 1. has metastasized to the lung, liver, bone, and
brain.
○ 2. involves the kidney but is not resectable.
○ 3. is limited to the kidney and is completely
resected.
○ 4. extends beyond the kidney but is completely
resected.

**80.** The left nephrectomy went well and Henry is
returned to his room. In which of the following
positions should the nurse place Henry?
○ 1. Semi-Fowler's.
○ 2. Prone.

○ 3. Supine.

○ 4. Modified Trendelenburg.

**81.** In planning postoperative teaching for Henry's parents, the nurse is aware that the optimum treatment protocol for Wilms' tumor at stage II should include chemotherapy and

○ 1. radiation.

○ 2. bone marrow transplantation.

○ 3. leukapheresis.

○ 4. hyperthermia.

**82.** Based on knowledge of the potential postoperative complication that Henry is *most likely* to develop after abdominal surgery, the nurse should assess him for increased

○ 1. urinary output.

○ 2. blood pressure.

○ 3. bowel sounds.

○ 4. abdominal distention.

**83.** Henry is to receive dactinomycin (Actinomycin-D) and vincristine. The nurse teaches Henry's parents about the side effects of chemotherapy and asks them how many weeks after the initial treatment hair loss usually occurs. Which of the following answers indicates they have understood the teaching?

○ 1. Two weeks.

○ 2. Four weeks.

○ 3. Six weeks.

○ 4. Eight weeks.

**84.** The nursing care plan for discharge would include teaching Henry's parents how to care for him while he is receiving chemotherapy. Given the chemotherapeutic agents that Henry is to receive, it is *most important* that the nurse teach Henry's parents to

○ 1. keep him out of the sun.

○ 2. monitor the color of his urine.

○ 3. encourage him to drink.

○ 4. observe him for drowsiness.

**85.** Additional discharge planning should involve identifying interventions that will prevent damage to the remaining kidney and

○ 1. minimize the severe pain.

○ 2. prevent the development of dependent edema.

○ 3. restrict the dietary intake of protein.

○ 4. prevent urinary tract infection.

# CORRECT ANSWERS AND RATIONALES

Numbers appear in parentheses following the rationales. The numbers identify textbooks listed in the references at the end of Part III, where correct answers can be verified.

## The Patient with Cryptorchidism

1. 2. Testicles should normally descend by the time the infant is 6 weeks old. Testicles that have not descended into the scrotal sac after the infant is 6 weeks old may indicate a problem with the patency of the inguinal canal or a hormonal imbalance. (11)

2. 3. A cold environment can cause the testes to retract. Cold and touch stimulate the cremasteric reflex, which causes normal retraction of the testes. (11)

3. 4. The nurse needs much more information about the father's perceptions and feelings before providing any information or taking any action. It is important to determine the exact nature of the father's concern rather than making an assumption about it. Telling the father not to worry devalues his concern; the testes may not descend spontaneously. (11)

4. 2. An undescended testis is unlikely to produce sperm normally, is usually smaller than one that has descended, and is more prone to develop a malignancy after puberty. A patient with an undescended testis is not more prone to develop epididymitis in adolescence. (7, 21)

5. 1. An inguinal hernia, hydrocele, or upper urinary tract anomaly may occur on the same side as the undescended testis. These three genitourinary conditions are often associated with cryptorchidism. One anomaly in a system warrants a more focused assessment of that system. (7)

6. 4. A trial of human chorionic gonadotrophic hormone (HCG) may be given parenterally to stimulate descent of the affected testis. Cryptorchidism is not treated with growth, adrenocorticotropic, or thyroid hormone. (11)

7. 3. Preschool children must be told what to expect after surgery, because they fear mutilation. The child undergoing an orchiopexy must be told that his body part will not be removed but will be moved to the correct place. Although the child will be unable to see the testis in the scrotum, he will see the tension device attached to his scrotum and leg, so surgery will be evident. (11)

8. 2. In surgery, a rubber band or similar device is attached by a suture to the testis to maintain a moderate, steady tension. Then the rubber band is taped to the inner thigh. This traction device prevents the testis, which is now in the scrotum, from ascending. The traction device is removed 5 to 7 days after surgery. (20)

9. 2. A priority goal at this time is preventing infection at the operative site. Relief of postoperative comfort is achieved collaboratively by the nurse and the parents. Protecting healthy skin surfaces and promoting a positive self-image are important but are not the priority of teaching at this time. (11)

10. 2. Testicular tumors, although rare, occur at least 14 times more frequently in undescended testes than in descended testes. Unless signs and symptoms of hormonal deficiency appear, hormonal levels do not need to be checked. Scrotal scarring after an orchiopexy is usually minimal and plastic surgery is not required. Accumulation of fluid in the scrotum is not a long-term sequela of orchiopexy. (20)

## The Patient with Hydrocele

11. 4. A hydrocele is a collection of fluid in the tunica vaginalis of the testicle or along the spermatic cord. It is caused by failure of the processus vaginalis to be obliterated. In a noncommunicating hydrocele, peritoneal fluid remains within the tunica vaginalis, and the proximal portion of the processus vaginalis has been obliterated. A hydrocele of the spermatic cord may be evident if there has been segmental closure of the processus vaginalis. In a communicating hydrocele, the processus vaginalis is patent and the hydrocele communicates with the peritoneal cavity. (7, 21)

12. 2. A distended hydrocele can be transilluminated. Inguinal hernias can be reduced unless incarcerated (which is a medical emergency); hydroceles cannot be reduced. Hydroceles and hernias can both be either unilateral or bilateral. Scrotal size does not differentiate hydrocele from hernia. (7, 11)

13. 1. Since the fluid is steadily being absorbed, and more fluid is not accumulating, the best treatment is time. The fluid will be absorbed spontaneously. Massage and gravity do little to hasten reabsorption. (11)

14. 1. Slight swelling and bruising are normal postoperatively. The swelling and bruising usually resolve spontaneously without further medical intervention. (21)

**15.** 4. Hydroceles are often associated with inguinal hernia, because the inguinal canal may be involved in a communicating hydrocele (fluid passes up and down the processus vaginalis through the inguinal canal). Inguinal hernias usually develop when a child is 2 to 3 months old. Hydrocele is not associated with bowel obstruction, sterility, or endocrine deficiency and has few, if any, sequelae. (11)

## *The Patient with Hypospadias*

**16.** 2. In hypospadias, the urethra opens on the ventral surface of the penis or the perineum. In congenital chordee, a fibrous band of tissue extends from the scrotum up the penis and pulls it ventrally in an arc; congenital chordee may or may not be associated with hypospadias. In epispadias, the urethra opens on the dorsal surface of the penis. In exstrophy of the bladder, the bladder is turned out and the urethral orifices are visible. (7, 17, 21)

**17.** 4. The foreskin is used to repair the urethra. Circulatory development is unimpaired. Circumcision involves removal of the end of the prepuce of the penis. Chordee necessitates straightening of the penis. Urethral meatal stenosis, which can occur in circumcised infants, is a result of meatal ulceration and can lead to symptoms of urinary obstruction. (7, 17)

**18.** 1. The preferred time for surgery is 6 to 18 months, before the child develops castration and body-image anxiety. Pain is different for each patient and is not related to the preferred time for surgery. Surgical repair will disrupt toilet-training, but this does not affect the preferred time for repair of hypospadias and/or chordee. The reconstructed tissue will grow with the child, regardless of the child's age. (21)

**19.** 3. An alternate urinary elimination route is important because the surgical site needs to be kept dry, clean, and free from the pressure of a full bladder. Pressure from a full bladder might cause urine to leak around the urethral catheter or might disrupt the delicate plastic surgery. The bladder is rarely irrigated. Measuring urinary output and noting the color of the urine are important, but are not the primary purpose for the suprapubic catheter. (7)

**20.** 2. The main purpose of the urethral catheter is to maintain patency of the reconstructed urethra. The catheter prevents the new tissue inside the urethra from healing upon itself, but it can cause bladder spasms. The penis does not have to be completely immobilized. Urinary output can be measured via the suprapubic catheter. (7)

**21.** 1. The penis may appear somewhat misshapen or bumpy because of the intermediate phase of reconstruction. The penis is *not* likely to appear "normal" at this stage. Swelling and some local bruising are normal. Blood supply to the penis should be adequate. (7)

**22.** 4. Having parents comfort the child and administering analgesics are the most effective means of minimizing postoperative pain in a 12-month-old child. Playing with other children and with age-appropriate toys and having adequate rest may contribute to minimizing the pain, but are not the most effective methods. (11)

**23.** 2. It is most important that the catheters not be removed, as this could disrupt the surgical reconstruction. Twelve-month-old infants like to explore their world, so the catheters must be protected. Being held and comforted and playing with favorite toys are appropriate nursing interventions, but are not the most important. (21)

**24.** 2. Handwashing is the most effective infection control measure. Hands should be washed before and after changing diapers, manipulating drainage tubes, and touching the faces and hands of others. (20, 21)

**25.** 4. A white blood cell count of 25 per high-powered field indicates urinary tract infection. Specific gravity ranges from 1.002 to 1.030 and with normal fluid intake is from 1.015 to 1.030. Red blood cells, indicating hematuria, are normal due to urologic surgery. Normal urinary pH is 4.6 to 8. (17, 20, 21)

## *The Patient with a Urinary Tract Infection*

**26.** 3. Abdominal pain frequently accompanies urinary tract infections in young children. Other signs and symptoms of urinary tract infection in young children include decreased appetite, vomiting, fever, and irritability. Flank or back pain is associated with urinary tract infections in older children and adults. A skin rash is unrelated to urinary tract infection, but may indicate an allergy or contagious disease such as measles. (17)

**27.** 4. A clean-voided specimen indicates bacteriuria when the bacterial colony count is more than 100,000/ml. Counts between 10,000 and 100,000 indicate that the test should be repeated, and counts less than 10,000/ml are negative. (11)

**28.** 1. In the presence of bacteria, the urine is usually positive for protein and the pH is more than 8.0 (alkaline). Dark amber-colored urine indicates concentrated urine, not bacteriuria. Urine specific gravity reflects the kidney's ability to concentrate urine. The normal range of urine specific gravity is 1.002 to 1.030. (17, 21)

29. 3. Emptying the bladder frequently and at the first urge to void prevents urinary stasis and reduces the chance that infection will ascend to the kidneys. Increased fluid intake promotes frequent urination, which flushes bacteria out of the urinary tract. Although warm baths may stimulate voiding, bubble baths are irritating to the vulva and urethra. Simply wiping the perineum from front to back after voiding and defecating prevents urethral contamination. (17)

30. 3. A repeat clean-voided urine specimen after 72 hours is cultured to determine the effectiveness of the antibiotic treatment. Antibiotic treatment must be continued for the full 10 days to eliminate the bacteria. The medication does not affect the color of the urine. Adding unpalatable medications to milk or food may change the flavor of the food and cause the patient to dislike a nutritious food. (11)

31. 2. A 3-year-old needs to have psychosocial development maintained as much as possible during illnesses. Family routines and rewards and discipline should be kept as normal as possible. (15)

32. 2. The absence of bacterial growth indicates that the urinary tract infection has been eradicated. The infection could exist in the absence of symptoms such as abdominal pain and irritability. The 10-day course of antibiotic therapy would have eliminated the infection only if the organism were sensitive to that particular antibiotic. (15, 20)

## The Patient With Acute Chronic Glomerulonephritis

33. 4. Oliguria is defined as the subnormal production of urine (less than about 20 ml of urine per hour, or less than about 400 to 600 ml in a 24-hour period). Anuria refers to the total suppression of urine production. Dysuria is painful urination. Enuresis refers to involuntary urination that occurs during sleep. (12, 21)

34. 3. An infection of the throat with streptococci (usually group A betahemolytic streptococci) is usually present in the history of a patient who has acute glomerulonephritis. Much less commonly, infection with pneumococci or varicella viruses have been linked to acute glomerulonephritis. (7, 21)

35. 2. Nocturnal emissions, or wet dreams, occur in about 85% of men. They may occur at any age but usually begin during the teen years. A relatively common misconception is that wet dreams are a sign of a sexual disorder. They do not ensure the presence of sperm and are not a sign of disease. (7, 21)

36. 1. The rate of human growth is complex and varies among individuals. The tempo is uneven and different aspects of growth occur at different rates. Nevertheless, there is an underlying continuous and orderly pattern. Although each individual develops in his or her unique way, certain qualifications can be made concerning all normal human growth. (7, 21)

37. 1. Swelling that occurs below the bandage on an extremity suggests that circulation is poor below the level of the bandage. The bandage is very probably applied too tightly and should be removed to prevent tissue damage. Applying a circular bandage on an extremity while using a figure-of-eight turn, having the knee slightly flexed, and using elasticized bandaging material describe appropriate techniques. (12)

38. 4. Half-strength hydrogen peroxide is most often recommended for cleansing the mouth and lips of crusted mucus, or sordes. The foaming action that results when the hydrogen peroxide releases oxygen and the moisture of the solution act to remove the debris. Hydrogen peroxide should not be used for regular and frequent cleansing of the mouth because repeated exposure to hydrogen peroxide may damage tooth enamel. (12)

39. 1. It is best to serve the patient who has a limited fluid intake ice chips to help prevent thirst. Ice chips help moisten the mouth and lips while keeping the fluid intake low. Salty beverages, such as bouillon, and sweet beverages, such as ginger ale, tend to add to thirst. Tap water is less likely than ice chips to relieve thirst while still maintaining a low fluid intake. (12)

40. 1. The patient described in this item has edema on admission and therefore is most likely to have his sodium intake limited. Ham has a high salt content and would be contraindicated for this patient. The amount of protein in the diet of a patient with acute glomerulonephritis varies and depends on the amount of renal insufficiency and nitrogen retention. Carbohydrates are ordinarily offered in generous amounts to provide energy and decrease the catabolism of protein in the body. (6, 21)

41. 1. Generally, teenagers enjoy activities with their peers in preference to socializing with younger persons and parents. Clannish peer relationships are common and normal during adolescence. They work to help the teenager develop self-identity. (6, 21)

42. 1. A teenager who handles and solves daily prob-

lems with relative ease and seems to have a good idea of where he is going usually is demonstrating a good sense of self-identity. According to the psychologist Erik Erikson, the adolescent is concerned in his psychosocial development with developing self-identity. When this does not occur successfully, the youngster suffers from identity diffusion. An adolescent's success in developing self-identity is not related to intelligence. While poor relationships with parents may have effects on a teenager, his establishing self-identity is not necessarily a result of that type of relationship. The patient described in this item is not demonstrating independence from his family by appearing to develop his self-identity, although teenagers do work normally toward independence from the family. (6, 21)

**43.** 2. Teenagers tend to be moody, concerned with personal appearance, and interested in members of the opposite sex. They are least likely to demonstrate submissive behavior. As they develop self-identity and begin to work toward independence from family ties, they are likely to be assertive and often tend to defy authority as they try to become their own persons. (6, 21)

**44.** 4. Neurologic status should be assessed and seizure precautions instituted because hypertensive encephalopathy is a major potential complication of the acute phase of glomerulonephritis. Hypertensive encephalopathy can result in transient loss of vision and/or hemiparesis, disorientation, and grand mal seizures. Acute cardiac decompensation and acute renal failure are other complications associated with the acute phase of glomerulonephritis. A low-sodium diet is encouraged but is not most important initially. Bed rest is advocated during the acute phase of glomerulonephritis to decrease the glomerular filtration rate. Fluids are restricted in the patient experiencing oliguria. (15, 21)

**45.** 1. Urinary pH, an indication of the renal tubules' ability to maintain normal hydrogen ion concentration in plasma and extracellular fluid, does not need to be measured daily. Glomerulonephritis results in proteinuria. However, the patient should be weighed and intake and output recorded daily. Vital signs, including blood pressure, are recorded every 4 hours. (15, 21)

**46.** 3. No diet restrictions are imposed during convalescence from glomerulonephritis. Fatigue is to be avoided and participation in sports is usually restricted until there is no microscopic evidence of hematuria or proteinuria. Infections of all types are to be avoided. (15, 21)

**47.** 3. Ambulation is usually not restricted. Treatment for chronic glomerulonephritis is appropriate to the underlying disease and is largely symptomatic. Efforts are directed toward optimum conditions for the patient's physical, psychological, and social development. As few restrictions as possible are imposed. The patient is taught measures to prevent infection, intake and output are recorded, and vital signs are monitored routinely. (15, 21)

**48.** 1. Chronic glomerulonephritis (CGN) affects primarily adolescents and includes a variety of different disease processes. Unless accompanied by other diseases, CGN may remain undetected for years. It is relatively asymptomatic until there is marked reduction in renal function due to kidney destruction. CGN may or may not be preceded by several attacks of acute glomerular disease. Renal tubular acidosis, a syndrome of sustained metabolic acidosis, does not herald CGN. (15, 21)

## The Patient with Nephrotic Syndrome

**49.** 4. The blood pressure of a child with nephrotic syndrome is characteristically normal or slightly low. In contrast, the blood pressure of a child with acute glomerulonephritis tends to be mildly to moderately elevated. The other vital signs are likely to be normal, unless edema causes respiratory distress, in which case respirations will tend to be rapid and labored. The temperature and pulse rate can be expected to be elevated if the child has an infection. (21)

**50.** 1. There is altered glomerular permeability in the presence of nephrotic syndrome, which results in the excretion of large amounts of protein in the urine. Normally, the kidneys retain proteins and only wastes are filtered out into the urine. Such signs as retaining red blood cells, excreting urine of a low specific gravity, and retaining albumin in the bloodstream are not associated with nephrotic syndrome. (6, 21)

**51.** 2. The child with nephrotic syndrome gains weight insidiously over a period of days or weeks. The usual course is one of progressive weight gain, until either a rapid or gradual increase in the edema prompts the family to seek medical attention for the child. The volume of urine is decreased, and the urine appears frothy. Edema of the intestinal mucosa may result in loss of appetite and diarrhea. (15, 21)

**52.** 2. The generalized edema associated with nephrotic syndrome develops so slowly that parents may consider it a sign of healthy growth and may not seek medical advice. Thus, when the diagnosis is made, most parents feel guilty. They believe they should have recognized the symptoms earlier and sought advice sooner. (21)

**53.** 3. Diet therapy for a child with nephrotic syndrome tends to be conservative, but most authorities favor at least some salt restriction and a diet high in protein. During periods when the child is edematous, his appetite is poor and he may not tolerate a high-protein diet well. Malnutrition is common because the child is losing large amounts of protein from the urinary system. Therefore, it is particularly important to obtain information from a caretaker concerning the food likes and dislikes of a child with nephrotic syndrome so that as appealing a diet as possible can be offered. Information concerning the child's rest and sleeping habits, elimination pattern, and favorite playtime activities is also important but is not as critical as obtaining the dietary history of a child with nephrotic syndrome. (6, 21)

**54.** 3. Sodium is restricted in the therapeutic management of nephrotic syndrome during periods of massive edema. Food is not salted at the table and all foods with a high sodium content are avoided. Water is seldom restricted but is not encouraged in excess. Fluid intake greater than 500 ml/kg of body weight is excessive. Somatotropic hormone (STH), the growth hormone that promotes growth of bone and soft tissues, is not used in the treatment of nephrotic syndrome. Surgical excision of the diseased glomeruli is not a means of treatment in nephrotic syndrome. (6, 21)

**55.** 3. Admission nursing orders for a child with nephrotic syndrome are most likely to include weighing the patient daily, offering fluids as the child desires, and measuring fluid intake and output. Weighing is done to determine changes in the amount of edema the child has. Most often, fluids are not restricted, but it is important to record the fluid intake and output. Activity for a child with nephrotic syndrome who is edematous is ordinarily not restricted. The child usually is lethargic and lies quietly in bed because of discomfort. Nursing care should then include changing the patient's position and preventing skin breakdown. (6, 21)

**56.** 1. It is best to elevate the head of the bed of a patient with edematous eyelids. The force of gravity tends to increase the downward flow of fluids in the body and away from the face. Such measures as limiting television, irrigating the eyes, and applying cool compresses to the eyes may be comforting but will not reduce the edema. (11)

**57.** 2. The use of prednisone (Deltra) has been found effective for treating many children with nephrotic syndrome. The reason for its effectiveness is not clearly understood, but it is credited with reducing the mortality rate markedly. (6, 21)

**58.** 3. Children with nephrotic syndrome who are sensitive to steroids or have frequent relapses are candidates for therapy with a cytotoxic agent such as cyclophosphamide (Cytoxan). Common side effects include a decrease in the white blood cell count (leukopenia), increased susceptibility to infections, cystitis from bladder irritation when the drug accumulates in the bladder prior to excretion, and possibly hair loss and sterility. Because a child with nephrotic syndrome is susceptible to infections, it is particularly important to monitor the white blood cell count of a patient receiving cyclophosphamide and take necessary precautions to eliminate as many sources of infection from the patient's environment as possible. Cyclophosphamide is an alkylating agent and is also often used in cancer chemotherapy. (6, 16, 21)

**59.** 4. The daily weight record is often the best way to determine the accumulation of fluid. Strict records of intake and output are important, but accuracy may be difficult in young children. Measuring abdominal girth and assessing urine specific gravity provide data about fluid retention but are not the best means of evaluating it. (10, 21)

**60.** 2. A school-aged child with nephrotic syndrome may attend school but should avoid contact with infected playmates. Urine should be tested for albumin, not pH. The physician should be notified about a decrease in urinary output because this could indicate a relapse. Pain is not associated with nephrotic syndrome. (7, 21)

## The Patient with Acute/Chronic Renal Failure

**61.** 4. A person on peritoneal dialysis has few dietary restrictions, whereas a person on hemodialysis usually has fluid and food restrictions. During peritoneal dialysis, plasma proteins, amino acids, and polypeptides diffuse into the dialysate because of the permeability of the peritoneal membrane. Peritoneal dialysis removes the fluid less rapidly than does hemodialysis. Infection is associated with both hemodialysis and peritoneal dialysis. The risk of peritonitis is the major disadvantage of peritoneal dialysis. (15)

**62.** 1. Until healed, the catheter exit site is particularly vulnerable to invasion by pathogenic organisms. Therefore, the site is examined for signs of infection. Holding the catheter taut or pulling on it may cause irritation of the skin at the exit site, which could lead to infection. Site care may be done any time, but the patient may experience abdominal discomfort if the peritoneal space is dry during site care. An occlusive dressing is not needed because there is no danger of air being sucked in or out of the peritoneal space. Furthermore, the catheter used is designed with a cuff, so the skin grows around the catheter. (20)

**63.** 4. With minimal or absent kidney function, serum phosphate levels rise, and the level of ionized calcium falls in response. This causes an increased secretion of parathyroid hormone, which releases calcium from bones. Renal failure results in decreased erythropoietin production, and increased iron intake is needed. Caloric intake needs to be maintained to prevent catabolism of body tissue. Fluid intake is usually not restricted because excess fluid will be removed with dialysate drains. (20)

**64.** 2. Compliance with the medical regime indicates a positive self-image. Social withdrawal from activities may indicate depression. Diffuse somatic complaints could indicate anxiety. (15)

**65.** 1. Increase in weight is the best indicator of unrecovered dialysate. Activity level does not usually change in direct response to incomplete recovery. Abdominal distention and fullness may be due to gastrointestinal factors such as constipation. (15)

**66.** 1. Body image is an important concern to an adolescent, and the patient needs opportunities to discuss feelings about an altered body image. Other developmental needs of an adolescent are increasing appropriate independence and maintaining social activities. The patient may choose to confide in friends for both psychological health and physical safety. (15)

**67.** 2. Tissue swelling, pain, redness, and the presence of exudate indicate infection. Granulation tissue indicates healing around the exit site. Dialysate leakage is associated with improper catheter function, incomplete healing at the insertion site, or excessive instillation of dialysate. Rebound tenderness is a manifestation of peritonitis. (20)

**68.** 1. With peritonitis, large numbers of bacteria, white blood cells, and fibrin cause the dialysate to appear cloudy. A weight increase indicates fluid excess or a gain in true body weight. Shortness of breath is associated with fluid excess. Abdominal distention is unrelated to peritonitis. (11)

**69.** 4. The nurse notifies the physician so that a change in medical management can be made. A sample of peritoneal fluid is sent for culture and sensitivity. The results indicate those antibiotics effective against the causative agent. Discontinuing perito-

neal dialysis promotes infection and also leads to fluid and electrolyte imbalances. Dialysate positive for occult blood is not associated with peritonitis. Adequate nutrition is important during an infectious process. Peritonitis can cause an ileus; therefore, fluid intake is not increased. (7, 21)

**70.** 3. In the presence of edema, pallor can occur due to hemodilution. Other indications of edema include a higher than normal blood pressure, pulmonary rales, and decreased dialysate outflow. (11)

**71.** 2. The weight loss, the inability to sleep, and the worrying indicate anxiety. Discussion of the problem with the public health nurse and husband indicates trust and adequate communication skills. There is no evidence of overprotectiveness (that is, keeping the child from age-appropriate activities and expectations). (15)

**72.** 2. Normal inflow and drain times are about 10 minutes each. (11)

**73.** 1. Tensing the abdominal muscles decreases drain time. Peritonitis and catheter exit site infection do not affect flow of the dialysate. Warming the dialysate to body temperature promotes patient comfort and prevents abdominal pain. It does not affect drain time. (11)

**74.** 2. The accumulation of hard stool in the bowel can cause the distended intestine to block the holes of the catheter. Consequently, the dialysate cannot flow freely through the catheter. Increasing the amount of dialysate infused can cause pain and possible leakage at the exit site. Adjusting the dialysis schedule to accommodate the increased inflow and drain times may make the dialysis less effective. Altering the fluid, electrolytes, and waste products removed can cause fluid and electrolyte imbalances and elevated blood urea nitrogen (BUN) and creatinine levels. Shoulder pain can be caused by air in the peritoneal space and diaphragmatic irritation. (8, 11)

## *The Patient with Wilms' Tumor*

**75.** 3. Wilms' tumor, or nephroblastoma, is the most common type of intra-abdominal tumor of childhood. It is the most common type of renal cancer and is highly malignant. Anemia, which is secondary to hemorrhage within the tumor, results in pallor, anorexia, and lethargy. The most common presenting sign of Wilms' tumor is swelling of the abdominal mass. Other signs and symptoms are the result of compression from the tumor mass, metabolic alterations secondary to the tumor, or metastasis. Hypertension occurs occasionally and is probably the result of excess excretion of renin by the tumor. Other effects of malignancy include weight loss and fever. Petechiae are not associated with Wilms' tumor. (15, 21)

**76.** 3. The abdomen of a child with Wilms' tumor should not be palpated because of the danger of disseminating tumor cells. Techniques such as testing for reflex activity, upright positioning, and measuring chest circumference are not necessarily contraindicated. However, a child with Wilms' tumor should be handled gently and carefully. (15, 21)

**77.** 1. A chest x-ray is done to determine pulmonary metastasis at the time of diagnosis. In a child suspected of having Wilms' tumor, an intravenous pyelogram, ultrasonography, and computerized tomography are done to determine the tumor's position, size, and relationship to the involved kidney and to assess the status of the uninvolved kidney. (10, 21)

**78.** 3. Teaching the parents about the staging of Wilms' tumor has the lowest priority because staging is done at the time of diagnosis. Preoperative explanations should be kept simple and should focus on what the child will experience. Vital signs, including blood pressure, must be monitored frequently because hypertension from excess renin production is possible. Careful bathing and handling are essential to prevent trauma to the tumor. As with all diagnoses of cancer, Wilms' tumor is a shock to the family. The parents may feel guilty for not finding the mass sooner, and with the swiftness of the diagnosis will need emotional support. (15, 21)

**79.** 4. A stage II tumor extends beyond the kidney but is completely resected. The tumor is staged during surgery to maximize treatment protocols. The following criteria for staging are most commonly used:
*Stage I:* Tumor is limited to kidney and completely resected.
*Stage II:* Tumor extends beyond the kidney but is completely resected.
*Stage III:* Residual nonhematogenous tumor is confined to abdomen.
*Stage IV:* Hematogenous metastases; deposits be-

yond stage III, namely to lung, liver, bone, and brain.
*Stage V:* Bilateral renal involvement is present at diagnosis. (15, 21)

**80.** 1. The patient who has had abdominal surgery is usually placed in a semi-Fowler's position to facilitate draining of abdominal contents and to promote pulmonary expansion. The prone position is likely to be uncomfortable because of the large transabdominal incision. The supine position, without the head elevated, can cause aspiration. The modified Trendelenburg position is used for patients in shock. (15, 21)

**81.** 1. The optimum treatment protocol for Wilms' tumor at stage II is abdominal radiation and chemotherapy. Postoperative radiotherapy is indicated for all children with Wilms' tumor except those with stage I disease and favorable histology. Chemotherapy is indicated for all stages. (15, 21)

**82.** 4. A postoperative complication for which children with abdominal surgery are at risk is intestinal obstruction from adynamic ileus. Indications of intestinal obstruction include abdominal distention, decreased or absent bowel sounds, and vomiting. Later signs of intestinal obstruction include tachycardia, fever, hypotension, or shock, with decreased urinary output. (10, 21)

**83.** 1. Hair loss or alopecia does not occur until 2 weeks after the initial chemotherapy treatment. Chemotherapy for Wilms' tumor is begun immediately after surgery. (21)

**84.** 3. Dactinomycin (Actinomycin-D) and vincristine both cause nausea and vomiting. Oral fluids are encouraged and antiemetics are given to prevent dehydration. It is unnecessary to avoid exposure to the sun. Drowsiness and changes in urine color are not associated with dactinomycin or vincristine. (15, 21)

**85.** 4. Because the child has only one kidney, measures are recommended to prevent urinary tract infection and injury to the remaining kidney. Severe pain and dependent edema are not associated with postoperative Wilms' tumor patients. Dietary protein is not restricted because function in the remaining kidney is not impaired. (15, 21)

# test 7

*The Patient with Myelomeningocele*
*The Patient with Hydrocephalus*
*The Patient with a Seizure Disorder*
*The Patient with Meningitis*
*The Patient with Reye Syndrome*
*The Patient with Infectious Polyneuritis*
*(Guillain-Barré Syndrome)*
*The Patient with a Head Injury*
*The Patient with a Brain Tumor*
*The Patient with a Spinal Cord Injury*
*Correct Answers and Rationales*

Select the one *best* or *correct* answer and indicate your choice by filling in the circle with a pencil in front of the option you have chosen. If the answer you would prefer is not given, select the one you think is *most appropriate*.

## THE PATIENT WITH MYELOMENINGOCELE

Myles O'Donovan is admitted to the neonatal unit following delivery and is placed in an isolette. He has a 3 cm × 5 cm sac in the lumbar area of his back. His diagnosis is upper lumbar myelomeningocele.

**1.** A myelomeningocele can *most accurately* be described as
○ 1. a soft sac containing spinal fluid, meninges, spinal cord, and/or nerve roots protruding through a bony defect in the spine.
○ 2. a soft sac containing spinal fluid and meninges located anywhere on the spine.
○ 3. a skin-covered sac containing bits of hair located on the low lumbar or sacral area of the spine.
○ 4. a cyst containing serosanguineous fluid and fatty tissue located on any area of the spinal column.

**2.** Given the clinical manifestations associated with upper lumbar myelomeningocele, which of the following would the nurse anticipate finding when assessing Myles?
○ 1. Minimal movement of the lower extremities and dribbling of urine.
○ 2. Paralysis of the lower extremities and rectal prolapse.
○ 3. Minimal movement of the lower extremities and dribbling of urine and feces.
○ 4. Paralysis of the upper and lower extremities and dribbling of feces.

**3.** The doctor tells Mr. and Mrs. O'Donovan that their infant has a myelomeningocele. The nurse arranges for them to see Myles as soon as possible.

While they are looking at Myles for the first time, the nurse should *initially*
○ 1. reinforce the doctor's explanation of the defect.
○ 2. emphasize his normal and positive features.
○ 3. tell them they can hold him in a few minutes.
○ 4. encourage them to discuss their fears and concerns.

**4.** Mrs. O'Donovan asks if infants with myelomeningocele, like Myles, are likely to have other defects. The nurse bases her answer on the fact that myelomeningocele is frequently associated with
○ 1. microcephaly.
○ 2. anencephaly.
○ 3. hydrocephalus.
○ 4. craniosynostosis.

**5.** The parents ask the nurse if Myles will be retarded. What would be the nurse's *best* response?
○ 1. "Most infants with myelomeningocele are significantly retarded."
○ 2. "Probably not, because he is very alert now."
○ 3. "Approximately one-third are mentally retarded, but it is too early to tell."
○ 4. "You will need to talk with the physician about that later."

**6.** Myles is experiencing urinary retention with overflow incontinence. Which of the following nursing interventions would be *most appropriate* to facilitate emptying the bladder?
○ 1. Insert an indwelling urethral catheter.
○ 2. Initiate an intermittent clean catheterization program.
○ 3. Apply gentle pressure to the suprapubic area.
○ 4. Perform a suprapubic aspiration.

**7.** Myles is scheduled for corrective surgery tomorrow. Until then, nursing care of the sac would include

○ 1. covering it with moist, sterile saline dressings.
○ 2. leaving it exposed to the air.
○ 3. covering it with a dry, nonadherent dressing.
○ 4. applying thin layers of tincture of benzoin.

**8.** A nursing goal is to protect the sac from pressure and potential infection prior to closure. In order to achieve this goal, in what position would it be *best* for the nurse to position Myles?
○ 1. Supine, with the upper body slightly elevated.
○ 2. Low Trendelenburg, with the hips slightly flexed.
○ 3. Side-lying, with support behind the sac.
○ 4. Prone, with slight elevation of the lower extremities.

**9.** At 36 hours of age, Myles undergoes surgery to close the sac. He tolerates the procedure well, but postoperatively has shown no movement in his lower legs. To prevent musculoskeletal deformity, the postoperative nursing care plan should include which of the following interventions?
○ 1. Perform passive range-of-motion exercises to the legs.
○ 2. Maintain the feet in a flexed position.
○ 3. Maintain the legs in an adducted position.
○ 4. Maintain the hips in moderate adduction.

**10.** Postoperatively, the nurse monitors Myles' vital signs frequently and assesses him for clinical manifestations of hydrocephalus. The *earliest* signs and symptoms of hydrocephalus in the infant are
○ 1. frontal bossing and sunset eyes.
○ 2. increasing head circumference and bulging fontanels.
○ 3. irritability and shrill cry.
○ 4. distended scalp veins and vomiting.

**11.** Because of increasing hydrocephalus and increasing intracranial pressure, 7-day-old Myles undergoes surgery for placement of a ventriculoperitoneal shunt. Nursing care of Myles postoperatively should include
○ 1. checking the urine for glucose and ketones.
○ 2. administering narcotics to control postoperative pain.
○ 3. testing cerebral fluid leakage for the presence of protein.
○ 4. monitoring for manifestations of cerebrospinal fluid infection.

**12.** To facilitate positive family functioning and child development, the nurse would help the family
○ 1. identify facilities for future residential placement of their child.
○ 2. find a local support group such as the Spina Bifida Association of America.

○ 3. identify financial resources to help with the medical expenses.
○ 4. find a counselor or psychologist for ongoing therapy.

**13.** The nurse has been preparing Mr. and Mrs. O'Donovan for Myles' discharge home. Which of the following statements indicates that they have understood the teaching?
○ 1. "We will apply a heating pad to his lower back."
○ 2. "We will prevent him from rolling over."
○ 3. "We will keep him away from other children."
○ 4. "We will notify the doctor if the urine has a bad odor."

## ●THE PATIENT WITH HYDROCEPHALUS

Mrs. Sharmet has taken her 6-week-old son Matthew for a well child visit.

**14.** The nurse weighs Matthew and measures his length, head circumference, and chest circumference. His weight, length, and chest circumference are all at the 50th percentile for his age, and his head circumference is at the 85th percentile. What should the nurse do?
○ 1. Have him return in 1 month for follow-up.
○ 2. Examine his fontanels and sutures.
○ 3. Assess the motor and sensory function of his legs.
○ 4. Obtain a signed consent for transillumination.

**15.** Matthew is admitted to the hospital, and following diagnostic evaluation a diagnosis of aqueductal stenosis is made. What type of hydrocephalus is caused by blockage of the aqueduct of Sylvius?
○ 1. Communicating.
○ 2. Extraventricular.
○ 3. Noncommunicating.
○ 4. Subarachnoid.

**16.** Matthew is to have a ventriculoperitoneal shunt placed to relieve the hydrocephalus. Preoperatively, Matthew is irritable, lethargic, and difficult to feed. The *best* way to maintain his nutrition is to
○ 1. leave him flat in the crib while feeding him.
○ 2. feed him just before doing procedures.
○ 3. schedule his feedings for every 6 hours.
○ 4. give him small feedings every 3 hours.

**17.** Mrs. Sharmet asks the nurse if Matthew will have any long-term problems because of the hydrocephalus. The nurse would explain that

○ 1. Matthew should do very well and will have normal intelligence.

○ 2. Matthew will have some sensory and motor deficits.

○ 3. it is impossible to predict Matthew's outcome at this point.

○ 4. the physician can answer this question after the shunt has been placed.

18. Surgery is performed and a ventriculoperitoneal shunt is inserted on the right side. Immediately postoperatively, the nurse should position Matthew on his

○ 1. left side, with the foot of the crib elevated.

○ 2. back, with the head of the crib elevated.

○ 3. back, with the head of the crib flat.

○ 4. right side, with the head of the crib elevated.

19. Two days after surgery, Matthew shows signs of increasing intracranial pressure. The physician asks the nurse to compress the valve of the shunt. A valve that depresses easily but does not refill indicates

○ 1. a properly functioning shunt.

○ 2. blockage of the ventricular catheter.

○ 3. blockage of the distal end of the catheter.

○ 4. reverse flow of cerebrospinal fluid through the catheter.

20. When preparing Matthew's parents for home care, the nurse teaches them to watch for signs that indicate obstruction of the shunt. These signs are the same as those seen with

○ 1. bacterial or viral meningitis.

○ 2. increased intracranial pressure.

○ 3. spinal cord shock.

○ 4. Reye syndrome.

21. The parents also need to know the signs of an infected shunt. These signs are the same as those seen with

○ 1. bacterial or viral meningitis.

○ 2. increased intracranial pressure.

○ 3. spinal cord shock.

○ 4. Reye syndrome.

22. Matthew is the Sharmets' first child and they talk with the nurse about having other children. They ask if their other children could have the same problem. The nurse bases her response on the knowledge that

○ 1. the probability of their having a second child with hydrocephalus is very unlikely.

○ 2. their children would have an increased risk of hydrocephalus.

○ 3. their male children would be at increased risk of hydrocephalus.

○ 4. the probability of their children and grandchildren developing hydrocephalus is high.

## THE PATIENT WITH A SEIZURE DISORDER

Gary Young, age 7, experienced a generalized tonic-clonic (grand mal) seizure at school. Gary has no history of seizure disorders or of any other chronic health problems.

23. The school nurse is called to Gary's classroom and arrives when Gary is still in the clonic phase of the seizure. The nurse's *first* priority is to

○ 1. have the other children leave the room.

○ 2. move furniture and other objects out of the way.

○ 3. obtain a description of the events preceding the seizure.

○ 4. place a padded tongue blade between Gary's teeth.

24. Immediately following the seizure, the school nurse notices that Gary has been incontinent of urine and is very difficult to arouse. Based on this information, the nurse would

○ 1. perform a complete neurologic check every 3 to 5 minutes.

○ 2. awaken him every 3 to 5 minutes in order to assess his mentation.

○ 3. ask the teacher if Gary has had previous problems with urinary incontinence.

○ 4. place him on his side, stay with him, and allow him to sleep.

25. Gary is hospitalized for a diagnostic workup. The physician orders phenobarbital (Luminal) for Gary. What pharmacologic action of this drug makes it useful in treating seizures?

○ 1. It increases neuronal activity.

○ 2. It lowers the seizure threshold.

○ 3. It raises the seizure threshold.

○ 4. It stimulates hepatic microsomal enzymes.

26. Gary continues to experience generalized seizures while in the hospital, and he is started on a second anticonvulsant, phenytoin sodium (Dilantin). Mrs. Young asks the nurse why the phenobarbital (Luminal) is still being given since it was ineffective. The nurse's response should be based on which of the following facts?

○ 1. Phenytoin sodium controls seizures most effectively when given with phenobarbital.

○ 2. Phenobarbital is least useful in combination with other drugs.

○ 3. The usual protocol for seizure control is to use only one drug at a time.

○ 4. When one drug alone does not control seizures, then a second drug is added.

27. Gary is unable to swallow the phenytoin sodium (Dilantin) capsules and does not like the chewable form of the medication. Mrs. Young asks if he could have a liquid form of the medication. What fact should form the basis for the nurse's response?
    - ○ 1. Phenytoin sodium loses its potency when mixed with liquids.
    - ○ 2. A person Gary's age should learn to swallow capsules.
    - ○ 3. Inaccurate dosage can occur with the liquid suspension form of phenytoin sodium.
    - ○ 4. Liquid suspensions of phenytoin sodium discolor the teeth.

28. When teaching Gary and his family about long-term care, the nurse should emphasize that Gary
    - ○ 1. should never abruptly stop taking his medication.
    - ○ 2. will need to take the medication for the rest of his life.
    - ○ 3. should cut back on his medications when side effects occur.
    - ○ 4. will need less medication as he becomes older.

29. Which of the following statements made by Mrs. Young indicates that she understands Gary's medication therapy?
    - ○ 1. "I should make sure that he takes his medication every other day."
    - ○ 2. "I should not give him other medications without asking the doctor."
    - ○ 3. "I should not worry about giving him his medication if he is vomiting."
    - ○ 4. "I should call to refill the prescriptions as soon as the bottles are empty."

30. Mr. and Mrs. Young ask the nurse what they should do if Gary has a seizure at home. What is the *most appropriate* response for the nurse to make?
    - ○ 1. Tilt his neck forward so that his tongue will not fall back.
    - ○ 2. Restrain his arms and legs so he will not hurt himself.
    - ○ 3. Stay with him during the seizure and after it is over.
    - ○ 4. Try to get him to swallow an extra dose of the phenobarbital.

31. Mr. and Mrs. Young are concerned that Gary will not be able to keep up in school. In helping the Youngs plan for Gary's return to school, the nurse should advise them that children with seizure disorders
    - ○ 1. are physically impaired and benefit from attending a school for handicapped children.
    - ○ 2. most frequently have normal intelligence and can attend regular school.
    - ○ 3. suffer from social stigma and should not attend public school.
    - ○ 4. have a learning disability and need tutoring to help them reach their grade level.

32. When Gary is 9 years old, he still has occasional generalized seizures. His parents want to know whether he can attend summer camp. The nurse explains that he can attend summer camp but should *avoid*
    - ○ 1. archery.
    - ○ 2. tennis.
    - ○ 3. horseback riding.
    - ○ 4. hiking.

Two-year-old Ashwin Patel has a simple generalized seizure that is tentatively diagnosed as a febrile seizure. He is hospitalized for diagnostic workup and treatment.

33. Which of the following statements from Ashwin's nursing history would be indicative of febrile seizures?
    - ○ 1. The patient's family history is negative for febrile convulsions.
    - ○ 2. The patient has had a low-grade fever for several weeks.
    - ○ 3. The seizure lasted more than 20 minutes.
    - ○ 4. The seizure occurred when the patient had an upper respiratory infection.

34. Phenobarbital (Luminal) and antibiotics are administered for several days, but Ashwin is to be discharged home with only antibiotic therapy. Mrs. Patel asks the nurse if Ashwin should be on continuous anticonvulsant drugs. The nurse should base her response on the fact that children who have febrile seizures
    - ○ 1. do not usually need long-term anticonvulsant therapy.
    - ○ 2. need long-term anticonvulsant therapy.
    - ○ 3. need anticonvulsants only when they have upper respiratory infections or tonsillitis.
    - ○ 4. need anticonvulsants if the seizures lasted less than 15 minutes.

35. Mrs. Patel tells the nurse she is concerned that Ashwin will be intellectually or neurologically impaired because of the seizure. Which of the following responses is *most appropriate* for the nurse to make?
    - ○ 1. "It will not be possible to assess Ashwin's intelligence until he is older."
    - ○ 2. "Ashwin may well have some neurologic impairment, so closely observe the development of his motor skills."

3. "It would be a good idea to have Ashwin evaluated for neurologic impairment yearly."
4. "The probability of Ashwin having any impairments is very slight."

36. A 16-year-old girl who has a seizure disorder that is controlled with phenytoin sodium (Dilantin) and carbamazepine (Tegretol) asks the nurse about getting married and having children. Which of the following statements would be accurate for the nurse to make?
1. "Your children will have no increased risk of seizure disorders."
2. "It is best not to consider having children until your seizures are cured."
3. "Women who have seizure disorders have a difficult time conceiving."
4. "When you decide to have children, ask your physician to change your medication."

37. When administering phenytoin sodium (Dilantin) intravenously to a child with status epilepticus, the nurse gives the drug slowly. This is essential because the drug can cause
1. cardiotoxicity
2. hepatotoxicity.
3. venous irritation.
4. hyperglycemia.

## THE PATIENT WITH MENINGITIS

Four-year-old Laura Lopez is brought to the hospital by her parents. Her temperature is 39° C, and a diagnosis of meningitis is suspected.

38. When measured on the Fahrenheit scale, Laura's temperature of 39° C is equivalent to
1. 101.3° F.
2. 102.2° F.
3. 103.1° F.
4. 104.0° F.

39. The nurse weighs Laura when she is admitted to the hospital. The *primary* reason for weighing Laura is to help
1. calculate drug doses for the patient.
2. evaluate the patient's nutritional status.
3. estimate whether the patient is edematous.
4. determine the patient's developmental status.

40. During the neurologic examination, the nurse notes that Laura's Kernig's sign is positive. Which of the following responses to stimuli indicates a *positive* Kernig's sign?
1. A loud noise causes extension followed by flexion of the arms.

2. Passive flexion of the neck causes bending of the hips and knees.
3. The large toe extends and the other toes fan when the bottom of the foot is stroked.
4. Straightening of the legs at the knees is met with resistance when the hip and leg are flexed.

41. The nurse is to administer an intravenous infusion to Laura. Approximately how many drops per minute of solution should Laura receive if 500 ml of intravenous solution is to be infused over a 12-hour period when the drop factor is 60 drops per ml?
1. 32 drops.
2. 42 drops.
3. 52 drops.
4. 62 drops.

42. Laura is restless and irritable during the acute stage of her illness. Which of the following nursing measures should assume *top priority* at this time?
1. Omit bathing the patient.
2. Limit conversation with the patient.
3. Perform the patient's treatments as quickly as possible.
4. Keep extraneous noise in the patient's room at a minimum.

43. The nurse observes Laura for signs of increased intracranial pressure. In addition to a change in level of consciousness, a sign of increased intracranial pressure is
1. dyspnea.
2. deafness.
3. seizure activity.
4. an unusually rapid pulse rate.

44. Which of the following nursing observations would help *most* to assist in determining that Laura has developed disseminated intravascular coagulation (DIC)?
1. The patient is cyanotic.
2. The patient has swollen glands.
3. The patient is dyspneic on exertion.
4. The patient has a hemorrhagic skin rash.

45. Laura is found to have pneumococcal meningitis. Which of the following illnesses *most often* predisposes a person to this type of meningitis?
1. Mumps.
2. Septic arthritis.
3. A bladder infection.
4. A middle-ear infection.

46. When discontinuing Laura's intravenous therapy, the nurse allows her to apply a dressing to the area where the needle is removed. The nurse bases her action on knowledge that Laura has a need to
1. find more diversional activities.

○ 2. protect her image of an intact body.

○ 3. relieve the anxiety of separation from her home.

○ 4. enhance her confidence in personnel caring for her.

47. Laura recuperates and is readied for discharge. She becomes angry when she cannot go home on the planned day. Which of the following play activities will help Laura *most* to relieve pent-up hostilities?

○ 1. Stacking blocks.

○ 2. Pounding a peg board.

○ 3. Painting with watercolors.

○ 4. Having a story read aloud to her.

48. The nurse has previously cared for a child of Laura's age who had viral meningitis. An infectious disease that *most commonly* predisposes a person to viral meningitis is

○ 1. mumps.

○ 2. hepatitis.

○ 3. chicken pox.

○ 4. whooping cough.

## THE PATIENT WITH REYE SYNDROME

Jessica, age 11, is admitted to the pediatric intensive care unit with a tentative diagnosis of Reye syndrome. Two days ago she developed severe and persistent vomiting and diarrhea and complained of increasing fatigue. Now she is combative. Her pulse and respiratory rates are elevated and she has a fever.

49. Jessica's mother tells the nurse all of the following facts. Which fact is associated with Reye syndrome?

○ 1. Jessica's brother had a streptococcal infection 2 weeks ago.

○ 2. Jessica had an upper respiratory tract infection 1 week ago.

○ 3. Jessica spent 2 weeks at summer camp a month ago.

○ 4. Jessica is allergic to both penicillin and tetracycline.

50. Results of laboratory studies confirm a diagnosis of Reye syndrome. Given this diagnosis and Jessica's signs and symptoms, interventions are aimed *primarily* at preventing

○ 1. grand mal seizures.

○ 2. central nervous system damage.

○ 3. fluid and electrolyte imbalances.

○ 4. fatty infiltration of the liver.

51. The nurse assesses Jessica's neurologic status and vital signs frequently. In addition, she carefully monitors the infusion rate of the 10% glucose solution and records output from the Foley catheter and nasogastric tube. When the nurse observes that Jessica's response to pain is decorticate posturing, what would be her *priority* action?

○ 1. Increase the infusion rate.

○ 2. Decrease the infusion rate.

○ 3. Notify the physician.

○ 4. Check the pupillary responses.

52. In what position should the nurse place Jessica?

○ 1. Side-lying with the head of the bed flat.

○ 2. Supine with the head of the bed flat.

○ 3. Left side-lying with the head of the bed elevated 45°.

○ 4. Supine with the head of the bed elevated 30°.

53. The nurse explains Jessica's care to her parents. The care plan contains the following intervention: "Speak softly to Jessica and keep her environment quiet and dimly lit." Jessica's parents ask the nurse why this is necessary. The nurse would explain that

○ 1. excessive noise or light may cause agitation.

○ 2. sensitivity to light is a common problem with Reye syndrome.

○ 3. the nurses need to be able to assess the patient's ability to hear.

○ 4. the room must be dimly lit in order to be able to do neurologic checks.

54. Jessica's condition stabilizes and begins to improve. During this time, her parents tell the nurse that they feel guilty because they did not bring Jessica to the hospital sooner. Which of the responses would be *most appropriate* for the nurse to make?

○ 1. "I can understand why you would feel guilty about her getting so sick, but Reye syndrome comes on quickly."

○ 2. "You had no way of knowing that Reye syndrome is a medical emergency."

○ 3. "Tell me more about your feeling guilty."

○ 4. "You really shouldn't feel guilty, because she's going to be all right."

55. Jessica's parents are concerned that her 15-year-old brother will also contract Reye syndrome. On which of the following facts should the nurse base her response?

○ 1. The period of communicability for Reye syndrome is 10 to 14 days.

○ 2. Siblings do have an increased risk for developing Reye syndrome.

○ 3. Fifteen-year-olds are unlikely to contract Reye syndrome.

○ 4. There is an association between Reye syndrome and the use of acetaminophen (Tylenol).

# THE PATIENT WITH INFECTIOUS POLYNEURITIS (GUILLAIN-BARRÉ SYNDROME)

Theresa Box, age 5, has had progressive pain and weakness in her feet and legs for 2 days. She is admitted to the hospital with the diagnosis of infectious polyneuritis or Guillain-Barré syndrome.

**56.** During the first 2 days of hospitalization, Theresa develops motor paralysis of her legs. While assessing her, the nurse asks Theresa, who is lying in bed, to squeeze her hands and to raise her arms and legs as high as she can. The purpose of these requests is to

○ 1. assess the patient's ability to follow simple commands.

○ 2. evaluate the patient's bilateral muscle strength.

○ 3. make the patient's range-of-motion exercises into a game.

○ 4. provide the patient with a diversional activity.

**57.** Both the volume and clarity of Theresa's speech decreases and she has difficulty coughing voluntarily. The nurse reports these changes to the physician because they indicate that Theresa is

○ 1. entering a serious phase of separation anxiety.

○ 2. experiencing an increase in intracranial pressure.

○ 3. experiencing involvement of facial and cranial nerves.

○ 4. regressing to an earlier developmental level.

**58.** The nurse establishes goals for Theresa's nursing care during the acute phase of Guillain-Barré syndrome. The *first* priority would be to

○ 1. maintain adequate respiratory function.

○ 2. promote skin integrity.

○ 3. reduce anxiety.

○ 4. maintain mobility of joints in the affected limbs.

**59.** Theresa is transferred to the pediatric intensive care unit, where she rapidly develops respiratory paralysis. She is intubated and placed on mechanical ventilation. Intravenous therapy and nasogastric tube feedings are started. In addition, Theresa is attached to a cardiac monitor. The rationale for use of the cardiac monitor is that patients with Guillain-Barré syndrome can experience

○ 1. autonomic dysfunction.

○ 2. brain stem edema.

○ 3. hypokalemia.

○ 4. hypoglycemia.

**60.** While being mechanically ventilated, Theresa should be

○ 1. receiving vigorous passive range-of-motion exercises to prevent loss of muscle function in the extremities.

○ 2. maintained in a supine position to prevent unnecessary nerve stimulation.

○ 3. moved to a bedside chair twice a day to prevent orthostatic hypotension.

○ 4. turned slowly and gently from side to side to prevent respiratory complications.

**61.** After 6 days, Theresa is successfully weaned from the ventilator but continues to receive nasogastric tube feedings. Her parents ask the nurse when Theresa will be able to eat normally. Which of the following observations would indicate that Theresa is ready for oral feedings?

○ 1. The patient moves her hands to her mouth.

○ 2. The patient can sit up in a chair without help.

○ 3. The patient gags when the nasogastric tube is repositioned.

○ 4. The patient tells her parents that she is hungry.

**62.** After several weeks, Theresa is transferred from the intensive care unit to the general pediatric unit. The nurse develops a discharge plan for Theresa with her parents. Which of the following interventions would be appropriate for the nurse to include in the discharge plan?

○ 1. Develop a rehabilitation plan that includes orthopedic care.

○ 2. Limit the patient's contact with peers until she has fully recovered.

○ 3. Locate a school for handicapped children in the patient's neighborhood.

○ 4. Have the patient return to her kindergarten class immediately.

**63.** Theresa refuses to do her arm exercises. Which of the following nursing actions would be *most appropriate* to implement?

○ 1. Give the patient ice cream if she promises to do her exercises.

○ 2. Have the patient color or read her a favorite story before having her do her exercises.

○ 3. Play a game of catch with the patient with a large ball.

○ 4. Have the patient watch her peers while they exercise.

## THE PATIENT WITH A HEAD INJURY

Eight-year-old Johnny Selwyn was hit by a car while riding his bicycle. He was unconscious at the scene of the accident and was taken to the hospital emergency department.

**64.** Upon Johnny's arrival at the hospital, the nurse's *first* priority in caring for Johnny would be to
○ 1. assess his neurologic status.
○ 2. determine the presence of abdominal injuries.
○ 3. establish ventilation.
○ 4. establish intravenous access.

**65.** A diagnosis of closed head injury is made and Johnny is admitted to the intensive care unit. In what position is it *best* for the nurse to place Johnny?
○ 1. Flat on his right side.
○ 2. Flat on his left side.
○ 3. Prone with his head turned to the right.
○ 4. Supine with his head elevated 30°.

**66.** The nurse evaluates Johnny's neurologic status using the Glasgow coma scale. She observes and records his eye opening response to stimuli. Lack of response to which of the following stimuli would yield the *lowest* or *least* desirable score?
○ 1. Having his arm moved.
○ 2. Having his mother stroke his face.
○ 3. Having the nurse speak to him.
○ 4. Having an IV started.

**67.** Johnny's admission orders include insertion of a nasogastric tube. The purpose of inserting a naso-gastric tube *at this time* would be to
○ 1. provide adequate nutrition.
○ 2. administer medications.
○ 3. obtain gastric specimens for analysis.
○ 4. decompress the stomach.

**68.** Although comatose, Johnny is breathing on his own. He has an endotracheal tube in place to ensure a patent airway. The nurse evaluates his vital signs and neurologic status every half hour. When assessing the size and reactivity of Johnny's pupils, the nurse is evaluating the function of the
○ 1. cerebral cortex.
○ 2. cerebellum.
○ 3. third cranial nerve.
○ 4. brain stem.

**69.** Johnny is to receive dexamethasone (Decadron) intravenously. He is to receive 7.2 mg and the drug comes in a vial containing 4 mg per ml. What volume of the drug contains 7.2 mg?
○ 1. 0.4 ml.
○ 2. 0.72 ml.
○ 3. 1.8 ml.
○ 4. 7.2 ml.

**70.** Johnny's parents ask the nurse if Johnny is going to be all right. Which of the following responses would be *most* appropriate for the nurse to make?
○ 1. "Children usually don't do very well after head injuries like this."
○ 2. "I'm sure he will be fine; children can recover rapidly from head injuries."
○ 3. "It's hard to tell this early, but we'll keep you informed of his progress."
○ 4. "That's something you'll have to talk to the doctors about."

**71.** Johnny is coming out of the coma. He is restless, irritable, and confused about where he is. What is the nurse's *priority* action when he begins pulling at the endotracheal and nasogastric tubes?
○ 1. Ask his parents to leave.
○ 2. Encourage his parents to stay.
○ 3. Restrain all four extremities.
○ 4. Apply a chest restraint.

**72.** As Johnny's level of consciousness improves, the nurse involves Johnny's parents in his care. This is important *primarily* because it enables the nurse to
○ 1. involve them in discharge planning.
○ 2. evaluate their coping strategies.
○ 3. remind them to care for their own health.
○ 4. teach them the basics of child safety.

## THE PATIENT WITH A BRAIN TUMOR

Cindy Thomas, age 8, has been going to the school nurse frequently with complaints of nausea, headaches, and difficulty seeing.

**73.** When interviewing Cindy, the school nurse observes that Cindy tilts her head to one side and has a wide-based gait when walking. The nurse decides to talk with the Thomases about Cindy's behavior. The *best* reason for making this decision is that Cindy shows signs of
○ 1. a brain tumor.
○ 2. Reye syndrome.
○ 3. school phobia.
○ 4. a seizure disorder.

**74.** After being examined by her physician, Cindy is hospitalized for possible infratentorial (cerebellar) brain tumor. During Cindy's admission to the pediatric unit, it would be *most important* for the nurse to

○ 1. alleviate the parents' anxiety.

○ 2. implement seizure precautions.

○ 3. introduce the patient to other children her own age.

○ 4. prepare the patient and her parents for diagnostic procedures.

75. A diagnosis of probable cerebellar astrocytoma is made, and surgical removal is scheduled. Preoperatively, it would be important for the nurse to tell Cindy and her parents about the

○ 1. patient's postoperative appearance.

○ 2. patient's long-term prognosis.

○ 3. long-term therapy for this type of tumor.

○ 4. side effects of the planned chemotherapy.

76. An infratentorial craniotomy is performed and the diagnosis of cerebellar astrocytoma, stage I, is confirmed. Postoperatively, Cindy is admitted to the intensive care unit. The nurse's *first priority* of care should be to ensure adequate

○ 1. analgesia for pain control.

○ 2. cardiorespiratory function.

○ 3. fluid and electrolyte balance.

○ 4. protection from infection.

77. Cindy's parents want to know what "stage I" means. The nurse would explain that stage I is a way of classifying tumors and means the tumor

○ 1. is localized.

○ 2. is undifferentiated.

○ 3. has extended.

○ 4. has metastasized.

78. In what position should the nurse place Cindy immediately postoperatively?

○ 1. Reverse Trendelenburg.

○ 2. Prone.

○ 3. Side-lying.

○ 4. Trendelenburg.

79. Cindy shows signs of decreased level of consciousness, and the physician orders manual hyperventilation to keep the $PaCO_2$ between 25 and 29 mm Hg and the $PaO_2$ between 80 and 100 mm Hg. The purpose of maintaining the blood gas values within these ranges is to

○ 1. ensure a patent airway.

○ 2. decrease intracranial pressure.

○ 3. lower the arousal level.

○ 4. produce hypercapnia.

80. The nurse notes clear drainage on Cindy's dressing and the linen under her head. An appropriate nursing action would be to test the drainage for the presence of

○ 1. bacteria.

○ 2. glucose.

○ 3. lipids.

○ 4. protein.

81. Cindy progresses well postoperatively and is transferred to the pediatric unit. Although she was told preoperatively that her head would be shaved, Cindy is very upset when the dressing is removed and she sees her shaved head. The *most appropriate* nursing intervention would be to

○ 1. ask the patient if she would like a hat or wig.

○ 2. assure the patient that her hair will grow back quickly.

○ 3. suggest that the patient's parents buy a wig as a surprise.

○ 4. explain that this is a normal reaction.

82. Which of the following statements made by Cindy's mother would warrant further exploration by the nurse?

○ 1. "After this, I will never allow Cindy out of my sight again."

○ 2. "I hope that Cindy will be able to go back to school soon."

○ 3. "Cindy's best friend, Sara, is coming to lunch when we get home."

○ 4. "I wonder how long it will be before Cindy can ride her bike."

## THE PATIENT WITH A SPINAL CORD INJURY

Paul Carson, age 17, is involved in a motorcycle accident. He is thrown about 40 feet from the motorcycle.

83. A nurse arrives at the scene of the accident and finds that Paul is alert. He is lying on his back and says his back hurts. He is unable to move his legs. While waiting for the emergency medical service to arrive, the nurse should

○ 1. roll the patient onto his left side.

○ 2. remove the patient's helmet immediately.

○ 3. flex the patient's knees to relieve stress on his back.

○ 4. leave the patient as he is and stay with him.

84. Paul arrives at the emergency department with a diagnosis of suspected thoracic spinal cord injury. The *first* priority of care should be to

○ 1. provide the patient with emotional support.

○ 2. maintain cardiorespiratory function.

○ 3. obtain a signed consent from the patient's parents.

○ 4. prevent fluid and electrolyte imbalance.

85. In the emergency department, Paul remains conscious and is agitated and anxious. The nurse observes that his pulse and respirations are increasing and that his blood pressure is decreasing.

The nurse suspects that Paul is developing

○ 1. autonomic dysreflexia.

○ 2. increased intracranial pressure.

○ 3. metabolic alkalosis.

○ 4. spinal shock.

**86.** A diagnosis of a T3 spinal cord injury is made. Following insertion of an IV, nasogastric tube, and Foley catheter, Paul is admitted to the intensive care unit. The nurse notes that Paul's feet and legs are cool to the touch. An appropriate nursing action would be to

○ 1. cover the patient's legs with blankets.

○ 2. reposition the patient's legs.

○ 3. sit the patient up to aid circulation.

○ 4. report the change to the physician immediately.

**87.** Over the past several days, Paul's parents have noticed nurses auscultating his abdomen and finally ask the purpose of this procedure. The nurse explains that this is done because spinal cord injured patients often develop

○ 1. abdominal cramping.

○ 2. projectile vomiting.

○ 3. hyperactive bowel sounds.

○ 4. paralytic ileus.

**88.** Which of the following findings would indicate that spinal shock is resolving?

○ 1. Hyperactive reflexes.

○ 2. Atonic urinary bladder.

○ 3. Return of sensation.

○ 4. Flaccid paralysis.

**89.** After Paul's condition stabilizes, he is moved to the rehabilitation unit. The nurses describe his behavior as "uncooperative and hostile" but recognize that this type of behavior indicates a

○ 1. normal stage of grief reaction.

○ 2. severe separation anxiety.

○ 3. phase of adolescent rebellion.

○ 4. reaction to sensory overload.

**90.** Adjustment to paraplegia will be especially difficult for 17-year-old Paul because of his developmental stage. According to Erikson, Paul is in a developmental stage that involves establishing independence and

○ 1. ego integrity.

○ 2. industriousness.

○ 3. self-definition.

○ 4. sense of generativity.

**91.** Three months after Paul's T3 spinal cord injury, the nurse enters his room and Paul says he has a pounding headache. The nurse notes that his arms and face are flushed and that he is diaphoretic. The nurse should immediately

○ 1. check the patency of the patient's Foley catheter.

○ 2. lower the patient's head.

○ 3. place the patient in a supine position.

○ 4. prepare to administer epinephrine.

**92.** Paul is to be discharged to his parents' home and will be living with them. Before Paul is discharged, the nurse assesses the ability of Paul's parents to perform his activities of daily living, Paul's ability to meet his self-care needs independently, and the physical design of his parent's home. These assessments are important because once Paul is at home *high priority* will be placed on

○ 1. having his activities of daily living met by his parents.

○ 2. meeting all his self-care needs independently.

○ 3. being able to maneuver independently inside the house.

○ 4. being able to leave the house.

# CORRECT ANSWERS AND RATIONALES

Numbers appear in parentheses following the rationales. The numbers identify textbooks listed in the references at the end of Part III, where correct answers can be verified.

## *The Patient with Myelomeningocele*

**1.** 1. A myelomeningocele has three components (bony defect, spinal fluid, and nerve tissue) and protrudes over the vertebrae, usually in the lower back. A meningocele is a soft sac containing only spinal fluid and meninges located anywhere on the spine. A pilonidal cyst is a skin-covered sac containing bits of hair located on the low lumbar or sacral area of the spine. A simple cyst contains serosanguineous fluid and fatty tissue located on any area of the spinal column. (14)

**2.** 3. Clinical manifestations of myelomeningocele are related to the anatomic level of the defect and the nerves involved. An upper lumbar (L1-2) myelomeningocele is associated with minimal movement of the lower extremities and dribbling of urine and feces. The upper lumbar area of the spinal cord controls leg flexion at the hip and adduction of the thigh. The sacral area of the spinal cord controls foot and toe movement, as well as sphincter and perineal muscle contraction. (14, 21)

**3.** 2. The parents should see their infant as soon as possible, and the infant's normal and positive features should be emphasized. The longer parents have to wait to see the infant, the more anxiety they feel. Since the parents are acutely aware of the deficit, emphasizing the infant's normal and positive features is more important than reinforcing the doctor's explanation of the defect. The parents should spend time with or care for their infant after birth because mother-father-infant contact is necessary for attachment to occur. They cannot hold the infant before the defect is repaired, but they can fondle and stroke him. Although parents need to discuss their fears and concerns, the nurse initially emphasizes the infant's normal and positive features. (7, 21)

**4.** 3. Hydrocephalus is the anomaly most frequently associated with myelomeningocele. Microcephaly, or an abnormally small head, and craniosynostosis, premature fusion of the cranial sutures with skull deformity, are rarely associated with myelomeningocele. Anencephaly, congenital absence of the cranial vault, is a different neural tube defect. (21)

**5.** 3. Approximately one-third of infants with myelomeningocele are mentally retarded, but it is particularly difficult to predict intellectual functioning in newborns. The parents are asking for an answer now and should not be told to talk with the physician later. (15, 21)

**6.** 3. Overflow incontinence with constant dribbling is common in infants with myelomeningocele. Applying gentle pressure to the suprapubic area helps empty the bladder, thus preventing urinary tract infection. Catheterization is used most frequently when a specimen is urgently needed or when the child is unable to void. Intermittent clean catheterization is an appropriate technique for management of urinary retention in older infants. Suprapubic aspiration is useful in clarifying the diagnosis of suspected urinary tract infection in very ill infants. (15, 21)

**7.** 1. If corrective surgery is to be done immediately, the sac is kept moist by covering it with sterile saline dressings. If corrective surgery is not to be done immediately, the sac may be exposed to the air or covered with a dry, sterile, nonadherent dressing. This facilitates drying and epithelialization of the sac. Similarly, applications of tincture of benzoin make the covering of the sac firmer and more resistant to injury, if corrective surgery is delayed. (7, 21)

**8.** 2. A low Trendelenburg position is ideal, because it reduces spinal fluid pressure in the sac; slight hip flexion reduces tension on the defect. The side-lying position is also acceptable, but support is placed behind the head and buttocks, not the sac. Prone position with the legs slightly elevated is acceptable. The supine position is unacceptable because it causes pressure on the defect. (7, 15, 21)

**9.** 1. Passive range-of-motion exercises help prevent contractures. The potential for fracture secondary to osteoporotic bone mandates gentleness. Feet are maintained in a neutral position, and because of the potential for hip dislocation the legs should be slightly abducted and the hips maintained in slight to moderate abduction. (7, 15, 21)

**10.** 2. In infants with open cranial sutures, increasing head circumference is the predominant and *earliest* sign of increased intracranial pressure and hydrocephalus. Some infants may have bulging fontanels without head enlargement. Other early signs and symptoms are frontal bossing or enlargement with depressed eyes and a "setting-sun" sign. In the latter, the sclera is visible above the iris. Distended scalp veins, especially when the infant cries, and irritability may also occur. A brief, shrill, and high-pitched cry occurs if the hydrocephalus progresses. (15, 21)

**11.** 4. Infection is the greatest hazard postoperatively after the placement of a ventriculoperitoneal shunt and the nurse monitors for manifestations of cerebrospinal fluid infection. Neither glucosuria nor ketonuria is associated with placement of a ventriculoperitoneal shunt. Pain is minimal postoperatively and mild analgesics are given. Narcotics and sedatives are not given because they alter the level of consciousness. Any fluid leakage is tested for glucose, an indication of cerebrospinal fluid. (7, 14, 21)

**12.** 2. Local parent support groups such as the Spina Bifida Association of America are helpful to the parents. While financial problems can influence family functioning, support groups can help parents cope with the wide range of problems that the family may encounter. Referrals for counseling and residential placement can be made when appropriate. (21)

**13.** 4. Children with myelomeningocele are prone to urinary tract infections; because of sensory impairment, the child is unaware of bladder discomfort. Similarly, the child is insensitive to pressure and other sources of tissue damage such as heat. Activities that encourage body consciousness, such as rolling over, are encouraged. The child needs the stimulation of others and has a competent immune system. (21)

## The Patient with Hydrocephalus

**14.** 2. Head circumference usually parallels the percentile for length. The discrepancy found requires close and immediate attention because it could indicate hydrocephalus, with the possibility of brain damage. In infants, bulging fontanels and widening cranial sutures are signs of increasing intracranial pressure. Transillumination is a noninvasive procedure and does not require signed consent. Difficulty walking may indicate hydrocephalus in an older child. (6, 8, 20)

**15.** 3. Two important anatomic types of hydrocephalus are noncommunicating and communicating. In noncommunicating (intraventricular or obstructive) hydrocephalus, a blockage between the ventricular and subarachnoid systems interferes with the circulation of cerebrospinal fluid. In communicating or extraventricular hydrocephalus, the communication between the ventricles and the spinal

subarachnoid space is normal. However, the cerebrospinal fluid is inadequately circulated or reabsorbed in the subarachnoid space, or there is an overproduction of cerebrospinal fluid by the choroid plexus. (6, 7, 8)

**16.** 4. Small, frequent feedings given when the infant is relaxed and calm are tolerated best. Infants with hydrocephalus are difficult to feed because of poor sucking, lethargy, and vomiting, which are associated with increased intracranial pressure. Ideally, the infant is held during feeding with the neck supported. (20)

**17.** 3. The outcomes for children with hydrocephalus vary and range from normal growth and development to delayed motor and cognitive development. The degree of impairment is difficult to predict. The nurse should respond now to the inquiry rather than refer the patient's mother to the physician at a later time. (14, 20)

**18.** 3. The infant is positioned flat for at least the first 24 hours after surgery. Lying on the operative side is avoided because it puts pressure on the shunt valve. Elevating the head increases cerebrospinal fluid drainage and reduces cerebrospinal fluid pressure. But rapid reduction in the size of the ventricles may cause a subdural hematoma. Infants are often not turned to the unoperative side (the side opposite the shunt) in order to prevent rapid decompression. Elevating the foot of the crib could increase intracranial pressure. (6, 7, 8, 11, 14)

**19.** 2. Shunts used to treat hydrocephalus consist of a ventricular catheter, a one-way valve, and a distal catheter. The one-way valve prevents reflux of cerebrospinal fluid back into the ventricles. When the valve is depressed, cerebrospinal fluid flows into the distal end of the catheter. If the ventricular portion of the shunt is free flowing, the valve should refill when released. (6, 8, 14, 20)

**20.** 2. Obstruction of the shunt used to treat hydrocephalus results in increased intracranial pressure. In an infant these signs would be tense fontanels, increased head circumference, irritability, lethargy, poor sucking, vomiting, and decreased level of consciousness. (6, 8, 20)

**21.** 1. Signs of a shunt infection include fever, irritability, stiff neck, nausea, and vomiting. These are the same signs as those seen with meningitis. (6, 8, 20)

**22.** 3. The incidence of hydrocephalus is approximately 1 in 1,000 live births. Some types of abnormalities, especially stenosis of the aqueduct of Sylvius, can be inherited as an X-linked trait. Aqueductal stenosis may also be related to infectious diseases. Genetic counseling is indicated if parents wish to have other children. (3, 7, 20)

## The Patient with a Seizure Disorder

**23.** 2. During a generalized tonic-clonic seizure, the first priority is to protect the individual from injury. Although obtaining information about events surrounding the seizure and providing privacy are important considerations, they are not the first priority during a seizure. After a seizure has begun, nothing should be forced into the mouth, as this can cause severe damage to the teeth and mouth. The child's classmates need an opportunity to discuss this incident and to learn about seizures. (6, 8)

**24.** 4. It is normal for a child to sleep and be difficult to arouse during the postictal period of a generalized tonic-clonic seizure. During this time, the child should be allowed to sleep until he awakens. Sleep and drowsiness do not follow other forms of generalized seizures. Obtaining information about neurologic status following the seizure is important, but awakening the child every 3 to 5 minutes would not be helpful. Urinary incontinence during a seizure is common. (14)

**25.** 3. Phenobarbital (Luminal) raises the seizure threshold. People with a seizure disorder experience seizures when their level of neuronal excitability exceeds a critical point. Anticonvulsant drugs prevent seizures by raising this point or threshold. Lowering the seizure threshold or increasing neuronal activity increases the probability of a seizure. Phenobarbital (Luminal) is metabolized in the liver and does stimulate microsomal enzymes. However, this effect is not a pharmacologic action associated with seizure control. (1)

**26.** 4. The goal of anticonvulsant drug therapy is to control or decrease the frequency of seizures. Therapy is begun with a single anticonvulsant drug known to be effective for the type of seizure experienced. If the single drug is ineffective, a second drug is added to the regimen. Phenobarbital (Luminal) and phenytoin sodium (Dilantin) are both effective in treatment of generalized seizures, either alone or in combination. Phenobarbital is most useful in combination with other drugs. (14, 21)

**27.** 3. Although many anticonvulsants are available as liquid extracts and emulsions, the drug can be unequally distributed in the solvent. This unequal distribution can result in inaccurate dosages, even when the medication is shaken well before pouring. If necessary, the contents of the capsule can be mixed with a small amount of jam or honey to make it palatable. (1)

**28.** 1. The most common cause for status epilepticus is sudden withdrawal of medications. Some children may be able to discontinue their anticonvulsant drugs, but only under carefully supervised conditions and only after being completely seizure-free on medication for several years. Physical growth, such as occurs during adolescence, frequently necessitates an increase in medication. The physician should be notified of troublesome side effects. (6, 8, 14)

**29.** 2. Many medications, including over-the-counter drugs such as antihistamines, central nervous system stimulants, and alcohol, can lower the seizure threshold. In order to maintain plasma drug levels within the threshold range, anticonvulsants are taken at least once daily, depending on the brand. When a child is unable to take an oral anticonvulsant, the physician should be notified. Prescriptions should be refilled *before* the bottle is empty so that the dosage is not interrupted. (6, 8, 14)

**30.** 3. Safety is the primary concern. It is a common misconception that people having a seizure swallow their tongues. However, flexing the neck could obstruct the airway. Trying to restrain a child during a seizure or attempting to have him swallow anything, including medications, can result in further injury or aspiration. (6, 8, 20)

**31.** 2. The majority of children who develop seizures after infancy are intellectually normal. Children with seizure disorders need the same experiences and opportunities to develop their intellectual, emotional, and social abilities as other children do. (6, 8, 14)

**32.** 3. Children who have generalized seizures should not participate in activities that are potentially hazardous. Even if accompanied by a responsible adult, a child could be seriously injured if he were to have a seizure while riding horseback. (14)

**33.** 4. Most febrile seizures occur in the presence of an upper respiratory infection, otitis media, or tonsillitis. There appears to be an increased susceptibility of febrile seizures within families. Febrile seizures, which occur during a temperature rise rather than after prolonged fever, last less than 20 minutes. (20)

**34.** 1. The child who is at low risk for recurrence is usually not treated with anticonvulsant drugs because the drugs' side effects frequently outweigh the benefits. Without anticonvulsant therapy, the likelihood that a child will experience a second febrile seizure is 30 to 40 percent, and about 15 percent for a third febrile seizure. Children for whom prophylactic treatment is indicated include those who have their first febrile seizure before 18 months of age, have a family history positive for seizures, and have seizures lasting more than 15 minutes. (20)

**35.** 4. The prognosis for febrile seizures is excellent.

Children who have only one uncomplicated febrile seizure do not experience intellectual or neurologic impairment secondary to the seizure. (20)

**36.** 4. Phenytoin sodium (Dilantin) is a known teratogenic agent, causing numerous fetal problems, and anticonvulsant requirements usually increase during pregnancy. There is a familial tendency for seizure disorders. Seizures are controlled, not cured. Seizure disorders and infertility are not related. (1, 14)

**37.** 1. Although phenytoin sodium (Dilantin) can produce cardiotoxicity, hepatotoxicity, venous irritation, and hyperglycemia, the most life-threatening during intravenous administration is cardiotoxicity. Bradycardia, hypotension, and cardiac arrest are potential cardiovascular problems associated with the intravenous administration of phenytoin sodium. Thus, it is important for the nurse to monitor the child's vital signs closely during and after intravenous administration of phenytoin sodium. (1)

## The Patient With Meningitis

**38.** 2. To convert centigrade to Fahrenheit, multiply the centigrade temperature by $9/5$ and add 32. Using this formula, the conversion is determined as follows:

$$39°C \times 9/5 = 70.2$$
$$70.2 + 32 = 102.2°F$$

To convert Fahrenheit to centigrade, subtract 32 from the Fahrenheit temperature and multiply the result by $5/9$, as follows:

$$102.2°F - 32 = 70.2$$
$$70.2 \times 5/9 = 39°C$$

(13)

**39.** 1. There is no standard dosage for medications for pediatric patients. Medication dosages are most commonly determined according to a child's weight or body surface. The child described in this situation is weighed primarily to help calculate proper dosages of medications. Weighing the patient may also be used to estimate fluid needs, but a child with meningitis is very unlikely to be weighed to determine whether edema is present. (6, 21)

**40.** 4. A positive Kernig's sign is present if there is pain and resistance when a flexed leg and hip are straightened. A positive Brudzinski's sign is present if there is pain and rigidity in the neck when the neck is flexed. Positive Kernig's and Brudzinski's

signs indicate meningeal irritation. A loud noise causing extension followed by flexion of the arms describes the Moro reflex of the newborn. Extension of the large toe with other toes fanning outward when the bottom of the foot is stroked describes the Babinski reflex. (6, 21)

**41.** 2. The number of drops the patient described in this item should receive each minute is determined as follows:

$$\frac{500 \text{ ml}}{12 \text{ hr}} = 41\text{–}42 \text{ ml approximately to be infused each hour}$$

$$\frac{42 \text{ ml} \times 60 \text{ (drop factor)}}{60 \text{ min}} = \frac{2520}{60}$$

= 42 drops to be infused every minute

(12, 13)

**42.** 4. During the time when a child with meningitis is acutely ill and irritable, the patient is hypersensitive to loud noises and prefers to remain undisturbed. Extraneous noises should be kept at a minimum. The child should be spoken to and bathed. Treatments should be done gently and calmly, and unnecessary noise and sudden movements should be avoided. (6, 21)

**43.** 3. One cause of seizure activity in a child with meningitis is increased intracranial pressure. The pulse rate tends to decrease. Edema of the optic papilla (papilledema), changes in respiratory patterns (but not dyspnea), and irritability are additional signs of increased cerebral pressure. Deafness is not associated with increased intracranial pressure. (21)

**44.** 4. Disseminated intravascular coagulation (DIC) is characterized by the presence of skin petechiae and a purpuric skin rash due to spontaneous bleeding into the tissues. An abnormal coagulation phenomenon causes this condition. Heparin therapy is often used to interrupt the clotting process. (6, 21)

**45.** 4. Organisms causing bacterial meningitis, such as pneumococcal meningitis, are commonly spread in the body by vascular dissemination from a middle-ear infection. The meningitis may also be a direct extension from the paranasal and mastoid sinuses. When the causative organism is a pneumococcus, a chronic draining ear is frequently also found. (21)

**46.** 2. Preschool-age children worry about having an intact body and become fearful when there is a threat to the body's integrity. Allowing a child to participate as possible with required care helps protect the child's image of an intact body. Finding more diversional activity, relieving the anxiety of separation from the home, and enhancing the patient's confidence in personnel caring for him are invalid reasons for allowing the child described in this item to place a dressing on the area where an intravenous needle has been positioned. (6, 21)

**47.** 2. An emotionally tense child with pent-up hostilities needs a physical activity that will release energy and frustration. Pounding on a peg board offers this opportunity. Such activities as stacking blocks and painting require concentration and fine movements that would be likely to aggravate the situation. Listening to a story does not allow the child to express emotions and casts the child in a passive role. (6, 21)

**48.** 1. Mumps is a viral disease that predisposes to viral meningitis. Other illnesses that predispose to viral meningitis include measles, herpes, and leukemia. (6, 21)

## The Patient with Reye Syndrome

**49.** 2. The etiology of Reye syndrome is unknown, but symptoms of Reye syndrome usually develop a few days to several weeks after the onset of a mild viral illness such as a respiratory tract infection or chicken pox. The other data provided are not associated with Reye syndrome. (7, 8, 20)

**50.** 2. Severe encephalopathy or cerebral edema accompanies Reye syndrome, so a primary goal is to prevent central nervous system damage. Seizures are characteristic of a child in stage V of Reye syndrome. A combined respiratory alkalosis and metabolic acidosis and fatty infiltration of the liver are associated with Reye syndrome. Preventing fluid and electrolyte imbalances is a goal of nursing care and is a factor in controlling cerebral edema to minimize central nervous system damage, which is the primary goal. (5, 7, 20)

**51.** 3. The physician should be notified, because decorticate posturing in response to pain indicates neurologic deterioration and is a characteristic of stage III Reye syndrome. Pupillary responses provide data about neurologic status, but checking them in this situation is not the priority action. The physician determines the rate of the infusion, depending on the fluid being administered and the patient's clinical status. (7, 8, 20)

**52.** 4. Elevating the head of the bed 30° and keeping the patient's head in a midline (supine) position help minimize increasing intracranial pressure. Flexion or rotation of the neck can obstruct venous return, which can increase intracranial pressure. (5, 20)

**53.** 1. Minimizing excessive and/or inappropriate stim-

ulation helps minimize the child's agitation. Photosensitivity and hearing loss are not associated with Reye syndrome. The only part of a neurologic check that requires a darkened room is a check of pupillary reflexes. (8, 20)

**54.** 3. Guilt is a common parental response, and the parents should be allowed to express their feelings. Reye syndrome does develop quickly and it is a medical emergency, but affirming, discounting, or denying the parents' guilt feelings is not helpful. (8, 20)

**55.** 3. Reye syndrome affects children from 2 months to adolescence, but the incidence peaks at 6 and 11 years. Reye syndrome is not a communicable disease and siblings are not at increased risk for contracting it. Although its cause is unknown, Reye syndrome seems to be associated with a viral infection. Research suggests that giving salicylates (aspirin) to children who have a viral illness can contribute to the development of Reye syndrome. (7, 8, 20)

## The Patient with Infectious Polyneuritis (Guillain-Barré Syndrome)

**56.** 2. Muscle paralysis seen in Guillain-Barré syndrome is usually progressive and ascending in nature. It can progress rapidly. Assessment of progressive muscle weakness helps determine the extent of involvement. (6, 8, 14)

**57.** 3. In children with Guillain-Barré syndrome, a decrease in the volume and clarity of speech and a decreased ability to cough voluntarily indicate ascending progression of neural inflammation. These are not signs and symptoms of increasing intracranial pressure, separation anxiety, or regression. (5, 14)

**58.** 1. The most serious complication in the acute stage of Guillain-Barré syndrome is respiratory failure. The mortality rate is estimated to be between 5% and 20%, with death most often due to respiratory and cardiac complications. Promoting skin integrity, reducing anxiety, and preventing contractures are important goals, but maintaining respiratory function is the primary goal. (5, 6, 8)

**59.** 1. Impairment of autonomic function in Guillain-Barré syndrome can result in cardiac dysrhythmias, which can result in cardiovascular shock and death. The vital centers in the medulla oblongata may be affected, not by edema, but by patchy demyelination. Neither hypokalemia nor hypoglycemia is associated with Guillain-Barré syndrome. (5, 6, 7, 8)

**60.** 4. Because the child with Guillain-Barré syndrome can experience muscular pain and be hypersensitive to touch, she should be turned with extreme gentleness. Even in the absence of respiratory problems or distress, the child needs frequent turning to prevent the pulmonary problems associated with immobility. During the acute phase of the disease, vigorous physiotherapy is contraindicated. (6, 8)

**61.** 3. Impaired gag and swallowing reflexes associated with cranial nerve involvement require nasogastric tube feedings in a child with Guillain-Barré syndrome. The presence of a gag reflex indicates the returning function of normal swallowing. (5, 6, 8)

**62.** 1. The family should be involved early in developing a rehabilitation plan. The convalescent period for a child with Guillain-Barré syndrome is lengthy, and full recovery may require 1 to 2 years. Most children recover completely; only 10% to 15% have neurologic sequelae. Maintaining peer relationships during convalescence is important for psychosocial development. Children with Guillain-Barré syndrome can attend regular school. (5, 6, 8)

**63.** 3. Developmentally appropriate activities and therapeutic use of play can be used as rehabilitation modalities. Inappropriate rewards or threats should not be used to coerce children into compliance. Significant persons for a child of this age are family members. Peer groups are the significant persons in early adolescence. (14)

## The Patient with a Head Injury

**64.** 3. The first priority in caring for a child who has sustained a head injury is to establish and maintain ventilation. All other activities are secondary to adequate oxygenation. (5)

**65.** 4. A supine position with the head of the bed elevated approximately 30° maximizes diaphragmatic excursion and aids cerebral venous return. (5, 20)

**66.** 4. Lack of response to pain yields the lowest score. From highest to lowest, the order of eye-opening response to stimuli on the Glasgow coma scale is spontaneous response, response to speech, response to pain, and no response. (5, 20)

**67.** 4. A nasogastric tube is initially placed following serious head trauma to decompress the stomach and to prevent vomiting and aspiration. The tube may also be used to administer tube feedings and medications and to obtain specimens for analysis, but in this situation it is inserted initially to decompress the stomach. (5)

**68.** 3. The third cranial nerve controls pupillary size, reaction to light, and accommodation. (5, 20)

**69.** 3. Using the ratio:proportion method, the answer is:

$$\frac{4 \text{ mg}}{1 \text{ ml}} = \frac{7.2 \text{ mg}}{x \text{ ml}}$$

$$4x = 7.2$$

$$x = \frac{7.2}{4}$$

$$x = 1.8 \text{ ml}$$

Therefore, 1.8 ml equals 7.2 mg of drug. (13)

**70.** 3. As a rule, children demonstrate more rapid and more complete recovery from coma than do adults, and spontaneous respirations indicate a favorable prognosis. However, it is extremely difficult to predict a specific outcome. (5)

**71.** 2. The parents' presence may help calm the child. Restraints can frighten and frustrate a child, and straining against them can lead to an increase in intracranial pressure. (6, 8)

**72.** 1. The family should be involved in planning for discharge and rehabilitation, although it is difficult to predict the outcome for their child. The child who has suffered head trauma may regain his previous level of functioning or may have permanent residual deficits. When helping the family plan for the child's discharge, the nurse may also be able, when appropriate, to assess the family's coping strategies, remind them to care for their own health, and teach them the basics of child safety. (6, 8)

## The Patient with a Brain Tumor

**73.** 1. Common signs and symptoms of infratentorial brain tumor in children are headache, visual disturbances, vomiting with or without nausea, and ataxia in the form of gait disturbances. (6, 8)

**74.** 4. When a brain tumor is suspected, the child and parents are likely to be very apprehensive and anxious. Preparation of both child and family during hospitalization can help them cope with their anxieties. It is unrealistic to expect to alleviate the parents' anxiety; rather, the goal is to decrease the anxiety. Children with infratentorial tumors do not usually have seizures. Introducing the patient to other children her own age is nice, but not the most important action for the nurse during the child's admission. (6, 8, 17)

**75.** 1. Both the child and parents should be told preoperatively about head shaving, bulky bandages, possible facial edema, and the intensive care unit stay. The prognosis and treatment plan cannot be determined until after surgery, when the type of tumor is diagnosed. (6, 8, 17)

**76.** 2. Postoperatively, the child undergoing neurosurgery for removal of a brain tumor is at risk for cardiorespiratory compromise due to anesthesia, surgical complications, or increased intracranial pressure. The other problems do not take first priority. (6, 8, 17)

**77.** 1. Stage I indicates localized disease without evidence of spread. Such a tumor has a favorable prognosis, if all tumor tissue is surgically removed. Poor prognosis, undifferentiation, extension, and metastasis characterize stage III and IV tumors. (6, 8, 17)

**78.** 3. Following surgery for an infratentorial tumor, the child is usually positioned flat and on either side with the head and neck in midline with the body and slightly extended. Pillows against the back, not the head, help maintain the desired position. Such a position avoids pressure on the operative site. After a supratentorial craniotomy, the head is usually elevated above the heart. This facilitates the drainage of cerebrospinal fluid and decreases excessive blood flow to the brain. Trendelenburg position is contraindicated in both infratentorial and supratentorial craniotomies because it increases intracranial pressure and the risk of hemorrhage. (17, 21)

**79.** 2. Hypercapnia, hypoxia, and acidosis are potent cerebral vasodilators that can cause increased intracranial pressure. Lowering the $CO_2$ level and increasing the $O_2$ level through hyperventilation is the most effective short-term method of reducing intracranial pressure. (5, 6, 8)

**80.** 2. Cerebrospinal fluid is a clear, colorless fluid. The presence of glucose in the drainage indicates that the drainage contains cerebrospinal fluid. (5, 17)

**81.** 1. It is not uncommon for the child to be concerned about the change in appearance, whether the entire head or only a part has been shaved. The school-aged child should participate in decisions about care when possible. Assuring the child that the hair will grow back quickly does not address the immediate change in appearance. Similarly, explaining that this is a normal reaction does not address the patient's change in appearance. (17)

**82.** 1. Parents of a child who has undergone neurosurgery can easily become overprotective, yet the parents must foster independence in the convalescing child. It is important for the child to resume age-appropriate activities, and parents play an important role in the child's resumption of these activities. (17, 20)

## The Patient with a Spinal Cord Injury

**83.** 4. The history and symptoms suggest a spinal cord injury. A person suspected of having a spinal cord injury should not be moved without the spine being immobilized. Turning the patient, removing the helmet, or flexing the knees could aggravate a spinal cord injury. (6, 17)

**84.** 2. The first priority in emergency care of the spinal-cord-injured patient is to maintain cardiovascular and respiratory function. Surgical intervention during the acute phase is usually avoided. Prevention of fluid and electrolyte imbalance and providing emotional support are important goals but are not the *first* priority. (6, 17)

**85.** 4. Spinal shock occurs 30 to 60 minutes after a spinal cord injury because of the sudden disruption of central and autonomic pathways. This disruption causes flaccid paralysis, lack of reflexes, vasodilation, hypotension, and increasing pulse and respiratory rates. Autonomic dysreflexia occurs only after the return of spinal reflexes and is characterized by hypertension. Increased intracranial pressure is associated with widening pulse pressure and decreasing pulse and respiratory rates. Metabolic alkalosis does not occur with spinal shock. (6, 17)

**86.** 1. In spinal cord injury, temperature regulation distal to the injury is lost. Body temperature is maintained by adjusting room temperature and/or bed linens. Changing position does not alleviate the problem with temperature regulation and could be harmful, considering the diagnosis. Reporting this finding to the physician is unnecessary because it is an expected development. (6)

**87.** 4. A thoracic-level spinal cord injury involves the muscles of the lower extremities, bladder, and rectum. Paralytic ileus often occurs and is evaluated by auscultating the abdomen. (6)

**88.** 1. Spinal cord shock causes a loss of reflex activity below the level of injury. The results are atonic urinary bladder and flaccid paralysis. When the reflex arc returns, it has a tendency to be overactive, resulting in spasticity. The bladder becomes hypertonic during this phase of spinal shock resolution. Sensation does not return. (6)

**89.** 1. Initially after a catastrophic injury, denial is common. With gradual awareness of the reality of the situation, anger is common. The four major stages of grief are denial, anger, depression, and acceptance. (17)

**90.** 3. Erikson's concept of identify is the task of adolescence. It includes components of self-definition and evaluation. A sudden accident with long-term consequences requires many adjustments in terms of self-concept. Industry is a task of children 6 to 12 years of age, whereas ego integrity and generativity are tasks of adult development. (6, 17)

**91.** 1. These are signs of autonomic dysreflexia, a generalized sympathetic response usually caused by bladder or bowel distention. Immediate treatment is removal of the cause. Since bladder distention is a common cause of this problem, the patency of the Foley catheter is immediately determined. The patient is assisted to a sitting position to lower the blood pressure. Epinephrine elevates blood pressure and thus would exacerbate the problem. (6, 17)

**92.** 4. A high priority is placed on leaving the house so that the patient can participate in his normal activities as much as possible. Although independent performance of activities of daily living is important, complete independence may be a long-term goal. (17)

# test 8

Select the one *best* or *correct* answer and indicate your choice by filling in the circle with a pencil in front of the option you have chosen. If the answer you would prefer is not given, select the one you think is most appropriate.

**Screening Patients for Musculoskeletal Dysfunction**

**The Patient with Cerebral Palsy**

**The Patient with Muscular Dystrophy**

**The Patient with Congenital Hip Dysplasia**

**The Patient with Congenital Clubfoot**

**The Patient with Juvenile Rheumatoid Arthritis**

**The Patient with a Fracture**

**The Patient with Osteomyelitis**

**Correct Answers and Rationales**

## SCREENING PATIENTS FOR MUSCULOSKELETAL DYSFUNCTION

A nurse is participating in a screening program for musculoskeletal disorders among schoolchildren.

1. A child who limps and is found to have pain is referred by the nurse for medical care. It is determined that the child has Legg-Calvé-Perthes disease (coxa plana, osteochondrosis). The right femur is involved. The *most important* aspect of this child's care while he is undergoing therapy is to
   ○ 1. prevent flexion of the right hip.
   ○ 2. control pain that is especially acute at night.
   ○ 3. prevent weight-bearing on the head of the right femur.
   ○ 4. encourage the child to walk despite discomfort at the right hip.

2. Most of the care of a child with Legg-Calvé-Perthes disease is conducted on an outpatient basis. In planning nursing care, the *major* emphasis in planning nursing care should be on teaching
   ○ 1. gentle stretching exercises for both legs.
   ○ 2. diet planning for weight reduction.
   ○ 3. management of the corrective appliance.
   ○ 4. relaxation techniques for pain control.

3. The nurse examines an adolescent who has kyphosis. This disease is characterized by
   ○ 1. an abnormal increased convex angulation in the curvature of the thoracic spine.
   ○ 2. a lateral curvature of the spine usually associated with a rotary deformity.
   ○ 3. an accentuation of the cervical or lumbar curvature beyond physiologic limits.

○ 4. an outgrowth of bone-like deposits on the vertebrae that may cause a distorted spine.

4. Which of the following body parts should the nurse examine to help determine whether a child may have torticollis (wry neck)?
   ○ 1. The clavicle.
   ○ 2. The trapezius muscle.
   ○ 3. The cervical vertebrae.
   ○ 4. The sternocleidomastoid muscle.

5. The nurse assesses a child who wears corrective shoes for flat feet. The *primary* purpose of prescribing corrective shoes for this youngster is to help
   ○ 1. strengthen the arches of the feet.
   ○ 2. keep the legs in proper alignment.
   ○ 3. prevent the development of pigeon toes.
   ○ 4. maintain proper weight-bearing balance on the feet.

6. A youngster the nurse examines is known to have muscular dystrophy, a disease caused by
   ○ 1. severe trauma.
   ○ 2. a hereditary factor.
   ○ 3. a hormonal factor.
   ○ 4. a generalized infection.

7. The nurse plans to screen only the *highest*-risk children between ages 10 and 14 for scoliosis. Of the following groups of children, she should screen the
   ○ 1. boys only.
   ○ 2. girls only.
   ○ 3. last-born children only.
   ○ 4. first-born children only.

8. Which position taken by the children will help *most* to detect scoliosis among those the nurse is screening?
   ○ 1. Lying flat on the floor while extending the legs straight from the trunk.

○ 2. Sitting in a chair while lifting the feet and legs to a right angle with the trunk.

○ 3. Standing against a wall while pressing the length of the back against the wall.

○ 4. Bending forward at the waist while allowing the head and arms to fall freely.

9. The nurse suspects that a youngster may have scoliosis when she observes that a child has a skeletal defect that results in
   - ○ 1. having a rib hump.
   - ○ 2. walking in a waddling manner.
   - ○ 3. having a longer-than-average trunk.
   - ○ 4. thrusting the body forward while walking.

10. One youngster is found to have scoliosis. Which of the following statements should the nurse use as a rationale for her response when the child is fitted for a Milwaukee brace and asks about the purpose for which it is prescribed?
    - ○ 1. The brace stretches soft tissue and muscle.
    - ○ 2. The brace applies countertraction to the pelvis.
    - ○ 3. The brace facilitates separation of the cervical vertebrae.
    - ○ 4. The brace provides longitudinal traction and lateral pressure.

11. The nurse *correctly* teaches the youngster wearing a Milwaukee brace that the *only* time the brace should be removed is when the youngster
    - ○ 1. eats, about 3 hours a day.
    - ○ 2. sleeps, about 10 hours a day.
    - ○ 3. is at school, about 7 hours a day.
    - ○ 4. carries out personal hygiene, about 1 hour a day.

12. Exercises are prescribed for the child wearing the Milwaukee brace for scoliosis *primarily* to help
    - ○ 1. prevent contractures of the spine.
    - ○ 2. decrease spasms in the back muscles.
    - ○ 3. improve the traction effect of the brace.
    - ○ 4. strengthen the muscles of the torso.

13. The nurse examines a youngster who complains of "growing pains." The nurse should plan to discuss ways to relieve the discomfort, which is *typically* described to be in the area of the tuberosity of the youngster's
    - ○ 1. tibia.
    - ○ 2. femur.
    - ○ 3. fibula.
    - ○ 4. calcaneus.

14. The nurse suspects that an obese adolescent may have a slipped femoral capital epiphysis (SFCE), or coxa vara. The *most common* clinical manifestations of this problem are limping and pain in the
    - ○ 1. hip.
    - ○ 2. ankle.

○ 3. spine.
○ 4. foot.

## THE PATIENT WITH CEREBRAL PALSY

The nurse in an outpatient cerebral palsy clinic meets Mr. and Mrs. Sean and their 15-month-old son, Ben. Ben has a history of neonatal anoxia and has increased tone in the calf muscle of his right leg and right elbow flexor. Ben is scheduled for a series of developmental screening tests.

15. Mrs. Sean asks about the primary purpose of developmental screening tests. The nurse should base her answer on the knowledge that the goal of developmental screening tests is to recognize primary developmental delays early, in order to
    - ○ 1. facilitate communication.
    - ○ 2. prevent secondary delays.
    - ○ 3. prevent secondary injury.
    - ○ 4. encourage health maintenance.

16. Based on the results of a complete neurologic history and examination, Ben is diagnosed as having cerebral palsy. Mrs. Sean asks the nurse to explain cerebral palsy. The nurse should base her response on the knowledge that cerebral palsy is
    - ○ 1. a specific term for impaired neurologic functioning due to progressive damage in the cerebellum.
    - ○ 2. a congenital malformation of the arteriovenous circulatory structure of the cerebellum.
    - ○ 3. a nonspecific term for impaired neuromuscular control as a result of nonprogressive damage to the cerebellum.
    - ○ 4. an acquired injury to the cerebellar portion of the brain secondary to viral infection.

17. Which of the following is a *universal* manifestation of cerebral palsy?
    - ○ 1. Mental retardation.
    - ○ 2. Perceptual deafness.
    - ○ 3. Perceptual blindness.
    - ○ 4. Delayed gross motor development.

18. Based on knowledge of the clinical types of cerebral palsy, the nurse would anticipate that Ben has which type of cerebral palsy?
    - ○ 1. Spastic.
    - ○ 2. Dyskinetic.
    - ○ 3. Ataxic.
    - ○ 4. Atonic.

19. Which of the following would the nurse identify as a *primary* goal of therapy for Ben?
    - ○ 1. Maintenance of joint mobility.

○ 2. Promotion of general health.

○ 3. Preparation for corrective surgery.

○ 4. Actualization of individual potential.

20. The nurse watches Ben as he attempts, unsuccessfully, to pick up his teddy bear with his right hand. The nurse would be correct in documenting this observation as right-sided

○ 1. quadriparesis.

○ 2. paraplegia.

○ 3. hemiparesis.

○ 4. diplegia.

21. After observing Mrs. Sean as she plays with Ben, the nurse encourages her to position him upright and to offer toys to his affected side. The nurse's rationale for making this suggestion would be to

○ 1. keep the infant occupied.

○ 2. challenge the use of the affected limb.

○ 3. test his visual acuity.

○ 4. increase the strength in the affected limb.

22. Mrs. Sean asks the nurse if Ben will be able to walk normally, since he is able to stand without help. The nurse's *most appropriate* response would be

○ 1. "He might, and he might not. How old were you when you walked?"

○ 2. "It's not easy to predict, but the fact that he's able to bear weight is a positive factor."

○ 3. "That all depends. If he really wants to walk, he probably will be able to do so eventually."

○ 4. "Ask the doctor what he thinks at your next appointment."

23. Ben's mother asks the nurse if medications can be used to decrease spasticity in cerebral palsy. The nurse would base her answer on the knowledge that drugs to decrease spasticity have been

○ 1. found to be minimally useful in improving function.

○ 2. shown to improve function.

○ 3. restricted to use with older children.

○ 4. effective in combination with anticonvulsants.

24. The nurse evaluates the Sean family's ability to cope with Ben's cerebral palsy. Information about which of the following factors would provide the *most accurate* indication of their ability to cope?

○ 1. Their understanding of cerebral palsy.

○ 2. Their financial ability to care for Ben.

○ 3. Their ability to meet Ben's physical needs.

○ 4. Their response to friends' reactions to Ben.

## THE PATIENT WITH MUSCULAR DYSTROPHY

A community health nurse visits the Moreno family because the brothers Bill, 4, and Ray, 5, were diagnosed several years ago as having Duchenne muscular dystrophy.

25. Duchenne muscular dystrophy is also known as

○ 1. myotonic muscular dystrophy.

○ 2. congenital muscular dystrophy.

○ 3. pseudohypertrophic muscular dystrophy.

○ 4. myoclonic muscular dystrophy.

26. The physician told Mrs. Moreno that an X-linked inheritance pattern is identified in 50% of cases of Duchenne muscular dystrophy. Mrs. Moreno asks what an "X-linked inheritance pattern" is. The nurse would *correctly* explain that it means

○ 1. females are affected almost exclusively.

○ 2. males are affected almost exclusively.

○ 3. males and females are affected equally.

○ 4. males are affected twice as often than females.

27. The nurse reviews the boys' medical histories with Mrs. Moreno. Which of the following assessment data would accurately reflect the *first* clinical manifestations of Duchenne muscular dystrophy?

○ 1. Small weak muscles.

○ 2. Lack of facial mobility.

○ 3. Abnormal gait on a level surface.

○ 4. Difficulty running.

28. The nurse observes Bill as he attempts to rise from a sitting position on the floor. After attaining a kneeling position, he "walks" his hands up his legs. The nurse would *correctly* identify this as

○ 1. Galleazzi sign.

○ 2. Gower sign.

○ 3. Good-enough sign.

○ 4. Goodell sign.

29. Mrs. Moreno tells the nurse she read that many children with Duchenne muscular dystrophy have intelligence quotients 20 points below normal. She asks if this means Bill and Ray will be mentally retarded. The nurse should base her answer on the knowledge that the approximate percentage of children with Duchenne muscular dystrophy that have a frank mental deficit is

○ 1. 10%.

○ 2. 15%.

○ 3. 20%.

○ 4. 25%.

30. The nurse develops nursing care plans for Bill and Ray. Which of the following would be the *primary* nursing goal for both boys at this time?

○ 1. Maintain function in unaffected muscles.

○ 2. Foster social interactions.

○ 3. Prevent circulatory impairment.

○ 4. Encourage early wheelchair use.

31. Because of the major orthopedic complication as-

sociated with muscular dystrophy, the nursing care plan should include interventions that prevent
- 1. contractures.
- 2. multiple fractures.
- 3. osteomyelitis.
- 4. clubfoot.

**32.** Mrs. Moreno feels guilty that both her sons have muscular dystrophy. Mrs. Moreno's guilt feelings are most likely due to the
- 1. dependent behavior of the children.
- 2. sudden onset of the disease.
- 3. congenital nature of the disease.
- 4. genetic mode of transmission.

**33.** Mrs. Moreno's sister asks the nurse what the usual cause of death is in children with muscular dystrophy. Which of the following would be the *most appropriate* response for the nurse to make?
- 1. "The usual cause of death is respiratory tract infection or cardiac failure."
- 2. "Are you concerned about the death of the children?"
- 3. "Do you know other children who have muscular dystrophy?"
- 4. "Most children with muscular dystrophy die from renal failure."

**34.** Mrs. Moreno's sister asks about the usual life span of children with Duchenne muscular dystrophy. The nurse bases her answer on the knowledge that death for the child with Duchenne muscular dystrophy usually occurs between
- 1. 3 and 5 years of age.
- 2. 6 and 9 years of age.
- 3. 10 and 12 years of age.
- 4. 15 and 25 years of age.

**35.** The nurse teaches Mr. and Mrs. Moreno about muscular dystrophy, including therapeutic management and nursing considerations. Which of the following statements would *most likely* indicate that Mr. Moreno has understood the teaching?
- 1. "The boys will probably be unable to walk independently by the time they are 9 to 11 years of age."
- 2. "I understand that muscle relaxants can be effective in some children."
- 3. "When the boys are a little older, they can have surgery to improve their ability to walk."
- 4. "We will help the boys be as active as possible so as to prevent progression of the disease."

**36.** Parents of children with muscular dystrophy may inappropriately expend energy in therapy while denying or failing to understand the
- 1. progressive nature of the disease.
- 2. appropriate drug therapy for the disease.
- 3. appropriate surgery to treat the disease.
- 4. appropriate ways to prevent progression.

## THE PATIENT WITH CONGENITAL HIP DYSPLASIA

The nurse performs a newborn assessment on Tanya May. While gently abducting the hips, the nurse feels the femoral head slip into the acetabulum.

**37.** The nurse correctly documents this as a *positive*
- 1. Ortolani sign.
- 2. Barlow test.
- 3. Jackson sign.
- 4. Trendelenburg sign.

**38.** Other signs of congenital hip dysplasia are asymmetric thigh folds and a positive Galleazzi sign. The nurse *correctly* defines a Galleazzi sign as
- 1. broadening of the perineum.
- 2. symmetric gluteal folds.
- 3. shortening of the limb on the affected side.
- 4. severely limited abduction of the affected leg.

**39.** Tanya is diagnosed as having congenital hip dysplasia and is placed in a Pavlik harness. Mrs. May asks the nurse how effective this treatment is. The nurse should base her answer on the knowledge that the device's effectiveness depends on *all* of the following *except*
- 1. adequate follow-up care.
- 2. informed parental care.
- 3. concurrent use with a spica cast.
- 4. a well-constructed device.

**40.** It is important that Tanya's parents know how to use the Pavlik harness properly. Which of the following would be the nurse's *most appropriate initial* step in teaching Tanya's parents how to use the device?
- 1. Give them written instructions.
- 2. Assess their coping strategies.
- 3. Determine their knowledge about the device.
- 4. Provide a list of community resources.

**41.** Neonate Allison Perez has congenital hip dysplasia and has a plaster hip spica cast applied. When teaching Allison's parents about the spica cast, the nurse would explain that the abduction stabilizer bar can be
- 1. used as a handle for turning when completely dry.
- 2. used as a lifting aid.
- 3. covered with linen.
- 4. adjusted by only the physician.

**42.** Allison's mother has been breast-feeding successfully and asks if she will be able to continue now that Allison is in a spica cast. Which of the following responses would be *most appropriate* for the nurse to make?
- ○ 1. "Do you want to continue to breast-feed?"
- ○ 2. "Yes, but you may need to try different nursing positions."
- ○ 3. "It's possible, but very difficult because of the cast."
- ○ 4. "How would you feel if you couldn't breast-feed?"

## THE PATIENT WITH CONGENITAL CLUBFOOT

During assessment, newborn Mikhail Soroka was found to have a bilateral clubfoot deformity.

**43.** Which treatment can the nurse anticipate that the physician will order for Mikhail in the nursery?
- ○ 1. Elevation of both legs.
- ○ 2. Gentle passive foot exercises.
- ○ 3. Application of corrective shoes.
- ○ 4. Attachment of a footboard to the crib.

**44.** Mikhail's parents tell the nurse they feel guilty about Mikhail's deformity. They are anxious about how the problem will be treated and feel helpless. Which nursing intervention is likely to be most helpful for them *initially?*
- ○ 1. Discuss the problem and explain how clubfoot deformities are usually corrected.
- ○ 2. Arrange a meeting with other parents whose infants have had successful clubfoot treatments.
- ○ 3. Suggest that they make an appointment with a counselor.
- ○ 4. Ask them what concerns them most about the situation.

**45.** Plaster casts are applied to Mikhail's lower legs to hold the feet in a corrected position. Which nursing measure is appropriate in the *immediate* post-application period?
- ○ 1. Handle the casts with the fingertips only.
- ○ 2. Change the infant's position at least every 2 hours.
- ○ 3. Dry the casts rapidly with a hair dryer.
- ○ 4. Coat the casts with a clear acrylic spray finish.

**46.** The parents ask why the casts are applied when Mikhail is only a few days old. The nurse's reply should be based on the knowledge that

- ○ 1. the neonate's ligaments are more supple now than they will be later.
- ○ 2. early casting improves parental acceptance of the deformity.
- ○ 3. the abnormality can be exacerbated by the infant's leg movements.
- ○ 4. nerve damage can occur if the condition is not immediately corrected.

**47.** Mikhail is ready to be discharged home and the nurse has been teaching his parents about cast care. Which of the following statements indicates they have understood the teaching?
- ○ 1. "We will clean the casts with soap and water carefully when they become soiled."
- ○ 2. "We will remove the petals from the edges of the casts after 24 hours."
- ○ 3. "We will observe the color and temperature of the toes frequently."
- ○ 4. "We will elevate the casts on pillows so that the legs will be above the level of the heart."

**48.** The Sorokas are told to bring Mikhail to the orthopedic clinic for a cast change 1 week after discharge. Mrs. Soroka asks why the cast must be changed so soon. The nurse bases her answer on knowledge that frequent cast changes for infants with a clubfoot
- ○ 1. inhibit the growth of microorganisms beneath the casts.
- ○ 2. facilitate assessment of the neurovascular status of the legs.
- ○ 3. allow the circumference of the legs to be measured and compared to norms.
- ○ 4. accommodate the increasing size of the infant's legs.

**49.** After the clubfoot deformity is overcorrected by serial casting, Mikhail is to wear a Denis Browne splint. The purpose of this splint is to
- ○ 1. prevent kicking.
- ○ 2. help maintain the feet in the desired position.
- ○ 3. prevent possible bone deformities.
- ○ 4. assess the strength of the calf and ankle muscles.

**50.** The nurse has been teaching Mikhail's parents to maintain the function of the Denis Browne splint. Which of their actions during the return demonstration indicates that they have understood the teaching?
- ○ 1. They reposition the angle of the shoes on the bar.
- ○ 2. They slip Mikhail's feet into the shoes without socks.
- ○ 3. They use the bar to help lift Mikhail.
- ○ 4. They tighten a loose shoe against the splint.

**51.** Mrs. Soroka telephones the nurse at the orthopedic clinic and reports that Mikhail is able to wobble across the floor on his hands and knees while wearing the Denis Browne splint. The nurse should suggest that Mrs. Soroka

○ 1. put Mikhail in a playpen to restrict his movement.

○ 2. remove the splint so Mikhail can be more mobile.

○ 3. notify the physician so that corrective shoes can be prescribed.

○ 4. remove the tablecloths from all rooms to which Mikhail has access.

## *THE PATIENT WITH JUVENILE RHEUMATOID ARTHRITIS*

Jean Isles, age 4, is admitted to the pediatric unit. For the past 5 days she has had an intermittent fever of 101.5° F. She has a diffuse skin rash, and her knee joints are swollen, warm, and painful. Juvenile rheumatoid arthritis (JRA) is suspected.

52. Jean is scheduled for a series of tests to establish the diagnosis. Her father asks which test is specific for JRA. The nurse should base her answer on the knowledge that

○ 1. no specific laboratory test exists for JRA.

○ 2. the erythrocyte sedimentation rate is 0 to 10 mm/hr using the Westergren method.

○ 3. the synovial fluid contains increased amounts of protein.

○ 4. the hemoglobin is 11.5 to 15.5 g/dl.

53. The diagnosis of JRA is made. Jean's parents tell the nurse the diagnosis frightens them because they know nothing about its prognosis. The nurse should explain that

○ 1. the disease usually progresses to crippling rheumatoid arthritis as the child reaches adulthood.

○ 2. in most children the disease will be in permanent remission by adolescence.

○ 3. the majority of children recover completely within a few years.

○ 4. many children go into long remissions but have severe deformities and loss of function.

54. After the diagnosis is made, drug therapy is begun. What is the *primary* group of drugs used to treat JRA?

○ 1. Nonsteroidal anti-inflammatory drugs (NSAIDs).

○ 2. Adrenocorticosteroids.

○ 3. Slower-acting antirheumatic drugs (SAARDs).

○ 4. Cytotoxic drugs.

55. Jean's mother tells the nurse that Jean enjoys preschool and attends from 7:30 a.m. to noon daily. Mrs. Isles is worried that Jean will have to stop going to preschool because of the arthritis. The nurse should explain that Jean

○ 1. should be kept home from preschool whenever she has joint discomfort.

○ 2. should be encouraged to attend preschool, but will need time to reduce the early-morning joint stiffness.

○ 3. will need to wear splints or knee braces while at preschool to give her more support.

○ 4. may find it difficult to attend preschool because of side effects from the medications.

56. The nurse prepares Mr. and Mrs. Isles for Jean's discharge home. Since joint stiffness is a problem for children with JRA, the nurse develops a care plan that promotes joint movement. Which of these interventions is related to attainment of this goal?

○ 1. Restriction of the daily intake of dietary purine.

○ 2. Application of moist heat to affected joints.

○ 3. Repetitive weight-bearing exercises involving the affected joints.

○ 4. Application of cool compresses to affected joints.

57. Mr. and Mrs. Isles talk with the nurse about the effect of Jean's chronic illness on their family. Mr. Isles explains that Jean has a 5-year-old brother and a 3-year-old sister, both of whom have no health problems. The Isleses have always been a close family and do not want a chronic disease to disrupt their family unit. The nurse helps the Isleses develop a plan that will enable them to continue to function as a strong family unit. Which of the following interventions should the nurse consider *most* important?

○ 1. Contacting community resources.

○ 2. Ensuring that Jean has appropriate equipment.

○ 3. Discussing Jean's illness with her siblings.

○ 4. Providing parental education and support.

58. Two months later, Mrs. Isles brings Jean to the clinic for a follow-up visit. Mrs. Isles reports that Jean has become withdrawn. Which statement *best* explains this behavior?

○ 1. It is most likely a reaction to the disease.

○ 2. It is a side effect of the medication.

○ 3. It is a normal stage of development.

○ 4. It is an indication of sibling rivalry.

59. Mrs. Isles explains that she and her husband are very concerned about Jean's behavior, but are

unsure what to do. The nurse should suggest that they

○ 1. have Jean's older brother read to her.
○ 2. obtain psychological counseling for Jean.
○ 3. introduce Jean to other children with arthritis.
○ 4. be supportive and understanding of Jean.


# THE PATIENT WITH A FRACTURE

One-year-old Kenneth Farmer is admitted to the hospital with a fracture of the left femur. He is accompanied by his parents, both of whom appear healthy. Mr. and Mrs. Farmer give different descriptions of the accident that caused Kenneth's fracture. Child abuse is suspected.

**60.** Bryant's traction is ordered for Kenneth. The nurse should explain to Kenneth's parents that the *primary* purpose for the use of this traction is to
○ 1. maintain muscle strength.
○ 2. minimize demineralization of the femur.
○ 3. prevent infection at the fracture site.
○ 4. keep the broken bone in proper alignment.

**61.** When Kenneth is placed in Bryant's traction, he should be positioned on his back and his legs should be
○ 1. straight in line with his body resting flat on the bed.
○ 2. flexed at a 90° angle at his hips, and his hips should be slightly off the bed.
○ 3. flexed at a 45° angle at his hips, and his hips should be resting flat on the bed.
○ 4. separated, with the affected leg at a right angle to his body and the unaffected leg in any comfortable position.

**62.** After Kenneth has been placed in Bryant's traction, the nurse should indicate on the child's nursing care plan that he should be observed *especially* carefully for
○ 1. decubitus ulcer formation.
○ 2. regression in toilet-training.
○ 3. drainage at the skeletal pin sites.
○ 4. decreased circulation in the lower extremities.

**63.** Which of the following actions in relation to Kenneth's traction is considered an *appropriate* nursing measure?
○ 1. Allowing the weights on the traction to hang freely.
○ 2. Decreasing the amount of weight on the traction slightly each day.
○ 3. Changing the moleskin used on his legs for obtaining traction each day.

○ 4. Removing the weights while inspecting his legs for evidence of friction over bony prominences.

**64.** If the nurse notes that Kenneth displays the following behaviors while being cared for, which one *most strongly* suggests that he has been experiencing child abuse?
○ 1. The child sucks his thumb.
○ 2. The child eats his lunch without urging.
○ 3. The child is underdeveloped for his age.
○ 4. The child appears happy when personnel work with him.

**65.** The nurse observes Kenneth carefully and interviews his parents. To which of the following factors should the nurse assign *most* significance when she tries to determine the potential for child abuse in the Farmer family?
○ 1. The severity of the child's physical injuries.
○ 2. The estimated degree of competency the parents display in their parenting ability.
○ 3. The amount of child abuse reported in the geographic area in which the family resides.
○ 4. The degree of inappropriateness in the parent's comments about their child's health needs.

**66.** If the following findings were obtained during interviews with Mr. and Mrs. Farmer, which should the nurse judge *most typical* of parents who abuse their children?
○ 1. The parents each were previously married.
○ 2. The parents were themselves abused children.
○ 3. The parents had children whose births were separated by very brief intervals.
○ 4. The parents were under 20 years of age when married.

**67.** When the nurse suspects that Kenneth has been abused by his parents, it would be *best* for her to
○ 1. inform the parents that she suspects that Kenneth has been abused.
○ 2. ensure that her findings are reported to the designated authorities in the state in which she practices.
○ 3. keep the findings confidential because they are considered legal privileged communication between a nurse and her patient.
○ 4. report her findings to the physician because, legally, reporting evidence of child abuse falls within the province of medical practice.

**68.** It is established that Kenneth is an abused child. When working with abusive parents such as the Farmers, the nurse should take into account that a very common finding concerning abusive parents is that they
○ 1. are unemployed.
○ 2. have a low self-esteem.

○ 3. are members of a low socioeconomic group.

○ 4. have lost emotional attachments in the family.

Five-year-old Sally Hanson is brought to the emergency room by her parents. She has fallen from a tree and broken her right humerus.

69. Sally demonstrates fear and cries, "Mommy, I want to go home. Is the doctor going to cut into my arm? Will it hurt? I hate the nurse!" Which of the following courses of action is the *most appropriate* for the nurse to take in this situation?

○ 1. Have another nurse care for the child because of the child's reaction to the first nurse.

○ 2. Ask the child's parents to leave the room for a while until the nurse has had a chance to calm the child.

○ 3. Suggest to the child that she will be acting like a big girl if she is quiet while the doctor fixes her arm.

○ 4. Explain to the child what the doctor will be doing during the procedure in language the child can readily understand.

70. Sally, a normally developing preschooler, is *most likely* feeling anxiety because of a fear of

○ 1. being separated from her mother.

○ 2. losing control over what is happening.

○ 3. being mutilated and disfigured.

○ 4. feeling pain when the arm is being cared for and casted.

71. Sally is prepared to be sent home after her fracture is reduced and her arm is casted. Her parents should be instructed to bring Sally back to the emergency room promptly if she

○ 1. is irritable and insists the cast is too heavy.

○ 2. complains of nausea before her evening meal.

○ 3. notices that the cast is damp as long as 6 hours after application.

○ 4. complains that her fingers below the cast feel cold and are bluish in color.

72. When the nurse explains that healing can be expected in about 4 to 6 weeks, Mr. Hanson expresses surprise and says, "My father broke his arm and it took much longer than that to heal!" The nurse's response to this comment should be based on the knowledge that a youngster's fracture normally heals more rapidly than an adult's because a child's bones

○ 1. are more pliable than an adult's bones.

○ 2. have epiphyseal plates, whereas an adult's plates are closed.

○ 3. have a more abundant blood supply than an adult's bones.

○ 4. rarely sustain a comminuted fracture, whereas an adult's bones almost always comminute.

73. Sally is tired and says she wants to sleep. Mrs. Hanson should be taught to allow Sally's cast to dry when Sally sleeps by placing the casted arm on

○ 1. a soft pillow.

○ 2. a firm mattress.

○ 3. the top of a bedside nightstand.

○ 4. a block made from a cardboard box.

Three-year-old Alexander Hopke is brought to the emergency room because he refuses to walk after falling off a chair an hour ago. His mother explains that prior to falling off the chair, Alexander had no problems walking. Alexander can move his left leg, but says it hurts.

74. Alexander's refusal to walk after falling off the chair *most likely* indicates

○ 1. traumatic paralysis.

○ 2. paresthesia.

○ 3. fracture.

○ 4. behavioral regression.

75. When examining Alexander, the nurse recalls that the *weakest* point of long bones is the

○ 1. diaphysis.

○ 2. epiphyseal plate.

○ 3. periosteum.

○ 4. medullary canal.

76. The nurse assesses Alexander's left leg. Which of the following findings would the nurse correctly associate with a long-bone fracture?

○ 1. Flabby muscles.

○ 2. Unchanged muscles.

○ 3. Relaxed muscles.

○ 4. Contracted muscles.

77. The nurse notices that Alexander's left thigh is quite swollen. Based on this finding, the nurse's *next* priority action would be to

○ 1. document the findings in the nurse's notes.

○ 2. assess the neurologic status of the toes.

○ 3. notify the physician immediately.

○ 4. determine the circulatory status of the upper thigh.

78. Mrs. Hopke asks the nurse, "How will the doctor know if Alexander's leg is broken?" The nurse would base the answer on knowledge that diagnosis is determined by x-ray of the affected leg and

○ 1. palpation.

○ 2. patient history.

○ 3. x-ray views of the uninjured leg.

○ 4. appearance of the affected leg.

79. A diagnosis of a left fractured femur is made. The physician says that Alexander's fracture is complete. The nurse would *most accurately* interpret this to mean that the bone fragments are

○ 1. oblique.

○ 2. compressed.

○ 3. separated.

○ 4. twisted.

80. Alexander is to be placed in Buck's extension. Mrs. Kopke asks the nurse what Buck's extension is. The nurse would explain that it is a type of traction used to

○ 1. immobilize the fracture until realignment occurs.

○ 2. provide assistance in range-of-motion exercises.

○ 3. increase muscle spasms, thus enhancing circulation.

○ 4. allow for adequate time in arranging for surgery.

81. When setting up the traction, the nurse recalls that the three *essential* components of traction management are traction, countertraction, and

○ 1. friction.

○ 2. pressure.

○ 3. gravity.

○ 4. suction.

82. Because Alexander is immobilized, the nurse anticipates diversional deficit needs. Which of the following toys would be *most appropriate* for 3-year-old Alexander?

○ 1. Marbles.

○ 2. Hand puppets.

○ 3. Blocks.

○ 4. A ball.

83. Alexander experiences a temporary setback in self-toileting and resumes a previous pattern of incontinence. Mrs. Hopke tells the nurse Alexander has not had an "accident" in several months and asks why this is happening. The nurse should base her answer on knowledge that the accidents are an example of

○ 1. remission.

○ 2. regression.

○ 3. depression.

○ 4. sublimation.

84. The nurse notices that Alexander has a low-grade fever and considers the possibility of Alexander's developing osteomyelitis. Which of the following pathogens is *most commonly* involved in osteomyelitis?

○ 1. Cytomegalovirus.

○ 2. *Streptococcus vieridans*.

○ 3. *Candida albicans*.

○ 4. *Staphylococcus aureus*.

85. If Alexander suddenly developed chest pain and dyspnea while being turned, the nurse should suspect

○ 1. respiratory paralysis.

○ 2. pulmonary emboli.

○ 3. pneumonia.

○ 4. pulmonary edema.

86. When Alexander's parents visit their son, they are unable to stay very long because of the needs of their other five children. Mrs. Hopke candidly tells the nurse that she feels guilty about not being able to stay longer. Which of the following responses would *most likely* alleviate Mrs. Hopke's guilt?

○ 1. "Not all parents can stay all the time."

○ 2. "It is important that you visit when you can."

○ 3. "I am sure that you feel very guilty."

○ 4. "You and your husband could take turns visiting."

87. Mr. Hopke asks the nurse how long it usually takes for a 3-year-old's bones to heal. The nurse would correctly answer

○ 1. "2 weeks."

○ 2. "4 weeks."

○ 3. "8 weeks."

○ 4. "10 weeks."

88. After a few days, a spica cast is applied. In the immediate postcasting hours, a *primary* nursing goal would be to prevent

○ 1. respiratory impairment.

○ 2. neurovascular impairment.

○ 3. altered skin integrity.

○ 4. urinary stasis.

89. Alexander is to be discharged home in a few days. The nurse prepares Mr. and Mrs. Hopke for his discharge. Which of the following indicates that Mrs. Hopke *most likely* needs more teaching about preventing skin irritation?

○ 1. She checks the smoothness of the cast edges.

○ 2. She covers the cast around the perineum with plastic film.

○ 3. She inspects inside the cast.

○ 4. She applies lotion to the skin beneath the cast.

90. The nurse continues the discharge planning. Mr. and Mrs. Hopke have understood the teaching if they say they will bring Alexander to the emergency room immediately if

○ 1. his temperature remains less than 100.4° F.

○ 2. he refuses to eat dinner.

○ 3. the toes on the left foot look blue.

○ 4. his cast becomes loose.

# THE PATIENT WITH OSTEOMYELITIS

Steven Knaft, age 8, is admitted to the pediatric unit with a diagnosis of osteomyelitis in the left tibia. While taking the admission history, the nurse learns that 5 days ago Steven sustained a penetrating wound to his anterior left leg in a bicycle accident. He says the leg is painful, especially when he moves it.

**91.** As part of the initial assessment, the nurse examines the area over the left tibia. Which of the following clinical findings is associated with osteomyelitis?
- ○ 1. Diffuse tenderness.
- ○ 2. Localized swelling.
- ○ 3. Increased warmth.
- ○ 4. Increased pallor.

**92.** Given the nature of osteomyelitis, what other clinical manifestations would the nurse expect Steven to have?
- ○ 1. Fever.
- ○ 2. Bradycardia.
- ○ 3. Bradypnea.
- ○ 4. Pulse deficit.

**93.** The nurse reviews the preliminary laboratory results. Which of the following findings is consistent with the diagnosis of osteomyelitis?
- ○ 1. An erythrocyte sedimentation rate of 17 mm/hr.
- ○ 2. A white blood cell count of 12,000/mm³.
- ○ 3. A hematocrit of 30%.
- ○ 4. A serum potassium of 5.0 mEq/L.

**94.** Mrs. Knaft asks about the medical care plan for Steven. The nurse explains that medical therapy will include long-term antibiotic therapy, bed rest, immobilization of the affected leg, and
- ○ 1. abduction of the affected leg.
- ○ 2. passive range-of-motion exercises to the unaffected leg.
- ○ 3. elevation of the affected leg.
- ○ 4. application of cool moist packs to the affected leg.

**95.** Mrs. Knaft asks when Steven's antibiotic therapy will start. The nurse tells her it will start as soon as blood is drawn for
- ○ 1. creatinine.
- ○ 2. culture.
- ○ 3. leukocyte count.
- ○ 4. hemoglobin.

**96.** Based on knowledge of the most common etiologic microorganism of osteomyelitis in the school-aged child, which of the following antibiotics does the nurse anticipate will be ordered for Steven intravenously?
- ○ 1. Kanamycin and ampicillin.
- ○ 2. Methicillin and ampicillin.
- ○ 3. Penicillin G and methicillin.
- ○ 4. Gentamicin and ampicillin.

**97.** The nurse knows that Steven will be receiving high-dose intravenous antibiotic therapy for at least 3 to 4 weeks. Because of the nature of this therapy, the nurse plans to monitor his
- ○ 1. blood glucose levels.
- ○ 2. urinary output.
- ○ 3. prothrombin times.
- ○ 4. urinary glucose levels.

**98.** Steven's left leg is immobilized using a fiberglass splint and Ace wraps. Two days after application of the splint, the nurse notices swelling and diminished capillary refill of the toes on the left foot. Steven says he had decreased feeling in his toes. The nurse knows that these findings indicate circulatory impairment and *correctly* attributes it to
- ○ 1. increased infection in the leg.
- ○ 2. immobilization of the leg.
- ○ 3. development of a deep vein thrombosis.
- ○ 4. too-tight application of the splint and wraps.

**99.** Given the developmental needs of an 8-year-old, which of the following interventions would the nurse include in Steven's care plan?
- ○ 1. Make a referral to occupational therapy.
- ○ 2. Encourage communication with schoolmates.
- ○ 3. Encourage his parents to visit often.
- ○ 4. Talk to him about his interests each day.

**100.** Bed rest and immobilization of the affected leg increases Steven's risk for skin breakdown. Therefore, a nursing goal is to maintain skin integrity. All of the following nursing interventions are included in Steven's care plan. Which is likely to be *most* effective in attaining this goal?
- ○ 1. Turn him every 2 hours.
- ○ 2. Attach a trapeze to his bed.
- ○ 3. Encourage fluid intake.
- ○ 4. Inspect his skin every 8 hours.

**101.** Which of the following menus would be an appropriate diet for Steven?
- ○ 1. Hamburger on a bun, French fries, and an apple.
- ○ 2. An egg, whole-wheat toast, and bacon.
- ○ 3. Hot dog on a bun, baked beans, and baked custard.
- ○ 4. Tuna-fish sandwich, tomato, and a fresh peach.

**102.** During the second week of treatment, Steven responds to a request to begin his bath by throwing the soap and refusing to bathe. Steven is *most likely* responding to
- ○ 1. lack of control.
- ○ 2. separation from his friends and classmates.
- ○ 3. a dislike for the nurse providing care that day.
- ○ 4. the doctor having checked his leg a few minutes earlier.

# CORRECT ANSWERS AND RATIONALES

Numbers appear in parentheses following the rationales. The numbers identify textbooks listed in the references at the end of Part III, where correct answers can be verified.

## Screening Patients for Musculoskeletal Dysfunction

**1.** 3. Legg-Calvé-Perthes disease is also known as coxa plana or osteochondrosis. It is characterized by aseptic necrosis at the head of the femur when blood supply to the area is interrupted. Avoiding weight-bearing is especially important to prevent the head of the femur from leaving the acetabulum. Various devices are used, such as an abduction brace, a leg cast, or a harness sling, to protect the affected joint while revascularization and bone healing occur. Surgical procedures are used in some cases. (6, 21)

**2.** 3. Since most of the child's care takes place on an outpatient basis, the *major emphasis* for nursing care is to teach the family the care and management of the corrective appliance. Corrective devices, such as abduction braces, leg casts, and leather harness slings, are used to keep the head of the femur "contained" in the acetabulum. Traction to stretch tight abductor muscles is used in some cases. Legg-Calvé-Perthes disease does occur in obese children because they are more prone to orthopedic problems. However, weight reduction is not the major emphasis of teaching in the majority of children with Legg-Calvé-Perthes disease. Pain is not usually a problem once therapy has been initiated. (15, 21)

**3.** 1. Kyphosis is an abnormally increased convex angulation in the curvature of the thoracic spine. The most common form of kyphosis in children is postural. It is usually a result of bizarre sitting and standing positions. Scoliosis, the most common spinal deformity, is a lateral curvature of the spine. It is usually associated with a rotary deformity that eventually causes cosmetic and physiologic alterations in the spine, chest, and pelvis. Accentuation of the cervical or lumbar curvature beyond physiologic limits is lordosis. Lordosis is often associated with flexion contractures of the hip, obesity, congenital dislocated hip, and slipped femoral capital epiphysis. An outgrowth of bone-like deposits on the vertebrae that may fuse and cause a rigid and distorted spine is called spondylitis deformans. (15, 21)

**4.** 4. The sternocleidomastoid muscle appears to be contracted, or shortened, when torticollis is present. Range of motion is limited. The condition is often called wry neck. It causes the head to turn laterally to one side with the chin directed to the opposite side. (6, 21)

**5.** 2. There is no treatment for flat feet. However, corrective shoes are often prescribed to help keep the legs in proper alignment. Being pigeon-toed is not associated necessarily with flat feet, and corrective shoes will not change weight-bearing or strengthen the arches. (6, 21)

**6.** 2. Muscular dystrophy is a genetically determined, sex-linked condition. It is a progressive degenerative disease of the skeletal muscles. There are several different forms of muscle involvement. The various deviations that involve progressive weakness of muscle groups form the largest group of muscular diseases of childhood. (6, 21)

**7.** 2. Scoliosis is a lateral curvature of the spine, usually associated with a rotary deformity. If the condition is not properly cared for, eventually cosmetic and physiologic alterations in the chest, spine, and pelvis are likely. Scoliosis occurs about five to seven times more often in girls than in boys. Order of birth does not appear to affect the incidence of scoliosis. (6, 21)

**8.** 4. The recommended position of the child while being screened for scoliosis is to bend forward at the waist while allowing the head and arms to fall freely. (6, 21)

**9.** 1. A characteristic sign of scoliosis is a rib hump. This hump is best observed when the child, undressed to the waist, bends over while allowing the arms and head to hang freely and is viewed from the back and front. The rib hump and flank asymmetry then become obvious. A slight limp, a crooked hemline, and complaints of back pain are other common findings when a child has scoliosis. (6, 21)

**10.** 4. The Milwaukee brace, which has been found to be the most effective spinal brace for correcting scoliosis, extends from the pelvis to the occiput. It provides longitudinal traction and lateral pressure, which help to decrease the curvature. Children who for some reason cannot use the brace often require surgical procedures for correction of the curvature. (6, 21)

**11.** 4. The common procedure is to have the patient wear the Milwaukee brace at all times except while carrying out personal hygiene measures. (6, 21)

**12.** 4. Exercises are prescribed for the child with scoliosis who wears a Milwaukee brace to help strengthen muscles that will help overcome the spinal curvature. Exercise also helps improve the correction of the spine and ribs and improves the child's stamina. (6, 21)

**13.** 1. The osteochondroses are a group of diseases affecting various parts of the body, the most common one of this group being Osgood-Schlatter disease. This disease is frequently referred to as growing pains. This condition occurs mostly in males between about 13 and 15 years of age, when epiphyseal growth is very rapid. This growth places stress on muscles and tendons and eventually produces a tendonitis, usually at the tibial tuberosity. Osgood-Schlatter disease is ordinarily self-limiting and usually responds to rest. Warm compresses placed over the painful area are often used to promote comfort. (6, 21)

**14.** 1. Slipped femoral capital epiphysis (SFCE) or coxa vara is the spontaneous displacement of the proximal femoral epiphysis. The most common clinical manifestations of SFCE are limping and intermittent or continuous hip pain. The pain is frequently referred to the groin, the knee, or the anteromedial aspect of the thigh or knee. (15, 21)

## The Patient with Cerebral Palsy

**15.** 2. The goal of early recognition of primary developmental delays is to prevent secondary and tertiary delays. For example, a young infant who is unable to reach or focus on objects would be unable to attain the various levels of sensory-perceptual development described by Piaget. Facilitating communication, preventing physical injury, and encouraging health maintenance are all nursing goals for the child with cerebral palsy, but are not the goal of early recognition of primary developmental delays. (7, 21)

**16.** 3. Cerebral palsy is a collective term applied to nonprogressive cerebellar damage that results in a variety of alterations in neuromuscular tone/function. (7, 21)

**17.** 4. An overall delay in gross motor development is a universal manifestation of cerebral palsy. There is a discrepancy between expected achievement and motor ability, and this discrepancy increases with successive developmental milestones. One-third of children with cerebral palsy have normal or above-normal intelligence; two-thirds are mildly or moderately retarded. Perceptual deficits may occur but are not a universal manifestation. (7, 21)

**18.** 1. Spastic cerebral palsy is the most common clinical type. It represents an upper motor neuron muscular impairment in which there may be altered

tone, persistent primitive reflexes, and a lack or delay of postural control. Dyskinetic movements are involuntary and may be manifested in athetoid movements. Ataxia is the least common type of cerebral palsy, and atonic is very uncommon. (7, 21)

**19.** 4. The goals of therapy for children with cerebral palsy are early recognition and promotion of optimal development so that the child can realize his potential. (7, 21)

**20.** 3. The term "hemiparesis" refers to a half of the body; in this case, the affected side is the right side. Hemiparesis is the most common form of spastic cerebral palsy. Quadriparesis refers to spastic cerebral palsy in which all four extremities are involved. Paraplegia is pure cerebral paralysis of the lower extremities. In the diplegia type of spastic cerebral palsy, similar parts on both sides of the body are involved. (7, 21)

**21.** 2. Challenging the use of the affected limb facilitates increased function. Positioning the child upright and handing toys to his affected side will keep him occupied and may test his visual acuity, but neither of these is the reason for the activity. Similarly, this activity is not done to increase the strength of the affected limb. (7, 21)

**22.** 2. In the hemiparesis type of spastic cerebral palsy, most children are able to walk. The motor deficit is usually greater in the upper extremity. The nurse should answer the mother's questions honestly and with sensitivity. The will to walk is important, but without neurologic stability the child may be unable to do so. There is no need for the nurse to refer the mother to the physician for an answer to the question. (7, 21)

**23.** 1. Drugs to decrease spasticity have little use in improving function in cerebral palsy. Skeletal muscle relaxants may be used on a short-term basis for older children and adolescents. Anticonvulsants are used routinely for children who have seizures. (7, 21)

**24.** 4. The parents' response to friends' reactions to a child with cerebral palsy provides the most accurate information about the parents' ability to cope with the cerebral palsy. The ability of the family to cope with the reactions and responses of friends outweighs other factors. (7, 21)

## The Patient with Muscular Dystrophy

**25.** 3. Duchenne muscular dystrophy is also known as pseudohypertrophic muscular dystrophy. The term "pseudohypertrophy" is derived from the characteristic muscular enlargement. Myotonic dystrophies are hereditary diseases characterized by muscular wasting and myotonia. The term "myotonic" refers to difficulty in relaxing muscles after contraction. Myoclonic muscular dystrophy is not a disease. (7, 21)

**26.** 2. In all X-linked disorders, males are affected almost exclusively because the mother carries the gene that is expressed in males. (7, 21)

**27.** 4. Usually the first clinical manifestations of Duchenne muscular dystrophy are difficulty running, riding a bicycle, and climbing stairs. Abnormal gait on a level surface becomes apparent later. Occasionally, enlarged calves may be noticed. Lack of facial mobility is associated with facioscapulohumeral muscular dystrophy. (7, 21)

**28.** 2. Gower sign is the term given to "walking" the hands up the legs in an attempt to stand. Galleazzi sign refers to the shortening of the affected limb in congenital dislocation of the hip. Good-enough refers to a test of mental age. Goodell sign refers to the softening of the cervix and is considered a sign of probable pregnancy. (7, 21)

**29.** 4. The mean intelligence quotient for the child with muscular dystrophy is about 20 points below normal, and frank mental deficit is present in 25% of these children. (7, 21)

**30.** 1. The primary goal is to maintain function in unaffected muscles for as long as possible. There is no effective treatment for childhood muscular dystrophy. Children who remain active are able to avoid wheelchair confinement for a longer period. Children with muscular dystrophy become socially isolated as their condition deteriorates and they can no longer keep up with friends. Maintaining function helps prevent social isolation. Circulatory impairment is not associated with muscular dystrophy. (7, 21)

**31.** 1. Contractures of hips, knees, and ankles occur as a result of selective muscle involvement. Fractures are not as common as contractures and osteomyelitis is not a complication of muscular dystrophy. Clubfoot is associated with muscular dystrophy, but nursing intervention is focused on preventing contractures. (7, 21)

**32.** 4. The guilt feelings that mothers of children with muscular dystrophy commonly experience are due to the mother-to-son transmission of the defective gene. Children with muscular dystrophy are typically passive, withdrawn, and emotionally immature but usually strive to be as independent as possible. Onset of muscular dystrophy is usually gradual. Congenital forms of muscular dystrophy are rare. (7, 21)

**33.** 1. The usual cause of death in children with muscular dystrophy is respiratory tract infection or cardiac failure. The sister is asking for information; nothing in the situation indicates the need to request additional information before answering the question. (7, 21)

**34.** 4. Death of children with Duchenne muscular dystrophy usually occurs between 15 and 25 years of age. Onset of the disease is usually between 3 and 5 years of age and the child is usually wheelchair-bound by age 10 or 11. (7, 21)

**35.** 1. Muscular dystrophy is a progressive disease and children are usually unable to walk independently by the time they are between 9 and 11 years of age. There is no effective treatment for childhood muscular dystrophy. Children who remain active are able to avoid wheelchair confinement for a longer period, but activity does not prevent progression of the disease. (7, 21)

**36.** 1. The erroneous thinking has to do with failure to comprehend the progressive nature of the disease. There is no curative treatment known, including drugs, surgery, or other modalities. Maintaining potential function for the longest possible time, while attempting to meet the family's needs as they cope with the disease and its effects, is the goal of therapy. (7, 21)

## The Patient with Congenital Hip Dysplasia

**37.** 1. Ortolani sign refers to the feeling of the femoral head slipping forward into the acetabulum when forward pressure is exerted from behind the greater trochanter and the knee is held laterally. This sign indicates dislocation of the hip. A positive Barlow test indicates that the hip is unstable with the possibility of being dislocatable. Jackson sign is the prolongation of the expiratory sound over the affected area in pulmonary tuberculosis. Trendelenburg sign refers to the downward tilting of the pelvis toward the normal side when a child with a dislocated hip stands on the affected side with the uninvolved leg elevated. (7, 21)

**38.** 3. Shortening of the limb on the affected side is called Galleazzi sign and indicates congenital hip dysplasia. Other signs of congenital hip dysplasia include broadening of the perineum in bilateral dislocation, asymmetric thigh and gluteal folds, and limited abduction of the affected leg. (7, 21)

**39.** 3. The Pavlik harness, an abduction device, is highly effective when the device is well-constructed, follow-up care is adequate, and the parents follow instructions in its use. The harness is not used concurrently with a spica cast. (7, 21)

**40.** 3. Assessing the learner's level of knowledge is the initial step in teaching. The assessment forms the basis for subsequent teaching. Giving parents written instructions and a list of community resources are appropriate teaching strategies but not the *most appropriate initial* steps. Assessing coping strategies can provide information that is helpful in developing a teaching plan, but it is not an initial step. (7, 21)

**41.** 3. The purpose of the abduction stabilizer bar is to maintain the proper degree of abduction. It should never be used as a handle for turning or lifting. The bar can be covered with linen and is not adjusted. (7, 21)

**42.** 2. The mother can continue to breast-feed the infant in a spica cast but may need to try alternate nursing positions to accommodate the cast. Since the mother was successful in breast-feeding and will be able to continue, it is not necessary to ask either if she wants to continue or how she would feel if she could not continue. Telling her that it is possible but very difficult is false and could create anxiety. (7, 21)

## The Patient with Congenital Clubfoot

**43.** 2. Management of the infant who has a clubfoot deformity starts as soon as possible after birth. Treatment in early infancy is conservative and, depending on the severity of the deformity, consists of manipulating the feet into a functional position and applying a series of casts until a marked overcorrection of the deformity is achieved. Corrective shoes may be used once the deformity has been corrected. Elevation of the extremities and use of a footboard are not modes used to treat clubfoot. (21)

**44.** 4. When an infant is born with an unexpected anomaly, parents are faced with questions, uncertainties, and possible disappointments. They may feel inadequate, helpless, and anxious. The nurse can help the family initially by assessing their concerns and then by providing appropriate information needed to help the family clarify and/or resolve the immediate problems. (15)

**45.** 2. Complete drying of a plaster cast takes several hours. Turning the child with a newly applied cast at least every 2 hours helps the cast dry uniformly. The drying cast must be handled with the palms only to prevent indentations from the fingers that

could cause pressure areas. Heated dryers are not used to dry the cast, because the cast dries on the surface but remains wet underneath. Furthermore, heat may be conducted to the tissues through the wet cast, causing burns. The cast must not be coated with any substance that would inhibit the evaporation of moisture from the plaster. (21)

**46.** 1. Because of the influence of maternal hormones, the tendons and ligaments of the neonate are more relaxed and more amenable to manipulation now than they will be later. Early casting is not done to promote parental acceptance of the deformity. Leg movements do not exacerbate a clubfoot deformity, nor does nerve damage result from an uncorrected clubfoot. (2, 20)

**47.** 3. A cast that is too tight can cause a tourniquet effect and compromise the neurovascular integrity of the extremity. Manifestations of neurovascular impairment include pain, edema, pulselessness, discoloration, coolness, altered sensation, and inability to move the distal exposed extremity. Therefore, the casted extremity should be assessed frequently. Wetting a cast softens the plaster, which may alter the cast's effectiveness. Adhesive tape petals are applied to cover the rough edges of the cast and should be left in place. There is no reason to elevate the casted extremities when a child is being treated for clubfoot. (21)

**48.** 4. Casts may have to be changed every 1 to 2 weeks in an infant with a clubfoot deformity because of the infant's rapid growth. Frequent cast changes allow tight muscles to stretch and flaccid muscles to tighten. The frequent cast changes have nothing to do with infection, but the cast itself may cause skin pressure and breakdown and thus infection. Infection is something that is always assessed. Neurovascular status is evaluated by assessing the extremity distal to the cast. With clubfeet, the legs are neither measured nor compared to norms. (21)

**49.** 2. The Denis Browne splint is an adjustable metal bar to which special shoes are attached. This splint provides an appropriate degree of eversion, dorsiflexion, and rotation to keep the feet in a slightly overcorrected position. When the infant kicks, the feet are automatically moved into a corrected position. (17)

**50.** 4. If the shoes become loose, they can be tightened against the Denis Browne splint. The shoes and footpieces are set at a particular angle to maintain the correction achieved through casting. The angle of the shoes on the bar should not be repositioned. Parents should put socks on the child's feet before applying the splint to decrease irritation. The splint should not be used as a weight-bearing device when lifting the child. (2, 20)

**51.** 4. When an infant begins to be mobile, child-proofing the home is necessary. One aspect of child-proofing is to remove tablecloths. This eliminates the child's pulling on them in an attempt to stand and either falling or pulling objects on top of him. The child in a Denis Browne splint needs opportunities to increase mobility to achieve developmental tasks. Increasing mobility is not an indication to remove the splint or to obtain corrective shoes. (15)

## The Patient with Juvenile Rheumatoid Arthritis

**52.** 1. No specific laboratory test exists for JRA. The erythrocyte sedimentation rate (ESR) may be elevated during active disease; normal ESR using the Westergren method is 0 to 10 mm/hr. The synovial fluid contains increased amounts of protein. Anemia is common; normal hemoglobin is 11.5 to 15.5 g/dl. (21)

**53.** 2. In most children with JRA, the disease will be in permanent remission by adolescence. Seventy-five percent of children with the disease go into long remissions without severe deformity or functional loss. Some children recover completely within a few years. (7, 21)

**54.** 1. The primary group of drugs used to treat JRA is nonsteroidal anti-inflammatory drugs (NSAIDs). These include aspirin, naproxen, and ibuprofen. They are used because of their analgesic, antipyretic, and anti-inflammatory effects. Adrenocorticosteroids are used only when arthritis does not respond to NSAIDs. Prolonged steroid therapy is avoided because these drugs suppress growth. Slower-acting antirheumatic drugs (SAARDs) compose the second group of drugs used to treat JRA. Drugs included in this group are gold, D-penicillamine, and hydroxychloroquine. Cytoxic drugs are used with patients who have severe debilitating disease and who have responded poorly to NSAIDs and SAARDs. (21)

**55.** 2. Activity and socialization should be encouraged, but mornings are the most difficult time for children with JRA. These children need time to "warm up" their joints. Children should be encouraged to attend school when they have joint pain as long as it is not prohibitive. Splints are worn during rest, not activity. If side effects of the medications prevent school attendance, the child should be evaluated for toxic blood levels. (21)

**56.** 2. The application of moist heat to affected joints at any time may facilitate joint movement. Heat increases circulation, decreases pain, and increases mobility. Exercise is important, but only after the joints are loosened by warmth. Weight-bearing exercises are temporarily restricted when joints are painful and swollen. Cool compresses constrict blood vessels and decrease circulation. Dietary purine is related to gouty arthritis, not JRA. (7, 21)

**57.** 4. Providing parental education and support is the most important intervention because this enables the parents to contact community resources, acquire necessary equipment, and provide information to their other children. This approach also enables the family to make informed decisions, solve problems, and seek alternatives that meet their needs. (21)

**58.** 1. Children with chronic diseases, regardless of their seriousness or the child's developmental stage, suffer a loss. Withdrawal and regression are two coping strategies that young children use. Side effects of nonsteroidal anti-inflammatory drugs include nausea, vomiting, and gastrointestinal distress. A 4-year-old is involved in Erikson's psychosocial stage of sense of initiative. Sibling rivalry is common in first-born children, particularly when there is a 2- to 4-year difference in age. (7, 21)

**59.** 4. Parents need to be supportive and understanding of the child while helping her deal with grief and loss associated with chronic illness. The child needs to feel valued. Psychological counseling is not needed at this time. Peer support is not effective with a 4-year-old because a child this age is developmentally egocentric. (21)

## The Patient with a Fracture

**60.** 4. The primary purpose of traction is the relief of painful muscle spasms so that the fracture can be reduced to achieve appropriate anatomic alignment. Traction immobilizes the bone fragments until sufficient healing has occurred to apply a cast on the leg. Muscle strength and mass are not maintained by traction. Demineralization of bone occurs with immobility, but traction does not prevent it. Infection at a fracture site most often occurs when the fracture is compound. Traction has no role in preventing infection. (6, 21)

**61.** 2. When placed in Bryant's traction, the child should be on his back and his legs should be flexed at a 90° angle at his hips. The hips should be slightly off the bed. This positioning provides adequate countertraction to reduce and immobilize the fracture. (6, 21)

**62.** 4. Blood vessel occlusion from constriction by the bandages around the legs can lead to muscle anoxia and reflex vasospasms. Damage to the muscles can occur within a day and permanent damage with contractions or paralysis in 5 to 10 days if circulation in the extremities is inadequate. Signs of adequate circulation include rapid capillary refilling and movement of the toes on request. If the child is too young to cooperate by moving his toes, his response to stimulation of the toes can be observed and pedal pulses can be palpated. When circulation is satisfactory, the skin will be free of cyanosis and pallor. Decubitus ulcers are unlikely to occur in the infant described in this item. Regression in toilet-training is common among hospitalized youngsters, but an infant of 1 year of age has probably not started toilet-training. No pins are used for Bryant's traction; the traction is applied directly to the skin. (6, 21)

**63.** 1. Weights used for traction must be allowed to hang freely to maintain a consistent traction. Changing the moleskins used for securing an infant's traction and decreasing the amount of weight could result in a return of the bone fragments to a misaligned position, and soft tissue damage would then most probably ensue. The bony prominences can be observed without releasing weights. Traction should be maintained unless a specific order is given with other directions. (6, 21)

**64.** 3. Although the descriptions of abused children vary, an almost universal finding is that the child is underdeveloped for his age. This may be reflected in body size, but usually there is also a decrease in skills and poor psychosocial development. A child who is not within the normal range of development for his age should be evaluated further until a plausible reason can be established. Children sucking their thumbs contentedly and eating food without urging are not typical in abusive families. Abused children are often suspicious and tend to shy away from personnel. (6, 21)

**65.** 4. The degree to which parents are concerned about their child's health needs is a significant factor in trying to determine whether child abuse is occurring. Usually, abusive parents show little apparent concern for their child's health needs. Characteristically, only one child in a family is abused, and usually it is the one parents perceive as being different from the others. The severity of a child's injuries, the degree of competency the parents demonstrate as parents, and the amount of child abuse in the family's neighborhood have not been found to be very significant in establishing whether child abuse is occurring. (6, 21)

**66.** 2. The family history of abused children illustrates a disturbance in the parent-child relationship. Parenting is believed to be learned behavior, not instinctive behavior. It has often been noted that parents who abuse their children were abused themselves and came from environments in which parent-child relationships were disturbed or distorted. (6, 21)

**67.** 2. Evidence of child abuse is reportable, and nurses should ensure that findings are reported. Most state laws require anyone who works with children to report suspicion of child abuse. The specific persons required to report and the specific policies concerning the reporting vary among agencies. These laws ordinarily provide immunity from legal action for persons reporting child abuse if it is reported in good faith. The nurse should document her findings carefully, being as specific as possible, when caring for an abused child and his family. (6, 21)

**68.** 2. A rather consistent finding is that abusive parents have low self-esteem and a poor self-image. Abusive parents are found in all socioeconomic groups. There may be no loss of emotional attachment in the family, and most of these parents feel strongly about their child and would object to giving up the child to a foster home. Whether the parents are employed or unemployed appears to have no significance in terms of child abuse. (6, 21)

**69.** 4. A 5-year-old child often responds to simple descriptions of what to expect in terms of what will be heard, seen, and felt. Telling the child how he can cooperate also is often effective. Such explanations often relieve fears. Most 5-year-old children fear mutilation, disability, and even death when an injury occurs. The nurse is interpreting the child's behavior as a personal rejection if she asks another nurse to care for the child because of a reaction to care. Sometimes this may be necessary, but such instances are rare. Asking the parents to leave the room while the child is being cared for is likely to result in increased distress. Suggesting that the child act as a "big girl" uses shame as a method of eliciting desired behavior and is not recommended. This technique may at times produce desired behavior, but explanations are recommended instead. (6, 21)

**70.** 3. The major fear of a preschooler is fear of bodily mutilation and disfigurement. Infants and toddlers fear most being separated from their mother. School-aged children fear loss of self-control most. (6, 21)

**71.** 4. A child should be seen promptly if the fingers below a casted arm feel cool and appear bluish. These signs indicate poor circulation in the extremity, and if poor circulation continues, tissue damage can occur. Such signs as complaining of nausea after a meal following a fracture, feeling irritable, believing the cast is too heavy, and noting that the cast is damp after 6 hours are fairly normal findings and are not grave. (6, 21)

**72.** 3. Bones heal more quickly in a child than in an adult because the child's bones have a better blood supply and a greater source of osteoblasts from a thicker periosteum. It is true that a child's bones are more pliable than an adult's bones, have epiphyseal plates, and rarely sustain a comminuted fracture. However, these characteristics do not influence healing of a fractured bone. (21)

**73.** 1. A wet cast should be placed on a soft surface, such as a pillow. Placing it on a hard and flat surface is likely to cause the cast to dent and flatten, which may cause pressure on tissues under the cast. (6, 21)

**74.** 3. A fracture should be suspected if a young child who previously walked without problems refuses to walk after injury. Pseudoparalysis from pain is found in young children with fractures. Paresthesia is characterized by numbness and lack of sensation. Behavioral regression usually does not take the form of refusing to walk. (7, 21)

**75.** 2. The epiphyseal growth plate is the weakest point of long bones. The diaphysis is the hard shaftlike portion constituting the major portion of the bone. The periosteum is the thin membrane that covers the bones. It contains blood vessels that nourish living bone and is not a growth plate. The medullary canal is found within the diaphysis and is composed of the bone marrow. (7, 21)

**76.** 4. Immediately after a fracture, the muscles contract and physiologically splint the injured area. This phenomenon also accounts for the deformity that results as the muscles pull the bone ends out of alignment. (7, 21)

**77.** 2. Assessing the neurologic and circulatory status of the toes, the tissues distal to the fracture, is important. Contusions of soft tissues, which frequently accompany femur fractures, can result in severe hemorrhage into the tissue and subsequent circulatory and neurologic impairment. The nurse can document the findings after assessing the leg. There is no need to notify the physician immediately. (7, 21)

**78.** 3. Radiographic examination is the most useful tool in diagnosing skeletal trauma. However, x-ray diagnosis is difficult because of the presence of non-ossified cartilage of the epiphysis and the growth plate. Therefore, x-ray views are taken of the uninjured limb for comparison. Palpation does not provide conclusive data about a fracture, nor does the appearance of the affected leg. Patient history is helpful, but children are not reliable informants. (7, 21)

**79.** 3. Fractures are either complete or incomplete. In a complete fracture, the bone fragments are separated. More information is needed to differentiate the type of complete fracture. An oblique fracture is a type of complete fracture in which the fracture line extends in a slanting but straight direction. In a greenstick fracture, the compressed side of the bone bends. In a torsion fracture, which is also a type of complete fracture, the bones have been twisted apart. (7, 21)

**80.** 1. Buck's extension is a type of skin traction used to align and immobilize bone fragments. It is also used to relieve muscle spasms, which enhances circulation and decreases pain. (7, 21)

**81.** 1. The frictional force between the patient and the bed, together with the countertraction, balance the traction. The countertraction is the backward force of the muscle pull, while the traction is the forward force produced by attaching weight to the distal bone fragment. Pressure, gravity, and suction are not essential components of traction management. (7, 21)

**82.** 2. Hand puppets would enable a 3-year-old child in Buck's traction to act out feelings within the constraints imposed by the traction. Marbles are unsafe because they could be swallowed. Blocks are more appropriate for a younger child, and with traction there is no flat surface on which to set them. A ball would encourage more movement than a child in Buck's traction is allowed. (7, 21)

**83.** 2. Regression is the temporary return to previous behavioral patterns and often occurs in young children because of the stress of illness or hospitalization. Remission refers to an abatement of symptoms. Depression refers to a condition in which the individual feels hopeless or inadequate. Sublimation refers to a coping mechanism in which the individual expresses socially or personally unacceptable impulses in constructive and acceptable forms. (7, 21)

**84.** 4. *Staphylococcus aureus* is the pathogen most commonly involved in osteomyelitis, although any bacterial organism can cause this infection. Cytomegalovirus is associated with congenital defects. *Streptococcus vieridans* is the most common causative agent of bacterial endocarditis. *Candida albicans* is associated with yeast infection. (7, 21)

**85.** 2. Chest pain and dyspnea in an immobilized child with a fractured femur suggest pulmonary emboli. Fat droplets from the marrow are transferred to the general circulation via the venous arterial route and eventually reach the lung or brain. Respiratory paralysis is not usually associated with a fracture. Pneumonia may occur but would not present as sudden chest pain. Pulmonary edema is not commonly associated with fractures. (7, 21)

**86.** 2. Stressing that the parents visit when they can will help alleviate the guilt they feel. Acknowledging the guilt gives the parent an opportunity to talk about it but does not help alleviate it. Suggesting that the parents take turns visiting implies that they should feel guilty because they may not be doing all they could. Comparing them to other parents does not alleviate guilt feelings. (7, 21)

**87.** 2. Children's bones usually heal within 4 to 6 weeks, a neonate's bones within 2 to 3 weeks. An adult's bones heal within 8 to 12 weeks. (7, 21)

**88.** 2. A too-tight cast, always a possibility in the immediate postcasting period, can cause neurovascular impairment. Respiratory impairment is not a problem associated with cast application. Impaired skin integrity and urinary stasis would not develop in the immediate postcasting hours. (7, 21)

**89.** 4. Lotion should not be applied to skin beneath the cast because it can cause irritation and skin breakdown. Checking the smoothness of the cast edges, covering the cast around the perineum, and inspecting inside the cast help prevent skin irritation. (7, 21)

**90.** 3. Bluish toes indicate compromised circulation, which requires immediate attention. A body temperature less than 100.4° F. is an expected outcome. Refusing to eat dinner does not warrant immediate attention. As edema in the casted leg subsides and as the cast dries, the cast may become more loose, but not so loose as to provide no support. (7, 21)

## The Patient with Osteomyelitis

**91.** 3. Findings associated with osteomyelitis usually include increased warmth, localized tenderness, and diffuse swelling over the involved bone. The area over affected bone is reddened, not pale. (7, 17, 21)

**92.** 1. Increased temperature and increased pulse and respiratory rates are clinical manifestations of osteomyelitis. Pulse deficit is associated with atrial fibrillation. (7, 17, 21)

**93.** 1. In osteomyelitis, the erythrocyte sedimentation rate (ESR) is elevated (for the child, normal is 0 to 13 mm/hr, depending on the method); the leukocyte count is 15,000 to 25,000/mm³; hematocrit and serum potassium levels should be normal. The ESR rises in the presence of severe localized or systemic inflammation. (7, 21)

**94.** 3. The affected leg is elevated and warm moist packs are applied to the affected area. This helps decrease the swelling and improves circulation. Good body alignment is maintained; neither leg is abducted. Active range-of-motion exercises are performed with the unaffected leg. (7, 21)

**95.** 2. Antibiotic therapy starts *after* blood cultures are drawn. The blood cultures will determine the causative organism, which in turn determines the appropriate antibiotic therapy. (7, 21)

**96.** 3. Large doses of penicillin G are given and augmented by methicillin or oxacillin because most cases of osteomyelitis in school-aged children are caused by staphylococci. Antibiotics such as kanamycin or gentamicin, together with ampicillin, are used with neonates who have osteomyelitis because the causative organisms are coliforms. Methicillin, nafcillin, or clindamycin, in conjunction with ampicillin, are used to treat osteomyelitis in children younger than 3 years. Infectious agents in this age group are likely to be penicillin-resistant staphylococci or gram-negative organisms. (21)

**97.** 2. Long-term high-dose intravenous antibiotic therapy can adversely affect renal, hepatic, and hematopoietic function. Therefore, these systems should be assessed carefully. Antibiotics do not usually affect blood glucose levels, prothrombin times, or urinary glucose levels. (21)

**98.** 4. Circulatory impairment is due to too-tight application of the splint and Ace wraps. Increased infection and immobilization of the leg do not affect capillary refill of the toes on the affected foot. In deep vein thrombosis, the entire affected leg is swollen, pale, and cold. The area along the vein is very tender. (21)

**99.** 2. Encouraging communication with schoolmates is important because the peer group is a major social factor in assisting the school-age child to achieve the various developmental tasks of this age group. Limited mobility and the length of hospitalization foster a sense of isolation. Parental visits, a referral to occupational therapy, and talking about the child's interests may be helpful but do not meet the developmental need of peer contact. (21)

**100.** 1. Turning the child every 2 hours is most effective in preventing skin breakdown. A trapeze may help the child move in bed and encouraging fluid intake may help prevent breakdown, but these interventions are not as effective as turning every 2 hours. Inspecting the skin provides feedback about goal attainment. (21)

**101.** 3. Children with osteomyelitis need a diet high in protein and calories. Milk, eggs, cheese, meat, fish, and vegetables such as beans are the best sources of these nutrients. (7, 14, 21)

**102.** 1. School-aged children have an increasing need for independence. Anger and resentment are common responses to dependence and loss of control over the environment, with minimal opportunity to participate in planning and decision-making. (15)

# test 9

● **The Patient Who is Preterm**

● **The Patient with Sepsis**

● **The Patient with Failure to Thrive**

● **The Patient with Atopic Dermatitis (Eczema)**

● **The Patient with Burns**

**The Patient with Hypothyroidism**

● **The Patient with Insulin-Dependent Diabetes Mellitus**

● **The Patient Who is Abused**

**Correct Answers and Rationales**

Select the one *best* or *correct* answer and indicate your choice by filling in the circle with a pencil in front of the option you have chosen. If the answer you would prefer is not given, select the one you think is *most appropriate*.

## THE PATIENT WHO IS PRETERM

John Carrington is delivered prematurely. He weighs 1,870 g (4 pounds, 2 ounces) at birth. After initial care is given in the delivery room, he is transferred to the intensive-care nursery in the pediatric department.

**1.** John is small for his gestational age as well as premature. During a physical assessment upon his admission to the nursery, the nurse can expect that John will display
  ○ 1. full areola with breast tissue.
  ○ 2. lanugo over the upper arms and back.
  ○ 3. firm cartilage to the edge of the ear pinna.
  ○ 4. prominent creases on the soles and heels of the feet.

**2.** During the physical assessment of John, the nurse should also expect that the infant will display
  ○ 1. dry, cracked skin.
  ○ 2. a thin, wasted appearance.
  ○ 3. an abundance of scalp hair.
  ○ 4. numerous rugae on the scrotum.

**3.** Because John is suffering from cold stress in addition to prematurity, the nurse should be *especially* alert in observing for
  ○ 1. jaundice.
  ○ 2. abdominal distention.
  ○ 3. slow, shallow respirations.
  ○ 4. hyperirritability.

**4.** John is to have a heel stick to obtain capillary blood. The blood specimen is *most likely* to be obtained to determine the infant's blood level of
  ○ 1. glucose.
  ○ 2. bilirubin.
  ○ 3. hematocrit.
  ○ 4. hemoglobin.

**5.** An important nursing responsibility when repeated blood specimens are obtained from John is to maintain a careful record of the
  ○ 1. amount of blood withdrawn from the infant for each specimen.
  ○ 2. color of the blood each time a specimen is taken from the infant.
  ○ 3. last time the infant was fed before obtaining each specimen of blood.
  ○ 4. infant's body temperature immediately before obtaining each specimen of blood.

**6.** John is to receive sodium bicarbonate intravenously. The nurse is correct when she judges that sodium bicarbonate is given to the infant *primarily* to alleviate
  ○ 1. edema.
   ○ 2. dehydration.
  ○ 3. metabolic acidosis.
  ○ 4. respiratory alkalosis.

**7.** John receives oxygen therapy. The nurse evaluates whether one desired effect of oxygen is being attained by monitoring John's
  ○ 1. pulse rate.
  ○ 2. blood pressure.
  ○ 3. respiratory rate.
  ○ 4. body temperature.

**8.** The nurse documents John's response to oxygen therapy and the amount he receives. The eye condition John is *very likely* to develop if oxygen therapy is used indiscriminately is
  ○ 1. glaucoma.
  ○ 2. cataracts.
  ○ 3. ophthalmia neonatorum.
  ○ 4. retrolental fibroplasia.

**9.** John is to receive formula using a bottle. Before giving John his first feeding of formula, the nurse gives the infant approximately 5 ml of sterile water. The *primary* purpose for giving John the sterile water before the formula is to

○ 1. initiate the infant's peristalsis.

○ 2. ascertain the patency of the infant's esophagus.

○ 3. determine whether or not the infant can retain the feeding.

○ 4. ensure that the infant has the energy to take oral feedings.

10. John is to be fed by gavage. Which of the following statements describes the method *most often* recommended to judge whether or not the nurse has introduced the catheter into John's stomach?

○ 1. Stomach contents are aspirated through the catheter with a syringe.

○ 2. The catheter is introduced the measured length without resistance.

○ 3. After water is introduced into the catheter with a syringe, the water returns easily with aspiration.

○ 4. While air is inserted into the catheter with a syringe, auscultation over the lungs reveals clear air sounds.

11. John's parents are concerned about the infant's condition. Which of the following measures is likely to be of *most* help to the parents at this time?

○ 1. Allowing the parents to see and touch the infant.

○ 2. Encouraging the parents to participate in feeding and bathing the infant.

○ 3. Arranging a visit between the parents and another couple with a premature infant.

○ 4. Explaining to the parents that their concerns are needless because the infant is doing well.

12. Although all the following techniques are beneficial, authorities generally agree that the *single most effective* way to control infection in a nursery housing high-risk infants such as John is to

○ 1. require personnel to wear gowns and masks.

○ 2. have personnel use frequent hand- and arm-washing techniques.

○ 3. keep each infant in an isolette that is opened as infrequently as possible.

○ 4. maintain a ventilation system in the nursery that provides for continuous clean-air exchange.

13. Lee Fong is a newborn premature infant who has idiopathic respiratory distress syndrome (surfactant deficiency disease). When surfactant is present in *normal* amounts, it affects respiratory functioning by

○ 1. keeping pulmonary capillaries well dilated.

○ 2. helping prevent the alveoli from collapsing.

○ 3. clearing mucus from the airway efficiently.

○ 4. stimulating the chest wall muscles to contract with exhalations.

14. Oxygen therapy is started for Lee and plans are made to monitor his arterial oxygen concentration. The artery *most likely* to be used to obtain blood samples is the

○ 1. carotid artery.

○ 2. femoral artery.

○ 3. brachial artery.

○ 4. umbilical artery.

## THE PATIENT WITH SEPSIS

Mr. and Mrs. Mondant bring their 10-day-old daughter, Sherri, to the hospital because she is lethargic. They explain that Sherri was fine until early this morning when she just "didn't look right" and began breathing very rapidly. Her pulse rate is 200 beats per minute. A tentative diagnosis of sepsis is made.

15. The physician tells Mr. and Mrs. Mondant that Sherri must be admitted to the hospital. The nurse should explain that because of Sherri's diagnosis, she will need to be placed

○ 1. in the special care nursery.

○ 2. on a general pediatric unit.

○ 3. in an isolation room.

○ 4. in the normal newborn nursery.

16. When examining Sherri, the nurse should *first* assess her

○ 1. appetite.

○ 2. hydrational status.

○ 3. stool consistency.

○ 4. sleep pattern.

17. As the nurse examines Sherri, Mrs. Mondant says, "I can't believe that Sherri is so sick. It all happened so quickly and Sherri didn't even have a fever. Did I miss something?" The nurse's response would be based on the fact that most neonatal infections are

○ 1. characterized by specific respiratory distress.

○ 2. commonly accompanied by fever.

○ 3. accompanied by a local inflammatory response.

○ 4. characterized by nearly imperceptible signs.

18. The nurse would explain that *early* manifestations of sepsis in neonates are *most likely* to include

○ 1. warm dry skin.

○ 2. abdominal distention.

○ 3. stiff neck.

○ 4. hypertension.

19. In an attempt to isolate the causative organism, blood studies are done. Which of the following findings should concern the nurse *most*?

○ 1. Anemia.

○ 2. Leukocytosis.

○ 3. Leukopenia.

○ 4. Hyperbilirubinemia.

20. The nurse should anticipate that Sherri's pharmacologic treatment will most likely include

○ 1. ampicillin and gentamicin.

○ 2. kanamycin and furosemide (Lasix).

○ 3. vitamin K and gentamicin.

○ 4. phenytoin sodium (Dilantin) and ampicillin.

21. The nurse monitors Sherri's vital signs frequently, including blood pressure. Blood pressure monitoring is included because a severe complication of sepsis is

○ 1. fluid imbalance.

○ 2. septic shock.

○ 3. necrotizing enterocolitis.

○ 4. sudden infant death syndrome.

22. Mr. and Mrs. Mondant are overwhelmed by Sherri's hospitalization and the seriousness of her condition. With tears in her eyes, Mrs. Mondant tells the nurse, "All of this is so difficult to understand. We tried to be such good parents." What would be the nurse's *best* response?

○ 1. "We're doing all we can for Sherri. Try not to worry."

○ 2. "What is most difficult to understand?"

○ 3. "Are you thinking that this is your fault?"

○ 4. "I know you are good parents; you love Sherri."

## THE PATIENT WITH FAILURE TO THRIVE

Amanda Frazier, age 5 months, is brought to the clinic because "she vomits a lot" and "cries too much." Her birth weight was 6 pounds, 10 ounces; her current weight is 7 pounds, 4 ounces. She is hospitalized with a diagnosis of failure to thrive.

23. Failure to thrive is the term used to describe infants or young children who

○ 1. fall below the 5th percentile in weight and height for their ages.

○ 2. gain weight at a rate of less than one-half ounce per week.

○ 3. are delayed in the attainment of their developmental milestones.

○ 4. have a history of vomiting and irritability over several weeks.

24. Which of the following information obtained from Mrs. Frazier during the nursing history is consistent with a diagnosis of failure to thrive?

○ 1. Amanda vomits frequently and cries during feedings.

○ 2. Amanda has difficulty eating, but has no problem sleeping.

○ 3. Amanda likes being held but does not protest when put down.

○ 4. Amanda fears strangers and avoids eye-to-eye contact.

25. The nurse develops a care plan for Amanda. What objective information would the nurse need *most* in order to plan the interventions?

○ 1. Multiple test results to rule out an organic cause of Amanda's condition.

○ 2. A history of Amanda's height and weight from birth until the present.

○ 3. A complete diet history for the past week.

○ 4. Parent-child interaction during feedings and waking hours.

26. "Alteration in nutrition: less than body requirements" is a nursing diagnosis formulated from the assessment data. Given this diagnosis, which of the following nursing interventions would the nurse include on Amanda's initial care plan?

○ 1. Have Amanda's nurse feed her.

○ 2. Ask Amanda's parents to feed her.

○ 3. Sit Amanda in a high chair to be fed.

○ 4. Provide scheduled, limited feedings of formula.

27. Which of the following outcomes *best* indicates that the nursing interventions implemented relative to the nursing diagnosis are effective?

○ 1. Amanda gains 2 ounces per day.

○ 2. Amanda responds positively to feeding practices.

○ 3. Amanda smiles at the nurses.

○ 4. Amanda responds positively to being held.

28. If 5-month-old Amanda did not have failure to thrive, her caloric intake should be

○ 1. 70 kcal/kg/day.

○ 2. 90 kcal/kg/day.

○ 3. 115 kcal/kg/day.

○ 4. 140 kcal/kg/day.

29. Based on assessment data, the nurse determines that Amanda's parents need a better understanding of Amanda's physical, developmental, and emotional needs. Which of the following interventions is likely to be *most* effective in reaching that understanding?

○ 1. Attending parenting classes after Amanda is discharged.

○ 2. Attending parenting classes before Amanda is discharged.

○ 3. Observing nurses appropriately caring for Amanda.

○ 4. Receiving verbal instructions supplemented by handouts.

**30.** Amanda is to be discharged home within the next few days. Her parents have improved in their ability to care for her, and the nurse wants to implement a plan that will provide continued support and education for the parents. Based on the knowledge of the *most effective* support mechanism, the nurse would arrange for
○ 1. twice-weekly clinic appointments.
○ 2. daily telephone follow-up by the primary nurse.
○ 3. weekly visits from the community health nurse.
○ 4. enrollment in community parenting classes.

## THE PATIENT WITH ATOPIC DERMATITIS (ECZEMA)

Eleven-month-old Sara Takis is hospitalized with a skin rash. It is determined that she has atopic dermatitis (eczema).

**31.** The nurse observes that Sara is irritable, fretful, and unable to sleep, which are signs due *primarily* to the infant's having
○ 1. diarrhea.
○ 2. persistent pruritus.
○ 3. a systemic subclinical infection.
○ 4. a disturbance in maternal-infant attachment.

**32.** The nurse studies Sara's family health history as part of her nursing assessment. Which of the following conditions, if there is repeated evidence in the family history, *most likely* plays a role in Sara's having eczema?
○ 1. Asthma.
○ 2. Hypertension.
○ 3. Malignant tumors.
○ 4. Febrile seizure activity.

**33.** Because infection is present, a penicillin preparation prescribed for Sara is given intramuscularly. Which of the following measures has been found to meet an infant's emotional needs *best* when the infant experiences an uncomfortable procedure such as an intramuscular injection?
○ 1. Allow the infant's mother to be present during the procedure.
○ 2. Rock the infant for a few minutes before beginning the procedure.
○ 3. Allow the infant to become familiar with the equipment to be used.
○ 4. Provide the infant with a bottle of formula during the procedure.

**34.** Which of the following types of nightclothes would be *best* for Sara?

○ 1. Nylon nightsack.
○ 2. One-piece cotton pajamas.
○ 3. Two-piece flannel pajamas.
○ 4. Woolen sleeper with feet and mittens.

**35.** When discussing the home care of Sara with Mrs. Takis, the nurse recommends that she give diphenhydramine (Benadryl), p.r.n., to Sara at bedtime. The *primary* reason for the nurse's recommendation is that this drug acts effectively as
○ 1. a sedative.
○ 2. an analgesic.
○ 3. an anti-inflammatory agent.
○ 4. a bronchial antispasmodic.

**36.** Dressings moistened in aluminum acetate solution (Burow's solution) are applied to Sara's eczematous areas. The nurse judges *correctly* that the desired effects of these moist dressings are being achieved when Sara's skin
○ 1. lesions decrease in size.
○ 2. lesions rupture and then dry.
○ 3. appears less red and inflamed.
○ 4. is lubricated and no longer dry.

**37.** A hypoallergenic diet is prescribed for Sara. Which food should the nurse teach Mrs. Takis to *avoid* in Sara's diet?
○ 1. Eggs.
○ 2. Pears.
○ 3. Carrots.
○ 4. Applesauce.

**38.** Which of the following toys should the nurse teach Mrs. Takis to *avoid* giving Sara?
○ 1. A large ball.
○ 2. Rubber blocks.
○ 3. A stuffed animal.
○ 4. Spools on a cord.

## THE PATIENT WITH BURNS

Five-year-old Bobby White is admitted to the hospital with burns received while playing with matches. His legs, head, and lower abdomen are burned most, but there is some burned surface on other parts of the body as well. Some smoke inhalation has occurred.

**39.** The nurse uses the "rule of nines" to estimate the burned area on Bobby's body. Which part of Bobby's body will be allocated a *larger* percentage of total surface area than would be allocated to a child over 12 years of age?
○ 1. The child's head and neck.
○ 2. The child's upper extremities.

○ 3. The child's lower extremities.

○ 4. The child's anterior and posterior chest wall.

**40.** Because Bobby's burns are evaluated as being serious, he requires large amounts of fluids for his age. The *initial primary* shift in the location of his body plasma is from

○ 1. interstitial to intracellular spaces.

○ 2. interstitial to intravascular spaces.

○ 3. intravascular to interstitial spaces.

○ 4. intracellular to intravascular spaces.

**41.** Bobby has an indwelling catheter in his urinary bladder. The *primary* reason for this measure is to help

○ 1. prevent urinary retention.

○ 2. decrease the workload of the kidneys.

○ 3. obtain regular urine specimens with ease.

○ 4. ensure accurate urinary output measurements.

**42.** An order for intravenous therapy for Bobby reads as follows: 5% dextrose in Ringer's lactate intravenously; 3 ml/kg per percentage of burn to be received in the first 24 hours. Bobby weighs 44 pounds (20 kg) and has second- and third-degree burns over approximately 44% of his body surface. How much intravenous fluid should he receive in the first 24 hours?

○ 1. 1,760 ml.

○ 2. 2,640 ml.

○ 3. 3,520 ml.

○ 4. 4,400 ml.

**43.** Which of the following blood value determinations is *most likely* to be used to evaluate the adequacy of Bobby's fluid replacement therapy?

○ 1. The creatinine level.

○ 2. The hematocrit level.

○ 3. The urea nitrogen level.

○ 4. The carbon dioxide tension.

**44.** The nurse is justified in judging that Bobby is *very probably* receiving too much intravenous fluid when she observes that he has

○ 1. dark urine.

○ 2. moist rales.

○ 3. abdominal distention.

○ 4. peripheral vasoconstriction.

**45.** Of the following signs, the one Bobby is *most likely* to demonstrate if he develops a sodium deficit, or water intoxication, is

○ 1. hoarseness.

○ 2. muscle twitching.

○ 3. a slow pulse rate.

○ 4. flushing of the skin.

**46.** The nurse is correct in judging that Bobby's intravenous fluid intake should *most probably* be increased if she observes that Bobby

○ 1. is becoming increasingly irritable.

○ 2. answers "no" when asked if he is thirsty.

○ 3. has a urinary output of 10 ml in the last hour.

○ 4. has had an increase in blood pressure within the last 3 hours.

**47.** Six hours after Bobby's intravenous infusion is begun, the nurse notes that the rate of infusion is less than prescribed and is approximately 3 hours behind the ordered schedule. Which of the following courses of action would be *best* for her to take?

○ 1. Consult the physician concerning a new schedule for the intravenous infusion.

○ 2. Calculate a new drip rate so that within a 24-hour period, the total amount of ordered solution will be infused.

○ 3. Increase the drip rate so that the total amount of ordered solution will be infused within the 8-hour period.

○ 4. Correct the drip rate to the prescribed rate even though less than the total ordered amount of solution for the 8-hour period will be infused.

**48.** Which of the following signs should suggest to the nurse that Bobby may be hemolyzing red blood cells?

○ 1. The child's stools are black.

○ 2. The child's eyes appear bloodshot.

○ 3. The child's intact skin appears flushed.

○ 4. The child's urine is dark brown.

**49.** The nurse notes that Bobby may be having an allergic reaction to the ampicillin he is receiving. Which of the following courses of action should the nurse take *first* in this situation?

○ 1. Stop administering the drug.

○ 2. Prepare for the administration of whole blood.

○ 3. Decrease the infusion rate of intravenous fluids.

○ 4. Place the patient in bed with his head lower than his body.

**50.** Which of the following signs should the nurse judge *most typical* if Bobby is having an allergic reaction to ampicillin?

○ 1. Joint swelling.

○ 2. Mental confusion.

○ 3. A rapid pulse rate.

○ 4. A skin rash.

**51.** Which of the following electrolytes will Bobby likely lose in the *largest* amounts during the first 48 hours following his burn, resulting in a plasma deficit?

○ 1. Sodium.

○ 2. Potassium.

○ 3. Magnesium.

○ 4. Phosphorus.

**52.** The nurse observes Bobby closely for signs of

metabolic acidosis. This acid-base imbalance is characterized by respirations that are

○ 1. deep and rapid.
○ 2. slow and labored.
○ 3. difficult and stridulous.
○ 4. interspersed with periods of no breathing.

53. Bobby is to receive tetanus prophylaxis. When the nurse learns that Bobby's tetanus immunization is up-to-date, she should anticipate that the biologic product that will be used to offer Bobby further protection will be

○ 1. a toxoid.
○ 2. a vaccine.
○ 3. an antitoxin.
○ 4. immune globulin.

54. After initial debridement of burned areas, mafenide acetate (Sulfamylon) is applied topically to burned areas every 8 hours. Because topical mafenide acetate therapy may affect certain normal blood values, the nurse should anticipate that Bobby's blood will need to be monitored for

○ 1. pH level.
○ 2. platelet level.
○ 3. leukocyte level.
○ 4. hemoglobin level.

55. In addition to its possible effects on Bobby's blood, another disadvantage of mafenide acetate (Sulfamylon) therapy is that the drug

○ 1. stains linen permanently.
○ 2. tends to disintegrate easily.
○ 3. has a strong, disagreeable odor.
○ 4. causes a burning sensation when applied.

56. When a child feels he has control of what is happening, he is more likely to cooperate. Which of the following nursing measures will allow Bobby to feel *most* in control during his mafenide acetate (Sulfamylon) treatments?

○ 1. Allowing him to help apply the cream.
○ 2. Telling him it is all right for him to cry.
○ 3. Arranging to have a parent support him during the treatments.
○ 4. Delaying the treatment for a short time if he seems unwilling to cooperate.

57. What recommendations do the Centers for Disease Control give concerning the use of sterile gloves when caring for Bobby's infected burn areas?

○ 1. Gloves are a desirable precautionary measure, but wearing them is optional.
○ 2. Gloves should be worn whenever any kind of care is being given to the burn victim.
○ 3. Gloves should be worn whenever giving direct care to burned areas; the same pair may be used for removing soiled dressings and applying new dressings.

○ 4. Gloves should be worn whenever giving direct care to burn areas; one pair is used for removing soiled dressings and another for applying new dressings.

58. Bobby has paralytic ileus with vomiting and abdominal distention. He is to have nothing by mouth and a nasogastric tube is inserted. The nurse judges *correctly* that Bobby can *most likely* tolerate oral fluids when she notes that the patient

○ 1. has no diarrhea.
○ 2. is no longer distended.
○ 3. is showing eagerness to take nourishment.
○ 4. has bowel sounds when the abdomen is auscultated.

59. When Bobby starts eating after being burned, it is *particularly* important that his diet have a high content of

○ 1. fats.
○ 2. proteins.
○ 3. minerals.
○ 4. carbohydrates.

60. If Bobby has a low blood potassium level, which of these beverages would provide him with the *most* potassium when he begins to take fluids orally?

○ 1. Ginger ale.
○ 2. Grape juice.
○ 3. Orange juice.
○ 4. Cranberry juice.

61. Which of the following measures is *least likely* to interest Bobby in eating?

○ 1. Allowing the child's mother to help feed him.
○ 2. Offering the child foods he can eat with his fingers.
○ 3. Serving the child small amounts of food at a time.
○ 4. Explaining to the child that dessert will be served after other foods are eaten.

62. Bobby's parents ask the nurse why Bobby is receiving "that white liquid medicine," which the nurse knows is an antacid. The *best* response for the nurse is

○ 1. "Bobby is receiving an antacid to counteract constipation."
○ 2. "The reason for giving Bobby the medication should be discussed with your doctor."
○ 3. "Many medications are used for a child who is severely burned, and because Bobby is doing so well it's best not to worry."
○ 4. "The antacid Bobby is receiving is used to help prevent the development of ulcers of the stomach and small intestine, which is a common complication of burns."

63. The nurse explains to Mr. and Mrs. White the skin grafting procedure that will be used for Bobby.

Bobby is to have a xenograft, which means that the grafting material comes from

○ 1. an animal.

○ 2. the patient's body.

○ 3. synthetic ingredients.

○ 4. another person's body.

64. The nurse should explain to the Whites that the *primary* purpose for using a xenograft on Bobby's burn areas is to

○ 1. decrease the child's pain.

○ 2. stimulate the growth of granulation tissue.

○ 3. facilitate the child's range of body motion.

○ 4. provide a covering for burned areas until another type of grafting material is available.

65. After Bobby has been hospitalized for 3 weeks, Mrs. White asks the nurse why she was asked to sign a permit for a tracheostomy shortly after Bobby's admission to the hospital. In this situation, it would be *best* for the nurse to respond by saying

○ 1. "You'll have to ask Bobby's doctor."

○ 2. "There's no need to worry about the permit for a tracheostomy because it becomes invalid after a few days."

○ 3. "Having a signed permit for a tracheostomy is a routine request of parents whose children are acutely ill, as Bobby was."

○ 4. "A permit for a tracheostomy for Bobby was requested because he may have developed swelling due to smoke inhalation that might have blocked his airway."

66. Silver nitrate solution is sometimes used for treating burns. If a silver nitrate solution is used carelessly, there is danger of upsetting the body's ability to maintain

○ 1. water balance.

○ 2. nitrogen balance.

○ 3. electrolyte balance.

○ 4. temperature control.

○ 2. has a normally functioning fetal thyroid gland that has failed to develop after birth.

○ 3. receives sufficient thyroxine through the mother's milk for the first few weeks after birth.

○ 4. receives sufficient hormone during fetal life from its mother to delay signs of thyroxine deficiency.

68. Kelly is ordered to receive desiccated thyroid, which acts in the body to help

○ 1. increase the metabolic rate.

○ 2. stimulate the thyroid to secrete thyroxine.

○ 3. limit excessive growth of the skeletal system.

○ 4. promote reabsorption of thyroxine in the kidney tubules.

69. Kelly's mother asks the nurse, "How will we know if the medicine is helping Kelly?" The nurse should respond by saying that in addition to certain blood tests, Kelly will also be evaluated by regular examinations of her

○ 1. metabolic rate.

○ 2. skeletal growth.

○ 3. muscular coordination.

○ 4. electrolyte blood levels.

70. The nurse is justified in judging that Kelly is demonstrating signs of toxicity from thyroid-replacement therapy when Kelly has

○ 1. an excessive gain in weight and edema.

○ 2. a rapid pulse rate, dyspnea, and sleeplessness.

○ 3. pain and fractures of long bones with minimal trauma.

○ 4. reduced responsiveness to common environmental stimuli.

71. If Kelly's cretinism is not properly diagnosed and treated, in addition to changes in physical appearance it can be anticipated that she will also be

○ 1. blind.

○ 2. epileptic.

○ 3. mentally retarded.

○ 4. emotionally unstable.

## THE PATIENT WITH HYPOTHYROIDISM

Kelly Walters appears normal at birth. Six weeks later, she begins to eat poorly, her skin becomes dry and scaly, and her tongue begins to protrude. She is being breast-fed. Kelly has cretinism.

67. Hypothyroidism, the cause of cretinism, would have been very difficult to detect when Kelly was born because the infant

○ 1. has little need for thyroxine until approximately 1 to 2 months of age.

## THE PATIENT WITH INSULIN-DEPENDENT DIABETES MELLITUS

Eight-year-old Andy Thompson is admitted to the hospital unconscious. He has ketoacidosis due to type I diabetes.

72. In which of the following positions is it *best* to place Andy upon admission?

○ 1. On his back.

○ 2. On either side.

○ 3. On his abdomen.

○ 4. In a low sitting position.

73. A *typical* sign Andy is *likely* to demonstrate on admission is

○ 1. dilated pupils.

○ 2. a slow pulse rate.

○ 3. excessive perspiration.

○ 4. deep, rapid respirations.

74. Which of the following substances accounts for the sweet, fruity odor that the nurse notes on Andy's breath when she admits him?

○ 1. Urea.

○ 2. Glycogen.

○ 3. Amino acids.

○ 4. Ketone bodies.

75. In addition to a high blood glucose level, Andy also can be expected to have

○ 1. overhydration.

○ 2. liver shutdown.

○ 3. an electrolyte imbalance.

○ 4. improper renal function.

76. The nurse begins a teaching program for the Thompsons when Andy begins to recuperate. Andy's parents ask the nurse why Andy has diabetes mellitus. Which of the following statements *most accurately* describes current opinion concerning the etiology of diabetes mellitus?

○ 1. It is most probably a hereditary disease.

○ 2. It has no known cause.

○ 3. It is most probably due to damage incurred by Andy's pancreas during a difficult birth.

○ 4. It is most probably due to Andy's mother's having a streptococcal infection early in her pregnancy.

77. When the nurse interviews Mr. and Mrs. Thompson, they describe Andy's behavior as having changed before he became acutely ill and unconscious. The sign that *most strongly* suggests Andy has hyperglycemia due to diabetes mellitus is that Andy has been

○ 1. irritable.

○ 2. bed-wetting.

○ 3. more active than usual.

○ 4. less hungry than usual.

78. The nurse teaches Andy and his parents the relationship between the results of urine tests for glucose and his blood glucose level. Glucose will initially appear in the urine when the blood glucose level reaches a value of approximately

○ 1. 120 mg/100 ml.

○ 2. 150 mg/100 ml.

○ 3. 180 mg/100 ml.

○ 4. 200 mg/100 ml.

79. Andy's parents ask the nurse why Andy cannot take insulin by mouth. The nurse should explain that insulin is not given by mouth because it is

○ 1. excreted before being absorbed.

○ 2. absorbed too slowly to be effective.

○ 3. too irritating to stomach mucous membranes.

○ 4. rendered inactive by gastrointestinal secretions.

80. A combination of NPH and regular insulin is prescribed for Andy. Which of the following techniques is *most often* recommended when preparing the two insulins for injection?

○ 1. Premix the insulins in a vial, then withdraw the amount needed in one syringe.

○ 2. Use two syringes, one for the regular insulin and one for the NPH insulin.

○ 3. Withdraw the regular insulin first, then withdraw the NPH insulin with the same syringe.

○ 4. Withdraw the NPH insulin first, then withdraw the regular insulin with the same syringe.

81. If Andy takes his insulins at 8 a.m., what time during the day should Andy and his parents be taught that the *onset* of action from the NPH insulin should be expected?

○ 1. Between 8:30 and 10:30 a.m.

○ 2. Between 10 a.m. and noon.

○ 3. Between noon and 2 p.m.

○ 4. Between 2 and 4 p.m.

82. Before preparing to remove insulin from its vial, what step should the nurse teach Andy and his parents to take *first*?

○ 1. Inject at least two times more air into the vial than the amount of insulin to be removed.

○ 2. Inject about the same amount of air into the vial as the amount of insulin to be withdrawn.

○ 3. Inject approximately half as much air into the vial as the amount of insulin to be withdrawn.

○ 4. Be sure the plunger is inserted completely into the barrel of the syringe so that no air can be injected into the vial.

83. The nurse teaches Andy and his parents to rotate the site for injecting insulin into the body. Which of the following sites is *inappropriate*?

○ 1. The thighs.

○ 2. The abdomen.

○ 3. The forearms.

○ 4. The upper arms.

84. Andy and his parents should be taught that of the following factors, the one that will *most often decrease* Andy's need for insulin is

○ 1. an infection.

○ 2. an emotional experience.

○ 3. an increase in exercise.

○ 4. preparing for hospitalization.

**85.** At what temperature should the Thompsons be taught to store Andy's insulin between uses?
○ 1. In a refrigerator, near freezing, about 35° F. (2° C.).
○ 2. In a refrigerator, between 45° and 50° F. (7° and 10° C.).
○ 3. In a warm place, between 95° and 100° F. (35° and 38° C.).
○ 4. At room temperature, between 68° and 75° F. (20° and 24° C.).

**86.** Which of the following foods should Andy be taught to *avoid?*
○ 1. Pizza.
○ 2. Yogurt.
○ 3. A hamburger and French fries.
○ 4. A peanut-butter-and-jelly sandwich.

**87.** Which of the following actions should Andy and his parents be taught to take *first* if Andy appears to be hyperglycemic?
○ 1. He should drink a cup of hot, well-sugared tea.
○ 2. His insulin should be withheld until he sees a physician.
○ 3. His blood should be checked to determine the glucose level.
○ 4. He should go to the nearest emergency room for intravenous therapy to prevent coma.

**88.** The Thompsons should be taught that if Andy presents signs or symptoms of hypoglycemia (insulin shock), the *best* course of action is *first* to
○ 1. have him increase his activity.
○ 2. call his physician for instructions.
○ 3. have him eat several cubes of sugar.
○ 4. have him rest in bed until his symptoms subside.

**89.** Andy and his parents should be taught that when he is an adult, his need for insulin (in terms of amount) will
○ 1. decrease, provided he keeps his diabetes under good control.
○ 2. decrease, so that eventually he can switch to an oral hypoglycemic agent.
○ 3. continue in a manner similar to his need for insulin during his childhood.
○ 4. continue until old age, when dietary discretion will most likely be sufficient to control his disease.

**90.** Which of the following suggestions in relation to activities of daily living would be *inappropriate* for the nurse to make to Andy and his parents?
○ 1. The patient should be particularly careful to wear properly fitting shoes.
○ 2. The patient should be treated in a manner similar to other 8-year-old boys.

○ 3. The patient should avoid especially strenuous physical activities, such as contact sports.
○ 4. The patient should be prepared to make insulin and dietary adjustments when he develops an infection.

**91.** The Thompsons should be taught that the food constituents Andy is failing to metabolize properly because of his diabetes are
○ 1. fats and proteins only.
○ 2. fats and carbohydrates only.
○ 3. proteins and carbohydrates only.
○ 4. fats, proteins, and carbohydrates.

# THE PATIENT WHO IS ABUSED

Michael Rehm, age 3, is brought to the emergency room by his parents. They explain that he hurt his arm when he got it caught in the rails of the crib. Physical examination and x-rays reveal a spiral fracture of the left distal humerus and multiple bruises on his back and buttocks. Some of the bruises have the shape of a handprint. Child abuse is suspected and Michael is admitted to the pediatric unit.

**92.** When obtaining the nursing history, the nurse may find that the parents
○ 1. give information about Michael's developmental achievements.
○ 2. show little concern about the extent of Michael's injury.
○ 3. blame themselves for Michael's injury.
○ 4. ask questions about Michael's hospitalization.

**93.** Which of the following factors should the nurse consider when deciding whether to report the suspicions of child abuse?
○ 1. Nurses who suspect child abuse are required by law to report their suspicions.
○ 2. Conclusive evidence is needed before reporting suspected child abuse.
○ 3. Physicians are primarily responsible for reporting suspected child abuse.
○ 4. The nurse may be sued when reporting only "suspected" child abuse.

**94.** When does primary prevention of child abuse and neglect begin?
○ 1. At the first well-baby visit.
○ 2. In the prenatal clinic.
○ 3. As soon as the first injury occurs.
○ 4. After the first injury has occurred.

**95.** The *primary* reason for admitting Michael to the hospital is to
○ 1. provide treatment for his injuries.

○ 2. gather additional information about his family.

○ 3. protect him from further injury.

○ 4. provide time to determine who injured him.

**96.** A factor common to the background of abusive parents is that they

○ 1. are of lower socioeconomic status.

○ 2. were abused themselves as children.

○ 3. have less than a high-school education.

○ 4. have realistic expectations of their children.

**97.** Which of the following statements made by Mrs. Rehm is *most likely* to be made by an abusive parent?

○ 1. "A good friend and I meet for coffee twice a week."

○ 2. "Michael likes books about things he knows."

○ 3. "My mother takes care of Michael on Saturday evening so my husband and I can go out together."

○ 4. "I think Michael should be able to tie his shoes by now."

**98.** When the nurse asks Michael how he hurt his arm, he replies, "It was my fault. I was bad." The nurse's *best* response would be

○ 1. "You'll have to behave better so this won't happen again."

○ 2. "Tell me what you did that made your father hit you."

○ 3. "Perhaps it wasn't your fault. Can we talk about what happened?"

○ 4. "We'll help you get better and see that this doesn't happen again."

**99.** When Michael has blood drawn, he does not respond to the pain. An appropriate response from the nurse would be

○ 1. "You sure were good not to cry."

○ 2. "That really didn't hurt much, did it?"

○ 3. "It's OK to cry or say 'ouch' if it hurts."

○ 4. "We're mean to hurt you that way, aren't we?"

**100.** When developing Michael's care plan, the nurse keeps Michael's needs in mind. Which of the following interventions is *most likely* to meet these needs?

○ 1. A program of attention based on play.

○ 2. Consistent management of inappropriate behavior.

○ 3. A program of restrictive limit-setting.

○ 4. Consistent reinforcement of his specialness as an abused child.

**101.** As part of Michael's nursing care, a primary nurse on each shift cares for him. The overall goal of this consistent relationship is to

○ 1. modify Michael's negative behavior.

○ 2. provide a role model for Michael's parents.

○ 3. guide Michael toward physical and mental wellness.

○ 4. discourage Michael's continuing relationship with his parents.

**102.** When developing a long-term care plan for Michael and his parents, the nurse keeps in mind the goal of improved family function. Interventions that are *most important* in attaining this goal include improved child-care skills, improved coping skills, and

○ 1. ongoing involvement in parenting classes.

○ 2. coordination with community services.

○ 3. increased trust in health-care professionals.

○ 4. improved family interaction patterns.

**103.** Several months later, the nurse who cared for Michael is called to testify in court about the case. Which of the following would it be *most important* for the nurse to have for the court proceedings?

○ 1. A clear recollection of Mr. and Mrs. Rehm's behavior when Michael was admitted.

○ 2. Well-formulated subjective opinions about the cause of Michael's injury.

○ 3. Well-thought-out answers to questions asked by the attorney.

○ 4. Documentation of physical findings and behavior observed when Michael was admitted.

**104.** Mr. Joiner telephones the clinic and explains that he is concerned about his 5-year-old daughter's change in behavior. He says that his daughter Betsy has become very clinging and no longer wants to visit her favorite aunt and uncle. Mr. Joiner asks the nurse for advice. What would be the nurse's *best* response?

○ 1. "Children at this age demonstrate strong attachment for the parent of the opposite sex."

○ 2. "Tell me more about your concerns."

○ 3. "Discuss the situation with Betsy's aunt and uncle."

○ 4. "Clinging behavior is normal for 5-year-olds."

During the past 2 months, Susan Cantrell, age 12, has frequently come to the school nurse's office with complaints of recurrent headaches. The nurse knows that Susan underwent a battery of tests to determine the cause of the headaches. All results were negative and no physiologic cause was found. The nurse spoke with Susan's teacher, who explains that Susan's grades have fallen sharply. She is aggressive with her peers and clings to her teacher at every opportunity. The nurse suspects sexual abuse.

**105.** Which of the following are potential manifestations of sexual abuse?
○ 1. Poor personal hygiene and lack of subcutaneous fat.
○ 2. Unexplained sudden illness and apprehension when hearing other children cry.
○ 3. Excessive day-dreaming and regressive behavior.
○ 4. Sleep disorders and lags in emotional and intellectual development.

**106.** One day when Susan comes to see the school nurse about her headaches, she tells the nurse she is being sexually abused by a family friend. What would the nurse's *best initial* response be?
○ 1. "I think you should tell your mother and father about this."
○ 2. "I believe you; you were right to tell me."
○ 3. "Can you tell me what happened?"
○ 4. "Who else have you told about this?"

**107.** If Susan were a 3-year-old who had been sexually abused, what technique would be *best* for the nurse to use in interviewing her?
○ 1. Ask her to describe the incident.
○ 2. Have her draw and describe pictures of the event.
○ 3. Have her "play out" the event with anatomically correct dolls.
○ 4. Ask the doll "victim" open-ended questions.

**108.** If Susan were the victim of physical neglect, a goal of working with her parents would be to determine
○ 1. the dynamics of family functioning.
○ 2. Susan's developmental history.
○ 3. the parent's response to a child's illness.
○ 4. a typical daily meal plan.

# CORRECT ANSWERS AND RATIONALES

Numbers appear in parentheses following the rationales. The numbers identify textbooks listed in the references at the end of Part III, where correct answers can be verified.

## The Patient Who is Preterm

1. 2. Lanugo covers the entire body until about 20 weeks of gestation, when it begins to disappear from the face, trunk, and extremities, in that order. It has disappeared in the full-term infant. Lanugo on the body is one of the consistent findings in premature infants. Firm cartilage to the edge of the ear pinna, full areola with breast tissue, and creases on the soles and heels of the feet are examples of physical characteristics found in infants born at term. (7, 21)

2. 2. Physical characteristics of the infant born prematurely include a thin, wasted appearance; scarce scalp hair; thin, pink, and smooth skin; and an absence of rugae on the scrotum. The testicles tend to be high in the inguinal canal. (7, 21)

3. 4. Hyperirritability and twitching are signs of hypoglycemia. Premature infants, as well as postmature, small-for-gestational-age, and large-for-gestational-age infants, are prone to develop hypoglycemia. When the infant has cold stress, he must produce heat through increased metabolism, causing oxygen use to increase and glycogen stores to be quickly depleted. Jaundice, abdominal distention, and slow, shallow respirations are not associated with neonatal hypoglycemia. (7, 21)

4. 1. The blood glucose level will reveal whether the infant described in this item is suffering from hypoglycemia, which is common in the premature infant suffering from cold stress (see the previous item). Capillary blood obtained with a heel prick is the common way to obtain the blood specimen for determining blood glucose levels. Hemoglobin, bilirubin, and hematocrit determinations are not used to confirm hypoglycemia. (7, 21)

5. 1. When repeated blood specimens are obtained from a premature infant, it is a nursing responsibility to keep a record of the amount of blood taken for each specimen. The total blood volume of a premature infant is small, and repeated blood collections can deplete blood volume. A record of the amount of blood taken for specimens is used as one guide when determining whether an infant may need a transfusion. The color of the blood is not a reliable measure for determining blood constitu-

ents or volume. The time the infant was last fed and his body temperature immediately before obtaining a specimen are not necessary in terms of determining whether the infant needs a transfusion. (21)

6. 3. Metabolic acidosis results from the metabolic changes associated with cold stress. End products of metabolism increase the acidity of the blood. Therefore, sodium bicarbonate is often used to combat metabolic acidosis. Sodium bicarbonate is not used to correct fluid imbalances such as edema and dehydration. Respiratory alkalosis results from the excess loss of carbon dioxide, a condition that would be very rare in an infant such as the one described in this item. (6, 21)

7. 4. The best way to help the infant described in this item, who has cold stress, is to increase his oxygen supply. Monitoring the infant's body temperature helps judge whether cold stress is being overcome. Oxygen is necessary to increase the body's metabolic rate through a complex process of increasing metabolism within the brown fat (see also the previous item). (9, 21)

8. 4. Oxygen administered indiscriminately to a premature infant often results in retrolental fibroplasia. The immature blood vessels in the eye constrict and then overgrow, resulting in edema and hemorrhage that produce scarring and retinal detachment. These conditions cause eventual blindness. Cataracts and glaucoma are congenital abnormalities in the newborn. Ophthalmia neonatorum is a gonorrheal infection of the eyes and is likely to occur if an infected mother has the gonorrheal organism in her birth canal. This infection is prevented by the administration of prophylactic agents instilled in infants' eyes soon after birth. (6, 21)

9. 2. Before the initial feeding of formula to the premature infant described in this item, sterile water is given to ascertain that the esophagus is patent and thus to prevent aspiration of formula if it is not. The nurse would need to allow a period of time to elapse to determine when the infant can retain the feeding and to ensure that the infant has the energy to take oral feedings; this would be contraindicated in the infant with hypoglycemia because the condition will progress if feedings are withheld. (9, 21)

10. 1. The method most often recommended to determine whether the catheter used for gavage is in the stomach is to aspirate stomach contents through the catheter with a syringe. The presence of stom-

ach contents upon aspiration tells the nurse that the catheter is in the stomach. Any stomach contents aspirated by this technique should be reintroduced to prevent depletion of gastric secretions and other substances. The ordered amount of feeding is decreased by the amount that has been aspirated so that the stomach is not overdistended with the introduction of a full amount of formula. Being able to insert the catheter without resistance for its measured length does not ensure that the catheter is in the stomach. Water inserted into the catheter before determining by aspiration that the catheter is in the stomach may cause the nurse to introduce water into the respiratory passageways. Auscultating over the lungs for clear air sounds while air is introduced into the catheter is not recommended. Auscultating over the stomach for the whooshing sounds of air while introducing air into the catheter is sometimes used; however, any air introduced into the catheter should be aspirated to prevent overdistention of the stomach and abdominal distention. (6, 21)

**11.** 1. Permitting the parents to see the high-risk infant allows for visual searching and information-gathering, one of the first steps in the bonding process. Fingertip-touching also helps promote the bonding process. Seeing and touching the infant often help the parents feel less concern and more comfortable with their child. The nurse should be present to help the parents understand therapeutic measures that may be in use for the infant while they see and touch him. The parents are likely to have even more concerns if, soon after the birth of their child, they visit other parents who have a premature infant. Although parents are generally encouraged to help care for an ill child, this may be unwise when the child is a high-risk premature infant because they lack the necessary skills to give safe care. Telling parents that their concerns are needless ignores their feelings and tends to cut off further conversation between the nurse and the parents. (6, 21)

**12.** 2. Authorities say the single most effective way to control the spread of infection is to have personnel use frequent hand- and arm-washing techniques, even though such practices as wearing gowns and masks, keeping infants in isolettes, and providing a clean-air exchange in a nursery also help control the spread of infection. (6, 12)

**13.** 2. Surfactant has a detergent effect on the walls of the alveoli in the lungs. The surfactant helps prevent their collapse. There is poor oxygen absorption and poor oxygen-carbon dioxide exchange in the lungs when alveoli are collapsed. This results in

hypoxia and, eventually, respiratory distress. (9, 21)

**14.** 4. A catheter is ordinarily inserted into the umbilical artery to obtain blood samples on a premature infant receiving oxygen therapy for respiratory distress syndrome. Other arteries *may* be used, but they are usually not as convenient as the umbilical artery and using them requires repeated needle insertion. Capillary blood samples are usually taken from the heel. (6, 21)

## The Patient with Sepsis

**15.** 3. Infants with sepsis are isolated from other infants. Separating infected people from noninfected ones prevents transmission of disease. Quarantine is the isolation of people with communicable disease or those exposed to a communicable disease during the contagious period. (21)

**16.** 2. Hydrational status is the first priority of assessment. Sepsis can alter fluid status through emesis and diarrhea. Dehydration can be life-threatening and can occur within hours in an infant. Diarrhea is only one possible source of altered fluid status. Changes in appetite and sleep patterns may occur with sepsis, but they are not immediately life-threatening. (15)

**17.** 4. Systemic infections in neonates are characterized by nearly imperceptible signs such as subtle changes in appearance and behavior. Often the only complaint is that the infant does not "look right" or has nonspecific respiratory distress. Fever, which is a universal feature of infection in older children, may be absent in neonates. Indication of a local inflammatory response is rarely present. (20, 21)

**18.** 2. Nonspecific early manifestations include changes in the feeding pattern, which leads to unabsorbed formula with abdominal distention, cool clammy skin, and hypotension. Stiff neck or nuchal rigidity occurs in the older child. (20, 21)

**19.** 3. Blood studies may show evidence of anemia, leukocytosis, leukopenia, or hyperbilirubinemia. Because of its association with high mortality, leukopenia is an ominous sign. Direct hyperbilirubinemia often occurs in infants with sepsis, especially gram-negative sepsis. (21)

**20.** 1. Antibiotic therapy is often begun before the causative organism is identified but after specimens for cultures have been obtained. Broad-spectrum antibiotic therapy effective against almost 90% of all potential organisms is used. Antibiotics such as ampicillin and an aminoglycoside are commonly ordered. (15)

**21.** 2. Septic shock or shock of septicemia is a potentially life-threatening complication of sepsis. Although it is difficult to differentiate signs and symptoms of shock from those of sepsis, blood pressure usually falls in shock. Fluid imbalance, if severe, may contribute to the severity of the shock syndrome but usually is not life-threatening. Neither necrotizing enterocolitis nor sudden infant death syndrome is associated with sepsis. (21)

**22.** 2. Asking an open-ended question gives the parents an opportunity to express their fears and concerns and avoids making assumptions about them. Telling the parents not to worry devalues their concern; telling them they are good parents does not give them the opportunity to express their concerns. (15)

## The Patient with Failure to Thrive

**23.** 1. Failure to thrive is the term used to describe infants or young children whose weight (and sometimes height) falls below the 5th percentile for their age. Characteristics of children with failure to thrive include eating disorders and developmental retardation. (21)

**24.** 1. Children with psychosocial failure to thrive vomit frequently and cry during feedings. Other clinical manifestations include difficulty eating and problems sleeping. These children characteristically dislike being held, protest when put down, are not fearful of strangers, and avoid eye-to-eye contact. (21)

**25.** 4. Observing parent-child interaction during feedings and waking hours provides information about the parent-child attachment. This is an important variable in the complex set of variables that are significant in failure to thrive. Multiple tests are unnecessary if improvement in intake and eating behavior results in rapid weight gain in a more nurturing environment. History of height and weight and a complete dietary history reflect parent-child interaction. (15, 21)

**26.** 1. A child with failure to thrive benefits from being fed by the same nurse. One of the first goals of care is to assess the child's negative feeding patterns and replace those with positive patterns. A consistent caretaker can assess these patterns and institute positive patterns. Because children with failure to thrive are very distractible, having only one adult in the feeding situation is advisable. Initially, the nurse feeds the child because of the difficulty in parent-child attachment. Parents are not encouraged to be present at mealtime until the child's caloric intake and weight gain are adequate. Younger children should be held while being fed and should have unlimited amounts of age-appropriate foods. (21)

**27.** 1. An expected outcome of the nursing interventions is that the child gains at least 1 to 2 ounces per day. Smiling at the nurses, responding positively to being held, and responding positively to feeding practices indicate that the nursing interventions are effective, but weight gain is the most definitive datum. (21)

**28.** 3. The average daily caloric intake for a normal 5-month-old is 115 kcal/kg/day. (7, 14)

**29.** 3. Teaching parents about the child's physical, developmental, and emotional needs is best accomplished through example, not lecture. (21)

**30.** 3. The community or home health nurse is the best resource for providing continuing support for the parents. The community health nurse's weekly visits facilitate a natural environment. (21)

## The Patient with Atopic Dermatitis (Eczema)

**31.** 2. The most characteristic and distressing feature of atopic dermatitis (eczema) is the persistent itching that interferes with the infant's sleeping and serves as a constant stressor. A disturbance in the maternal-infant attachment would more likely be the result of a lack of positive feedback from the infant to the mother and to chronic fatigue and distress of the mother and infant. Chronic subclinical infection and chronic diarrhea could be complications of eczema but are not part of the underlying problem in this condition. (7, 21)

**32.** 1. A family history of allergies predisposes a child to having allergies too. Asthma and atopic dermatitis are classified as allergic conditions. Such factors as a family history of hypertension, malignant tumors, and febrile seizure activity are important in a health history but do not influence the development of infantile eczema. (15, 21)

**33.** 1. An infant 11 months old will not be comforted by such actions as rocking him before beginning an unpleasant procedure or allowing him to become familiar with equipment to be used, but he will most often be more cooperative when the mother is present during the procedure. Giving the infant formula is not likely to distract him and may cause him to associate eating with an unpleasant experience. (4)

**34.** 2. Itching is worse when the patient is warm and perspiring and when he wears scratchy clothing, such as woolen garments. The best nightclothes would be a one-piece cotton garment; there is no elastic at the waist to irritate the skin, and cotton is cool and unlikely to be irritating. Nylon tends to be hot. (6, 21)

35. 1. Diphenhydramine (Benadryl) is an antihistamine often used for allergic conditions. An important side effect is that it produces drowsiness, and it would be used primarily for its sedative effect for the infant described in this item. Diphenhydramine is not an analgesic. It helps control bronchial spasms, but they are not a problem in this situation. A variety of drugs other than diphenhydramine are effectively used as anti-inflammatory agents. (11, 16, 21)

36. 3. Aluminum acetate solution (Burow's solution) is often used for moistening dressings applied to eczematous skin lesions. These dressings serve several purposes. The solution cools the skin as moisture in the dressings evaporates. This helps reduce inflammation and relieves itching. The solution also acts as a mild antiseptic on the skin and helps cleanse the skin as well. (6, 7)

37. 1. Eggs and cow's milk are major offending foods in the diets of infants with allergies. Instituting a very restricted hypoallergenic diet is generally the first step taken to remove offending allergens from the child's diet. This diet begins with a milk substitute, usually a commercially prepared soy formula, and adds hypoallergenic fruits and vegetables for children who are eating solids or table foods. Apples, apricots, pears, carrots, and rice cereals are used in hypoallergenic diets. (11, 21)

38. 3. Suitable toys for an 11-month-old infant include rubber blocks, stuffed animals, large balls, and spools on a cord. But a child with allergies should not be given stuffed toys because they tend to collect dust and are difficult to clean, factors that tend to aggravate allergies. (7, 21)

## The Patient with Burns

39. 1. For a child under 12 years of age, 9% plus 1% for each year under 12 is allocated to the head and neck when using the "rule of nines" to estimate the surface area of burns. For a child over 12, 9% is allocated to the head and neck. The percentage of burned areas are the same for children over and under 12 years of age for the upper extremities (9% each) and the posterior and anterior chest walls (18% each). For a child over 12, each lower extremity is allocated 18%, for a child under 12, 18% minus 0.5% for each year under 12. (6, 15)

40. 3. The primary fluid shift is from the intravascular spaces to interstitial spaces when burns occur. The first effect of a burn is to produce dilatation of capillaries and small vessels in the area, and capillary permeability increases. Plasma seeps into the surrounding tissues to produce blisters and edema. There is also an exchange of electrolytes between cells and interstitial spaces as sodium enters a cell in exchange for the electrolyte potassium. (6, 21)

41. 4. Accurate determination of urinary output is a crucial factor in the care of a burn victim. The benefits of using an indwelling catheter to measure urinary output to the nearest milliliter each hour outweigh the potential for infection and other problems associated with its use. An indwelling catheter does not decrease the workload of the kidneys. (15, 21)

42. 2. The amount of intravenous fluid given to a child with burns depends on body weight in kilograms and percentage of body surface with second- and third-degree burns. For the child described in this item, the formula used to determine the requirements for the first 24 hours is:

3 ml/kg of body weight $\times$ percent of burn = 3 $\times$ 20 $\times$ 44 = 2,640 ml in the first 24 hours. Other formulae used to determine fluid needs serve as good guides, but additional observations, especially blood volume estimates, are also used in conjunction with them. (21)

43. 2. Hematocrit levels, obtained as frequently as every 6 hours, are usually used to help judge intravascular volume requirements following severe burns. The erythrocytes do not shift from intravascular to interstitial spaces, and therefore an increased hematocrit value would reflect inadequate fluid replacement. A decreased hematocrit level suggests excessive fluid replacement. Carbon dioxide tension reflects changes in ventilation and pulmonary function. Changes in urea nitrogen and creatinine blood levels may occur from a variety of stressors on the body. An increase would most likely suggest high catabolism of body protein and decreased renal function. (6, 21)

44. 2. A patient receiving excessive fluids is most likely to have circulatory overload with the associated danger of pulmonary edema. The patient then has moist rales and will likely also develop dyspnea if the condition is not relieved. Such conditions as abdominal distention and peripheral vasoconstriction are not associated with fluid overload. The presence of dark urine suggests that the patient may be receiving inadequate fluids, causing urine to be concentrated. (10, 21)

45. 2. Signs of a sodium deficit, sometimes called water intoxication, include muscle twitching and tremors,

apathy, loss of visual acuity, headaches, diarrhea, scanty urine production, and, finally, generalized seizures. (10, 21)

**46.** 3. Insufficient urinary output in a burn patient indicates the need for more parenteral fluid. For a child between about 4 and 7 years of age, the urinary output should be between approximately 24 and 28 ml per hour. A blood pressure decrease suggests that too little fluid is being infused. Such subjective signs as irritability and a negative answer when the patient is asked if he is thirsty cannot be relied upon as accurate assessments of fluid intake in an acutely ill child. (15, 21)

**47.** 1. Because of the typically unstable condition of a child with extensive burns, the physician should be consulted to obtain a new schedule for an intravenous infusion when it is noted that the infusion is running behind schedule. The patient may receive the fluid too rapidly if the rate is advanced rapidly to catch up on fluid intake. If the drip rate is corrected to the prescribed rate, the child will then likely suffer for not receiving a sufficient amount of fluid. (11, 21)

**48.** 4. A sign of hemolysis is hemoglobinuria. The presence of hemolyzed red blood cells in the urine will cause the urine to appear dark brown. The condition can result from trauma, such as a severe burn. (21)

**49.** 1. The most effective method for managing an allergic reaction is to eliminate the cause. The nurse's first course of action should be to stop administering a drug when the patient demonstrates an allergy to the medication. An allergic reaction can be serious! Such actions as preparing for the administration of whole blood, decreasing the infusion rate of intravenous fluids, and placing the patient in bed with his head lowered are not indicated when a patient demonstrates signs of an allergic reaction to a drug. Anaphylactic shock is the most severe form of an allergic reaction. (12)

**50.** 4. A skin rash is the most common sign when a allergic reaction occurs following the use of ampicillin. A serum sickness–like reaction may also occur, often with joint pains, but this type of reaction is much less common than a skin rash. Such signs as mental confusion and a rapid pulse rate are not associated with an allergic reaction to ampicillin. (16)

**51.** 1. Severely burned patients are predisposed to many electrolyte imbalances. The most common ones during the first 48 hours are a sodium deficit (the electrolyte is lost in trapped edema fluid and exudate by a shift of sodium into cells) and a potassium excess (the electrolyte escapes from traumatized cells into extracellular fluid). (10, 21)

**52.** 1. Bicarbonate ions are lost when a patient is seriously burned. The result is metabolic acidosis. The patient's respirations are characteristically deep and rapid, illustrating the body's efforts to rid itself of excess carbon dioxide (carbonic acid). These respirations are called Kussmaul respirations. (10, 21)

**53.** 1. The nurse can anticipate that a toxoid will be used for the child described in this situation because he has had tetanus immunization previously. A toxoid is a toxin treated with formaldehyde to destroy the toxin's toxicity without changing its antigenicity. If the patient had never been immunized for tetanus, tetanus immune globulin (TIG) would ordinarily be given. This item illustrates the importance of obtaining an immunization history when a patient such as the child described in this item is admitted to a hospital. (11, 21)

**54.** 1. Mafenide acetate (Sulfamylon) is a carbonic anhydrase inhibitor that may adversely affect the blood pH level. The condition that will result with the indiscriminate use of this agent is systemic acidosis. To compensate for the acidosis, the patient tends to hyperventilate, and respiratory alkalosis is then likely to develop. (11, 16)

**55.** 4. Mafenide acetate (Sulfamylon) causes a burning sensation when applied. The discomfort can last as long as an hour in some patients. Silver nitrate, which is also used on burns, has the disadvantage of staining. (11, 16, 21)

**56.** 1. Allowing a child to participate in his care (for example, having him apply ointment to burned areas) increases his self-esteem and helps him feel in control. Delaying the treatment is contraindicated because the therapy is important for the child's well-being. It may help to have a parent nearby to offer the child support, and the child should know it is all right for him to cry if he wishes. But these measures will not accomplish the desired goal of helping a child feel in control. (21)

**57.** 4. The Centers for Disease Control recommend that sterile gloves should be used when any care is given to a patient's badly burned areas. However, the gloves' effectiveness will be limited unless they are changed after removing soiled dressings and before handling and applying new dressings. (10, 21)

**58.** 4. Paralytic ileus often occurs in burn patients. The signs and symptoms result from decreased or absent peristalsis. Auscultation of the abdomen with a stethoscope to assess for bowel sounds provides data to determine if peristalsis has returned. When bowel sounds are heard, oral fluids are ordinarily started. Diarrhea is unlikely to be present in a patient with burns. An absence of abdominal distention and an eagerness to take nourishment are not satisfactory evidence to judge whether peristalsis has returned following paralytic ileus. (6, 21)

**59.** 2. Hypoproteinemia is common following severe burns because protein is lost in the wound exudate. The patient's diet should be high in protein to compensate for protein loss and to promote tissue healing. The child will also almost always require a high-calorie diet that is rich in iron to help prevent anemia. (6, 21)

**60.** 3. Orange juice is rich in potassium; it contains at least 400 mg per cup. Grape juice and cranberry juice are poorer sources of potassium, and ginger ale has no potassium. Additional rich sources of potassium are bananas, cantaloupe, grapefruit juice, tomato juice, honeydew melon, nectarine, and boiled and baked potatoes. (10, 21)

**61.** 4. Such measures as allowing the mother of a child to help feed him, serving the child small amounts of food at a time, and offering the child finger foods are recommended when a child loses interest in eating. Punishment, such as denying the child dessert until other foods are eaten, is rarely a successful technique. (21)

**62.** 4. Stomach and duodenal ulcers, called stress or Curling's ulcers, occur relatively often after severe burns. Antacids have been found helpful in reducing their incidence. A child's therapy and the parents' questions should be discussed whenever possible. Explaining therapy to parents helps gain their support and cooperation and also helps them cope with fears and anxiety resulting from the unknown and from an unfamiliar environment. It is not helpful to the parents to tell them not to worry or to refer them to the physician when it is a nursing responsibility to teach parents of ill children. The antacid used following burns does not counteract constipation. (11, 21)

**63.** 1. Tissues taken from animal sources are called xenografts. Porcine (pig) skin is frequently used for xenografts. Tissues taken from the patient's body are called autografts. Tissues taken from another person are called allografts. (10, 21)

**64.** 4. The primary purpose of a xenograft is to cover the burned areas until the patient's skin (autograft) is available for grafting. The covering helps minimize the growth of granulation tissue and protects the wound from infection and trauma. It also decreases fluid loss from evaporation from the wounds. A xenograft may also help decrease discomfort and thus promote movement, but these are not the primary reasons for using a xenograft. (10, 21)

**65.** 4. A burn patient, such as the child described in this item, often has irritation and edema in respiratory passageways that will block the airway. Parents in such situations are asked to sign a permit for a tracheostomy so that it can be done quickly in an emergency. The nurse can assist parents of an acutely ill child by offering explanations they can understand. Telling them not to worry is nonsupportive and tends to cut off further questions and expressions of feelings. It is incorrect to tell the parents in this situation that obtaining a permit for a tracheostomy is a routine procedure or that the permit is no longer valid. (11, 21)

**66.** 3. A disadvantage of using moist silver nitrate dressings on a burned area is that the solution's hypotonicity causes a loss of the electrolytes sodium and chloride from the wound's surface. The dressings should be kept well moistened because drying increases the solution's concentration and it may then become toxic to new epithelium. Occlusive dressings are recommended because they help reduce fluid loss through evaporation. (11, 21)

## The Patient with Hypothyroidism

**67.** 4. Thyroxine can pass through the placenta to the fetus. This exogenous maternal hormone prevents the appearance of signs of hypothyroidism at birth for most newborns with cretinism. Failure of normal development occurs during the embryonic period, or an inborn error of metabolism prevents normal synthesis of thyroxine. These conditions are present at birth. The fetus and the newborn require thyroxine, but there is little need for the infant to produce its own thyroxine because the exogenous maternal hormone appears to be sufficient. Breast-feeding delays the onset of overt signs of hypothyroidism, but the thyroxine in breast milk is not sufficient for normal growth or sufficient during the entire period of usual breast-feeding in infancy. (6, 21)

**68.** 1. Desiccated thyroid is manufactured from the thyroid glands of animals slaughtered for food. Its function is equivalent to that of endogenous thyroxine. The metabolic rate is increased so that normal growth and development is possible. Secretion of thyroxine is stimulated by the thyroid-stimulating hormone (TSH), produced by the pituitary gland. Exogenous desiccated thyroid depresses thyroxine production by the infant's thyroid gland. Limiting growth of the skeleton is not a function of thyroxine. Thyroxine is metabolized primarily in the liver and excreted in bile into the intestines. Some health-care personnel prefer synthetic thyroid preparation to desiccated thyroid because the synthetic preparation's potency is more standardized. (6, 16, 21)

**69.** 2. When a child with cretinism is receiving thyroid-replacement therapy, regular examinations of the child's skeletal growth are done to determine the effectiveness of the therapy. X-ray examinations may be used to help determine skeletal growth. Tests to determine thyroid-blood levels and serum alkaline phosphatase levels are often done in conjunction with studies of skeletal growth. (6, 16, 21)

**70.** 2. Typical signs of toxicity from thyroid-replacement therapy are a rapid pulse rate, dyspnea, sleeplessness, irritability, sweating, and weight loss. These signs result from an increased metabolic rate. Fractures, poor responses to environmental stimuli, and fluid imbalance with weight gain are not associated with thyroid toxicity. (16, 21)

**71.** 3. The hallmark signs of cretinism when the disease is not effectively treated are mental retardation and poor physical development. Cretinism has been reported as the most common cause of preventable retardation in contemporary health care. The effects of cretinism can be prevented when effective therapy is begun *early* in the 1st year of life. Blindness, epilepsy, and emotional instability are not associated with cretinism. (6, 21)

## The Patient with Insulin-Dependent Diabetes Mellitus

**72.** 2. An unconscious patient should be placed on either side with a pillow propped at his back. The head of the bed may be slightly elevated. This position allows for the best drainage from the mouth and helps prevent aspiration. A comatose person should not be placed flat on his back in bed. Placing the patient on his abdomen may be dangerous because of the possibility of suffocation. (6, 21)

**73.** 4. Ketones, which are organic acids, readily release free hydrogen ions that cause the blood pH to fall. When ketoacidosis is present, the body attempts to compensate by activating the respiratory buffering process. This causes the patient to make extra efforts to rid himself of excess carbon dioxide. The patient will take deep, rapid breaths and breathe as though he is experiencing air hunger. This type of breathing is called Kussmaul's breathing. (6, 21)

**74.** 4. In the patient with ketoacidosis due to diabetes mellitus, fats break down into fatty acids and glycerol in fat cells and the liver. They convert to ketone bodies. Ketones accumulate in the blood (ketonemia) and are then expelled in the urine (ketonuria) and as acetone by the lungs. There are two main types of diabetes. The patient described in this situation has type I or insulin-dependent diabetes mellitus (IDDM); formerly, this type of diabetes was called juvenile diabetes, juvenile-onset diabetes, ketosis-prone diabetes, or brittle diabetes. Type II diabetes is non-insulin-dependent diabetes mellitus (NIDDM) and was formerly called adult-onset diabetes, maturity-onset diabetes, ketosis-resistant diabetes, stable diabetes, or maturity-onset diabetes. (6, 21)

**75.** 3. In the presence of a high blood glucose level, the tubules of the kidney do not reabsorb all the glucose, and glycosuria results. An osmotic diuresis follows with an excess loss of water and such electrolytes as sodium, chloride, potassium, and phosphate. Water and electrolyte imbalances require prompt treatment in the patient with ketoacidosis. (6, 21)

**76.** 1. Diabetes mellitus is most probably a genetic disease, but the genetic pattern is unclear. Diabetes may also be called a syndrome because a variety of factors may play a role in its etiology. Diabetes is not related to the process of birth or intrauterine influences. (6, 21)

**77.** 2. One sign that most certainly suggests the presence of hyperglycemia due to diabetes mellitus, especially in a child, is bed-wetting. It is due to the production of excessive amounts of urine (polyuria). Another typical sign is excessive thirst (polydipsia). Being hungry (polyphagia) and irritable may be observed with hypoglycemia as well as hyperglycemia. The patient's activity level does not help to differentiate well, although the hyperglycemic person may complain of being lethargic. (6, 21)

**78.** 3. Although renal threshold levels vary, glycosuria usually occurs when the blood glucose level reaches 180 mg/100 ml of blood. In addition to urine testing, many diabetics also monitor blood glucose levels at home with equipment that measures the blood glucose level on an electronic meter. (6, 21)

**79.** 4. Insulin cannot be given by mouth because it is rendered inactive by gastrointestinal enzymes. (6, 16, 21)

**80.** 3. It is recommended that the patient using regular insulin with an intermediate- or long-acting insulin use one syringe. Using two syringes is not recommended because the insulins can be mixed and using two syringes requires two injections. NPH does not remain stable for *extended* periods of time when mixed with regular insulin, so premixing is rarely recommended. When mixing regular insulin and an intermediate- or long-acting insulin from two vials, withdraw the regular insulin first. Then withdraw the intermediate- or long-acting insulin. Insulin preparations such as protamine zinc, globin zinc, or isophane (NPH) contain an additional modifying protein that slows absorption. A vial of insulin that does *not* contain the added protein (for example, regular insulin) should *never* be contaminated with insulin that does have the added protein. (6, 21)

**81.** 2. The onset of action of intermediate-acting insulin, such as NPH, is 2 to 4 hours after injection. The action will *peak* between 6 and 8 hours after injection. This information is important in terms of timing meals and snacks and of recognizing when insulin reactions are most likely to occur. (6, 16, 21)

**82.** 2. A vial has a cap that makes the vial airtight. A volume of air about the same as the amount of insulin to be withdrawn should be injected into the vial. If too little air is injected, the vial will develop a partial vacuum, making removal of insulin difficult. If too much air is injected, the vial will have positive pressure, and when a needle is inserted the pressure is likely to blow out the plunger or make it difficult to measure the amount of insulin desired. (12)

**83.** 3. The forearms are inappropriate sites for injecting insulin because subcutaneous tissue in the forearms is very sparse. Areas where subcutaneous tissue is more abundant, such as the thighs, abdomen, and upper arms, are advised for the injection of insulin. The sites must be rotated to prevent tissue damage and ineffective absorption of insulin. (6, 21)

**84.** 3. An increase in the usual amount of exercise will *decrease* the amount of insulin the body requires because exercise promotes the utilization of carbohydrates and enhances the action of insulin. Stress, such as experienced when preparing for hospitalization or when emotionally upset, and infection increase the body's usual needs for insulin. (6, 21)

**85.** 4. Insulin may be stored between uses at room temperature. Extremes in temperature are not recommended. Insulin manufactured today is stable for one year at room temperature. (6, 16, 21)

**86.** 4. Concentrated sweets are contraindicated in the diet of a person with diabetes. Examples of such foods include jellies, jams, honey, most desserts, and candy. Such foods as peanut butter, pizza, yogurt, hamburger, and French fries are satisfactory, provided dietary calculations are taken into account. (6, 21)

**87.** 3. To establish the possibility of impending diabetic acidosis, the first action is to check the blood for glucose level. If it is elevated, the patient should be prepared to take insulin. Taking sugar and withholding insulin are contraindicated and will aggra-

vate the situation. It may be necessary to take a patient with impending diabetic acidosis to the emergency room of a hospital for care, but the first action should be to determine the blood glucose level. (6, 21)

**88.** 3. Insulin shock is the result of hypoglycemia, which often occurs if the patient has had too much insulin or not enough food. It is best to relieve the symptoms by taking sugar (for example, eating several cubes of sugar or drinking a glass of orange juice). Eating a piece of hard candy and drinking a regular carbonated beverage will accomplish the same thing. Increasing activity will aggravate the situation. Resting in bed will not alleviate the signs. The physician may need to be consulted if conservative care does not help. (6, 21)

**89.** 3. Diabetes mellitus cannot be cured. This child can be expected to need insulin and dietary adjustments throughout life. The severity of the disease cannot be decreased. Type I insulin-dependent diabetes mellitus requires the use of insulin throughout life, whereas type II non-insulin-dependent diabetes mellitus can often be controlled with oral hypoglycemics, diet, and exercise. (6, 21)

**90.** 3. It would be inappropriate to recommend that a child with diabetes mellitus refrain from strenuous sports. Many diabetics lead completely normal lives and often do participate in various sporting activities. A teaching program for a diabetic should include such suggestions as wearing properly fitting shoes, anticipating that adjustments in diet and insulin requirements will change in the presence of an infection, and treating a diabetic in a manner similar to others his age. (6, 21)

**91.** 4. The person with diabetes mellitus fails to metabolize carbohydrates, fats, and proteins properly. This is an important teaching point because most laypersons believe that carbohydrates are the only food constituent important to watch in a diabetic diet. (6, 21)

## The Patient Who is Abused

**92.** 2. Parents of an abused child are typically unconcerned about the child's injury. They may blame the child or others for the injury, may not ask questions about treatment, and may not know developmental information. (7, 21)

**93.** 1. All states have mandatory reporting laws relating to child abuse and neglect. A nurse or other health-care professional who fails to report suspected abuse may be charged with a misdemeanor. Nurses who report suspected child abuse have immunity from being sued. (7, 15, 17, 21)

**94.** 2. Primary prevention of child abuse and neglect is initiated during pregnancy and involves steps designed to promote family well-being. A thorough prenatal assessment can help identify potential abusers. (15, 21)

**95.** 3. The primary goal in cases of child abuse is to protect the child from injury. This often means hospitalization. The child could probably be treated as an outpatient, but this does not protect the child. Those charged with investigating the situation can obtain additional information about the family, regardless of whether the child is hospitalized. It is not the role of the health-care team to determine "who did it," but rather to report the suspicion of or actual abuse to the appropriate agency. (21)

**96.** 2. Most abusive parents were themselves abused and are repeating a learned behavior. The incidence of child abuse cannot be correlated with social status, income level, or educational level. Abusive parents typically have very unrealistic expectations of their children. (7, 15, 21)

**97.** 4. Parents who are abusive typically lack knowledge about the child's development and needs. A 3-year-old does like books about things that he knows, but will be unable to tie his shoes until he is 5 years old. Abusive parents tend to be socially isolated, lacking friends and a support system. (7, 21)

**98.** 3. Encouraging the abused child to talk about or play out the events surrounding the "accident" can help the child and also provide assessment data. Abused children tend to feel they are at fault; if the parent is accused of abuse, the child may accept responsibility for the act. Promises that cannot be kept should not be made. (21)

**99.** 3. Abused children have become "immune" to pain and have found that crying may bring on more pain. They need to learn that appropriate emotional expression is acceptable. (14)

**100.** 2. Abused children need attention and affection as well as consistent management of inappropriate behavior. They have often learned undesirable behavior to get attention, cope with their environment, and relate to people. Behavior modification is used, and anger and any aggressive act is not rewarded. A program of attention based on group intervention with other children is planned. The child is treated as a child with normal interests and needs, not as a victim of child abuse. (21)

**101.** 2. The goal of the consistent nurse-child relationship is to provide a role model for the parents and to foster a therapeutic environment for the child. The nurse does attempt to modify negative behavior and guide the child toward physical and mental wellness, but these are secondary to the overall goal of providing a role model. The child's continuing relationship with the parents is encouraged. (21)

**102.** 4. Improved family functioning hinges on improved coping skills, child-care skills, and interaction patterns. Parenting classes may be helpful, but too many people or services may overwhelm a family. Coordinating with community agencies is also important. (15)

**103.** 4. It is most important for the nurse to have a patient's record that includes documentation of physical findings and behaviors observed. Court proceedings usually occur sometime after the nurse's involvement with the child and family, and memories fade. Thus, careful documentation of the facts, not hearsay or subjective opinion, is essential. (14, 21)

**104.** 2. A child's not wanting to visit a previously favorite place or relatives is a clue that something has happened in that setting to frighten or upset the child. Gathering more information is the first step in helping the parent and child. Four-year-old children demonstrate strong attachment for the parent of the opposite sex, and this response negates the father's expressed concern. Five-year-olds separate easily from parents and relate appropriately to adults outside the family. (7, 21)

**105.** 3. In masked sexual abuse, somatic complaints are the presenting symptoms as the child seeks help but cannot ask directly or is afraid to discuss the real problem. Another potential manifestation of sexual abuse is excessive day-dreaming. Poor personal hygiene and lack of subcutaneous fat may indicate physical neglect. Unexplained sudden illness and apprehension when hearing other children cry are potential indicators of physical abuse. Sleep disorders and lags in emotional and intellectual development are associated with emotional abuse. (15, 21)

**106.** 2. Children who report abuse must be believed. The nurse should deal with the child with sensitivity and discretion. When interviewing the child, the nurse should start with neutral questions and later ask the child for an account of the event. Often, the child has tried to tell the parents but has not been believed or has been rejected, or the child may be afraid to tell the parents. (15, 21)

**107.** 3. Young children are able to use play and anatomically correct dolls to describe what happened to them. Young children lack verbal skills for describing body parts adequately. Drawing, itself, can be used with both younger and older children, but younger children would have difficulty verbally describing the events. (15, 21)

**108.** 1. Determining the dynamics of family functioning is a goal of working with the parents of a physically neglected child. Some parents neglect their children intentionally. Some forget to feed them, while others are ignorant of their needs. Some parents lack needed resources and do not know how to obtain them. Information obtained about the child's developmental history, the parents' reactions to a child's illness or an accident, and a typical daily meal plan help determine the dynamics of family functioning. (15)

# REFERENCES FOR PART III
## The Nursing Care of Children

1. Baer CL, Williams BR. Clinical Pharmacology and Nursing. Springfield, PA: Springhouse, 1988.
2. Burtis G, Davis J, Martin S. Applied Nutrition and Diet Therapy. Philadelphia: WB Saunders, 1988.
3. Evans OW. Manual of Child Neurology. New York: Churchill Livingstone, 1987.
4. Govoni LE, Hayes JE. Drugs and Nursing Implications. 5th ed. New York: Appleton-Century-Crofts, 1985.
5. Hazinski MF. Nursing Care of the Critically Ill Child. American Association of Critical Care Nurses, St. Louis: CV Mosby, 1984.
6. James SR, Mott SR. Child Health Nursing: Essential Care of Children and Families. Menlo Park, CA: Addison-Wesley, 1988.
7. Marlow DR, Redding BA. Textbook of Pediatric Nursing. 6th ed. Philadelphia: WB Saunders, 1988.
8. Mott SA, Fazekas NF, James SR. Nursing Care of Children and Families: A Holistic Approach. Menlo Park, CA: Addison-Wesley, 1985.
9. Olds SB, London ML, Ludewig PA. Maternal Newborn Nursing, A Family-Centered Approach. 3rd ed. Menlo Park, CA: Addison-Wesley, 1988.
10. Phipps WJ, Long BC, Woods NF. Medical-Surgical Nursing Concepts and Clinical Practice. 3rd ed. St. Louis: CV Mosby, 1987.
11. Pillitteri A. Child Health Nursing: Care of the Growing Family. 3rd ed. Boston: Little Brown, 1987.
12. Potter PA, Perry AG. Basic Nursing Theory and Practice. St. Louis: CV Mosby, 1987.
13. Radcliff RK, Ogden SJ. Calculation of Drug Dosages: A Workbook. 3rd ed. St. Louis: CV Mosby, 1987.
14. Scipien GM, Barnard MU, Chard MA, Howe J, Phillips PJ. Comprehensive Pediatric Nursing. 3rd ed. New York: McGraw-Hill, 1986.
15. Servonsky J, Opas SR. Nursing Management of Children. Boston: Jones and Bartlett, 1987.
16. Skidmore-Roth L. Nursing Drug Reference. St. Louis: CV Mosby, 1988.
17. Smith M, Goodman J, Ramsey N. Child and Family: Concepts of Nursing Practice. New York: McGraw-Hill, 1987.
18. Sorenson KC, Luckmann J. Basic Nursing: A Psychophysiologic Approach. 2nd ed. Philadelphia: WB Saunders, 1986.
19. Stuart G, Sundeen SJ. Principles and Practice of Psychiatric Nursing. 3rd ed. St. Louis: CV Mosby, 1987.
20. Waechter EH, Phillips J, Holoday B. Nursing Care of Children. 10th ed. Philadelphia: JB Lippincott, 1985.
21. Whaley LF, Wong DL. Nursing Care of Infants and Children. 3rd ed. St. Louis: CV Mosby, 1987.
22. Zeman FJ, Neg DM. Application of Clinical Nutrition. Englewood Cliffs, NJ: Prentice Hall, 1988.

# PART IV

## The Nursing Care of Adults with Medical/Surgical Disorders

# test 1

*The Patient with Pneumonia*

*The Patient with Tuberculosis*

*The Patient with Chronic Obstructive Pulmonary Disease*

*The Patient with Lung Cancer*

*The Patient with Chest Trauma*

*Correct Answers and Rationales*

Select the one *best* or *correct* answer and indicate your choice by filling in the circle with a pencil in front of the option you have chosen. If the answer you would prefer is not given, select the one you think is *most appropriate.*

## ▲ THE PATIENT WITH PNEUMONIA

Ms. Bertha Litke, age 79, is admitted to the hospital with a diagnosis of bacterial pneumonia. She has a temperature of 102.6° F, a productive cough, and is experiencing difficulty breathing.

1. When the nurse obtains Ms. Litke's health history, she learns that the patient has long-standing osteoarthritis, follows a vegetarian diet, has never been seriously ill, and is very concerned with cleanliness. Ms. Litke says, "I hope I can take a bath each day. I feel so dirty if I don't bathe every day." Which of the following factors adds *most* to the danger of her illness?
   ○ 1. The patient's age.
   ○ 2. The history of osteoarthritis.
   ○ 3. Following a vegetarian diet.
   ○ 4. Bathing daily in cold water.
2. Considering Ms. Litke's clinical symptoms, what site should the nurse use to obtain her temperature?
   ○ 1. Oral.
   ○ 2. Groin fold.
   ○ 3. Rectal.
   ○ 4. Axillary.
3. Ms. Litke appears slightly cyanotic on admission. The cyanosis that accompanies bacterial pneumonia is primarily due to
   ○ 1. cardiac involvement.
   ○ 2. iron-deficiency anemia.
   ○ 3. inadequate circulation.
   ○ 4. poor oxygenation of blood.
4. Ms. Litke is to be started on intravenous antibiotics immediately. Which of the following must be completed *before* the nurse begins the antibiotic therapy?

   ○ 1. Urinalysis.
   ○ 2. Sputum examination.
   ○ 3. Chest x-ray.
   ○ 4. Complete blood count.
5. Ms. Litke is experiencing pleuritic chest pain. This type of chest pain is usually described as being
   ○ 1. a mild but constant aching in the chest.
   ○ 2. severe midsternal pain.
   ○ 3. moderate pain that worsens on inspiration.
   ○ 4. muscle spasm pain that accompanies coughing.
6. Which of the following nursing measures is *most likely* to be successful in reducing Ms. Litke's chest pain?
   ○ 1. Encourage her to breathe shallowly.
   ○ 2. Have her practice abdominal breathing.
   ○ 3. Offer her an incentive spirometer.
   ○ 4. Teach her to splint her rib cage during coughing.
7. Aspirin is administered to patients with pneumonia because of its antipyretic and
   ○ 1. analgesic effects.
   ○ 2. cholinergic effects.
   ○ 3. adrenergic effects.
   ○ 4. antihistamine effects.
8. Ms. Litke is coughing up tenacious purulent sputum. Which of the following nursing measures is *most likely* to help liquefy these viscous secretions?
   ○ 1. Postural drainage.
   ○ 2. Breathing humidified air.
   ○ 3. Clapping and percussion over the affected lung.
   ○ 4. Coughing and deep-breathing exercises.
9. Ms. Litke is extremely diaphoretic with her high fever. Considering her age, she is at particular risk for developing
   ○ 1. hyponatremia.
   ○ 2. hypokalemia.

**337**

   ○ 3. hypercalcemia.

   ○ 4. hyperphosphatemia.

**10.** Considering Ms. Litke's symptoms and personality, the nurse should include which of the following measures in her care?

   ○ 1. Frequent position changes.

   ○ 2. Regular bedside visits.

   ○ 3. Frequent linen changes.

   ○ 4. Frequent offers of the bedpan.

**11.** Which of the following behaviors could indicate that Ms. Litke is experiencing hypoxia?

   ○ 1. Anger.

   ○ 2. Apathy.

   ○ 3. Anxiety.

   ○ 4. Aggression.

**12.** Oxygen at 4 liters per minute is ordered for Ms. Litke. The *most effective* way to deliver the prescribed oxygen would be by

   ○ 1. nasal cannula.

   ○ 2. nasal prongs.

   ○ 3. face mask.

   ○ 4. tent.

**13.** Bed rest is prescribed for Ms. Litke during the acute phase of her illness. The purpose of bed rest in this situation is to

   ○ 1. reduce the cellular demand for oxygen.

   ○ 2. decrease the basal metabolic rate.

   ○ 3. promote patient safety.

   ○ 4. promote clearance of secretions.

**14.** After 3 days of therapy, a lab report indicates that Ms. Litke has a white blood cell count of 8,000/mm$^3$. Which action should the nurse take in response to this report?

   ○ 1. Notify the physician promptly.

   ○ 2. Omit the next dose of antibiotic.

   ○ 3. Initiate reverse isolation precautions.

   ○ 4. Continue with the current regimen.

**15.** Ms. Litke develops mild constipation and the nurse administers dioctyl sodium sulfosuccinate (Colace). This drug works by

   ○ 1. softening the stool.

   ○ 2. lubricating the stool.

   ○ 3. increasing stool bulk.

   ○ 4. stimulating peristalsis.

**16.** Ms. Litke says to the nurse, "It's terrible to grow old. I remember things I used to do and can do no more." Which of the following phenomena is considered to be an inevitable consequence of aging, even when health is good?

   ○ 1. An end to sexual activity.

   ○ 2. A general intellectual decline.

   ○ 3. A decrease in verbal skill.

   ○ 4. A slowing of thought and learning processes.

**17.** As Ms. Litke is preparing for discharge, she asks the nurse if there is anything she can do to prevent the recurrence of pneumonia. It is *least* important for the nurse to teach Ms. Litke about

   ○ 1. avoiding possible contact with ill people.

   ○ 2. continuing her current diet habits.

   ○ 3. receiving the annual flu vaccine.

   ○ 4. seeking prompt antibiotic therapy for viral infections.

## THE PATIENT WITH TUBERCULOSIS

Mr. Hector Valquez, age 48, has just been diagnosed with tuberculosis. He had been feeling unwell for the last several weeks, but sought medical attention when he began coughing up bloody secretions.

**18.** *All* of the following symptoms are commonly experienced by persons with active tuberculosis *except*

   ○ 1. anorexia and weight loss.

   ○ 2. fatigue and malaise.

   ○ 3. high fever and shaking chills.

   ○ 4. afternoon fever and night sweats.

**19.** The nurse obtains a sputum specimen from Mr. Valquez for laboratory study. Which of the following laboratory techniques is used *most commonly* to identify tubercle bacilli in sputum?

   ○ 1. Acid-fast staining.

   ○ 2. Sensitivity testing.

   ○ 3. Agglutination testing.

   ○ 4. Darkfield illumination.

**20.** Mr. Valquez's sputum is positive for tubercle bacilli. The nurse should teach Mr. Valquez that the *most common* means of transmitting tubercle bacilli from person to person is by contaminated

   ○ 1. dust particles.

   ○ 2. droplet nuclei.

   ○ 3. water.

   ○ 4. eating utensils.

**21.** The nurse teaches Mr. Valquez various ways to decrease the spread of all microorganisms. Most authorities believe that the single *most effective* way to decrease the spread of microorganisms is by

   ○ 1. washing the hands frequently.

   ○ 2. having separate personal-care items for each person.

   ○ 3. using disposable equipment to the greatest extent possible.

   ○ 4. isolating persons known to be harboring disease-causing microorganisms.

22. An antituberculous drug that may damage the eighth cranial nerve is prescribed for Mr. Valquez. Eighth cranial nerve damage is a common side effect of which drug?
    ○ 1. Streptomycin.
    ○ 2. Isoniazid (INH).
    ○ 3. Aminosalicylic acid (PAS).
    ○ 4. Ethambutol hydrochloride (Myambutol).

23. If Mr. Valquez experiences eighth cranial nerve damage, he will *most likely* report which symptom?
    ○ 1. Vertigo.
    ○ 2. Facial paralysis.
    ○ 3. Impaired vision.
    ○ 4. Difficulty swallowing.

24. Many patients with tuberculosis take two antitubercular drugs simultaneously. The *primary* reason for administering two or more drugs at one time is to
    ○ 1. potentiate the actions of the drugs.
    ○ 2. reduce undesirable side effects of the drugs.
    ○ 3. allow lower dosages of the drugs to be given.
    ○ 4. delay resistance of the causative organisms to the drugs.

25. Mr. Valquez is to be discharged home with community health nursing follow-up. The nursing goals listed below are all important to home care of tuberculosis patients, but which goal has the *highest* priority?
    ○ 1. To offer patients emotional support.
    ○ 2. To teach patients about their disease.
    ○ 3. To coordinate various agency services the patients require.
    ○ 4. To assess the environments of patients for standards of sanitation.

26. In teaching Mr. Valquez about self-care at home, the nurse will include all of the following measures. Which of the measures has the *highest* priority?
    ○ 1. Getting enough rest.
    ○ 2. Eating a nourishing diet.
    ○ 3. Taking medications as prescribed.
    ○ 4. Living where there is clean fresh air.

27. Mr. Valquez's family and friends must undergo tuberculosis screening, and arrangements are made for them to receive the Mantoux skin test. Which of the following techniques is *incorrect* when administering the Mantoux test?
    ○ 1. The needle and syringe are held almost parallel to the patient's skin.
    ○ 2. The skin is kept slightly taut when the needle is inserted.
    ○ 3. The needle is inserted with the bevel side up.

    ○ 4. The injected area is massaged after introducing the solution.

28. Which member of Mr. Valquez's family is at *highest risk* for contracting tuberculosis?
    ○ 1. His 45-year-old wife.
    ○ 2. His teenaged children.
    ○ 3. His grade-school children.
    ○ 4. His 76-year-old mother.

29. Two members of the Valquez family exhibit positive Mantoux tests. What is the nurse's *best* interpretation of this finding?
    ○ 1. They have clinical tuberculosis.
    ○ 2. They have had contact with the tubercle bacilli.
    ○ 3. They have developed a resistance to the tubercle bacilli.
    ○ 4. They have developed a passive immunity to tuberculosis.

30. In view of the positive skin tests, the physician will probably recommend that Mr. Valquez's family members
    ○ 1. be evaluated every 6 months for clinical signs of tuberculosis.
    ○ 2. have a skin test every 6 months.
    ○ 3. take isoniazid (INH) for approximately 9 months.
    ○ 4. take isoniazid (INH) until their skin tests revert back to negative.

31. To prevent the development of the peripheral neuropathies that are a common side effect of isoniazid (INH) administration, patients are usually advised to
    ○ 1. follow special foot care regimens.
    ○ 2. supplement their diet with pyridoxine (vitamin B$_6$).
    ○ 3. get extra rest.
    ○ 4. avoid excessive sun exposure.

32. The nurse should caution sexually active female patients who are taking isoniazid (INH) that the drug
    ○ 1. increases the risk of vaginal infections.
    ○ 2. has mutagenic effects on ova.
    ○ 3. decreases the effectiveness of oral contraceptives.
    ○ 4. inhibits ovulation.

33. Mr. Valquez needs to understand that he will be at risk for recurrence of tuberculosis during periods of
    ○ 1. hot, humid and cool, damp weather.
    ○ 2. active exercise and exertion.
    ○ 3. physical and emotional stress.
    ○ 4. rest and inactivity.

34. In which areas of the United States does tuberculosis *most commonly* occur?
    ○ 1. Rural farming areas.

○ 2. Inner-city areas.
○ 3. Areas where clean water standards are low.
○ 4. Suburban areas with significant industrial pollution.

## THE PATIENT WITH CHRONIC OBSTRUCTIVE PULMONARY DISEASE

Mr. Peter Whitney, age 65, is admitted to the hospital with an acute exacerbation of long-standing COPD brought on by an upper respiratory infection. He is tachypneic and acutely short of breath. Both Mr. Whitney and his wife are extremely anxious.

35. Mr. Whitney is admitted to room 13. He states that he does not want to remain in the room because the number will bring him bad luck. Personnel in the admitting office say a change can be made if the nurse feels it is wise to do so. Which of the following statements offers the best guide for the nurse in this situation?
○ 1. Move the patient; the patient's fears, even when unfounded, can impede recovery.
○ 2. Move the patient; superstitions have a good chance of coming true for those who believe them.
○ 3. Do not move the patient; having the patient use the room will help him overcome an unwarranted fear.
○ 4. Do not move the patient; the patient may become unmanageable and demanding when he knows he can have his way.

36. Which of the following physical assessment findings is typical in a patient with advanced obstructive pulmonary disease?
○ 1. Increased anterior posterior chest diameter.
○ 2. Underdeveloped neck muscles.
○ 3. Collapsed neck veins.
○ 4. Increased chest excursions with respiration.

37. Oxygen at the rate of 1.5 L/min via nasal prongs is prescribed for Mr. Whitney. Which of the following statements best describes why Mr. Whitney's oxygen therapy is maintained at a relatively low level of concentration?
○ 1. The oxygen will be lost at the patient's nostrils if given at a higher level in nasal prongs.
○ 2. The patient's long history of a respiratory problem indicates that he would be unable to absorb oxygen given at a higher rate.
○ 3. The cells in the alveoli are so damaged by the patient's long history of a respiratory problem

that higher levels of oxygen and reduced levels of carbon dioxide are likely to cause the cells to burst.
○ 4. The patient's respiratory center is so accustomed to high carbon dioxide and low blood oxygen concentrations that changing these concentrations with oxygen therapy may eliminate the patient's stimulus for breathing.

38. Mr. Whitney becomes acutely anxious and short of breath. Which of the following nursing interventions is most likely to reduce the dyspnea?
○ 1. Increase his oxygen flow rate to 6 L/min.
○ 2. Lower the head of his bed.
○ 3. Have him breathe into a paper bag.
○ 4. Encourage him to breathe rhythmically.

39. The nurse teaches Mr. Whitney to purse his lips while breathing. The primary purpose of pursed-lip breathing is to help
○ 1. promote oxygen intake.
○ 2. strengthen the diaphragm.
○ 3. strengthen the intercostal muscles.
○ 4. promote carbon dioxide elimination.

40. The nurse teaches Mr. Whitney measures to conserve energy when performing activities of daily living. The nurse should teach Mr. Whitney to lift objects
○ 1. while inhaling through pursed lips.
○ 2. while exhaling through pursed lips.
○ 3. after exhaling but before inhaling.
○ 4. after inhaling but before exhaling.

41. Mr. Whitney receives theophylline ethylene-diamine (aminophylline) intravenously every 6 hours. Which of the following changes in Mr. Whitney's condition would indicate to the nurse that the drug is exerting its primary desired effect?
○ 1. The patient sleeps better.
○ 2. The patient has less ankle edema.
○ 3. The patient breathes easier.
○ 4. The patient is more encouraged about his condition.

42. Chest percussion is ordered for Mr. Whitney q.i.d. The primary purpose of chest percussion for this patient is to
○ 1. stimulate deeper inhalations.
○ 2. improve ciliary action in the bronchioles.
○ 3. propel secretions along the respiratory tract.
○ 4. loosen secretions in congested areas of the lungs.

43. Arterial blood gases are drawn while Mr. Whitney is breathing room air. The results are pH, 7.32; PaO$_2$, 53 mm Hg; PaCO$_2$, 80 mm Hg. What conclusion can the nurse safely make from these findings?

○ 1. The patient is in metabolic acidosis.
○ 2. The patient is in respiratory acidosis.
○ 3. The patient is in metabolic alkalosis.
○ 4. The patient is in respiratory alkalosis.

**44.** What conclusion can the nurse safely make from the laboratory findings about Mr. Whitney's arterial blood carbon dioxide tension ($PaCO_2$)?
○ 1. The $PaCO_2$ level indicates that the patient is alkalotic.
○ 2. The $PaCO_2$ level indicates that the patient is hypoventilating.
○ 3. The $PaCO_2$ level indicates that the patient is hyperventilating.
○ 4. The $PaCO_2$ level indicates that the patient is using oxygen therapy.

**45.** What conclusion can the nurse safely make from the laboratory findings about Mr. Whitney's arterial blood oxygen tension ($PaO_2$)?
○ 1. The $PaO_2$ level indicates that the patient has increasing hypoxia
○ 2. The $PaO_2$ level indicates that the patient's $PaO_2$ level is low but poses no problem.
○ 3. The $PaO_2$ level indicates that the patient's $PaO_2$ level is within normal range.
○ 4. The $PaO_2$ level indicates that the patient requires therapy with very low concentrations of oxygen.

**46.** The nurse takes into account that Mr. Whitney has trouble raising respiratory secretions. Which of the following nursing measures will help reduce the tenacity of the patient's secretions?
○ 1. Ensuring that the patient's diet is low in salt.
○ 2. Making sure that the patient's oxygen therapy is continuous.
○ 3. Helping the patient maintain a high fluid intake.
○ 4. Keeping the patient in a semi-sitting position as much as possible.

**47.** Mrs. Whitney cares for her husband between hospitalizations and asks the nurse about his feelings of depression, irritability, and poor appetite. The nurse shows an understanding of Mr. Whitney's behavior when she explains that it is *most likely* the result of
○ 1. his current illness.
○ 2. the normal aging process.
○ 3. premonitions that death may be near.
○ 4. feelings of resentment toward health care personnel.

**48.** Mr. Whitney becomes angry when his dinner is delayed. Which of the following courses of action would be *most appropriate* for the nurse to take *first* when Mr. Whitney becomes angry?
○ 1. Ignore the patient's behavior until his anger subsides.

○ 2. Listen to the patient as he expresses his anger.
○ 3. Tell the patient that his anger is interfering with his recovery.
○ 4. Ask the patient if he would like to discuss the problem with the dietitian.

**49.** Mr. Whitney has been steadily losing weight. He explains that the dyspnea interferes with his eating. Which of the following measures would minimize the effect of dyspnea on Mr. Whitney's dietary intake?
○ 1. Eating large frequent meals.
○ 2. Avoiding between-meal snacks.
○ 3. Avoiding gas-producing foods.
○ 4. Encouraging him to use oxygen intermittently at mealtimes.

**50.** In order to have Mr. Whitney maintain adequate nutrition, the nurse should advise him to eat a diet
○ 1. high in protein and low in calories.
○ 2. high in protein and high in calories.
○ 3. low in protein and high in carbohydrates.
○ 4. high in calories and low in carbohydrates.

**51.** Mrs. Whitney says her husband often uses postural drainage at home. What causes the greatest amount of movement of debris from the lower to the upper respiratory tract when the patient is using postural drainage?
○ 1. Friction between the cilia.
○ 2. The force of gravity.
○ 3. The sweeping motion of cilia.
○ 4. Involuntary muscular contractions.

**52.** Mr. Whitney is often bedridden at home and gets little exercise. Which of the following is a *normal* physiologic reaction of the body to prolonged periods of bed rest and inactivity?
○ 1. Sodium retention is increased.
○ 2. Calcium excretion is increased.
○ 3. Insulin utilization is increased.
○ 4. Red blood cell production is increased.

**53.** When developing Mr. Whitney's discharge plan, the nurse should be guided by an understanding that Mr. Whitney is *most likely* to
○ 1. develop infections easily.
○ 2. maintain his current status.
○ 3. require less supplemental oxygen.
○ 4. show permanent improvement.

## THE PATIENT WITH LUNG CANCER

Ms. Maureen Rand is a 49-year-old stockbroker who was admitted with a diagnosis of lung cancer. She enjoyed good health until 2 months ago, when she developed a persistent cough that became productive of blood-tinged sputum 1 week ago. She has also experienced increasing fatigue over the last month. She had no anorexia and appears well nourished (5-foot-7, 140 pounds). She has smoked a pack of cigarettes a day for 28 years. A chest x-ray and sputum cytology done a week ago are the basis for the diagnosis.

54. A major intervention nurses can carry out as a means of preventing lung cancer is to
    ○ 1. encourage cigarette smokers to have yearly chest x-rays.
    ○ 2. emphasize the causative relationship of cigarette smoking to lung cancer.
    ○ 3. recommend that people have their houses and apartments checked for asbestos leakage.
    ○ 4. encourage people to install central air cleaners in their homes.

55. As part of her diagnostic work-up, Ms. Rand is to have a bronchoscopy under local anesthesia. Her preoperative medication will be atropine sulfate 0.4 mg and meperidine hydrochloride (Demerol) 100 mg IM. Which of the following nursing interventions should the nurse carry out after the test?
    ○ 1. Irrigate the nasogastric tube with 30 ml of normal saline every 2 hours.
    ○ 2. Offer her 200 ml of oral fluids every hour to liquefy lung secretions.
    ○ 3. Observe her abdomen for signs of distention and boardlike rigidity.
    ○ 4. Position her on her side and keep her n.p.o. for several hours.

56. The bronchoscopy confirmed the diagnosis of cancer of the left lower lobe. A lobectomy is scheduled in 2 days. Several tests are ordered for Ms. Rand that will provide data useful in planning and guiding medical and nursing care. Which of the following tests will give the nurse the *most* valuable information in planning Ms. Rand's participation in her postoperative nursing care?
    ○ 1. Hematocrit and hemoglobin.
    ○ 2. Arterial blood gases.
    ○ 3. Pulmonary function tests.
    ○ 4. Lung tomograms.

57. Considering the fact that Ms. Rand is to have a left lung lobectomy, certain data become more important than others in planning her postoperative nursing care. The following assessments were obtained in the nurse's admission interview and nursing history of Ms. Rand. *All* will play an important part in her care *except* that she
    ○ 1. is 5-foot-7 and weighs 140 pounds.
    ○ 2. tends to keep her real feelings to herself.
    ○ 3. ambulates and can climb one flight of stairs without dyspnea.

○ 4. has difficulty maintaining her normal bowel pattern when stressed.

58. A nursing diagnosis the nurse identifies for Ms. Rand is "knowledge deficit related to postoperative expectations and self-care." The nursing care plan addressing that diagnosis should include which of the following interventions?
    ○ 1. Informing her about the nasogastric tube she will have and explaining its purpose.
    ○ 2. Explaining the reasons for and demonstrating the range-of-motion exercises she will do with her left arm.
    ○ 3. Explaining that given her type of lung surgery, she will be allowed to lie only on her back.
    ○ 4. Explaining that she will have one or two chest tubes that will be irrigated every 8 hours.

59. Major teaching interventions for Ms. Rand prior to her lobectomy include explaining the need to cough and deep-breathe every hour postoperatively and demonstrating the techniques. Coughing expels secretions. Why is deep-breathing so important?
    ○ 1. It causes the diaphragm to ascend, which enlarges the thorax and increases the lung surface available for gas exchange.
    ○ 2. It expands the alveoli, stimulates surfactant, and increases the lung surface available for gas exchange.
    ○ 3. It decreases the blood flow to the lungs and increases the lung surface available for ventilation.
    ○ 4. It controls the rate of air flow to the remaining lobe so that it will not become hyperinflated.

60. The night before surgery, the nurse notices that Ms. Rand looks sad and is quieter than usual. The nurse shares with her the perception of her behavior, and Ms. Rand says, "I'm scared of having cancer. It's so horrible and I brought it on myself. I should have quit smoking years ago." What would be the nurse's *best* response to Ms. Rand?
    ○ 1. "It's okay to be scared. What is it about cancer that you're afraid of?"
    ○ 2. "It's normal to be scared. I would be, too. We'll help you through it."
    ○ 3. "Don't be so hard on yourself. You don't know if your smoking caused the cancer."
    ○ 4. "Do you feel guilty because you smoked?"

61. The preoperative medications ordered for Ms. Rand are atropine sulfate 0.4 mg and morphine sulfate 10 mg IM. Before giving the medications, the nurse tells Ms. Rand some of the normal things to expect from them. Which statement reflects an effect of atropine sulfate?
    ○ 1. "You'll begin to feel sleepy, even drowsy."
    ○ 2. "Your skin will feel slightly cool and moist."

○ 3. "You'll begin to feel tingling in your fingertips."
○ 4. "Your mouth will feel dry, like cotton."

Ms. Rand had a left lower lobectomy this morning. She is now alert and responsive. Her vital signs are stable, and her skin is warm and dry. She has two chest tubes attached to water-seal drainage with −20 cm $H_2O$ suction applied to the system. The nurse notes that she has a posterolateral incision, and a Foley catheter is draining clear yellow urine. Her orders include: check vital signs every hour; measure urine and chest drainage every hour; cough and deep-breathe every hour; turn every 2 hours; meperidine hydrochloride (Demerol), 100 mg IM, every 4 hours p.r.n.

**62.** Ms. Rand has been out of surgery for several hours now. Which of the following signs and symptoms would alert the nurse to the fact that she may be bleeding?
○ 1. An increase in blood pressure and a decrease in pulse and respirations.
○ 2. Sanguineous drainage from the chest tube at a rate of 50 ml per hour over the last 3 hours.
○ 3. Restlessness and shortness of breath.
○ 4. A urine output of 180 ml over the last 3 hours.

**63.** Ms. Rand complains of moderately severe pain in her left thorax that worsens when she coughs. As a means of controlling the pain during this activity, the nurse
○ 1. places the bed in a slight Trendelenburg position and helps Ms. Rand turn to her operative side to splint the incision.
○ 2. raises the bed to a semi-Fowler's position and places one hand on Ms. Rand's left back and one hand under the incision.
○ 3. keeps the bed flat and tells Ms. Rand to place her hands over the incision before taking a deep breath.
○ 4. raises the bed to complete Fowler's position and helps Ms. Rand turn to her operative side to splint the incision.

**64.** Pain is a major postoperative problem for Ms. Rand that needs to be minimized. Which of the following interventions should the nurse use to accomplish this goal?
○ 1. Plan care efficiently so Ms. Rand can rest at least 30 minutes each hour.
○ 2. Have Ms. Rand deep-breathe and cough vigorously every 2 hours.
○ 3. Begin passive range-of-motion exercises to Ms. Rand's left arm 24 hours after surgery.
○ 4. Give Ms. Rand meperidine hydrochloride (Dem-

erol), 100 mg IM, 15 minutes before any anticipated activity such as sitting up, turning, or deep-breathing.

**65.** Postoperatively, the nurse identifies "impaired gas exchange" as a potential nursing diagnosis. *All* of the following factors contribute to this diagnosis *except*
○ 1. the use of meperidine hydrochloride (Demerol).
○ 2. possible phrenic nerve damage.
○ 3. incisional pain.
○ 4. the amount of chest tube suction.

**66.** The goal for the nursing diagnosis "impaired gas exchange" is to promote optimal ventilation. *All* of the following criteria indicate attainment of this goal *except*
○ 1. tachypnea.
○ 2. bilateral vesicular breath sounds.
○ 3. $PaO_2$ 90 mm Hg; $PaCO_2$ 40 mm Hg.
○ 4. resonance of the thorax on percussion.

**67.** The nurse assesses Ms. Rand's incisional area and the chest tube exit sites. She feels a crackling sensation under her fingertips along the whole incision. The nurse's *first* action should be to
○ 1. lower the head of the bed and call the physician.
○ 2. check Ms. Rand's blood pressure and get an aspiration tray ready.
○ 3. mark the area with a skin pencil at the outer periphery of the crackling.
○ 4. turn off the suction of the chest drainage system.

**68.** The nurse's assessment of Ms. Rand also includes the gastrointestinal tract because a complication that can develop following a lobectomy is acute gastric dilatation. This complication is serious because
○ 1. the patient's nutritional status is threatened.
○ 2. the mediastinum shifts, causing compression of the vena cava.
○ 3. the suture line where the lobe was removed can tear.
○ 4. diaphragmatic movement is impaired.

**69.** While caring for Ms. Rand, the nurse remembers the basic rules to follow when caring for a patient with a chest tube and water-seal drainage system. Which statement contains one of these rules?
○ 1. Be sure the air vent on the water-seal drainage system is capped when the suction is off.
○ 2. Strip the chest and drainage tubes frequently if a pneumothorax is present.
○ 3. Be sure the collection and suction bottles are at the patient's chest level at all times.
○ 4. When stripping the chest tube and drainage system, strip only small segments.

**70.** When the fluid in the chest and drainage tubes stops fluctuating or "swinging," it generally means that the
○ 1. lung has fully expanded.
○ 2. lung has collapsed.
○ 3. chest tube is in the pleural space.
○ 4. mediastinal space has decreased.

**71.** The nurse notices a constant gentle bubbling in the water-seal bottle. This observation should prompt the nurse to
○ 1. continue monitoring as usual; this is a normal expectation.
○ 2. check the connectors between the chest and drainage tubes and where the drainage tube enters the collection bottle.
○ 3. decrease the suction to −15 cm $H_2O$.
○ 4. drain half the water in the water-seal chamber.

**72.** The nurse notices that Ms. Rand is breathing with a little more effort and at a faster rate than she was an hour ago. Her pulse rate is also increased. Based on an understanding of the pathophysiology involved in Ms. Rand's situation and of chest tube function, which of the following nursing actions would be appropriate?
○ 1. Check the tubing to be sure she is not lying on it or kinking it.
○ 2. Increase the suction.
○ 3. Lower the drainage bottles 2 to 3 feet below the level of the chest.
○ 4. Be sure the chest tube has two clamps on it to prevent air leaks.

## THE PATIENT WITH CHEST TRAUMA

After a serious automobile accident, Mr. Henry Taylor, age 74, is transported by ambulance to the emergency department. He complains of severe pain in his right chest where he struck the steering wheel. He also experienced a compound fracture of his right tibia and fibula and multiple lacerations and contusions.

**73.** The primary nursing goal at this point should be to
○ 1. reduce patient anxiety.
○ 2. maintain effective respirations.
○ 3. decrease chest pain.
○ 4. maintain adequate circulating volume.

**74.** Mr. Taylor undergoes a complete respiratory, neurologic, musculoskeletal, and abdominal assessment. Which of the following findings would confirm the presence of a right pneumothorax?
○ 1. Pronounced rales.
○ 2. Inspiratory wheezes.
○ 3. Dullness to percussion.
○ 4. The absence of breath sounds.

**75.** Mr. Taylor's respiratory rate is 40/min and his blood pressure has fallen to $^{100}/_{60}$ with a weak, rapid pulse at 96/min. With a diagnosis of right rib fracture and closed pneumothorax, he should be placed in
○ 1. modified Trendelenburg position with his lower extremities elevated.
○ 2. reverse Trendelenburg with his head down.
○ 3. left side-lying position with his head elevated 15° to 30°.
○ 4. semi- to high-Fowler's position, tilted toward his right side.

**76.** On admission, Mr. Taylor's blood gases were pH 7.20, $PaO_2$ 64 mm Hg, $PaCO_2$ 60 mm Hg, and $HCO_3^-$ 22 mEq/L. A chest tube is inserted. Thirty minutes later, his repeat blood gases are pH 7.30, $PaO_2$ 76, $PaCO_2$ 50, and $HCO_3^-$ 22 mEq/L. This change indicates
○ 1. impending respiratory failure.
○ 2. improving respiratory status.
○ 3. the development of respiratory alkalosis.
○ 4. obstruction in the chest tubes.

**77.** The nurse administers oxygen to Mr. Taylor by nasal cannula at 3 L/min. Approximately what percentage of oxygen is Mr. Taylor receiving through the cannula at this prescribed rate?
○ 1. 5% to 10%.
○ 2. 15% to 20%.
○ 3. 30% to 35%.
○ 4. 50% to 60%.

**78.** A central line is inserted with orders to measure and record Mr. Taylor's central venous pressure hourly. His readings are 2 cm and 6 cm respectively for the first and second measurements. The nurse should interpret these values as reflecting
○ 1. fluid loss.
○ 2. normal pressure.
○ 3. fluid overload.
○ 4. a nonfunctioning manometer.

**79.** Mr. Taylor's morphine sulfate order allows for the administration of 1 to 2 mg/hour IV as needed for pain. The principal objective of this order is adequate pain control to allow the patient to breathe effectively. Which of the following outcomes indicates successful achievement of the objective?
○ 1. Patent chest tube.
○ 2. Decreased patient anxiety.
○ 3. A respiratory rate of 26 breaths/min.
○ 4. Normal blood gas values.

**80.** The nurse believes that Mr. Taylor is experiencing

a side effect from the morphine sulfate. Which of the following clinical manifestations would lead the nurse to this conclusion?
- ○ 1. Increased blood pressure.
- ○ 2. Transient visual disturbances.
- ○ 3. Decreased respiratory rate.
- ○ 4. Inhibited secretion of mucus.

**81.** Mrs. Taylor has been out of town and arrives on the unit 6 hours after her husband's accident. She is distraught because she was not with her husband when he needed her. The most appropriate initial nursing intervention would be to
- ○ 1. allow Mrs. Taylor to verbalize her feelings and concerns.
- ○ 2. describe Mr. Taylor's medical treatment since admission.
- ○ 3. explain the nature of the injury and reassure Mrs. Taylor that her husband's condition is stable.
- ○ 4. reassure Mrs. Taylor that the important fact is she is here now.

**82.** Mr. Taylor goes to surgery for repair of his fractures. His postoperative orders include the transfusion of a unit of packed cells at a rate of 60 ml/hour. Approximately how long should it take to infuse one unit of blood? *1 U = 250*
- ○ 1. 2 hours.
- ○ 2. 4 hours.
- ○ 3. 6 hours.
- ○ 4. 8 hours.

**83.** The *primary* reason for infusing the blood at a rate of 60 ml/hour is to help prevent
- ○ 1. emboli formation.
- ○ 2. pulmonary edema.
- ○ 3. hemolysis of red blood cells.
- ○ 4. allergic reactions to the blood.

**84.** When teaching Mr. Taylor to cough effectively, it would be *best* for the nurse to teach him to
- ○ 1. contract his abdominal muscles.
- ○ 2. swallow immediately before coughing.
- ○ 3. exert pressure with his hands on his voice box.
- ○ 4. hold his breath for a few seconds before coughing.

**85.** Which of the following items should be readily available at the bedside because Mr. Taylor has a chest tube in place?
- ○ 1. A nasopharyngeal airway.
- ○ 2. A tracheostomy tray.
- ○ 3. Rubber-capped hemostats.
- ○ 4. A spirometer.

**86.** On the 4th postoperative day, the nurse hears some scattered rales bilaterally. Which of the following interventions are *most appropriate?*
- ○ 1. Encourage coughing and check the water-seal system.
- ○ 2. Encourage fluids, deep-breathing, and coughing.
- ○ 3. Initiate endotracheal suctioning once per shift and ask the physician to order an expectorant.
- ○ 4. Reduce the frequency of the morphine administration and increase the suction in the water-seal bottle.

**87.** Which of the following rehabilitative measures would the nurse instruct a patient who has had chest surgery to perform in order to prevent the development of a "frozen shoulder"?
- ○ 1. Turn from side to side.
- ○ 2. Raise and lower his head.
- ○ 3. Raise the arm on the affected side over his head.
- ○ 4. Flex and extend the elbow on the affected side.

**88.** On Mr. Taylor's 5th postoperative day, the water level in the long glass tube in the chest drainage bottle stops fluctuating. The nurse is justified in judging that the *most probable* cause for this occurrence is that the
- ○ 1. tubing is kinked.
- ○ 2. lung has re-expanded.
- ○ 3. water seal is leaking.
- ○ 4. tubing is blocked with mucus plugs.

**89.** Mr. Taylor's chest tube is removed on the 6th postoperative day. Which of the following items should the nurse have ready to be placed directly over the wound when the chest tube is removed?
- ○ 1. A butterfly dressing.
- ○ 2. A Montgomery strap.
- ○ 3. A fine-mesh gauze dressing.
- ○ 4. A petrolatum gauze dressing.

**90.** Twelve hours after Mr. Taylor's chest tube is removed, his arterial blood gases are drawn. The $PaO_2$ value is 90 mm Hg. The nurse should interpret this value as indicating that
- ○ 1. Mr. Taylor needs additional oxygen.
- ○ 2. Mr. Taylor should be encouraged to cough and deep-breathe.
- ○ 3. Mr. Taylor's physician should be notified immediately.
- ○ 4. Mr. Taylor's response is adequate.

# CORRECT ANSWERS AND RATIONALES

Numbers appear in parentheses following the rationales. The numbers identify textbooks listed in the references at the end of Part IV, where correct answers can be verified.

## The Patient With Pneumonia

1. 1. The patient described in this item is 79 years old; the pneumonias most commonly strike the aged and debilitated. Having arthritis, being a vegetarian, and bathing in cold water are unlikely predisposing factors for pneumonia. (5, 31)

2. 3. The most commonly recommended site for obtaining the temperature of a patient with pneumonia who is coughing and having difficulty breathing is the rectum. The groin and axillary sites are usually used when the oral and rectal sites are contraindicated. (24, 36)

3. 4. A patient with pneumonia has a ventilation problem that causes poor oxygenation of blood due to infection and congestion in the lungs. This will cause the patient to become cyanotic because blood pumped from the lungs to the heart and thence to the general circulation is being poorly oxygenated. (25, 31)

4. 2. A sputum specimen is obtained for culture to determine the causative organism. After the organism is identified, an appropriate antibiotic can be prescribed. (25, 31)

5. 3. Chest pain in a patient with pneumonia is generally caused by friction between the pleural layers. It is more severe on inspiration than expiration due to chest movement. (5, 26)

6. 4. The pleuritic pain is triggered by chest movement and is particularly severe during coughing. (Splinting the chest wall will help reduce the discomfort of coughing.) Deep-breathing is essential to prevent further atelectasis; an incentive spirometer facilitates effective deep-breathing. (25, 31)

7. 1. Aspirin acts in several ways. It is an analgesic because it helps control pain, an antipyretic because it helps reduce fever, and an anti-inflammatory agent because it reduces inflammation. The drug also reduces blood platelet aggregation and sometimes *may* be used to help prevent clotting in persons prone to heart attacks and strokes. (12, 16)

8. 2. Humidified air helps liquefy respiratory secretions and then makes them easier to raise and expectorate. Postural drainage, vibration and percussion of the chest wall, and coughing and deep-breathing exercises may be helpful for respiratory hygiene but will not affect the nature of secretions as humidified air will. (25, 31)

9. 1. The electrolyte lost in largest amounts through perspiration is sodium. This accounts for the salty taste of perspiration. (26, 31)

10. 3. All of the interventions are appropriate, but frequent linen changes take priority for this patient. The patient has shared her concern for feeling clean. Diaphoresis will produce general discomfort. (25, 31)

11. 3. Patients characteristically show evidence of anxiety when hypoxia is present. Less frequently will they demonstrate anger, apathy, or aggression. (25, 31)

12. 3. A face mask delivers the most accurate amount of oxygen and is the desired route. Often, however, patients cannot tolerate face masks, and alternate delivery methods must be used. (25, 31)

13. 1. The process of pneumonia interferes with ventilation. It is essential to reduce the body's need for oxygen at the cellular level, and bed rest is the most effective method for reducing the body's need for oxygen. (25, 31)

14. 4. The patient described in this item has a white blood cell count of 8,000/mm$^3$. Normal total white blood cell count is between 5,000 and 10,000/mm$^3$ in adults. Because this patient's white blood cell count is within normal limits, there is no need to take action other than to continue her current regimen. (26, 31)

15. 1. Dioctyl sodium sulfosuccinate (Colace) is a stool softener. It acts in a manner similar to a detergent; that is, it allows fluid and fatty substances to enter the stool and soften it. (12, 16)

16. 4. The thought process slows with advancing age. Older people are perfectly capable of learning, but it takes a little longer. Intelligence survives intact and older people in good health do not lose their judgment, their ability to think abstractly, or their knowledge. Sexual activity need not end with advancing age. (5, 23)

17. 4. Antibiotics are usually ineffective in the treatment of viral infections. Avoiding possible contact with ill people and following good nutritional habits are general health promotion measures. Receiving an annual flu vaccine directly reduces the patient's risk of pneumonia. (25, 31)

## The Patient with Tuberculosis

**18.** 3. Tuberculosis typically produces symptoms such as anorexia and weight loss, pronounced fatigue, afternoon fevers, and night sweats. High fevers and shaking chills are characteristic of pneumonia rather than tuberculosis. (25, 31)

**19.** 1. The most commonly used technique to identify tubercle bacilli is acid-fast staining. The bacilli have a very waxy surface, which makes them difficult to stain in the laboratory. But when stained, the colorization is very resistant to removal, even with acids. Therefore, tubercle bacilli are often called acid-fast bacilli. (20, 25)

**20.** 2. Tubercle bacilli may be spread in various ways, the most common being by droplet nuclei. Droplet nuclei are carried in air currents. They are residue of evaporated droplets containing the bacilli. They remain suspended and are circulated in the air. (25, 31)

**21.** 1. Authoritative opinion is that unclean hands spread most organisms. Many techniques can be used to help control the spread of organisms, such as having separate personal-care items, using disposable equipment, and isolating persons known to be harboring disease-causing organisms, but most important is washing the hands thoroughly and frequently. (25, 26)

**22.** 1. Streptomycin is an aminoglycoside, and eighth cranial nerve damage is a common side effect of aminoglycosides. Common side effects of isoniazid (INH), aminosalicylic acid (PAS), and ethambutol hydrochloride (Myambutol) are peripheral neuritis, gastrointestinal intolerance, and optic neuritis, respectively. (12, 25)

**23.** 1. The most common side effect of streptomycin is vertigo, a result of damage to part of the eighth cranial nerve. Other symptoms of eighth cranial nerve toxicity include tinnitus, hearing loss, and ataxia. (12, 16)

**24.** 4. Using a combination of antitubercular drugs slows the rate at which organisms develop a resistance to the drugs. Combination therapy also appears to be more effective than single drug therapy. (25, 30)

**25.** 2. Offering patients emotional support, teaching patients about their disease, coordinating agency services, and assessing environments all play a part in the care of patients with tuberculosis. However, ensuring that patients are well educated about their disease has highest priority. (25, 31)

**26.** 3. It is essential that patients with tuberculosis take medications exactly as prescribed. Sufficient rest, a nourishing diet, and living where air is clean are important but do not rate the same high priority that drug therapy does for patients with tuberculosis. (25, 31)

**27.** 4. The area into which an intradermal injection is made is not massaged. Appropriate techniques include holding the needle and syringe almost parallel to the patient's skin, keeping the skin slightly taut when the needle is inserted, and inserting the needle with the bevel side up. (24, 36)

**28.** 4. Tuberculosis was once a disease that affected primarily the young; currently, the elderly are believed to be at higher risk. Immigrants are another high-risk group. (25, 31)

**29.** 2. A positive Mantoux skin test indicates that the person has had contact with tubercle bacilli. It does *not* mean that the patient has active tuberculosis, nor does it mean the person has developed a resistance to tubercle bacilli or a passive immunity to tuberculosis. (25, 31)

**30.** 3. Patients with newly positive skin tests are aggressively treated with a course of isoniazid (INH) for approximately 9 months. Repeat skin testing should not be performed and skin tests do not convert to negative once a positive response has been obtained. (25, 31)

**31.** 2. Isoniazid (INH) competes for the available vitamin $B_6$ in the body and leaves the patient at risk for developing neuropathies related to vitamin deficiency. Supplemental $B_6$ is routinely prescribed. (12, 25)

**32.** 3. Isoniazid (INH) interferes with the effectiveness of oral contraceptives, and patients should be counseled to use an alternate form of birth control while taking the drug. (12, 16)

**33.** 3. Tuberculosis can be controlled but is never completely eradicated from the body. Periods of intense physical or emotional stress increase the chances of its recurrence. (25, 31)

**34.** 2. Statistics show that of the four geographic areas described in this item, most cases of tuberculosis are found in inner-core residential areas of large cities, where health and sanitation standards tend to be low. These city areas are generally also characterized by substandard housing and poverty. (25, 31)

## The Patient with Chronic Obstructive Pulmonary Disease

**35.** 1. Fear, even when unfounded, can stand in the way of recovery. When the patient described in this item expresses a fear of being in room 13 because he thinks the number would bring him bad luck, it would be best for the nurse to eliminate the reason for the patient's fears. Refusing to move the patient to another room fails to take the patient's fears into account. Moving the patient because superstitions have a good chance of coming true relies on an unproven phenomenon. A superstition becomes truth only on the basis of chance. (11, 38)

**36.** 1. An increased anteroposterior chest diameter is characteristic of advanced obstructive pulmonary disease. Air is trapped in the overextended alveoli and the ribs are fixed in an inspiratory position. The result is the typical barrel-chested appearance. Other physical changes associated with COPD are overly developed neck muscles, distended neck veins, and diminished chest excursions with respiration. (25, 30)

**37.** 4. Relatively low concentrations of oxygen are administered to patients with COPD so as not to eliminate their respiratory drive. Carbon dioxide content in the blood normally regulates respirations. However, patients with COPD are often accustomed to high carbon dioxide and low oxygen blood levels. If they receive excessive oxygen and experience a drop in the blood carbon dioxide, they may stop breathing. (25, 31)

**38.** 4. Rhythmic breathing helps a patient regain control over his breathing pattern and reduces dyspnea. Increasing the oxygen concentration can cause respiratory arrest, and breathing into a paper bag will dangerously increase the $CO_2$ levels. Sitting up facilitates breathing. (25, 31)

**39.** 4. Pursed-lip breathing increases pressure within the alveoli and makes it easier for a patient to empty the air in the lungs, thereby promoting carbon dioxide elimination. By lowering the expiratory rate and helping the patient relax, pursed-lip breathing helps the patient learn to control the rate and depth of his respirations. (25, 30)

**40.** 2. Exhaling normally requires less energy than inhaling. Therefore, lifting while exhaling saves energy and reduces perceived dyspnea. (25, 31)

**41.** 3. Theophylline ethylenediamine (aminophylline), a xanthine derivative, is a direct-acting bronchodilator and relieves bronchial constriction and spasms. When the drug exerts its primary desired effect, dyspnea and shortness of breath decrease. Aminophylline also acts as a mild diuretic, but it acts primarily as a bronchodilator. (25, 31)

**42.** 4. Percussion helps loosen mucus. Deeper inhalations may sometimes result, but this is not the primary purpose of percussion. Percussion itself neither improves ciliary action nor propels secretions along respiratory passages. (25, 31)

**43.** 2. The patient's pH is acidotic and the $PaCO_2$ is grossly elevated above normal. The resulting condition is respiratory acidosis. The $PaO_2$ level has little direct bearing on acid-base status. (25, 31)

**44.** 2. The $PaCO_2$ level indicates that the patient is hypoventilating. Normal arterial blood carbon dioxide ($PaCO_2$) levels are between 35 and 45 mm Hg. Alveolar hypoventilation is considered present when the $PaCO_2$ level exceeds 50 mm Hg. (25, 31)

**45.** 1. Normal arterial blood oxygen levels are between about 80 and 100 mm Hg. This range drops with age, and between the ages of about 60 and 70 years $PaO_2$ levels are normally between about 70 and 80 mm Hg. When the patient's values fall to 53 mm Hg, as described in this item, the nurse should be alert for signs of hypoxia, which, if unabated, would pose a problem with metabolic acidosis. (25, 31)

**46.** 3. A fluid intake of 2 to 3 L/day, in the absence of cardiovascular or renal disease, helps liquefy bronchial secretions. A low-salt diet, continuous oxygen therapy, and the use of a semi-sitting position will not help reduce the viscosity of mucus. (25, 31)

**47.** 1. Patients with diseases that alter normal breathing are very likely to experience behavioral changes such as depression, irritability, and a poor appetite. The behavior of the patient described in this item is most probably due to his illness, rather than to a normal aging process, premonitions of death, or resentment toward health-care personnel. (25, 31)

**48.** 2. By listening to a patient express his anger, the nurse helps the patient overcome his feelings of frustration and anger. Furthermore, listening helps the nurse understand the cause of the patient's feelings. Once the patient and nurse have identified the problem, they can identify and implement interventions that address it. (11, 38)

**49.** 3. Avoiding gas-producing foods decreases dyspnea because the gas elevates the diaphragm. Dyspnea increases during eating because the stomach pushes against the diaphragm. Eating small frequent meals rather than large frequent meals minimizes dyspnea. Between-meal snacks augment the patient's nutritional status and do not affect dyspnea. Oxygen should be used continuously at mealtimes. (25, 31)

**50.** 2. Patients with COPD need a diet high in protein and calories. Protein deficiency decreases colloid osmotic pressure, which predisposes the patient to pulmonary edema. Increased calories are needed because of the increased work of breathing. (25, 37)

**51.** 2. Gravity helps move secretions from smaller to larger airways in postural drainage. It is best used after percussion when secretions have been loosened. (25, 31)

**52.** 2. Prolonged periods of inactivity cause the body to excrete larger-than-normal amounts of calcium. This leads to a breakdown of bone tissue, and as a result the bones become brittle and fracture easily. The condition is referred to as osteoporosis. (26, 31)

**53.** 1. A patient with COPD is subject to respiratory infections. COPD is slowly progressive; therefore, maintaining current status, requiring less supplemental oxygen, and showing permanent improvement are unrealistic expectations. (25, 31)

## The Patient With Lung Cancer

**54.** 2. Epidermoid cancer involving the larger bronchi is almost entirely associated with heavy cigarette smoking. The American Cancer Society reports that smoking is responsible for 83% of lung cancers in men and women. The prevalence of lung cancer is related to the length of time and intensity of the smoking, so nurses can best prevent lung cancer by persuading patients to stop smoking. Chest x-rays detect lung cancer; they do not prevent it. Exposure to asbestos has been implicated as a risk to developing lung cancer, but cigarette smoking is the *major* risk. (26, 31)

**55.** 4. Positioning on the side allows any vomitus to roll out by gravity, thereby preventing aspiration. A nasogastric tube is not placed after a bronchoscopy because the gastrointestinal tract is not entered. Oral fluids are withheld until the gag and swallow reflexes return. Preoperative sedation and the local anesthesia impair swallowing and the laryngeal reflex, which is protective in nature. The trachea can be perforated inadvertently, not the bowel; abdominal distention and rigidity would indicate bowel perforation. (5, 26)

**56.** 3. By assessing the ability of the remaining lung tissue to provide adequate oxygenation, pulmonary function tests determine if the patient can tolerate removal of the lobe. Hemoglobin and hematocrit indicate the oxygen-carrying capacity of the blood. Arterial blood gas values provide information about oxygenation of the blood. Tomograms help localize the tumor. (5, 26)

**57.** 1. Normal weight does not affect postoperative nursing care. Obesity increases the potential for developing postoperative pulmonary complications. The lobectomy reduces the lung volume, which means there is less surface for gas exchange. The decrease in available oxygen leads to decreased energy. The body gradually adjusts to this decrease in respiratory capacity. Knowledge of preoperative activity tolerance is needed, as is knowl-

edge of any behavior that could increase oxygen need. Keeping feelings inside can increase stress and cause anxiety, which increases oxygen need. Becoming constipated can lead to an increase in intraabdominal pressure that would impinge on the diaphragm, preventing ventilatory excursion and leading to microatelectasis. (5, 26)

**58.** 2. Range-of-motion exercises prevent shoulder ankylosis, stiffness, and contractures of the arm on the affected side. Muscles involving the shoulder girdle and those maintaining posture are cut. Adhesions can occur between them. A nasogastric tube is not routinely placed following a lobectomy. After a lobectomy, a patient can lie on either side and on the back. Following a pneumonectomy, the patient can be tilted only slightly to either side at first because the mediastinum is no longer held by both sides of the lung. Chest tubes are very rarely irrigated, and then only for specific reasons. (5, 26)

**59.** 2. Deep-breathing helps prevent microatelectasis and pneumonitis and also helps force air/fluid out of the pleural space into the chest tubes. The diaphragm is the major muscle of respiration and deep-breathing causes it to descend, thereby increasing the ventilating surface. More than half the ventilatory process is accomplished by the rise and fall of the diaphragm. Deep-breathing increases blood flow to the lungs. The remaining lobe will naturally hyperinflate to fill the space created by the resected lobe. This is an expected phenomenon. (5, 26)

**60.** 1. Acknowledging the basic feeling that the patient expressed and asking an open-ended question enables the patient to explain her fear. The first option addresses the main feeling expressed—fear of cancer—and attempts to explore it further. The second option does not focus on the basic feeling; it gives reassurance. The third option does not acknowledge the feeling at all. The fourth option assumes guilt, which might be present, and evades the basic feeling. (25, 31)

**61.** 4. Atropine sulfate is an anticholinergic drug that decreases mucus secretions in the respiratory tract and dries the mucous membranes of the mouth, nose, pharynx and bronchi. Atropine does not cause drowsiness; in large doses it causes excitement and maniacal behavior. It causes the skin to become hot and dry and, in doses less than 0.5 mg, can cause bradycardia. Moderate to large doses cause tachycardia and palpitations. (12, 16)

**62.** 3. Restlessness indicates cerebral hypoxia due to decreased circulating volume. Shortness of breath occurs because blood collecting in the pleural space faster than suction can remove it prevents the lung from re-expanding. Increased blood pressure and decreased pulse and respirations are signs of increased intracranial pressure. Decreasing blood pressure and increasing pulse and respirations occur with hypovolemic shock. Sanguineous drainage that changes to serosanguineous drainage at a rate less than 100 ml/hour is normal early postoperatively. A urine output of 180 ml over the last 3 hours indicates normal kidney perfusion (60 ml of urine/hour). (5, 26)

**63.** 2. The semi-Fowler's position allows for downward displacement of the diaphragm and relaxation of the abdominal muscles, which are needed for good ventilatory excursion. The hand placement supports the operative area and splints it without causing pain from pressure. The Trendelenburg position is contraindicated because abdominal contents pushing against the diaphragm decrease effective lung volumes. Keeping the bed flat does not allow diaphragm descent. Positioning on the operative side prevents maximum inflation of the left lung, and placing hands on the operative area before inhalation can restrict thoracic movement. (5, 26)

**64.** 1. By being efficient in her work, the nurse can plan 30 minutes of rest per hour for the patient. Fatigue increases the perception of pain, so decreasing fatigue decreases pain perception. Deep-breathing helps prevent microatelectasis and pneumonitis and facilitates re-expansion of the left lung. Coughing helps remove secretions. Thus, although they are painful, deep-breathing and coughing need to be done every hour. During surgery, muscle groups that move the shoulder and maintain posture are cut. To prevent a frozen left shoulder joint and to decrease muscle use of the left back, passive range-of-motion exercises are usually started 4 hours after recovery from anesthesia. The peak action of intramuscular meperidine hydrochloride (Demerol) is 30 to 60 minutes. (5, 26)

**65.** 4. This is a normal amount of suction applied to the intrapleural space. Its purpose is to reexpand the lung and reestablish normal negative intrapleural pressure. Meperidine hydrochloride (Demerol) depresses respiratory rate and depth. The phrenic nerve innervates the diaphragm. If the nerve is damaged, the diaphragm rises and becomes immobile. The lung does not inflate well on the affected side. Pain causes splinting of the thorax and makes it difficult to deep-breathe and cough. (5, 26)

**66.** 1. Increased respiratory rate is a sign of hypoxia. The other criteria are normal findings that indicate good ventilation. Breath sounds will be absent where the lobe was removed. (5, 26)

**67.** 3. Subcutaneous emphysema is not an unusual finding and is not dangerous if confined. Progression of the emphysema can be serious, especially if the neck is involved. A tracheotomy may be needed. If the emphysema progresses more than one hand-width per hour, the physician should be called. Lowering the head of the bed and taking the blood pressure will not arrest the progress or provide any further information. A tracheotomy tray, not an aspiration tray, would be useful if the emphysema progressed to the neck. The emphysema may progress if the chest drainage system does not adequately remove air and fluid. Therefore, the system would not be turned off. (5, 26)

**68.** 4. A distended stomach causes upward pressure on the diaphragm, preventing the diaphragm from descending and causing poor ventilatory excursion. Gastric distention is treated by making the patient n.p.o. and by administering intravenous fluids to prevent volume depletion. Being n.p.o. for a few days will not threaten this patient's nutritional status. Acute gastric dilatation does not affect the mediastinum or left thorax. The stomach is not in the thorax, since the diaphragmatic foramen is intact. (5, 26)

**69.** 4. Stripping a chest tube causes excessive negative intrapleural pressure and may cause complications. The amount of pressure created is directly related to the length of the tube stripped, so stripping only shorter segments causes less pressure. Stripping is done only when a chest tube is clogged with a clot and milking is unsuccessful. Air does not clot, so stripping is unnecessary in the pleural pneumothorax. The air vent must always be open in the closed chest drainage system to allow air from the patient to escape. The drainage apparatus is always kept *below* chest level to prevent back flow of fluid into the pleural space. (25, 31)

**70.** 1. When the fluctuating or "swinging" of fluid in the tubing stops, it can mean one of several things: the lung has fully expanded and negative intrapleural pressure has been reestablished; the chest tube is occluded; or the chest tube is not in the pleural space. Fluctuating or "swinging" is due to the fact that during inspiration intrapleural pressure exceeds the negative pressure generated in the water-seal system. Therefore, drainage moves toward the patient. During expiration, the pleural pressure exceeds that generated in the water-seal system and fluid moves away from the patient. (5, 26)

**71.** 2. Constant bubbling in the water-seal bottle indicates an air leak. There should never be constant bubbling in the water-seal bottle. A leak means that less negative pressure is being exerted on the pleural space. Decreasing the suction will not reduce the leak, nor will draining part of the water in the water-seal chamber. (5, 26)

**72.** 1. There might be some obstruction to the flow of air and fluid out of the pleural space and these are collecting, building up pressure. This prevents the remaining lung from re-expanding and can cause a mediastinal shift to the opposite side. Increasing the suction will not improve the removal of air and fluid. The set amount in the suction control bottle is $-20$ cm $H_2O$, and will not get any higher if increased. The normal position of the drainage bottles is 2 to 3 feet below chest level. Clamping the tubes obstructs the flow of air and fluid out of the pleural space. (5, 26)

## The Patient with Chest Trauma

**73.** 2. Blunt chest trauma is of special concern in elderly patients with chronic conditions that may decrease vital capacity. Respiratory failure may develop more quickly in these patients. Although pain is distressing to the patient and can increase anxiety and decrease respiratory effectiveness, pain control is secondary to maintaining effective respirations. Decreasing the patient's anxiety is related to maintaining effective respirations. Maintaining adequate circulatory volume is also secondary to maintaining effective respirations. (5, 26)

**74.** 4. Pneumothorax indicates that the lung has collapsed and is not functioning. There will be no sounds of air movement upon auscultation. (25, 31)

**75.** 4. A pneumothorax will cause a patient to feel extremely short of breath. A semi- or high-Fowler's position will facilitate ventilation by the unaffected lung. A flat or reverse Trendelenburg position places additional pressure on the chest and inhibits ventilation. Likewise, the patient should not be positioned on his unaffected side, which would compromise the remaining functional lung. (25, 31)

**76.** 2. Admission blood gas values reveal respiratory acidosis and are consistent with a diagnosis of pneumothorax. The blood gas values after chest tube insertion are returning to normal, indicating the effectiveness of the treatment. The respiratory acidosis would worsen from $CO_2$ retention if the patient were experiencing an asthma attack. The patient is not alkalotic because the pH values are less than 7.35. If the chest tubes were obstructed, the patient's respiratory status would deteriorate. (25, 31)

**77.** 3. The percentage of oxygen a patient receives when oxygen is given by cannula at 3 L/min is between 30% and 35%. If a patient requires a high concentration of oxygen, a mask or a mask with a reservoir bag is used. (25, 31)

**78.** 1. Normal central venous pressure readings range between 4 and 12 cm of water. Lower-than-normal readings suggest fluid loss and decreased circulating volume. A higher-than-average reading is likely to mean fluid overload and increased circulating volume or poor cardiac contractility. No information given in this item suggests that the manometer is not functioning. (5, 26)

**79.** 4. Normal blood gas values are the best indicator of effective respirations and attainment of the stated nursing objective. Chest tube patency relates to the patient's overall status but does not indicate successful attainment of the objective. Decreased patient anxiety is not related only to the stated objective; decreased anxiety could also be related to pain relief. A respiratory rate within normal limits is a factor in effective breathing, but blood gas values indicate attainment of the objective. (25, 31)

**80.** 3. Morphine sulfate depresses the respiratory center. Other side effects include hypotension, nausea, vomiting, and constipation. Morphine sulfate does not cause transient visual disturbances or inhibit the secretion of mucus. (12, 24)

**81.** 1. Verbalization of feelings and concerns helps decrease anxiety and allows the family member to move on to understanding the current situation. Describing events or explaining equipment is appropriate when the individual is not distraught and is ready to learn. Reassuring the family member does not allow verbalization of feelings and discounts the family member's feelings. (13, 41)

**82.** 2. There are approximately 250 ml in one unit of packed red blood cells. If the blood is delivered at a rate of 60 ml/hour, it will take about 4 hours to infuse the entire unit. (24, 36)

**83.** 2. Too-rapid infusion of blood, or any intravenous fluid, is likely to cause pulmonary edema. Emboli formation, hemolysis of red cells, and allergic reactions to blood are not related to rapid infusion. (24, 36)

**84.** 1. Contracting (pulling in) the abdominal muscles helps produce a forceful and productive cough. The patient should be taught to cough twice with each effort while his mouth is open and his tongue is out. Coughing should be done after the patient takes several short breaths followed by a deep inspiration. Such measures as swallowing before coughing, exerting pressure on the larynx, and holding the breath before coughing do not produce effective coughing. (24, 36)

**85.** 3. Clamps should be readily available and in view when a patient has chest drainage. Although used infrequently, clamps may be used to locate a source of malfunctioning of the equipment. Occasionally, they may be used when transporting a patient. (5, 31)

**86.** 2. Shallow breathing is a common problem after chest injury due to the pain associated with deep-breathing. Fluids prevent the buildup of viscous secretions. Assisting the patient to cough and deep-breathe should clear the lungs regularly and effectively. There is no indication of malfunction in the water-seal system. Reducing pain medication would simply make effective coughing more difficult. Endotracheal suctioning is not indicated at this time. (5, 31)

**87.** 3. A patient who has had chest surgery should be taught to raise his arm on the affected side over his head to help prevent "frozen shoulder." The exercise helps restore normal shoulder movement, prevents stiffening of the shoulder joint, and improves muscle tonus and power. (25, 31)

**88.** 2. Fluctuation of the water level in the long glass tube when the patient has a closed chest drainage system is related to the patient's inspirations and expirations. When the fluctuations stop on the 5th postoperative day for the patient described in this item, the most probable cause is that the patient's lung has reexpanded. Other possible causes if the fluid in the tubing stops fluctuating include an obstruction or a dependent loop in the tube, but for the patient described in this item these are less likely causes. (25, 31)

**89.** 4. A petrolatum gauze is placed over the wound immediately following chest tube removal. This gauze, which is covered with a dry sterile dressing, serves as an airtight seal to prevent air leakage or movement of air in either direction. Bandages or straps are not used directly over wounds. Mesh gauze would allow air movement. (25, 31)

**90.** 4. The normal range for $PaO_2$ is 80 to 100 mm Hg. The patient's current value is within normal limits and no additional interventions are warranted. This blood gas value indicates that his lung has remained adequately expanded following removal of the chest tube and that oxygen delivery to the tissues is adequate. (25, 31)

# *test* 2

**The Patient with Myocardial Infarction**
**The Patient with Congestive Heart Failure**
**The Patient with Valvular Heart Disease**
**The Patient with Hypertension**
**The Patient with Angina**
**Correct Answers and Rationales**

Select the one *best* or *correct* answer and indicate your choice by filling in the circle with a pencil in front of the option you have chosen. If the answer you would prefer is not given, select the one you think is *most appropriate*.

## THE PATIENT WITH MYOCARDIAL INFARCTION

Mrs. Myra Hall, age 60, is admitted through the emergency department with crushing substernal chest pain that radiates to her shoulder, jaw, and left arm. The admission diagnosis is acute myocardial infarction. The patient is extremely restless and frightened.

1. Immediate admission orders for Mrs. Hall include oxygen by nasal cannula at 4 L/min, blood work, a chest x-ray, a 12-lead EKG, and 2 mg of morphine sulfate IV. Which intervention has the priority and should be accomplished *first?*
   ○ 1. Administer the morphine.
   ○ 2. Obtain an EKG.
   ○ 3. Start the oxygen.
   ○ 4. Obtain the blood work and the chest x-ray.
2. The pain associated with Mrs. Hall's myocardial infarction is due to
   ○ 1. an overloaded left ventricle.
   ○ 2. impending circulatory collapse.
   ○ 3. imbalances in extracellular electrolytes.
   ○ 4. insufficient oxygen reaching the heart muscle.
3. Mrs. Hall is admitted to the coronary care unit for constant monitoring. She is observed closely for complications. The complication responsible for most deaths following an acute myocardial infarction is
   ○ 1. a pulmonary embolism.
   ○ 2. a cardiac dysrhythmia.
   ○ 3. congestive heart failure.
   ○ 4. rupture of the myocardium.
4. An intravenous infusion is ordered to run at a "keep open" rate for Mrs. Hall *primarily* in order to
   ○ 1. help keep the patient well hydrated.
   ○ 2. help keep the patient well nourished.
   ○ 3. prevent the possibility of kidney failure.
   ○ 4. be prepared to give drugs in an emergency.
5. Cardiac monitoring is done on a continuous basis for Mrs. Hall. If the nurse notes that the patient has eight premature ventricular contractions (PVCs) in a minute's time, the nurse's *first* course of action should be to
   ○ 1. increase the rate of the patient's intravenous infusion.
   ○ 2. notify the patient's physician promptly.
   ○ 3. increase the concentration of the patient's oxygen therapy.
   ○ 4. administer an analgesic prescribed for the patient.
6. If Mrs. Hall develops cardiogenic shock, which *characteristic* sign of the condition should the nurse expect to observe?
   ○ 1. Pulmonary rales.
   ○ 2. A slow pulse rate.
   ○ 3. Low blood pressure.
   ○ 4. A sudden onset of fever.
7. The results of Mrs. Hall's admission blood laboratory studies are available. Which is a *typical* finding of a myocardial infarction?
   ○ 1. An elevated cholesterol value.
   ○ 2. An elevated creatinine phosphokinase (CPK) value.
   ○ 3. A below-normal sedimentation rate.
   ○ 4. A below-normal white blood cell count.
8. Mrs. Hall continues to have episodes of chest pain during the first 8 hours following her admission. During periods of pain, Mrs. Hall's arterial blood pressure rises as high as 200 mm Hg; between attacks, it remains between 110 and 120 mm Hg. It is *most likely* that the increase in arterial blood pressure during attacks of pain is due to
   ○ 1. the patient's anxiety.

**353**

○ 2. excessive activity by the patient.

○ 3. a poor oxygen supply to the heart.

○ 4. an accumulation of sodium ions in heart muscle tissues.

9. After one attack of pain, Mrs. Hall says to the nurse, "My husband died of a heart attack, and I suppose I will too." Which of the following comments would be the *most appropriate* response for the nurse to make?

○ 1. "Tell me more about what you are feeling."

○ 2. "Are you thinking that you won't recover from this illness?"

○ 3. "You have a fine doctor. Everything will be all right soon, I am sure."

○ 4. "Would you agree that this would be very unlikely?"

10. Which of the following activities is *contraindicated* for Mrs. Hall on her 2nd day of hospitalization?

○ 1. Filing her fingernails.

○ 2. Lying on her stomach for a backrub.

○ 3. Using the commode for a bowel movement.

○ 4. Reaching into the lower compartment of her bedside stand for reading material.

11. Nursing measures for Mrs. Hall include helping her avoid activity that results in the Valsalva maneuver (bearing down against a closed glottis). Which of the following nursing orders should appear on the patient's care plan to help prevent the Valsalva maneuver?

○ 1. Have the patient take fewer but deeper breaths.

○ 2. Have the patient clench her teeth while moving in bed.

○ 3. Have the patient take oral fluids through a straw.

○ 4. Have the patient avoid holding her breath during activity.

12. Oral furosemide (Lasix) is prescribed for Mrs. Hall. Which of the following signs/symptoms documents the need for this medication?

○ 1. The patient is anxious.

○ 2. The patient is restless.

○ 3. The patient has anterior chest pain.

○ 4. The patient has rales in the lower lobes of the lungs.

13. Mrs. Hall is taught to move her legs about while resting in bed. This type of exercise is recommended *primarily* in order to help

○ 1. prepare the patient for ambulation.

○ 2. promote urinary and intestinal elimination.

○ 3. prevent thrombophlebitis and blood clot formation.

○ 4. decrease the likelihood of decubitus ulcer formation.

14. Which of the following diet instructions *accurately* reflects the principles upon which Mrs. Hall's diet is most likely to be based during the *acute* phase of myocardial infarction?

○ 1. Coffee and other liquids as desired.

○ 2. Small frequent feedings.

○ 3. Three meals daily that include high-fiber foods.

○ 4. Nothing by mouth.

15. Gradually, when Mrs. Hall's condition is stable, she is allowed increased activity. Of the following criteria, the *best* one on which to judge whether her activity is appropriate is to note her

○ 1. degree of edema.

○ 2. degree of cyanosis.

○ 3. amount of dyspnea.

○ 4. amount of weight loss.

16. Nursing care for Mrs. Hall includes measures to prevent sensory deprivation while in the cardiac care unit. Which of the following activities would be *least appropriate* for this patient?

○ 1. Watching television.

○ 2. Visiting with her daughter.

○ 3. Reading the daily newspaper.

○ 4. Keeping her door closed to provide privacy.

17. After obtaining Mrs. Hall's blood pressure on one occasion, the nurse determines that the patient's *diastolic* pressure is 88 mm Hg. The nurse should understand that the diastolic blood pressure is *best* described as the *minimum* pressure

○ 1. within the left ventricle.

○ 2. exerted on the walls of the veins.

○ 3. exerted on the walls of the arteries.

○ 4. within the entire circulatory system.

18. As her convalescence continues, Mrs. Hall wonders what could have caused her heart attack. She says, "I've always been so healthy." Of the following factors related to Mrs. Hall's daily living, the one that appears *most closely* linked to the development of coronary artery disease is

○ 1. diet.

○ 2. climate.

○ 3. air pollution.

○ 4. excessive exercise.

19. Mrs. Hall loses 3.2 kg of weight while hospitalized. How many pounds has she lost?

○ 1. Approximately 1.5 pounds.

○ 2. Approximately 3 pounds.

○ 3. Approximately 5.25 pounds.

○ 4. Approximately 7 pounds.

20. Mrs. Hall has the equipment and skills to obtain her vital signs. She is walking and is taught to continue walking on a progressive basis after discharge. Which of her vital signs should Mrs. Hall be

taught to monitor to determine whether to increase or decrease her exercise?

○1. Pulse rate.

○2. Blood pressure.

○3. Body temperature.

○4. Respiratory rate.

21. If Mrs. Hall displays behavior detrimental to her health such as smoking cigarettes, eating a diet high in saturated fat, or leading a sedentary lifestyle, techniques of behavior modification may be used to help her change. The nurse can *best* reinforce new adaptive behaviors by

○1. explaining how the old behavior leads to ill health.

○2. withholding praise until the new behavior is well established.

○3. rewarding the patient whenever she performs acceptable behavior.

○4. discussing the advantages of developing healthful behavior.

## THE PATIENT WITH CONGESTIVE HEART FAILURE

Mrs. Frances Bomar, age 69, has a history of congestive heart failure. Her physician recently increased her daily digoxin (Lanoxin) dose as her condition was deteriorating. Ten days ago Mrs. Bomar stopped taking all her medications, which she blamed for her frequent headaches. She is admitted now to the emergency department with congestive heart failure complicated by pulmonary edema. She is edematous and cyanotic, in acute respiratory distress, extremely anxious, and complaining of nausea.

22. Mrs. Bomar receives morphine sulfate IV soon after admission. When evaluating Mrs. Bomar's response to the morphine sulfate, the nurse should assess the morphine's effect on the patient's

○1. nausea.

○2. blood pressure.

○3. cyanosis.

○4. anxiety.

23. When auscultating Mrs. Bomar's lungs, the type of sounds the nurse will *most likely* hear are

○1. wheezing sounds.

○2. crackling sounds.

○3. metallic tingling sounds.

○4. louder inspiratory than expiratory sounds.

24. In which of the following positions in bed is Mrs. Bomar likely to be *most* comfortable?

○1. Semi-sitting (low Fowler's position).

○2. Lying on her right side (Sims' position).

○3. Sitting nearly upright (high Fowler's position).

○4. Lying on her back with her head somewhat lowered (Trendelenburg position).

25. Mrs. Bomar receives oxygen therapy. The nurse can *best* evaluate the effectiveness of oxygen therapy by observing changes in Mrs. Bomar's

○1. electrocardiogram.

○2. arterial blood gases.

○3. central venous pressure.

○4. serum electrolyte values.

26. Mrs. Bomar is to have rotating tourniquets applied, the *primary* purpose being to help

○1. promote diuresis.

○2. strengthen ventricular heartbeats.

○3. prevent venous congestion in the extremities.

○4. reduce blood volume in the central circulation.

27. When rotating tourniquets are used, how many of Mrs. Bomar's extremities should have compression applied at one time?

○1. One.

○2. Two.

○3. Three.

○4. Four.

28. Blood pressure cuffs are used as tourniquets for Mrs. Bomar. The *best* guide for determining the amount of inflation each cuff should have is that in relation to the patient's blood pressure, inflation should be

○1. at about the systolic pressure.

○2. slightly above the systolic pressure.

○3. slightly above the diastolic pressure.

○4. slightly below the diastolic pressure.

29. When rotating tourniquets are used for Mrs. Bomar, each tourniquet is rotated so that the maximum number of minutes the blood flow is decreased in any one extremity will be

○1. 15 minutes.

○2. 30 minutes.

○3. 45 minutes.

○4. 60 minutes.

30. Which of the following assessments would be *best* for the nurse to use *regularly* to determine that the pressure in Mrs. Bomar's tourniquets is not too great?

○1. The patient's sense of orientation.

○2. The color of the skin in each extremity.

○3. The patient's pulse at an artery distal to each tourniquet.

○4. The neurovascular status of each extremity.

31. When the procedure of rotating tourniquets is completed for Mrs. Bomar, in which of the following orders should the cuffs be removed?

○ 1. From the legs first, then the arms.
○ 2. From the arms first, then the legs.
○ 3. One at a time at 15-minute intervals.
○ 4. All at one time as quickly as possible.

**32.** Digoxin (Lanoxin) is administered intravenously to Mrs. Bomar *primarily* because the drug helps
○ 1. dilate coronary arteries.
○ 2. strengthen the heartbeat.
○ 3. decrease cardiac dysrhythmias.
○ 4. decrease the electrical conductivity of the myocardium.

**33.** Furosemide (Lasix) is administered to Mrs. Bomar intravenously. How soon after the intravenous administration of this drug should the nurse begin to see results of the drug's desired effect?
○ 1. After 5 to 10 minutes.
○ 2. After 30 minutes to 1 hour.
○ 3. After 2 to 4 hours.
○ 4. After 6 to 8 hours.

**34.** Mrs. Bomar will require careful skin care *primarily* because an edematous patient is prone to develop
○ 1. itchy skin.
○ 2. decubitus ulcers.
○ 3. electrolyte imbalance.
○ 4. distention of weakened veins.

**35.** Mrs. Bomar has been receiving daily doses of digoxin (Lanoxin) since her admission. Which of the following symptoms should cause the nurse to suspect that Mrs. Bomar is *most likely* experiencing an undesirable side effect of digoxin?
○ 1. A skin rash.
○ 2. Constipation.
○ 3. Lightheadedness.
○ 4. Loss of appetite.

**36.** Of the following signs, the one the nurse is *most likely* to notice first if Mrs. Bomar is developing digitalis toxicity is a
○ 1. heart murmur.
○ 2. slow respiratory rate.
○ 3. slow apical pulse rate.
○ 4. drop in blood pressure.

**37.** The nurse should be *especially* alert to assess for signs and symptoms of digitalis toxicity if laboratory blood findings indicate that Mrs. Bomar has a
○ 1. low sodium level.
○ 2. high glucose level.
○ 3. high calcium level.
○ 4. low potassium level.

**38.** Mrs. Bomar is being prepared for discharge from the hospital. She will continue to take oral furosemide (Lasix) at home. To help Mrs. Bomar evaluate the effectiveness of furosemide therapy, the nurse should teach her to

○ 1. weigh herself daily.
○ 2. take her blood pressure daily.
○ 3. take a specimen of her urine to the laboratory for analysis each week.
○ 4. have a specimen of her arterial blood obtained for blood gas determinations each week.

**39.** The nurse teaches Mrs. Bomar to take the oral furosemide (Lasix) in the morning. The *primary* reason for teaching her to take the furosemide in the morning is to help
○ 1. decrease gastrointestinal irritation.
○ 2. retard the rapid absorption of the drug.
○ 3. excrete fluids accumulated during the night.
○ 4. prevent disturbances of rest during the night.

**40.** Which of the following foods should Mrs. Bomar be taught to avoid or restrict because of her prescribed moderate sodium-restricted diet?
○ 1. Apples.
○ 2. Tomatoes.
○ 3. Hard cheeses.
○ 4. Cornish game hen.

**41.** Because of Mrs. Bomar's moderate sodium-restricted diet, she should be taught to *avoid* using
○ 1. dill.
○ 2. wine.
○ 3. garlic.
○ 4. catsup.

**42.** To help maintain a normal blood level of potassium, Mrs. Bomar should be encouraged to include in her diet such foods as bananas, orange juice,
○ 1. beans, and celery.
○ 2. tomatoes, and asparagus.
○ 3. processed and soft cheeses.
○ 4. honeydew melons, and cantaloupe.

**43.** Which of the following is *most often* recommended in the nutritional management of patients with congestive heart failure?
○ 1. Decreased potassium intake.
○ 2. Avoidance of excess alcohol.
○ 3. Increased caloric intake.
○ 4. Increased sodium intake.

# THE PATIENT WITH VALVULAR HEART DISEASE

Mrs. Teresa Alden, age 71, is scheduled to undergo mitral valve replacement for severely calcific mitral stenosis and mitral regurgitation. Although the diagnosis was made during childhood, Mrs. Alden had been asymptomatic until 4 years ago. Recently she has noticed an increase in symptoms despite daily doses of digoxin (Lanoxin) and furosemide (Lasix).

**44.** Which of the following symptoms would *least likely* be found in a patient with combined mitral stenosis and regurgitation?
- ○1. Exertional dyspnea.
- ○2. Weight gain.
- ○3. Fatigue.
- ○4. Peripheral edema.

**45.** During the initial interview with Mrs. Alden, the nurse is *most likely* to learn that the patient's childhood health history includes having had
- ○1. scarlet fever.
- ○2. poliomyelitis.
- ○3. rheumatic fever.
- ○4. meningitis.

**46.** The nurse can expect that because Mrs. Alden has mitral stenosis, she will *most likely* demonstrate symptoms typical of those associated with congestion in the
- ○1. aorta.
- ○2. right atrium.
- ○3. superior vena cava.
- ○4. pulmonary circulation.

**47.** Mrs. Alden has been taking digoxin (Lanoxin) and furosemide (Lasix) and has been maintained on quinidine sulfate to control atrial dysrhythmias. A problem that Mrs. Alden may experience because of the quinidine is
- ○1. constipation.
- ○2. hypertension.
- ○3. digoxin toxicity.
- ○4. tachycardia.

**48.** Because Mrs. Alden is a prospective valve recipient, the nurse preoperatively assesses Mrs. Alden's past compliance with medical regimens. Lack of compliance with which of the following regimens poses the greatest health hazard for Mrs. Alden?
- ○1. Medication therapy.
- ○2. Diet modification.
- ○3. Activity restrictions.
- ○4. Lifestyle modifications.

**49.** In preparing Mrs. Alden and her family for her postoperative intensive care unit stay, the nurse explains that
- ○1. visiting hours are unrestricted for members of the immediate family.
- ○2. the patient will sleep most of the time while in the intensive care unit.
- ○3. noise and activity within the intensive care unit are minimal.
- ○4. patients may experience transient disorientation and confusion.

**50.** Mrs. Alden undergoes a mitral valve replacement and experiences persistent bleeding from her surgical incision during the early postoperative

hours. In this situation, which of the following pharmaceutical agents should the nurse be prepared to administer?
- ○1. Vitamin C.
- ○2. Protamine sulfate.
- ○3. Quinidine sulfate.
- ○4. Warfarin sodium (Coumadin).

**51.** When Mrs. Alden develops multiple premature ventricular contractions (PVCs), the physician orders lidocaine hydrochloride (Xylocaine), 1,000 mg in 500 ml of 5% dextrose in water IV at the rate of 3 mg of lidocaine hydrochloride per minute. If the equipment used for administering the drug and solution indicates that 60 microdrops are equal to 1 ml, how many microdrops would provide 3 mg of lidocaine hydrochloride each minute?
- ○1. 12 microdrops.
- ○2. 24 microdrops.
- ○3. 60 microdrops.
- ○4. 90 microdrops.

**52.** After Mrs. Alden experiences some initial excitation, the nurse judges *correctly* that she is demonstrating a *typical* toxic reaction to lidocaine hydrochloride (Xylocaine) when she complains of
- ○1. dyspnea.
- ○2. dizziness.
- ○3. ringing in the ears.
- ○4. numbness in the extremities.

**53.** Mrs. Alden is ordered to have her central venous pressure (CVP) monitored. The purpose for determining her CVP is to help assess the
- ○1. circulatory volume in her arteries.
- ○2. blood pressure in the left ventricle.
- ○3. heart's ability to receive and pump blood.
- ○4. oxygen and carbon dioxide pressure in the blood.

**54.** Mrs. Alden asks the nurse to adjust the bed so that her knees will be supported in a flexed position. The nurse should explain that the position Mrs. Alden requests is *contraindicated primarily* to avoid
- ○1. placing the feet in a dropped position.
- ○2. causing the knees to ankylose ("freeze").
- ○3. causing stagnation of blood in her lower extremities.
- ○4. placing pressure on nerves in the area under her knees.

**55.** Mrs. Alden's chest tube is accidentally disconnected from the drainage tube when she is turning onto her side. Of the following courses of action, the one the nurse should take *first* is to
- ○1. notify the physician.
- ○2. reconnect the tube.
- ○3. raise the level of the drainage bottle.

4. apply a petrolatum-imbedded dressing to the chest wall.

56. Of the following practices of asepsis the nurse should observe when changing Mrs. Alden's dressings, which is usually credited as being the *most effective* in helping prevent a wound infection?
    1. Careful handwashing before beginning the procedure.
    2. Cleansing the incisional area with an antiseptic solution.
    3. Using prepackaged sterile dressings to cover the incision.
    4. Placing the soiled dressings in a waterproof bag before disposing of them.

57. If Mrs. Alden's body excretes calcium in excessive amounts during the postoperative period, which of the following measures should the nurse institute to help prevent a complication associated with the excessive excretion of calcium?
    1. Ensure a liberal fluid intake.
    2. Provide an alkaline-ash diet.
    3. Prevent constipation.
    4. Enrich the patient's diet with dairy products.

58. During visiting hours one day, Mrs. Alden's children discuss their plans for caring for Mrs. Alden at her home after discharge. The nurse notes that Mrs. Alden seems withdrawn and is not participating in the conversation. The nurse is probably correct in evaluating that Mrs. Alden's behavior is caused by
    1. anxiety about her possible death.
    2. concern about her sudden role changes.
    3. anxiety that her children consider her a burden.
    4. fear that she may end up in a nursing home.

59. To prevent thromboembolic complications associated with mechanical valves, Mrs. Alden will be maintained indefinitely on warfarin sodium (Coumadin). To prevent side effects of Coumadin anticoagulation, the nurse needs to know that
    1. the partial thromboplastin time (PPT) determines the dosages of warfarin sodium.
    2. protamine sulfate is used to reverse the effect of warfarin sodium.
    3. other medications and medical conditions can alter the anticoagulant effect of warfarin sodium.
    4. warfarin sodium is started after heparin is discontinued.

60. Good dental care is an important strategy for reducing the risk of endocarditis. A teaching plan to promote good dental care in Mrs. Alden's situation includes demonstrating the proper use of
    1. a manual toothbrush.
    2. an electric toothbrush.
    3. an irrigation device.
    4. dental floss.

61. Before Mrs. Alden's discharge, the nurse should evaluate her understanding of postcardiac surgery activity restrictions. Which of the following should Mrs. Alden *not* engage in until after her 1-month postdischarge appointment with the surgeon?
    1. Showering.
    2. Lifting anything heavier than 10 pounds.
    3. A program of gradual progressive walking.
    4. Light housework.

62. Mrs. Alden needs to be aware of the signs and symptoms of possible complications after discharge. Which of the following would be *least* indicative of valve dysfunction?
    1. Weakness, paresthesia, and speech dysfunction.
    2. Dyspnea, peripheral edema, and weight gain.
    3. Chills, fever, and leukocytosis.
    4. Chest wall pain, shoulder pain, or back discomfort.

## THE PATIENT WITH HYPERTENSION

*12/7/93*

Marting Manufacturing Company sponsors a blood pressure screening program. The industrial health nurse finds Mr. Sam Guadelupe's blood pressure to be elevated on two occasions a month apart and refers him to his private physician. Mr. Guadelupe, age 40, works as a machinist. He is about 25 pounds overweight and has smoked a pack of cigarettes daily for over 20 years.

63. Essential hypertension would be diagnosed in a man Mr. Guadelupe's age if his blood pressure were consistently at or above what level?
    1. 120/90 mm Hg.
    2. 130/85 mm Hg.
    3. 140/90 mm Hg.
    4. 160/80 mm Hg.

64. The nurse completes a thorough patient history and examination. The *primary purpose* of gathering this information is to
    1. assess the patient's ability to participate in various therapies such as a stress reduction class.
    2. complete the insurance forms and payment vouchers.
    3. develop a baseline for treatment evaluation.
    4. identify other current or potential health problems.

**65.** During the assessment process, Mr. Guadelupe says, "I don't really know why I'm here. I feel fine and haven't had any symptoms." The nurse realizes it will be important to explain to Mr. Guadelupe that symptoms related to hypertension
○ 1. are seldom present.
○ 2. signify a high risk of stroke.
○ 3. occur only with malignant hypertension.
○ 4. begin when the kidneys have suffered irreversible damage.

**66.** Mr. Guadelupe's physician starts him on therapy with methyldopa (Aldomet) and hydrochlorothiazide (HydroDIURIL). The industrial nurse will monitor Mr. Guadelupe's blood pressure. The nurse recognizes that Mr. Guadelupe must be monitored frequently during the first days of therapy because methyldopa frequently causes which side effects?
○ 1. Drowsiness and an inability to concentrate.
○ 2. Nausea and facial flushing.
○ 3. Tremors and incoordination.
○ 4. Hyperexcitability and aggression.

**67.** Patient teaching for Mr. Guadelupe about his antihypertensive drug therapy should include *all* of the following *except*
○ 1. avoid taking prolonged hot baths or showers.
○ 2. wear support stockings.
○ 3. take the medications at bedtime with a full glass of water.
○ 4. nasal stuffiness may result from the drugs.

**68.** The nurse teaches Mr. Guadelupe about his diet restrictions. The physician wants him to follow a low-calorie, low-fat, 2-gram sodium diet. Which of the following menu selections *best* meets his needs?
○ 1. Mixed green salad with bleu cheese dressing, crackers, and cold cuts.
○ 2. Ham sandwich on rye bread and an orange.
○ 3. Cold chicken, an apple, and a slice of white bread.
○ 4. Hot dogs, baked beans, and celery and carrot sticks.

**69.** In an attempt to help Mr. Guadelupe comply with his dietary restrictions, what other information should the nurse give him?
○ 1. Use lemon juice or vinegar as a seasoning.
○ 2. Canned vegetables are less expensive than frozen vegetables.
○ 3. Limit the daily amount of leafy green vegetables.
○ 4. Substitute diet cola for coffee.

**70.** Mr. Guadelupe is also advised to include potassium-rich foods in his diet. The nurse reviews his eating habits and gives him information about high-potassium foods. Which of the following lunches, if chosen by Mr. Guadelupe, would indicate his understanding of this dietary intervention?
○ 1. Coffee, tuna sandwich, and grapes.
○ 2. Apple juice, hamburger, and fruit salad.
○ 3. Cherry cola, egg salad, and gelatin.
○ 4. Tomato juice, cheese sandwich, and butter cookies.

**71.** Mr. Guadelupe's job involves working in a warm, dry room and frequently bending and crouching to check the underside of the press. The press runs at high speed and the operator always wears eye guards. Given this information, for which side effect of hydrochlorothiazide (HydroDIURIL) would the nurse monitor Mr. Guadelupe?
○ 1. Muscle aches.
○ 2. Thirst.
○ 3. Lethargy.
○ 4. Postural hypotension.

**72.** Mr. Guadelupe asks whether he should begin an exercise program. Patient teaching about exercise in this situation should include which of the following?
○ 1. Avoid acute exercise; it will increase the heart's workload.
○ 2. Follow exercise sessions with soaks or steam baths to prevent cramping.
○ 3. Use isometric exercises to reduce the heart's workload.
○ 4. Practice muscle pump exercises for the legs whenever prolonged standing is required.

**73.** Mr. Guadelupe realizes the importance of quitting or cutting back on cigarettes. The nurse develops a plan to help Mr. Guadelupe achieve his goal. Which of the following nursing interventions should be the *initial* step in this plan?
○ 1. Review the negative effects of smoking on the body.
○ 2. Discuss the effects of passive smoking on environmental pollution.
○ 3. Establish the patient's daily smoking pattern.
○ 4. Explain how smoking worsens the problem of blood pressure control.

**74.** The *most important* long-term goal for Mr. Guadelupe would be for him to
○ 1. learn how to avoid stress.
○ 2. explore a job change or early retirement.
○ 3. make a commitment to long-term therapy.
○ 4. control his blood pressure.

**75.** Mr. Guadelupe has been keeping his regularly scheduled appointments for follow-up blood pressure readings. Which factor *best* supports the nurse's decision to increase the interval between Mr. Guadelupe's appointments?

○ 1. Regular attendance at stress reduction classes.
○ 2. Preference for having his blood pressure checked.
○ 3. Consistently stable blood pressure.
○ 4. Being symptom-free for 2 consecutive months.

## THE PATIENT WITH ANGINA

12/6/93

Mrs. Mary Serpe, age 57, is an extremely active woman who cares for her house and yard and is an avid gardener. Over the last few months she has noticed brief twinges of chest pain while she is working. She comes to the hospital when she experiences severe anterior chest pain while raking leaves. Her workup shows the presence of angina pectoris.

76. Which of the following are generally considered to be risk factors for the development of atherosclerosis?
○ 1. Family history of early myocardial infarct, hypertension, and anemia.
○ 2. Diabetes, smoking, and late onset of puberty.
○ 3. Male gender, total blood cholesterol of more than 240 mg/dl, and low protein intake.
○ 4. Physical inactivity, hypertension, and diabetes.

77. Under the age of about 50 years, many more men than women suffer from coronary artery disease as a result of atherosclerosis. It is generally believed that this difference is due to the fact that women have
○ 1. lifestyles with fewer stressors than men.
○ 2. higher blood levels of estrogen than men.
○ 3. lifestyles with more activity and exercise than men.
○ 4. diets that result in lower blood cholesterol levels than men.

78. Which of the following questions included in the nurse's initial assessment of Mrs. Serpe elicits the *most significant* information?
○ 1. "How severe was the pain?"
○ 2. "Do you smoke cigarettes?"
○ 3. "What medications are you taking?"
○ 4. "Can you describe the pain and when it occurred?"

79. Mrs. Serpe says, "I really thought I was having a heart attack. How can you tell the difference?" Which response by the nurse would provide the patient with the *most accurate* information about the difference between the pain of angina and myocardial infarction?
○ 1. "The pain associated with a heart attack is much more severe."

○ 2. "The pain associated with a heart attack radiates into the jaw and down the left arm."
○ 3. "It is impossible to differentiate anginal pain from that of a heart attack without an EKG."
○ 4. "The pain of angina is usually relieved by resting or lying down."

80. Mrs. Serpe asks the nurse, "What information is gained from an EKG?" The nurse would respond based on the knowledge that an EKG primarily gives information about the
○ 1. electrical conduction of the myocardium.
○ 2. oxygenation and perfusion of the heart.
○ 3. contractile status of the ventricles.
○ 4. physical integrity of the heart muscle.

81. As an initial step in Mrs. Serpe's treatment, nitroglycerin tablets 0.4 mg sublingually for anginal pain are prescribed. The principal effects of this drug are produced by
○ 1. antispasmodic effects on the pericardium.
○ 2. stimulation of alpha and beta receptor sites.
○ 3. vasodilatation of the peripheral vasculature.
○ 4. improved conductivity in the myocardium.

82. The nurse teaches Mrs. Serpe about the common expected side effects of nitroglycerin. These side effects include which of the following?
○ 1. Headache, hypotension, and dizziness.
○ 2. Hypertension, flushing, and fainting.
○ 3. Hypotension, shock, and shortness of breath.
○ 4. Stomach cramps, flushing, and dizziness.

83. Nitroglycerin begins to work within 1 to 2 minutes. How should the nurse instruct Mrs. Serpe to use the drug when chest pain occurs?
○ 1. Take 1 tablet every 2 to 5 minutes until the pain stops.
○ 2. Take 1 tablet and rest for 10 minutes. Call the physician if pain is still present.
○ 3. Take 1 tablet and then an additional tablet every 5 minutes for 3 doses. Call the physician if pain is still present.
○ 4. Take 1 tablet. If pain persists after 5 minutes, take 2 tablets. If pain is still present 5 minutes later, call the physician.

84. The nurse would provide Mrs. Serpe with *all* of the following additional information about sublingual nitroglycerin *except*
○ 1. the pill will cause a burning or tingling sensation under the tongue.
○ 2. store the tablets in a tight light-resistant container.
○ 3. try to use the tablets only when the pain is severe.
○ 4. the shelf life of nitroglycerin is short.

85. Nitroglycerin is also available in ointment or paste

not be prevented by such activities as taking deep breaths, clenching the teeth, or taking fluids through a drinking tube. (26, 31)

**12.** 4. Furosemide (Lasix) is a diuretic and is often used when pulmonary rales are present. The rales occur when fluid accumulates in lung tissues. The drug is ineffective for controlling discomfort, anxiety, and restlessness. (26, 31)

**13.** 3. Exercise helps prevent stasis of blood. Stasis predisposes to thrombophlebitis and blood clot formation. (5, 26)

**14.** 2. Recommended dietary principles in the acute phase of myocardial infarction include: avoid ingestion of myocardial stimulants, such as caffeine; avoid large meals, because small frequent feedings are better tolerated; and avoid foods that contribute to constipation. Fluids are given according to the patient's needs, and salt restrictions may be prescribed, especially for patients with manifestations of heart failure. (37, 41)

**15.** 3. Physical activity is gradually increased following a myocardial infarction while the patient is still hospitalized and through a period of rehabilitation. This type of progression in activity requires adjustments, however, if the patient has suffered complications. One of the best ways to judge progression of activity is to determine the effects of activity on degree of fatigue. The patient is becoming fatigued and progressing too rapidly if activity causes dyspnea, chest pain, a rapid heartbeat, or feelings of tiredness. When any of these symptoms appear, the patient should reduce his activity and progress more slowly. (26, 31)

**16.** 4. Keeping the patient's door closed is likely to contribute to feelings of isolation and sensory deprivation. Such activities as watching television, visiting with a relative, and reading a newspaper help prevent sensory deprivation and do not require physical effort. Television programs of a violent nature are usually contraindicated. (10, 23)

**17.** 3. Diastole is the period when the heart's ventricles are relaxed and filling with blood from the atria. Diastolic blood pressure describes the minimum pressure exerted on the walls of the arteries, which occurs when the heart is relaxed between beats. (26, 31)

**18.** 1. Among environmental factors, diet appears to be linked to coronary heart disease most significantly. (26, 31)

**19.** 4. There are about 2.2 pounds per kilogram; 3.2 × 2.2 = about 7 pounds. (24, 36)

**20.** 1. Patients who continue on a progressive exercise program at home after having a myocardial infarction should be taught to monitor their pulse rate. It can be expected that the pulse will increase with exercise, but exercise should not be increased if the rate increases more than about 25 beats per minute from baseline or exceeds 100 to 125 beats per minute. Patients should also be taught to decrease exercise if chest pain or dyspnea occurs. The patient's physician usually spells out the exact guidelines for pulse increases and when to notify the physician. (26, 31)

**21.** 3. A basic principle of behavior modification is that behavior that is learned and continued is behavior that has been rewarded. Other reinforcement techniques have not been found to be as effective as reward. (10, 23)

## The Patient with Congestive Heart Failure

**22.** 4. Morphine sulfate is given to help alleviate the anxiety that is ordinarily present when patients are suffering from acute pulmonary edema and associated distress. It does not affect nausea, blood pressure, and cyanosis. (26, 31)

**23.** 2. The characteristic sound when lungs are congested with fluid is a crackling or bubbling sound (rales) on auscultation. (26, 31)

**24.** 3. Sitting in bed with the feet and legs resting on the mattress decreases venous return to the heart, thus helping to lower the right ventricle's output and lung congestion. Also, the sitting position allows maximum space for lung expansion. (26, 31)

**25.** 2. Oxygen is administered to a patient with congestive heart failure to help overcome hypoxia and dyspnea. The best way to evaluate the effectiveness of oxygen therapy is to observe changes in arterial blood gases. This is most often done by determining the pressure of oxygen dissolved in the blood ($PaO_2$). When the $PaO_2$ is high, hemoglobin is carrying large amounts of oxygen, and oxygen therapy should cause the $PaO_2$ to increase. When the $PaO_2$ is low, the patient has hypoxia. (26, 31)

**26.** 4. The use of rotating tourniquets helps remove blood from the central circulation by temporarily pooling blood in the extremities. This decreases the venous return and the output of blood from the right ventricle, thereby helping relieve pulmonary edema. (26, 31)

**27.** 3. One extremity is free of a tourniquet while three extremities have tourniquets applied. This technique of allowing one extremity to be free of a tourniquet helps avoid tissue damage and emboli formation by providing full circulation in each extremity for 15 minutes every hour. (26, 31)

**28.** 3. When a blood pressure cuff is used for rotating tourniquets, the amount of inflation should be slightly above the patient's diastolic pressure. Venous flow should be occluded but arterial flow should *not* be impeded. (26, 31)

**29.** 3. Authorities recommend that no one extremity have a decreased blood flow for longer than 45 minutes, to help avoid tissue damage in the extremity. Longer periods may compromise circulation in the extremity. In some elderly patients or patients with poor circulation, the tourniquets may be rotated as often as every 5 minutes to prevent complications. (26, 31)

**30.** 3. When the pressure is correct during the application of rotating tourniquets, the venous blood supply, not the arterial blood supply, is impeded. Being able to determine pulses at arteries distal to the tourniquets ensures that arterial blood is entering the extremity. The nurse can expect the skin below the tourniquets to appear cyanotic and feel cool. The patient's blood pressure should also be assessed regularly because some patients become hypotensive during the procedure of applying rotating tourniquets. (25, 31)

**31.** 3. Releasing tourniquets one at a time at 15-minute intervals helps prevent central circulatory overload and recurring pulmonary edema. The first tourniquet applied should be the first one removed. (25, 31)

**32.** 2. Digoxin (Lanoxin) is a glycoside used to help strengthen myocardial contractions and increase output of blood from the left ventricle. As a result, there is less oozing of fluid into the lung fields. Digoxin is not used primarily to decrease the electrical conductivity of the myocardium, dilate coronary arteries, or decrease dysrhythmias. (26, 31)

**33.** 1. After the intravenous injection of furosemide (Lasix), diuresis normally begins in about 5 minutes and reaches its peak within about a half-hour. The effect of the medication lasts from 2 to 4 hours. When furosemide is given intramuscularly or orally, the action begins more slowly and lasts longer than when the drug is given intravenously. (12, 16)

**34.** 2. Edematous areas are subject to the development of decubitus ulcers because there is interference with the proper blood supply to the skin and underlying tissues. The primary cause of decubitus ulcers is unrelieved pressure over an area that results in poor circulation to tissue cells. (26, 31)

**35.** 4. Anorexia, sometimes with nausea and vomiting, is a common undesirable side effect of a digitalis preparation. It *may* be due to local gastric irritation, in which case the symptoms are often self-limiting, or digoxin toxicity may be occurring. Other undesirable side effects are diarrhea, restlessness or lethargy, irritability, and dysrhythmias. (26, 31)

**36.** 3. A very slow apical pulse rate indicates digoxin toxicity. A pulse rate as low as 50 or less (or 60 or less in some agencies) should be reported promptly, and the drug should be withheld until further orders are received. A heart murmur, slow respiratory rates, and a drop in blood pressure are not associated with digoxin toxicity. (26, 31)

**37.** 4. A low potassium blood level predisposes the patient to digoxin toxicity. Therefore, the nurse should be especially alert to assess for signs and symptoms of toxicity if the patient's blood findings reveal hypokalemia. Because potassium inhibits cardiac excitability, a low level of blood potassium increases cardiac excitability. (26, 31)

**38.** 1. A study of daily weights will help determine the effectiveness of diuretic therapy. If the patient gains weight without changes in her diet, it can be assumed that she is most probably retaining fluids and her diuretic therapy needs adjusting. Taking blood pressure readings, having regular urinalyses, and having blood studies for blood gas levels are not used to determine the effectiveness of diuretic therapy. (26, 31)

**39.** 4. When diuretics are given early in the day, the patient's need to void more frequently will not disturb nighttime rest. (26, 31)

**40.** 3. Hard (processed) cheeses are high in sodium and should be avoided or limited in a diet with moderate sodium restriction. Such foods as apples, tomatoes, and Cornish game hens are very low in sodium or contain no sodium. (25, 26)

**41.** 4. Catsup contains a considerable amount of salt and should not be included in a diet for a patient with sodium restrictions. Various herbs, except celery leaves and seeds, may be used; wine and lemon juice are other satisfactory seasoning agents. (25, 26)

**42.** 4. Rich sources of potassium include bananas, orange juice, and melons, such as honeydew, cantaloupe, and watermelons. Other rich sources of potassium are grapefruit juice, nectarines, potatoes, canned tomato juice, dried prunes, raisins, figs, and spinach. (37, 41)

**43.** 2. Alcohol can depress myocardial contractility, so excessive intake should be avoided. Sodium restriction is used to reduce fluid retention and cardiac workload. Caloric intake is restricted to control obesity and reduce cardiac workload. Potassium intake should not be reduced because hypokalemia is associated with digitalis toxicity. (37, 41)

## The Patient with Valvular Heart Disease

**44.** 2. While weight gain may signal acute fluid retention and worsening heart failure, weight loss and cachexia are often found in patients with long-standing mitral stenosis and regurgitation. The rise in left atrial pressure that accompanies mitral valve disease is transmitted backwards to the pulmonary veins, capillaries, and arterioles, and eventually to the right ventricle. Signs and symptoms of pulmonary and systemic venous congestion follow. (1, 15)

**45.** 3. Most patients with mitral stenosis have a history of rheumatic fever or bacterial endocarditis. Such infectious diseases as scarlet fever, poliomyelitis, and meningococcal meningitis are not associated with mitral stenosis. (5, 26)

**46.** 4. When mitral stenosis is present, the left atrium has difficulty emptying its contents into the left ventricle. Hence, since there is no valve to prevent backward flow into the pulmonary vein, the pulmonary circulation is under pressure. Functioning of the aorta, the right atrium, and the superior vena cava are not immediately influenced by mitral stenosis. (5, 26)

**47.** 3. Quinidine sulfate may cause elevated serum digoxin levels. Furosemide (Lasix) may induce hypokalemia, which sensitizes the myocardium to the development of digoxin toxicity. Quinidine sulfate may cause diarrhea and hypotension. Both quinidine sulfate and digoxin (Lanoxin) slow the heart rate. (1, 15)

**48.** 1. Preoperatively, anticoagulants may be prescribed for the patient with advanced valvular heart disease to prevent embolic phenomena. Postoperatively, all patients with mechanical valves, and some patients with bioprostheses, are maintained indefinitely on anticoagulant therapy. Adhering strictly to a dosage schedule and observing specific precautions are necessary to prevent hemorrhage or thromboembolism. Some patients are maintained on life-long antibiotic prophylaxis to prevent a recurrence of rheumatic fever. Episodic prophylaxis is required to prevent infective endocarditis following dental procedures or instrumentation or surgery of the upper respiratory, gastrointestinal, or genitourinary tract. (1, 15)

**49.** 4. Altered levels of consciousness, including hallucinations, confusion, delusions, depression, excitement, and disorientation, are common after cardiac surgery. Sensory deprivation and overload, high noise levels, and disruption of normal sleep-rest patterns are some environmental factors implicated in postcardiotomy delirium. Restricting the number of visitors and the amount of time they spend with the patient may be necessary to allow frequent rest periods. (1, 15)

**50.** 2. Protamine sulfate is used to help combat persistent bleeding in a patient who has had open-heart surgery. Warfarin sodium (Coumadin) is an anticoagulant, as is heparin, and these two agents would tend to cause the patient to bleed even more. Vitamin C and quinidine sulfate do not influence blood clotting. (12, 16)

**51.** 4. The solution to this problem is as follows:

$$1,000 \text{ mg} : 500 \text{ ml} :: 3 \text{ mg} : x \text{ ml}$$

$$1,000\, x = 1,500$$

$$x = \frac{1,500}{1,000} = 1.5 \text{ ml of solution/minute}$$

$$1.5 \text{ ml} \times 60 \text{ (microdrops)} = 90 \text{ microdrops/minute}$$

(24, 36)

**52.** 2. Typical adverse side effects of lidocaine hydrochloride (Xylocaine) include such neurologic signs and symptoms as dizziness, blurred vision, and excessive perspiration. Other adverse effects are hypotension, convulsions, and finally coma. The *desired* effect of lidocaine hydrochloride is to depress the myocardium and thereby decrease heart excitability. (5, 16)

**53.** 3. Central venous pressure (CVP) determination is used to assess the heart's ability to receive and pump blood. It represents filling pressure within the right atrium or great veins in the thorax. CVP helps test the right side of the heart's ability to manage fluid load and reflects right ventricular failure when it cannot handle its load. CVP may be used to help assess the patient's cardiovascular status, but in the situation described in this item its use to determine blood volume is not of primary concern. (5, 26)

**54.** 3. Every effort should be made to prevent stagnation of blood in the lower extremities during the postoperative period. Having the knees flexed by using a gatched bed or by placing pillows under the knees in the popliteal area promotes stagnation of blood and is contraindicated. If the patient wants some support near the knees while lying on her back or while in the Fowler's position, a *small* roll or *small* pillow may be placed at the area under the lower thigh just above the knees. This placement of support prevents interference with circulation in the legs. (24, 36)

**55.** 2. When a chest tube becomes disconnected, the

nurse should take immediate steps to prevent air from entering the chest cavity, which may cause the lung to collapse. Therefore, when a chest tube is accidentally disconnected from the drainage tube, quickly wipe the exposed end of the tubes with an antiseptic solution and immediately reconnect the tubes, or cut off the contaminated tips of the chest tube and tubing, insert a sterile connector in the chest tube and drainage tubing, and reattach to the drainage system. Observe the system to make sure it is functioning. Taping the tubing at the site of all connections prevents accidental disconnection. (5, 26)

56. 1. Many factors help prevent wound infections, including washing hands carefully, using sterile pre-packaged supplies and equipment, cleansing the incisional area well, and disposing of soiled dressings properly. However, most authorities say that the single most effective measure in preventing wound infections is to wash the hands *carefully* before and after changing dressings. Careful hand-washing is also important in helping reduce other infections often acquired in hospitals, such as urinary and respiratory infections. (24, 36)

57. 1. When a person is immobilized, calcium leaves the bone and concentrates in the extracellular fluid. When a large amount of calcium passes through the kidneys, calcium can precipitate and form calculi. Nursing interventions that help prevent calculi include ensuring a liberal fluid intake, unless contraindicated; providing a diet rich in acid to keep the urine acid, which increases the solubility of calcium; and limiting foods rich in calcium, such as dairy products. (6, 13)

58. 2. Because of the nature of her illness, the patient's usual family role is likely to change, at least temporarily. A role change often is accompanied by withdrawal, concern, and fear. The family members should be helped to understand this type of behavior so they do not misinterpret it. No information is given in this item to indicate the patient is withdrawn because of a fear of death, anxiety that her children consider her a burden, or fear that she may end up in a nursing home. (5, 26)

59. 3. Hepatic disease, heart failure, vitamin K deficiency, and broad-spectrum antibiotics are only a few of the factors that may increase the effects of warfarin sodium (Coumadin). The anticoagulant action may be decreased by vitamin K, antacids, and many other preparations. Coumadin dosage is determined by prothrombin time (PT) determinations. Because it takes 36 to 72 hours to obtain peak effects, Coumadin is usually begun while the patient is still receiving heparin. Fresh frozen plasma or vitamin K is used to reverse Coumadin's anticoagulant effect. (1, 19)

60. 1. Daily dental care and frequent checkups by a dentist who is informed about the patient's condition are required to maintain a healthy mouth. Irrigation devices, electric toothbrushes, or flossing may cause gums to bleed and allow bacteria to enter mucous membranes and the bloodstream, risking endocarditis. (1, 19)

61. 2. Most cardiac surgical patients have median sternotomy incisions, which take about 3 months to heal. Measures that assist the healing process include avoiding lifting heavy objects; muscle reconditioning; and exercising caution when driving. Showering or bathing is allowed as long as incisions are well approximated without open areas or drainage. While the patient is usually able to return to work after 1 month, activities should gradually be resumed upon discharge. (1, 19)

62. 4. Generalized discomfort due to immobility and the presence of drainage tubes is common following cardiac surgery. Mitral valve prostheses are more commonly associated with systemic embolization than are valves in the aortic position. Signs of embolization include weakness, paresthesia, speech dysfunction, dyspnea, and stroke. Valve wear and dysfunction are manifested by worsening angina, dyspnea, significant heart failure, and increasing hemolysis. Infective endocarditis, 2 or more months after replacement, is accompanied by chills, fever, leukocytosis, and the development of a new murmur. (15, 19)

## The Patient with Hypertension

63. 3. American Heart Association standards define hypertension as a consistent, systolic blood pressure level above 140 mm Hg and a consistent diastolic blood pressure level above 90 mm Hg. The diastolic value is more meaningful than the systolic value, which is affected by external variables such as stress, emotion, and exercise. (25, 31)

64. 3. Establishing a baseline for treatment evaluation is essential if the nurse is to monitor and evaluate the patient's progress. Completing insurance forms is secondary to successful treatment. Identifying other problems is a nonspecific reason to gather patient history and physical examination data. The data gathered will eventually be used to determine the patient's ability to participate in various treatment options. (5, 26)

65. 1. Most patients with hypertension are completely asymptomatic and may continue to be so even with

dangerous elevations in blood pressure. Therefore, the presence of symptoms is not an accurate reflection of the patient's status. Symptoms are not directly related to the status of the kidney. The severity of the hypertension, rather than the presence or absence of symptoms, determines the risk of complications such as stroke. (25, 31)

**66.** 1. Methyldopa (Aldomet) often produces drowsiness and an inability to concentrate during the first days of therapy or whenever the dosage is adjusted. This can be extremely dangerous for persons who drive or operate machinery and must be closely monitored. (12, 16)

**67.** 3. Antihypertensive medications cause significant side effects that frequently lead to noncompliance with the regimen. Orthostatic hypotension is a common problem, and patients should avoid prolonged standing, if possible, as well as hot baths and showers. Support stockings may help venous return. Nasal stuffiness is another common complaint with methyldopa (Aldomet). A drug such as Aldomet may be given at bedtime, but diuretics should not be given at bedtime because they would seriously interrupt the patient's sleep. (16, 25)

**68.** 3. Processed and cured meat products such as cold cuts, ham, and hot dogs are all high in both fat and sodium and should be avoided on a low-calorie, low-fat, low-salt diet. Diet restrictions of all types are complex and difficult to implement with patients who are basically asymptomatic. (31, 37)

**69.** 1. Lemon juice and vinegar make excellent seasonings for sodium-restricted diets, which are otherwise bland and tasteless to many patients. Canned foods are typically high in sodium. Green vegetables should be eaten liberally; most cola drinks have large amounts of both sodium and caffeine. (31, 37)

**70.** 2. All the food choices in this menu are rich sources of potassium. The other menus include only some foods that contain potassium. Tomato juice is high in sodium and potassium and therefore not recommended on a sodium-restricted diet. Sources of potassium include potatoes, peanut butter, dried fruit, apple juice, oranges, melon, tomatoes, squash, dried beans, bananas, and celery. The patient should know a variety of potassium-rich foods so that he does not limit himself to a small selection and tire of these foods. (25, 31)

**71.** 4. The risk of dizziness from postural hypotension when rising from a crouched or bent position increases the patient's risk of being injured by the equipment. The nurse should take the patient's blood pressure in all three positions (lying, sitting, and standing) at all routine visits. The other side effects listed could also cause complications in the work environment but are not as potentially dangerous as postural hypotension. (5, 26)

**72.** 4. A regular exercise program will be prescribed for the patient to assist in weight control and to improve cardiac fitness. The program will be initiated slowly to avoid heart damage. Isometric exercises increase muscle tone but do not meet the goals of aerobic fitness. Postural hypotension is an ongoing problem that requires muscle pump exercises for standing. Steam baths should be avoided because they can induce hypotensive fainting and injury. (26, 31)

**73.** 3. A plan to reduce or stop smoking begins with establishing the patient's personal daily smoking pattern and activities associated with smoking. It is important that patients understand the associated health risks, but this knowledge has not been shown to successfully help patients change their smoking behavior. (5, 26)

**74.** 3. Compliance is the most critical element of hypertension therapy. Once diagnosed as hypertensive, most patients require life-long treatment and cannot be managed successfully without drug therapy. Stress and weight management are important components of hypertension therapy, but the priority goal is related to compliance. (25, 31)

**75.** 3. Actual blood pressure readings are the only accurate way to monitor hypertension. Patient compliance is critical in management but is not the only measure of effectiveness. The nurse should consider a patient's preference about the monitoring schedule, but the patient's physical status is the major factor that determines the schedule. (25, 31)

## The Patient with Angina

**76.** 4. Risk factors for atherosclerosis include the following: Being male, a family history of atherosclerosis, hypertension, high blood cholesterol, abnormal electrocardiogram, diabetes, an excess calorie and/or fat intake, and physical inactivity. (7, 13)

**77.** 2. It is generally agreed, and increasing evidence supports the theory, that estrogen helps protect the female from atherosclerotic changes. Such factors as a difference in lifestyles, exercise, activity, and diets have not been found significant in determining why more men than women under age 50 have coronary heart disease. (26, 31)

**78.** 4. Pain is an individual and subjective experience that is difficult to evaluate objectively. The nurse must help the patient describe the pain experience and the circumstances surrounding it objectively.

This information is used for planning therapy and patient teaching about the disease and its management. Exploring the patient's smoking and medication history are important but peripheral issues. (26, 31)

**79.** 4. The essential element of anginal pain that helps differentiate it from the pain of a heart attack is the fact that anginal pain is transient and usually alleviated by resting and/or lying down. Anginal pain is not always less severe than that of a myocardial infarction and may radiate down the arm or into the jaw. (26, 31)

**80.** 1. An EKG directly reflects the transmission of the electrical cardiac impulse through the heart. This information makes it possible to evaluate indirectly the functional status of the heart muscle and the contractile response of the ventricles. However, these elements are not measured directly. (26, 31)

**81.** 3. Nitroglycerin produces peripheral vasodilatation, which reduces myocardial oxygen consumption and demand. Vasodilatation in coronary arteries and collateral vessels *may* also increase blood flow to the ischemic areas of the heart. Nitroglycerin affects neither alpha nor beta receptors. It does not affect pericardial spasticity or conductivity of the myocardium. (26, 31)

**82.** 1. Because of its widespread vasodilating effects, nitroglycerin often produces such side effects as headache, hypotension, and dizziness. The patient should sit or lie down to avoid fainting. Nitroglycerin does not cause shortness of breath or stomach cramps. (16, 25)

**83.** 3. The correct protocol for nitroglycerin use involves its immediate administration with subsequent doses taken at 5-minute intervals as needed, for a total dose of three tablets. Sublingual nitroglycerin appears in the bloodstream within 2 to 3 minutes and is metabolized within approximately 10 minutes. (16, 25)

**84.** 3. Patients should be instructed to use nitroglycerin at the first indication of chest pain and not wait before using the drug. Sublingual nitroglycerin should cause a tingling sensation under the tongue; it should be kept in a tight, dark container; and it should be replenished frequently because it deteriorates rather rapidly. (16, 25)

**85.** 2. When applying nitroglycerin ointment on a patient's skin, the nurse should be very careful to avoid getting any ointment on her skin. She can absorb the nitroglycerin through her skin and receive medication in her bloodstream the same way the patient does. No dangerous fumes arise from the ointment. The ointment should *not* be massaged into the skin, and the application site should be rotated to avoid irritating the skin in one area. (16, 25)

**86.** 3. Nitroglycerin may be used prophylactically before stressful physical activities such as stair-climbing to help the patient remain pain-free. Resting before or after an activity is not likely to help prevent an activity-related pain episode. (25, 26)

**87.** 2. Physical activity can precipitate angina pectoris, but total curtailment of a favorite activity is an overreaction that can lead to psychosocial disturbances such as depression or decreased self-esteem. Appropriate education should reassure the patient that life need not stop due to angina. There is no reason to assume that the patient will gradually increase her activity level. Because physical activity is only one factor precipitating angina, the need for nitroglycerin is not eliminated. (25, 31)

**88.** 4. Eating a large meal can precipitate an anginal attack, particularly if physical activity follows the meal. Avoiding large meals and large portions at meals help prevent anginal attacks. The other dietary modifications are unrelated to angina. (5, 26)

**89.** 2. Cold weather tends to aggravate angina pectoris. Dry, warm, or humid weather has not been noted to influence the condition. (5, 31)

**90.** 1. Verapamil (Calan), a calcium channel blocker, decreases the heart rate by decreasing the rate of depolarization and automaticity. The patient monitors her pulse rate to detect bradycardia. The other monitoring procedures are unrelated to verapamil's side effects. (5, 26)

**91.** 1. A change in the pattern of chest pain is an essential sign that the patient should be instructed to report. It may indicate a deterioration in the status of the myocardium. Pain occurring during stress or sexual activity would not be unexpected. (26, 31)

**92.** 2. Cardiac catheterization is used with angina patients primarily to assess the extent and severity of the blockage in the coronary arteries. A decision about medical management, angioplasty, or coronary artery bypass surgery will be made from these data. (5, 26)

# test 3

The Patient with Peptic Ulcer Disease
The Patient with Cholecystitis
The Patient with Cancer of the Stomach
The Patient with Pancreatitis
The Patient with Hiatal Hernia
Correct Answers and Rationales

Select the one *best* or *correct* answer and indicate your choice by filling in the circle with a pencil in front of the option you have chosen. If the answer you would prefer is not given, select the one you think is *most appropriate*.

## THE PATIENT WITH PEPTIC ULCER DISEASE

Mr. George Small, a 54-year-old sales executive, is admitted through the emergency department with a bleeding duodenal ulcer. He has been treated for peptic ulcer disease over the last 3 years and has recently noticed an increase in the frequency and severity of his pain. He was brought to the hospital when he vomited bright-red blood.

1. The physician orders a nasogastric tube to be inserted for irrigation of the stomach. Which of the following insertion techniques would most likely make it *more* difficult for the nurse to insert the tube?
   - ○ 1. Lubricating the tube with a water-soluble lubricant.
   - ○ 2. Asking the patient to swallow while the tube is passed to the stomach.
   - ○ 3. Firming the tube by placing it in ice chips a few minutes before inserting it.
   - ○ 4. Having the patient tilt his head toward his chest while inserting the tube into the nose.

2. Which of the following techniques is considered the *best* way to determine whether the tube is in Mr. Small's stomach?
   - ○ 1. Applying suction to the tube and observing for the return of gastric contents.
   - ○ 2. Irrigating the tube with normal saline and observing for the return of solution.
   - ○ 3. Placing the free end of the tube in water and observing for air bubbles.
   - ○ 4. Instilling air into the tube and palpating over the epigastric area for the presence of the tube.

3. While Mr. Small is bleeding, it will be essential for the nurse to assess him frequently for signs of early shock. *All* of the following are important indicators of early shock *except*
   - ○ 1. tachycardia.
   - ○ 2. cool clammy skin.
   - ○ 3. increased urine output.
   - ○ 4. restlessness.

4. Which of the following clinical manifestations is Mr. Small *most likely* to demonstrate if his ulcer perforates?
   - ○ 1. Projectile vomiting.
   - ○ 2. Frequent belching.
   - ○ 3. Diarrhea.
   - ○ 4. Boardlike abdomen.

5. The nurse correctly judges that Mr. Small was probably ignoring an important warning sign of bleeding when he reports that prior to admission the color of his stools was
   - ○ 1. gray.
   - ○ 2. black.
   - ○ 3. dark green.
   - ○ 4. light brown.

6. Mr. Small has been taking propantheline bromide (Pro-Banthine) at home. This medication is ordered for patients with peptic ulcer disease *primarily* because it
   - ○ 1. suppresses gastric secretions.
   - ○ 2. neutralizes acid in the stomach.
   - ○ 3. shortens the time required for digestion in the stomach.
   - ○ 4. improves the mixing of foods and gastric secretions.

7. Although Mr. Small appears calm, the nurse believes he is experiencing anxiety. The nurse bases her judgment on knowledge that a clinical manifestation of anxiety is
   - ○ 1. flushed skin.
   - ○ 2. decreased heart rate.

○ 3. dry lips and mouth.

○ 4. decreased blood pressure.

**8.** Mr. Small is to have an examination of his upper gastrointestinal tract (GI series). Which of the following should Mr. Small receive after the examination?

○ 1. A laxative.

○ 2. A clear liquid diet.

○ 3. An enema.

○ 4. An intravenous infusion.

**9.** Aluminum hydroxide (Amphojel), 30 ml every 2 hours, is prescribed for Mr. Small. A problem often associated with the use of aluminum hydroxide is

○ 1. anorexia.

○ 2. nausea.

○ 3. constipation.

○ 4. belching.

**10.** At what time do duodenal ulcers usually cause epigastric pain?

○ 1. At mealtime.

○ 2. 30 minutes after eating.

○ 3. 2 to 4 hours after eating.

○ 4. 4 to 6 hours after eating.

**11.** Mr. Small tells the nurse that when he first had ulcers some years ago, he was on a diet of milk and cream. He asks, "Why don't they use that type of diet now?" The nurse should explain that milk and cream are no longer commonly used because they

○ 1. stimulate gastric acid secretion.

○ 2. cause renal calculi.

○ 3. precipitate lactose intolerance.

○ 4. produce biliary stones.

**12.** While he is in the hospital, Mr. Small is served a modified bland diet. If the nurse notes the following items on Mr. Small's dinner tray, which one should she remove before serving the tray?

○ 1. Salt.

○ 2. Sugar.

○ 3. Mayonnaise.

○ 4. Pepper.

**13.** After dinner, the nurse asks Mr. Small, "Did you have a good dinner?" Which of the following is the patient *most likely* to give?

○ 1. A brief "yes" or "no" answer.

○ 2. A description of the food served.

○ 3. A complaint about the food served.

○ 4. A comparison with the patient's usual dinner.

**14.** Which of the following beverages should the nurse instruct Mr. Small to *avoid* after discharge?

○ 1. Carbonated mineral water.

○ 2. Low-sodium skim milk.

○ 3. Wine coolers.

○ 4. Fruit juice.

**15.** Which of the following statements *best* describes current opinion about diet during convalescence for patients with peptic ulcers?

○ 1. A bland diet is most effective for the patient with a peptic ulcer.

○ 2. The type of diet appears to be less important than including foods the patient tolerates.

○ 3. Eliminating specific foods from the diet is no longer recommended, as long as the patient eats frequently.

○ 4. Dietary restrictions appear to be most helpful among elderly persons but are rarely helpful among young and middle-aged adults.

**16.** Mr. Small is to undergo an upper GI endoscopy to help the physician visualize the location and severity of the ulcer. When Mr. Small returns to the unit, what should the nurse evaluate in addition to his vital signs?

○ 1. The return of the gag reflex.

○ 2. Bowel sounds.

○ 3. Breath sounds.

○ 4. Intake and output.

**17.** Mr. Small's treatment plan includes modified bed rest. One afternoon the nurse finds him surrounded by papers from his briefcase and arguing on the telephone with a co-worker. The nurse's interaction with Mr. Small should be based on knowledge that

○ 1. involvement with his job will keep Mr. Small from becoming bored in the hospital.

○ 2. rest is an essential component of ulcer healing.

○ 3. not keeping up with his job will increase Mr. Small's stress level.

○ 4. setting limits on a patient's behavior is an essential aspect of the nursing role.

**18.** Mr. Small will not be able to avoid stress in his job. Therefore, it is *most* important that he

○ 1. consider changing jobs.

○ 2. identify stressors at work.

○ 3. set his goals a little lower.

○ 4. improve his ability to cope with stress.

**19.** Mr. Small smokes about two packs of cigarettes a day. The nurse recommends that Mr. Small try to stop smoking because of the effects of nicotine. Nicotine increases the body's secretion of

○ 1. thyroxin.

○ 2. epinephrine.

○ 3. pancreatic juices.

○ 4. gastrointestinal mucus.

**20.** Mr. Small has been stabilized on cimetidine (Tagamet) and will take the drug at home. The nurse teaches Mr. Small about the proper administration of the drug. The nurse knows that Mr. Small has understood the teaching when he says he will take the drug

○ 1. before meals.
○ 2. with meals.
○ 3. after meals.
○ 4. when pain occurs.

# THE PATIENT WITH CHOLECYSTITIS

Mrs. Florence Metcalf, age 56, is admitted to the hospital with acute upper right quadrant pain that radiates to her back. She is extremely nauseated and has vomited several times. Her diet is high in fat and although she has been experiencing discomfort after fatty meals for several months, this attack is much more severe. Mrs. Metcalf is accompanied by the oldest of her five children. On assessment, Mrs. Metcalf appears as an overweight middle-aged woman with extremely pale skin who is in obvious distress.

**21.** Mrs. Metcalf's admitting diagnosis is cholecystitis with cholelithiasis. *All* of the following factors predispose Mrs. Metcalf to cholelithiasis *except* her
○ 1. age.
○ 2. weight.
○ 3. sex.
○ 4. diet.

**22.** Which of the following nursing interventions should have *highest* priority during the *first* hour after Mrs. Metcalf's admission?
○ 1. Administering pain medication.
○ 2. Completing the admission history.
○ 3. Maintaining hydration.
○ 4. Teaching about planned diagnostic tests.

**23.** Nitroglycerine (glyceryl trinitrate) is ordered in addition to meperidine hydrochloride (Demerol). The rationale for using nitroglycerine is that it
○ 1. relaxes smooth muscle.
○ 2. reduces nausea and vomiting.
○ 3. enhances the action of meperidine hydrochloride.
○ 4. decreases the secretion of gastric hydrochloric acid.

**24.** Mrs. Metcalf is to have an intravenous infusion started. Before inserting the needle into a vein, the nurse applies a tourniquet to Mrs. Metcalf's arm. The purpose of the tourniquet is to
○ 1. distend the veins.
○ 2. stabilize the veins.
○ 3. immobilize the arm.
○ 4. occlude arterial circulation.

**25.** If a gallstone becomes lodged in the common bile duct, the nurse should anticipate that the color of Mrs. Metcalf's stools would *most likely* be
○ 1. green.
○ 2. gray.
○ 3. black.
○ 4. yellow.

**26.** When the common bile duct is obstructed, the nurse should monitor the patient for signs of
○ 1. respiratory distress.
○ 2. circulatory overload.
○ 3. urinary tract infection.
○ 4. prolonged bleeding time.

**27.** Mrs. Metcalf is scheduled for a cholecystogram. In preparation for the test she is to take iopanoic acid (Telepaque) tablets after her evening meal. Before administering the tablets, the nurse should ask Mrs. Metcalf if she is allergic to
○ 1. eggs.
○ 2. iodine.
○ 3. food colorings.
○ 4. organ meats.

**28.** Mrs. Metcalf's x-rays show the presence of gallstones and she is prepared for a cholecystectomy and choledochotomy. This procedure indicates that the surgeon will remove the gallbladder and
○ 1. drain the gallbladder.
○ 2. open the common bile duct.
○ 3. remove the common bile duct.
○ 4. insert a drainage tube into the cystic duct.

**29.** Preoperatively, the nurse instructs Mrs. Metcalf in the correct use of an incentive spirometer. This treatment is essential following gallbladder surgery because
○ 1. the patient is on bed rest for several days.
○ 2. ambulation is restricted by the presence of a T-tube.
○ 3. the operative incision is quite near the diaphragm.
○ 4. the presence of a nasogastric tube makes it difficult for the patient to cough effectively.

**30.** The incentive spirometer is used primarily to
○ 1. stimulate circulation.
○ 2. prepare for ambulation.
○ 3. strengthen abdominal muscles.
○ 4. increase respiratory effectiveness.

**31.** Mrs. Metcalf's surgery is scheduled for tomorrow and is to be done under general anesthesia. Mrs. Metcalf receives no oral food or fluids after midnight tonight. The nurse should understand that the primary reason for withholding food and fluids from patients like Mrs. Metcalf is to help prevent
○ 1. constipation during the immediate postoperative period.

○ 2. vomiting and possible aspiration of vomitus during surgery.

○ 3. pressure on the diaphragm with poor lung expansion during surgery.

○ 4. gas pains and distention during the immediate postoperative period.

32. The nurse administers Mrs. Metcalf's preoperative intramuscular medication at the ventrogluteal site. The muscle into which the nurse will inject the medication is the

○ 1. rectus femoris muscle. *anterior aspect of thigh*

○ 2. gluteus minimus muscle. *ventro gluteal site*

○ 3. vastus lateralis muscle. *lateral thigh*

○ 4. gluteus maximus muscle. *dorso buttocks*

33. Mrs. Metcalf undergoes a cholecystectomy and choledochotomy and returns to her room with an intravenous infusion, a Penrose drain, and a T-tube in place. In order to evaluate the effectiveness of the T-tube, the nurse should understand that the *primary* reason for using a T-tube with this patient is to

○ 1. promote wound drainage.

○ 2. provide a means to irrigate the biliary tract.

○ 3. minimize the passage of bile into the duodenum.

○ 4. prevent bile from entering the peritoneal cavity.

34. How much bile would the nurse expect the T-tube to drain during the first 24 hours after surgery?

○ 1. 50 to 100 ml.

○ 2. 150 to 250 ml.

○ 3. 300 to 500 ml.

○ 4. 500 to 600 ml.

35. Mrs. Metcalf's intake and output are measured postoperatively. To maintain accurate records, the nurse should measure the amount of drainage from Mrs. Metcalf's T-tube and record it by

○ 1. adding it to the patient's urinary output.

○ 2. charting it separately on the output record.

○ 3. adding it to the amount of wound drainage.

○ 4. subtracting it from the total intake for each day.

36. The presence of the T-tube makes it important for the nurse to give extra attention to

○ 1. skin around the insertion site.

○ 2. intake and output.

○ 3. electrolyte imbalance.

○ 4. acid-base imbalance.

37. Prochlorperazine dimaleate (Compazine) is prescribed for Mrs. Metcalf on her first postoperative day. The nurse judges that the drug has had a therapeutic effect when the patient no longer complains of

○ 1. nausea.

○ 2. dizziness.

○ 3. abdominal spasms.

○ 4. abdominal distention.

38. During the first few weeks after cholecystectomy, Mrs. Metcalf would probably be more comfortable if she restricted her diet in which of the following ways?

○ 1. Decrease intake of fruits, vegetables, whole grains, nuts, and seeds to increase fiber and minimize pressure within the small intestine.

○ 2. Consume at least 4 or 5 servings of meats, cheese, and peanut butter daily to boost protein and essential amino acids for healing the surgical incision.

○ 3. Distribute intake of fat in small portions throughout the day so that there is not an excessive amount in the intestine at any one time.

○ 4. Use pancreatic extracts with meals to replace the enzymes that would normally have been secreted by the organ that was surgically removed.

39. Mrs. Metcalf is to follow a low-fat diet. Which of the following foods would be *most* appropriate for Mrs. Metcalf's lunch?

○ 1. Cheese omelette and vanilla pudding.

○ 2. Egg-salad sandwich and fresh fruit cup.

○ 3. Ham-salad sandwich and baked custard.

○ 4. Roast beef and green beans.

## THE PATIENT WITH CANCER OF THE STOMACH

Mr. Sam Bolten, age 70, came to his physician with a 2-month history of fatigue and vague digestive complaints. He reported a progressive weight loss, occasional nausea and vomiting, anorexia, and a sensation of feeling full after eating small amounts of food. He is very thin and weak. An upper GI series was done, and a lesion on the lesser curvature of the stomach was seen. A endoscopic examination with a biopsy of the lesion confirmed the diagnosis of adenocarcinoma of the stomach. A subtotal gastric resection is planned.

40. On admission to the hospital, it is determined that Mr. Bolten's nutritional status is severely compromised. Which of the following therapies would be *most* effective in correcting his nutritional deficits prior to surgery?

○ 1. High-protein between-meal nourishment 4 times a day.

○ 2. Tube feedings at 200 ml/hour.

○ 3. Total parenteral nutrition (TPN) for several days.

○ 4. Intravenous infusion of normal saline at 125 ml/hour.

**41.** Preoperatively, Mr. Bolten expresses anxiety and apprehension about the surgery. Which of the following nursing interventions would help achieve the goal of reducing Mr. Bolten's anxiety?

○ 1. Provide Mr. Bolten with information, but only if he requests it.

○ 2. Tell Mr. Bolten what to expect in the postoperative period.

○ 3. Reassure Mr. Bolten about the high percentage of patients who live 5 years or more following surgery for gastric cancer.

○ 4. Impress on Mr. Bolten the importance of seeing a doctor before symptoms become as severe as his did.

**42.** Mr. Bolten is scheduled to have a subtotal gastrectomy (Billroth II). When teaching the patient preoperatively, the nurse should explain that the surgical procedure he is to have allows stomach contents to bypass the

○ 1. ileum.

○ 2. duodenum.

○ 3. cardiac sphincter.

○ 4. fundus of the stomach.

Mr. Bolten has his surgery. Postoperative orders include: keep n.p.o.; nasogastric tube to low intermittent suction; IV fluids at 125 ml/hour; turn, cough, and deep-breathe patient every 2 hours; meperidine hydrochloride (Demerol) 100 mg IM every 3 to 4 hours p.r.n. for pain.

**43.** The care of patients who have had a subtotal gastrectomy differs in several ways from that of patients who have had other types of gastric resections. Which of the following events would be anticipated in the care of the patient undergoing a *subtotal gastrectomy,* but would not apply to the care of patients undergoing other types of gastric resections?

○ 1. With a subtotal gastrectomy, there will be less drainage through the nasogastric tube.

○ 2. With a subtotal gastrectomy, oral feedings can be resumed earlier but must progress very slowly.

○ 3. With a subtotal gastrectomy, vitamin $B_{12}$ injections are required as life-long replacement therapy.

○ 4. With a subtotal gastrectomy, the patient will

not have chest tubes because the chest cavity is not entered.

**44.** Mr. Bolten will have a nasogastric tube in place for several days postoperatively. A major reason for inserting this tube is to

○ 1. prevent excessive pressure on suture lines.

○ 2. prevent the development of ascites.

○ 3. allow for feeding the patient in the immediate postoperative period.

○ 4. allow for the administration of antacids to promote healing of the anastomosis.

**45.** The nurse should anticipate that drainage from Mr. Bolten's nasogastric tube would be what color for the first 12 to 24 hours after surgery?

○ 1. Brown.

○ 2. Green.

○ 3. Bright red.

○ 4. Cloudy white.

**46.** The care of Mr. Bolten's nasogastric tube and drainage system should include which of the following nursing interventions?

○ 1. Irrigate the tube with 30 ml of sterile water every hour, if needed.

○ 2. If the tube is not draining well, reposition it.

○ 3. Observe Mr. Bolten for nausea, vomiting, and abdominal distention.

○ 4. If the drainage is sluggish on low suction, turn the machine to high suction.

**47.** The nurse uses 30 ml of solution to irrigate Mr. Bolten's nasogastric tube and notes that 20 ml returns promptly into the drainage container. When the nurse records the results of the irrigation, how much solution should she record as intake?

○ 1. 10 ml.

○ 2. 20 ml.

○ 3. 30 ml.

○ 4. 50 ml.

**48.** Mr. Bolten complains of sore nares while the nasogastric tube is in place. Which of the following nursing measures is *most appropriate* to help alleviate the patient's discomfort?

○ 1. Repositioning the tube in the nares.

○ 2. Irrigating the tube with cool solution.

○ 3. Applying a water-soluble lubricant to the nares.

○ 4. Having the patient change his position more frequently.

**49.** Because Mr. Bolten has a nasogastric tube attached to low suction, he will receive intravenous replacement therapy postoperatively *primarily* to

○ 1. stabilize blood gas levels.

○ 2. facilitate osmotic diuresis.

○ 3. equalize intake and output.

○ 4. maintain fluid and electrolyte balance.

50. From an analysis of the data collected about Mr. Bolten and his surgery (subtotal gastrectomy), the nurse identifies the nursing diagnosis "potential for alteration in respiratory function postoperatively." *All* of the following factors contribute to this diagnosis *except* the

    ○ 1. presence of a high abdominal incision.

    ○ 2. patient's weakness and fatigue.

    ○ 3. possibility of aspiration of gastric contents.

    ○ 4. postoperative semi-Fowler's position.

51. A major goal for Mr. Bolten's postoperative nursing care is to prevent atelectasis and pneumonia. Which of the following measures would *best* accomplish this?

    ○ 1. Give meperidine hydrochloride (Demerol) sparingly to prevent depressing the cough reflex and respirations.

    ○ 2. Offer meperidine hydrochloride (Demerol) 30 minutes before having Mr. Bolten cough and deep-breathe.

    ○ 3. Encourage coughing, deep-breathing, and turning in bed once every 4 hours.

    ○ 4. Maintain bed rest for at least 48 hours to minimize incisional pain and splinting of the chest.

52. Mr. Bolten begins to complain of abdominal distention. Which of the following measures should the nurse implement *first?*

    ○ 1. Call the physician.

    ○ 2. Irrigate the nasogastric tube.

    ○ 3. Check the functioning of the suction equipment.

    ○ 4. Reposition the nasogastric tube.

53. Mr. Bolten's serum electrolyte values are obtained postoperatively. The nurse should interpret a potassium level of 4.2 mEq/L to mean that Mr. Bolten's potassium level is

    ○ 1. above normal.

    ○ 2. within the normal range.

    ○ 3. slightly below normal.

    ○ 4. life-threateningly low.

54. Which of the following signs/symptoms is an *early* indication that Mr. Bolten's serum potassium level is below normal?

    ○ 1. Diarrhea.

    ○ 2. Sticky mucous membranes.

    ○ 3. Muscle weakness in the legs.

    ○ 4. Tingling in the fingers.

55. Mr. Bolten will be observed for complications common to all surgical patients as well as those specific to gastric resections. Which of the following signs and symptoms would alert the nurse to the development of a leaking anastomosis?

○ 1. Pain, fever, and dyspnea when oral fluids are begun.

○ 2. Diarrhea with the presence of fat in the stool.

○ 3. Palpitations, pallor, and diaphoresis after eating.

○ 4. Feeling of fullness and nausea after eating.

56. As part of Mr. Bolten's discharge planning, the nurse has identified "alteration in nutrition: less than body requirements" as a major nursing diagnosis. In order to help Mr. Bolten and his family meet his nutritional goals, the nurse should

    ○ 1. instruct Mr. Bolten to increase the amount of food eaten at each meal by doubling that of the previous meal.

    ○ 2. encourage Mr. Bolten to eat smaller amounts more frequently and to stop when he feels full.

    ○ 3. explain that if he should vomit after a meal, he should eat nothing more that day.

    ○ 4. inform Mr. Bolten that bland foods may cause gastric distress and to introduce them into his diet gradually.

57. As a result of his gastric resection, Mr. Bolten is at risk for developing dumping syndrome. This problem occurs primarily from

    ○ 1. excess secretion of digestive enzymes in the intestine.

    ○ 2. rapid emptying of stomach contents into the small intestine.

    ○ 3. excess glycogen production by the liver.

    ○ 4. the loss of the gastric juices.

58. Which of the following symptoms would strongly suggest that Mr. Bolten is experiencing dumping syndrome?

    ○ 1. Constipation.

    ○ 2. Extreme hunger.

    ○ 3. Feeling faint.

    ○ 4. Abdominal cramps.

59. To reduce the incidence of dumping syndrome in Mr. Bolten, the nurse should teach him *all* the following strategies *except*

    ○ 1. lie down on the left side after meals.

    ○ 2. avoid drinking fluids with meals.

    ○ 3. increase the protein content of meals.

    ○ 4. increase the carbohydrate content of meals.

60. *All* the following data indicate that Mr. Bolten's nutritional goal is being achieved *except*

    ○ 1. a gradual increase in the intake and tolerance of food.

    ○ 2. the absence of nausea and vomiting.

    ○ 3. the ingestion of an iron and vitamin supplement daily.

    ○ 4. a rapid weight gain in 1 week.

# THE PATIENT WITH PANCREATITIS

Mrs. Mildred Ottinger, age 62, is admitted to the medical unit with a diagnosis of acute pancreatitis. She has severe left upper quadrant pain, nausea, and vomiting. This is her second admission with this diagnosis.

61. Pancreatitis is most accurately described as an
    ○ 1. inherited degenerative disease process that causes gradual pancreatic breakdown.
    ○ 2. autoimmune response to an unidentified viral or bacterial agent.
    ○ 3. acute inflammation of the pancreas that produces obstruction and edema.
    ○ 4. infectious disease triggered by the hepatitis virus.

62. Which of the following describes a function of the pancreas as an exocrine gland?
    ○ 1. Secretion of insulin.
    ○ 2. Secretion of digestive enzymes.
    ○ 3. Facilitation of glycogen storage by the liver.
    ○ 4. Promotion of glucose transport into the cells.

63. The initial diagnosis of pancreatitis would be confirmed if Mrs. Ottinger's blood work shows a significant elevation in serum
    ○ 1. amylase.
    ○ 2. glucose.
    ○ 3. potassium.
    ○ 4. trypsin.

64. Mr. Ottinger tells the nurse, "This is the second time this has happened and I still don't understand it." The nurse bases her response on the knowledge that although the disease process is complicated, the basic pathophysiology of pancreatitis involves
    ○ 1. spasm of the sphincter of Oddi.
    ○ 2. increased gastric secretions.
    ○ 3. autodigestion of the pancreas.
    ○ 4. severe volume depletion.

65. Because the Ottingers rarely drink due to religious convictions, Mr. Ottinger becomes upset when the physicians persist in asking his wife about alcohol intake. The nurse should explain that the reason for these questions is
    ○ 1. there is a strong link between alcohol use and acute pancreatitis.
    ○ 2. alcohol intake can interfere with some of the tests used to diagnose pancreatitis.
    ○ 3. alcoholism is a major health problem and any hospitalized patient is questioned about alcohol intake.
    ○ 4. the physicians must obtain the pertinent facts and religious beliefs cannot be considered.

66. Pain control is an important nursing goal for Mrs. Ottinger. Which of the following medications would be the drug of choice in this situation?
    ○ 1. Meperidine hydrochloride (Demerol).
    ○ 2. Cimetidine (Tagamet).
    ○ 3. Morphine sulfate.
    ○ 4. Codeine sulfate.

67. The nurse monitors Mrs. Ottinger's vital signs frequently, observing for early signs of shock. Shock is extremely difficult to manage in pancreatitis primarily because of the
    ○ 1. frequency and severity of gastrointestinal hemorrhage.
    ○ 2. vasodilating effects of kinin peptides.
    ○ 3. tendency toward congestive heart failure.
    ○ 4. frequent incidence of acute tubular necrosis.

68. Which of the following assessment features would be an *unexpected* finding in Mrs. Ottinger?
    ○ 1. Hypoglycemia.
    ○ 2. Abdominal distention and tenderness.
    ○ 3. Nausea and vomiting.
    ○ 4. Hyperlipidemia.

69. While helping her change position in bed, the nurse notices muscle twitching in Mrs. Ottinger's hands and forearms. She should report these symptoms immediately because patients with pancreatitis are at serious risk for
    ○ 1. hypermagnesemia.
    ○ 2. hypoglycemia.
    ○ 3. hyperkalemia.
    ○ 4. hypocalcemia.

70. Mrs. Ottinger's *initial* treatment plan is most likely to focus on
    ○ 1. resting the gastrointestinal tract.
    ○ 2. ensuring adequate nutrition.
    ○ 3. maintaining fluid and electrolyte balance.
    ○ 4. treating infection.

71. Which of the following medications is *most likely* to be prescribed to augment efforts to control Mrs. Ottinger's pain?
    ○ 1. Ibuprofen (Motrin).
    ○ 2. Magnesium hydroxide (Maalox).
    ○ 3. Propantheline bromide (Pro-Banthine).
    ○ 4. Propranolol (Inderal).

72. During the acute period, Mrs. Ottinger's diet order will most likely be
    ○ 1. bland low fat.
    ○ 2. 1,800 calorie ADA.
    ○ 3. clear liquids.
    ○ 4. n.p.o.

73. Mrs. Ottinger's condition becomes chronic. What is the appropriate diet for a patient with chronic pancreatitis?

○ 1. A low-protein, high-fiber diet distributed over 4 to 5 moderate meals.

○ 2. A low-fat, bland diet distributed over 5 to 6 small feedings.

○ 3. A high-calcium, soft diet distributed over 3 meals and an evening snack.

○ 4. A diabetic exchange diet distributed over 3 meals and 2 snacks.

74. Pancreatic enzyme replacements are ordered for Mrs. Ottinger. The nurse should instruct her to take them

○ 1. 3 times daily between meals.

○ 2. with each meal and snack.

○ 3. in the morning and at bedtime.

○ 4. every 4 hours at specified times.

75. How should the nurse teach Mrs. Ottinger to monitor the effectiveness of the pancreatic enzyme replacement?

○ 1. Monitor her fluid intake.

○ 2. Perform regular fingersticks for glucose.

○ 3. Observe her stools for steatorrhea.

○ 4. Test her urine for ketones.

## THE PATIENT WITH HIATAL HERNIA

Ms. Janice Fox, age 45, is being worked up for a possible hiatal hernia. She has been self-medicating with antacids for symptoms of gastric acidity that have become progressively worse over the last 6 months. Ms. Fox works as a baker and her job involves lifting and carrying heavy pans and sacks of flour. She is 5-foot-1 and weighs 160 pounds.

76. In taking Ms. Fox's health history, the nurse would expect her to report that her symptoms are worse when she is

○ 1. lying down.

○ 2. physically active.

○ 3. upset or angry.

○ 4. sitting.

77. An upper GI series confirms that Ms. Fox has a sliding hiatal hernia. She asks what this means. Which of the following is the *most accurate* description?

○ 1. A hernia that develops at the lower esophageal sphincter, allowing stomach contents to regurgitate.

○ 2. A portion of the stomach is herniated into the thorax alongside the esophageal sphincter.

○ 3. A herniation in the diaphragm where the esophagus passes through it.

○ 4. Movement of the esophagogastric junction into the thorax or back to the abdomen in response to changing body positions.

78. Factors that may have contributed to the development of a hiatal hernia in Ms. Fox include *all* of the following *except* her

○ 1. age.

○ 2. weight.

○ 3. occupational activities.

○ 4. sex.

79. Self-care is the cornerstone of the management of hiatal hernia. Which of the following nursing interventions is *most* likely to promote Ms. Fox's self-care behaviors?

○ 1. Introduce her to other people who are successfully managing their care.

○ 2. Include her daughter in the teaching so she can help implement the plan.

○ 3. Ask her to identify other situations in which she demonstrated responsibility for herself.

○ 4. Assure her that she will be able to implement all aspects of the plan successfully.

80. Ms. Fox has been taking magnesium hydroxide (Milk of Magnesia) at home in an attempt to control her symptoms. The nurse should be aware that the most common complaint associated with the ongoing use of magnesium-based antacids is

○ 1. anorexia.

○ 2. weight gain.

○ 3. diarrhea.

○ 4. constipation.

81. Life-style modification is an important aspect of treatment for hiatal hernia. Which of the following should Ms. Fox include in her daily routine?

○ 1. Daily aerobic exercise.

○ 2. Eliminating smoking and alcohol.

○ 3. Carefully spacing activity periods with rest.

○ 4. Avoiding high-stress situations.

82. The nurse assess Ms. Fox's understanding of the relationship between body position and gastroesophageal reflux. Which response indicates that Ms. Fox understands measures to take to avoid problems with reflux while sleeping?

○ 1. "I elevate the foot of the bed 4" to 6"."

○ 2. "I sleep on my stomach with my head turned to the left."

○ 3. "I sleep on my back without a pillow under my head."

○ 4. "I elevate the head of the bed 4" to 6"."

83. In developing a teaching plan for Ms. Fox, the nurse's assessment of which work-related factors is *most* useful?

○ 1. Number and length of breaks.

○ 2. Body mechanics used in lifting.

○ 3. Temperature in work area.

○ 4. Cleaning solvents used.

**84.** Ms. Fox attends two sessions with the dietitian to learn about dietary modifications that will minimize problems with gastroesophageal reflux. The teaching would be successful if Ms. Fox says she will decrease her intake of

○ 1. fats.

○ 2. sodium-rich foods.

○ 3. carbohydrates.

○ 4. high-calcium foods.

**85.** Which of the following dietary measures can also be useful in preventing esophageal reflux?

○ 1. Eating small frequent meals; avoiding overeating.

○ 2. Belching frequently to reduce abdominal distention.

○ 3. Avoiding air-swallowing with meals.

○ 4. Reducing the size of the evening meal and adding a bedtime snack.

**86.** Ms. Fox reports that all of the following activities are part of her usual routine. Which is *most likely* to be associated with esophageal reflux and should be eliminated?

○ 1. Spending evenings sitting and watching television.

○ 2. Snacking at bedtime.

○ 3. Sampling her products at the bakery.

○ 4. Frequent attempts at dieting.

**87.** The physician prescribes metoclopramide hydrochloride (Reglan) for Ms. Fox. This drug is used in hiatal hernia therapy to

○ 1. increase the resting tone of the esophageal sphincter.

○ 2. neutralize gastric secretions.

○ 3. delay gastric emptying.

○ 4. reduce the secretion of digestive juices.

**88.** The nurse teaches Ms. Fox about metoclopramide hydrochloride (Reglan). Which of the following side effects has the potential to interfere with Ms. Fox's work?

○ 1. Constipation.

○ 2. Drowsiness.

○ 3. Restlessness.

○ 4. Transient hypertension.

**89.** Cimetidine (Tagamet) may also be used in the treatment of hiatal hernia. This drug is used to prevent

○ 1. esophageal reflux.

○ 2. the feeling of fullness after meals.

○ 3. esophagitis.

○ 4. ulcer formation.

**90.** Ms. Fox asks the nurse whether having a hernia means that she will need surgery to correct it. Which reply would be *most accurate* for the nurse to make?

○ 1. Surgery is usually required, although medical treatment is attempted first.

○ 2. The symptoms of hiatal hernia can usually be successfully managed through diet, medications, and life-style changes.

○ 3. Surgery is not performed for this type of hernia.

○ 4. A minor procedure to reduce the size of the diaphragmatic opening will probably be planned.

# CORRECT ANSWERS AND RATIONALES

Numbers appear in parentheses following the rationales. The numbers identify textbooks listed in the references at the end of Part IV, where correct answers can be verified.

## The Patient with Peptic Ulcer Disease

1. 4. Having the patient look toward the ceiling when the nurse inserts a nasogastric tube into the nostril facilitates tube insertion. When the tube reaches the nasopharyx, the patient should be instructed to bring his head forward a bit by flexing the neck. This technique closes the trachea and opens the esophagus to receive the tube. Correct techniques include firming a rubber tube for easier handling by placing it in ice chips for a few minutes (a plastic tube can be softened in warm water), lubricating the tube with a water-soluble lubricant, and having the patient swallow while the tube is passed into the stomach. (24, 36)

2. 1. The best way to determine whether a nasogastric tube is in the patient's stomach is to apply suction to the tube with a syringe and observe for the return of stomach contents. Another satisfactory method is to instill air into the tube with a syringe while auscultating over the epigastric area. Hearing the air enter the stomach helps ensure proper placement. If the tube is not in the stomach and solution is introduced, the solution will enter respiratory passages and harm the patient. Observing for air bubbles when the free end of the tube is placed under water and palpating for the presence of the tube are unacceptable methods of determining tube placement. (24, 36)

3. 3. In early shock, the body attempts to meet its perfusion needs through tachycardia, vasoconstriction, and fluid conservation. The patient may experience increased restlessness and anxiety from hypoxia. Urine output in early shock may be normal or slightly decreased. (25, 31)

4. 4. The body reacts to perforation of an ulcer by immobilizing the area as much as possible. This results in boardlike rigidity of the abdomen, and the abdomen is usually extremely tender. This may occur over several hours or days. Projectile vomiting, belching, and diarrhea are not associated with perforated ulcer. (25, 31)

5. 2. The digested blood in the stool causes it to be black. The odor of the stool is very offensive. (25, 31)

6. 1. Propantheline bromide (Pro-Banthine) is an anticholinergic drug. Anticholinergic drugs act to reduce the rate of secretion by the gastric, salivary, bronchial, and sweat glands. Anticholinergic drugs act by blocking ganglionic action in the autonomic nervous system. (12, 25)

7. 3. Clinical manifestations of anxiety include pale skin, rapid heart rate, dry lips and mouth, and increased blood pressure. These manifestations are the result of epinephrine. (30, 38)

8. 1. A laxative is administered following an upper GI series. This examination involves the administration of barium, which must be eliminated from the body because it may harden and cause an obstruction. (25, 31)

9. 3. Aluminum products, such as aluminum hydroxide, form insoluble salts in the body. They precipitate and accumulate in the intestines to cause constipation. (12, 25)

10. 3. Pain associated with duodenal ulcers usually occurs within 2 to 4 hours after eating. Food passes through the duodenum and the action of digestive juices on exposed nerve endings triggers the pain. (25, 31)

11. 1. Milk and cream are not considered central to peptic ulcer therapy because they increase the secretion of gastric acids. They do, however, neutralize the resulting acidity and are not contraindicated for use. (6, 25)

12. 4. Pepper is to be avoided because it seems to irritate the gastrointestinal mucosa. (6, 25)

13. 1. A simple "yes" or "no" question, such as the nurse posed in this situation, tends to elicit a noncommittal response that usually discourages further conversation. In general, a cliché-type question, such as that posed in this item, should be avoided because of its limited value in eliciting useful information concerning the patient's possible problems. (11, 38)

14. 3. Alcohol can stimulate gastric acid secretion and break down the gastric mucosal barrier, resulting in gastritis. If foods that are thought to increase gastric acid, such as cola, coffee, and tea, lead to discomfort, they should be avoided. (25, 41)

15. 2. Current nutritional therapy for patients with peptic ulcers is best expressed by the statement, "The type of diet appears to be less important than including foods the patient tolerates." There is no evidence that special diets promote healing of an uncomplicated peptic ulcer regardless of the patient's age. Eating frequent small meals was once

suggested, but because eating stimulates acid production, most authorities now recommend eating three meals a day consisting of foods the patient tolerates well. (25, 41)

**16.** 1. The patient who has had an upper GI endoscopy should be monitored for return of the gag reflex. An upper GI endoscopy does not affect bowel sounds or breath sounds. (25, 31)

**17.** 2. Rest is an essential component of ulcer healing. Nurses can help patients understand the importance of rest and find ways to balance work and family demands so permanent healing is possible. Nurses cannot demand these changes; patients must choose them. (25, 31)

**18.** 4. Although patients cannot eliminate stress from their lives, they can improve their ability to cope with it. Identifying stressors at work, setting goals a little lower, and considering a job change may help a patient deal with stress, but improving the ability to cope with stress is most important. (25, 31)

**19.** 2. One of nicotine's effects on the body is to increase the secretion of epinephrine, which causes vasoconstriction. In addition, cigarette smoking has carcinogenic effects on the lungs. Chronic dyspepsia often results from cigarette smoking, and therefore the already irritated gastrointestinal mucosa in patients with peptic ulcers appears to be further irritated by heavy smoking. (25, 31)

**20.** 2. Cimetidine (Tagamet) acts to decrease gastric acid secretion and should be taken regularly with meals. (12, 16)

## The Patient with Cholecystitis

**21.** 4. A high-fat diet is not a risk factor in the development of cholelithiasis. The condition occurs most commonly in overweight middle-aged women who have experienced multiple pregnancies, although the etiologic relationships are unclear. (25, 31)

**22.** 1. Administering pain medication has the highest priority during the first hour after the patient's admission. Completing the admission history, maintaining hydration, and teaching about planned diagnostic tests are part of the patient's care but do not have the highest priority. (25, 31)

**23.** 1. Nitroglycerin relaxes all smooth muscles, and the pain associated with cholecystitis and cholelithiasis is most probably caused by spasms of smooth muscles in the biliary tract. Although used most commonly in the treatment of angina pectoris because it relaxes and dilates the large arteries in the heart, nitroglycerin also relaxes biliary, renal, bronchial, uterine, and gastrointestinal smooth

muscle. Nitroglycerin does not relieve nausea and vomiting, enhance the action of meperidine hydrochloride (Demerol), or decrease the secretion of gastric acids. (5, 26)

**24.** 1. Applying a tourniquet obstructs venous blood flow and distends the veins. (24, 36)

**25.** 2. When bile is not reaching the intestine, the feces will not contain bile pigments. The stool then becomes gray, claylike, or putty-like in color. Black stool can be caused by upper gastrointestinal bleeding and by medications such as iron. (25, 31)

**26.** 4. A patient with an obstruction of the common bile duct should be monitored for prolonged bleeding time. Such an obstruction prevents bile from entering the intestinal tract. An absence of bile in this tract prevents absorption of fat-soluble vitamins A, D, E, and K. Vitamin K is necessary for the formation of prothrombin. Prothrombin deficiency causes delayed clotting of the blood, which results in prolonged bleeding time. (25, 31)

**27.** 2. Several common iodine compounds are used as radiographic contrast media, one being iopanoic acid (Telepaque). These compounds should not be administered to the patient with iodine and seafood allergies because anaphylaxis may occur. (25, 31)

**28.** 2. Choledochotomy means an opening into the common bile duct. The suffix "otomy" means incision. The root "choledocho" means the common bile duct. A choledochotomy may be done to remove stones, but the removal of stones is not implied in the term itself. (26, 31)

**29.** 3. The high incision used for gallbladder surgery is quite near the diaphragm and makes deep-breathing very painful. Incentive spirometry is essential to prevent the development of atelectasis after surgery. (25, 31)

**30.** 4. Incentive spirometry promotes lung expansion and increases respiratory function. When used properly, an incentive spirometer causes sustained maximal inspiration and increases cardiac output. (25, 31)

**31.** 2. Oral food and fluids are withheld prior to surgery when a patient has general anesthesia primarily to help prevent vomiting. When vomiting occurs during surgery, the patient may aspirate stomach contents. Withholding food and fluids prior to surgery does not prevent constipation, gas pains, or distention in the postoperative period, nor does it relieve pressure on the diaphragm. (25, 31)

**32.** 2. The muscle into which the nurse will inject the medication when using the ventrogluteal site is the gluteus minimus muscle. The rectus femoris muscle is on the anterior aspect of the thigh. The gluteus maximus muscle is located on the buttock and is used for injecting the dorsogluteal site. The vastus lateralis muscle is located on the lateral aspect of the thigh. (24, 36)

**33.** 4. A T-tube is used after exploration of the common duct to help prevent bile from spilling into the peritoneal cavity. The tube also helps maintain patency of the common duct and helps ensure drainage of bile out of the body until the edema in the common duct subsides sufficiently for bile to drain into the duodenum. A Penrose drain promotes blood and serosanguineous drainage from a wound. A T-tube is not used to irrigate the biliary tract or to minimize passage of bile into the duodenum. (26, 31)

**34.** 3. The T-tube usually drains 300 to 500 ml in the first 24 hours after surgery. After 3 to 4 days, the amount decreases to less than 200 ml per 24 hours. (25, 31)

**35.** 2. T-tube drainage is recorded separately on the output record. Adding it to other output makes it difficult to determine the amount of bile drainage. The patient's total intake will be incorrect if drainage is subtracted from it. (24, 36)

**36.** 1. Bile is erosive and extremely irritating to the skin. Therefore, it is essential that skin around the T-tube be kept clean and dry. (25, 31)

**37.** 1. Prochlorperazine dimaleate (Compazine) is used to control nausea, vomiting, and retching. In doses larger than those used to control nausea and vomiting, prochlorperazine dimaleate is used in psychotherapy because of its effects on mood and behavior. (12, 16)

**38.** 3. Bile flows almost continuously into the intestine for the first few weeks after removal of the gallbladder. Limiting the amount of fat in the intestine at one time ensures that an adequate amount of bile will be available to facilitate digestion. There is no need to eliminate foods with fiber, and doing so would tend to increase (rather than decrease) pressure within the large intestine (not the small intestine). Eating large amounts of meats, cheese, and peanut butter would be undesirable because they are often high in fat. Removing the gallbladder does not stop pancreatic secretions. (37, 41)

**39.** 4. Lean meats, such as beef, lamb, and veal, and *well-trimmed* lean ham and pork are low in fat. Ham and egg salad are high in fat because of the fat in salad dressings. Rice, pasta, and fresh, frozen, dried, and canned vegetables are low in fat when they are not served with butter, cream, or sauces containing whole milk, cream, or butter. Fruits are low in fat. (37, 41)

## The Patient with Cancer of The Stomach

**40.** 3. Total parenteral nutrition bypasses the enteral route and provides total nutrition: protein, carbohydrates, fats, vitamins, minerals, and trace elements. Oral and tube feedings would enter the stomach and could cause the symptoms of fullness, nausea, and vomiting that the patient had prior to admission. Intravenous isotonic saline provides incomplete nutrition: water, sodium, and chloride only. (26, 31)

**41.** 2. If the patient understands the reasons for prescribed treatments, he is more likely to participate and cooperate with the plan. Fear of the unknown can increase anxiety. Cancer of the stomach has a poor prognosis; 5% to 10% of all patients live 5 years. No useful purpose is served by making the patient feel guilty about delaying medical care. (5, 26)

**42.** 2. A Billroth II procedure bypasses the duodenum and anastomoses the stump of the stomach directly to the jejunum. The pyloric sphincter is sacrificed along with some of the stomach fundus. The cardiac sphincter remains intact. (5, 26)

**43.** 4. The surgical procedure usually involves an abdominal approach, and the chest cavity is not entered. There are more secretions and drainage, and they may contain some blood for the first 12 hours. Because the remaining part of the stomach produces secretions and acts as a reservoir, the feeding process is begun earlier and progresses more rapidly. Subtotal gastrectomy does not halt production of intrinsic factor, the gastric secretion needed for absorption of vitamin $B_{12}$ from the gastrointestinal tract. Therefore, life-long vitamin $B_{12}$ injections are not needed. (5, 26)

**44.** 1. Nasogastric suctioning is ordered to remove gas or fluid (secretions) that accumulate. Excessive fluid can cause pressure on suture lines, resulting in injury, rupture, or dislodgement. Ascitic fluid collects in the peritoneal space. The gastrointestinal tract should remain empty (no food or fluids) until peristalsis returns and suture lines have healed adequately, at which time the nasogastric tube is removed. Oral feedings are attempted before resorting to tube feeding. Antacids are not used to promote healing of suture lines postoperatively. (25, 31)

**45.** 1. Gastric drainage the first 12 to 24 hours after subtotal gastrectomy is normally brown, which indicates digested blood. Drainage during the first 6 to 12 hours contains some bright-red blood, but large amounts of blood or excessive bloody drainage should be reported to the physician promptly. Green or cloudy-white drainage is not expected the first 12 to 24 hours after subtotal gastrectomy. (25, 31)

**46.** 3. These symptoms indicate that gas and secretions are accumulating within the remaining gastric pouch due to impairment of peristalsis or edema at the operative site. These symptoms indicate that the drainage system is not working properly. Saline solution is used to irrigate nasogastric tubes. Hypotonic solutions (water) would increase electrolyte loss. A physician's order is needed to irrigate nasogastric tubes. Following gastric surgery, only the surgeon repositions the nasogastric tube because of the danger of rupturing or dislodging the suture line. The amount of suction varies with the type of tube used and is ordered by the physician. (25, 31)

**47.** 3. The nurse records the total amount of solution used to irrigate a gastric tube as intake. The total amount of return in the drainage bottle is recorded as output. (24, 36)

**48.** 3. Applying a water-soluble lubricant to the nares helps alleviate sore nares when a gastric tube is in place. Measures such as irrigating and repositioning the tube and having the patient change position do not relieve irritation from the tube. Also, repositioning the tube may cause further problems by dislodging a scab or breaking open an ulceration. (24, 36)

**49.** 4. The primary purpose of replacement therapy for a patient with gastric suction is to maintain fluid and electrolyte balance. Gastric suctioning interrupts the normal intake of fluids, and therefore intravenous replacement therapy is indicated. (5, 26)

**50.** 4. The semi-Fowler's position facilitates the drainage of the remaining stomach, thus decreasing the possibility of regurgitation, which could result in aspiration of gastric contents. The position also allows for greater expansion of the chest wall and contraction of the diaphragm. All other options are factors that contribute to respiratory problems. Breathing and coughing cause pain in patients with high abdominal incisions. Splinting of the chest occurs, which decreases coughing and deep-breathing efforts. Shallow breathing leads to hypoventilation and atelectasis. Weak and fatigued patients have a decreased cough effort and cannot move well. Secretions in the gastric stump may collect due to decreased peristalsis and edema around the anastomosis. This increases the risk of regurgitation and aspiration. (5, 31)

**51.** 2. Coughing and deep-breathing are more effective when pain is minimal. A patient tends to limit movement and breathe shallowly to decrease incisional pain. Enough pain medication should be given to decrease pain without depressing respirations; this allows the patient to cough effectively. Deep-breathing exercises should be done at least every 2 hours. Ambulation to increase ventilation and gas exchange should be encouraged as soon as possible postoperatively (usually the 1st postoperative day). (5, 31)

**52.** 3. When a patient with a nasogastric tube becomes distended, the nurse should first check the suction machine. If the equipment is functioning properly, she should then take other steps, such as checking the patency of the tube. (24, 36)

**53.** 2. The normal serum potassium level in an adult is between 3.5 and 5.5 mEq/L. (20, 25)

**54.** 3. An early indication of hypokalemia is muscle weakness in the legs. Potassium is essential for proper neuromuscular impulse transmission. When the mechanism is impaired, as in hypokalemia, leg muscles become weak and flabby. If hypokalemia progresses, respiratory muscles become involved, and the patient becomes apneic. Hypokalemia also causes electrocardiogram changes. Diarrhea is common in hyperkalemia. Tingling in the fingers and around the mouth occurs in hypocalcemia. Sticky mucous membranes are common in hypernatremia. (20, 25)

**55.** 1. Pain, fever, and dyspnea are symptoms of inflammation/peritonitis. An anastomotic leak becomes apparent when the ingestion of oral fluids challenges the integrity of the suture line. Diarrhea with fat in the stool is steatorrhea. Palpitations, pallor, and diaphoresis after eating are vasomotor symptoms of the dumping syndrome. Nausea and feeling full are symptoms of gastric retention. (25, 31)

**56.** 2. Because of the stomach's reduced capacity, frequent small feedings are recommended. Early satiety can result and large quantities of food are not well tolerated. Each patient should progress at his own pace; gradually increasing the amount of food eaten at each meal is the key. The goal is 3 meals a day *if possible*, but this can take 6 months or longer to achieve. Nausea can be episodic and can result from eating too fast or eating too much at one time. Eating less and more slowly, rather than not eating at all, can be a solution. Bland foods are recommended as starting foods because they are more easily digested and less irritating to the healing mucosa. (5, 26)

**57.** 2. Following a gastric resection, ingested food moves rapidly from the remaining stomach into the duodenum or jejunum. The food has not undergone adequate preliminary digestion in the stomach. It is concentrated, distends the intestine, and stimulates a significant secretion of insulin by the pancreas. The dumping syndrome is a result of these factors, which are initiated by the rapid movement of food out of the stomach. (25, 31)

**58.** 3. Faintness, weakness, a full feeling, dizziness, excessive perspiration, and diarrhea are characteristic symptoms of the dumping syndrome. (25, 31)

**59.** 4. Carbohydrates are restricted but protein is recommended because it digests more slowly. Fluids are restricted to reduce the bulk of food, and patients are encouraged to lie on their left side to decrease movement of the food bolus. (25, 31)

**60.** 4. Weight gain will be slow and gradual since less food can be eaten at one time due to the decreased size of the remaining stomach. Rapid weight gain over a short time may be due to fluid retention (1 pint = 1 pound). More food and fluid will be tolerated as edema at the suture line decreases and healing occurs. The remaining stomach may stretch over time to accommodate more food. Food intake will be greater if nausea and vomiting are absent. (5, 26)

## The Patient with Pancreatitis

**61.** 3. Pancreatitis is an acute inflammation of the pancreas that creates edema and congestion. Normal secretions are obstructed and the pancreatic enzymes may be activated within the pancreas itself, causing extensive autodigestion and destruction. (25, 31)

**62.** 2. The pancreas functions as both an endocrine and an exocrine gland. The exocrine cells of the pancreas secrete amylase, lipase, trypsinogen, and chymotrypsin, which aid in protein and fat digestion and the breakdown of starch. (25, 31)

**63.** 1. The primary diagnostic tests for pancreatitis are serum levels of amylase and lipase and urine levels of amylase. Serum amylase is the most commonly used test; the result may be above 200 Somogyi units/dL. (25, 31)

**64.** 3. Premature activation of pancreatic enzymes within the pancreas, rather than in the duodenum, causes the autodigestion process that produces pancreatitis. Spasm of the sphincter of Oddi is not the causative factor. Increased gastric secretions can aggravate pancreatitis by stimulating the pancreas. Volume depletion is a consequence of pancreatitis. (5, 26)

**65.** 1. Alcoholism is the major cause of acute pancreatitis in the United States. Since some patients are reluctant to discuss their alcohol use, staff may inquire about it in several ways. Alcohol intake does not interfere with the pertinent tests used to diagnose pancreatitis. However, acute alcohol ingestion may cause an increased serum amylase, and large amounts of ethyl and methyl alcohol may produce elevated urinary amylase levels. All hospitalized patients are asked about alcohol and drug use on admission but are not repeatedly asked about their use of alcohol and drugs. Physicians do seek all the facts, but this can be done with consideration of religious beliefs. Religious beliefs are pertinent to total patient care. (5, 26)

**66.** 1. Meperidine hydrochloride (Demerol), a strong narcotic analgesic, is effective for the pain of acute pancreatitis. Morphine sulfate and codeine sulfate are contraindicated in pancreatitis because they may cause spasm and increase the pain. Cimetidine (Tagamet), a histamine ($H_2$)-receptor antagonist, decreases gastric acidity. (26, 31)

**67.** 2. Life-threatening shock is a potential complication of pancreatitis. Kinin peptides activated by the trapped trypsin cause vasodilation and increased capillary permeability. These events worsen shock and are not easily reversed with pharmacologic agents such as vasopressors. (25, 31)

**68.** 1. Hypoglycemia would be unexpected. Pancreatitis interferes with beta cell functioning, and patients must be monitored carefully for the development of hyperglycemia. Hyperlipidemia and symptoms of gastrointestinal distress are also common. (25, 31)

**69.** 4. Hypocalcemia is one of the major potential complications of pancreatitis. Muscle twitching and irritability are primary symptoms of hypocalcemia. It is imperative that calcium replacement begin as soon as hypocalcemia is validated. Hypomagnesemia may occur due to vomiting in patients with pancreatitis, especially if they are malnourished. Serum glucose is elevated. Hypokalemia may occur with loss of gastric juice via vomiting or nasogastric suction. (26, 31)

**70.** 1. There is little definitive treatment for pancreatitis. It is important to suppress enzymes to reduce pancreatic stimulation. This is done by resting the gastrointestinal tract, and the patient is n.p.o. Preventing infections, ensuring nutrition and fluid and electrolyte balance are related issues but are not the focus of treatment. (25, 31)

**71.** 3. Antispasmodic drugs such as propantheline bromide (Pro-Banthine) may be administered in addition to narcotics to deal with the intense pain associated with pancreatitis. (25, 31)

**72.** 4. The patient is initially placed n.p.o. in an effort to provide complete rest for the gastrointestinal tract and reduce stimulation of the pancreas. (25, 31)

**73.** 2. The low-fat, bland diet prevents stimulation of the pancreas while providing adequate nutrition. While calcium is important, the low fat content is more significant. Dietary protein and fiber are not directly related to pancreatitis. The hyperglycemia of acute pancreatitis is usually transient and does not require long-term dietary modifications. (25, 31)

**74.** 2. Pancreatic enzymes are prescribed to facilitate the digestion of protein and fat and as such should be used in conjunction with every meal and snack. Specified hours for administration are ineffective, as the enzymes must be used in conjunction with food ingestion. (25, 31)

**75.** 3. If the dose and administration of pancreatic enzymes are adequate, the patient's stool will be relatively normal. Any increase in malodor or fat content would indicate that the dose needs to be adjusted. Stable body weight would be another indirect indicator. (5, 26)

## The Patient with Hiatal Hernia

**76.** 1. Hiatal hernia produces symptoms of esophageal reflux as the sphincter slides up into the negative-pressure environment of the thorax. The symptoms occur most commonly when patients are in a recumbent position. Neither emotions nor normal activity influence the incidence of reflux. (25, 32)

**77.** 4. In a sliding hiatal hernia, the esophagogastric junction slides between the abdomen and the thorax. It does not involve direct herniation of either the diaphragm or the esophageal sphincter. In the less common rolling hernia, the sphincter stays in position in the abdomen while a portion of the stomach moves up into the thorax. (25, 32)

**78.** 4. Any factor that increases intra-abdominal pressure can contribute to the development of hiatal hernia. Such factors include obesity, abdominal straining, and pregnancy. Hiatal hernia is also associated with aging and occurs in both males and females. (25, 31)

**79.** 3. Self-responsibility is the key to individual health maintenance. Using examples of situations in which the patient had demonstrated responsibility for herself can be very reinforcing and supporting. Meeting other people who are managing their care and involving family members can be helpful, but individual motivation is more important. Reassurance can be helpful but is less important than individualization of care. The individual has ultimate responsibility for personal health habits. (5, 26)

**80.** 3. The magnesium salts in magnesium hydroxide (Milk of Magnesia) are related to those found in laxatives and may cause diarrhea. Aluminum salt products can cause constipation. Many patients find that the use of a combination product is required to maintain normal bowel elimination. (12, 16)

**81.** 2. Smoking and alcohol use both reduce the tone of the esophageal sphincter and can result in reflux. These should be eliminated or reduced by patients with hiatal hernia. The other factors may increase the patient's general health and well-being but are not associated directly with hiatal hernia. (25, 31)

**82.** 4. Sleeping with the head of the bed elevated encourages the movement of food through the esophagus by gravity. By fostering esophageal acid clearance, gravity helps keep the acidic pepsin and alkaline biliary secretions from contacting the esophagus. Neither elevating the foot of the bed nor sleeping flat without a pillow under the head enhances this clearance. Sleeping on the right side minimizes problems for some people. (25, 31)

**83.** 2. Bending, especially after eating, can cause gastroesophageal reflux; lifting heavy objects increases intra-abdominal pressure. Knowing the patient's lifting technique enables the nurse to assess the patient's understanding of factors contributing to hiatal hernia and to methods that prevent complications. The other factors are not directly related to hiatal hernia. (25, 31)

**84.** 1. Fats decrease the lower esophageal sphincter pressure, which increases reflux. Since obesity contributes to the development of hiatal hernia, a low-fat diet might also aid in weight loss. Fat is the most concentrated source of calories. The other choices do not affect reflux. (25, 31)

**85.** 1. Esophageal reflux worsens when the stomach is overdistended with food. An important intervention, therefore, is to eat small frequent meals. Food intake in the evening should be strictly limited to reduce the incidence of nighttime reflux. (25, 31)

**86.** 2. Bedtime snacking increases the incidence of reflux at night. These episodes are the most severe and damaging and are worsened by the recumbent position of sleep. Bedtime snacking should be eliminated. (25, 31)

**87.** 1. Metoclopramide hydrochloride (Reglan) increases sphincter tone and facilitates gastric emptying; both actions reduce the incidence of reflux. Antacids or histamine receptor antagonists may also be prescribed to help control reflux and esophagitis. (12, 16)

**88.** 2. Drowsiness, restlessness, and anxiety are common side effects of metoclopramide hydrochloride (Reglan). A person whose job requires alertness

*antacid*

needs to avoid activities requiring alertness for 2 hours after each dose. The other side effects listed are not likely to interfere with the patient's work. (12, 16)

**89.** 3. Cimetidine (Tagamet) is a histamine receptor antagonist that decreases the quantity of gastric secretions. It may be used in hiatal hernia therapy to prevent or treat the esophagitis and heartburn symptoms associated with reflux. (12, 16)

**90.** 2. Surgery for hiatal hernia is extensive and produces frequent complications. It is used only when medical therapy fails to control the symptoms. Most patients can be successfully treated with a combination of diet, medications, weight control, and life-style modifications. The Nissen fundoplication is the surgery usually performed for intractable hiatal hernia. (25, 31)

# test 4

The Patient with Cancer of the Colon

The Patient with Hepatitis A

The Patient with Hemorrhoids

The Patient with Inflammatory Bowel Disease

The Patient with an Intestinal Obstruction

The Patient with Cirrhosis

Correct Answers and Rationales

Select the one *best* or *correct* answer and indicate your choice by filling in the circle with a pencil in front of the option you have chosen. If the answer you would prefer is not given, select the one you think is *most appropriate*.

## THE PATIENT WITH CANCER OF THE COLON

Mrs. Karla Long, 66, is admitted to the hospital for a diagnostic workup and probable surgery for a suspected diagnosis of cancer of the colon. She has been experiencing cramping pain in her lower abdomen and has noticed a gradual change in her elimination pattern.

1. Mrs. Long is scheduled for a barium enema. As part of her preparation, she is ordered to receive 60 ml of castor oil orally. Castor oil facilitates cleansing of the bowel *primarily* by
   - ○ 1. softening the feces.
   - ○ 2. lubricating the feces.
   - ○ 3. increasing the volume of intestinal contents.
   - ○ 4. irritating the nerve endings in the intestinal mucosa.

2. Following the barium enema, the nurse should be prepared to administer which type of medication to Mrs. Long?
   - ○ 1. A laxative.
   - ○ 2. An emetic.
   - ○ 3. An antacid.
   - ○ 4. A digestant.

3. The diagnosis of cancer is confirmed and Mrs. Long is scheduled for an abdominoperineal resection with permanent colostomy. Bowel preparation begins and includes an order for succinylsulfathiazole (Sulfasuxidine). Drugs of this type are used in bowel preparation *primarily* to help reduce
   - ○ 1. electrolyte disturbances.
   - ○ 2. bacterial content in the colon.
   - ○ 3. peristaltic action in the colon.
   - ○ 4. inflammation caused by the tumor.

4. If the position of the tumor permits a choice, the *preferred* site for creating a permanent colostomy for Mrs. Long would be in the
   - ○ 1. hepatic flexure.
   - ○ 2. splenic flexure.
   - ○ 3. lower portion of the descending colon.
   - ○ 4. middle portion of the transverse colon.

5. Mrs. Long requires a transfusion on her 2nd postoperative day and is ordered to receive 2 units of packed red blood cells. The nurse assembles a blood administration set-up in which the blood is hung in tandem with which solution?
   - ○ 1. Distilled water.
   - ○ 2. 0.9% saline solution.
   - ○ 3. 5% dextrose in distilled water.
   - ○ 4. 10% dextrose in normal saline.

6. Which of the following actions should the nurse take *first* when Mrs. Long complains of a headache and tingling sensations in her fingers shortly after the blood transfusion is started?
   - ○ 1. Notify the physician.
   - ○ 2. Check for infiltration.
   - ○ 3. Slow the rate of the infusion.
   - ○ 4. Stop the infusion of blood.

7. Which of the following nursing interventions would be *inappropriate* during Mrs. Long's postoperative period?
   - ○ 1. Encourage the patient to practice diaphragmatic breathing.
   - ○ 2. Teach the patient to cough against a closed glottis.
   - ○ 3. Raise the knee gatch of the bed to prevent the patient from sliding down in bed.
   - ○ 4. Apply thigh-high antiembolism stockings.

8. Mrs. Long had a nasogastric tube inserted at the time of surgery. This tube will *most likely* be removed when the patient demonstrates

○ 1. absence of bowel sounds.

○ 2. passage of mucus from the rectum.

○ 3. passage of flatus and feces from the colostomy.

○ 4. absence of stomach drainage for about 24 hours.

9. After Mrs. Long's nasogastric tube is removed, the doctor orders a clear liquid diet for her. Which of the following foods would be *inappropriate* on this diet?

○ 1. Beef broth.

○ 2. Apple juice.

○ 3. Tea with sugar.

○ 4. Vanilla ice cream.

10. Mrs. Long indicates that she is ready to learn about her colostomy. Which of the following nursing interventions is *most likely* to be effective in preparing Mrs. Long to look at her colostomy?

○ 1. Telling the patient how normal body functions will continue.

○ 2. Encouraging the patient to ask questions about the colostomy.

○ 3. Asking a member of the local ostomy club to visit the patient.

○ 4. Using illustrative material during teaching sessions with the patient.

11. A colostomy irrigation is ordered for Mrs. Long on her 5th postoperative day. The *primary* purpose of this first irrigation is to

○ 1. cleanse the colon.

○ 2. regulate the bowel.

○ 3. dilate the sphincter.

○ 4. stimulate peristalsis.

12. If Mrs. Long complains of abdominal cramping after receiving approximately 150 ml of solution during the colostomy irrigation, the nurse should temporarily

○ 1. stop the flow of solution.

○ 2. have the patient sit up in bed.

○ 3. remove the irrigating cone or tube.

○ 4. insert the cone or tube further into the colon.

13. If the nurse uses the following measures while changing Mrs. Long's soiled colostomy bag, which would be *least likely* to convey acceptance of the patient's altered body image?

○ 1. Putting on gloves before starting the procedure.

○ 2. Discussing subjects of interest with the patient.

○ 3. Encouraging the patient to assist to the extent that she wishes.

○ 4. Explaining that the patient will be taught the procedure when she is ready.

14. A clue that Mrs. Long is ready to participate in her care would be present if, while the nurse is changing the patient's colostomy bag and dressing, the patient

○ 1. asks what time her physician will visit that day.

○ 2. asks about the supplies used during the dressing change.

○ 3. talks about something she read in the morning newspaper.

○ 4. complains about the way the night nurse changed the dressing.

15. Appropriate skin care will be an important aspect of patient teaching for Mrs. Long. Which of the following preparations would be *best* to apply around her colostomy?

○ 1. Karaya.

○ 2. Petrolatum.

○ 3. Cornstarch.

○ 4. Antiseptic cream.

16. Which of the following measures would most effectively promote wound healing after Mrs. Long's perineal drains have been removed?

○ 1. Taking sitz baths.

○ 2. Taking daily showers.

○ 3. Applying warm moist dressings to the area.

○ 4. Applying a protected heating pad to the area.

17. When planning diet teaching for Mrs. Long, the nurse should develop a teaching plan based on the knowledge that

○ 1. foods containing roughage should be eliminated from the diet of a person with a colostomy.

○ 2. liquids are best limited in the diet of a patient with a colostomy to prevent diarrhea.

○ 3. patients with colostomies must experiment to determine the balance of food best for them.

○ 4. a constipating diet will produce a formed stool that can be passed with more regularity through a colostomy.

## THE PATIENT WITH HEPATITIS A

Charles Hardy, a 22-year-old college student, is admitted to the hospital. He is acutely ill with hepatitis A (infectious hepatitis).

18. The nurse would expect Mr. Hardy to exhibit *all* of the following symptoms during the acute phase of hepatitis *except*

○ 1. loss of appetite.

○ 2. yellowing of the sclera.

○ 3. shortness of breath.

○ 4. dark frothy urine.

19. Which of the following precautions has the *lowest priority* in planning appropriate care for Mr. Hardy?

○ 1. Using disposable dishes.

○ 2. Double-bagging and tagging his soiled linens.

○ 3. Assigning him to a private room.

○ 4. Wearing a gown and gloves when giving direct care.

**20.** The nurse prepares a nursing care plan for Mr. Hardy. Nursing orders should reflect that the *primary* treatment for Mr. Hardy will be concerned with ensuring that he receives

○ 1. adequate bed rest.

○ 2. a generous fluid intake.

○ 3. regular antibiotic therapy.

○ 4. daily intravenous electrolyte therapy.

**21.** Which of the following test results would the nurse monitor to assess Mr. Hardy's liver function?

○ 1. Glucose tolerance.

○ 2. Creatinine clearance.

○ 3. Serum transaminase.

○ 4. Serum electrolytes.

**22.** Which of the following diets is *most likely* to be prescribed for Mr. Hardy?

○ 1. A high-fat diet.

○ 2. A high-protein diet.

○ 3. A high-carbohydrate diet.

○ 4. A well-balanced diet.

**23.** Mr. Hardy's prescribed activity level is bed rest with bathroom privileges. The *primary* purpose of bed rest for Mr. Hardy is to

○ 1. reduce the body's need for oxygen.

○ 2. reduce metabolic demands on the liver.

○ 3. control the spread of the disease.

○ 4. prevent the breakdown of stored fat.

**24.** Although it is present in other secretions, the virus causing hepatitis A will be excreted from Mr. Hardy's body *primarily* through his

○ 1. skin.

○ 2. feces.

○ 3. urine.

○ 4. mucus.

**25.** Contaminated hands are often responsible for the transmission of hepatitis. In addition, the virus that caused Mr. Hardy's hepatitis is *very often* spread by

○ 1. infected insects.

○ 2. infected rodents and birds.

○ 3. contaminated food and liquids.

○ 4. contaminated clothing and eating utensils.

**26.** Mr. Hardy expresses concern because he fears members of his fraternity may also acquire hepatitis. Which of the following is *most commonly* used for prophylactic treatment of persons exposed to hepatitis A?

○ 1. Penicillin.

○ 2. Sulfadiazine (Microsulfon).

○ 3. Immune serum globulin.

○ 4. Hepatitis A vaccine.

**27.** Mr. Hardy's convalescence will continue at home for a number of weeks. A very *typical* symptom that he is likely to experience during this period is

○ 1. fatigue.

○ 2. insomnia.

○ 3. constipation.

○ 4. a low-grade fever.

**28.** In preparing Mr. Hardy for his extended convalescence, the nurse teaches him about problems that may occur. The nurse knows that Mr. Hardy has understood the teaching when he tells her that he is *most likely* to have difficulty

○ 1. controlling his pain.

○ 2. maintaining a regular bowel elimination pattern.

○ 3. preventing respiratory complications.

○ 4. maintaining a positive, optimistic outlook.

**29.** As a result of having had hepatitis A, Mr. Hardy should be instructed *never* to

○ 1. drink alcohol.

○ 2. donate blood.

○ 3. smoke.

○ 4. eat fatty foods.

**30.** The nurses caring for Mr. Hardy are concerned about the increasing incidence of both hepatitis A and hepatitis B among hospitalized patients. Research shows that nurses are at the *highest risk* for acquiring hepatitis B in which patient care area?

○ 1. Operating room.

○ 2. Emergency department.

○ 3. Intensive-care units.

○ 4. Kidney dialysis units.

**31.** Which of the following *best* explains the marked increase in the number of cases and carriers of hepatitis B in the United States today?

○ 1. Widespread use of marijuana.

○ 2. Sexual permissiveness.

○ 3. Low standards for testing blood donors.

○ 4. Growing numbers of intravenous drug abusers.

## THE PATIENT WITH HEMORRHOIDS

Mrs. Lorene O'Day, 36, is admitted for an elective hemorrhoidectomy. She has had increasing problems with hemorrhoids over the last 5 years and her physician is concerned that the hemorrhoids may become thrombosed.

**32.** If Mrs. O'Day reports that she experiences a small amount of rectal bleeding every time she has a

bowel movement, the nurse would recognize that Mrs. O'Day has
○ 1. internal hemorrhoids.
○ 2. external hemorrhoids.
○ 3. prolapsed hemorrhoids.
○ 4. strangulated hemorrhoids.

33. Which of the following factors in Mrs. O'Day's nursing history is most likely a *primary* cause of her hemorrhoids?
○ 1. Her age.
○ 2. Three pregnancies with vaginal deliveries.
○ 3. Her job as a schoolteacher.
○ 4. Varicosities in her legs.

34. Although Mrs. O'Day has elected to have surgery, her hemorrhoids could also be effectively treated by *all* of the following methods *except*
○ 1. rubber-band ligation.
○ 2. injection of sclerosing substance.
○ 3. cryosurgery.
○ 4. inducing fibrosis and shrinkage with phenol in oil.

35. Prior to surgery, the nurse would expect which of the following diets to be prescribed for Mrs. O'Day?
○ 1. High-protein, soft.
○ 2. Low-roughage, high-fiber.
○ 3. High-roughage, high-fiber.
○ 4. Bland, soft.

36. Mrs. O'Day is to have a cleansing enema before surgery. In which of the following positions should the nurse place Mrs. O'Day prior to administering the enema?
○ 1. The prone position.
○ 2. The knee-chest position.
○ 3. The left lateral position.
○ 4. The right lateral position.

37. Meperidine hydrochloride (Demerol) and diazepam (Valium) are to be given to Mrs. O'Day preoperatively. How should the nurse prepare these drugs for intramuscular injection?
○ 1. Draw up each drug in a separate syringe and give two injections.
○ 2. Draw up the diazepam first in a syringe and then draw up the meperidine hydrochloride in the same syringe.
○ 3. Draw up the meperidine hydrochloride first in a syringe and then draw up diazepam in the same syringe.
○ 4. Draw up both drugs in one syringe; it makes no difference which drug is drawn up first.

38. Mrs. O'Day is 5-foot-6 and weighs 115 pounds. When all of the following needles are available, which should be the nurse's *first* choice for administering Mrs. O'Day's preoperative medications intramuscularly?

○ 1. A 19G, 1½″ needle.
○ 2. A 20G, 1″ needle.
○ 3. A 22G, 1½″ needle.
○ 4. A 26G, 1″ needle.

39. Immediately after surgery, the *priority* goal of nursing care for Mrs. O'Day should be to
○ 1. prevent venous stasis.
○ 2. promote ambulation.
○ 3. control pain.
○ 4. prevent infection.

40. Which position would be *ideal* for Mrs. O'Day in the early postoperative period?
○ 1. High Fowler's.
○ 2. Supine.
○ 3. Prone.
○ 4. Trendelenburg.

41. Mrs. O'Day says she feels the urge to void but cannot empty her bladder. Urinary retention often occurs after hemorrhoidectomy and is usually directly related to
○ 1. anesthesia.
○ 2. reflex spasm.
○ 3. perineal edema.
○ 4. anxiety.

42. Warm sitz baths are prescribed three or four times a day after surgery. Implementation should be delayed until at least 12 hours postoperatively to avoid inducing
○ 1. hemorrhage.
○ 2. rectal spasm.
○ 3. urinary retention.
○ 4. constipation.

43. Mrs. O'Day is to continue sitz baths after discharge, and the nurse has been teaching her the proper procedure for taking them. The nurse believes that she has understood the teaching when she says that it is *most important* to take a sitz bath
○ 1. first thing each morning.
○ 2. as needed for discomfort.
○ 3. after a bowel movement.
○ 4. at bedtime.

44. Mrs. O'Day says she feels the urge to have her first postoperative bowel movement but is very concerned about the potential pain. Which of the following responses indicates the nurse's understanding of appropriate pain-alleviation techniques?
○ 1. "I'll get you a pain pill right away."
○ 2. "As soon as you've had a bowel movement, take a warm sitz bath."
○ 3. "After the bowel movement, cleanse the rectal area with warm water."
○ 4. "You may have some pain, but I'll give you pain medication."

45. The nurse has been teaching Mrs. O'Day how to avoid a recurrence of hemorrhoids and has explained the importance of a high-fiber diet. Mrs. O'Day's selection of which breakfast menu indicates that she understands the instructions?
    ○ 1. Danish pastry, prune juice, coffee, and milk.
    ○ 2. Oatmeal, milk, grapefruit wedges, and bran muffin.
    ○ 3. Corn flakes, milk, white toast, and orange juice.
    ○ 4. Scrambled eggs, bacon, English muffin, and apple juice.
46. Mrs. O'Day is discharged with instructions to take psyllium hydrophilic mucilloid (Metamucil) twice daily. This preparation will help prevent constipation during the healing period by
    ○ 1. increasing the bulk of the stool.
    ○ 2. softening the stool.
    ○ 3. controlling irritating flatus.
    ○ 4. stimulating peristalsis through contact irritation.

## THE PATIENT WITH INFLAMMATORY BOWEL DISEASE

Mr. Samuel Goldstein, 24, has suffered from ulcerative colitis for the last 5 years. He is currently in his final year of law school and has recently begun a clerkship with a local law firm. He is admitted to the hospital with an exacerbation of his disease with which he has attempted to cope at home for the last 10 days.

47. From her knowledge of ulcerative colitis, the nurse would expect that Mr. Goldstein's *primary* symptom has been
    ○ 1. anorexia.
    ○ 2. abdominal cramping.
    ○ 3. profuse diarrhea.
    ○ 4. bloating.
48. It has been several years since Mr. Goldstein had a complete physical examination and his physician orders a proctosigmoidoscopy. The nurse realizes that adjustments will be necessary in the routine preparation for this test because
    ○ 1. routine preparation is needed only for patients over 40 years of age.
    ○ 2. administration of cathartics to a person with severe diarrhea may aggravate electrolyte imbalances.
    ○ 3. routine preparation would be too uncomfortable for a patient with ulcerative colitis.
    ○ 4. routine preparation would make it more difficult to locate the source of mucus and pus.

49. Which of the following factors was most likely of *greatest* significance in causing an exacerbation of Mr. Goldstein's disease?
    ○ 1. He reports that the law clerkship is very demanding and he's worried about "measuring up."
    ○ 2. He has recently begun following a modified vegetarian diet.
    ○ 3. He has been working out with weights for the last 3 months.
    ○ 4. He has begun attending a holistic health group with his girlfriend.
50. Which goal for Mr. Goldstein's care will take *priority* during the initial portion of his hospitalization?
    ○ 1. Promoting self-care and independence.
    ○ 2. Stopping the diarrhea.
    ○ 3. Maintaining adequate nutrition.
    ○ 4. Promoting rest and comfort.
51. Mr. Goldstein is following orders for bed rest with bathroom privileges. What is the *primary* rationale for his activity restriction?
    ○ 1. To conserve energy.
    ○ 2. To reduce intestinal peristalsis.
    ○ 3. To promote rest and comfort.
    ○ 4. To prevent injury.
52. Mr. Goldstein's symptoms have been present for over a week. The nurse recognizes that he should be assessed carefully for signs of
    ○ 1. congestive heart failure.
    ○ 2. deep vein thrombosis.
    ○ 3. hypokalemia.
    ○ 4. hypocalcemia.
53. The nurse should include *all* of the following measures in Mr. Goldstein's care *except*
    ○ 1. encouraging deep-breathing.
    ○ 2. suggesting sitz baths p.r.n.
    ○ 3. keeping a bedpan at the bedside.
    ○ 4. wearing a gown to provide direct care.
54. Mr. Goldstein is quite thin and has lost 12 pounds since the exacerbation of his disease. The physician decides on a short course of hyperalimentation to correct Mr. Goldstein's nutritional deficiencies. The site of choice for administering total parenteral nutrition is the
    ○ 1. subclavian vein.
    ○ 2. innominate vein.
    ○ 3. superior vena cava.
    ○ 4. internal jugular vein.
55. The basic component of Mr. Goldstein's total parenteral nutrition solution is *most likely* to be
    ○ 1. an isotonic glucose solution.
    ○ 2. a hypertonic glucose solution.
    ○ 3. a hypotonic dextrose solution.
    ○ 4. a low-molecular-weight dextrose solution.
56. The nurse regularly assesses Mr. Goldstein's abil-

ity to metabolize the total parenteral nutrition solution adequately by monitoring his
- ○ 1. pulse rate.
- ○ 2. blood pressure.
- ○ 3. temperature.
- ○ 4. urine.

**57.** Which of the following interventions should the nurse include in Mr. Goldstein's care in order to prevent complications associated with total parenteral nutrition administered via a central line?
- ○ 1. Use strict clean technique for all dressing changes.
- ○ 2. Tape all connections of the system.
- ○ 3. Encourage bed rest.
- ○ 4. Cover the insertion site with a moisture-proof dressing.

**58.** Which of the following would be the *best* indication that the goals for total parenteral nutrition are being achieved for Mr. Goldstein?
- ○ 1. Urine negative for glucose.
- ○ 2. A serum potassium level of 4.0.
- ○ 3. A serum glucose level of 96.
- ○ 4. A weight gain of one-half pound per day.

**59.** When Mr. Goldstein is able to tolerate oral fluids and food, he is started on an elemental diet. The purpose of an elemental diet is to
- ○ 1. allow rapid nutrient absorption from the upper gastrointestinal tract.
- ○ 2. enrich the amino acid content of the diet.
- ○ 3. provide mineral and electrolyte supplements.
- ○ 4. provide readily digestible forms of fat.

**60.** The doctor prescribes sulfasalazine (Azulfidine) for Mr. Goldstein and he is to continue taking it at home. What instructions should the nurse give Mr. Goldstein about taking this medication?
- ○ 1. "Avoid taking it with food."
- ○ 2. "Take the total dose at bedtime."
- ○ 3. "Take it with a full glass (240 ml) of water."
- ○ 4. "Stop taking it if your urine turns orange-yellow."

**61.** Mr. Goldstein expresses serious concerns about his career as an attorney because of the effects of stress on ulcerative colitis. Which course of action would it be *best* for the nurse to suggest?
- ○ 1. Review current coping mechanisms and develop alternatives, if needed.
- ○ 2. Consider a less stressful career that would use his current education.
- ○ 3. Ask his colleagues to help decrease the stress by giving him the easier cases.
- ○ 4. Prepare family members for the fact that he will need to work part-time.

**62.** Mr. Goldstein is to follow a well-balanced high-protein, high-calorie, low-residue diet. In addition, the nurse counsels him to minimize the use of which food group that typically is poorly tolerated by patients with ulcerative colitis?
- ○ 1. Eggs and egg products.
- ○ 2. High-fat foods.
- ○ 3. Milk and milk products.
- ○ 4. Highly seasoned foods.

**63.** Which of the following menu selections would be *most appropriate*, given Mr. Goldstein's diet restrictions?
- ○ 1. Roast beef sandwich.
- ○ 2. Strawberry shortcake.
- ○ 3. Fresh peaches.
- ○ 4. Caesar salad.

## THE PATIENT WITH AN INTESTINAL OBSTRUCTION

Mrs. Esther Martin, a 48-year-old line worker in an automobile plant, goes to the industrial nurse complaining of abdominal pain that occurs in waves. While in the office, Mrs. Martin becomes acutely nauseated and vomits. She is sent to the hospital; a bowel obstruction is suspected.

**64.** During the initial assessment of Mrs. Martin, high-pitched tinkling bowel sounds are heard on auscultation and dull sounds are heard on percussion. What is the rationale for the dull sounds?
- ○ 1. Hyperactive peristalsis.
- ○ 2. Excessive gas trapped in the intestine.
- ○ 3. The presence of a mass or tumor in the bowel.
- ○ 4. Fluid trapped in the intestine.

**65.** All of the following are symptoms of bowel obstruction. Which symptom is related *primarily* to small-bowel obstruction rather than large-bowel obstruction?
- ○ 1. Profuse vomiting.
- ○ 2. Crampy abdominal pain.
- ○ 3. Abdominal distention.
- ○ 4. High-pitched bowel sounds above the obstruction.

**66.** The physician orders intestinal decompression for Mrs. Martin using a Cantor tube. The *primary* purpose of intestinal tubes such as a Cantor tube is to
- ○ 1. remove fluid and gas from the intestine.
- ○ 2. prevent fluid accumulation in the stomach.
- ○ 3. break up the obstruction.
- ○ 4. provide an alternative route for drug administration.

**67.** As soon as the Cantor tube has been inserted, the nurse should instruct Mrs. Martin to

○ 1. lie still on her back.

○ 2. lie on her right side.

○ 3. lie on her left side.

○ 4. get up and sit in a chair.

**68.** *All* of the following statements about a Cantor tube are correct *except*

○ 1. it can be attached to suction.

○ 2. it contains a soft rubber bag filled with mercury.

○ 3. it is taped securely to the patient's cheek after insertion.

○ 4. its placement can be determined by fluoroscopy.

**69.** Which of the following measures would *most likely* be included in Mrs. Martin's care as soon as the Cantor tube has passed into the duodenum?

○ 1. Bed rest with bathroom privileges.

○ 2. Advance the tube 2″ to 4″ every 4 hours.

○ 3. Provide frequent mouth care.

○ 4. Provide ice chips for the patient to suck.

**70.** An intravenous cannula is inserted in order to replace fluid and electrolytes. What, in addition to vomiting, causes the volume depletion associated with intestinal obstruction?

○ 1. Fluid retention in the obstructed intestine.

○ 2. Increased skin permeability and vascularity.

○ 3. Increased insensible fluid loss.

○ 4. Compensatory increase in urinary output.

**71.** Mrs. Martin continues to have pain even though the Cantor tube is patent and draining. The doctor wants to delay administering pain medication. When Mrs. Martin asks for pain medication, what would be the nurse's best explanation?

○ 1. "Narcotics trigger the vomiting center and would cause more fluid loss."

○ 2. "Narcotics may mask symptoms of increased obstruction or complications."

○ 3. "There is some risk of becoming addicted to narcotics, so it is best to take them only when necessary."

○ 4. "Narcotics will interfere with the anesthetic if surgery is needed."

**72.** The Cantor tube has reached the desired point in the intestine, and Mrs. Martin tells the nurse that the tube is causing her discomfort. The nurse includes *all* of the following interventions in her plan to increase Mrs. Martin's comfort *except*

○ 1. applying a water-soluble lubricant to the external nares.

○ 2. encouraging her to brush her teeth every 4 hours.

○ 3. coiling extra tubing on the bed.

○ 4. taping the tube securely to the forehead.

**73.** Intestinal decompression has been successful but Mrs. Martin needs surgery to relieve the obstruc-

tion. The day before surgery, the nurse finds the following set of orders for Mrs. Martin. Which order should the nurse question before performing?

○ 1. Tap-water enemas until clear.

○ 2. Out of bed as tolerated.

○ 3. Neomycin sulfate 1 g every 4 hours.

○ 4. Betadine scrub to abdomen b.i.d.

**74.** Mrs. Martin will be going to surgery soon. The nurse monitors Mrs. Martin's urinary output and finds that the total output for the last 2 hours is 35 ml. This indicates

○ 1. successful intestinal intubation.

○ 2. inadequate pain relief.

○ 3. extension of the obstruction.

○ 4. inadequate fluid replacement.

**75.** Mrs. Martin undergoes a bowel resection and is in the postanesthesia recovery unit for 1 hour. She returns from the recovery room with an intravenous infusion, a nasogastric tube, and a Foley catheter in place. As the nurse performs the postoperative assessment, Mrs. Martin complains of pain and asks for medication. What action should the nurse take *first?*

○ 1. Administer the ordered narcotic.

○ 2. Establish the location and severity of the pain.

○ 3. Determine if she was medicated for pain in the postanesthesia recovery unit.

○ 4. Reposition her and give her a backrub.

**76.** During the evening shift on the day of her surgery, Mrs. Martin's nasogastric tube drains 500 ml of greenish-brown fluid. What action should the nurse take?

○ 1. Call the physician immediately.

○ 2. Increase the intravenous infusion rate.

○ 3. Record the amount on the patient's chart.

○ 4. Irrigate the tube with normal saline.

**77.** Five days after surgery, Mrs. Martin begins to have temperature spikes and a fever with chills and diaphoresis, and she complains of increased incisional pain. Her white blood count is elevated. Which of the following postoperative complications does the nurse suspect?

○ 1. Pneumonia.

○ 2. Urinary tract infection.

○ 3. Wound infection.

○ 4. Atelectasis.

# THE PATIENT WITH CIRRHOSIS

Mr. Howard Carter, a 55-year-old factory worker, has a long history of cirrhosis related to chronic alcoholism. He has been experiencing a slow but steady decline in his general health. Recent blood work shows Mr. Carter to have hypokalemia, anemia, elevated liver function studies, a prolonged prothrombin time, and an increase in his level of circulating estrogens.

78. Because of the elevation in circulating estrogens, the nurse would expect Mr. Carter to exhibit *all* of the following symptoms *except*
    ○ 1. gynecomastia.
    ○ 2. decreased chest and body hair.
    ○ 3. impotence.
    ○ 4. increased libido.

79. Mr. Carter complains that his skin always seems to be itchy and he scratches himself raw while he sleeps. The nurse should recognize that the itching is the result of which abnormality associated with cirrhosis?
    ○ 1. Folic acid deficiency.
    ○ 2. Prolonged prothrombin time.
    ○ 3. Increased bilirubin levels.
    ○ 4. Hypokalemia.

80. During this stage of his illness, Mr. Carter should be encouraged to follow which diet?
    ○ 1. High-calorie, restricted protein, low-sodium.
    ○ 2. Bland, low-protein, low-sodium.
    ○ 3. Well-balanced normal nutrients, low-sodium.
    ○ 4. High-protein, high-calorie, high-potassium.

81. Mr. Carter's wife asks the nurse about health-promoting activities that she could help her husband include in his daily routine. The nurse would appropriately suggest *all* of the following measures *except*
    ○ 1. supplement the diet with daily multivitamins.
    ○ 2. reinforce all efforts to avoid alcohol.
    ○ 3. take a sleeping pill at bedtime.
    ○ 4. avoid contact with ill persons when possible.

82. Mr. Carter's weight has not changed over the last 6 months, but he has noticed that his abdominal girth has increased. The nurse recognizes that the pathological basis for the development of ascites is the presence of portal hypertension and
    ○ 1. excess serum sodium and increased aldosterone excretion.
    ○ 2. increased aldosterone excretion and decreased serum albumin.
    ○ 3. decreased colloid osmotic pressure and lymphatic obstruction.
    ○ 4. decreased serum albumin and decreased colloid osmotic pressure.

83. The position of choice for a patient with severe ascites would be
    ○ 1. high Fowler's.
    ○ 2. side-lying.
    ○ 3. modified Trendelenburg.
    ○ 4. any position as long as frequent position changes are ensured.

84. The physician decreases Mr. Carter's sodium restricted to 1 g daily and orders a diuretic for him. The diuretic that facilitates sodium excretion while conserving body potassium is
    ○ 1. furosemide (Lasix).
    ○ 2. spironolactone (Aldactone).
    ○ 3. hydrochlorothiazide (HydroDIURIL).
    ○ 4. ethacrynic acid (Edecrin).

85. Mr. Carter receives 100 ml of 25% serum albumin IV. Which factor would *best* indicate that the albumin was having its desired effect?
    ○ 1. Increased urine output.
    ○ 2. Increased serum albumin levels.
    ○ 3. Decreased anorexia and itching.
    ○ 4. Increased ease of breathing.

86. Four months later, Mr. Carter is admitted through the emergency department. He is vomiting bright-red blood. The physician suspects bleeding esophageal varices. The nurse realizes that the varicosities develop primarily in response to
    ○ 1. pronounced abdominal ascites.
    ○ 2. portal hypertension.
    ○ 3. chronic arterial hypertension.
    ○ 4. elevated central venous pressure.

87. An intravenous infusion is started immediately as is oxygen, 4 L/minute via nasal prongs. In addition, the physician decides to insert a Sengstaken-Blakemore tube. Mr. Carter asks what the purpose of the tube is. The nurse bases her response on the knowledge that the tube acts by
    ○ 1. providing a large diameter for effective gastric lavage.
    ○ 2. applying direct pressure to gastric bleeding sites.
    ○ 3. blocking the blood flow to the stomach and esophagus.
    ○ 4. applying direct pressure to the esophagus.

88. Once the Sengstaken-Blakemore tube is successfully inserted, Mr. Carter will need constant nursing care. Which of the following nursing interventions would be appropriate for Mr. Carter?
    ○ 1. Provide him with an emesis basin to expectorate secretions.
    ○ 2. Get an order for lozenges to counteract dry mouth.
    ○ 3. Moisten the internal nares with a petroleum-based lubricant.
    ○ 4. Get an order for viscous xylocaine to decrease the discomfort of swallowing.

89. Approximately 30 minutes after the tube is inserted, the nurse observes that Mr. Carter appears

to be having difficulty breathing. The nurse's *first* action should be to

○ 1. remove the tube.

○ 2. deflate the esophageal portion of the tube.

○ 3. determine whether the tube is obstructing the airway.

○ 4. raise the head of the bed and increase the oxygen flow rate.

90. Mr. Carter's condition stabilizes and the Sengstaken-Blakemore tube is removed. The doctor orders oral neomycin for Mr. Carter as well as a neomycin enema. The purpose of this therapy is to

○ 1. reduce abdominal pressure and prevent further bleeding.

○ 2. prevent the patient from straining at stool and stimulating rebleeding.

○ 3. remove intestinal contents and block ammonia formation.

○ 4. reduce the irritating effect of blood on the intestinal mucosa.

91. Mr. Carter will be observed carefully for the development of portal systemic encephalopathy. The nurse should be alert for changes in Mr. Carter's

○ 1. level of consciousness.

○ 2. vital signs.

○ 3. urine output.

○ 4. respiratory status.

92. Mr. Carter's serum ammonia level begins to rise and his physician orders 30 ml of lactulose (Cephulac). Which of the following effects would be expected?

○ 1. Increased urine output.

○ 2. Improved level of consciousness.

○ 3. Diarrhea.

○ 4. Nausea and vomiting.

93. Mr. Carter recovers slowly. He is to be discharged home with a prescription for lactulose (Cephulac). The nurse teaches Mr. and Mrs. Carter proper administration of this medication. Which of the following statements indicates that Mrs. Carter has understood the teaching?

○ 1. "I'll administer it with some Maalox."

○ 2. "I'll mix it with some apple juice."

○ 3. "I'll administer it with a laxative."

○ 4. "I'll mix the crushed tablets in some gelatin."

Lactulose SE Diarrhea

# CORRECT ANSWERS AND RATIONALES

Numbers appear in parentheses following the rationales. The numbers identify textbooks listed in the references at the end of Part IV, where correct answers can be verified.

## The Patient with Cancer of the Colon

1. 4. Castor oil breaks down in the intestines to form ricinoleic acid. This acid irritates nerve endings in the intestinal mucosa, producing evacuation. Mineral oil is a laxative that acts to soften and lubricate the stool. Saline cathartics, such as magnesium sulfate and citrate, act to increase the volume of intestinal content, thus stimulating evacuation. (12, 16)

2. 1. Following a barium enema, a laxative is ordinarily prescribed for the patient. This is done to assist with the expulsion of the barium because if retained, it predisposes the patient to constipation and fecal impaction. (25, 31)

3. 2. The reason for giving the patient chemical agents prior to surgery for an abdominoperineal resection and colostomy is to reduce the bacterial count in the colon. Every effort is made to render the bowel as free of stool and bacteria as possible preoperatively. Thus, the likelihood of postoperative infection in the operative area is reduced. (25, 31)

4. 3. When there is a choice, the preferred site for a permanent colostomy is in the lower portion of the descending colon. The colon normally absorbs large quantities of water. Hence, when the colostomy is as near the end of the colon as possible, the colostomy is easier to manage because the stool will be near-normal consistency. (5, 26)

5. 2. The solution of choice for administering blood in a tandem setup is a 0.9% saline solution. This solution is isotonic and will not disturb the electrolyte balance or damage red blood cells. Solutions of dextrose are not recommended because dextrose tends to cause stickiness and clumping of red blood cells. If the intravenous solution that is used is hypertonic, crenation is likely. If the solution is hypotonic, hemolysis may occur. (24, 36)

6. 4. When a patient complains of headache and tingling sensations in the fingers while receiving a blood transfusion, the nurse should first stop the infusion of blood. The patient may be having an adverse reaction to the blood. The intravenous line should be kept open. Proper personnel should then be notified. Headache and tingling of the fingers are

not symptomatic of infiltration or of too-rapid infusion. (23, 25)

7. 3. Raising the knee gatch to prevent the patient from sliding down in bed is contraindicated because it contributes to venous stasis. Patients who have had abdominoperineal resections should practice diaphragmatic breathing, should cough if secretions are present, and may wear antiembolism stockings. (26, 31)

8. 3. A sign that indicates a patient's colostomy is open and ready to function is passage of feces and flatus. When this occurs, gastric suction is ordinarily discontinued and the patient is allowed to start taking fluids and food orally. Absence of bowel sounds would indicate the tube should remain in place because peristalsis has not yet returned. Passage of mucus from the rectum will not occur in the patient described in this item because of the nature of the surgery. Absence of stomach drainage is not a criterion for judging whether gastric suction is necessary. (26, 31)

9. 4. Vanilla ice cream is not considered a clear liquid. It may be used in a full liquid diet. Foods allowed on a clear liquid diet include water, ice chips, clear fruit juices such as apple and grape juice, clear broth, consommé or bouillon, plain gelatin desserts, and soft drinks. (6, 41)

10. 4. When a patient demonstrates readiness to learn about a colostomy, it is usually best to start with such simple techniques as using illustrative material during teaching sessions. This will help the patient learn how the colostomy will appear. Telling the patient how normal body functions will continue and encouraging him to ask questions are recommended, but these measures will do less to prepare the patient for the sight of a colostomy than using illustrative material. Visits from members of an ostomy club are also recommended, but usually these visits are more beneficial when the patient has knowledge of the colostomy and how it looks and functions. (25, 31)

11. 4. The primary purpose of the colostomy irrigation on a patient's 5th postoperative day is to stimulate peristalsis. It is not done to flush the colon. Stimulating peristalsis so that the colon will empty naturally is an early step in controlling elimination from a colostomy. There is no sphincter to control elimination from the colostomy. (25, 31)

12. 1. The abdominal cramping that may occur during a colostomy irrigation is due to stimulation of the colon by the irrigating solution. The best course of

action is to stop the flow of solution temporarily until the cramping subsides. Having the patient sit up in bed or inserting the cone or tube farther will not help stop cramping. There is no need to remove the cone or tube because this will mean having to reinsert it again when the irrigation is continued. (25, 31)

**13.** 1. When properly changing a colostomy bag, the nurse need not wear gloves, because her hands should not become contaminated with feces. If she wears gloves unnecessarily, the patient may feel unclean, infectious, or undesirable. The nurse should discuss subjects of interest with a patient, encourage the patient to assist with colostomy care as possible, and explain that the procedure of changing a colostomy bag will be taught whenever the patient feels ready. (5, 26)

**14.** 2. When a patient asks about supplies used for dressings, the patient may be ready to participate in self-care. Such activities as inquiring about the physician's visit, discussing news events, and complaining about a dressing change are behaviors that avoid the subject of the colostomy. (25, 31)

**15.** 1. Karaya and Stomahesive are both effective agents for protecting the skin around a colostomy. They keep the skin healthy and prevent enzymatic action on skin by drainage from the stoma. Petrolatum, cornstarch, and antiseptic creams do not adequately protect the skin. (25, 31)

**16.** 1. An effective way to cleanse the operative area following an abdominoperineal resection is to have the patient take sitz baths. They bring heat to the area, improve circulation, and promote healing and cleanliness. Most patients find them very comfortable and relaxing. (25, 31)

**17.** 3. Experience has shown that it is best to adjust the diet of a patient with a colostomy in a manner that best suits the patient rather than trying special diets. Limiting roughage and liquids and using a constipating diet are not recommended. (25, 31)

### The Patient with Hepatitis A

**18.** 3. The inflammation and obstruction in the liver block the normal flow of bile. Excess bilirubin turns the skin and sclera yellow and the urine dark and frothy. Profound anorexia is also common, but shortness of breath would be unexpected. (25, 31)

**19.** 3. Enteric precautions are recommended for patients with hepatitis A, but a private room for an adult patient is unnecessary. These recommendations are made by the Centers for Disease Control. (25, 31)

**20.** 1. Treatment during the acute phase of hepatitis

consists primarily of bed rest with bathroom privileges. When activity is gradually resumed, the patient should be taught to rest before he feels overly tired. (25, 31)

**21.** 3. Bilirubin levels and liver enzymes, such as serum glutamic pyruvic transaminase (SGPT) and serum glutamic oxaloacetic transaminase (SGOT), are carefully monitored during hepatitis. Their levels provide important data about liver function. Blood glucose, creatinine clearance, and serum electrolytes provide no information about liver function. (25, 31)

**22.** 4. Unlike the hepatitis of alcoholism, viral forms of hepatitis are not usually associated with nutritional depletion. Therefore, a well-balanced diet to ensure nutritional status is advocated. It is a challenge to ensure that patients with hepatitis A ingest a balanced diet with sufficient calories because these patients are generally anorexic and have little interest in eating. (37, 40)

**23.** 2. There is no definitive treatment for hepatitis. Bed rest is used during the acute period to reduce the metabolic demand on the liver, thus increasing its blood supply and supporting cell regeneration. (25, 31)

**24.** 2. The organism causing hepatitis A leaves the body primarily through feces. The respiratory route has not been ruled out entirely as a possible portal but is not considered the most common route of exit. (25, 31)

**25.** 3. The hepatitis A virus is transmitted through the fecal-oral route. The common vehicles spreading the virus are contaminated hands, water, and food, especially shellfish growing in contaminated water. Certain animal-handlers are at risk for hepatitis A, particularly those handling primates. (25, 31)

**26.** 3. Immune serum globulin, an immune serum, is used for prophylactic purposes for persons exposed to hepatitis A. There are no vaccines for hepatitis A, and antibiotics are ineffective. (25, 31)

**27.** 1. It may take months for a patient who has been acutely ill with hepatitis A to recover completely. A common symptom during convalescence is fatigue. Such symptoms as insomnia, constipation, and fever are not associated with convalescence following hepatitis. (26, 31)

**28.** 4. The convalescent period following hepatitis may take weeks or even months. Boredom and depression are extremely common problems that the patient should anticipate. Pain, maintaining a regular bowel elimination pattern, and preventing respiratory complications are unlikely. Bed rest is not prescribed, but activity is strictly limited to support healing. (5, 26)

**29.** 2. Uncomplicated hepatitis A does not require any particular life-style modifications once healing has occurred. Moderation in alcohol consumption is recommended. Patients should, however, never donate blood. (22, 26)

**30.** 4. Nurses working in kidney dialysis units are at highest risk for acquiring hepatitis B from their patients. (25, 31)

**31.** 4. Hepatitis B is most often spread by blood and plasma and by contaminated instruments used to puncture the skin. Its incidence is not related to the use of marijuana or sexual activity, but it occurs in alarming numbers among intravenous drug abusers. (26, 31)

## The Patient with Hemorrhoids

**32.** 1. Internal hemorrhoids typically produce bleeding and pain with defecation. The amount of bleeding is usually small but can produce iron-deficiency anemia over time. External hemorrhoids rarely cause bleeding. Thrombosed or prolapsed hemorrhoids are acute hematomas causing painful anal lumps. (25, 31)

**33.** 2. The development of hemorrhoids is associated with prolonged sitting or standing, portal hypertension, chronic constipation, and prolonged increases in intra-abdominal pressure, as associated with pregnancy and the strain of vaginal delivery. (25, 31)

**34.** 3. Cryosurgery is not yet a viable treatment for hemorrhoids, but alternatives to surgery exist for otherwise healthy persons. Rubber-band ligation of internal hemorrhoids is particularly effective, and a variety of sclerosing substances, such as 5% phenol in oil, may be injected to induce fibrosis and shrinkage. (5, 25)

**35.** 2. A low-roughage, high-fiber diet will produce a soft stool that is not irritating to the inflamed hemorrhoidal area. (40, 41)

**36.** 3. The left lateral position is usually recommended so that the sigmoid colon is below the rectum. This position facilitates instillation of the enema fluid. (24, 36) .

**37.** 1. Injectable diazepam (Valium) should not be mixed or diluted with other solutions or drugs and should not be added to intravenous fluid. Injectable diazepam is a colorless crystalline compound, insoluble in water. (12, 16)

**38.** 3. For a patient who is 5-foot-6 and weighs 115 pounds, a 22G, 1½″ needle is preferable for an intramuscular injection. A 1″ needle is ordinarily too short to reach deep muscle tissue, and a needle larger than 22G will tend to cause unnecessary trauma and discomfort. A 26G needle is not recommended for intramuscular injections. (24, 36)

**39.** 3. Rectal surgery is accompanied by severe pain resulting from spasms of sphincters and muscles. Therefore, controlling pain is a priority goal of post-hemorrhoidectomy nursing care. Preventing venous stasis, promoting ambulation, and preventing infection are important goals but are not the priority goal given the nature of the surgery. (25, 31)

**40.** 3. Positioning in the early post-hemorrhoidectomy phase should avoid stress and pressure on the operative site. The prone or side-lying positions are ideal from a comfort perspective. Any sitting position is less than ideal and there is no need for the Trendelenburg position. (5, 25)

**41.** 2. Voiding is often a problem due to a reflex spasm of the sphincter at the outlet of the bladder and muscle-guarding from apprehension and pain. Anesthesia, perineal edema, and anxiety can potentially cause urinary retention but are not directly related to urinary retention following hemorrhoidectomy. (5, 26)

**42.** 1. Applying heat during the *immediate* postoperative period may cause hemorrhage at the surgical site. Moist warm heat may relieve rectal spasms following bowel movements. Urinary retention caused by reflex spasm may also be relieved by warm moist heat. Constipation is prevented by increasing fiber and fluid in the diet. (5, 26)

**43.** 3. Adequate cleansing of the anal area is difficult but essential. After rectal surgery, sitz baths assist in this process, so the post-hemorrhoidectomy patient should take a sitz bath after defecating. Other times are dictated by patient comfort. (25, 31)

**44.** 2. The first bowel movement after hemorrhoidectomy is often painful because of sphincter spasm. A warm sitz bath or warm compresses relieve the painful sphincter spasm quickly. Oral analgesics take longer to be effective. Cleansing the rectal area with warm water after a bowel movement promotes hygiene and comfort, but warm sitz baths relieve sphincter spasm. (5, 31)

**45.** 2. Oatmeal, grapefruit wedges, and bran muffins are all high-fiber foods. Processed foods such as pastries, processed cereals, and white bread are low in fiber. Protein foods contain little if any fiber. Prune juice is not high in fiber but has a laxative effect caused by dihydroxyphenyl isatin. (13, 41)

**46.** 1. Psyllium hydrophilic mucilloid (Metamucil) is a bulk-forming laxative that promotes peristalsis and prevents constipation. It does not prevent flatus. Excessive use can cause diarrhea. (12, 16)

## *The Patient with Inflammatory Bowel Disease*

**47.** 3. Diarrhea is the primary symptom of ulcerative colitis. It is profuse and severe, and the patient may have as many as 15 to 20 watery stools per day. They may contain blood, mucus, and pus. The frequent diarrhea is often accompanied by anorexia and nausea. Cramping and abdominal pain are the characteristic features of Crohn's disease. (25, 31)

**48.** 2. Diarrhea causes fluid and electrolyte imbalances; cathartics may worsen the problem and may even cause shock. Routine preparations are appropriate for patients of all ages. Individualization is important for all patients and should always be considered. Lack of adequate preparation interferes with visualization. (25, 31)

**49.** 1. Stressful and emotional events have been clearly linked to exacerbations of ulcerative colitis, although their role in the etiology of the disease has been refuted. Diet and exercise are unlikely causes of an acute exacerbation. (25, 31)

**50.** 2. Diarrhea is the primary symptom, and stopping it is the first goal of treatment. The other goals are ongoing and will be best achieved by halting the exacerbation. The patient may receive antidiarrheal agents, antispasmodics, bulk hydrophilic agents, and/or anti-inflammatory drugs. (5, 31)

**51.** 2. Modified bed rest helps conserve energy and promote comfort, but its primary purpose is to help reduce the hypermotility of the colon. (5, 31)

**52.** 3. Massive diarrhea causes significant depletion of the body's stores of sodium and potassium, as well as fluid. The patient should be closely monitored for hypokalemia and hyponatremia. (25, 31)

**53.** 4. Anal excoriation is inevitable with profuse diarrhea, and meticulous perianal hygiene is essential. Sitz baths are comforting and cleansing. Urgency in defecation requires the ready availability of a bedpan. Deep-breathing is an important measure for any patient on bed rest. A gown is not indicated because no infectious agent is involved. (25, 31)

**54.** 3. The superior vena cava is preferred for introducing hyperalimentation nutrients. It is a large, rapid-flow vein, and the concentrated solution will dilute quickly. The superior vena cava is generally entered through the right or left subclavian vein; it may be entered through the internal jugular vein. (5, 26)

**55.** 2. The solution introduced when total parenteral nutrition is used is ordinarily a hypertonic glucose solution. If a commercial preparation is unavailable, the solution is best prepared in a pharmacy under strict aseptic conditions. Electrolytes may be added to meet a particular patient's needs. (5, 31)

**56.** 4. The urine should be regularly examined for glycosuria when a patient is receiving total parenteral nutrition. If the patient is not metabolizing the nutrients well, glucose tends to be eliminated in the urine. Very often, the patient may require small amounts of insulin to improve glucose metabolism. The patient should also be observed for signs of hypoglycemia, which may occur if the body overproduces insulin in response to a high glucose intake or if too much insulin is administered to help improve glucose metabolism. (26, 31)

**57.** 2. Complications associated with total parenteral nutrition administered via a central line include infection and air embolism. In order to prevent these complications, strict aseptic technique is used for all dressing changes, the insertion site is covered with an air-occlusive dressing, and all connections of the system are taped. Ambulation and activities of daily living are encouraged. (25, 31)

**58.** 4. A steady and progressive weight gain is the best indication that nutritional goals are being met for a patient receiving total parenteral nutrition. The laboratory values stated in this item are within normal limits but do not indicate attainment of nutritional goals. (5, 36)

**59.** 1. An elemental diet is easily and rapidly absorbed in the upper portion of the gastrointestinal tract, allowing the colon to continue to rest and heal. The major difficulty with this diet is its lack of palatability; it is usually best tolerated chilled. (25, 31)

**60.** 3. Adequate fluid intake prevents crystalluria and stone formation with sulfasalazine (Azulfidine). This drug can cause gastrointestinal distress and is best taken after meals. Sulfasalazine should be taken in equally divided doses. It colors alkaline urine orange-yellow. (16, 31)

**61.** 1. Patients with chronic diseases need not curtail their career goals. Self-care is the cornerstone of long-term management, and learning to cope with and modify stressors enables a person to live with the disease. Giving up a desired career could discourage and even depress the patient. Placing the responsibility for minimizing stressors at work in the hands of others leads to a feeling of loss of control and stunts the sense of responsibility needed for sound self-care. Working part-time rather than full-time is unnecessary. (25, 31)

**62.** 3. The foods most commonly associated with an exacerbation of ulcerative colitis symptoms are milk and milk products, and patients are encouraged to minimize their use. The etiologic nature of this food intolerance is not well understood. (25, 31)

**63.** 1. The meat sandwich provides protein and calories and a limited amount of fiber. Fruits are high in fiber and low in protein. Because salads lack protein and calories and are high in fiber, they are not good choices for a low-residue diet. (13, 41)

## The Patient with an Intestinal Obstruction

**64.** 4. Air produces a resonant sound and fluid produces a dull sound on percussion. An intestinal obstruction causes large amounts of fluid to be trapped in the intestine. Hyperperistalsis would be apparent on auscultation. (5, 28)

**65.** 1. Profuse vomiting is the classic sign of small-bowel obstruction. Abdominal distention and discomfort tend to be more pronounced with large-bowel obstruction. The high-pitched bowel sounds indicate hyperperistalsis and will be present early in obstruction. (25, 31)

**66.** 1. Intestinal decompression is accomplished via a Cantor, Harris, or Miller-Abbott tube. These 6- to 10-foot-long tubes are passed through the gastrointestinal tract to the site of obstruction. They remove accumulations of fluid and gas at the site of the obstruction, thereby relieving pressure. (25, 31)

**67.** 2. The patient is placed on her right side to facilitate the movement of the mercury-weighted tube through the pyloric sphincter. After the tube is in the intestine, the patient will be turned from side to side or encouraged to ambulate to facilitate movement of the tube through the intestinal loops. (25, 31)

**68.** 3. An intestinal tube is not taped in position until it has reached the site of the obstruction. A Cantor tube is attached to suction and has a small balloon at its tip that is injected with mercury. Because the tube has a radiopaque strip, its progress through the intestinal tract can be followed by x-ray. (26, 31)

**69.** 3. Once the intestinal tube has passed into the duodenum, it is usually advanced, as ordered, 2″ to 4″ every 30 to 60 minutes. This enables peristalsis to carry the tube forward. The patient is encouraged to walk, which also facilitates progression of the tube. Frequent mouth care is essential to stimulate saliva secretion, to maintain a healthy oral cavity, and to promote comfort. Ice chips are contraindicated because hypotonic fluid will draw extra fluid into an already distended bowel. (5, 31)

**70.** 1. Normally, 7 to 8 liters of electrolyte-rich fluid are secreted and reabsorbed by the bowel daily. Intestinal obstruction causes increased retention of this fluid in the bowel. Fluid moves from the plasma and interstitial space into the distended bowel. Intesti-

nal obstruction does not increase skin permeability and vascularity, or increase insensible fluid loss. Severe volume depletion can cause acute renal failure and decrease urinary output. (5, 26)

**71.** 2. Medications that mask symptoms may delay accurate diagnosis and appropriate treatment. Narcotics are thought to stimulate a chemoreceptor emetic trigger zone in the medulla, resulting in nausea and vomiting. Potential fluid loss is not the reason that such medications are not administered to patients with suspected intestinal obstruction; a patent intestinal tube minimizes vomiting. Addiction is unlikely when pain medication is administered in the presence of pain. Narcotics are often used to facilitate the induction of anesthesia. (5, 26)

**72.** 4. Nursing measures that increase the comfort of a patient who has an intestinal tube in place include applying water-soluble lubricant to the external nares and encouraging or helping the patient to brush her teeth every 4 hours. As soon as the tube has reached the desired position, the tube is taped to the patient's nose or cheek and extra tubing is coiled on the bed or pinned to the patient's gown. The tube is *never* taped to the patient's forehead because this would increase pressure on the patient's nares. (24, 36)

**73.** 1. High colon irrigation can increase the risk of perforation in a distended and inflamed colon. Tap water is hypotonic in the bowel and would draw increased fluid into the area. The other measures are standard preparation for intestinal surgery. (5, 26)

**74.** 4. The kidney is very sensitive to circulating fluid volume. Urinary output of less than 30 ml per hour indicates that the kidney is concentrating urine and fluid replacement needs to be increased. The intestinal tube removes sequestered fluid in the bowel, not fluid in the general circulation. The effect of pain on renal function is not this dramatic. (5, 26)

**75.** 2. Assessing pain, including location and severity, is essential before administering pain medication. Since the patient in this situation spent an hour in the postanesthesia recovery unit, the nurse would next determine if the patient had been medicated for pain in that unit. The pain is most likely incisional but could be from positioning, a too-tight dressing, or anxiety. (23, 36)

**76.** 3. Since peristalsis has not been reestablished, this amount of gastric drainage would not be unexpected. The color is also as expected. The only action required is to chart the amount and color of the output accurately and continue to monitor the patient. (5, 36)

**77.** 3. Temperature spikes, fever with chills and diaphoresis, and an elevated white blood count are associated with pneumonia, urinary tract infection, and atelectasis, but increased incisional pain is associated specifically with wound infection. (5, 26)

## *The Patient with Cirrhosis*

**78.** 4. The normal liver acts to metabolize and inactivate hormones. Loss of this function increases the levels of circulating hormones. Excess estrogen in the male may cause gynecomastia; loss of axillary, chest, and pubic hair; testicular atrophy; and impotence; but will not increase libido. Palmar erythema and spider angiomas are also common results of hormone excess. (25, 31)

**79.** 3. Excess retained bilirubin produces an irritating effect on the peripheral nerves, causing intense itching. Folic acid, prothrombin, and potassium imbalances cause varied symptoms, but itching is not directly related to these imbalances. (25, 31)

**80.** 3. Cirrhosis is a slowly progressive disease. Inadequate nutrition is the primary ongoing problem. Patients are encouraged to eat normal, well-balanced diets, restricting sodium to prevent fluid retention. Protein is not restricted until the liver actually fails, which is usually very late in the disease. (25, 31)

**81.** 3. General health-promotion measures include good nutrition, avoiding infection, and abstaining from alcohol. Rest and sleep are essential, but an impaired liver may not be able to detoxify sedatives and barbiturates. Such drugs must be used cautiously, if at all, by patients with cirrhosis. (25, 31)

**82.** 4. The development of ascites is the result of increased pressure in the venous system, low levels of serum albumin (which contribute to a decreased colloid osmotic pressure), and sodium retention, resulting in part from decreased aldosterone clearance. It is a complex and difficult condition to manage. (5, 31)

**83.** 1. Ascites can compromise the action of the diaphragm and increase the patient's risk of respiratory problems. Frequent position changes are important, but the preferred position is high Fowler's. Ascites also tremendously increases the risk of skin breakdown. (25, 31)

**84.** 2. Hypokalemia is an ongoing problem for patients with cirrhosis. When a diuretic is needed, the ideal choice is a potassium-sparing product. Spironolactone (Aldactone) is the diuretic of choice for patients with cirrhosis because it facilitates sodium excretion while conserving potassium. Furosemide (Lasix), hydrochlorothiazide (HydroDIURIL), and ethacrynic acid (Edecrin) are thiazide diuretics and, as such, waste potassium. (16, 31)

**85.** 1. Normal serum albumin is administered to reduce ascites. Hypoalbuminemia, a mechanism underlying ascites formation, results in decreased colloid osmotic pressure. Administering serum albumin increases the plasma colloid osmotic pressure, which causes fluid to flow from the tissue space into the plasma. An increased urine output is the best indication that the albumin is having the desired effect. Patients receiving albumin should be monitored for complications such as fluid overload and pulmonary edema. (25, 31)

**86.** 2. As the structural integrity of the liver is compromised, blood flow through this highly vascular organ can be obstructed. Collateral vessels attempt to bypass the obstruction, but as pressures rise varicosities can develop in these thin-walled collateral vessels. (25, 31)

**87.** 4. The Sengstaken-Blakemore tube has a small gastric balloon that anchors the tube and applies pressure to the area of the cardiac sphincter. The large esophageal balloon applies direct pressure on the bleeding sites in the esophagus. A tube through the balloons allows for aspiration and irrigation. (25, 31)

**88.** 1. Inflation of the esophageal balloon prevents swallowing. Therefore, the nurse provides the patient with tissues and encourages him to spit into the tissues and/or an emesis basin. If the patient is unable to manage his secretions, gentle oral suctioning will be required. Mouth and nasal care is provided every 1 to 2 hours. A water-soluble lubricant is applied to the external nares. (26, 31)

**89.** 3. If the gastric balloon should rupture or deflate, the esophageal balloon can move and partially or totally obstruct the airway. The patient needs close observation. No direct action should be taken, however, until the condition is accurately diagnosed. (5, 31)

**90.** 3. Neomycin is administered to decrease the bacterial effect on digested blood in the intestines, which results in ammonia production. This ammonia, if not detoxified by the liver, can result in hepatic coma. (25, 31)

**91.** 1. Ammonia has a toxic effect on the tissue of the central nervous system and produces changes in level of consciousness, drowsiness and irritability. If this process is unchecked, the patient may lapse into coma. (25, 31)

**92.** 3. Lactulose (Cephulac) increases intestinal motility, thereby decreasing ammonia formation in the intestine. An expected effect, therefore, would be diarrhea. (16, 31)

**93.** 2. The taste of lactulose (Cephulac) is a problem for some patients, and mixing it with fruit juice can make it more palatable. For patients whose dietary sodium is not restricted, lactulose can also be mixed with milk. Lactulose should not be given with antacids because they may inhibit its action. Lactulose *is* a laxative that expels the trapped ammonia from the colon. Lactulose is a syrup for oral or rectal administration. (12, 16)

# test 5

- *The Patient with Hyperthyroidism*
- *The Patient with Diabetes Mellitus*
- *The Patient with a Pituitary Adenoma*
- *The Patient with Addison's Disease*
- *The Patient with Cushing's Disease*
- *Correct Answers and Rationales*

Select the one *best* or *correct* answer and indicate your choice by filling in the circle with a pencil in front of the option you have chosen. If the answer you would prefer is not given, select the one you think is *most appropriate*.

## THE PATIENT WITH HYPERTHYROIDISM

Mrs. Muriel Torry, a 32-year-old homemaker and mother of three children, visits her physician because of nervousness, irritability, and difficulty sleeping. A tentative diagnosis of hyperthyroidism is made.

1. *All* of the following are also typical symptoms of hyperthyroidism *except*
   - ○ 1. anorexia.
   - ○ 2. tachycardia.
   - ○ 3. heat intolerance.
   - ○ 4. fine hand tremors.

2. Which symptom related to Mrs. Torry's menstrual cycle is she very likely to report on the initial assessment?
   - ○ 1. Dysmenorrhea.
   - ○ 2. Metrorrhagia.
   - ○ 3. Oligomenorrhea.
   - ○ 4. Menorrhagia.

3. A radioactive iodine uptake (RAIU) test and a protein-bound iodine (PBI) test are planned for Mrs. Torry. These two tests will be *falsely* elevated if Mrs. Torry has recently been taking medications containing
   - ○ 1. iodine.
   - ○ 2. digitalis.
   - ○ 3. ferrous salts.
   - ○ 4. antihistamines.

4. Propylthiouracil (PTU) is prescribed for Mrs. Torry. Which of the following symptoms should the nurse teach Mrs. Torry to report *immediately* if they occur?
   - ○ 1. A sore throat and fever.
   - ○ 2. Painful and excessive menstruation.
   - ○ 3. Constipation and abdominal distention.
   - ○ 4. Increased urinary output and itchy skin.

5. Mrs. Torry also exhibits early signs of exophthalmos. Which of the following symptoms would be typical of this condition?
   - ○ 1. Poor depth perception.
   - ○ 2. Poor pupillary responses.
   - ○ 3. Protrusion of the eyeballs.
   - ○ 4. Inability to distinguish colors.

6. Mr. Torry has accompanied his wife to the physician's office. He says to the nurse, "My wife has become so irritable. She's yelling at the children all the time. Our house is in chaos." Which of the following responses provides Mr. Torry with the *most accurate* explanation of Mrs. Torry's behavior?
   - ○ 1. "Your wife's behavior is caused by temporary confusion brought on by her illness."
   - ○ 2. "Your wife's behavior is caused by the excess thyroid hormone in her system."
   - ○ 3. "Your wife's behavior is caused by her worry over the seriousness of her illness."
   - ○ 4. "Your wife's behavior is caused by the stress of trying to manage your home and still cope with her illness."

7. Mrs. Torry's eyelids do not completely close at rest due to her exophthalmos. Which of the following measures would be *most helpful* in preventing damage to her eyes while she sleeps?
   - ○ 1. Massaging the eyes.
   - ○ 2. Instilling an ophthalmic anesthetic.
   - ○ 3. Taping the eyelids shut with nonirritating tape.
   - ○ 4. Covering both eyes with moistened gauze pads.

8. Mrs. Torry's hyperthyroidism cannot be controlled by medications and she elects to have surgery. She is admitted to the hospital and scheduled for a subtotal thyroidectomy. If the following hospital rooms are available, which would be *best* for the nurse to select for Mrs. Torry?

○ 1. A private room located in an area where the patient has privacy and quiet.

○ 2. A semiprivate room that the patient can share with another patient who has had nasal surgery.

○ 3. A private room next to the nurse's station so that the patient can be observed frequently.

○ 4. A semiprivate room that is currently empty but has one bed used only for emergency admissions.

9. Saturated solution of potassium iodide (SSKI) is prescribed for Mrs. Torry preoperatively. The *primary* reason for using this drug is that it helps

○ 1. decrease the progression of exophthalmos.

○ 2. reduce the vascularity of the thyroid gland.

○ 3. decrease the body's ability to store thyroxin.

○ 4. increase the body's ability to excrete thyroxin.

10. Which of the following nursing measures is *most often* recommended to prepare a saturated solution of potassium iodide (SSKI) for administration?

○ 1. Pour the solution over ice chips.

○ 2. Mix the solution with an antacid.

○ 3. Dilute the solution with water, milk, or fruit juice.

○ 4. Disguise the solution in a pureed fruit or vegetable.

11. A friend who visits Mrs. Torry before surgery expresses concern to the nurse by saying, "She seems worse and can't sit still and concentrate, even for a minute." Which of the following responses would be *best* for the nurse to make to the patient's friend?

○ 1. "Thank you for telling me. I'll check on Mrs. Torry immediately."

○ 2. "Mrs. Torry had a bad night but she'll be better, we're sure, after some rest."

○ 3. "Mrs. Torry's behavior is part of her illness, but she's receiving medication that will help her."

○ 4. "Unfortunately, I can't discuss Mrs. Torry's condition with you since you are not a family member."

12. Mrs. Torry undergoes a subtotal thyroidectomy. As soon as Mrs. Torry regains consciousness postoperatively, the nurse asks her to state her name and repeats this request from time to time. The nurse carries out this activity *primarily* to monitor for signs of

○ 1. internal hemorrhage.

○ 2. decreasing level of consciousness.

○ 3. laryngeal nerve damage.

○ 4. upper airway obstruction.

13. Certain items should be kept in Mrs. Torry's room to treat postoperative complications if they de-

velop. Which of the following items is *least likely* to be necessary?

○ 1. Suction equipment.

○ 2. Cutdown tray.

○ 3. Tracheostomy equipment.

○ 4. Equipment for administering oxygen.

14. Which of the following symptoms might indicate that Mrs. Torry was developing tetany postoperatively?

○ 1. Backache and joint pains.

○ 2. Tingling of the fingers.

○ 3. Hoarseness and weakness of the voice.

○ 4. Retraction of neck muscles with inspiration.

15. Which of the following medications should be available to provide emergency treatment if Mrs. Torry develops tetany?

○ 1. Sodium phosphate.

○ 2. Calcium gluconate.

○ 3. Phospholine iodide.

○ 4. Sodium bicarbonate.

16. Which of the following techniques would *best* enable the nurse to assess Mrs. Torry's wound for bleeding?

○ 1. Gently slip her hand behind the patient's neck and check for blood on the back of the neck and bed linens.

○ 2. Carry out a routine dressing change every 2 hours for at least 12 hours and then every 4 hours for the next day or two.

○ 3. Carefully loosen the dressings on both ends and have the patient turn her head to one side while observing for blood on the dressings.

○ 4. Check the patient's blood pressure, pulse, and respiratory rate every hour for the first 24 hours and then every 2 hours for the next 24 hours.

17. To minimize tension on the incision line, the nurse should teach Mrs. Torry to follow which technique when she moves herself to a sitting position?

○ 1. Pressing her chin against her chest while moving to the sitting position.

○ 2. Supporting her head by placing both hands behind it while moving to the sitting position.

○ 3. Rolling to her side first and then moving to the sitting position while holding her head perfectly still.

○ 4. Grasping her flexed knees with both arms while in the back-lying position and then rocking forward to the sitting position.

18. Mrs. Torry could develop hypothyroidism following surgery. The nurse teaches her to notify her physician if she develops typical signs of hypothyroidism. These symptoms might include

○ 1. joint pain.

○ 2. weight loss.
○ 3. general fatigue.
○ 4. oily skin.

## THE PATIENT WITH DIABETES MELLITUS

Mrs. Rosa Lonzo, 55, has recently been diagnosed with non-insulin-dependent diabetes mellitus (NIDDM) and is being started on the sulfonylurea compound tolbutamide (Orinase). She is very concerned about her diagnosis and says she knows nothing about diabetes. She needs a lot of teaching and support.

**19.** Tolbutamide (Orinase) is believed to lower Mrs. Lonzo's blood glucose level by
○ 1. potentiating the action of insulin.
○ 2. lowering the renal threshold of glucose.
○ 3. stimulating pancreatic cells to release insulin.
○ 4. combining with glucose to render it inert.

**20.** The nurse learns through her assessment that Mrs. Lonzo ordinarily wears the articles of clothing described below. The nurse should recommend that Mrs. Lonzo *discontinue* wearing
○ 1. a girdle.
○ 2. pantyhose.
○ 3. nylon stockings.
○ 4. knee-high stockings.

**21.** Mrs. Lonzo tells the nurse that her feet often feel cold and her skin is very dry. Which of the following factors is *least likely* to be contributing to the patient's having cold feet?
○ 1. Smoking cigarettes.
○ 2. Wearing round garters.
○ 3. Wearing low-heeled shoes.
○ 4. Crossing her legs when sitting.

**22.** When Mrs. Lonzo asks the nurse to recommend something to remove corns from her toes, the nurse should advise her to
○ 1. apply a high-quality corn plaster.
○ 2. consult her physician about removing the corns.
○ 3. apply iodine to the corns before peeling them off.
○ 4. soak her feet in borax solution to peel off the corns.

**23.** The nurse teaches Mrs. Lonzo about foot care. Which of the following should the nurse teach Mrs. Lonzo to avoid?
○ 1. Going barefoot.
○ 2. Wearing hard-soled shoes.
○ 3. Applying toenail polish.
○ 4. Using bar detergents to wash her feet.

**24.** The nurse observes that Mrs. Lonzo has several small bandages covering cuts on her hands. Mrs. Lonzo says, "I'm so clumsy. I'm always cutting or burning myself in the kitchen." Which of the following responses would be *most appropriate?*
○ 1. "Don't worry about it, but keep all your cuts clean and covered."
○ 2. "Even small cuts can be serious for diabetics and need special care."
○ 3. "Why do you think you injure yourself so frequently?"
○ 4. "You really should have your doctor check all injuries, even small ones."

**25.** Mrs. Lonzo is taught that an especially desirable constituent in her diet that has been observed to minimize a rise in blood glucose levels after meals is
○ 1. dietary fibers.
○ 2. dairy products.
○ 3. foods fortified with vitamins.
○ 4. organ meats.

**26.** Mrs. Lonzo says, "If I could just avoid what you call carbohydrates in my diet, I guess I would be OK." The nurse should base her response to the patient's comment on knowledge that diabetes affects the metabolism of
○ 1. carbohydrates only.
○ 2. fats and carbohydrates only.
○ 3. protein and carbohydrates only.
○ 4. proteins, fats, and carbohydrates.

**27.** Mrs. Lonzo says her family eats a lot of pasta products, such as macaroni and spaghetti. She asks if she can still eat them. Which of the following would be the nurse's *best* response?
○ 1. "Because you're overweight, it's better to eliminate pasta from your diet."
○ 2. "Pasta products can be included in your diet. They are included in the bread and cereal exchange."
○ 3. "Pasta products can be included in your diet, but they should not be served with sauces."
○ 4. "Eating pasta products predisposes to various complications, so it's better to eliminate them from your diet for the time being."

**28.** Mrs. Lonzo says, "My husband and I are not heavy drinkers, but we do like to have wine with our evening meal. Is that all right?" The nurse should caution Mrs. Lonzo that alcoholic beverages must be included in calculating total caloric intake and, if used in excess by someone taking tolbutamide (Orinase), tend to cause symptoms of
○ 1. hypokalemia.
○ 2. hyperkalemia.

3. hyperglycemia.
4. hypoglycemia.

29. If the nurse notes the following factors in Mrs. Lonzo's health history, which should the nurse judge as having been *most important* in predisposing her to diabetes mellitus?
1. Being overweight.
2. Smoking cigarettes.
3. Having had six children.
4. Being of Italian ancestry.

30. To which of the following diseases is Mrs. Lonzo most predisposed because of the diabetes?
1. Arthritis.
2. Otitis media.
3. Osteoporosis.
4. Atherosclerosis.

31. The nurse recommends moderate exercise for Mrs. Lonzo. In which of the following ways does exercise affect the body's physiologic functioning?
1. Exercise helps avoid hypoglycemia.
2. Exercise stimulates an overproduction of insulin.
3. Exercise decreases the renal threshold for glucose.
4. Exercise increases the use of glucose by muscles.

32. After five years of treatment, Mrs. Lonzo, now age 60, needs to switch to insulin therapy. The oral hypoglycemic agent is discontinued and isophane insulin suspension (NPH insulin) is prescribed for her. Mrs. Lonzo is taught to take her insulin at 8 a.m. each day. At which time is Mrs. Lonzo at *greatest risk* for hypoglycemia?
1. About 11 a.m., shortly before lunch.
2. About 1 p.m., shortly after lunch.
3. About 5 p.m., shortly before dinner.
4. About 11 p.m., shortly before bedtime.

33. The nurse teaches Mrs. Lonzo to administer her own insulin. Learning goals are mostly likely to be attained when they are established by the
1. nurse and physician, so the nurse knows the physician's wishes.
2. physician, because he is the manager of the patient's care.
3. patient, because she is best able to identify her needs.
4. patient and nurse, so the patient can participate in her care.

34. The *most accurate* indication that Mrs. Lonzo has learned how to give herself insulin correctly is that the patient can
1. perform the procedure faultlessly.
2. critique the nurse's performance of the procedure.

3. explain all steps of the procedure correctly.
4. answer correctly questions about the procedure.

35. The nurse teaches Mrs. Lonzo about hypoglycemia. Mrs. Lonzo says, "I'm not sure I'd recognize it if it happened." The nurse should teach her that the *most common* symptoms of hypoglycemia are
1. nervousness and weakness.
2. anorexia and incoherent speech.
3. Kussmaul respirations and mental confusion.
4. bradycardia and blurred vision.

36. According to a blood test, Mrs. Lonzo has an elevated blood glucose level, but her urine specimen is negative when tested for the presence of glucose. Which of the following factors should the nurse *most certainly* consider when evaluating this phenomenon of hyperglycemia without glycosuria?
1. The patient's need for glucose most probably has increased with advanced age.
2. The patient's renal threshold for glucose most probably has increased with advanced age.
3. The patient's exercise program most probably has become too strenuous because of her advanced age.
4. The patient's response to stress has been impaired by aging.

37. The nurse examines Mrs. Lonzo's urine for the presence of ketones. The nurse would *correctly* interpret ketonuria as indicating that the body is deriving most of its energy from the metabolism of
1. fats.
2. minerals.
3. proteins.
4. carbohydrates.

38. The nurse teaches Mrs. Lonzo how to manage her disease during episodes of minor illness such as colds or the flu. The nurse should include *all* the following measures in the teaching plan *except*
1. increase the frequency of blood and urine testing.
2. try to convert the ordered diet to liquids.
3. call the physician if ketones appear in the urine.
4. stop taking the long-acting insulin.

39. Vascular changes that occur in the diabetic patient may affect all organs of the body. Vascular changes will have their *most serious* effects on Mrs. Lonzo's life when they become prevalent in her
1. liver.
2. lungs.
3. kidneys.
4. pancreas.

**40.** If Mrs. Lonzo develops eye problems, the problem *least likely* to be related to her diabetes mellitus is
○ 1. cataracts.
○ 2. blindness.
○ 3. astigmatism.
○ 4. blurred vision.

## THE PATIENT WITH A PITUITARY ADENOMA

Mr. Peter Saunders, 42, is admitted for surgery to treat a pituitary tumor. On admission, he says he is happy the physician finally discovered what was wrong with him. He had been experiencing symptoms for the last 5 months.

**41.** Mr. Saunders reports, with some embarrassment, that he has been experiencing mild galactorrhea. The nurse knows that this problem is caused by overproduction of which hormone?
○ 1. Prolactin.
○ 2. Adrenocorticotropic hormone (ACTH).
○ 3. Growth hormone (GH).
○ 4. Thyroid-stimulating hormone (TSH).

**42.** The nurse would anticipate that Mr. Saunders' *primary* symptoms were probably
○ 1. severe lethargy and fatigue.
○ 2. decreased libido and impotence.
○ 3. bony proliferation of the hands, jaw, and feet.
○ 4. deepening or coarsening of the voice.

**43.** A CT scan shows that Mr. Saunders' tumor is a macroadenoma. The nurse would therefore expect that he also experienced which symptoms?
○ 1. Changes in facial features.
○ 2. Memory loss.
○ 3. Visual defects.
○ 4. Impaired glucose tolerance.

**44.** Mr. Saunders is scheduled for a transsphenoidal hypophysectomy. The nurse tells Mr. Saunders that the surgery will be performed through an incision in the
○ 1. back of the mouth.
○ 2. nose.
○ 3. sinus channel below the right eye.
○ 4. space between the upper gums and lip.

**45.** To help minimize the possibility of postoperative respiratory complications, the nurse would focus Mr. Saunders' preoperative teaching on the importance of
○ 1. using blow bottles.
○ 2. frequent position changes.
○ 3. deep-breathing.
○ 4. coughing.

**46.** Mr. Saunders undergoes hypophysectomy. In the immediate postoperative period, the nurse should monitor him closely for signs of
○ 1. decreasing intracranial pressure.
○ 2. cerebral edema.
○ 3. thyroid storm.
○ 4. hyperglycemic shock.

**47.** Which of the following is a *major* focus of nursing care for the patient following transsphenoidal hypophysectomy?
○ 1. Monitoring for cerebrospinal fluid leak.
○ 2. Monitoring for fluctuations in blood glucose.
○ 3. Monitoring for Cushing's syndrome.
○ 4. Monitoring for respiratory complications.

**48.** Mr. Saunders complains of postnasal drip and a cerebrospinal fluid (CSF) leak is suspected. The nurse would confirm that his nasal drainage contains CSF by testing the drainage for
○ 1. acidity.
○ 2. protein.
○ 3. glucose.
○ 4. blood.

**49.** Mr. Saunders asks the nurse how they closed the incision made in the dura. The nurse would respond based on the knowledge that
○ 1. dissolvable sutures are used to close the dura.
○ 2. the nasal packing provides pressure until normal wound healing occurs.
○ 3. a patch is made with a piece of fascia.
○ 4. a synthetic mesh is placed to facilitate healing.

**50.** *Initial* treatment for a cerebrospinal fluid (CSF) leak will most likely consist of
○ 1. repacking the nose.
○ 2. returning the patient to surgery.
○ 3. bed rest with the head of the bed elevated.
○ 4. high-dose corticosteroid therapy.

**51.** Mr. Saunders is monitored for the development of diabetes insipidus. For which symptom should the nurse observe?
○ 1. Urine specific gravity greater than 1.030.
○ 2. Urine output between 5 and 10 L or more.
○ 3. Blood glucose greater than 300 mg/100 ml.
○ 4. Urine negative for glucose and ketones.

**52.** Diabetes insipidus is usually managed conservatively, but Mr. Saunders develops signs of dehydration. The nurse would expect the physician to order which medication?
○ 1. Corticotropin (ACTH).
○ 2. Vasopressin (Pitressin).
○ 3. Oxytocin.
○ 4. Cosyntropin (Cortrosyn).

**53.** Nursing care of Mr. Saunders' incision will include *all* of the following *except*

1. rinsing his mouth with saline.
2. frequent tooth-brushing.
3. cleaning his teeth with toothettes.
4. rinsing his mouth with half-strength peroxide.

**54.** Mr. Saunders' physician expects him to make a complete recovery, but he will be monitored for the development of which potential complication?
1. Acromegaly.
2. Cushing's disease.
3. Diabetes mellitus.
4. Hypopituitarism.

**55.** Mr. Saunders expresses concern about the effect that surgery will have on his sexual ability. Which of the following provides the *most accurate* information concerning the physiologic effects of hypophysectomy?
1. Removal of the source of excess hormone will restore the patient's natural potency and fertility.
2. Potency will be restored but the patient will remain infertile.
3. Fertility will be restored but decreased libido and potency will persist.
4. Exogenous hormones will be needed to restore potency now that the adenoma has been removed.

## THE PATIENT WITH ADDISON'S DISEASE

Mr. George Chang, a 48-year-old salesman, came down with what appeared to be a routine case of the flu. He awakened during the night extremely ill, anxious, and very weak. Afraid that her husband was dying, Mrs. Chang drove him to the emergency room, where he is tentatively diagnosed as having Addison's disease and being in crisis.

**56.** Which of the following is the *priority* nursing goal for Mr. Chang in the emergency room?
1. Controlling hypertension.
2. Preventing irreversible shock.
3. Preventing infection.
4. Relieving anxiety.

**57.** *All* of the following would be expected findings in Mr. Chang *except*
1. hypoglycemia.
2. nausea.
3. edema.
4. hypotension.

**58.** Mr. Chang is believed to have primary Addison's disease. Which of the following accurately describes this process?
1. Insufficient secretion of adrenocorticotropic hormone (ACTH).
2. Hypothalamic pituitary dysfunction.
3. Idiopathic atrophy of the adrenal gland.
4. Oversecretion of the adrenal medulla.

**59.** Neither Mr. nor Mrs. Chang had realized that he was ill. However, the nurse might expect that Mr. Chang had been exhibiting which symptoms recently?
1. Weight gain and irritability.
2. Hunger and double vision.
3. Lethargy and depression.
4. Muscle spasms and tetany.

**60.** In completing a visual inspection of Mr. Chang's skin, the nurse would expect it to exhibit which changes?
1. Abdominal striae.
2. Dry skin.
3. Bruised patches.
4. Deeper pigmentation.

**61.** Blood is sent for routine tests. *All* of the following results would be typical of Addison's disease *except*
1. hyperkalemia.
2. hyponatremia.
3. hyperglycemia.
4. elevated BUN.

**62.** During the management of the addisonian crisis, which nursing action would be appropriate?
1. Encourage frequent visitors to provide diversion for the patient.
2. Encourage the patient to assume responsibility for his care.
3. Permit as much activity as the patient's energy level can tolerate.
4. Keep the patient at absolute rest, providing no self-care.

**63.** Mr. Chang has an IV of 5% dextrose in normal saline running at 125 ml/hour. When hanging a new bottle of fluid, the nurse notes swelling and hardness at the needle site. Which action should she take?
1. Discontinue the infusion.
2. Apply a warm dressing to the site.
3. Stop the flow of solution temporarily.
4. Irrigate the needle with normal saline.

**64.** Mrs. Chang asks the nurse if the intravenous infusion meets her husband's nutritional needs, since he has vomited several times. The nurse's response should be based on the knowledge that one liter of 5% dextrose in normal saline delivers

1. 170 calories.
2. 200 calories.
3. 340 calories.
4. 500 calories.

**65.** Mr. Chang is admitted to the medical unit. A nursing diagnosis is "fluid volume deficit due to inadequate fluid intake and to fluid loss secondary to inadequate adrenal hormone secretion." As his oral intake increases, which of the following fluids would be *most* appropriate for Mr. Chang?
1. Milk and diet soda.
2. Water and eggnog.
3. Bouillon and juice.
4. Coffee and milkshakes.

**66.** Mr. Chang has been receiving glucocorticoid replacement. On what principle should Mr. Chang base his medication administration at home?
1. Various circumstances increase the need for glucocorticoids, so dosage adjustments will be needed.
2. The need for glucocorticoids stabilizes and a predetermined dose is taken every 3rd day.
3. Glucocorticoids are cumulative, so a dose is taken every 3rd day.
4. Because of the pattern of glucocorticoid secretion, a dose is taken every 6 hours.

**67.** Mr. Chang is prescribed cortisone acetate (Cortone) and fludrocortisone acetate (Florinef) as replacement. Which administration schedule will be followed?
1. Take both drugs three times a day.
2. Take the entire dose of both drugs first thing in the morning.
3. Take all the Florinef and two-thirds of the Cortone in the morning, the remaining Cortone in the afternoon.
4. Take half of each drug in the morning and at bedtime.

**68.** All patients taking glucocorticoids should be instructed to take them
1. with a full glass of water.
2. on an empty stomach.
3. between meals.
4. with meals or an antacid.

**69.** Mr. Chang must learn to interpret his own body cues and determine whether he is receiving the correct amount of glucocorticoid replacement. Fluid balance is one important cue. As part of patient teaching, the nurse should inform Mr. Chang that the *best* indicator of fluid balance is
1. skin turgor.
2. temperature.
3. thirst.
4. daily weight.

**70.** Which of the following would be an important indication that Mr. Chang is receiving too much glucocorticoid replacement?
1. Anorexia.
2. Dizziness.
3. Rapid weight gain.
4. Poor skin turgor.

**71.** Mr. Chang is attending a stress-management class because stress can precipitate addisonian crisis. The nurse discusses dietary modification that can be implemented during times of stress, since some stress is unavoidable. Selecting which of the following dietary modifications indicates that Mr. Chang has understood the teaching?
1. Increased sodium intake.
2. Restricted protein intake.
3. Restricted carbohydrate intake.
4. Increased potassium intake.

**72.** The nurse should teach Mr. Chang to include *all* of the following in his daily pattern of activities *except*
1. keeping his medications available at all times.
2. minimizing his daily activities to avoid overstressing his body.
3. following a regular activity and sleep pattern as much as possible.
4. monitoring his body's responses to the hormones daily.

**73.** Mr. Chang should anticipate a need for increased glucocorticoid supplementation in which situation?
1. Returning to work after a weekend.
2. Going on vacation.
3. Having dental work performed.
4. Having a routine medical checkup.

# THE PATIENT WITH CUSHING'S DISEASE

Mrs. Sally Spencer, 42, noticed that she had gained weight and that her face and body were round, while her legs and arms had become thinner. A tentative diagnosis of Cushing's disease is made.

**74.** The nurse knows that Cushing's disease causes multiple signs and symptoms. In taking the patient's history, the nurse would anticipate that Mrs. Spencer would report *all* of the following *except*
1. weight gain.
2. toughening of the skin.
3. slow healing of cuts.
4. periods of depression or euphoria.

75. When examining Mrs. Spencer, the nurse would expect to find
    ○ 1. orthostatic hypotension.
    ○ 2. muscle hypertrophy in the extremities.
    ○ 3. bruised areas on the skin.
    ○ 4. decreased body hair.

76. The symptoms of Cushing's disease can result from several different causes. Possible etiologies would include *all* of the following *except*
    ○ 1. atrophy of the adrenal cortex.
    ○ 2. pituitary oversecretion of adrenocorticotropic hormone (ACTH).
    ○ 3. tumor of the adrenal glands.
    ○ 4. prescription use of high-dose steroids.

77. Mrs. Spencer undergoes multiple laboratory tests. Which of the following test results would be consistent with a diagnosis of Cushing's disease?
    ○ 1. Postprandial hypoglycemia.
    ○ 2. Hypokalemia.
    ○ 3. Hyponatremia.
    ○ 4. Decreased urinary calcium.

78. Mrs. Spencer tells the nurse that the physician said her morning serum cortisol level was within normal limits. She asks, "How can that be? I'm not imagining all these symptoms!" The nurse's response should be based on the knowledge that
    ○ 1. some patients are very sensitive to the effects of cortisol and develop symptoms even with normal levels.
    ○ 2. a single random blood test cannot provide reliable information about endocrine levels.
    ○ 3. the excess cortisol in Cushing's disease is often a result of a loss of the normal diurnal secretion pattern.
    ○ 4. tumors tend to secrete hormones irregularly and the hormones are often not present in the blood.

79. Which of the following nursing goals should have the *highest* priority during Mrs. Spencer's preoperative care?
    ○ 1. Maintain adequate nutrition.
    ○ 2. Increase fluid intake.
    ○ 3. Ensure rest.
    ○ 4. Promote adequate activity.

80. Mrs. Spencer's diet needs to be modified to control her symptoms. Which diet would be *most appropriate?*
    ○ 1. A high-protein, high-calorie, restricted-sodium diet.
    ○ 2. A high-protein, low-calorie, restricted-sodium diet.
    ○ 3. A high-protein, high-calorie, high-potassium diet.
    ○ 4. A low-protein, restricted-sodium, high-potassium diet.

81. Mrs. Spencer has been found to have an adrenal tumor and she is scheduled for bilateral adrenalectomy. The nurse begins extensive preoperative teaching, which includes the importance of coughing and deep-breathing. Which of the following represents the *most accurate* teaching?
    ○ 1. "Sit in an upright position, take a deep breath, and then cough."
    ○ 2. "Hold your abdomen firmly, take several deep breaths, and then cough."
    ○ 3. "Tighten your stomach muscles as you inhale, and then cough forcefully."
    ○ 4. "Raise your shoulders to expand your chest and then give a deep cough."

82. Mrs. Spencer undergoes a bilateral adrenalectomy. Which of the following nursing interventions will take *priority* during the first day of Mrs. Spencer's postoperative care?
    ○ 1. Starting oral nutrition.
    ○ 2. Administering pain medication.
    ○ 3. Monitoring vital signs.
    ○ 4. Ensuring frequent position changes.

83. Mrs. Spencer's postoperative orders include an order for hydromorphone hydrochloride (Dilaudid) 2 mg subcutaneously every 4 hours p.r.n. for pain. This drug is administered in relatively small doses *primarily* because it is
    ○ 1. less likely to cause dependency.
    ○ 2. less irritating to subcutaneous tissues.
    ○ 3. as potent as most other analgesics in larger doses.
    ○ 4. excreted before accumulating in the body.

84. Which of the following factors would be *most important* in selecting the length of needle the nurse should use for Mrs. Spencer's subcutaneous injection?
    ○ 1. The diameter of the needle.
    ○ 2. The circumference of the patient's arm.
    ○ 3. The viscosity of the solution to be injected.
    ○ 4. The amount of medication to be administered.

85. On the day after surgery, Mrs. Spencer has a slightly elevated temperature. The nurse recognizes that the *most probable* cause of temperature elevation in the early postoperative period is
    ○ 1. dehydration.
    ○ 2. poor lung excursion.
    ○ 3. wound infection.
    ○ 4. urinary tract infection.

86. Mrs. Spencer is kept on bed rest for several days to stabilize her body's need for steroids postoperatively. Which of the following exercises has been found to be especially helpful in preparing a client for ambulation after a period of bed rest?
    ○ 1. Alternately flexing and extending the knees.
    ○ 2. Alternately abducting and adducting the legs.

3. Alternately tensing and relaxing the Achilles' tendons.

4. Alternately flexing and relaxing the quadriceps femoris muscles.

87. As the nurse helps Mrs. Spencer out of bed, she complains of gas pains in her abdomen. The nurse knows that the *most effective* way of relieving this discomfort would be to
    1. encourage the patient to ambulate.
    2. insert a rectal tube.
    3. insert a nasogastric tube.
    4. encourage the patient to drink carbonated liquids.

88. The nurse observes Mrs. Spencer's surgical incisions frequently. Because of Mrs. Spencer's steroid excess, she is at an increased risk for
    1. fistula formation.
    2. suture line dehiscence.
    3. wound infection.
    4. keloid scar formation.

89. Mrs. Spencer is nearing discharge. She tells the nurse that she is concerned about persistent body changes and the fact that her moods are still so unpredictable. She says, "I thought surgery was supposed to fix all that." The *most appropriate* nursing goal for this patient is to help her accept that
    1. the body changes are permanent.
    2. her body and mood will gradually return to near normal.
    3. the physical changes are permanent but the mood swings will disappear.
    4. the physical changes are temporary but the mood swings are permanent.

90. Which of the following should the nurse include in Mrs. Spencer's discharge teaching?
    1. Emphasizing that the patient will need steroid replacement for the rest of her life.
    2. Instructing the patient about the importance of tapering steroid medication carefully to prevent crisis.
    3. Informing the patient that steroids will be required only until her body is able to manufacture sufficient quantities on its own.
    4. Emphasizing that the patient will need to take steroids whenever her life involves physical or emotional stress.

91. Bone resorption is a complication of Cushing's disease. To counter the damage done by the disease, the nurse should encourage Mrs. Spencer to
    1. increase the amount of calcium in her diet.
    2. maintain a regular program of weight-bearing exercise.
    3. limit her dietary phosphate.
    4. include isometric exercise in her daily routine.

92. The physician has told Mrs. Spencer that she needs periodic testosterone injections. She asks the nurse, "What is that for? Did he forget I'm a female?" What is the nurse's correct response?
    1. "Androgens are needed to balance the reproductive cycle."
    2. "Androgens are necessary to restore the body's sodium and potassium balance."
    3. "Androgens are given to stimulate protein anabolism."
    4. "Androgens are given to stabilize mood swings."

# CORRECT ANSWERS AND RATIONALES

Numbers appear in parentheses following the rationales. The numbers identify textbooks listed in the references at the end of Part IV, where correct answers can be verified.

## The Patient with Hyperthyroidism

1. 1. Hyperthyroidism is a state of hypermetabolism. The increased metabolic rate generates heat and produces tachycardia and fine muscle tremors. It also causes weight loss and increased appetite. Anorexia would not be an expected finding. (25, 31)

2. 3. A change in the menstrual interval, diminished menstrual flow (oligomenorrhea), or even the absence of menstruation (amenorrhea) is likely to occur with the hormonal imbalances of hyperthyroidism. Dysmenorrhea is painful menstruation. Metrorrhagia is loss of blood during intermenstrual periods and menorrhagia is excessive loss of blood. (25, 31)

3. 1. A patient is likely to have falsely elevated radioactive iodine uptake (RAIU) and protein-bound iodine (PBI) tests if she has taken medications containing iodine within the past month or so. A relatively large variety of medications can falsely elevate or depress test results, but a medication containing iodine is most commonly used by a patient with hyperthyroidism. Digitalis, antihistamines, and ferrous sulfate are among medications that do not influence these tests. The RAIU and PBI uptake tests are used to evaluate thyroid function. (26, 31)

4. 1. Two serious side effects of propylthiouracil (Propacil) are leukopenia and agranulocytosis. The patient should be taught to report promptly any signs of an infection, such as a sore throat and fever, because the drug must be discontinued if untoward reactions occur. Other side effects include skin rash, edema, and enlargement of the salivary and lymph nodes. Such symptoms as painful menstruation, constipation, abdominal distention, increased urinary output, and itching are not associated with propylthiouracil therapy. (12, 16)

5. 3. Exophthalmos is characterized by protrusion of the eyeballs with a typical fixed stare. The condition is due to an accumulation of fluid in the fat pads behind the eyeballs. Exophthalmos may become so severe that the patient is unable to close the eyes. Such signs and symptoms as poor depth perception, poor pupillary responses, and inability to distinguish color are not associated with exophthalmos. (25, 31)

6. 2. A typical sign of hyperthyroidism is irritability due to the high level of thyroid hormone in the body. Such behavior decreases as the patient responds to therapy. Other explanations for the behavior of the patient described in this item are neither satisfactory nor correct. (25, 31)

7. 3. Because the eyelids tend not to close completely during sleep when exophthalmos is present, they should be taped shut to prevent drying. Sleeping masks have also proved helpful for some patients. Massaging the eyes, instilling ointment into the eyes, and covering the eyes with moist gauze pads are not satisfactory nursing measures to protect the eyes of a patient with exophthalmos while the patient sleeps. (25, 31)

8. 1. The best guideline in caring for a patient with hyperthyroidism is to provide an environment that promotes maximum physical and mental rest. A private room located in an area where the patient has privacy and quiet is best. The patient is likely to be disturbed if her room is near the noise and activity of the nurses' station. (25, 31)

9. 2. Potassium iodide (SSKI) is frequently administered before a thyroidectomy because it helps decrease the vascularity of the thyroid gland. A highly vascular thyroid gland is very friable, a condition that presents a hazard during surgery. Potassium iodide does not decrease the progression of exophthalmos, decrease the body's ability to store thyroxin, or increase the body's ability to excrete thyroxin. (25, 31)

10. 3. A saturated solution of potassium iodide (SSKI) should be well diluted in milk, water, juice, or a carbonated beverage before administering it to the patient to help disguise the strong, unpleasant, bitter taste. Also, this drug is very irritating to mucosa if taken undiluted. The diluted medication should be taken by the patient through a drinking straw to help prevent staining of the teeth. (12, 16)

11. 3. When a nurse discusses a patient's condition with a friend of the patient, as described in this item, she should offer an accurate description of the patient's condition without revealing confidential information. The statement should be as supportive of the friend as possible. Dismissing the friend by saying the nurse will check the patient, suggesting that the patient will be better after resting, and refusing to say anything about the patient are nonsupportive and ignore the friend's feelings. (11, 38)

**12.** 3. Laryngeal nerve damage is a potential complication of thyroid surgery because of the proximity of the thyroid gland and the recurrent laryngeal nerve. Asking the patient to speak helps monitor for signs of laryngeal nerve damage. Level of consciousness can be partially assessed by asking a patient to speak, but in this situation is not the primary reason for doing so. (25, 31)

**13.** 2. It is unlikely that a cutdown tray will be necessary for a patient who has had a thyroidectomy. Suctioning equipment, tracheostomy equipment, and equipment for administering oxygen should be readily available following a thyroidectomy in case the patient is unable to breathe properly. (25, 31)

**14.** 2. Tetany may occur following a thyroidectomy if the parathyroid glands are accidentally injured or removed during surgery. This would cause a disturbance in calcium metabolism. An early sign of tetany is numbness with tingling of the fingers and the circumoral region. (25, 31)

**15.** 2. The patient with tetany is suffering from hypocalcemia, which is treated by administering a preparation of calcium, such as calcium gluconate. (25, 31)

**16.** 1. The patient is most often placed in the Fowler's position following a thyroidectomy. The dressings are rather bulky. To check for hemorrhage, it is best for the nurse to slip her hand behind the patient's neck and check for blood on the back of the neck and on bed linens. Considerable bleeding can occur before it is discovered, if such measures as changing dressings, loosening dressings, and routinely checking the patient's vital signs are used to check for bleeding. (26, 31)

**17.** 2. To minimize tension on the incision when moving into the sitting position, the post-thyroidectomy patient should place both hands behind the head. (5, 25)

**18.** 3. Typical symptoms of hypothyroidism include fatigue and apathy, weight gain, brittle nails, dry skin, and numbness and tingling in the fingers. (25, 31)

## The Patient with Diabetes Mellitus

**19.** 3. Oral hypoglycemic agents of the sulfonylurea group, such as tolbutamide (Orinase), lower the blood glucose level by stimulating pancreatic cells to release insulin. These agents also increase insulin's ability to bind to the body's cells, thereby increasing the number of insulin receptors in the body. (25, 31)

**20.** 4. Knee-high stockings have circular elastic tops and are contraindicated because they obstruct circulation in the lower legs and feet. A person with diabetes is prone to serious foot problems when circulation is impaired. A diabetic should be taught to wear pantyhose, a garter belt, loose-top anklets, or a girdle with snap garters attached to it. Nylon stockings are not contraindicated, but if the patient's feet perspire freely cotton stockings, which absorb moisture better than nylon, are recommended. Nylon stockings are also contraindicated for those allergic to nylon. Well-fitting low-heeled shoes are recommended. (26, 31)

**21.** 3. Smoking cigarettes, wearing round garters, and crossing the legs when sitting predispose to poor circulation in the feet, causing them to feel cold. Wearing low-heeled shoes does not predispose to poor circulation in the feet. The diabetic patient is prone to serious foot problems when circulation is impeded and should be taught the importance of proper foot care. (26, 31)

**22.** 2. The diabetic patient should be advised to consult her physician when corns occur. Removing corns is serious for a diabetic because of the danger of traumatizing foot tissue. (25, 31)

**23.** 1. To minimize foot injury, a patient with diabetes mellitus should avoid going barefoot. (25, 31)

**24.** 2. Proper and careful first-aid treatment is important when a diabetic has a skin break, and the patient should be taught to consult a physician promptly if there are any signs of infection, such as redness, swelling, pain, or blistering. It is essential to teach the diabetic that any skin break, no matter how small, is worthy of concern. (25, 31)

**25.** 1. Foods high in dietary fibers are recommended by the American Diabetic Association because they tend to blunt the rise in blood glucose levels after meals. Dietary fibers are the part of food not broken down and absorbed during digestion. Most fibers come from plants. Good sources of fiber are whole grains, legumes, vegetables, fruit, and nuts. Poor sources of fiber include dairy products and meat, including organ meats. Foods fortified with vitamins are satisfactory if they also contain fiber. However, many foods fortified with vitamins either contain no dietary fiber, such as fortified milk, or contain very little fiber, such as products fortified with vitamins but made with refined grains. (26, 31)

**26.** 4. Diabetes mellitus is a disease of *glucose intolerance*. It is a disorder affecting the metabolism of carbohydrates, fats, and proteins. The diet of a diabetic should contain appropriate amounts of all three food nutrients, plus minerals and vitamins. (25, 31)

**27.** 2. Special foods are no longer required for a diabetic, nor should certain foods (except refined sugars) be eliminated entirely from the diet. More important is that mealtimes, meal size, and meal composition are consistent. Pasta products may be included in the diabetic's diet as part of the bread and cereal exchange. For example, one-half cup of pasta is equivalent to one slice of bread. Pasta sauces may be used if they are taken into account in the total diet. Food preferences of persons with various ethnic, religious, and cultural backgrounds should be taken into account in meal planning. If these preferences are not considered, patients may eat foods they prefer without making proper adjustments, or they may reject the diet entirely. (26, 31)

**28.** 4. Patients using tolbutamide (Orinase) should be cautioned about drinking alcohol. The two in combination, if alcohol is used excessively, tend to cause hypoglycemia. (12, 25)

**29.** 1. Factors predisposing to the development of non-insulin-dependent diabetes mellitus include obesity and decreased physical activity, which accentuates obesity. Smoking cigarettes, having had several children, and being of Italian ancestry are not factors predisposing to the development of non-insulin-dependent diabetes mellitus. (5, 31)

**30.** 4. The person with diabetes mellitus is especially prone to atherosclerosis. Such atherosclerotic complications as myocardial infarctions, cerebrovascular accidents, uremia, and gangrene are reported to cause 70% of deaths among diabetics. Death from cardiovascular and renal complications is rising among diabetics. (25, 31)

**31.** 4. Exercise increases the use of blood glucose by the muscles and therefore reduces the body's insulin requirements. Exercise also tends to lower cholesterol and triglyceride blood levels, which is especially important for diabetics because they are prone to cardiovascular diseases. In addition, exercise is a healthful diversional activity, is a good way to help control weight, and promotes circulation. The patient should be taught the effects of exercise on blood glucose levels and the importance of

snacking before exercise, unless the amount and time of exercise is the same every day and has already been taken into account when determining the dosage of hypoglycemic agents. (26, 31)

**32.** 3. The patient in this item uses NPH insulin; if hypoglycemia occurs, it is most likely to occur shortly before her evening meal (see table below). (25, 31)

**33.** 4. Learning goals are most likely to be attained when they are established mutually by the patient and the nurse. Learning is motivated by perceived problems or goals arising out of unmet needs. The perception of the unmet needs must be the patient's; the nurse helps the patient arrive at his own perception of the need or reason to learn. (31, 34)

**34.** 1. Learning has occurred when there is evidence of a change in behavior. A patient who performs a procedure faultlessly demonstrates that he has acquired a skill. Evaluating skill acquisition requires performance of that skill. (31, 34)

**35.** 1. The four signs of hypoglycemia most commonly reported by patents are nervousness, weakness, perspiration, and mental confusion. Other signs and symptoms include hunger, incoherent speech, tachycardia, and blurred vision. Anorexia and Kussmaul respirations are clinical manifestations of hypoglycemia or ketoacidosis. (26, 31)

**36.** 2. The renal threshold tends to rise with age. Therefore, the elderly patient may have an elevated blood glucose level without spilling glucose in the urine. (26, 31)

**37.** 1. Ketonuria indicates that the body is deriving most of its energy from the metabolism of fats rather than from carbohydrates. Glucose fails to enter body cells, and the body turns to fat as an alternate source of energy. Free fatty acids from fat tissues are acted upon by the liver to produce ketone bodies. The body's cells are limited in their ability to metabolize ketone bodies, and they then accumulate in the bloodstream and are excreted in the urine. (26, 31)

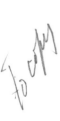

**TABLE: Insulin Therapy (see answer 32)**

| Type of Insulin | | Onset of Action (hrs) | Peak Action (hrs) | Duration of Action (hrs) |
|---|---|---|---|---|
| Regular-acting | Regular crystalline insulin | 1/2 to 1 | 2 to 4 | 6 to 8 |
| Intermediate-acting | Insulin zinc suspension (Lente) | 1 to 3 | 8 to 12 | 18 to 24 |
| | Isophane insulin suspension (NPH) | 2 to 4 | 8 to 12 | 18 to 28 |
| Long-acting | Protamine zinc insulin suspension (PZI) | 4 to 6 | 14 to 24 | 24 to 36 |

**38.** 4. Colds and the flu present special challenges to the diabetic because the body's need for insulin increases during illness. Therefore, the patient must take the prescribed dose of insulin, increase the frequency of blood and urine testing, attempt to maintain an adequate fluid intake to counteract the dehydrating effect of hyperglycemia, and contact the physician if urine ketone levels become significant. (26, 31)

**39.** 3. Renal failure frequently results from the vascular changes associated with diabetes mellitus. Deaths among diabetics due to renal and cardiovascular diseases are increasing. Heart disease and stroke are twice as common among diabetics than among non-diabetics. Damage to organs such as the liver, lungs, and pancreas is less life-threatening. (26, 31)

**40.** 3. The leading cause of blindness in the United States is diabetes mellitus, and the major cause of blindness in diabetics is diabetic retinopathy. Corneal problems, cataracts, refractive changes, and extraocular muscle changes also are noted. Astigmatism has not been associated with diabetes. (26, 31)

## The Patient with a Pituitary Adenoma

**41.** 1. Galactorrhea, the flow of breast milk, is caused by an overproduction of prolactin. Pituitary tumors can cause oversecretion of adrenocorticotropic hormone (ACTH), growth hormone (GH), and thyroid-stimulating hormone (TSH). Prolactin-secreting tumors account for 30% to 50% of the pituitary adenomas. (25, 31)

**42.** 2. Excess secretion of prolactin in males results in decreased libido and impotence; these are often the only significant symptoms until the tumor becomes quite large. Bony alterations and voice changes are associated with excess growth hormone. (25, 31)

**43.** 3. A macroadenoma of the pituitary extends beyond the confines of the sella turcica and may produce traditional symptoms of space-occupying lesions of the cranium indicative of intracranial pressure. Typical symptoms include headache and visual defects as the tumor encroaches on the optic nerve. (25, 31)

**44.** 4. With transsphenoidal hypophysectomy, the sella turcica is entered from below through the sphenoid sinus. There is no external incision; the incision is made between the upper lip and gums. (25, 31)

**45.** 3. Deep-breathing helps prevent atelectasis, but coughing is contraindicated because it increases intracranial pressure. Increased intracranial pressure should be avoided because it increases pressure on the graft site. The opening made in the dura mater on entering the sella turcica is frequently patched with a piece of fascia from the leg. Blow bottles are not effective in preventing atelectasis because they do not promote sustained alveolar inflation to maximal lung capacity. Frequent position changes help loosen lung secretions, but deep-breathing is *most important* in preventing atelectasis. (26, 31)

**46.** 2. Immediately after a hypophysectomy, the patient should be carefully monitored for signs of cerebral edema and increasing intracranial pressure (elevated blood pressure, widening pulse pressure, bradycardia, pupil changes, and altered respiratory pattern). Target gland deficiencies such as hypothyroidism and diabetes insipidus may result. Hypoglycemia may also occur. (26, 31)

**47.** 1. A major focus of nursing care following transsphenoidal hypophysectomy is preventing and monitoring for a CSF leak. Hypoglycemia and adrenocortical insufficiency may occur. Monitoring for postoperative respiratory complications is always important but is not related specifically to transsphenoidal hypophysectomy. (25, 31)

**48.** 3. CSF contains glucose, so the presence of glucose differentiates cerebrospinal fluid from nasal secretions. Frequent swallowing and complaints of postnasal drip may indicate a CSF leak. (25, 31)

**49.** 3. The dural opening is typically repaired with a patch of muscle or fascia taken from the leg. The patient should be prepared preoperatively for the presence of a leg incision. (25, 31)

**50.** 3. Significant or persistent CSF leaks are treated initially with bed rest with the head of the bed elevated to decrease pressure on the graft site. Most leaks heal spontaneously, but occasionally surgical repair is needed. (25, 31)

**51.** 2. Two major manifestations of diabetes insipidus are polyuria and polydipsia. The patient may drink and excrete 5 to 40 L of fluid daily. The urine specific gravity is low (between 1.001 and 1.006). Diabetes insipidus does not affect metabolism. Blood glucose greater than 250 mg/100 ml is associated with ketoacidosis. Urine negative for sugar and acetone is normal. (22, 25)

**52.** 2. Diabetes insipidus is usually self-limiting and can be managed by fluid replacement, but if a patient develops signs of dehydration vasopressin (Pitressin) is administered to promote fluid retention. Corticotropin (ACTH) and cosyntropin (Cortrosyn) are used to diagnose primary adrenal insufficiency. Oxytocin is used to induce or stimulate labor. (25, 31)

**53.** 2. After transsphenoidal surgery, the patient must be careful not to disturb the suture line while healing occurs. Frequent oral care will be provided with rinses of saline, peroxide, or other solutions and the teeth may be gently cleaned with toothettes, but vigorous tooth-brushing is contraindicated. (25, 31)

**54.** 4. Most patients who undergo removal of adenomas experience a gradual return to normal pituitary secretion, but the development of hypopituitarism is a possibility that should be monitored. There would be no reason for the excess secretion of other hormones. (25, 31)

**55.** 1. The patient's sexual problems are directly related to the excess quantities of prolactin. Removing the source of the excess hormone should allow the patient to return gradually to a normal physiologic pattern, but psychological effects may persist. (25, 31)

## The Patient with Addison's Disease

**56.** 2. Addison's disease is caused by a deficiency of adrenocortical hormones. Causes of this deficiency include surgical removal of the adrenal cortex or its destruction as a result of infections such as histoplasmosis. Immediate treatment for the patient in addisonian crisis is directed toward combating shock by restoring circulating volume and administering hydrocortisone. Hypotension is present due to the shock. Relieving anxiety is appropriate when the patient's condition is stabilized, but the calm, competent emergency department staff will be initially reassuring. Preventing infection is not an appropriate goal in this situation. (5, 26)

**57.** 3. The deficiency of adrenal hormones can cause profound changes. Inhibited gluconeogenesis produces hypoglycemia in many patients and the decreased ability to retain sodium causes decreased fluid volume and hypotension. Edema would not be expected. Gastrointestinal disturbances are expected findings in Addison's disease. (25, 31)

**58.** 3. Primary disease refers to a problem in the gland itself. Primary Addison's disease occurs from idiopathic atrophy of the glands. The process is believed to be autoimmune in nature. Pituitary dysfunction can cause Addison's disease, but this is not a primary disease process. (25, 31)

**59.** 3. The onset of Addison's disease is usually insidious and patients are relatively asymptomatic until a major stressor such as illness throws them into crisis. Although many of the disease symptoms are vague and nonspecific, lethargy and depression are early symptoms experienced by most patients. Other early symptoms include irritability, weight loss, nausea, and vomiting. (25, 31)

**60.** 4. A bronzing or general deepening of skin pigmentation is a classic sign of Addison's disease. Uncontrolled adrenocorticotropic hormone (ACTH) release occurs along with beta lipoprotein, which is hydrolyzed to melanocyte-stimulating hormone (MSH). The skin responds with deeper pigmentation. Dry skin is associated with hypothyroidism, and abdominal striae and bruised patches are associated with hypersecretion of the adrenal cortex. (25, 31)

**61.** 3. Hyperkalemia and hyponatremia are characteristic of Addison's disease. There is decreased renal perfusion and excretion of waste products. Decreased hepatic gluconeogenesis and increased tissue glucose uptake cause patients to experience hypoglycemia, not hyperglycemia, which is associated with cortisol excess. (25, 31)

**62.** 4. During addisonian crisis, patients should be kept at absolute rest, minimizing the body's psychological and physiologic stress. Patients should not participate in self-care during this period and the stimulation of social visiting should be minimized. (25, 31)

**63.** 1. Signs of infiltration include slowing of the infusion, swelling, pain, hardness, pallor, and coolness of the skin at the site. When these signs are present, the IV should be discontinued and restarted elsewhere. (16, 36)

**64.** 1. Each liter of 5% dextrose in normal saline contains 170 calories. (16, 36)

**65.** 3. The electrolyte imbalances found in Addison's disease are hypoglycemia, hyponatremia, and hyperkalemia. Salted bouillon and fruit juices provide glucose and sodium to replenish these deficits. Free water could cause further sodium dilution. Coffee would aggravate the fluid deficit because of its diuretic effect. Milk contains potassium and sodium, and diet soda does not contain sugar. (5, 26)

**66.** 1. The need for glucocorticoids changes with circumstances. The basal dose is established when the patient is discharged, but this dose covers only normal daily needs and does not provide for additional stressors. As the manager of the medication schedule, the patient needs to know signs of excessive and insufficient dosages. Glucocorticoids are not cumulative and must be taken daily. They are never discontinued suddenly, because in the absence of endogenous production an addisonian crisis could result. Glucocorticoids are taken daily, two-thirds of the dose at about 8 a.m. and the remainder at about 4 p.m. This schedule stimulates the diurnal pattern of normal secretion, with highest levels between 4 and 6 a.m. and lowest levels in the evening. (5, 31)

**67.** 3. Florinef can be administered once a day, but the administration of the glucocorticoid replacement should follow the body's natural diurnal pattern of secretion with greater amounts secreted during the day to meet increased demand. Typically baseline administration is 25 mg of cortisone acetate in the morning and 12.5 mg in the afternoon. (25, 31)

**68.** 4. Oral steroids have pronounced ulcerogenic properties and should consistently be administered with meals if possible or otherwise with antacid. They should never be taken on an empty stomach. (12, 31)

**69.** 4. Measuring daily weight is a reliable, objective method of monitoring fluid balance. Rapid variations in weight reflect changes in fluid volume. Tongue turgor is a more reliable indicator of fluid volume changes than skin turgor in older persons because their skin is less elastic. Temperature is not a direct measurement of fluid balance. (5, 26)

**70.** 3. Patients taking glucocorticoids walk a fine line between underdosage and overdosage. Fluid balance is an important indicator of the adequacy of hormone replacement. Rapid weight gain is a warning sign that the patient is receiving too much hormone replacement. (25, 31)

**71.** 1. Low serum sodium can occur if levels of adrenocortical hormones are low. Dietary protein intake is not affected. Because hypoglycemia is also associated with Addison's disease, restriction of carbohydrates is counterproductive. Hyperkalemia accompanies hyponatremia, so increased potassium intake would not be helpful. (5, 26)

**72.** 2. Self-care is an essential part of the management of Addison's disease. Patients must learn to adjust their glucocorticoid doses in response to the normal and unexpected stresses of daily living. Regularity in daily habits will make adjustment easier, but patients should not be encouraged to withdraw from normal activities to avoid stress. (25, 31)

**73.** 3. Episodes of illness or surgery place tremendous stress on the body, and increased glucocorticoids will be needed. Dental work is a good example. Extreme emotional or psychological stress will also require dosage adjustment. (25, 31)

## The Patient with Cushing's Disease

**74.** 2. Excess cortisol secretion causes rapid protein catabolism, depleting the collagen support of the skin. The skin is thin and fragile and bruises easily. Striae appear on the abdomen and hips. Weight gain, mood swings, and slow wound healing are all typical symptoms of Cushing's disease. (25, 31)

**75.** 3. Skin bruises from skin and blood vessel fragility are classic signs of Cushing's disease. Muscle wasting occurs in the extremities and fluid retention causes hypertension. Hair on the head typically thins, while body hair increases. (25, 31)

**76.** 1. Cushing's disease is caused by hormone oversecretion, which can be caused by a tumor, overstimulation from the pituitary, or the use of prescription steroids. It cannot occur from glandular atrophy. (25, 31)

**77.** 2. Sodium retention is typically accompanied by potassium depletion. Patients with Cushing's disease exhibit postprandial or persistent hyperglycemia, and bone resorption of calcium increases the urine calcium load. Kidney stones are possible. (25, 31)

**78.** 3. The most prominent feature of Cushing's disease is often the loss of the diurnal secretion pattern. Random morning cortisol levels may be within normal limits, but secretion continues at that level throughout the entire day. Twenty-four-hour urine collections are often useful in identifying the cumulative excess. (25, 31)

**79.** 3. During the acute period for a patient with excessive cortisol secretion, a major nursing goal is to prevent potential complications. These include electrolyte imbalance, hypertension, and glucose imbalance. These problems could be dangerous for the patient and/or could delay surgery. While all of these goals are important, ensuring adequate rest to avoid stress is the most basic way to prevent complications. (25, 31)

**80.** 2. The primary dietary interventions are to reduce weight by restricting total calories and reducing water weight by restricting sodium. Excess protein catabolism requires supplemental protein intake. In addition, the patient should be encouraged to eat potassium-rich foods, as serum levels are typically depleted. (25, 31)

**81.** 2. Effective splinting for a high incision reduces stress on the incision line, reduces pain, and increases the ability of the patient to cough and deep-breathe effectively. Deep-breathing should always precede coughing. (24, 36)

**82.** 3. The primary concern following adrenalectomy is to identify and prevent adrenal crisis. Vital signs are the most important evaluation measure; the other interventions are secondary concerns. (25, 31)

**83.** 3. Dilaudid is about five times more potent than morphine sulfate, from which it is prepared. It is therefore administered in small doses. It has the same but generally fewer side effects than morphine. (12, 16)

**84.** 2. The length of the needle depends on the amount of adipose tissue at the site and the angle used to administer the injection. Viscosity of the medication would determine the needle diameter. The amount of medication could influence the site of the injection, which in turn could affect the length of the needle; however, this is not the most important factor in this situation. (24, 36)

**85.** 2. Pulmonary problems become evident in the early postoperative period. Poor lung excursion from bed rest, pain, and retained anesthesia are all common causes of slight postoperative temperature elevations. Would infections typically appear 4 to 7 days after surgery. (5, 26)

**86.** 4. Alternately flexing and relaxing the quadriceps muscles helps prepare the patient for ambulation. The other exercises listed will do nothing to increase a patient's readiness for walking. (26, 36)

**87.** 1. Decreased mobility is one of the most common causes of distention. Ambulation increases peristaltic activity and helps move gas. (5, 36)

**88.** 2. Persistent cortisol excess undermines the collagen matrix of the skin, and wound healing is impaired. There is an increased risk of infection, but nonunion of the surgical incision is the most likely complication. (25, 31)

**89.** 2. As the body readjusts to normal cortisol levels, mood and many physical changes will gradually return to the individual's near-normal state. (5, 26)

**90.** 1. Bilateral adrenalectomy requires lifelong replacement of the adrenal hormones. If unilateral surgery is performed, most patients gradually re-establish a normal secretion pattern. (25, 31)

**91.** 2. Osteoporosis is a serious outcome of prolonged cortisol excess because the calcium is resorbed out of the bone. Regular daily weight-bearing exercise is the most effective way to drive calcium back into the bones. (25, 31)

**92.** 3. The testosterone is needed not to support sexual functioning but to support protein anabolism. It is therefore required by both males and females. (25, 31)

# test 6

*The Patient with Cancer of the Bladder*
*The Patient with Renal Calculi*
*The Patient with Acute Renal Failure*
*The Patient with Cystitis*
*The Patient with Chronic Renal Failure*
*Correct Answers and Rationales*

Select the one *best* or *correct* answer and indicate your choice by filling in the circle with a pencil in front of the option you have chosen. If the answer you would prefer is not given, select the one you think is *most appropriate*.

## THE PATIENT WITH CANCER OF THE BLADDER

Mr. Arthur Cooper, 57, is admitted to the outpatient surgery unit for a cystoscopy to rule out cancer of the bladder.

**1.** The *most common* symptom associated with bladder cancer is
○ 1. painless hematuria.
○ 2. decreasing urine output.
○ 3. burning on urination.
○ 4. frequent infections.

**2.** Which of the following symptoms would indicate that Mr. Cooper has developed a complication following the cystoscopy?
○ 1. Dizziness.
○ 2. Chills.
○ 3. Pink-tinged urine.
○ 4. Bladder spasms.

**3.** If Mr. Cooper develops lower abdominal pain, the nurse should instruct him to
○ 1. apply an ice pack to his pubic area.
○ 2. massage his abdomen gently.
○ 3. ambulate as much as possible.
○ 4. sit in a tub of warm water.

**4.** The diagnosis of cancer is made and Mr. Cooper is scheduled for an ileal conduit. Preoperatively, the nurse tells Mr. Cooper that he will have a nasogastric tube after surgery. The *primary* purpose of the nasogastric tube is to
○ 1. prevent the aspiration of stomach contents.
○ 2. provide a means for enteral feeding.
○ 3. prevent the accumulation of gas until peristalsis returns.
○ 4. allow the stomach to rest until healing occurs.

**5.** Mr. Cooper has an ileal conduit created and tolerates the surgery well. Which of the following postoperative complications is a patient undergoing pelvic surgery such as an ileal conduit at increased risk for developing?
○ 1. Bleeding.
○ 2. Infection.
○ 3. Thrombophlebitis.
○ 4. Atelectasis.

**6.** The nurse would expect Mr. Cooper's urine to contain
○ 1. pus.
○ 2. feces.
○ 3. glucose.
○ 4. mucus.

**7.** The nurse assesses Mr. Cooper's stoma regularly for edema. Which symptom would indicate that excessive stomal edema is probably occurring?
○ 1. The patient's temperature is elevated.
○ 2. The patient's stoma is dribbling urine.
○ 3. The patient complains of discomfort around the stoma.
○ 4. The patient's urinary output falls below 30 ml/hour.

**8.** The nurse begins teaching Mr. Cooper to care for his ileal conduit. She instructs him to empty the appliance frequently to help prevent
○ 1. tearing of the ileal conduit.
○ 2. interruption of urine production.
○ 3. forcing urine into the kidneys.
○ 4. separation of the appliance from the skin.

**9.** To prevent urine leakage when changing the appliance, the nurse should teach Mr. Cooper to
○ 1. insert a gauze wick into the stoma.
○ 2. close the opening temporarily with a cellophane seal.
○ 3. suction the stoma for a few minutes before changing the appliance.
○ 4. avoid oral fluids for several hours before changing the appliance.

10. Mr. Cooper will be using a reusable appliance at home. The nurse should teach him to clean it routinely with
    ○ 1. baking soda.
    ○ 2. soap.
    ○ 3. hydrogen peroxide.
    ○ 4. alcohol.
11. Which solution will be useful in helping control odor in the collecting bag after it has been cleaned?
    ○ 1. Salt solution.
    ○ 2. Vinegar solution.
    ○ 3. Ammonia solution.
    ○ 4. Bleaching solution.
12. Which of the following preparations would be *most effective* in protecting the skin around Mr. Cooper's stoma from irritation?
    ○ 1. Baking soda.
    ○ 2. Cornstarch.
    ○ 3. Stomahesive.
    ○ 4. Karaya.
13. The nurse teaches Mr. Cooper to attach his appliance to a standard urinary collection bag at night. The *most important* reason for doing this is to
    ○ 1. prevent reflux of urine into the stoma.
    ○ 2. avoid appliance separation.
    ○ 3. prevent leakage of urine.
    ○ 4. eliminate the need to restrict fluids.
14. The nurse teaches Mr. Cooper measures to prevent the development of urinary tract infection. Which of the following measures would likely be *most effective?*
    ○ 1. Avoiding persons with respiratory tract infections.
    ○ 2. Maintaining a daily fluid intake of 2,000 to 3,000 ml.
    ○ 3. Using sterile technique to change the appliance.
    ○ 4. Irrigating the stoma daily.
15. Which of the following juices is most often recommended as a means of maintaining urine acidity?
    ○ 1. Apple juice.
    ○ 2. Carrot juice.
    ○ 3. Pineapple juice.
    ○ 4. Cranberry juice.

## THE PATIENT WITH RENAL CALCULI

Ms. Madeline Crawford, 46, is admitted to the hospital with a diagnosis of renal calculi (stones). She developed renal calculi several years ago. She is experiencing severe flank pain and is nauseated, and her temperature is 100.6° F.

16. Given an understanding of renal calculi and Ms. Crawford's assessment data, the nurse's *immediate* goal should be to
    ○ 1. prevent urinary complications.
    ○ 2. alleviate the nausea.
    ○ 3. alleviate the pain.
    ○ 4. maintain fluid and electrolyte balance.
17. Ms. Crawford is to have a kidney, ureter, and bladder (KUB) x-ray. Which of the following would be ordered to prepare Ms. Crawford for the x-ray?
    ○ 1. Fluids and food will be withheld the morning of the examination.
    ○ 2. A tranquilizer will be ordered to be given prior to the examination.
    ○ 3. An enema will be ordered to be given prior to the x-ray examination.
    ○ 4. There is ordinarily no special preparation required for the x-ray examination.
18. Intravenous fluids are ordered for Ms. Crawford. When the nurse starts the patient's intravenous therapy, she applies a tourniquet and selects the site for inserting the needle. When should the tourniquet be removed?
    ○ 1. When the skin has been cleansed.
    ○ 2. As soon as the needle is in the vein.
    ○ 3. As soon as the needle is positioned under the skin.
    ○ 4. When the needle has been secured with tape.
19. Ms. Crawford's veins in all of the following areas appear easy to enter. Which area should the nurse use *first?*
    ○ 1. The back of the hand.
    ○ 2. The inner aspect of the elbow.
    ○ 3. The inner aspect of the forearm.
    ○ 4. The outer aspect of the forearm.
20. In addition to being nauseated and experiencing severe flank pain, Ms. Crawford is experiencing pain in her groin and bladder. The nurse should judge that these symptoms are *most likely* the result of
    ○ 1. nephritis.
    ○ 2. referred pain.
    ○ 3. urinary retention.
    ○ 4. additional stone formation.
21. Ms. Crawford is scheduled for an intravenous pyelogram (IVP) to determine the location of the stone. Which of the following would be *most important* to include in her pretest preparation?
    ○ 1. Ensuring adequate fluids the day of the test.
    ○ 2. Preparing her for the possibility of bladder spasms during the test.

○ 3. Checking for allergies to iodine.

○ 4. Determining when she had her last bowel movement.

**22.** The intravenous pyelogram indicates that Ms. Crawford has a 2-cm stone in her left kidney pelvis. Hydronephrosis is also present. If hydronephrosis goes unchecked, pyelonephritis is likely to develop due to

○ 1. low urine acidity.

○ 2. stagnation of urine in the renal pelvis.

○ 3. impaired circulation to the renal pelvis.

○ 4. poor filtration of blood in the nephrons.

**23.** Ms. Crawford undergoes a left nephrectomy after it is determined that her left kidney is nonfunctional. Her postoperative orders state that a daily urine specimen is to be sent to the laboratory. Ms. Crawford has an indwelling Foley catheter attached to a urinary drainage system. Which procedure for collecting a urine specimen is most often recommended?

○ 1. Open the spigot on the collecting bag and allow urine to empty into the specimen container.

○ 2. Disconnect the drainage tube from the collecting bag and allow urine to flow from the tubing into the specimen container.

○ 3. Disconnect the drainage tube from the indwelling catheter and allow urine to flow from the catheter into the specimen container.

○ 4. Remove urine from the drainage tube with a sterile needle and syringe and place urine from the syringe into the specimen container.

**24.** Which of the following changes is *most likely* to occur in the urine, if the nurse allows the urine specimen she has collected from Ms. Crawford to stand at room temperature for several hours?

○ 1. Its color will fade.

○ 2. It will become alkaline.

○ 3. It will develop a sweet odor.

○ 4. Its specific gravity will decrease.

**25.** Ms. Crawford also has a ureteral catheter in place. A priority nursing action is to

○ 1. irrigate the catheter with 30 ml of saline every 8 hours.

○ 2. ensure that the catheter is draining freely.

○ 3. clamp the catheter every 2 hours for 30 minutes.

○ 4. ensure that the catheter drains at least 30 ml per hour.

**26.** Where should the nurse tape Ms. Crawford's indwelling Foley catheter in order to reduce urethral irritation?

○ 1. To the patient's inner thigh.

○ 2. To the patient's gown.

○ 3. To the patient's lower abdomen.

○ 4. To the patient's lower thigh.

**27.** Paralytic ileus is a frequent complication of renal surgery. Which of the following orders would be *inappropriate* for Ms. Crawford if she develops paralytic ileus?

○ 1. Encourage the patient to ambulate every 2 to 4 hours.

○ 2. Offer the patient 3 to 4 ounces of carbonated beverage every hour.

○ 3. Encourage the patient to use the incentive spirometer every 2 hours while awake.

○ 4. Continue intravenous therapy with 1,000 ml of 5% dextrose in water every 8 hours.

**28.** Which of the following nursing assessments *best* indicates that Ms. Crawford's peristaltic activity is returning to normal?

○ 1. The patient passes flatus.

○ 2. The patient is thirsty.

○ 3. Bowel sounds are absent upon auscultation.

○ 4. Peristalsis can be felt when the abdomen is palpated.

**29.** Ms. Crawford develops thrombophlebitis postoperatively. A major goal of nursing care is to prevent

○ 1. arteriole collapse.

○ 2. pulmonary emboli.

○ 3. cerebrovascular aneurysm.

○ 4. contractures of the leg.

**30.** Which of the following pharmaceutical agents is *most likely* to be ordered to decrease blood clotting?

○ 1. Folic acid (Folvite).

○ 2. Heparin sodium.

○ 3. Vitamin $B_{12}$ (cyanocobalamin).

○ 4. Vitamin K (AquaMEPHYTON).

**31.** Warfarin sodium (Coumadin) is ordered for Ms. Crawford. After she receives the drug for a few days, the following medications are also prescribed for her in normal average adult doses. Which of these medications should the nurse question before administering it?

○ 1. Ampicillin (Amcill).

○ 2. Secobarbital (Seconal).

○ 3. Ascorbic acid (vitamin C).

○ 4. Dioctyl sodium sulfosuccinate (Colace).

**32.** All of the following findings appear in Ms. Crawford's nursing history. Which finding is *least likely* to have predisposed her to renal calculi?

○ 1. Having had several urinary tract infections in the past 2 years.

○ 2. Having taken large doses of vitamin C in the past several years.

○ 3. Drinking less than the recommended amount of milk.

○ 4. Having been on prolonged bed rest following an accident the previous year.

33. What information should the nurse include in Ms. Crawford's discharge teaching because of her history of stone formation?
    ○ 1. Her daily fluid intake should be at least 2 to 3 L.
    ○ 2. She should strain her urine at home regularly.
    ○ 3. She should eliminate dairy products from her diet.
    ○ 4. She should follow measures to alkalinize her urine.

34. Because Ms. Crawford's stone was found to be composed of uric acid, she is to eat a low-purine, alkaline-ash diet. The nurse has been reinforcing the dietitian's teaching. Ms. Crawford's selection of which food items indicates that she understands the dietary modification?
    ○ 1. Milk, apples, tomatoes, and corn.
    ○ 2. Eggs, spinach, dried peas, and gravies.
    ○ 3. Salmon, chicken, caviar, and asparagus.
    ○ 4. Grapes, corn, cereals, and liver.

35. Allopurinol (Zyloprim) 200 mg daily is prescribed for Ms. Crawford. Which of the following side effects are associated with this medication?
    ○ 1. Abdominal pain, retinopathy, and anorexia.
    ○ 2. Drowsiness, maculopapular rash, and anemia.
    ○ 3. Nausea, vomiting, and nasal congestion.
    ○ 4. Dizziness, erythema, and palpitations.

36. Ms. Crawford has a clinic appointment 10 days after discharge. Which laboratory finding indicates that allopurinol (Zyloprim) has had a therapeutic effect?
    ○ 1. The urinary alkaline phosphatase level has decreased.
    ○ 2. The urinary calcium excretion has increased.
    ○ 3. The serum calcium level has increased.
    ○ 4. The serum uric acid level has decreased.

## THE PATIENT WITH ACUTE RENAL FAILURE

Ms. Lois Janske suffered a severe anaphylactic response to a dose of penicillin. She develops acute renal failure over the next 72 hours.

37. Ms. Janske developed acute renal failure *primarily* because of
    ○ 1. spasms of the renal arteries.
    ○ 2. blood clots in the loops of Henle.
    ○ 3. inadequate cardiac output.
    ○ 4. acute tubular necrosis.

38. The *most significant* sign of acute renal failure is
    ○ 1. a rise in blood pressure.
    ○ 2. an elevation in body temperature.
    ○ 3. a decrease in urine output.
    ○ 4. an increase in urine specific gravity.

39. Ms. Janske's blood urea nitrogen (BUN) level is elevated. This *most probably* occurred because of
    ○ 1. destruction of kidney cells.
    ○ 2. hemolysis of red blood cells.
    ○ 3. below-normal metabolic rate.
    ○ 4. reduction in renal blood flow.

40. Ms. Janske's potassium blood level is elevated and she is to receive sodium polystyrene sulfonate (Kayexalate). Ms. Janske is receiving the drug because of its ability to
    ○ 1. increase potassium excretion from the colon.
    ○ 2. release hydrogen ions for sodium ions.
    ○ 3. increase calcium absorption in the colon.
    ○ 4. exchange sodium for potassium ions in the colon.

41. If Ms. Janske's potassium level were to continue to rise, the nurse should be prepared for which of the following emergency situations?
    ○ 1. Cardiac arrest.
    ○ 2. Pulmonary edema.
    ○ 3. Circulatory collapse.
    ○ 4. Hemorrhage.

42. A high-carbohydrate, low-protein diet is prescribed for Ms. Janske. The rationale for serving the patient a diet high in carbohydrates is that carbohydrates will
    ○ 1. act as a diuretic.
    ○ 2. reduce demands on the liver.
    ○ 3. help maintain urine acidity.
    ○ 4. prevent the development of ketosis.

43. Ms. Janske says, "The doctor says I am to have a low-protein diet. Why must I have that kind of a diet?" The nurse should base her explanation on knowledge that a low-protein diet helps minimize
    ○ 1. water retention.
    ○ 2. protein breakdown.
    ○ 3. sodium intoxication.
    ○ 4. metabolic alkalosis.

44. Ms. Janske asks the nurse what kinds of foods are classified as proteins of "high biologic value." Which response is correct?
    ○ 1. Soybeans, legumes, and beans.
    ○ 2. Whole grains, peanut butter, and corn.
    ○ 3. Breads, cereals, and nuts.
    ○ 4. Eggs, red meat, and poultry.

45. Ms. Janske asks the nurse for a snack. Because the patient's potassium level is elevated, which of the following snacks is *most appropriate* for the nurse to serve Ms. Janske?
    ○ 1. A gelatin dessert.
    ○ 2. Yogurt.

○ 3. An orange.

○ 4. Dried peanuts.

46. Ms. Janske is on a 24-hour fluid restriction of 500 ml, plus replacement for urine output. Since her 24-hour urine output yesterday was 150 ml, the total fluid allotment for the next 24 hours is 650 ml. What change-of-shift report information given by the nurse who worked from 7:30 a.m. to 3:30 p.m. indicates an understanding of how to distribute this fluid?

○ 1. The fluid allotment for this shift was supplemented with gelatin and ice cream.

○ 2. One-half of this shift's fluid allotment was given with both breakfast and lunch.

○ 3. The fluid allotment for this shift was given in small amounts throughout the entire shift.

○ 4. The entire fluid allotment for this shift was given in the morning to minimize the patient's thirst.

47. Mr. Janske expresses anxiety concerning his wife's recovery, even though prompt treatment was given. The nurse should base her response on knowledge that the patient's prognosis is *most likely*

○ 1. poor.

○ 2. fair.

○ 3. good.

○ 4. very good.

48. Ms. Janske has an external cannula inserted in her forearm for hemodialysis. Which of the following measures should the nurse *avoid* when caring for Ms. Janske?

○ 1. Using the unaffected arm for blood pressure measurements.

○ 2. Ensuring that clamps are at the bedside at all times.

○ 3. Auscultating the cannula for a bruit each shift.

○ 4. Injecting heparin into the cannula each shift.

49. An arteriovenous fistula is usually considered to be preferable to a cannula for long-term hemodialysis. What is the *primary* advantage of an arteriovenous fistula?

○ 1. It causes less discomfort.

○ 2. It can be used immediately after being created.

○ 3. It causes fewer problems with clotting or hemorrhage.

○ 4. It leaves no visible sign of the need for dialysis.

50. Ms. Janske undergoes her first hemodialysis treatment. It is essential that the nurse assess her carefully for signs of disequilibrium syndrome. Classic symptoms would include

○ 1. headache, confusion, and nausea.

○ 2. fever, rales, and shortness of breath.

○ 3. fever, chills, and chest pain.

○ 4. hypotension, tachycardia, and shortness of breath.

51. If disequilibrium syndrome should occur during dialysis, the *priority* nursing action is to

○ 1. start nasal oxygen.

○ 2. slow the rate of dialysis.

○ 3. reassure the client.

○ 4. place the patient in the Trendelenburg position.

52. Ms. Janske is heparinized while on dialysis. Which of the following statements about the anticoagulation that occurs with dialysis is correct?

○ 1. Regional anticoagulation can be achieved through the use of heparin for the machine and protamine sulfate for the patient.

○ 2. Warfarin sodium (Coumadin) is used to maintain anticoagulation between treatments.

○ 3. Heparin does not enter the patient's body, so there is no risk of bleeding.

○ 4. The patient's clotting time is seriously prolonged for several hours after each treatment.

53. Which of the following abnormalities in blood values will *not* be improved by Ms. Janske's dialysis treatment?

○ 1. Elevated serum creatinine.

○ 2. Hyperkalemia.

○ 3. Low hemoglobin.

○ 4. Hypernatremia.

## THE PATIENT WITH CYSTITIS

Mrs. Mary Jane Turner, 24, comes to a walk-in clinic in moderate distress with a probable diagnosis of acute cystitis. She is on her honeymoon and is accompanied by her husband.

54. Which of the following symptoms would the nurse expect Mrs. Turner to report during the assessment?

○ 1. Fever and chills.

○ 2. Burning and frequency with urination.

○ 3. Suprapubic pain and nausea.

○ 4. Dark, concentrated urine.

55. A midstream urine specimen is ordered and the nurse tells Mrs. Turner how to collect the specimen correctly. Which of the following should the nurse include in the instructions?

○ 1. Void directly into the sterile specimen container.

○ 2. Save the first urine that you void.

○ 3. Stop the collection of urine after the bladder is empty.

4. Cleanse the urethral meatus after obtaining the specimen.

56. The specimen is sent for a sensitivity test. The *primary* purpose for this test is to help
    1. detect drugs to which the patient may be allergic.
    2. determine whether the infection is located in the bladder or in the kidneys.
    3. identify the microorganisms found in the culture of the patient's urine.
    4. select drugs to which microorganisms in the patient's urine are susceptible.

57. Mrs. Turner asks the nurse, "How did I get this infection?" The nurse should explain that in most instances, cystitis is caused by
    1. congenital strictures in the urethra.
    2. an infection elsewhere in the body.
    3. a stasis of urine in the urinary bladder.
    4. an ascending infection from the urethra.

58. The nurse can anticipate to a reasonable degree of certainty that the microorganism *most likely* responsible for Mrs. Turner's cystitis is
    1. *Escherichia coli.*
    2. *Candida albicans.*
    3. *Staphylococcus aureus.*
    4. *Enterobacter aerogenes.*

59. The physician tells Mrs. Turner that the infection has probably been precipitated by sexual intercourse and that he will order an antibiotic for her. Before he can continue, she becomes emotionally upset, crying that her honeymoon is ruined. A urine specimen obtained after an emotional outburst of this type is most likely to contain
    1. serum.
    2. glucose.
    3. ketone bodies.
    4. microscopic casts.

60. The nurse helps calm Mrs. Turner, who tearfully asks if this means she should abstain from intercourse for the rest of her honeymoon. What advice should the nurse offer her?
    1. "Avoid intercourse until you've completed the antibiotic therapy and then limit intercourse to once a week."
    2. "Limit intercourse to once a day in the early morning after the bladder has rested."
    3. "As long as you're comfortable, you can have intercourse as often as you wish, but void within 15 minutes after intercourse."
    4. "You and your husband can enjoy intercourse as often as you wish. Just make sure he wears a condom and uses a spermicide."

61. Mrs. Turner is afraid to discuss this sexual issue with her husband. She feels that she is a failure because she got sick on her honeymoon and asks the nurse to speak to her husband for her. Which would be the *most* reasonable approach for the nurse?
    1. Have a group meeting with Mr. and Mrs. Turner, the doctor, the nurse, and the pharmacist to support Mrs. Turner.
    2. Insist that Mrs. Turner talk with her husband alone, as good communication is the basis for a successful marriage.
    3. Talk first with Mr. Turner alone and then with Mr. and Mrs. Turner to share Mr. Turner's reactions.
    4. Spend time with Mrs. Turner to increase her comfort and then stay with her while she talks with her husband.

62. Mrs. Turner is given a prescription for co-trimoxazole (Bactrim-DS) for her infection. Which of the following statements would indicate that Mrs. Turner understands the principles related to taking antibiotics?
    1. "I will take the pills until I feel better and keep the remainder for recurrence."
    2. "I will take all the pills and then return to my doctor."
    3. "I will take the pills until the symptoms subside and then taper the dose to one pill a day."
    4. "I will take all the pills and then have the prescription renewed once."

63. The nurse teaches Mrs. Turner methods to relieve her discomfort until the antibiotic takes effect. Which of the following responses by Mrs. Turner would indicate that she understands?
    1. "I'll place ice packs on my perineum."
    2. "I'll take hot tub baths."
    3. "I'll drink a cup of warm tea every hour."
    4. "I'll void every 5 to 6 hours."

64. Mrs. Turner is also given a prescription for phenazopyridine hydrochloride (Pyridium). This drug is used in urinary tract infection to
    1. release formaldehyde and provide bacteriostatic action.
    2. potentiate the action of the antibiotic.
    3. provide an analgesic effect on the bladder mucosa.
    4. prevent the crystallization that can occur with sulfa drugs.

65. Before using phenazopyridine hydrochloride (Pyridium), Mrs. Turner should be taught that the drug has which side effect?
    1. It turns the urine bright orange-red.
    2. It causes some burning on urination.
    3. It produces gastric distress.
    4. It causes slight drowsiness.

66. Which of the following statements by Mrs. Turner would indicate that she is at high risk for a recurrence of cystitis?
    ○ 1. "I can usually go 8 to 10 hours without needing to empty my bladder."
    ○ 2. "I shower every morning."
    ○ 3. "I wipe from front to back after voiding."
    ○ 4. "I drink a lot of water during the day."
67. To prevent recurrences of the cystitis, Mrs. Turner should be encouraged to include *all* of the following in her daily routine *except*
    ○ 1. wearing cotton underpants.
    ○ 2. avoiding prolonged wear of tight pants.
    ○ 3. douching regularly with 0.25% acetic acid.
    ○ 4. avoiding the use of bubble baths and vaginal sprays.
68. The nurse explains to Mrs. Turner the importance of drinking large quantities of fluid. To help Mrs. Turner understand, the nurse should tell her to drink
    ○ 1. twice as much fluid as she usually drinks.
    ○ 2. at least 1 quart more fluid than she usually drinks.
    ○ 3. a lot of water, juice, and other fluid throughout the day.
    ○ 4. at least 3 quarts of fluids each day.
69. Mrs. Turner had a blood specimen drawn as part of her infection workup and she is found to have iron-deficiency anemia. Typically, this means that the patient has
    ○ 1. high hemoglobin and hematocrit levels.
    ○ 2. an elevated white cell count and a low platelet count.
    ○ 3. a decreased white cell count and a high platelet count.
    ○ 4. a hemoglobin level proportionately lower than the hematocrit level.
70. Oral ferrous sulfate (Feosol) is prescribed for Mrs. Turner to take at home. The nurse's teaching plan indicates that Mrs. Turner should drink a half-glass of orange juice when taking the medication. What is the nurse's rationale for teaching the patient to take orange juice with the iron preparation?
    ○ 1. The orange juice decreases the toxicity of the medication.
    ○ 2. The orange juice helps prevent the development of mouth ulcers.
    ○ 3. The orange juice reduces the bitter taste caused by the enteric-coated tablet.
    ○ 4. The orange juice acts as a reducing agent to increase the absorption of the medication.
71. The nurse's teaching plan also indicates that Mrs. Turner should be told about an effect that the oral iron preparation will likely have on one of her body excretions. Which of the following effects is Mrs. Turner *most likely* to note?
    ○ 1. Her urine will become bright orange.
    ○ 2. Her perspiration will become excessive.
    ○ 3. Her stool will become dark red or black.
    ○ 4. Her sputum will become yellow or light green.

## THE PATIENT WITH CHRONIC RENAL FAILURE

Mr. Leroy Brown, a 48-year-old mail carrier, has been treated for hypertension since age 22. He developed renal insufficiency 5 years ago and went into chronic failure last year. He had a permanent peritoneal catheter inserted at that time. He was extremely reluctant to accept hemodialysis and has so far been successfully managed with peritoneal dialysis.

72. Common clinical manifestations of uremia include *all* of the following *except*
    ○ 1. dry, itchy skin.
    ○ 2. fatigue.
    ○ 3. anorexia.
    ○ 4. hypotension.
73. Which of the following laboratory results would be *unexpected* in a patient with chronic renal failure?
    ○ 1. Serum potassium 6.0 mEq/L.
    ○ 2. Serum creatinine 4.9 mg/dl.
    ○ 3. Blood urea nitrogen 15 mg/dl.
    ○ 4. Serum phosphate 5.2 mg/dl.
74. The primary disadvantage of using standard peritoneal dialysis for the long-term management of chronic renal failure is the fact that
    ○ 1. the danger of hemorrhage is very high.
    ○ 2. it cannot correct severe imbalances.
    ○ 3. it is a slow method of treatment.
    ○ 4. the chance of contracting hepatitis is very high.
75. Mr. Brown complains that he feels nauseated at least part of every day. The nurse should explain that the nausea is the result of
    ○ 1. the acidosis caused by his medications.
    ○ 2. the accumulation of waste products in his blood.
    ○ 3. chronic anemia and fatigue.
    ○ 4. his excess fluid load.
76. The dialysis solution is warmed before use in peritoneal dialysis *primarily* to
    ○ 1. encourage the removal of serum urea.
    ○ 2. force potassium back into the cells.
    ○ 3. add extra warmth to the body.
    ○ 4. promote abdominal muscle relaxation.

**77.** The *chief* characteristic of the peritoneum that makes peritoneal dialysis possible for patients such as Mr. Brown is that the peritoneal membrane is
○ 1. serous.
○ 2. convoluted.
○ 3. double-sided.
○ 4. semipermeable.

**78.** During Mr. Brown's dialysis, the nurse observes that the solution draining from his abdomen is consistently blood-tinged. Which interpretation of this observation would be correct?
○ 1. It is common when the patient has a permanent peritoneal catheter.
○ 2. It indicates abdominal blood vessel damage.
○ 3. It can indicate kidney damage.
○ 4. It is caused by too rapid infusion of the dialysate.

**79.** During Mr. Brown's dialysis, the nurse observes that the flow of dialysate stops before the full amount of solution has drained out. What would be the appropriate nursing intervention?
○ 1. Have the patient get out of bed and sit in a chair.
○ 2. Turn the patient from side to side.
○ 3. Reposition the peritoneal catheter.
○ 4. Have the patient get up and walk.

**80.** Which of the following nursing interventions would *not* be included in Mr. Brown's care plan while he is being dialyzed?
○ 1. Encourage visitors.
○ 2. Monitor his blood pressure.
○ 3. Observe his behavior.
○ 4. Keep him n.p.o.

**81.** The *most* potentially dangerous complication that may occur with peritoneal dialysis is
○ 1. abdominal pain.
○ 2. gastrointestinal bleeding.
○ 3. peritonitis.
○ 4. muscle cramps.

**82.** Following completion of dialysis, the nurse would expect Mr. Brown to exhibit
○ 1. hematuria.
○ 2. weight loss.
○ 3. hypertension.
○ 4. increased urinary output.

**83.** Aluminum hydroxide (Amphojel) is prescribed for Mr. Brown. The purpose of using this drug with patients who have chronic renal failure is to
○ 1. relieve the pain of gastric hyperacidity.
○ 2. prevent Curling's stress ulcers.
○ 3. bind phosphate in the intestine.
○ 4. reverse metabolic acidosis.

**84.** The nurse teaches Mr. Brown when to take the aluminum hydroxide (Amphojel). Which statement indicates that he understands the teaching?

○ 1. "I will take it every 4 hours around the clock."
○ 2. "I will take it between meals and at bedtime."
○ 3. "I will take it when I have a sour stomach."
○ 4. "I will take it with meals and bedtime snacks."

**85.** A medication history reveals that Mr. Brown takes magma (Milk of Magnesia) for constipation. Why does the nurse suggest that he switch to psyllium hydrophilic mucilloid (Metamucil)?
○ 1. Magnesium intoxication can occur.
○ 2. Milk of Magnesia is too harsh on the bowel.
○ 3. Metamucil is more palatable.
○ 4. Milk of Magnesia is high in sodium.

**86.** In planning patient teaching strategies for Mr. Brown, the nurse must keep in mind the neurologic impact of uremia. Which strategy is *most appropriate*?
○ 1. Providing all needed teaching in one extended session.
○ 2. Validating frequently Mr. Brown's understanding of the material.
○ 3. Conducting a one-on-one session with Mr. Brown.
○ 4. Using videotapes to reinforce the material as needed.

**87.** Mr. Brown is quite anemic. Anemia occurs in chronic renal failure primarily as a result of a deficiency in
○ 1. iron.
○ 2. erythropoietin.
○ 3. folic acid.
○ 4. vitamin $B_{12}$.

**88.** Sexual problems can be very troublesome to patients with chronic renal failure. *All* of the following strategies could be useful in helping patients cope with such problems *except* suggesting
○ 1. using vinegar-and-water mouthwash to control breath odor.
○ 2. using alternate forms of intimacy during periods of impotence.
○ 3. planning rest periods before sexual activity.
○ 4. avoiding sexual activity to prevent the embarrassment of impotency.

**89.** Mr. Brown has asked to be evaluated for a home continuous ambulatory peritoneal dialysis (CAPD) program. The *major advantage* of this approach to chronic renal failure is that it
○ 1. is relatively low in cost.
○ 2. allows the patient to be more independent.
○ 3. is faster and more efficient than standard peritoneal dialysis.
○ 4. has fewer potential side effects and complications.

**90.** Mr. Brown asks if his diet would change on continuous ambulatory peritoneal dialysis (CAPD).

Which of the following would be the nurse's *most accurate* response?

○ 1. Diet restrictions are more rigid with CAPD because standard peritoneal dialysis is a more effective technique.
○ 2. Diet restrictions are the same for both CAPD and standard peritoneal dialysis.
○ 3. Diet restrictions with CAPD are fewer than with standard peritoneal dialysis because dialysis is constant.
○ 4. Diet restrictions with CAPD are fewer than with standard peritoneal dialysis because it works more quickly.

**91.** Peritoneal infection is the most serious potential complication of CAPD. Which of the following manifestations is the *most significant* indication of peritoneal infection?
○ 1. Cloudy dialysate fluid.
○ 2. Swelling in the legs.
○ 3. Poor drainage of the dialysate fluid.
○ 4. Redness at the catheter insertion site.

# CORRECT ANSWERS AND RATIONALES

Numbers appear in parenthesis following the rationales. The numbers identify textbooks listed in the references at the end of Part IV, where correct answers can be verified.

## The Patient with Cancer of the Bladder

1. 1. Painless hematuria is the most common symptom associated with bladder cancer. Bleeding from the lesions occurs fairly early in the disease process, but bladder cancer is basically asymptomatic in the early stages. Bladder cancer is not related to infection or renal function. (25, 31)

2. 2. Pink-tinged urine and bladder spasms are common following cystoscopy, but the presence of chills could indicate the onset of acute infection that can progress to septic shock. (26, 31)

3. 4. Lower abdominal pain following cystoscopy is frequently caused by bladder spasms. Sitz baths provide comfort and relax the spasms. Ice is not effective in dealing with spasms. Ambulation may increase bladder irritability. (25, 26)

4. 3. The primary purpose of a nasogastric tube after surgery for an ileal conduit is to prevent the accumulation of gas and fluids (gastric secretions) and to prevent abdominal distention. Distention causes pressure on the intestinal anastomosis. By preventing abdominal distention, a nasogastric tube prevents aspiration; however, in this patient, the tube's primary purpose is to prevent abdominal distention. (25, 31)

5. 3. Patients undergoing pelvic surgery are at increased risk for developing thrombophlebitis postoperatively. Extensive pelvic surgery such as that involved in an ileal conduit removes lymph nodes from the pelvis and results in circulatory congestion from edema and stasis. Bleeding, infection, and atelectasis are not unique to this type of surgery. (25, 31)

6. 4. The urine causes some local irritation on the intestine, and hence the patient with an ileal conduit can be expected to excrete urine that contains mucus. Pus, or feces, in the urine are abnormal signs, and if they occur they should be reported promptly. There is no reason to expect that glucose will be found in the patient's urine. (25, 31)

7. 4. Urinary output of less than 30 ml/hour could indicate stomal edema, which obstructs urinary output. An elevated temperature should be noted but is not related to stomal edema. Discomfort around the stoma is common postoperatively after construction of an ileal conduit. Dribbling of urine from the stoma is normal. (22, 26)

8. 4. If the appliance becomes too full, it is likely to pull away from the skin completely or leak urine onto the skin. A full appliance will not tear the ileal conduit, interrupt urine production, or force urine into the kidneys. (5, 25)

9. 1. Inserting a gauze wick into the stoma helps prevent urine leakage when changing the appliance. The stoma should not be sealed or suctioned, and oral fluids should not be avoided. (25, 31)

10. 2. A reusable appliance should be routinely cleaned with soap and water. (25, 31)

11. 2. A distilled vinegar solution acts as a good deodorizing agent after an appliance has been cleansed well with soap and water. If the patient prefers, a commercial deodorizer may be used. Salt solution does not deodorize. Ammonia and bleaching agents may damage the appliance. (26, 31)

12. 3. Skin around a urinary stoma can be protected with Stomahesive. Karaya is not used because urine erodes it. Baking soda and cornstarch are not as effective as Stomahesive. (24, 36)

13. 1. The most important reason for attaching the appliance to a standard urinary collection bag at night is to prevent reflux of urine into the stoma and ureters. Use of a standard collection bag also prevents separation of the appliance from the skin and urinary leakage. A patient with an ileal conduit should drink 3,000 ml of fluid daily, unless contraindicated. (22, 25)

14. 2. Maintaining a daily fluid intake of 2,000 to 3,000 ml is likely to be most effective in preventing urinary tract infection. A high fluid intake results in high urinary output, which prevents urinary stasis and bacterial growth. Clean, not sterile, technique is used to change the appliance. An ileal conduit stoma is not irrigated. (22, 25)

15. 4. Cranberry juice helps increase urine acidity, as do vitamin C and an acid-ash diet. (31, 37)

## The Patient with Renal Calculi

16. 3. The immediate nursing goal for this patient with renal calculi is to alleviate the pain, which can be excruciating. The other goals are appropriate throughout the patient's hospitalization but are not immediate. (22, 31)

**17.** 4. A KUB x-ray examination ordinarily requires no preparation. It is usually done while the patient lies on her back. A KUB does not involve the use of radiopaque substances. (22, 26)

**18.** 2. When starting an intravenous infusion, the nurse should remove the tourniquet as soon as the needle is in the vein. Until then, the tourniquet keeps the vein distended so that it is more visible and easier to enter. After the needle is in the vein, the tourniquet should be removed before applying tape so that fluid will start to enter the vein promptly. (24, 36)

**19.** 1. When starting an intravenous infusion, the nurse initially uses veins low on the hand or arm. Should the vein be damaged, veins higher on the arm are still available for use. After a vein higher up on the arm has been damaged, veins below it on the arm cannot be used. (24, 36)

**20.** 2. The pain associated with renal colic due to calculi is often referred to the groin and bladder in the female and to the testicles in the male. Nausea, vomiting, abdominal cramping, and diarrhea may also be present. Unlikely causes of pain during renal colic in the groin and bladder or testicles include urinary retention or nephritis. The type of pain described in this situation is unlikely to be due to additional stone formation. (22, 25)

**21.** 3. A patient scheduled for an IVP should be assessed for allergies to iodine and shellfish. Patients with such allergies may be allergic to the IVP dye and be at risk for an anaphylactic reaction. Bowel preparation is important before an IVP to allow visualization of the ureters and bladder, but checking for allergies is most important. (25, 26)

**22.** 2. Residual urine in the calyces of the kidneys predisposes to pyelonephritis. Hence, an obstruction that causes urine to accumulate in the kidneys requires prompt treatment. Such factors as urine acidity and poor filtration of blood in the kidney nephrons do not play a role in the development of pyelonephritis when an obstruction in the urinary tract is present. (25, 26)

**23.** 4. When a urine specimen is to be obtained from a patient who has an indwelling Foley catheter attached to a closed urinary drainage system, the urine specimen should be removed from the drainage tube using a sterile needle and syringe. This technique is least likely to predispose to a urinary tract infection because the drainage system is not opened to the air. Furthermore, this urine specimen is fresh, unlike the urine collected in the drainage bag. (25, 26)

**24.** 2. Urine is normally acidic, but upon standing at room temperature it becomes alkaline. If water evaporates from the specimen, the specimen will become darker in color and the specific gravity will increase. The odor will not change appreciably in several hours. (25, 31)

**25.** 2. The ureteral catheter should drain freely without bleeding at the site. The catheter is rarely irrigated and is never clamped. The patient's *total* urine output, ureteral catheter plus voiding or Foley catheter output, should be 30 ml per hour or 60 ml per 2 hours. (22, 25)

**26.** 1. To reduce urethral irritation, the nurse tapes the Foley catheter to the inside of a female patient's thigh or to the thigh or abdomen of a male patient. Taping the catheter to the patient's gown does not prevent urethral irritation and may result in accidental removal of the catheter as the patient moves. (24, 36)

**27.** 2. Patients with paralytic ileus are n.p.o. until peristalsis returns. Ambulation stimulates the return of peristalsis. Intravenous fluids and incentive spirometry are routine postoperative orders. (22, 26)

**28.** 1. Passing of flatus indicates the return of peristalsis, as do active bowel sounds. Peristalsis is difficult to palpate and palpation is not an appropriate method of assessing bowel activity. Thirst is related to dehydration, not peristalsis. (5, 25)

**29.** 2. Pulmonary emboli are the greatest danger of thrombophlebitis. A clot may break loose and travel to a vital organ, such as the lungs, heart, or brain. (25, 26)

**30.** 2. An anticoagulant such as heparin sodium is the drug of choice when a patient develops thrombophlebitis. Anticoagulants prevent thrombi from forming and existing clots from extending, but do not dissolve existing clots. Vitamin K hastens blood clotting and is contraindicated in thrombophlebitis. Vitamin $B_{12}$ and folic acid do not affect blood clotting. (25, 26)

**31.** 2. Barbiturates such as secobarbital (Seconal) decrease anticoagulant activity. Barbiturates act to increase the liver synthesis of enzymes that metabolize anticoagulants. Therefore, if secobarbital must be used, the dosage of warfarin sodium (Coumadin) may need to be increased. (25, 26)

**32.** 3. A high, rather than low, milk intake predisposes to renal calculi formation. Such conditions as urinary tract infections, low fluid intake, periods of immobility, and large daily doses of vitamins C and D tend to predispose to stone formation. Men age 30 to 50 experience calculi more often than women. Patients who have had renal calculi twice often experience recurrence. People living in hot climates can develop calculi due to an increased insensible fluid loss combined with an inadequate fluid intake. This results in concentrated urine and precipitation of urinary salts. (25, 26)

**33.** 1. A high daily fluid intake is essential in patients at risk for calculi formation because it prevents urinary stasis, which can cause crystallization. Depending on the composition of the stone, the patient *may* be instructed to limit calcium intake or acidify the urine. (25, 31)

**34.** 1. Because a high-purine diet contributes to the formation of uric acid, a low-purine diet is advocated. An alkaline-ash diet is also advocated because uric acid crystals are more prone to develop in acid urine. Foods that may be used as desired on a low-purine diet include milk, fruits of all kinds, tomatoes, cereal and cereal products, and corn. Foods containing very large amounts of purines include liver, caviar, and gravies. Foods containing moderate to large amounts of purine include spinach, dried peas, salmon, chicken, and asparagus. Foods allowed on an alkaline-ash diet are milk; fruits, except cranberries, plums, and prunes; vegetables, especially legumes and green vegetables; and minimal amounts of ham, beef, trout, and salmon. (4, 26)

**35.** 2. Side effects associated with allopurinol (Zyloprim) include drowsiness, maculopapular rash, anemia, abdominal pain, retinopathy, nausea, vomiting, and erythema multiforme. (12, 16)

**36.** 4. By inhibiting the synthesis of uric acid, allopurinol (Zyloprim) decreases its excretion. The effectiveness of allopurinol is assessed using serum uric acid levels. The goal is to lower the serum level. (22, 25)

## The Patient with Acute Renal Failure

**37.** 4. There are three categories of acute renal failure: prerenal, renal, and postrenal. Causes of prerenal failure occur outside the kidney and include poor perfusion and a decrease in circulating volume due to such factors as trauma, septic shock, and dehydration. Causes of renal failure, such as hypersensitivity (allergic disorders), obstruction of renal vessels, and nephrotoxic agents, result in structural damage to the kidney due to acute tubular necrosis. Postrenal failure, or obstruction within the urinary tract, is a result of kidney stones, tumors, or benign prostatic hypertrophy. (25, 31)

**38.** 3. A sudden alteration in the amount of urinary output is typical of acute renal failure. Most commonly, the initial alteration is a very low urinary output. Later in the course of acute renal failure, the patient may have marked diuresis (nonoliguric failure). Other common signs and symptoms of acute renal failure include lethargy, nausea and vomiting, diarrhea, headaches, muscle twitching, and convulsions. Serum creatinine and urea nitrogen levels are elevated. The specific gravity of urine is usually within a low-normal range because the kidneys have difficulty concentrating urine. High body temperatures and sudden rises in blood pressure are not typically associated with acute renal failure. (25, 31)

**39.** 4. Reduction in renal blood flow causes an elevated blood urea nitrogen level. Urea is an end product of protein metabolism and is normally excreted by the kidneys. Any impairment in renal function causes an increase in the plasma urea level. (25, 31)

**40.** 4. Polystyrene sulfonate (Kayexalate), a cation-exchange resin, causes the body to excrete potassium through the gastrointestinal tract. In the intestines, particularly the colon, the sodium of the resin is partially replaced by potassium. The potassium is then eliminated when the resin is eliminated with feces. Polystyrene sulfonate may be administered orally or rectally and is used specifically to treat hyperkalemia. (25, 31)

**41.** 1. Hyperkalemia is *dangerous* because it predisposes to serious cardiac dysrhythmias and cardiac arrest. Therefore, the nurse should be prepared to treat cardiac arrest when caring for a hyperkalemic patient. (25, 31)

**42.** 4. High-carbohydrate foods meet the body's caloric needs during acute renal failure. Protein is limited because its breakdown may result in an accumulation of toxic waste products. (25, 31)

**43.** 2. A low-protein diet helps minimize protein breakdown (catabolism), one of the causes of hyperkalemia in a patient with acute renal failure. Whatever protein is allowed should be of high biologic value and should contain essential amino acids. (25, 31)

**44.** 4. Proteins of high biologic value are those that contain all the essential amino acids required for tissue building and repair. Meat, poultry, fish, eggs, and milk are good examples. These foods are important in renal disease because the total quantity of protein must be so severely restricted. (6, 41)

**45.** 1. Gelatin desserts contain little or no potassium and can be served to a patient whose potassium intake is limited. Foods high in potassium include bran and whole grains; most dried, raw, and frozen fruits and vegetables; most milk and milk products; chocolate, nuts, raisins, coconut, and strong brewed coffee. Highly refined foods, fruits and vegetables cooked in generous amounts of water, butter, cream, and hard candies are generally low in potassium content. (6, 41)

**46.** 3. Thirst is a strong motivator to drink. Giving small amounts of fluid during an 8-hour shift helps minimize thirst. Gelatin and ice cream are inappropriate supplements because they are foods that become liquid at room temperature. Some fluids should be given with meals, but not the entire 8-hour allotment. (25, 31)

**47.** 4. The kidneys have a remarkable ability to recover from serious insult. In view of the prompt and effective treatment, the patient's prognosis should be very good. Effective treatment for acute renal failure consists primarily of restoring normal fluid and electrolyte balances so the body can restore renal functioning and repair renal tissue. (25, 31)

**48.** 4. Heparin is not injected into the cannula. This intervention is used to maintain the patency of a heparin lock. Because it is part of the general circulation, the cannula cannot be heparinized. The external cannula must be handled carefully and protected from injury and disruption. The arm with the cannula is not used for blood pressure measurements, intravenous therapy, or venipunctures. A tourniquet or clamps should be at the bedside because dislodgement of the cannula would cause arterial hemorrhage. Patency is assessed by auscultating for a bruit every shift. (25, 31)

**49.** 3. The internal fistula causes fewer problems with clotting, and the risk of hemorrhage is minor. It requires fewer precautions for care and usually has significant longevity. It must heal and mature after surgery, however, and cannot be used immediately. The anastomosis is fairly prominent, but appearance is not a primary consideration. (25, 31)

**50.** 1. Typical symptoms of disequilibrium syndrome include headache, nausea and vomiting, confusion, and even seizures. Disequilibrium syndrome typically occurs near the end or after the completion of hemodialysis treatment. (25, 31)

**51.** 2. If disequilibrium syndrome occurs during dialysis, the most appropriate intervention is to slow the rate of dialysis. The syndrome is believed to result from the too-rapid removal of urea and excess electrolytes from the blood; this causes transient cerebral edema, which produces the symptoms. (25, 31)

**52.** 1. Regional anticoagulation can be achieved by using heparin in the dialyzer and protamine sulfate, its antagonist, in the patient. The patient's clotting time is not seriously affected, although some rebound effect may occur. The clotting time is monitored carefully. Coumadin is not used in dialysis treatment. (5, 26)

**53.** 3. Dialysis will correct electrolyte imbalances and clear metabolic waste products from the body, but it has no effect on anemia. Because some red cells are injured during the procedure, dialysis aggravates a low hemoglobin. (5, 26)

## The Patient with Cystitis

**54.** 2. The classic symptoms of cystitis are severe burning, urgency, and frequent urination. Some patients also have fever or may experience hematuria and suprapubic pain. Systemic symptoms are more likely to accompany pyelonephritis than cystitis. (25, 31)

**55.** 1. When collecting a midstream urine, the patient voids directly into a sterile specimen container. Other correct techniques include discarding the first 30 ml, stopping the collection before the bladder is empty, and cleaning the urethral meatus before obtaining the specimen. (24, 36)

**56.** 4. The culture helps identify the organisms that are causing the infection. The sensitivity test assists in the selection of the appropriate drugs for treatment. (20, 36)

**57.** 4. Although a variety of conditions may result in cystitis, the most common cause is an ascending infection from the urethra. (5, 25)

**58.** 1. *Escherichia coli* have been found to be responsible for approximately 80% to 90% of urinary tract infections. (5, 25)

**59.** 2. Emotional stress causes the body to secrete epinephrine, which causes an elevation in the blood glucose level. When the level of blood glucose surpasses the renal threshold concentration, glycosuria (glucose in the urine) can be expected. (20, 27)

**60.** 3. Intercourse is not contraindicated in cystitis. Voiding immediately after intercourse flushes bacteria from the urethra, which should help prevent recurrences of cystitis. There is no reason to wait until the antibiotic therapy is completed or to limit the frequency of intercourse. A condom and spermicide do not prevent cystitis because it is caused by the introduction of the patient's own organisms (usually *Escherichia coli*) into the urethra. (5, 26)

**61.** 4. As newlyweds, the patient and her husband need to develop a strong communication base. The nurse facilitates the development of this base by preparing the patient and being there for support. Being present also allows the nurse to intervene, if necessary, to facilitate the discussion of a difficult topic. Given this situation, an interdisciplinary conference is inappropriate and would not promote intimacy for the patient and her husband. Insisting that the patient talk with her husband alone is not complying with her request. Having the nurse speak first with the husband alone shifts responsibility away from the couple. (5, 26)

**62.** 2. Antibiotics are prescribed for a definite length of time and all the pills should be taken. A urine culture should be done after the course of antibiotic therapy to be sure the urine is bacteria-free. Stopping the medication early may cause a recurrence of the infection. Tapering the dosage is inappropriate with antibiotics because it lowers the therapeutic blood level. Refilling the prescription would be indicated only after urine culture indicates that the urine is not bacteria-free and the physician prescribes another course of antibiotics. (5, 26)

**63.** 2. Hot tub baths promote relaxation and help relieve urgency, discomfort, and spasm. Heat to the perineum is more helpful than cold because heat reduces inflammation. While liberal amounts of fluids are to be encouraged, tea, coffee, and cola can be irritating to the bladder and should be avoided. Voiding at least every 2 to 3 hours should be encouraged because it reduces urinary stasis. (5, 26)

**64.** 3. Phenazopyridine hydrochloride (Pyridium) is a urinary analgesic that works directly on the bladder mucosa to relieve the distressing symptoms of dysuria. (12, 16)

**65.** 1. Patients should be told that phenazopyridine hydrochloride (Pyridium) causes the urine to turn bright orange-red, which may stain underwear. It can be quite frightening for a patient to see bright orange-red urine without having been forewarned. (12, 16)

**66.** 1. Stasis of urine in the bladder is one of the chief causes of bladder infection, and individuals who void infrequently are at greater risk of reinfection. Generous fluid intake (unless contraindicated) and scrupulous hygiene are excellent preventive measures, but patients should also be taught to void every 2 to 3 hours during the day. (5, 25)

**67.** 3. A woman can adopt multiple health-promotion measures to prevent the recurrence of cystitis, including *avoiding* too-tight pants, non-cotton underpants, and irritating substances such as bubble baths and vaginal soaps and sprays. Regular douching is not recommended and can alter the pH of the vagina, increasing the risk of infection. (25, 31)

**68.** 4. The instruction should be as specific as possible and avoid general statements such as "a lot." A specific goal is most useful. A mix of fluids will increase the chances of compliance. (5, 26)

**69.** 4. Many women of child-bearing age are anemic. Anemia refers to the hemoglobin content of the red cells, which will be low in proportion to the hematocrit. Anemia does not involve white cells or platelets. (5, 26)

**70.** 4. The ascorbic acid in orange juice is believed to act as a reducing agent to promote better absorption of oral iron preparations from the gastrointestinal tract. (12, 16)

**71.** 3. Oral iron preparations typically cause the stools to become black or dark red. This is a common side

effect and patients should be prepared for it. Oral iron preparations affect neither the color of urine or sputum nor the amount of perspiration. (12, 16)

## The Patient with Chronic Renal Failure

**72.** 4. Hypertension, not hypotension, is typical of uremia. Hypertension occurs because renin is secreted in response to renal ischemia and elevates the blood pressure. Uremic patients typically have dry, itchy skin and are troubled by chronic fatigue, anorexia, and even nausea. (5, 31)

**73.** 3. The stated BUN level is within the normal limits of 10 to 15 mg/dl and therefore would be *unexpected* in renal failure. The BUN level is usually significantly elevated in chronic renal failure because chronic renal failure causes retention of waste products and electrolytes. Elevated serum potassium (normal 3.5 to 5.0 mEq/L), elevated serum creatinine (normal 0.8 to 1.7 mg/dl for males, 0.6 to 1 mg/dl for females), and hyperphosphatemia (normal 2.5 to 4.8 mg/dl) are normal in chronic renal failure. (26, 31)

**74.** 3. A disadvantage of standard peritoneal dialysis in long-term management of chronic renal failure is that it requires large blocks of time. Peritoneal dialysis is quite effective in maintaining a patient's fluid and electrolyte balance. Neither the danger of hemorrhage nor of contracting hepatitis is high with peritoneal dialysis. (26, 31)

**75.** 2. Nausea is typically the result of the chronic presence of retained waste products in the body. The patient can control the nausea most effectively by following his diet regimen strictly and avoiding wide swings in blood values between treatments. (25, 26)

**76.** 1. The primary reason for warming the solution used for peritoneal dialysis is that the warm solution helps dilate peritoneal vessels, which increases urea clearance. Warmed dialyzing solution also adds to the patient's comfort by preventing chilly sensations, but this is a secondary reason for warming the solution. (26, 31)

**77.** 4. The peritoneal membrane is semipermeable. Diffusion of molecules from the side of higher concentration to the side of lower concentration occurs across the semipermeable membrane. The membrane also allows for the exchange of fluids by osmosis. Peritoneal dialysis therefore allows for the removal of unwanted waste products from the body, such as urea, uric acid, creatinine, creatine, and excess water, sodium chloride, and ammonia. (26, 31)

**78.** 1. Because the patient has a permanent catheter in place, blood-tinged drainage should not occur. Persistent blood-tinged drainage could indicate damage to the abdominal vessels and the physician should be notified. However, blood-tinged drainage is common with the first few dialysis runs immediately after a peritoneal catheter has been inserted. (5, 31)

**79.** 2. Fluid return with peritoneal dialysis is accompanied by gravity flow. Actions that enhance gravity flow include turning the patient from side to side, raising the head of the bed, or gently massaging the abdomen. The nurse should not attempt to reposition the catheter. The patient is usually confined to a recumbent position for the duration of the dialysis. (5, 26)

**80.** 4. A patient on peritoneal dialysis need not be n.p.o. Because hypotension is a complication associated with peritoneal dialysis, the nurse records intake and output, monitors vital signs, and observes the patient's behavior. The nurse also encourages visiting and other diversional activities. (5, 25)

**81.** 3. Peritonitis is a very serious risk associated with peritoneal dialysis. Aseptic technique should be practiced during the procedure. Minor abdominal cramping may occur with dialysis and gastrointestinal bleeding is an extremely rare complication. (25, 31)

**82.** 2. Weight loss is expected and blood pressure usually decreases as well. The patient's weight before and after dialysis is one measure of evaluating the effectiveness of treatment. Dialysis minimally affects the ability of damaged kidneys to manufacture urine. Hematuria would not occur upon completion of peritoneal dialysis. (5, 26)

**83.** 3. Renal failure patients develop hyperphosphatemia that causes a corresponding excretion of the body's calcium stores. To decrease this loss, aluminum hydroxide (Amphojel) is prescribed to bind phosphates in the intestine and facilitate their excretion. (25, 31)

**84.** 4. Aluminum hydroxide (Amphojel) is administered to bind the phosphates in ingested foods and so must be given with or immediately after meals and snacks. Amphojel is not administered to treat hyperacidity in patients with chronic renal failure

and therefore is not prescribed between meals or p.r.n. (16, 25)

**85.** 1. Magnesium is normally excreted by the kidney. The major source of magnesium is medications, so when the kidneys fail, magnesium can accumulate and cause severe neurologic problems. Magnesium magna (Milk of Magnesia) is harsher than Metamucil, but magnesium toxicity is a more serious problem. Patients may find both Milk of Magnesia and Metamucil unpalatable. Milk of Magnesia is not high in sodium. (16, 25)

**86.** 2. Uremia can cause a decrease in mental alertness, so the nurse needs to validate the patient's comprehension frequently. The patient's ability to concentrate is limited, so short lessons are most effective. If family members are present at the sessions, they can reinforce material. Written materials that the patient can review are superior to videotapes. (25, 31)

**87.** 2. Anemia occurs in chronic renal failure because the kidney fails to manufacture erythropoietin. Erythropoietin stimulates bone marrow to produce hemoglobin. Hemolysis during dialysis worsens the condition. (25, 31)

**88.** 4. Altered sexual functioning occurs in chronic renal failure and can stress marriages and relationships. The patient should not avoid sexual activity, but instead should modify it. Effective coping strategies include removing uremic fetor and resting before sexual activity. (25, 31)

**89.** 2. The major benefit of CAPD is that it frees the patient from daily dependence on dialysis centers, health-care personnel, and machines for life-sustaining treatment. This independence is a treasured outcome for some people. (25, 31)

**90.** 3. Dietary restrictions with CAPD are fewer than with standard peritoneal dialysis because dialysis is constant, not intermittent. The constant slow diffusion of CAPD helps prevent the accumulation of toxins and allows for a more liberal diet. (25, 31)

**91.** 1. Cloudy drainage indicates bacterial activity in the peritoneum. Other signs and symptoms of infection are fever, hyperactive bowel sounds, and abdominal pain. Swollen legs and inadequate dialysate drainage are unrelated to infection. Redness at the insertion site indicates local infection, not peritonitis. If untreated, however, a local infection can progress to the peritoneum. (5, 26)

# test 7

- The Patient with Uterine Fibroids
- The Patient with Breast Cancer
- The Patient with Benign Prostatic Hypertrophy
- The Patient with a Sexually Transmitted Disease
- The Patient with Cancer of the Cervix
- The Patient with Testicular Cancer

*Correct Answers and Rationales*

Select the one *best* or *correct* answer and indicate your choice by filling in the circle with a pencil in front of the option you have chosen. If the answer you would prefer is not given, select the one you think is *most appropriate*.

## THE PATIENT WITH UTERINE FIBROIDS

Mrs. Connie Shaw, 51, has been experiencing intermittent vaginal bleeding for the last several months. Her physician tells her she has uterine fibroids and recommends an abdominal hysterectomy.

1. The nurse is completing Mrs. Shaw's admission routine when Mrs. Shaw expresses fear about the surgery. Which of the following statements offers the *best guide* for the nurse's response?
   ○ 1. The nurse should assure the patient of her physician's competence.
   ○ 2. The nurse should allow the patient opportunities to express her fears.
   ○ 3. The nurse should teach the patient that fear impedes recovery.
   ○ 4. The nurse should change the subject of conversation to pleasantries when fear appears to be present.

2. Mrs. Shaw's nursing care plan includes nursing orders to teach the patient to deep-breathe and cough in preparation for her postoperative period. Which of the following techniques should Mrs. Shaw be taught to use while she coughs?
   ○ 1. Lie on her abdomen with her knees flexed.
   ○ 2. Lie flat in bed with her hands behind her head.
   ○ 3. Support her rib cage with her hands.
   ○ 4. Support her abdomen with a pillow or her hands.

3. Which of the following early signs or symptoms is Mrs. Shaw *most likely* to experience if she hyperventilates while practicing deep-breathing exercises?
   ○ 1. Dyspnea.
   ○ 2. Dizziness.
   ○ 3. Blurred vision.
   ○ 4. Mental confusion.

4. Mrs. Shaw is ordered to have 0.4 mg of atropine sulfate and 75 mg of meperidine hydrochloride (Demerol) IM 1 hour before surgery. The stock ampule of atropine contains 0.8 mg/ml. The stock ampule of meperidine hydrochloride contains 100 mg/ml. The two drugs are compatible and can be drawn up in one syringe. How many milliliters will be in the syringe to give the ordered doses?
   ○ 1. 0.75 ml.
   ○ 2. 1.75 ml.
   ○ 3. 1.25 ml.
   ○ 4. 1.50 ml.

5. Eight hours after her abdominal hysterectomy, Mrs. Shaw has still not voided. Which of the following measures is *least likely* to help the patient void?
   ○ 1. Offering her a cool bedpan.
   ○ 2. Running water in a nearby sink.
   ○ 3. Having her use a bedside commode.
   ○ 4. Pouring warm water over her perineal area.

6. Mrs. Shaw requires catheterization when she is unable to void. As the nurse prepares to insert the catheter into the urinary meatus, she locates the anatomic structures between the labia minora. Starting from the area nearer the pubic bone and moving downward toward the anus, in which of the following order do the clitoris, vaginal opening, and urinary meatus lie?
   ○ 1. Clitoris, vaginal opening, urinary meatus.
   ○ 2. Urinary meatus, vaginal opening, clitoris.
   ○ 3. Vaginal opening, clitoris, urinary meatus.
   ○ 4. Clitoris, urinary meatus, vaginal opening.

7. Eight hours after catheterization, Mrs. Shaw has the urge to void frequently but voids only a few milliliters of urine each time. This symptom is *most commonly* associated with

○ 1. bladder damage.

○ 2. a kidney infection.

○ 3. inadequate fluid intake.

○ 4. urinary retention with overflow.

8. On the 2nd postoperative day, Mrs. Shaw tells the nurse, "I'm uncomfortable in this position but my incision hurts too much to move. Will you turn me, please?" Which of the following responses would be *best* for the nurse to make?

○ 1. "Gladly! I know your incisional area must still be very uncomfortable."

○ 2. "I'll help you get started, but it's good for you to move yourself as much as possible."

○ 3. "Let me get a medication for your pain. That will help you more than changing position."

○ 4. "I noted that you were up to the bathroom about an hour ago. Let's rest a while before moving more just now."

9. Mrs. Shaw complains of gas pains postoperatively. If none of the following nursing measures is contraindicated for the patient, the abdominal distention could *most often* be expected to be relieved by

○ 1. offering the patient a hot beverage.

○ 2. providing extra warmth with a blanket.

○ 3. applying a snugly fitting abdominal binder.

○ 4. helping the patient walk.

10. If Mrs. Shaw has an elevated temperature on her 2nd postoperative day, the *most likely* cause would be

○ 1. a wound infection.

○ 2. a bladder infection.

○ 3. atelectasis.

○ 4. phlebitis.

11. Mrs. Shaw's nursing care plan includes nursing orders intended to help reduce the risk of developing thrombophlebitis. An order that would be *contraindicated* would be to

○ 1. ambulate the patient.

○ 2. massage the patient's legs.

○ 3. have the patient wear elasticized stockings.

○ 4. have the patient exercise her legs in bed.

12. The nurse is about to change the dressing on Mrs. Shaw's abdomen. Which of the following nursing measures is *best* for the nurse to use when the dressing sticks to Mrs. Shaw's incisional area?

○ 1. Pull off the dressing quickly and then apply slight pressure over the area.

○ 2. Lift an easily moved portion of the dressing and then remove it slowly.

○ 3. Moisten the dressing with sterile normal saline and then remove it.

○ 4. Remove part of the dressing and then remove the remainder gradually over a period of several minutes.

13. The nurse applies fluffed dressings to Mrs. Shaw's wound, which is draining. The *primary* reason for applying fluffed dressings to a draining wound is that they

○ 1. incorporate air that helps keep the dressing dry.

○ 2. are more comfortable than flatly packed dressings.

○ 3. allow drainage to be lifted from its source by capillary action.

○ 4. permit drainage to leave its source readily by the force of gravity.

14. Mrs. Shaw is walking and feels a sudden "giving away" sensation in her incision. She has experienced a wound dehiscence. The nurse helps her back to bed and then takes immediate steps to

○ 1. replace the tissues carefully while wearing gloves.

○ 2. apply a snugly fitting sterile abdominal binder over the wound.

○ 3. approximate the wound edges by applying strips of adhesive over the wound.

○ 4. cover the exposed tissues with sterile dressings moistened with sterile normal saline.

15. Mrs. Shaw is an Orthodox Jew and refuses to eat hospital food. Hospital policy discourages food from being brought into the hospital. What step should the nurse take *first* in this situation?

○ 1. Teach the patient that it is important for her to eat what she is served.

○ 2. Discuss the situation and possible courses of action with the dietitian.

○ 3. Encourage the patient's family to bring food for the patient because of the special circumstances.

○ 4. Explain to the patient that if she does not eat, her physician will have to order intravenous therapy.

16. Mrs. Shaw's ovaries and fallopian tubes have been removed as well as her uterus. Which of the following hormones may be prescribed for her?

○ 1. Estrogen.

○ 2. Thyroxin.

○ 3. Prolactin.

○ 4. Testosterone.

## THE PATIENT WITH BREAST CANCER

A lump is discovered in Mrs. Ruth Murray's right breast during a routine physical examination. She is admitted for a breast biopsy and possible surgery.

17. During her admission workup, Mrs. Murray is extremely anxious and has many questions. Which of the following statements offers the *best* guide for the nurse when she answers questions raised by this apprehensive preoperative patient?
    - ○ 1. It is usually best to tell the patient as much as she wants to know and is able to understand.
    - ○ 2. It is usually best to delay discussing the patient's questions with her until she is convalescing.
    - ○ 3. It is usually best to delay discussing the patient's questions with her until her apprehension subsides.
    - ○ 4. It is usually best to explain to the patient that she should discuss her questions first with the physician.

18. *All* of the following would be considered risk factors for the development of breast cancer *except*
    - ○ 1. menopause after age 50.
    - ○ 2. a family history of breast cancer.
    - ○ 3. being childless.
    - ○ 4. breast-feeding.

19. Mrs. Murray asks the nurse, "Where is cancer usually found in the breast?" If the nurse sketches a diagram of a left breast, in which quadrant of the breast do most malignant tumors occur?

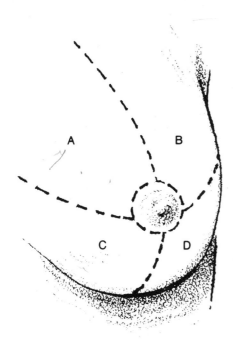

- ○ 1. Quadrant A.
- ○ 2. Quadrant B.

- ○ 3. Quadrant C.
- ○ 4. Quadrant D.

20. Mrs. Murray's biopsy is positive and her physician provides her with information about various treatment options. He recommends a modified radical mastectomy and she agrees. Atropine sulfate is included in her preoperative orders. The *primary* reason for giving this drug preoperatively is that it helps
    - ○ 1. promote general muscular relaxation.
    - ○ 2. decrease the pulse and respiratory rates.
    - ○ 3. decrease nausea.
    - ○ 4. inhibit secretions in the mouth and respiratory tract.

21. Which of the following observations should the recovery-room nurse plan to make *first* upon receiving Mrs. Murray from the operating room?
    - ○ 1. Obtaining and recording the patient's vital signs.
    - ○ 2. Observing that drainage tubes are patent and functioning.
    - ○ 3. Noting that the patient's airway is free of obstruction.
    - ○ 4. Checking the patient's dressings for drainage.

22. Which of the following positions is *best* for Mrs. Murray's right arm when she returns to her room from the recovery room?
    - ○ 1. Across her chest wall.
    - ○ 2. At her side at the same level as her body.
    - ○ 3. In the position that affords her the greatest comfort.
    - ○ 4. On pillows, with her hand higher than her elbow and her elbow higher than her shoulder.

23. Mrs. Murray has a drainage tube in her incision that is attached to suction. The *primary* purpose of this tube is to help
    - ○ 1. decrease intrathoracic pressure and facilitate breathing.
    - ○ 2. increase collateral lymphatic flow toward the operative area.
    - ○ 3. remove accumulations of serum and blood in the operative area.
    - ○ 4. prevent the formation of adhesions between the skin and chest wall in the operative area.

24. On the 3rd postoperative day, the drainage tube is removed and the dressings are changed. Mrs. Murray appears shocked when she sees the operative area and exclaims, "I look horrible! Will it ever look better?" Which of the following responses would be *best* for the nurse to make?
    - ○ 1. "After it heals and you're dressed, you won't know you had surgery."

○ 2. "Don't worry. You know the tumor is gone and the area will heal very soon."

○ 3. "Would you like to meet Ms. Paul? She looks just great and she had a mastectomy, too."

○ 4. "You're shocked by the sudden change in your appearance as a result of this surgery, aren't you?"

**25.** The nurse is doing discharge teaching with Mrs. Murray. As a result of the surgery, which of the following activities may Mrs. Murray need to modify or avoid?

○ 1. Shampooing her dog.

○ 2. Caring for her tropical fish.

○ 3. Working in her rose garden.

○ 4. Taking a late-evening swim.

**26.** The nurse finds that Mrs. Murray does not practice breast self-examination and is unsure of the technique. The nurse should teach Mrs. Murray that the *best* time in the menstrual cycle to examine her breasts is during the

○ 1. week ovulation occurs.

○ 2. week menstruation occurs.

○ 3. first week after menstruation.

○ 4. week before menstruation occurs.

**27.** Which of the following positions is the one of *choice* for palpating tissues during self-examination of the breasts?

○ 1. A sitting position.

○ 2. A standing position.

○ 3. Flat on the back with a pillow under the head.

○ 4. Flat on the back with a pillow under the shoulder on the side being examined.

**28.** Mrs. Murray asks the nurse what the firm ridge is that she feels under the lower part of her breast. The nurse should base her response on knowledge that this ridge is

○ 1. tumorous tissue, which requires further investigation.

○ 2. connective tissue, which is a normal part of the lower breast.

○ 3. glandular tissue, which normally enlarges prior to menstruation.

○ 4. muscular tissue, which normally develops with exercise and work.

**29.** Mrs. Murray says she has always noticed that her brassiere fits more snugly at certain times of the month. She asks the nurse if this is a sign of breast disease. The nurse should base her reply on knowledge that

○ 1. benign cysts tend to cause the breasts to vary in size.

○ 2. it is normal for the breasts to increase in size prior to menstruation.

○ 3. a change in breast size is sufficiently uncommon to warrant further investigation.

○ 4. differences in the sizes of the breasts are related to normal growth and development.

**30.** Mrs. Murray is to have radiation therapy following discharge from the hospital. When caring for the skin at the site of therapy, Mrs. Murray should avoid *all* of the following practices *except*

○ 1. washing the area with water.

○ 2. exposing the area to sunlight.

○ 3. applying an ointment to the area.

○ 4. using talcum powder on the area.

**31.** The nurse *correctly* teaches Mrs. Murray that a normal local tissue response to radiation *most often* appears as

○ 1. atrophy of the skin.

○ 2. scattered pustule formation.

○ 3. redness of the surface tissue.

○ 4. sloughing of two layers of skin.

**32.** Mrs. Murray asks the nurse why a friend of hers had to have her ovaries removed after having a mastectomy. The nurse should be guided in her response by knowledge that an oophorectomy helps control the growth of malignant cells by eliminating the body's source of the hormone

○ 1. estrogen.

○ 2. prolactin.

○ 3. testosterone.

○ 4. progesterone.

**33.** The nurse arranges for a member of the Reach to Recovery program to visit Mrs. Murray. The *primary* purpose of this American Cancer Society program is to

○ 1. help rehabilitate patients who have had mastectomies.

○ 2. raise funds to support early breast cancer detection programs.

○ 3. provide free dressings for patients who have had radical mastectomies.

○ 4. collect statistics for research from patients who have had mastectomies.

## THE PATIENT WITH BENIGN PROSTATIC HYPERTROPHY

Mr. James Ricker, 72, is brought to the emergency room by his son. He is extremely uncomfortable and has been unable to void for the last 12 hours. He has known for some time that he has an enlarged prostate but has wanted to avoid surgery.

**34.** The *best* method for the nurse to use to assess Mr. Ricker for a distended bladder is to check for a
○ 1. rounded swelling above the pubis.
○ 2. dullness in the lower left quadrant.
○ 3. rebound tenderness below the symphysis.
○ 4. urinary discharge from the urethral meatus.

**35.** Mr. Ricker is to be catheterized. The *primary* reason for lubricating the catheter very generously before inserting it is that this technique helps reduce
○ 1. spasms at the orifice of the bladder.
○ 2. friction along the urethra when the catheter is being inserted.
○ 3. the number of organisms gaining entrance to the bladder.
○ 4. the formation of encrustations that may occur at the end of the catheter.

**36.** Mr. Ricker's bladder is emptied gradually. The *best* rationale for the nurse's action is that emptying an overdistended bladder completely at one time tends to cause
○ 1. renal collapse and failure.
○ 2. abdominal cramping and pain.
○ 3. hypotension and possible shock.
○ 4. weakening and atrophy of bladder musculature.

**37.** The nurse should recognize that Mr. Ricker may have hydronephrosis because he has a long history of urinary retention. Which of the following mechanisms would *most likely* account for the hydronephrosis?
○ 1. Abnormally high retention of blood urea and nitrogen.
○ 2. Atrophy of the muscle fibers along the walls of the ureters.
○ 3. Gradual backing-up of stagnant urine into the pelvis of the kidneys.
○ 4. Insufficient arterial blood pressure, resulting in poor kidney circulation.

**38.** While taking Mr. Ricker's history, the nurse could anticipate that the patient will *most likely* report having experienced *all* of the following symptoms *except*
○ 1. voiding at more frequent intervals.
○ 2. difficulty starting the flow of urine.
○ 3. frequent voiding at night.
○ 4. having a urinary stream of greater force than usual.

**39.** A Foley catheter was inserted into Mr. Ricker's bladder. After inserting the catheter, the nurse tapes it to the patient's thigh as illustrated below. The *primary* reason for taping the catheter in this particular manner is to help

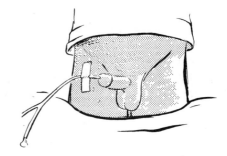

○ 1. eliminate pressure at the penoscrotal angle.
○ 2. prevent the catheter from kinking in the urethra.
○ 3. prevent the catheter from being removed accidentally.
○ 4. allow the patient to turn without kinking the catheter.

**40.** Mr. Ricker is prepared for admission to the hospital. Which of the following reports that the emergency-room nurse could make would be *most helpful* to the nurse responsible for admitting Mr. Ricker?
○ 1. "A urine specimen was obtained from Mr. Ricker and sent to the laboratory for analysis."
○ 2. "Mr. Ricker was catheterized for 1,100 ml of urine. The urine appeared cloudy, and a specimen was sent to the laboratory."
○ 3. "Mr. Ricker is a very cooperative patient. He is comfortable now that his bladder has been emptied. He had no ill effects from catheterization."
○ 4. "Mr. Ricker was in the emergency room for 3 hours because of bladder distention. He is fine now but is being admitted as a possible candidate for surgery."

**41.** The report on a culture of Mr. Ricker's urine indicates that numerous white and red blood cells are present and there is a moderate amount of bacterial growth. The nurse evaluates these findings accurately when she deduces that Mr. Ricker *most probably* has a
○ 1. urethral stricture.
○ 2. decreased renal filtration rate.
○ 3. urinary tract infection.
○ 4. malignancy of the prostate gland.

**42.** Mr. Ricker is scheduled for a transurethral resection of the prostate gland and a bilateral vasectomy. The procedure is to be done under spinal anesthesia. Postoperatively, the nurse should be *particularly* alert to observe the patient for evidence of his developing
○ 1. convulsions.
○ 2. cardiac arrest.
○ 3. renal shutdown.
○ 4. respiratory paralysis.

43. Mr. Ricker returned from his transurethral resection 3 hours ago. In which of the following instances should the nurse increase the flow rate of his continuous bladder irrigation?
    ○ 1. When the drainage is continuous but slow.
    ○ 2. When the drainage appears cloudy and dark yellow.
    ○ 3. When the drainage has become brighter red.
    ○ 4. When there is no drainage of urine and irrigating solution.

44. A nursing assistant tells the nurse, "I think Mr. Ricker is confused. He keeps telling me he has to void, but that isn't possible because he has a catheter in place." Which of the following possible responses to the nursing assistant is *most appropriate* for the nurse to make?
    ○ 1. "His catheter is probably plugged. I'll irrigate it in a few minutes."
    ○ 2. "That's a common complaint after prostate surgery. The urge to void is being imagined."
    ○ 3. "The urge to void is usually created by the large catheter, and he may be having some bladder spasms."
    ○ 4. "I think he may be somewhat confused and possibly may be having some internal bleeding."

45. Mr. Ricker's indwelling catheter is removed. The nurse should teach Mr. Ricker that a temporary symptom he can expect to experience after removal of the catheter is
    ○ 1. urinary retention.
    ○ 2. dribbling incontinence.
    ○ 3. loss of urine while straining.
    ○ 4. suppression of urinary output.

46. Mr. Ricker is to receive bethanechol chloride (Urecholine) postoperatively, as necessary. The nurse should give the patient this drug when he demonstrates signs of
    ○ 1. painful voiding.
    ○ 2. urinary retention.
    ○ 3. frequent urination.
    ○ 4. urinary tract infection.

47. Mr. Ricker's son asks the nurse why a vasectomy was performed on his father. The nurse's response should be guided by knowledge that a vasectomy is sometimes done when a prostatectomy is performed *primarily* to help
    ○ 1. reduce the risk of epididymitis.
    ○ 2. decrease the possibility of traumatic urethritis.
    ○ 3. eliminate hormone stimulus to the prostate gland.
    ○ 4. prevent future prostatic gland enlargement.

48. Mr. Ricker's son says to the nurse, "Men seem almost doomed to have problems with the prostate gland. What purpose does that gland serve?" The nurse should base her response on knowledge that the prostate gland serves *primarily* to
    ○ 1. store underdeveloped sperm prior to ejaculation.
    ○ 2. regulate the acidity/alkalinity environment for proper sperm development.
    ○ 3. produce a secretion that helps in the nourishment and passage of sperm.
    ○ 4. secrete a hormone that stimulates the production and maturation of sperm.

49. While Mr. Ricker is convalescing, which of the following measures should the nurse encourage him to use to help him regain full urinary control?
    ○ 1. Taking a sitz bath twice a day.
    ○ 2. Wearing a scrotal support while awake.
    ○ 3. Alternately tensing and relaxing the perineal muscles.
    ○ 4. Ambulating at least 10 to 15 minutes every hour while awake.

50. If Mr. Ricker's prostate enlargement had been malignant, which of the following blood examinations should the nurse have anticipated to be ordered when the physician wanted to assess whether there had been metastasis?
    ○ 1. Serum creatinine level.
    ○ 2. Serum acid phosphatase level.
    ○ 3. Total nonprotein nitrogen level.
    ○ 4. Endogenous creatinine clearance time.

51. In many instances, older men with prostatic hypertrophy, such as Mr. Ricker, do not seek medical attention until urinary obstruction is almost complete. Investigations have found that the *primary* reason for their delay in seeking attention is that they
    ○ 1. tend to feel too self-conscious to seek help when reproductive organs are involved.
    ○ 2. expect that it is normal to have to live with some urinary problems as they grow older.
    ○ 3. are fearful that sexual indiscretions in earlier life may be the cause of their problem.
    ○ 4. have little discomfort in relation to the amount of pathology, as responses to pain stimuli fade with age.

## THE PATIENT WITH A SEXUALLY TRANSMITTED DISEASE

The local public health department operates a sexually transmitted disease clinic twice a week. The nurse does all the basic assessment, screening, and teaching following established protocols for disease management.

52. Mr. Victor Walter comes to the clinic because he has developed a "sore" on his penis that he fears might be syphilis. The typical chancre of syphilis appears as
  ○ 1. a grouping of small tender pimples.
  ○ 2. an elevated wart.
  ○ 3. a painless, moist ulcer.
  ○ 4. an itching, crusted area.

53. As the nurse interviews Mr. Walter, she should anticipate that the *most difficult* problem is likely to be
  ○ 1. motivating the patient to undergo treatment.
  ○ 2. obtaining a list of the patient's sexual contacts.
  ○ 3. increasing the patient's knowledge of the disease.
  ○ 4. assuring the patient that records are confidential.

54. Mr. Walter is prescribed penicillin as the primary treatment for the syphilis. He is also prescribed probenecid (Benemid) to be taken in conjunction with the penicillin. It is prescribed because it helps to
  ○ 1. delay detoxification of penicillin.
  ○ 2. inhibit the excretion of penicillin.
  ○ 3. maintain sensitivity of organisms to penicillin.
  ○ 4. decrease the likelihood of an allergic reaction to penicillin.

55. The organism responsible for causing Mr. Walter's syphilis is classified as a
  ○ 1. virus.
  ○ 2. fungus.
  ○ 3. rickettsia.
  ○ 4. spirochete.

56. If Mr. Walter had not received therapy and eventually experienced the four stages of syphilis, during which stage would he *most likely* have been free of symptoms?
  ○ 1. The primary stage.
  ○ 2. The secondary stage.
  ○ 3. The latent stage.
  ○ 4. The noninfectious stage.

57. During which stage of the disease would Mr. Walter *most likely* have had a negative reaction to commonly used serologic tests for syphilis?
  ○ 1. The primary stage.
  ○ 2. The secondary stage.
  ○ 3. The latent stage.
  ○ 4. The noninfectious stage.

58. Ms. Liza Manley attends the clinic because she has herpes genitalis. She receives acyclovir (Zovirax), a drug that acts to help
  ○ 1. destroy the causative organism.
  ○ 2. improve the body's production of antibodies.
  ○ 3. reduce the healing time for lesions.
  ○ 4. neutralize toxins produced by the causative organism.

59. Ms. Manley is counseled by the nurse concerning follow-up care for herpes genitalis. Women who have this disease have been noted to be at risk for developing
  ○ 1. sterility.
  ○ 2. cervical cancer.
  ○ 3. uterine fibroid tumors.
  ○ 4. irregular menses.

60. Mr. Harry Day comes to the clinic for treatment of gonorrhea. Mr. Day's presenting symptom is *most likely* to be
  ○ 1. impotence.
  ○ 2. scrotal pain.
  ○ 3. urinary retention.
  ○ 4. urethral discharge.

61. The clinic nurse is planning a community program to help control the spread of sexually transmitted diseases. She studies the disease incidence statistics. Which of the following groups of people has experienced the greatest rise in the incidence of sexually transmitted diseases in the last two decades?
  ○ 1. Teenagers.
  ○ 2. Divorced persons.
  ○ 3. Young married couples.
  ○ 4. Infants.

62. In planning her program, the nurse should be aware that a major difficulty in preventing the spread of gonorrhea is that many women who have the disease
  ○ 1. are unaware that they have it.
  ○ 2. have a milder form of the disease than most men.
  ○ 3. are more reluctant to seek health care than men.
  ○ 4. acquire the disease without having sexual intercourse.

63. As part of her program, the nurse takes into account the fact that the most effective method known for controlling the spread of sexually transmitted diseases is
  ○ 1. premarital serological screening.
  ○ 2. ongoing sex education in the schools.
  ○ 3. laboratory screening of pregnant women.
  ○ 4. prophylactic treatment of exposed individuals.

## THE PATIENT WITH CANCER OF THE CERVIX

Mrs. Jennifer Olson, 27, makes an appointment with her gynecologist for an examination and Pap smear. She has always been in good health.

**64.** Mrs. Olson tells the nurse that she is always very nervous about these examinations because "there has been a lot of cancer in my family." The nurse should be aware that an *early* sign of cervical cancer is
- ○ 1. a thick, foul-smelling vaginal discharge.
- ○ 2. bleeding after intercourse.
- ○ 3. a change in the menstrual cycle.
- ○ 4. watery vaginal discharge.

**65.** Which of the following is *not* considered to be a risk factor for cervical cancer?
- ○ 1. Sexual experiences with multiple partners.
- ○ 2. History of venereal disease.
- ○ 3. Positive family history for cervical cancer.
- ○ 4. Adolescent pregnancy.

**66.** Which of the following responses would be *best* for the nurse to make when Mrs. Olson tells her that she is nervous about the pelvic examination?
- ○ 1. "Can you tell me more about how you're feeling?"
- ○ 2. "You're not alone. Most women feel uncomfortable about this exam."
- ○ 3. "You're not worried about Dr. Smith, are you? He's a specialist in female problems."
- ○ 4. "We'll do everything we can to avoid embarrassing you."

**67.** Correct preparation of a patient for a Pap smear would include which of the following?
- ○ 1. The test should be scheduled while the patient is menstruating.
- ○ 2. The patient should not bathe prior to the exam.
- ○ 3. The patient should not douche prior to the exam.
- ○ 4. The patient should take a laxative the night before the exam.

**68.** The nurse helps Mrs. Olson onto the examining table. The position of choice for a patient undergoing a vaginal examination is the
- ○ 1. Sims' position.
- ○ 2. lithotomy position.
- ○ 3. genupectoral position.
- ○ 4. dorsal recumbent position.

**69.** Mrs. Olson asks the nurse to explain the meaning of the results of a Pap smear. Which of the following should the nurse include in her response?
- ○ 1. A typical Pap smear means that abnormal, but not neoplastic, cells were found in the smear.
- ○ 2. An atypical Pap smear means that cancer cells were found in the smear.
- ○ 3. A positive Pap smear alone is not very important diagnostically because there are many false positives.
- ○ 4. Abnormal cells in a Pap smear may be caused by conditions other than cancer.

**70.** Mrs. Olson tells the nurse that she has considered using the "do-it-yourself" Pap test kits. She asks whether the kits are reliable. The nurse's *best* response would be that
- ○ 1. the kits are not very reliable because an expert is needed to take an accurate smear.
- ○ 2. it is dangerous to bypass an expert's knowledge by doing this test at home.
- ○ 3. the kits are quite reliable but the directions must be followed carefully.
- ○ 4. skillful use of the test can replace expensive gynecologic examinations.

**71.** The American Cancer Society recommends that the average adult woman follow which schedule for Pap smear screening?
- ○ 1. Annually after age 18.
- ○ 2. Annually if sexually active; every 5 years if sexually abstinent.
- ○ 3. Every 3 years after 3 initial negative tests taken annually.
- ○ 4. Every 3 years until age 40 and annually thereafter.

**72.** Mrs. Olson is diagnosed with cancer of the cervix in situ and a conization is scheduled. Which intervention would have the priority during the first 24 hours after the procedure?
- ○ 1. Monitoring vital signs hourly.
- ○ 2. Maintaining strict bed rest.
- ○ 3. Monitoring vaginal bleeding.
- ○ 4. Medicating the patient for pain.

**73.** Mr. Olson says to the nurse, "The doctor told Jennifer that her cancer is curable. Is he just trying to make us feel better?" Which would be the *most accurate* response for the nurse to make?
- ○ 1. "When cervical cancer is detected early and treated aggressively, it has an almost 100% cure rate."
- ○ 2. "The 5-year survival rate is about 75%, which makes the odds pretty good."
- ○ 3. "Saying a cancer is curable means that 50% of all patients survive at least 5 years."
- ○ 4. "Cancers of the female reproductive tract tend to be slow growing and respond well to treatment."

**74.** Mrs. Olson's cancer recurs and internal radiation treatment with a radium implant is planned. On admission, Mrs. Olson says she is concerned about being radioactive and has been having nightmares about Hiroshima. What is a reasonable explanation for the nurse to give her?
- ○ 1. "The radioactive material is controlled and stays with the source; once the material is removed, no radioactivity will remain."

○ 2. "The radioactivity will gradually decrease and you will be discharged when the radioactive material reaches its half-life."

○ 3. "These nightmares indicate that you are in the denial phase of accepting the diagnosis."

○ 4. "Careful shielding prevents the area above your waist from radioactivity."

**75.** What activity orders would be appropriate for Mrs. Olson while the radium implant is in place?

○ 1. Out of bed as tolerated within the room.

○ 2. Bed rest with bathroom privileges.

○ 3. Bed rest in position of comfort.

○ 4. Bed rest with the head of the bed flat.

**76.** Jennifer's mother asks why so many nurses are involved in her daughter's care, and says, "The doctor said I can be in the room for up to 2 hours each day, but the nurses say they're restricted to 30 minutes." The nurse explains that this variation is based on the fact that nurses

○ 1. touch the patient, which increases their exposure to radiation.

○ 2. work with many patients and could carry infection to a person receiving radiation therapy, if exposure is prolonged.

○ 3. work with radiation on an ongoing basis, while visitors have infrequent exposure to radiation.

○ 4. are at greater risk from the radiation because they are younger than the mother is.

**77.** A lead-lined container and a pair of long forceps are kept in Jennifer's room. What is the purpose of this equipment?

○ 1. Disposal of emesis or other bodily secretions.

○ 2. Handling of the dislodged radiation source.

○ 3. Disposal of patient utensils.

○ 4. Storage of the radiation booster dose.

**78.** Which of the following would be standard nursing care for Mrs. Olson while the implant is in place?

○ 1. Offer the bedpan every 2 hours.

○ 2. Provide perineal care twice daily.

○ 3. Check the position of the applicator hourly.

○ 4. Offer a low-residue diet.

**79.** The nurse should also carefully observe Mrs. Olson for typical side effects associated with radiation therapy to the cervix. These effects include

○ 1. cramping pain and severe vaginal itching.

○ 2. confusion and sleep disturbances.

○ 3. high fevers in the afternoon or evening.

○ 4. nausea, vomiting, and a foul discharge.

**80.** Mrs. Olson's implant is a sealed radiation source. Which of the following guidelines should the nurse follow in her care?

○ 1. Labeling soiled linens as a radiation hazard.

○ 2. Collecting urine in special lead containers for disposal.

○ 3. Collecting all body excreta in special containers for disposal.

○ 4. Handling linen and excreta without special precautions.

## THE PATIENT WITH TESTICULAR CANCER

Mr. Albert Cravitz is a 28-year-old printer who is diagnosed with acute epididymitis.

**81.** The nurse would expect that the classic symptoms of epididymitis that caused Mr. Cravitz to seek medical help were

○ 1. burning and pain on urination.

○ 2. severe tenderness and swelling in the scrotum.

○ 3. foul-smelling ejaculate and severe scrotal swelling.

○ 4. foul-smelling urine and pain on urination.

**82.** *All* of the following are appropriate interventions for Mr. Cravitz *except*

○ 1. bed rest.

○ 2. elevating the testes.

○ 3. increased fluid intake.

○ 4. hot packs.

**83.** Once the inflammation has subsided, the nurse teaches Mr. Cravitz to perform testicular self-examination. When should he be taught to perform the exam?

○ 1. After intercourse.

○ 2. First thing in the morning.

○ 3. After a warm bath or shower.

○ 4. After active exercise.

**84.** The normal testis can be described by *all* of the following *except*

○ 1. smooth.

○ 2. egg-shaped.

○ 3. spongy.

○ 4. lump-free.

**85.** A year later Mr. Cravitz returns to the physician, saying that he thinks the epididymitis has returned. The physician examines him and makes a preliminary diagnosis of testicular cancer. Which clinical manifestation helps differentiate testicular cancer from epididymitis?

○ 1. The inability to achieve or sustain a erection.

○ 2. Scrotal pain.

○ 3. A dragging sensation in the scrotum.

○ 4. Scrotal swelling.

**86.** Although the cause of testicular cancer is unknown, it is associated with a history of

○ 1. undescended testis.
○ 2. sexual relations at an early age.
○ 3. seminal vesiculitis.
○ 4. epididymitis.

87. The diagnosis of testicular cancer is confirmed. Mr. Cravitz is scheduled for a right orchiectomy. The day before surgery, Mr. Cravitz tells the nurse that he is concerned about the effect that losing a testicle will have on his "manhood." Which of the following facts about orchiectomy should form the basis for the nurse's comments?
○ 1. Testosterone levels are decreased.
○ 2. Sexual drive and libido are unchanged.
○ 3. Sperm count increases in the remaining testicle.
○ 4. Secondary sexual characteristics change.

88. Since Mr. Cravitz will have a high inguinal incision, a nursing goal for his immediate postoperative care would be to
○ 1. prevent bladder spasms.
○ 2. monitor the alphafetoprotein level.
○ 3. control the pain.
○ 4. monitor hematuria.

89. The orchiectomy is performed and the pathology report reveals a diagnosis of malignant seminoma. External radiotherapy is ordered. The nurse teaches Mr. Cravitz about the potential side effects of radiotherapy to the lower abdomen. Which of the following side effects is Mr. Cravitz *most likely* to experience?
○ 1. Alopecia.
○ 2. Diarrhea.
○ 3. Dysphagia.
○ 4. Nausea.

90. Efforts are made to protect the healthy testicle during treatment, but some irradiation is inevitable. Which of the following would provide the patient with accurate information about its effects?
○ 1. Sterility is an almost inevitable outcome of the treatment.
○ 2. Sperm-banking is essential if future parenthood is desired.
○ 3. Fertility will return, but the danger of genetic defects is very high.
○ 4. Sperm production will be decreased for months or even years.

# CORRECT ANSWERS AND RATIONALES

Numbers appear in parentheses following the rationales. The numbers identify textbooks listed in the references at the end of Part IV, where correct answers can be verified.

## *The Patient with Uterine Fibroids*

1. 2. The best guide when a patient is fearful about having surgery is for the nurse to allow the patient opportunities to express her fears. Such courses of action as assuring a patient of the physician's competence, saying that fear impedes recovery, and changing the subject are nonsupportive of the patient and deny the patient an opportunity to express her feelings. (31, 25)

2. 4. The patient who has had abdominal surgery is most likely to experience incisional-area discomfort postoperatively when she coughs. This discomfort can be minimized by splinting the operative area with a pillow or with her hands. (31, 25)

3. 2. Hyperventilation occurs when the patient breathes so rapidly and deeply that she exhales excessive amounts of carbon dioxide. A characteristic symptom of hyperventilation is dizziness. Such symptoms as dyspnea, blurred vision, and mental confusion are not associated with hyperventilation. (10, 23)

4. 3. The correct amount to administer is determined by using ratios as follows:

$$0.8 \text{ mg}:1 \text{ ml}::0.4 \text{ mg}:x \text{ ml}.$$
$$0.8\,x = 0.4$$
$$x = .50 \text{ ml of atropine/sulfate}$$
$$100 \text{ mg}:1 \text{ ml}::75 \text{ mg}:x \text{ ml}.$$
$$100\,x = 75$$
$$x = .75 \text{ ml of meperidine hydrochloride (Demerol)}$$

0.5 ml. of atropine + 0.75 ml of meperidine hydrochloride (Demerol) = 1.25 ml total (24, 36)

5. 1. Using a cool bedpan usually makes voiding difficult. It is better to offer the patient a warm bedpan and use such techniques as running water in a nearby sink, having the patient use a commode when possible, and pouring warm water over the perineal area to promote voiding. (25, 31)

6. 4. From the area nearer the pubic bone and moving toward the anus, the anatomic positions are clitoris, urinary meatus, and vaginal opening. (2, 27)

7. 4. The nurse should suspect that a patient has retention with overflow when the urge to void is present but the patient voids only small amounts of urine at one time. Retention with overflow is not associated with bladder damage, kidney infection, or an inadequate fluid intake. (25, 31)

8. 2. Moving about in bed, coughing, deep-breathing, and turning are indicated for the postoperative patient because they help prevent various postoperative complications, such as atelectasis, respiratory infections, thrombophlebitis, and problems with elimination. Such activity also helps the patient maintain muscle tone and general well-being. Offering to move the patient will defeat the purpose of moving in bed. Pain medication may relieve discomfort and make it easier for the patient to move, but medication does not replace the patient's need to move. (10, 23)

9. 4. Usually, the discomfort associated with gas pains is likely to be helped when the patient ambulates. The gas will be more easily expelled with exercise. Another technique that is often helpful to promote the passage of flatus is to have the patient assume a knee-chest position, if she can do so. In this position, the rectum is higher than the large intestine. Gas, which is lighter than intestinal content, rises in the intestine toward the elevated rectum for expulsion. Such techniques as applying an abdominal binder, offering the patient a hot beverage, and providing the patient with extra warmth are not recommended and may even aggravate the discomfort of gas pains postoperatively. (25, 31)

10. 3. An elevated temperature on the 2nd postoperative day is most suggestive of a respiratory tract infection. Respiratory infections most often occur during the first 48 hours after surgery. Signs of infection, if present in the wound or urinary tract, are likely to occur later in the postoperative period; so, also, will signs of phlebitis, which is an inflammatory process in a vein. (25, 31)

11. 2. Massaging the legs postoperatively is contraindicated because it may dislodge small clots of blood, if present, and cause even more serious problems. Such measures as ambulating the patient, having the patient wear elasticized stockings, and having the patient move her legs about in bed have been found helpful in reducing the incidence of postoperative thrombophlebitis. (25, 31)

**12.** 3. When a dressing sticks to a wound, it is best to moisten the dressing with sterile normal saline and then remove it carefully. Trying to remove the dressing when it is dry is likely to irritate the skin and wound. (24, 36)

**13.** 3. The property of surface tension exhibited by liquids and the forces of cohesion and adhesion causes a column of liquid to rise on threads that form dressing materials. This phenomenon is called capillarity. Capillarity will cause the drainage to be lifted up and away from the wound when dressings are fluffed and loosely placed on the wound. Incorporating air will not help keep the dressings dry. Fluffed dressings *may* be more comfortable, but that is not the primary reason for fluffing them. If drainage leaves the wound by gravity, it is likely to flow down and around the dressing onto the skin, which will irritate the patient's skin and will feel uncomfortable. (24, 36)

**14.** 4. The opening of a wound is called dehiscence. The nurse should cover the exposed tissues with sterile dressings moistened with sterile normal saline if a patient's wound opens and tissues are exposed. If the wound opens and abdominal organs are exposed and escape from the wound, it is called wound evisceration. The nurse should also cover an eviscerated wound with sterile dressings moistened with sterile normal saline. The physician should be notified immediately when a wound dehisces or eviscerates. Such measures as trying to replace the exposed tissues or organs, applying an abdominal binder, or trying to approximate the wound edges with adhesive strips are contraindicated and are likely to aggravate the problem. (25, 31)

**15.** 2. The best course of action when a patient refuses to eat food that is contrary to her religious beliefs is to discuss the situation with a dietitian. Members of the health team may need to confer about this patient's needs. Telling the patient that it is important for her to eat what is served is unlikely to help because she has already refused the food. Encouraging the patient's family to bring suitable food to the hospital for the patient is ordinarily against agency policy and should not be considered until the situation has been discussed with an agency dietitian. Threatening a patient by saying that if she does not eat, intravenous therapy will be necessary is nonsupportive of the patient and is unlikely to gain her cooperation. (10, 23)

**16.** 1. The primary hormone of the ovaries is estrogen. It is one hormone that is likely to be prescribed for a patient whose ovaries, fallopian tubes, and uterus have been surgically removed. Many authorities now use both estrogen and progesterone cyclically when using hormonal replacement therapy postoperatively. (25, 31)

## The Patient with Breast Cancer

**17.** 1. An important nursing responsibility is preoperative teaching, and the most frequently recommended guide for teaching is to tell the patient as much as she wants to know and is able to understand. Delaying discussing those things about which the patient has concerns is likely to aggravate the situation and cause the patient to feel distrust. (24, 36)

**18.** 4. A family history of breast cancer, early onset of menstruation, delayed onset of menopause, and being childless all appear to increase a woman's risk of breast cancer. Breast-feeding does not. (25, 31)

**19.** 2. Approximately 50% of malignant tumors in the breast occur in the upper outer quadrant of the breast. Interestingly, but for no known reason, cancer appears in the left breast more often than in the right breast. (25, 31)

**20.** 4. Atropine sulfate, a cholinergic blocking agent, is given preoperatively primarily to reduce secretions in the mouth and respiratory tract. The drug is not used to promote muscle relaxation, decrease the pulse and respiratory rates, or decrease nausea and vomiting. (12, 16)

**21.** 3. The highest priority when a nurse receives a patient from the operating room is to assess the patency of the patient's airway. If the airway is not clear, immediate steps should be taken so that the patient is able to breathe. After the nurse notes that the airway is clear and the patient is breathing well, she should proceed with such measures as obtaining the vital signs, observing that drainage tubes are functioning properly, and checking the patient's dressing. (26, 31)

**22.** 4. Lymph nodes are ordinarily removed from the axillary area when a modified radical mastectomy is done. Therefore, to facilitate drainage from the arm on the affected side, the arm should be elevated on pillows with the patient's hand higher than her elbow and her elbow higher than her shoulder. Other techniques for positioning the arm on the affected side do not facilitate drainage from the arm. (26, 31)

**23.** 3. A drainage tube is placed in the wound following a modified radical mastectomy to help remove accumulations of serum and blood in the area. Drainage tubes placed in a wound do not decrease intrathoracic pressure, increase collateral lymphatic flow, or prevent the formation of adhesions. (26, 31)

**24.** 4. When a patient appears shocked by her appearance following surgery, such as after having a mastectomy, the nurse should help the patient express her feelings and offer supportive care, which she needs at this time. Telling the patient not to worry or that her disfigurement will not show when she is dressed are nonsupportive and are likely to cause more concerns. Having the patient meet someone who has had breast surgery is often helpful but is better used later, when the patient is convalescing and used to the appearance of the operative site. The patient needs the nurse's support when the dressings are removed, not sometime later. (11, 38)

**25.** 3. Every effort should be made to avoid cuts, bruises, burns, and the like on the affected arm following a mastectomy because normal circulation has been impaired. Working in a rose or cactus garden is contraindicated because of the danger of skin pricks. Such activities as caring for pets and swimming are not contraindicated for the postmastectomy patient. (26, 31)

**26.** 3. It is generally recommended that the breasts be examined during the first week after menstruation. During this period the breasts are least likely to be tender or swollen, since the secretion of estrogen, which prepares the uterus for implantation, is lowest. (26, 31)

**27.** 4. For self-breast examination, a pillow or towel under the shoulder on the side being examined elevates the chest wall while the woman lies flat on her back. This positioning allows for better distribution of breast tissue over the chest wall and provides for the best examination of tissues by palpation. A standing position, with the woman facing a mirror, is used to examine the breasts for changes in size and shape, for dimpling of skin, and for nipple changes. The standing or sitting positions are not appropriate for palpating breast tissues. (26, 31)

**28.** 2. The firm connective tissue under the breast is normal. It is a supportive structure and is no cause for alarm. It is not tumorous, muscular, or glandular tissue, nor does it change in size due to exercise. Some women may also feel their ribs and need to be instructed to differentiate this from abnormal structures. (25, 31)

**29.** 2. The breasts are normally approximately the same size. They may vary in size somewhat prior to menstruation, due to breast engorgement caused by hormonal changes. A woman may then note that her bra fits more tightly than usual. (25, 31)

**30.** 1. Patients receiving radiation therapy should avoid lotions, ointments, and anything that may cause irritation to the skin, such as exposure to sunlight and talcum powder. The area may safely be washed with water if this is done gently and if care is taken not to injure the skin. (25, 31)

**31.** 3. The most common reaction of the skin to radiation therapy is redness of the surface tissues. Dryness, desquamation, tanning, and dilatation of the capillaries are also common. (25, 31)

**32.** 1. The ovaries are often removed when a radical mastectomy has been performed because of the patient's having breast cancer. The reason is to eliminate the body's source of estrogen, which tends to stimulate the growth of tumors. (26, 31)

**33.** 1. The American Cancer Society's Reach to Recovery is a rehabilitation program for women who have had breast surgery. It is designed to meet their physical, psychological, and cosmetic needs but does not provide funds or dressings, nor is research part of the program. (26, 31)

## The Patient with Benign Prostatic Hypertrophy

**34.** 1. The best way to assess for a distended bladder is to check for a rounded swelling above the pubis. This swelling is the distended bladder rising above the pubis into the abdominal cavity. (5, 26)

**35.** 2. Lubricating the catheter *well* before catheterizing a male decreases friction along the urethra and reduces irritation and trauma to urethral tissues. Because the urethra of the male is tortuous, a liberal amount of lubrication is advised to make the passage of the catheter as easy as possible. The female urethra is not tortuous and although the catheter should be lubricated before being inserted, the generous amount of lubricant recommended when a male is catheterized is unnecessary. (5, 26)

**36.** 3. Rapidly emptying an overdistended bladder may cause the patient to have hypotension and shock due to the sudden change of pressure within the abdominal viscera. Renal collapse is not likely, nor are such signs and symptoms as abdominal cramping and a weakening and atrophy of the bladder. (5, 26)

**37.** 3. When a patient has a history of urinary retention, hydronephrosis is likely to develop as a result of the gradual backing up of stagnant urine into the pelvis of the kidneys. There are no true sphincters at the ureteral openings in the bladder, so that sufficient pressure will cause the urine to back up into the kidneys. (25, 31)

**38.** 4. It is unlikely that the patient with prostatic hypertrophy will report having a urinary stream of greater force than usual. Typical symptoms of prostatic hypertrophy include frequency of urination, hesitancy in starting urination, a decrease in the size and force of the urinary stream, interruptions in the urinary stream when voiding, and frequent voiding at night (nocturia). The various symptoms of benign prostatic hypertrophy of the prostate are often referred to as prostatism. (25, 31)

**39.** 1. The primary reason for taping an indwelling catheter to a male patient so that the penis is held in a lateral position, as illustrated in this item, is to prevent pressure at the penoscrotal angle. Prolonged pressure at the penoscrotal angle is likely to cause a ureterocutaneous fistula. (5, 26)

**40.** 2. A report about a patient's condition should be as clear, pertinent, and concise as possible, and it should be free of subjective information that could be interpreted differently by different people. In the situation described in this item, the nurse should indicate how much urine had been drained from the patient's bladder and how the urine looked. She should also report that a urine specimen has been sent to the laboratory for analysis. (5, 26)

**41.** 3. The presence of red and white blood cells in the urine is most typical of a urinary tract infection. (25, 31)

**42.** 4. If paralysis of vasomotor nerves occurs in the upper spinal cord when spinal anesthesia is used, the patient is likely to develop respiratory paralysis. Artificial ventilation is required until the effects of anesthesia subside. Other complications that may occur with spinal anesthesia include hypotension, nausea and vomiting, postanesthesia headache, and neurologic complications, such as muscle weakness in the legs. (25, 31)

**43.** 3. When a patient has continuous bladder irrigation following a prostatectomy, the rate at which the solution enters the bladder should be increased when the drainage becomes brighter red. The color indicates the presence of blood. Increasing the flow of irrigating solution helps flush the catheter well so that clots do not plug it. There would be no reason to increase the flow of solution when the return is continuous or appears cloudy and dark yellow. Increasing the flow would be contraindicated if there were no return of urine and irrigating solution. (25, 31)

**44.** 3. The presence of the Foley catheter creates the urge to void and may also cause bladder spasms. Less likely reasons for the patient's having an urge to void include having a plugged catheter, imagining the urge, being confused, and bleeding internally. (25, 31)

**45.** 2. After an indwelling catheter is removed, the patient experiences some dribbling incontinence.

This is normal and temporary. The problem usually resolves itself as perineal muscles are strengthened by exercise. (25, 31)

**46.** 2. Bethanechol chloride (Urecholine) is a cholinergic drug that stimulates the parasympathetic nervous system. It acts to increase the tone and motility of the smooth muscles of the urinary and gastrointestinal tracts. The drug is frequently used when the patient lacks bladder tone and cannot empty the bladder completely. It is contraindicated when urinary retention is caused by an obstruction in the urinary system. The drug is administered to the patient described in this item to overcome urinary retention and to prevent the risk of urinary tract infection due to catheterization. (12, 16)

**47.** 1. A vasectomy is frequently performed at the time of a prostatectomy to decrease urinary tract infections and epididymitis. This procedure helps prevent retrograde spread of infection from the prostatic urethra through the vas and into the epididymis. (22, 25)

**48.** 3. The prostate gland serves one primary purpose: it produces a secretion that helps in the nourishment and passage of sperm. (22, 25)

**49.** 3. The patient should be taught to alternately tense and relax the perineal muscles to help regain control of urination. This exercise may be performed as many as 20 to 30 times every hour. (25, 31)

**50.** 2. The most specific examination to determine whether a malignancy extends outside of the prostatic capsule is a study of the serum acid phosphatase level. The level increases when a malignancy has metastasized. (25, 31)

**51.** 2. It has been found that older men tend to believe that it is normal to have to live with some urinary problems. As a result, symptoms are often overlooked and simply attributed to aging. (26, 31)

## The Patient with a Sexually Transmitted Disease

**52.** 3. The chancre of syphilis is characteristically a painless, moist ulcer. Its serous discharge is very infectious. The chancre is most often seen on the penis but may also be present on the anus, rectum, lips, and mouth. It occasionally also occurs on the skin where the causative organism entered the body. (25, 31)

**53.** 2. An important aspect of venereal disease control is to obtain a list of the sexual contacts of patients with venereal diseases. These people in turn should be encouraged to obtain immediate care. Many patients with a venereal disease are reluctant to reveal their sexual contacts, a factor that makes controlling venereal diseases difficult. There are no reported difficulties with motivating patients with venereal diseases to have treatment after they know they have a disease, increasing their knowledge of the disease, and assuring patients that records are confidential. (18, 31)

**54.** 2. The kidneys clear penicillin from the blood very effectively. Probenecid (Benemid) inhibits the excretion of penicillin and thereby helps maintain high blood plasma levels of penicillin. (12, 16)

**55.** 4. *Treponema pallidum,* the organism that causes syphilis, is classified as a spirochete because of its corkscrew appearance. (25, 31)

**56.** 3. Syphilis has four stages. The primary stage is characterized by the presence of a chancre; this stage is the most infectious stage of syphilis. The secondary stage is characterized by the presence of enlarged lymph nodes and painful joints. A skin eruption may also occur. The latent stage, sometimes called the tertiary stage, is symptom-free, and the patient appears healthy. The latent stage generally occurs several years after the primary stage and may last as long as 50 years. The fourth stage, the noninfectious stage, is also called late clinical syphilis and is characterized by a variety of symptoms due to complications that are irreversible. The complications may include inflammation of bones and joints, cardiovascular problems, and problems associated with the central nervous system. (25, 31)

**57.** 1. Common serologic tests are most likely to be negative during the primary stage of syphilis because antibodies have not yet had time to develop. During the primary stage, a darkfield examination is used to identify the causative organism. (25, 26)

**58.** 3. Acyclovir (Zovirax) acts to help reduce the healing time for lesions of herpes genitalis. There is no known cure for the infection, which is caused by a virus. (25, 26)

**59.** 2. Women who have herpes genitalis are more likely to develop cervical cancer than women who have never had the disease. Regular examinations, including Pap tests, are recommended. (25, 31)

**60.** 4. Gonorrhea in the male is characterized by a mucopurulent urethral discharge. Gonorrhea is the most common reportable communicable disease in the United States today. (25, 31)

**61.** 1. Statistics reveal that the incidence of venereal diseases among teenagers is rising more rapidly than among any other age group. Many reasons have been given for this trend, one being a change in morals and increasing sexual activity among teenagers. (26, 31)

**62.** 1. Many females are unaware that they have gonorrhea because they are free of symptoms or experience only very mild symptoms. These women make up a large pool of unsuspecting carriers of the disease. (25, 31)

**63.** 4. Treating the individual who has been exposed to a venereal disease has done more to control the spread of venereal diseases than other measures. This is why it is important to obtain a complete list of sexual contacts, who may then be encouraged to have treatment. (26, 31)

## The Patient with Cancer of the Cervix

**64.** 4. In its early stages, cancer of the cervix is usually asymptomatic, which underscores the importance of regular Pap smears. A watery vaginal discharge is often the first noticeable symptom. Discomfort, foul-smelling discharge, and weight loss are late signs. (25, 31)

**65.** 4. The incidence of cervical cancer is closely linked to sexual experience with multiple partners and a history of venereal disease. A positive family history is an associated risk. Pregnancy at an early age does not alone increase the risk. (25, 31)

**66.** 1. Asking the patient to describe her nervousness gives her the opportunity to express her concerns and allows the nurse to understand her better. Responses that make assumptions about the source of the concern or offer clichéd reinforcement are nonsupportive and block successful communication. (11, 38)

**67.** 3. Douching within 24 to 48 hours before a Pap smear may wash away cells and secretions needed for an accurate test. The test is scheduled for a time when the patient is not menstruating. No bowel preparation is needed and a patient may bathe as desired. (5, 26)

**68.** 2. Although other positions may be used, the preferred position for a patient undergoing a vaginal examination is the lithotomy position because it is convenient for the examiner and offers the best visualization. (24, 36)

**69.** 4. The Pap smear identifies atypical cervical cells that may be present for a variety of reasons. Cancer is the most common cause, but not the only one. An adequate smear provides quite accurate diagnostic data. The false-positive rate is 5%. (25, 31)

**70.** 3. The home kits are quite reliable, but the directions must be followed carefully. Use of this test does not replace the need for expert evaluation of the general health of the reproductive organs. (26, 31)

**71.** 3. Current American Cancer Society guidelines advocate Pap smears every 3 years after an initial negative pattern is established. Annual screening is recommended for any woman in a high-risk category. (25, 31)

**72.** 3. Uncontrolled vaginal bleeding is the priority concern during the first 24 hours after conization of the cervix. This is best monitored by keeping an accurate pad count, which assesses the extent of bleeding. Hourly vital signs and strict bed rest are unnecessary unless complications develop. Medicating the patient is important but is not the priority action in this situation. (25, 31)

**73.** 1. When cervical cancer is detected early and treated aggressively, the cure rate approaches 100%. (25, 31)

**74.** 1. The radioactivity comes from a radioactive material such as radium or cesium. The radioactivity affects tissues but does not make them radioactive. Once the radioactive source is removed, no radioactivity will remain. Accurate information can help alleviate ungrounded fears. The time required for a radioactive substance to be half-dissipated is called its half-life, but this does not determine discharge time. The patient receiving sealed internal radiotherapy is not discharged until the radioactive source is removed. Nightmares probably indicate the patient's concern about the therapy. There is no way to shield the area above the waist from radiation with cervical implants. (5, 26)

**75.** 4. The patient with a cervical implant is kept on strict bed rest, flat in bed. This limitation in movement is designed to prevent accidental displacement or even dislodgement of the implant. Patient knowledge and understanding are critical to compliance with these restrictions. (25, 31)

**76.** 3. The three factors related to radiation safety are time, distance, and shielding. Nurses on the unit work with radiation frequently and so must limit their contact. Nurses are physically closer to patients than are visitors, who are often asked to sit 6 feet away. Touching the patient does not increase the amount of radiation exposure; distance does. Aseptic technique and/or isolation prevent the spread of infection. Age is a risk factor for persons involved in reproduction. (25, 31)

**77.** 2. Dislodged radioactive materials should not be touched with bare or gloved hands. Forceps are used to place the material in the lead-lined container, which shields the radiation. Exposure to radiation can occur only by direct exposure to the encased radioactive substance. Exposure cannot result from contact with emesis or urine or from touching the patient. Radioactive materials are kept only in the radiation department. It is not usual to boost an applicator. (25, 31)

**78.** 4. Bowel movements can be difficult with the radium applicator in place. The purpose of the low-residue diet is to decrease the need for a bowel movement. To prevent dislodging the applicator, patients with internal radiation are on strict bed rest and only allowed to turn from side to side. Perineal care is omitted during radium implant therapy, although any vaginal discharge should be reported to the doctor. It is rare for the applicator to extrude, so checking need not be done every hour. (25, 31)

**79.** 4. Nausea, vomiting, and foul vaginal discharge are common side effects of internal radiation therapy for cervical cancer. Cramping pain is also common, but itching is uncommon. Fever and confusion would not be expected, although sleep disturbances may occur. (26, 31)

**80.** 4. A sealed source does not cause contamination of linens and does not enter body secretions and excretions. Therefore, special precautions are not required for dealing with these items. (25, 31)

## *The Patient with Testicular Cancer*

**81.** 2. Epididymitis causes acute tenderness and pronounced swelling of the scrotum. It is occasionally but not routinely associated with urinary tract infection. (25, 31)

**82.** 4. Rest is the foundation of treatment. Elevation of the scrotum may increase patient comfort. Intermittent ice will be prescribed for comfort and to reduce swelling. Hot packs will not be used, as the temperature in the scrotum should remain below body temperature. Excessive exposure to heat can cause destruction of sperm cells. (25, 31)

**83.** 3. After a warm bath or shower, the testes hang low and relaxed and are in ideal position for manual evaluation and palpation. (26, 31)

**84.** 3. Normal testes feel smooth, egg-shaped, and firm to the touch, without lumps. They should not be soft or spongy to the touch. (26, 31)

**85.** 3. A dragging sensation in the scrotum is associated with testicular cancer, not with epididymitis. The manifestations of testicular cancer are less dramatic than those of epididymitis. Other clinical manifestations of testicular cancer include a lump or swelling of the testis, a dull ache in the lower abdomen or inguinal area, and occasional pain. Sexual performance is unaffected. (26, 31)

**86.** 1. Cryptorchidism (undescended testicle) has a relative three- to fourteen-fold increased risk for testicular cancer. Other suspected causes include chemical carcinogens, trauma, orchitis, and environmental factors. There is no association of testicular cancer to early sexual relations in men, but in women early sexual relations are associated with cervical cancer. (14, 26)

**87.** 2. The remaining testicle undergoes hyperplasia and produces enough testosterone to maintain sexual drive, libido, and secondary sexual characteristics. Sperm count can decrease after a unilateral orchiectomy; this is attributed to the stress of the surgery. (14, 26)

**88.** 3. Due to the location of the incision, a nursing goal for immediate postoperative care is pain control. Bladder spasms and hematuria are associated with prostatic surgery. Alphafetoprotein (AFP) levels are monitored throughout therapy to determine the efficacy of therapeutic regimens. (14, 26)

**89.** 2. The side effects of radiotherapy to the lower abdomen are related to the site treated and to the exposure of the underlying organs to radiation. Thus, diarrhea is common with radiation to the retroperitoneal region since the gastrointestinal tract lies within the treatment field. Alopecia and dysphagia are not associated with radiotherapy to the retroperitoneal area. Nausea is experienced by patients undergoing radiation but is not related to radiotherapy to the retroperitoneal area. (14, 26)

**90.** 4. Sperm production is typically decreased and the effects may be significant. The duration of effect can be anywhere from 6 months to 5 years. Sexual potency is not adversely affected and the risk of genetic defect, although present, is not highly significant. (25, 31)

# test 8

- The Patient with a Head Injury
- The Patient with Seizures
- The Patient with a Cerebrovascular Accident
- The Patient with Parkinson's Disease
- The Patient with Multiple Sclerosis
- The Unconscious Patient

**Correct Answers and Rationales**

Select the one *best* or *correct* answer and indicate your choice by filling in the circle with a pencil in front of the option you have chosen. If the answer you would prefer is not given, select the one you think is *most appropriate*.

## THE PATIENT WITH A HEAD INJURY

Mr. John Marlen, 22, is brought to the emergency room about 20 minutes after being involved in a serious motor vehicle accident. Mr. Marlen was the driver of the car and experienced a head injury. He is unconscious upon arrival and exhibits signs of increasing intracranial pressure. He is accompanied by his fiancée and an adult friend, who were both wearing seat belts and escaped with minor injuries.

**1.** Which of the following methods is best, from a legal point of view, for obtaining permission to treat Mr. Marlen since he is unconscious?
- ○ 1. Having his fiancée sign the consent form.
- ○ 2. Having three physicians agree on treatment the patient requires.
- ○ 3. Receiving a verbal consent by telephone from a responsible relative.
- ○ 4. Obtaining written consent from the adult friend who accompanied the patient to the emergency room.

**2.** When Mr. Marlen arrives in the emergency room, to which of the following considerations should the nurse give *highest* priority in his care?
- ○ 1. Establishing an airway.
- ○ 2. Replacing blood losses.
- ○ 3. Stopping bleeding from open wounds.
- ○ 4. Determining whether the patient has a fractured neck.

**3.** Mr. Marlen's initial blood pressure is 124/80 mm Hg. As his condition worsens, Mr. Marlen's pulse pressure increases. Which of the following blood pressure readings illustrates a pulse pressure greater than the patient's initial pulse pressure?
- ○ 1. 102/60 mm Hg.
- ○ 2. 110/90 mm Hg.
- ○ 3. 140/100 mm Hg.
- ○ 4. 160/100 mm Hg.

**4.** The nurse assesses Mr. Marlen frequently for signs of increasing intracranial pressure. *All* of the following are typical signs of increasing intracranial pressure *except*
- ○ 1. unequal pupils.
- ○ 2. a rising systolic blood pressure.
- ○ 3. tachycardia.
- ○ 4. a rising body temperature.

**5.** Which of the following respiratory signs would be an indication of increasing intracranial pressure in the brain stem?
- ○ 1. Slow irregular respirations.
- ○ 2. Rapid shallow respirations.
- ○ 3. Asymmetric chest movements.
- ○ 4. Nasal flaring.

**6.** The nurse checks Mr. Marlen's gag reflex. The recommended technique to test the gag reflex is for the nurse to
- ○ 1. touch the back of the patient's throat with a tongue depressor.
- ○ 2. observe the patient for evidence of spontaneous swallowing when the neck is stroked.
- ○ 3. place a few milliliters of water on the patient's tongue and note whether the patient swallows.
- ○ 4. observe the patient's response to the introduction of a catheter for endotracheal suctioning.

**7.** Which of the following nursing assessments of Mr. Marlen's eyes is *least helpful* when the patient is assessed for signs of increased intracranial pressure?
- ○ 1. The color of the irises.
- ○ 2. The size of the pupils.
- ○ 3. The pupils' reaction to light.
- ○ 4. The reaction of the corneas to touch.

**8.** The nurse obtains a specimen when she observes clear fluid draining from Mr. Marlen's nose. A test that will determine whether the fluid is mucus or cerebrospinal fluid is one that tests for the

○ 1. pH level.
○ 2. specific gravity.
○ 3. presence of glucose.
○ 4. presence of microorganisms.

9. Mr. Marlen is taken to the operating room for surgery to relieve intracranial pressure. Which of the following nursing actions would be *least helpful* in supporting the family and friends while the patient is in the operating room?

○ 1. Suggest that they wait at home where they can relax in comfort.
○ 2. Tell them where the patient will be cared for when surgery is completed.
○ 3. Explain that they will be notified when the patient's surgery is completed.
○ 4. Prepare them for equipment that will be used during the patient's postoperative period.

10. Mr. Marlen receives mannitol (Osmitrol) during surgery to help decrease intracranial pressure. Which of the following nursing observations is *most likely* to indicate that the drug is having its desired effect?

○ 1. Urinary output increases.
○ 2. Pulse rate decreases.
○ 3. Blood pressure decreases.
○ 4. Muscular relaxation increases.

11. Which of the following comments that the nurse could make would help Mr. Marlen *most* to become oriented following surgery when he regains consciousness?

○ 1. "I am your nurse and will take care of you."
○ 2. "Can you tell me your name and where you live?"
○ 3. "Can you move your hands and feet a few inches from side to side?"
○ 4. "You are in a hospital where you had an operation after your accident."

12. As Mr. Marlen gradually regains consciousness, he becomes very restless and attempts to pull out his IV. Which action should the nurse take to protect the patient without increasing his intracranial pressure?

○ 1. Place the patient in a jacket restraint.
○ 2. Wrap the patient's hands in soft "mitten" restraints.
○ 3. Hold the patient's hands firmly in place at his sides.
○ 4. Apply a wrist restraint to each of the patient's arms.

13. When Mr. Marlen is fully conscious, it would be *best* for the nurse to assess his motor strength by having him

○ 1. squeeze the nurse's hands.
○ 2. feed himself with a spoon.
○ 3. demonstrate his ability to move his legs.
○ 4. signal as soon as pressure applied to the soles of his feet becomes discernible.

14. Which of the following postoperative care measures is *contraindicated* for a patient at risk for increasing intracranial pressure?

○ 1. Deep-breathing.
○ 2. Turning.
○ 3. Coughing.
○ 4. Passive range-of-motion exercises.

15. If the following nursing orders appear on Mr. Marlen's care plan, which would be *most helpful* in determining whether Mr. Marlen may be developing diabetes insipidus?

○ 1. Obtain vital signs every 2 hours.
○ 2. Measure urine specific gravity hourly.
○ 3. Determine arterial blood gases every other day.
○ 4. Test a urine specimen every morning for glucose.

16. The nurse helps Mr. Marlen eat. After the meal, which of the following nursing measures should the nurse plan to carry out next?

○ 1. Offer the patient a urinal.
○ 2. Give the patient a back rub.
○ 3. Help the patient with oral hygiene.
○ 4. Prepare the patient for a rest period.

17. During Mr. Marlen's recovery period, the nurse notes at 4 p.m. that Mr. Marlen seems uninterested in his visitors and is more lethargic than usual. If the following notations appear on the patient's record, which indicates the *most probable* reason for his lethargy?

○ 1. 12:30 p.m. Refused lunch; drank glass of milk only.
○ 2. 3 p.m. Placed in side-lying position after being in semisitting position for 2 hours.
○ 3. 3 p.m. Meperidine hydrochloride (Demerol) 100 mg given IM for pain.
○ 4. 3:30 p.m. Intake 800 ml and output 300 ml since 8 a.m.

## THE PATIENT WITH SEIZURES

Mr. Ronald Nyquist, a 25-year-old accountant, is admitted to the hospital for diagnostic studies after he experiences a grand mal seizure at his office.

18. Mr. Nyquist is placed on seizure precautions. Which of the following measures would be *contraindicated?*

○ 1. Encourage him to perform his own personal hygiene.

○ 2. Allow him to wear his own clothing.

○ 3. Obtain an oral temperature with a glass thermometer.

○ 4. Encourage him to be out of bed.

19. After an analysis of Mr. Nyquist's admission data, it is decided that computed tomography (CT scan) would help determine whether his seizure disorder is the result of

○ 1. genetic factors.

○ 2. toxic disturbances.

○ 3. metabolic problems.

○ 4. congenital abnormalities.

20. Plans are made to teach Mr. Nyquist about the CT scan that will be done at noon the next day. Which of the following statements the nurse could make is *most accurate* in relation to readying the patient for the scan?

○ 1. "You must shampoo your hair tonight to remove oil and dirt thoroughly."

○ 2. "You may drink fluids until about 8 a.m. Then we will give you a cleansing enema."

○ 3. "We will partially shave your head tonight so that electrodes can be attached securely to your scalp."

○ 4. "There is no special preparation necessary. You will need to hold your head very still during the examination."

21. An electroencephalogram (EEG) is ordered for Mr. Nyquist. What action should the nurse take when she observes that Mr. Nyquist has been served a breakfast consisting of a soft-boiled egg, toast with butter and marmalade, orange juice, and coffee on the morning of the EEG?

○ 1. Remove all the food.

○ 2. Remove the coffee.

○ 3. Remove the toast, butter, and marmalade only.

○ 4. Substitute vegetable juice for the orange juice.

22. An interdisciplinary conference is conducted to discuss Mr. Nyquist's seizures and possible causes. The *most common* cause of generalized convulsions in a person over 20 years of age is a

○ 1. brain tumor.

○ 2. birth injury.

○ 3. febrile state.

○ 4. structural lesion in the brain.

23. The nurse enters Mr. Nyquist's room as Mr. Nyquist, who is sitting in a chair, begins to have a seizure. Which of the following actions should the nurse take *first?*

○ 1. Lift the patient onto his bed.

○ 2. Ease the patient to the floor.

○ 3. Restrain the patient's body movements.

○ 4. Insert an airway into the patient's mouth.

24. In which position in bed should the nurse place Mr. Nyquist after his seizure has ended?

○ 1. Side-lying position.

○ 2. Supine position.

○ 3. Low Fowler's position.

○ 4. Modified Trendelenburg position.

25. After Mr. Nyquist's seizure has subsided, the nurse can expect that the patient is behaving in a *typical* manner if he

○ 1. becomes restless and agitated.

○ 2. sleeps for a period of time.

○ 3. says he is thirsty and hungry.

○ 4. is most comfortable walking and moving about.

26. Mr. Nyquist's roommate says that Mr. Nyquist "let out a strange cry" when the seizure began. A characteristic "cry" often heard at the beginning of a seizure is caused by

○ 1. the pain of the initial clonic movement.

○ 2. anxiety as the patient realizes a seizure is starting.

○ 3. air being expelled through the larynx that is partially closed by a spastic glottis.

○ 4. air expelled from the lungs in sudden bronchospasm.

27. Which of the following observations would be *unexpected* in a patient who has experienced a grand mal seizure?

○ 1. The patient was drowsy after the seizure.

○ 2. The patient was unable to talk after the seizure.

○ 3. The patient was incontinent of urine during the seizure.

○ 4. The patient failed to respond to stimuli during the clonic phase of the seizure.

28. Phenytoin (Dilantin) is prescribed for Mr. Nyquist. He asks the nurse how the medication will help him. The *best* response to the patient's question should be based on knowledge that the drug is thought to act by

○ 1. correcting the abnormal synthesis of norepinephrine in the body.

○ 2. depressing transmission of abnormal impulses in the spinal cord.

○ 3. reducing the responsiveness of neurons in the brain to abnormal impulses.

○ 4. interrupting the flow of abnormal impulses from the viscera to the brain.

29. The nurse plans a teaching program for Mr. Nyquist about the use of phenytoin (Dilantin). She teaches the patient to avoid substances that affect the action of the drug. Which of the following substances potentiates the action of phenytoin?

○ 1. Aspirin.

○ 2. Barbiturates.

○ 3. Antihistamines.

○ 4. Alcohol (when used chronically).

30. Mr. Nyquist tells the nurse that he is afraid he will not be able to drive a car again because of his seizures. The nurse responds *correctly* by telling him that driving will depend on local laws but most laws require
    ○ 1. that the person drive only during daytime hours.
    ○ 2. evidence that the seizures are under medical control.
    ○ 3. evidence that seizures occur no more often than every 6 months.
    ○ 4. that the person carry a medical identification card at all times.

31. Mr. Nyquist is studying about seizures and tells the nurse that he is unclear about what an aura is. The nurse *correctly* defines an aura when she explains that it is
    ○ 1. a postseizure state of amnesia.
    ○ 2. the occurrence of hallucinations during a seizure.
    ○ 3. a symptom that occurs just before a seizure.
    ○ 4. a feeling of relaxation as the seizure begins to subside.

32. When Mr. Nyquist is discharged from the hospital, the nurse instructs him to continue taking the phenytoin (Dilantin) as prescribed. One week after discharge, Mr. Nyquist calls his physician's office and tells the nurse he has a skin rash. In this situation, it would be *best* for the nurse to tell the patient to
    ○ 1. come to the office that day for consultation with the physician.
    ○ 2. decrease the amount of medication by taking one less pill each day.
    ○ 3. stop the medication but keep his regular appointment next week.
    ○ 4. continue the prescribed dosage of the medication but increase his fluid intake to at least 3,000 ml daily.

33. Mr. Nyquist takes phenytoin (Dilantin) for a considerable period of time. Which of the following findings should suggest to the nurse that the patient is having a *typical* reaction to the long-term use of phenytoin?
    ○ 1. The patient has gained considerable weight.
    ○ 2. The patient says he is having trouble with insomnia.
    ○ 3. The patient has an excessive growth of his gum tissue.
    ○ 4. The patient says that he now has to wear eyeglasses for proper vision.

## THE PATIENT WITH A CEREBROVASCULAR ACCIDENT

Mr. Homer Bacon, a 72-year-old retired engineer, experiences a thrombotic cerebrovascular accident while he is relaxing with his wife and reading the Sunday paper one morning. He is taken to the hospital in an ambulance.

34. Mr. Bacon has experienced a left cerebrovascular accident with flaccid hemiplegia of his right side. While the nurse initiates his care plan, she should keep in mind that rehabilitation for the stroke patient begins
    ○ 1. as soon as anticoagulant therapy begins for the patient.
    ○ 2. when the patient is admitted to his hospital room.
    ○ 3. when the patient is first able to work cooperatively with health-care personnel.
    ○ 4. as soon as a physical therapist can be brought into the patient's health-care team.

35. Regular oral hygiene is an essential intervention for Mr. Bacon. Which of the following oral hygiene techniques would be *inappropriate* for the nurse to use when providing Mr. Bacon's oral hygiene?
    ○ 1. The nurse places the patient on his back with a small pillow under his head.
    ○ 2. The nurse has portable suctioning equipment at the bedside.
    ○ 3. The nurse opens the patient's mouth with a padded tongue blade.
    ○ 4. The nurse cleans the patient's mouth and teeth with a toothbrush.

36. What characteristic of glycerin and lemon swabs make them *unsatisfactory* for long-term use?
    ○ 1. They take up water and cause dryness.
    ○ 2. They stain the teeth.
    ○ 3. They adhere poorly to oral mucosa.
    ○ 4. They alter the pH of the mouth.

37. The nurse changes Mr. Bacon's position in bed regularly. Which of the following techniques used to change the patient's position is *most likely* to cause friction and predispose the patient to decubitus ulcer formation?
    ○ 1. Rolling the patient onto his side.
    ○ 2. Sliding the patient to move him up in bed.
    ○ 3. Lifting the patient on a drawsheet when moving him up in bed.
    ○ 4. Having the patient help by lifting himself off the bed using a trapeze.

38. The nurse is concerned about the development of footdrop. Which of the following measures has

been found to be the *most effective* means of preventing footdrop in a stroke patient?

○ 1. Placing the feet against a firm footboard.
○ 2. Repositioning the patient every 2 hours.
○ 3. Having the patient wear ankle-high tennis shoes at intervals throughout the day.
○ 4. Massaging the feet and ankles regularly.

**39.** Because the cerebrovascular accident affected the left side of Mr. Bacon's brain, the nurse should anticipate that he will *most likely* experience

○ 1. expressive aphasia.
○ 2. dyslexia.
○ 3. apraxia.
○ 4. agnosia.

**40.** Mr. Bacon has an irritated cornea for which the nurse instills sterile eye drops. To which of the following causes is the patient's corneal irritation *most likely* due?

○ 1. The careless shaking of linens near his face.
○ 2. The continuous glare of overhead lighting in his room.
○ 3. The temporary loss of his blink reflex in the eye on his affected side.
○ 4. Paralysis involving the tear ducts of the affected eye, causing dryness.

**41.** Mr. Bacon has difficulty with dysphagia. *All* of the following measures would help decrease the risk of aspiration while Mr. Bacon is eating *except*

○ 1. ensuring that he is in an upright position.
○ 2. restricting his diet to liquids until swallowing improves.
○ 3. introducing foods on the unaffected side of his mouth.
○ 4. keeping distractions to a minimum.

**42.** Mr. Bacon experiences urinary incontinence following the cerebrovascular accident. Which of the following nursing interventions is likely to be *most successful* in helping Mr. Bacon re-establish urinary continence?

○ 1. Get an order for a Foley catheter.
○ 2. Apply an external urinary catheter.
○ 3. Make sure the urinal is within the patient's reach.
○ 4. Help the patient stand to void every 2 hours.

**43.** The nurse helps Mr. Bacon learn self-care skills. Which of the following interventions would be *appropriate* for the nurse to use when helping Mr. Bacon learn to dress himself?

○ 1. Encourage the patient to wear clothing designed especially for people who have had strokes.
○ 2. Dress the patient, explaining each step of the process as it is completed.
○ 3. Teach the patient to put clothing on the affected side first.

○ 4. Encourage the patient to ask his wife for help when dressing.

**44.** If Mr. Bacon is experiencing expressive aphasia, which of the following techniques would help the nurse successfully communicate with him?

○ 1. Speak in a clear normal voice.
○ 2. Use gestures instead of words to communicate.
○ 3. Speak in a voice that is louder than usual.
○ 4. Use pictures as cue cards for communication.

**45.** The cerebrovascular accident has caused Mr. Bacon to experience homonymous hemianopsia, blindness in half of his visual field. Homonymous hemianopsia would probably manifest itself in which of the following food-related behaviors?

○ 1. Increased preference for foods high in salt.
○ 2. Eating food on only half the plate.
○ 3. Forgetting the names of foods he likes.
○ 4. Inability to swallow liquids.

**46.** Although all of the following measures might be useful in reducing Mr. Bacon's visual disability, which measure should the nurse teach him *primarily* as a safety precaution?

○ 1. Wear a patch over one eye.
○ 2. Place his personal items on his sighted side.
○ 3. Lie in bed with his unaffected side toward the door.
○ 4. Turn his head from side to side when ambulating.

**47.** Mr. Bacon is experiencing mood swings and often has "crying jags" that are very distressing to his family. It would be *best* for the nurse to instruct the family to do which of the following when the "crying jags" occur?

○ 1. Sit quietly until the episode is over.
○ 2. Ignore the behavior and continue what they were doing.
○ 3. Attempt to divert the patient's attention.
○ 4. Tell the patient that this behavior is unacceptable.

**48.** Mr. Bacon is aware of and discouraged by his physical handicaps. The nurse can *best* help him overcome a negative self-concept by showing an attitude of

○ 1. helpfulness and sympathy.
○ 2. concern and charity.
○ 3. direction and firmness.
○ 4. encouragement and patience.

**49.** Mr. Bacon recalls the day his cerebrovascular accident occurred. Which of the following symptoms is a *typical* symptom of an impending stroke?

○ 1. Palpitations.
○ 2. Muscle cramps.
○ 3. Light-headedness.
○ 4. Euphoria.

12/93

## THE PATIENT WITH PARKINSON'S DISEASE

Mr. Vincent Kingly, 67, is admitted to the hospital for a diagnostic workup for probable Parkinson's disease.

50. When assessing Mr. Kingly, the nurse can anticipate that the patient is likely to exhibit *all* of the following symptoms *except*
    ○ 1. accumulation of saliva in the mouth.
    ○ 2. a low-pitched, monotonous voice.
    ○ 3. an exaggerated sense of euphoria.
    ○ 4. a stiff, masklike facial expression.

51. The nurse who admits Mr. Kingly to the hospital documents that the patient has a shuffling and propulsive gait. If the nurse is using the term "propulsive gait" *correctly*, she has observed that Mr. Kingly's walk is characterized by his
    ○ 1. slumping forward while walking.
    ○ 2. carrying himself erect on the balls of the feet.
    ○ 3. moving with increasingly quicker steps.
    ○ 4. having a tendency to lean backward while walking.

52. When the nurse asks Mr. Kingly to undress, she observes that his upper arm tremors disappear as he unbuttons his shirt. Which of the following statements would *best* guide the nurse when she analyzes her observations of the patient?
    ○ 1. The tremors are probably psychological and can be controlled by will.
    ○ 2. The tremors sometimes disappear with purposeful and voluntary movements.
    ○ 3. The tremors often increase in severity when attention is diverted by some activity.
    ○ 4. There is no explanation for the observation, which is probably a chance happening.

53. The nurse should understand that Mr. Kingly's signs and symptoms result because his body suffers from
    ○ 1. a depletion of a neurotransmitter.
    ○ 2. a sustained relaxation of nerve impulse activities.
    ○ 3. a blockage of depolarization at motor nerve plates.
    ○ 4. an absence of histamine in the central nervous system.

54. Which of the following goals is *most realistic* and *appropriate* in terms of planning Mr. Kingly's nursing care?
    ○ 1. To cure the disease.
    ○ 2. To stop the progression of the disease.
    ○ 3. To begin preparations for terminal care.
    ○ 4. To maintain optimal body function.

55. The physical therapy regimen developed for Mr. Kingly is aimed primarily at
    ○ 1. maintaining joint flexibility and relaxing muscles.
    ○ 2. building muscle strength.
    ○ 3. improving muscle endurance.
    ○ 4. reducing ataxia.

56. Parkinson's disease puts Mr. Kingly at risk for episodes of akinesia or "freeze-ups." The nurse must be particularly conscious of this possibility when she
    ○ 1. leaves Mr. Kingly sitting in a chair.
    ○ 2. helps Mr. Kingly with morning care.
    ○ 3. supervises Mr. Kingly's meals.
    ○ 4. teaches Mr. Kingly about his medications.

57. Mr. Kingly is started on levodopa (L-dopa). The nurse would judge that the drug is exerting its desired effect when Mr. Kingly experiences an improvement in
    ○ 1. moods.
    ○ 2. muscle rigidity.
    ○ 3. appetite.
    ○ 4. alertness.

58. To maintain the therapeutic effects of levodopa (L-dopa), most patients require gradually increasing dosages. Mr. Kingly's family should be taught that important symptoms of levodopa toxicity are
    ○ 1. lethargy and sleepiness.
    ○ 2. anorexia and nausea.
    ○ 3. diarrhea and cramping.
    ○ 4. delusion and hallucination.

59. A combination of levodopa (L-dopa) and carbidopa (Sinemet) is often the drug of choice in Parkinson's disease. One of the major advantages of this drug combination is that when combined with carbidopa, levodopa can be
    ○ 1. prescribed in lower doses.
    ○ 2. predicted to be free of side effects.
    ○ 3. expected to eliminate problems of tolerance.
    ○ 4. discontinued safely after a shorter period of therapy.

60. Mr. Kingly may be able to function effectively with less levodopa if he follows which dietary restriction?
    ○ 1. High-fiber diet.
    ○ 2. Low-fiber diet.
    ○ 3. High-protein diet.
    ○ 4. Low-protein diet.

61. Mr. Kingly requires a great deal of time to complete his morning hygiene, but he becomes quite annoyed when the nurse offers assistance, and he refuses all help. Which is the *best initial* response for the nurse to make in this situation?

1. Tell him firmly that he needs assistance and help him with his care.
2. Praise him for his desire to be independent and provide him with extra time and encouragement.
3. Tell him that he is being unrealistic about his abilities and must accept the fact that he needs help.
4. Suggest that if he insists on self-care, he should at least modify his routine.

**62.** The nurse asks Mr. Kingly to read the menu aloud each day. What is the purpose of this intervention?
1. To develop control of the tongue.
2. To decrease rigidity in the facial muscles.
3. To exercise the temporomandibular joint.
4. To increase awareness of voice intonation.

*12/93*

## THE PATIENT WITH MULTIPLE SCLEROSIS

Mrs. Norma Morley, a 48-year-old homemaker, is admitted to the hospital with a bladder infection and incontinence. She has had multiple sclerosis for the last 15 years.

**63.** The many and varied symptoms of multiple sclerosis are *primarily* the result of
1. patchy destruction of the myelin sheaths in the central nervous system.
2. disturbances in the synapses of the myoneural junction.
3. destruction of cells in the cerebellum.
4. degeneration of the peripheral nerves.

**64.** Patients with multiple sclerosis experience many different symptoms. Which of the following symptoms is *atypical* of multiple sclerosis?
1. Double vision.
2. Sudden bursts of energy.
3. Weakness in the extremities.
4. Muscle tremors.

**65.** Mrs. Morley's care plan includes nursing measures to help prevent complications commonly associated with multiple sclerosis. Which of the following complications is the patient *least likely* to experience?
1. Ascites.
2. Contractures.
3. Decubitus ulcers.
4. Respiratory infections.

**66.** Baclofen (Lioresal) is prescribed for Mrs. Morley. The nurse is justified in judging that the drug is

accomplishing its intended purpose when she observes that it is acting to help
1. induce sleep in the patient.
2. stimulate the patient's appetite.
3. relieve muscular spasticity in the patient.
4. reduce the bacterial count in the patient's urine.

**67.** Mrs. Morley has received varied drug therapies for her disease over the years. It is difficult to evaluate the effectiveness of any particular drug because patients with multiple sclerosis tend to
1. exhibit intolerances to many drugs.
2. experience spontaneous remissions from time to time.
3. require multiple drugs that are used simultaneously.
4. endure long periods of time before the illness responds to a particular drug.

**68.** Mrs. Morley is troubled with slurred speech. When the nurse is speaking with the patient, which of the following techniques is *contraindicated?*
1. Encouraging the patient to speak slowly.
2. Encouraging the patient to speak distinctly.
3. Asking the patient to repeat indistinguishable words.
4. Asking the patient to speak louder when tired.

**69.** Mrs. Morley walks unsteadily and in an uncoordinated manner. The term used to describe her gait is
1. ataxia.
2. vertigo.
3. paresis.
4. spasticity.

**70.** Mrs. Morley's right hand trembles severely whenever she attempts a voluntary action. She spills her coffee twice at lunch and cannot get her dress fastened securely. Which of the following nurses' notes offers the *best* account of these observations?
1. "Has an intention tremor of the right hand."
2. "Right-hand tremor worsens with purposeful acts."
3. "Needs assistance with dressing and eating due to severe trembling and clumsiness."
4. "Slight shaking of right hand increases to severe tremor when patient tries to button her clothes or drink from a cup."

**71.** Mrs. Morley is confined to a wheelchair when out of bed because of her general weakness and lack of coordination. Which of the following environmental conditions in the hospital is likely to be *most detrimental* to Mrs. Morley's well-being?
1. A drafty and cold main corridor.
2. An untidy and cluttered bedside stand.

○ 3. A wet area on the floor under the sink.

○ 4. A bag of soiled laundry near the doorway.

**72.** Mrs. Morley may eventually lose control of her bowels and require bowel retraining. In this event, which of the following measures is likely to be *least helpful?*

○ 1. Eating a diet high in roughage.

○ 2. Setting a regular time for elimination.

○ 3. Raising the toilet seat for easy access by wheelchair.

○ 4. Limiting fluid intake to 1,000 ml over a 24-hour period.

**73.** Mrs. Morley sometimes exhibits signs or symptoms of emotional distress. Patients with multiple sclerosis are *most likely* to exhibit

○ 1. mood disorders.

○ 2. thought disorders.

○ 3. psychosomatic illnesses.

○ 4. drug dependency problems.

**74.** During the rehabilitation program planned for Mrs. Morley, therapy and hobbies are used to help develop the patient's

○ 1. diligence and persistence.

○ 2. muscles and motivation.

○ 3. intellect and imagination.

○ 4. productivity and personality.

**75.** As the nurse helps prepare Mrs. Morley for discharge, she should encourage Mrs. Morley to

○ 1. accept the necessity for a quiet and inactive life-style.

○ 2. keep active while avoiding emotional upset and fatigue.

○ 3. follow good health habits to change the course of the disease.

○ 4. practice using the mechanical aids that will be needed when future disabilities arise.

**76.** Mrs. Morley has sensory impairments associated with her disease. *All* of the following are appropriate safety precautions that should be reinforced *except*

○ 1. carefully testing the temperature of bath water.

○ 2. avoiding kitchen activities due to the high risk of injury.

○ 3. avoiding the use of hot-water bottles or heating pads.

○ 4. inspecting her skin daily for injury or pressure.

**77.** Mrs. Morley's daughter and 3-year-old granddaughter live with her. The daughter asks the nurse what she can do to help her mother most at home. From which of the following measures would Mrs. Morley probably benefit *most* at home?

○ 1. A course of psychotherapy.

○ 2. A regular program of daily activities.

○ 3. A day-care center for the granddaughter.

○ 4. A weekly visit by another person who also has multiple sclerosis.

## THE UNCONSCIOUS PATIENT

Mr. Bill Evans, 38, is admitted to the emergency room after being found unconscious at the wheel of his car in the hospital parking lot. Mr. Evans is comatose and does not respond to stimuli. A drug overdose is suspected.

**78.** Which of the following assessment findings would lead the nurse to suspect that the coma is a result of a toxic overdose?

○ 1. Hypertension.

○ 2. Fever.

○ 3. Dilated pupils.

○ 4. Facial asymmetry.

**79.** Blood and urine analysis confirm the diagnosis of salicylate overdose. Mr. Evans is treated with gastric lavage. Which of the following positions would be *most appropriate* for Mr. Evans during this procedure?

○ 1. Lateral.

○ 2. Supine.

○ 3. Trendelenburg.

○ 4. Lithotomy.

**80.** In anticipation of further emergency treatment for Mr. Evans, which of the following medications would the nurse have available?

○ 1. Vitamin K (AquaMEPHYTON).

○ 2. Dextrose 50%.

○ 3. Activated charcoal powder.

○ 4. Sodium thiosulfate.

**81.** When Mr. Evans' wife and sister arrive at the hospital, they are distraught about his comatose condition as well as the possibility that this seems to be an intentional overdose. Which of the following would be an appropriate *initial* nursing intervention with this family?

○ 1. Explain that since Mr. Evans was found on hospital property, he was probably asking for help and did not intentionally overdose.

○ 2. Give Mr. Evans' wife and sister a big hug and assure them that he is in good hands.

○ 3. Encourage Mrs. Evans and her sister-in-law to ventilate their feelings and concerns and listen carefully.

○ 4. Allow Mrs. Evans and her sister-in-law to help care for Mr. Evans by rubbing his back when he is turned.

82. Mr. Evans is transferred to the intermediate care unit. His nursing care plan includes "turn every 2 hours." The major purpose of this turning schedule is to avoid pressure sores. Turning also provides stimulation of
    ○ 1. bronchial secretions.
    ○ 2. bladder function.
    ○ 3. deep tendon reflexes.
    ○ 4. proprioception.

83. Mr. Evans is at risk for developing a decubitus ulcer. The *first* warning of an impending decubitus ulcer is that the *initial* color of the skin when pressure is applied to it is
    ○ 1. bluish.
    ○ 2. reddish.
    ○ 3. whitish.
    ○ 4. yellowish.

84. Mr. Evans' skin care includes frequent massage over bony prominences. The *primary* reason for massage is to help
    ○ 1. relax tense muscles.
    ○ 2. improve blood circulation.
    ○ 3. allow the skin to stay dry.
    ○ 4. reduce the number of organisms on the skin.

85. At which of the following bony prominences has Mr. Evans the *least* potential for developing a decubitus ulcer?
    ○ 1. The heels.
    ○ 2. The knees.
    ○ 3. The coccyx.
    ○ 4. The back of the head.

86. Mr. Evans is placed in a right side-lying position. If the nurse uses the following techniques to position the patient, which is in *error*?
    ○ 1. The patient's head is placed on a small pillow.
    ○ 2. The patient's right leg is extended without pillow support.
    ○ 3. The patient's left arm rests on the mattress with the elbow flexed.
    ○ 4. The patient's left leg is supported on a pillow with the knee flexed.

87. To prevent external rotation of Mr. Evans' hips while he is lying on his back, it would be *best* for the nurse to place

○ 1. firm pillows under the length of his legs.
○ 2. sandbags alongside his legs from knees to ankles.
○ 3. trochanter rolls alongside his legs from ilium to midthigh.
○ 4. a footboard that supports his feet in the normal anatomic position.

88. A range-of-motion exercise program is initiated with Mr. Evans every 4 hours. The nurse alternately places his forearms and hands in the supine and prone positions. Mr. Evans' hand is pronated when it is
    ○ 1. held with the palm facing upward.
    ○ 2. held with the palm facing downward.
    ○ 3. closed into a fist.
    ○ 4. in the hand-shaking position.

89. The nurse *abducts* Mr. Evans' arm during range-of-motion exercises when she moves it so that the patient's arm is moved
    ○ 1. above the patient's head.
    ○ 2. below the level of the patient's body.
    ○ 3. toward the midline of the patient's body.
    ○ 4. away from the midline of the patient's body.

90. A Foley catheter is ordered for Mr. Evans. When lubricating the catheter before inserting it into the urinary meatus, the nurse should take precautions to *avoid*
    ○ 1. lubricating more than the tip of the catheter.
    ○ 2. contaminating her gloved hand with the lubricant.
    ○ 3. plugging the eye of the catheter with the lubricant.
    ○ 4. using so much lubricant that some may enter the bladder.

91. Of the following actions the nurse could take when giving catheter care to Mr. Evans, which should have the *highest* priority?
    ○ 1. Cleansing the area around the urethral meatus.
    ○ 2. Changing the catheter if it is not draining properly.
    ○ 3. Irrigating the catheter with several ounces of normal saline.
    ○ 4. Changing the location where the catheter is taped to the patient's leg.

# *CORRECT ANSWERS AND RATIONALES*

Numbers appear in parentheses following the rationales. The number identify textbooks listed in the references at the end of Part IV, where correct answers can be verified.

## *The Patient with a Head Injury*

**1.** 3. An operative permit must be signed before any surgical procedure is performed. If the patient is unable to sign a permit because of his condition, a responsible relative should be obtained to sign the permit. When a relative is not readily available and when time is of the essence, a letter, telephone call, or telegram is used to obtain permission. (10, 23)

**2.** 1. The highest priority of care when a person has multiple injuries is to establish an open airway so that there is effective ventilation and brain oxygenation. Unless the patient is breathing, other measures are likely to be futile. (25, 31)

**3.** 4. The pulse pressure is determined by subtracting the diastolic pressure from the systolic pressure. A widening pulse pressure is a sign of increased intracranial pressure. (25, 31)

| Blood Pressure | Pulse Pressure |
| --- | --- |
| 102/60 mm Hg | 42 |
| 110/90 mm Hg | 20 |
| 140/100 mm Hg | 40 |
| 160/100 mm Hg | 60 |
| 124/80 mm Hg (upon admission) | 44 |

**4.** 3. Increasing intracranial pressure causes unequal pupils from pressure on the third cranial nerve, rising body temperature from hypothalamic damage, and a rising systolic pressure, which reflects the additional pressure required to perfuse the brain. Pressure on the vagus nerve produces bradycardia, not tachycardia. (25, 31)

**5.** 1. The neural control of respiration takes place in the brain stem. Deterioration and pressure produce irregular respiratory patterns. Rapid shallow respirations, asymmetric chest movements, and nasal flaring are more characteristic of respiratory distress or hypoxia. (25, 31)

**6.** 1. The best technique for checking the gag reflex is to touch the back of the patient's throat in the pharyngeal area with a tongue depressor or cotton swab. The reflex is absent if the patient does not

gag. Reflexes are typically absent or sluggish in the presence of increased intracranial pressure. It is dangerous to place liquids in the mouth of an unconscious patient because of the danger of aspiration. (2, 28)

**7.** 1. In the presence of intracranial pressure, the pupils are likely to be unequal in size and to fail to react to light. There is absence of response when the corneas are touched. The color of the irises is not significant in the assessment of a patient for increased intracranial pressure. (25, 31)

**8.** 3. The constituents of cerebrospinal fluid are similar to the constituents found in blood plasma. An examination for glucose content is done to determine whether fluid from the body is mucus or cerebrospinal fluid. Mucus does not contain glucose; cerebrospinal fluid does. (25, 31)

**9.** 1. When relatives wait for a patient who is having surgery, it is least helpful to suggest that they wait at home. They want to be near their loved ones, and most agencies provide a waiting room for them. Telling the relatives they will be called when surgery is completed, where the patient will be cared for after surgery, and what equipment is likely to be used in the patient's care offers support and is recommended. (10, 23)

**10.** 1. Mannitol (Osmitrol) is an osmotic diuretic. It helps decrease intracranial pressure by its dehydrating effects. The drug is acting in the desired manner when the urinary output increases. It may be desirable for the pulse rate to decrease, the blood pressure to decrease, and the muscles to relax in certain situations, but mannitol will not be used to accomplish these goals. (25, 31)

**11.** 4. Explaining where a patient is and why he is there helps him become oriented after a period of unconsciousness. Asking the patient his name and to move his hands and feet are used to help determine the patient's state of orientation. (26, 31)

**12.** 2. It would be best to wrap a patient's hands in washcloths or to have him wear mitts when he becomes restless while regaining consciousness after brain surgery. Restraining him tends to increase his activity and restlessness and thus increases intracranial pressure. (25, 31)

**13.** 1. Having a patient squeeze the nurse's hand is a technique used to assess the patient's motor strength. Noting that the patient can feed himself verifies coordination as well as motor ability but does not help the nurse determine muscle strength. Being able to move the legs shows motor ability but not strength. Having the patient signal when pressure is applied to his feet tests sensory ability. (25, 31)

**14.** 3. Coughing is contraindicated for a patient at risk for increasing intracranial pressure because coughing increases intracranial pressure. Deep-breathing, turning, and passive range-of-motion exercises can be continued. (25, 31)

**15.** 2. Diabetes insipidus is due to a deficiency of antidiuretic hormone (ADH). The condition may occur in conjunction with head injuries as well as with other disease conditions. When the hormone is deficient, the patient is extremely thirsty and excretes large amounts of highly dilute urine. The degree of urine concentration is best assessed by measuring the specific gravity of urine samples. (26, 31)

**16.** 3. Debris from food and liquid does the most damage to teeth within the first 15 minutes after eating. To help prevent caries, it is important to give oral hygiene as soon after eating as possible. It is best to offer a patient the urinal before he eats. Giving a back rub and preparing the patient for rest can be done after giving oral hygiene. (24, 36)

**17.** 3. Meperidine hydrochloride (Demerol) is a narcotic analgesic. After receiving 100 mg intramuscularly, it is expected that an adult patient will be lethargic an hour later, owing to the drug's action. (26, 31)

## The Patient with Seizures

**18.** 3. A patient subject to seizure activity should have his temperature taken by a route other than the oral route when a mercury glass thermometer is used. A glass thermometer could break in the patient's mouth if a seizure occurs while an oral temperature is being obtained. (5, 26)

**19.** 4. Computed tomography (CT scan) reveals the detail and inner structure of an object. When a patient has seizure activity, a CT scan is used to help identify masses and vascular disorders in the brain. A congenital disorder usually involves a vascular disorder. Differences in tissue density help identify tumor masses. Disorders resulting from genetic factors, toxic disturbances, and metabolic problems would not be demonstrated with a CT scan. (25, 31)

**20.** 4. In general, there is no special preparation for a computed tomography (CT) scan. The patient will be asked to hold his head very still during the examination, which lasts about 30 to 60 minutes. In some instances, food and fluids *may* be withheld for 4 to 6 hours before the procedure if a contrast medium is used because the radiopaque substance sometimes causes nausea. (25, 31)

**21.** 2. Beverages containing caffeine, such as coffee, tea, and cola drinks, are withheld before an electroencephalogram (EEG) because of the stimulating effects of the caffeine. A meal should not be omitted before an EEG because low blood sugar could alter brain wave patterns. (25, 31)

**22.** 1. Generalized convulsions in patients over 20 years of age usually have an identifiable cause; the most common is a brain tumor. (25, 31)

**23.** 2. If a patient has a seizure while sitting in a chair, it is best to ease him to the floor and place a pillow under his head. No effort should be made to restrain him. The strong muscular contractions may cause the patient to suffer injury if he is restrained. The nurse is likely to hurt herself, as well as the patient, if she tries to lift him to a bed. It is not necessary or recommended that an airway be placed in the mouth of a patient while he is having a seizure. (26, 31)

**24.** 1. The position of choice during and following a seizure is the side-lying position because it facilitates drainage from the mouth and helps prevent aspiration. (25, 31)

**25.** 2. A brief period of confusion usually follows a seizure. Then, the patient typically sleeps for a period of time. (26, 31)

**26.** 3. The "cry" often heard when a seizure starts is caused by air that is being expelled through the larynx, which is partially closed by a spastic glottis. (26, 31)

**27.** 2. Patients are rarely able to respond to even painful stimuli during a seizure. They may be incontinent during the seizure and will be quite drowsy after the seizure. Despite drowsiness, however, the physical ability to speak should be preserved and its loss would be unexpected. (26, 31)

**28.** 3. It is uncertain exactly how phenytoin (Dilantin) helps control seizures. The most common theory is that it reduces the responsiveness of neurons in the brain to abnormal impulses (that is, it depresses neural activity). (25, 31)

**29.** 1. Many drugs affect the action of phenytoin (Dilantin). A few common ones that potentiate the effects of phenytoin are aspirin, estrogens, anticoagulants, and sulfonamides. Acute alcoholic intoxication also potentiates the action of the drug. Alcohol, antihistamines, and barbiturates are examples of substances that, used frequently, *inhibit* the action of phenytoin. (26, 31)

**30.** 2. Specific regulations and restrictions for persons who have seizures vary locally. Most commonly, laws require evidence that the seizures are under medical control before the person is given permission to drive a car. It is recommended that persons subject to seizures carry a card or wear an identification bracelet describing their illness so that in an emergency their condition can be quickly identified. (26, 31)

**31.** 3. An aura is a premonition of an impending seizure. The aura usually is of a sensory nature (that is, an olfactory, visual, gustatory, or auditory sensation). Some auras may be of a psychic nature. An aura may help identify the area of the brain from which the seizure originates. (26, 31)

**32.** 1. A skin rash may indicate a toxic effect of phenytoin (Dilantin). The patient should be instructed to come to the physician's office that day for a consultation. The nurse should not instruct the patient to adjust or stop the medication. (12, 16)

**33.** 3. A common effect of taking phenytoin (Dilantin) for prolonged periods of time is an overgrowth of gingival tissues. Problems may be minimized with good oral hygiene, but in some instances overgrown tissues may have to be removed surgically. (26, 31)

## The Patient with a Cerebrovascular Accident

**34.** 2. Rehabilitation for a patient who has a cerebrovascular accident, or stroke, should begin at the time the patient is admitted to the hospital. The first goal of rehabilitation should be to help prevent the patient from developing deformities. This goal is reached by such techniques as positioning the patient properly in bed, changing his position frequently, and supporting all parts of the body in proper alignment. Passive range-of-motion exercises may also be started unless there are orders to the contrary. (25, 31)

**35.** 1. A helpless patient should be positioned on his side, not on his back, with his head over a small pillow when being given oral hygiene. This positioning helps secretions escape from the throat and mouth and minimizes the danger of aspiration. Suctioning equipment should be available, the patient's mouth should be opened with a padded tongue blade, and the mouth and teeth can be cleaned with a toothbrush. (25, 31)

**36.** 1. Glycerin is hydrolytic (that is, it takes up water) and, when used over a period of time, tends to cause drying of the mucosa. Lemon juice helps increase salivation and decreases this drying effect, but dryness still occurs when a mixture of lemon juice and glycerin is used for a prolonged period. (24, 36)

**37.** 2. Sliding a patient on a sheet causes friction and should be avoided. Friction tends to injure skin tissues and then predisposes to the formation of decubitus ulcers. Rolling a patient, lifting him on a drawsheet, and having the patient help lift himself off the bed with a trapeze help prevent friction when a patient is being moved in bed. (24, 36)

**38.** 3. Regular repositioning and range-of-motion exercises are important interventions, but the use of ankle-high tennis shoes has been found to be most effective in preventing footdrop. Foot boards stimulate spasms and are not routinely recommended. (26, 31)

**39.** 1. Broca's area, which controls verbal, expressive speech, is located on the left side of the brain. Therefore, a person with a cerebrovascular accident in this area is likely to experience expressive or motor aphasia. Dyslexia is the inability of a person with normal vision to interpret written language. It is thought to be due to a central nervous system defect in the ability to organize graphic symbols. Apraxia is the inability to perform purposeful movements in the absence or loss of motor power, sensation, or coordination. Agnosia is the loss of comprehension of auditory, visual, or other sensations although the sensory sphere is intact. (25, 31)

**40.** 3. A stroke victim may have damage to nerves that control the blink reflex in the eye. This usually results in the eyelid's remaining open, which causes corneal drying and irritation. To prevent corneal irritation, sterile eye drops are used. Sterile mineral oil and artificial tears are common preparations used to protect the cornea. (26, 31)

**41.** 2. Patients who have dysphagia or difficulty swallowing frequently have the most difficulty ingesting liquids, which are easily aspirated. Measures that minimize the risk of aspiration in a patient who has dysphagia include positioning him in an upright position while eating, unless contraindicated, introducing foods on the unaffected side of the mouth, and keeping distractions to a minimum. (25, 28)

**42.** 4. Re-establishing urinary continence is a realistic goal for most stroke patients. Patients should be assisted to a normal voiding position and instructed to try to urinate. Foley catheters pose a serious infection risk and neither indwelling nor external catheters address the goal of re-establishing urinary continence. (25, 28)

**43.** 3. When dressing, a patient who has had a stroke should put clothing on the affected side first. He should wear normal clothing, if possible. Other people may help the patient dress, but the emphasis is on self-care. (28, 33)

**44.** 1. Expressive aphasia is a problem in speaking. Reception is intact and the nurse does not need to adjust her voice level or use other cues for communication. (25, 28)

**45.** 2. While many food behaviors may be disturbed after a cerebrovascular accident, eating food on half the plate would be the result of inability to coordinate visual images and spatial relationships. (37, 41)

**46.** 4. To increase the visual field, the partially sighted person should be taught to turn his head from side to side when walking. Neglecting to do so may result in accidents. This technique helps maximize the use of remaining sight. A patch does not address the problem of hemianopsia. Appropriate positioning of the patient and personal items will increase his ability to cope with the problem, but does not affect his safety. (22, 25)

**47.** 3. A patient who has brain damage may be emotionally labile and may cry or laugh for no explainable reason. "Crying jags" are best dealt with by attempting to divert the patient's attention. Ignoring the behavior or attempting to deal with it behaviorally will not affect it. (28, 33)

**48.** 4. The most positive method for the nurse to use when offering emotional support to a patient who is discouraged and has a negative self-concept because of physical handicaps is to display encouragement and patience. The patient should be praised when he shows progress in his efforts to overcome handicaps. Sympathy, charity, and firm discipline have little supportive value. (25, 28)

**49.** 3. Typical symptoms of an impending stroke include light-headedness, weakness, tiredness, transient paralysis of an extremity, speech and visual changes, dizziness, headache, mental confusion, and blackouts. (26, 31)

## The Patient with Parkinson's Disease

**50.** 3. Typical signs of Parkinson's disease include having saliva drool from the mouth, a low-pitched, monotonous voice, and a stiff, masklike facial expression. An exaggerated sense of euphoria would not be typical; more likely, the patient will exhibit depression, probably related to the progressive nature of the disease and the difficulties encountered by the patient in dealing with it. Many patients also often begin to show a decline in cognitive, memory, and perceptual abilities. (17, 25)

**51.** 3. A propulsive gait, which is a typical disorder of locomotion noted in persons with Parkinson's disease, is characterized by a tendency to take increasingly quicker steps while walking. This type of gait often causes the patient to fall or to have trouble when trying to stop walking. (26, 31)

**52.** 2. Voluntary and purposeful movements will often temporarily decrease or stop tremors associated with Parkinson's disease. Unfortunately, however, in some patients, tremors may increase with voluntary effort. Tremors are not psychological in nature and cannot be willfully controlled. (17, 31)

**53.** 1. The signs and symptoms of Parkinson's disease are caused by low levels of dopamine in the body. Dopamine is a neurotransmitter and has an inhibiting function in the central control of movement. (17, 25)

**54.** 4. Parkinson's disease progresses in severity and there is no known cure or way of stopping its progression. However, many patients live for years with the disease, and it would not be appropriate to start planning terminal care at this time for the patient described in this item. The most appropriate and realistic goal is to help the patient function at his best. (25, 26)

**55.** 1. Muscle rigidity, which can lead to contracture, is a major symptom of Parkinson's disease. Physical therapy is aimed at maintaining joint flexibility and relaxation of muscles. (25, 26)

**56.** 1. Akinesia or "freeze-ups" leave the individual completely unable to initiate movement. This is a particular concern when a patient is left unsupervised in a chair or on the commode. (8, 25)

**57.** 2. Levodopa (L-dopa) is prescribed to decrease severe muscle rigidity, and its effectiveness is primarily measured by the patient's response in this area. (8, 25)

**58.** 4. Increasing doses of levodopa (L-dopa) leaves a patient at serious risk for toxicity. Severe mental deterioration such as delusions or hallucinations frequently occur in the toxic state, and families must be instructed about this possibility. (12, 16)

**59.** 1. When levodopa (L-dopa) is used, much of it does not penetrate into the central nervous system well because of peripheral metabolism. Carbidopa helps prevent this process. As a result, a combination of levodopa and carbidopa means that the patient requires a lower dose of levodopa than when levodopa is used alone. Side effects still may occur, but they are not likely to be as severe. (12, 16)

**60.** 4. A high-protein diet reduces the effectiveness of levodopa (L-dopa). Patients on L-dopa therapy may be controlled more easily if they limit their dietary intake of protein, especially during the daytime hours when the effectiveness of the drug is most critical to normal functioning. (36, 41)

**61.** 2. Ongoing self-care is a major goal for patients with Parkinson's disease. They should be provided with additional time as needed and praised for their efforts to remain independent. (22, 25)

**62.** 4. The primary reason for having a patient with Parkinson's disease read aloud is to help the patient increase his awareness of the typical low-pitched, monotonous tone of his voice. Doing so makes it easier for the patient to modify intonation and speak more clearly. (8, 25)

## The Patient with Multiple Sclerosis

**63.** 1. Multiple sclerosis is characterized by demyelination, which means destruction of myelin sheaths. Demyelination occurs in the brain and the spinal cord. The lesions of multiple sclerosis are small patches where demyelination is present. The disease is a chronic and progressive one of the brain and spinal cord. The signs and symptoms of the disease are varied and depend on where demyelination in the central nervous system has occurred. The cause of demyelination is unknown. (25, 35)

**64.** 2. Visual disturbances, speech impairment, problems with walking associated with loss of muscle tone and tremors, spastic weakness in the extremities, and dizziness with nausea and vomiting are some common symptoms of multiple sclerosis. Hyperexcitability and euphoria may occur, but because of muscle weakness sudden bursts of energy are unlikely in patients with multiple sclerosis. (25, 35)

**65.** 1. Typical complications that the patient with multiple sclerosis encounters include contractures, decubitus ulcers, and respiratory infections, and nursing care should be directed toward the goal of preventing them. Ascites is not associated with multiple sclerosis. (8, 25)

**66.** 3. Baclofen (Lioresal) is a centrally acting skeletal muscle relaxant. It helps relieve spasms that patients with multiple sclerosis often experience. Methocarbamol (Robaxin) is another skeletal muscle relaxant also sometimes used for patients with multiple sclerosis; the nurse may encounter others in her practice. (12, 16)

**67.** 2. Evaluating drug effectiveness is difficult because a high percentage of patients with multiple sclerosis show remissions, exacerbations, and steady progress from time to time without apparent cause. (17, 31)

**68.** 4. Such practices as encouraging a patient with slurred speech to speak slowly and distinctly and asking her to repeat indistinguishable words tend to improve her ability to communicate effectively. Asking a patient to speak louder even when tired is an unsatisfactory practice and may aggravate the problem. (17, 35)

**69.** 1. Ataxia is an inability to coordinate walking movements. Vertigo is dizziness. Paresis is a type of paralysis. Spasticity is increased tone or contractions of muscles. (25, 29)

**70.** 4. Nurses' notes should be concise, objective, clearly stated, and relevant. The patient described in this item has trembling when she attempts voluntary action such as drinking a beverage or fastening clothing. This activity should be described exactly as it occurs so that the person who reads the note has no doubt about the nurse's observation of the patient's behavior. (8, 17)

**71.** 1. Patients with multiple sclerosis report an aggravation of symptoms when in a cold climate. It is also noted that the disease occurs more often in cold and temperate climates than in geographical areas nearer the equator. The reason for the effects of cold on multiple sclerosis is unknown. (8, 17)

**72.** 4. Limiting fluid intake is likely to aggravate, rather than help, symptoms when a bowel-training program is being used. Furthermore, water imbalance, as well as electrolyte imbalances, tends to aggravate symptoms of multiple sclerosis. (28, 33)

**73.** 1. Patients with multiple sclerosis often experience psychological disturbances that are best described as mood disorders. Emotional instability is typical. Thought disorders, psychosomatic illnesses, and drug dependency are not typical of patients with multiple sclerosis, unless the disorders are present independently. (8, 25)

**74.** 2. Care for the patient with multiple sclerosis is directed toward muscle rehabilitation and helping the patient remain motivated. The disease is chronic, and therefore goals should be those with the most benefit over a long period of time. (17, 25)

**75.** 2. The most positive approach is to encourage a patient with multiple sclerosis to keep active while avoiding emotional upset and fatigue. A quiet and inactive life-style is not necessarily indicated. Good health habits are not likely to alter the course of the disease, although they may avoid complications. Practicing the use of aids that will be needed for future disabilities may be helpful but also may discourage the patient. (17, 25)

**76.** 2. Safety concerns are essential with sensory impairment. Water temperature should be tested carefully, hot-water bottles should not be used, and patients should be taught to inspect their skin regularly. Independence and self-care are also important and patients should not be instructed to avoid kitchen activities out of fear of injury. (17, 35)

**77.** 2. A patient with multiple sclerosis usually does best and is least frustrated at home when a regular program of daily activities is planned. There is no information given in this item that suggests psychological counseling is necessary or that it would be helpful to have the granddaughter attend a day-care center. A weekly visit by a person who also has the disease may not be contraindicated but is less likely to benefit the patient as much as a regular program of planned activities. (28, 33)

## *The Unconscious Patient*

**78.** 3. Equal, normally reactive pupils indicate adequate neurologic functioning. Progressive dilatation indicates increased intracranial pressure, and fixed dilated pupils indicate injury at the midbrain. An overdose of amphetamines, alcohol, or cocaine also causes dilated pupils; an overdose of morphine and barbiturates results in constricted pupils. Blood pressure is regulated by various factors and hypertension would not pinpoint a toxic disorder. Fever is related either to infection or dehydration. Facial asymmetry indicates paralysis. (5, 26)

**79.** 1. An unconscious patient is best positioned in the lateral or semiprone position because it allows the jaw and tongue to fall forward, facilitates drainage of secretions, and prevents aspiration. If the patient is supine, there is a major risk of airway obstruction from the tongue falling back, vomitus, or nasopharyngeal secretions. In the Trendelenburg position, the head is lower than the heart. This position decreases effective lung volume and increases the risk of cerebral edema. The lithotomy position has no purpose in this situation. (5, 26)

**80.** 3. Activated charcoal powder is administered to absorb remaining particles of salicylate. Vitamin K (AquaMEPHYTON) is an antidote for warfarin (Coumadin). Dextrose 50% is an antidote for insulin. Sodium thiosulfate is an antidote for cyanide. (26, 31)

**81.** 3. The initial response to crisis is high anxiety. This must begin to dissipate before a person can deal with the actual situation. Allowing the family to ventilate provides some decompression. The reasons for the patient's actions are unknown; assumptions must be validated before they become facts. Touch can be appropriate but not when used as a form of false reassurance. Helping with the patient's care is appropriate at a later time. (5, 26)

**82.** 4. Proprioception is awareness of position, and a change in position increases the brain's awareness. Stimulation is needed to help overcome the profound sensory deprivation of the unconscious patient. Turning does not stimulate bronchial secretions, bladder function, or deep tendon reflexes. (5, 26)

**83.** 3. The *initial* reaction when pressure is applied to the skin is that the area becomes blanched, or whitish. If pressure is relieved, the body tends to carry excess amounts of blood to the area to make up for the temporary decrease in blood supply. This is called reactive hyperemia, and the skin then becomes red. A reddened area is a precursor of a pressure sore. (5, 23)

**84.** 2. Decubitus ulcers are caused by pressure on an area, which in turn decreases circulation to that area. The poorly oxygenated tissues then tend to break down, causing a decubitus ulcer. The primary reason for massaging areas at risk for decubitus ulcers is to improve circulation in the area. The massage may help relax muscles and may help the skin to dry, but these are of lesser importance in the situation described in this item. (5, 23)

**85.** 2. The knees are the least likely area on the body for developing decubitus ulcers, although bedsores can develop on knees too. The most common site for decubitus ulcers is the area over the coccyx. (5, 23)

**86.** 3. The patient will not be in proper body alignment if his left arm rests on the mattress with the elbow flexed when in the right side-lying position. This positioning of the arm pulls the left shoulder out of good alignment and, by so doing, restricts respiratory movements. The arm should be supported on a pillow. (5, 23)

**87.** 3. To prevent external rotation of the hips, trochanter rolls alongside the patient's legs from the ilium to midthigh are recommended. Using sandbags from the knees to the ankle will not effectively support the hips in proper alignment. Pillows can be used to support the legs properly, but they should be used only as a temporary measure because they do not hold the legs and hips in proper alignment over a period of time. A footboard does not help keep the legs and hips in proper alignment for the bedridden patient. (5, 23)

**88.** 2. The forearm is pronated when the palm of the hand faces downward; the body is pronated when the patient lies on his abdomen. In the supine position, the palm faces upward or the patient lies on his back. (5,23)

**89.** 4. Abduction refers to movement of a body part away from the midline of the body, such as when a patient's arm is moved laterally away from his body. The opposite movement, adduction, occurs when the arm is moved toward the midline of the person's body. Movements that place the arm above the head and below the level of the body exercise the shoulder joint with backward extension and forward flexion, respectively. (5, 23)

**90.** 3. When preparing to catheterize a patient, the nurse should avoid plugging the eye of the catheter with lubricant, in order to allow the free flow of urine when the catheter is in the bladder. The lubricant should be sterile, so if some of it is on the gloves it will not contaminate the nurse's hands. Approximately 1.5″ (3.7 cm) of the end of the catheter should be lubricated. This allows for sufficient lubricant to reduce friction as the catheter is inserted. If a little sterile lubricant enters the urinary bladder, it will do no harm. (5, 23)

**91.** 1. It is generally agreed that bladder infections that occur when a patient has an indwelling catheter are due to infections that ascend from the urethra and into the bladder. Giving catheter care that includes meticulous cleansing of the area around the urethral meatus has highest priority for the patient with an indwelling catheter. Antimicrobial solutions and ointments have been used to keep the meatus and surrounding area clean. More recently, cleaning the area *gently* with soap and water has been recommended. (5, 23)

# test 9

- The Patient with Rheumatoid Arthritis
- The Patient with a Hip Fracture
- The Patient with a Herniated Disc
- The Patient with Peripheral Vascular Disease
- The Patient with a Femoral Fracture
- The Patient with a Spinal Cord Injury

**Correct Answers and Rationales**

Select the one *best* or *correct* answer and indicate your choice by filling in the circle with a pencil in front of the option you have chosen. If the answer you would prefer is not given, select the one you think is *most appropriate*.

## THE PATIENT WITH RHEUMATOID ARTHRITIS

Mrs. Harriet Carter, 60, has had rheumatoid arthritis for 25 years, but the disease has worsened significantly over the last 5 years.

1. Mrs. Carter comes in for evaluation. She tells the nurse, "I never used to pay much attention to my arthritis. It was just a nuisance. I don't really understand the whole thing. What goes on in my joints to cause me all these problems?" The nurse should base her response on knowledge that the part of the joint in which pathophysiologic changes begin is the
   - ○ 1. bursa.
   - ○ 2. cartilage.
   - ○ 3. synovium.
   - ○ 4. ligaments.

2. Mrs. Carter takes aspirin to relieve her joint pain. Patients who take aspirin should be aware that an *important* symptom of aspirin toxicity is
   - ○ 1. dysuria.
   - ○ 2. tinnitus.
   - ○ 3. chest pain.
   - ○ 4. drowsiness.

3. Which statement by Mrs. Carter would indicate that she needs reteaching in order to receive maximum benefit from her aspirin therapy safely?
   - ○ 1. "I always take my aspirin with food to protect my stomach."
   - ○ 2. "Once I learned to take my aspirin with meals, I was able to start using the inexpensive generic brand."
   - ○ 3. "I always watch for bleeding of my gums or in my stool."
   - ○ 4. "I try to take aspirin only on days when the pain seems particularly bad."

4. Mrs. Carter asks the nurse, "Do only women get the kind of arthritis I have?" The nurse should explain that rheumatoid arthritis *most often* affects
   - ○ 1. men during middle life.
   - ○ 2. men during later life.
   - ○ 3. women during middle life.
   - ○ 4. women during later life.

5. Mrs. Carter tells the nurse, "My husband also has arthritis but our symptoms are completely different." Which of the following symptoms of arthritis is *unique* to rheumatoid arthritis?
   - ○ 1. Joint pain.
   - ○ 2. Joint stiffness.
   - ○ 3. Limited movement of joints.
   - ○ 4. Joint swelling.

6. If Mr. Carter has osteoarthritis, it would be reasonable to expect that the joints *least* likely to be affected by the disease would be those of the
   - ○ 1. hip.
   - ○ 2. knee.
   - ○ 3. finger.
   - ○ 4. shoulder.

7. Which of the following factors would be *most likely* to increase Mr. Carter's osteoarthritis joint symptoms?
   - ○ 1. A long history of smoking.
   - ○ 2. Excess alcohol use.
   - ○ 3. Obesity.
   - ○ 4. Emotional stress.

8. Mrs. Carter's doctor discontinues the aspirin and orders ibuprofen (Motrin). To minimize gastric mucosal irritation, the nurse should teach Mrs. Carter to take this medication
   - ○ 1. at bedtime.
   - ○ 2. upon arising.
   - ○ 3. immediately after a meal.
   - ○ 4. when her stomach is empty.

9. Mrs. Carter tells the nurse, "I have a friend who took gold shots and had a wonderful response. Why didn't my doctor let me try that?" Which of the following replies by the nurse would be *best?*
   - ○ 1. "It would be best if you asked the doctor. He doesn't always let me in on his thinking."
   - ○ 2. "Tell me more about your friend's arthritic condition. Maybe I can answer that question for you."
   - ○ 3. "That drug is used for cases that are worse then yours. It wouldn't help you."
   - ○ 4. "You shouldn't try to compare your condition with anyone else's. Every patient is different."

10. Mrs. Carter continues to have increasing disease involvement in her right knee and the physician recommends a total knee replacement. This type of procedure is called a
    - ○ 1. osteotomy.
    - ○ 2. arthrodesis.
    - ○ 3. arthroplasty.
    - ○ 4. osteosynthesis.

11. In planning postoperative care for Mrs. Carter, the nurse should consider that patients with rheumatoid arthritis should *usually* be positioned so as to
    - ○ 1. decrease edema around the joints.
    - ○ 2. promote maximum comfort.
    - ○ 3. prevent venous stasis.
    - ○ 4. prevent flexion deformities of the joints.

12. In the postoperative period, Mrs. Carter finds it very painful to move and she resists efforts to change her position in bed. Which nursing action is *most appropriate?*
    - ○ 1. Admonish the patient for her negative attitude toward therapy.
    - ○ 2. Explain to the patient why the turning and realignment are necessary.
    - ○ 3. Remind the patient that she is to blame if she develops complications.
    - ○ 4. Point out to the patient that she is not following health-care directions.

13. The nurse teaches Mrs. Carter to perform isometric exercises to re-educate her leg muscles after surgery. Isometric exercises are particularly effective with patients with rheumatoid arthritis because they
    - ○ 1. cost little in terms of time and money.
    - ○ 2. strengthen the muscles while keeping the joints stationary.
    - ○ 3. involve the patient in her own care and thus improve morale.
    - ○ 4. prevent joint stiffness.

14. When preparing Mrs. Carter to ambulate after her surgery, the nurse should explain the quadriceps setting exercises. These exercises are accomplished by
    - ○ 1. bending the knee to form a right angle.
    - ○ 2. rotating the leg slowly around in circles.
    - ○ 3. pressing the back of the knee into the mattress.
    - ○ 4. turning the leg inward toward the opposite thigh.

15. When helping Mrs. Carter plan her diet, the nurse should take into account that, when compared with younger adults, elderly persons require lesser amounts of
    - ○ 1. fats.
    - ○ 2. proteins.
    - ○ 3. calories.
    - ○ 4. carbohydrates.

16. Mrs. Carter wants to protect herself from quack treatments for her arthritis and asks the nurse, "How can I tell what is valid and good for me and what isn't?" The nurse should be guided in her reply by the fact that genuine and reputable products are *most often* sold through
    - ○ 1. testimonials inserted in leading magazines.
    - ○ 2. advertisements in circulars received in the mail.
    - ○ 3. prescriptions individually prescribed by physicians.
    - ○ 4. newspapers carrying advertisements as a direct sales campaign.

## THE PATIENT WITH A HIP FRACTURE

Mrs. Pearl Kwan, 73, is admitted to the hospital after falling in her home. She complains of right-hip pain and cannot move her right leg. The diagnosis is a fractured right hip.

17. The nurse assesses *correctly* that Mrs. Kwan has a *typical* sign of a hip fracture when she observes that the patient's right leg is
    - ○ 1. rotated internally.
    - ○ 2. held in a flexed position.
    - ○ 3. adducted.
    - ○ 4. shorter than the leg on the unaffected side.

18. The nurse assesses the area of Mrs. Kwan's fracture. Which of the following phenomenon is produced if broken bone fragments in Mrs. Kwan's hip are rubbing against each other?
    - ○ 1. Crepitation.
    - ○ 2. Ossification.
    - ○ 3. Proliferation.
    - ○ 4. Consolidation.

**19.** Mrs. Kwan's fracture is corrected by surgical internal fixation with the insertion of a pin. This procedure is the treatment of choice for most older persons because, in contrast to other surgical procedures, internal fixation with a pin
- ○ 1. is a simpler procedure.
- ○ 2. promotes more rapid healing.
- ○ 3. carries less danger of infection.
- ○ 4. makes earlier mobilization possible.

**20.** Mrs. Kwan returns from surgery with a drainage tube attached to suction in her incision. The nurse should understand that the *primary* purpose of this apparatus is to help
- ○ 1. detect a wound infection.
- ○ 2. eliminate the need for wound irrigations.
- ○ 3. prevent fluid from accumulating in the wound.
- ○ 4. provide a mechanism for instilling antibiotics into the wound.

**21.** Which of the following signs or symptoms is of *least importance* when the nurse evaluates Mrs. Kwan for postoperative peripheral nerve damage?
- ○ 1. Pain.
- ○ 2. Sensation.
- ○ 3. Bleeding.
- ○ 4. Pulselessness.

**22.** Which of the following pieces of equipment should the nurse use to help prevent external rotation of Mrs. Kwan's right leg?
- ○ 1. Sandbags.
- ○ 2. A high footboard.
- ○ 3. A rubber air ring.
- ○ 4. A metal bed cradle.

**23.** Which of the following measures should the nurse use to prevent flexion contractures of Mrs. Kwan's hips while she is bedridden?
- ○ 1. Place a bedboard under the patient's mattress.
- ○ 2. Obtain an overbed trapeze for the patient's use.
- ○ 3. Have the patient's feet rest against a footboard.
- ○ 4. Use an alternating pressure mattress on the patient's bed.

**24.** Before turning Mrs. Kwan onto her left side, two nurses first plan to move the patient as far as possible to the right side of the bed. The nurses can increase their own stability before moving Mrs. Kwan by
- ○ 1. bending at the waist.
- ○ 2. widening their base of support.
- ○ 3. leaning against the edge of the bed.
- ○ 4. moving the patient in a rocking manner.

**25.** When Mrs. Kwan is lying on her side, the nurse places a pillow between Mrs. Kwan's legs to prevent
- ○ 1. flexion of the knees.
- ○ 2. abduction of the thighs.

- ○ 3. adduction of the hip joint.
- ○ 4. hyperextension of the knees.

**26.** In which of the following chairs would it be *best* for Mrs. Kwan to sit postoperatively?
- ○ 1. A desk-type swivel chair.
- ○ 2. A padded upholstered chair.
- ○ 3. A high-backed chair with arm rests.
- ○ 4. A recliner with attached foot rest.

**27.** The nurse should teach Mrs. Kwan that, of the following leg positions, the one *contraindicated* for her while sitting in a chair is
- ○ 1. crossing her legs.
- ○ 2. elevating her legs.
- ○ 3. flexing her ankles.
- ○ 4. extending her knees.

**28.** Mrs. Kwan is being considered as a candidate for crutch walking. When assessing Mrs. Kwan, the nurse should take into account that for some elderly people, crutch walking is an *impractical* goal *primarily* because of their decreased
- ○ 1. visual acuity.
- ○ 2. reaction time.
- ○ 3. motor coordination.
- ○ 4. level of comprehension.

**29.** Mrs. Kwan is judged to be a good candidate for crutch walking. Which of the following activities should the nurse teach the patient to strengthen her hand muscles in preparation for the use of crutches?
- ○ 1. Brushing her hair.
- ○ 2. Squeezing a rubber ball.
- ○ 3. Alternately flexing and extending her wrists.
- ○ 4. Pushing her hands into the mattress while raising herself in bed.

**30.** Mrs. Kwan's home contains all of the following items. Which poses the *greatest* hazard to her safe use of crutches at home?
- ○ 1. A 4-year-old cocker spaniel.
- ○ 2. Scatter rugs.
- ○ 3. Snack tables.
- ○ 4. Rocking chairs.

**31.** Mrs. Kwan has been taking psyllium hydrophilic mucilloid (Metamucil) at home for occasional constipation. This agent stimulates peristalsis by
- ○ 1. moistening the fecal material.
- ○ 2. lubricating the fecal material.
- ○ 3. increasing the bulk within the intestinal tract.
- ○ 4. irritating the nerve endings in the intestinal mucosa.

**32.** If Mrs. Kwan fails to maintain an adequate fluid intake while she uses psyllium hydrophilic mucilloid (Metamucil), this preparation could
- ○ 1. cause dehydration.
- ○ 2. ulcerate the duodenum.

○ 3. cause a fecal impaction.
○ 4. produce an allergic reaction.

## THE PATIENT WITH A HERNIATED DISC

Ms. Beverly Sloan is hospitalized for a herniated lumbar disc at the L4-L5 interspace. She is to have a diagnostic workup and her physician has explained that surgery will probably be necessary to correct the problem.

33. During the initial patient interview, the nurse is *most likely* to learn that the symptom that first brought Ms. Sloan to seek health care was
○ 1. loss of urinary control.
○ 2. loss of voluntary muscle control.
○ 3. back pain that is relieved with resting.
○ 4. back pain that radiates to the shoulders.

34. Ms. Sloan may assume any position of comfort. Because hyperextension of the back causes Ms. Sloan discomfort, which of the following positions is *contraindicated*?
○ 1. Prone position.
○ 2. Supine position.
○ 3. Low Fowler's position.
○ 4. Right or left Sims' position.

35. Ms. Sloan is scheduled for a myelogram and asks the nurse about the procedure. The nurse would explain that x-rays will be taken of the patient's spine after an injection of
○ 1. sterile water.
○ 2. normal saline.
○ 3. liquid nitrogen.
○ 4. radiopaque dye.

36. Ms. Sloan returns from the myelogram, for which an iodized oil (Pantopaque) was used. *All* of the following measures should be included in Ms. Sloan's care *except*
○ 1. bed rest.
○ 2. unrestricted fluid intake.
○ 3. head of the bed elevated 45°.
○ 4. assessment of lower extremity movement and sensation.

37. Ms. Sloan is scheduled for a laminectomy. She asks the nurse to explain again what this surgery involves. The nurse's response should be based on knowledge that the herniated disc will be removed, as will
○ 1. the nerve roots affected by the cord compression.
○ 2. a major portion of the vertebra in the affected area.

○ 3. a portion of the involved vertebra's posterior arches.
○ 4. the spinous processes of the vertebra in the affected areas.

38. Spinal fusion is occasionally used as part of a laminectomy procedure to add stability. Spinal fusion immobilizes part of the spine by using a
○ 1. bone graft.
○ 2. metallic pin.
○ 3. skeletal clamp.
○ 4. chemical cement.

39. Ms. Sloan returns from surgery, and the recovery-room nurse reports that the patient received trimethobenzamide hydrochloride (Tigan) in the recovery room. The nurse would correctly judge that the drug is accomplishing its intended purpose if it acts to control Ms. Sloan's
○ 1. muscle spasms and anxiety.
○ 2. nausea and vomiting.
○ 3. shivering and dizziness.
○ 4. palpitations and dry mouth.

40. When Ms. Sloan complains of pain, the nurse chooses to use the deltoid muscle for a prescribed analgesic injection. Which area in the diagram illustrates the *best* site for injecting the drug into the deltoid muscle?

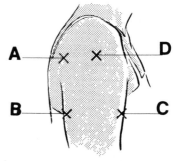

○ 1. Site A.
○ 2. Site B.
○ 3. Site C.
○ 4. Site D.

41. The nurse helps Ms. Sloan apply the back brace she is to wear. Which of the following positions should Ms. Sloan be helped to assume before starting to apply the brace?
○ 1. The standing position.
○ 2. Lying on her side in bed.
○ 3. Lying on her abdomen in bed.
○ 4. The sitting position in a straight chair.

42. To protect Ms. Sloan's skin under the brace, it would be *best* for the nurse to
○ 1. place padding as necessary for a snug fit.
○ 2. have the patient wear a thin cotton shirt under the brace.

○ 3. lubricate the areas where the patient's brace will contact skin surfaces.

○ 4. apply powder to the areas where the patient's brace will contact skin surfaces.

43. When Ms. Sloan walks for the first time, the nurse's arm is under the patient's arm, providing support. Ms. Sloan begins to feel faint. Which course of action would be *best* for the nurse to take until help arrives?

○ 1. Have the patient close her eyes for a few minutes.

○ 2. Maneuver the patient to a sitting position on the floor.

○ 3. Separate the nurse's feet to form a wide base of support and have the patient rest on the nurse's hip.

○ 4. Have the patient separate her feet to form a wide base of support and have her bend at the waist to place her head near her knees.

44. When Ms. Sloan is allowed to sit in a chair, in which of the following positions should the nurse instruct her to place her feet?

○ 1. Flat on the floor.

○ 2. On a low footstool.

○ 3. In any position of comfort while keeping her legs uncrossed.

○ 4. On a high footstool so that her feet are approximately at the same level as the chair seat.

45. Which of the following activities is *not* suitable for Ms. Sloan in the first postoperative days?

○ 1. Turning herself from side to side in bed.

○ 2. Lying flat on her back in bed.

○ 3. Walking in the hall.

○ 4. Sitting in her room to read or watch television.

46. Ms. Sloan complains of abdominal distention in the postoperative period. If all of the following medications have been prescribed for Ms. Sloan, which would be *best* to use to help relieve distention?

○ 1. Codeine sulfate.

○ 2. Diazepam (Valium).

○ 3. Neostigmine bromide (Prostigmin).

○ 4. Psyllium hydrophilic mucilloid (Metamucil).

## THE PATIENT WITH PERIPHERAL VASCULAR DISEASE

Mr. Bernard Kale, 65, is a retired mail carrier who is admitted with peripheral vascular disease of the lower extremities. He has mild hypertension that is controlled by sodium restriction. Mr. Kale smoked a pack of cigarettes a day for 40 years before quitting 1 month ago.

47. *All* of the following would be considered typical symptoms of peripheral arterial disease *except*

○ 1. ankle edema.

○ 2. intermittent claudication.

○ 3. decreased or absent pulses.

○ 4. cool skin.

48. As part of the admission assessment, the nurse palpates Mr. Kale's peripheral pulses. To assess the dorsalis pedis pulse the nurse should palpate the

○ 1. medial surface of the ankle.

○ 2. area behind the ankle.

○ 3. ventral aspect of the top of the foot.

○ 4. medial aspect of the dorsum of the foot.

49. Mr. Kale says, "I've really tried to manage this condition well." Which of the following routines should Mr. Kale have been following?

○ 1. Resting with the legs above the level of the heart.

○ 2. Walking slowly but steadily for 30 minutes twice a day.

○ 3. Minimizing activity.

○ 4. Wearing antiembolism stockings at all times when out of bed.

50. Mr. Kale's long smoking history was extremely detrimental to his condition *primarily* because smoking

○ 1. causes pronounced arterial vasoconstriction.

○ 2. interferes with pulmonary oxygenation of blood.

○ 3. causes polycythemia and pooling in the capillaries.

○ 4. accelerates the development of atherosclerosis.

Mr. Kale's workup reveals that the arterial obstruction in his left leg is complete. Early signs of gangrene are developing and the physicians inform him that an amputation will probably be necessary.

51. Since arterial obstruction in Mr. Kale's left leg is complete, which of the following clinical manifestations would the nurse *most likely* find on assessment?

○ 1. Aching pain.

○ 2. Burning sensations.

○ 3. Numbness and tingling.

○ 4. Coldness.

52. While the nurse is doing preoperative teaching with Mr. Kale, he says, "I hate the idea of being an invalid after they cut off my leg." The *most* therapeutic response for the nurse to make would be

○ 1. "You wouldn't be losing your leg if you hadn't smoked so heavily."

○ 2. "Tell me more about how you're feeling."

○ 3. "Let's finish the preoperative teaching."

○ 4. "You're fortunate to have a wife who can take care of you."

53. Mr. Kale asks the nurse, "Why can't the doctor tell me exactly how much of my leg he's going to take off? Don't you think I should know that?" The nurse should explain to Mr. Kale that the final decision on the level of the amputation will be based on *all* of the following *except*

○ 1. saving as much of the leg as possible.

○ 2. the adequacy of the blood supply to the tissues.

○ 3. the ease with which a prosthesis can be fitted.

○ 4. the patient's ability to walk with a prosthesis.

54. Mr. Kale returns from surgery for a below-the-knee amputation with the stump covered with dressings and a woven elastic bandage. Initially the bandage was dry, but now, 30 minutes later, the nurse notices a small amount of bloody drainage. What should be the *priority* action?

○ 1. Notify the physician.

○ 2. Mark the area of drainage.

○ 3. Replace the dressing.

○ 4. Reinforce the dressing.

55. Mr. Kale's room should contain which emergency equipment when he returns from surgery?

○ 1. Suction equipment.

○ 2. Emergency cart.

○ 3. Airway.

○ 4. Tourniquet.

56. What is the *most important* nursing intervention in caring for Mr. Kale's stump during the first 24 hours after surgery?

○ 1. Keeping the stump flat on the bed.

○ 2. Abducting the stump on a scheduled basis.

○ 3. Applying traction to the stump.

○ 4. Elevating the stump on a pillow.

57. Which of the following nursing goals takes *priority* when considering Mr. Kale's physical mobility following the amputation?

○ 1. Preventing contractures.

○ 2. Promoting comfort.

○ 3. Preventing edema.

○ 4. Preventing phantom-limb pain.

58. The second morning after surgery, Mr. Kale says, "This sounds crazy but I feel my left toes tingling." This statement indicates that Mr. Kale is experiencing a

○ 1. denial reaction.

○ 2. phantom-limb sensation.

○ 3. hallucination.

○ 4. body image disturbance.

59. Mr. Kale is to be fitted with a functioning prosthesis. The nurse has been teaching him stump care. Which behavior demonstrates that Mr. Kale has an understanding of *proper* stump care?

○ 1. Mr. Kale applies powder to the stump.

○ 2. Mr. Kale inspects the stump weekly with a mirror.

○ 3. Mr. Kale removes the prosthesis whenever he sits down.

○ 4. Mr. Kale washes and dries the stump daily.

60. Mr. Kale will use crutches while his prosthesis is being adjusted. Which of the following exercises will *best* prepare him for using crutches?

○ 1. Range-of-motion exercises of the shoulders.

○ 2. Isometric exercises of the biceps.

○ 3. Quadriceps and gluteal set exercises.

○ 4. Triceps exercises.

61. When using crutches Mr. Kale should support his weight *primarily* on his

○ 1. axillae.

○ 2. forearms.

○ 3. upper arms.

○ 4. palms.

62. Mr. Kale is to be discharged on a low-fat, low-cholesterol, low-sodium diet. Since Mrs. Kale prepares the meals, the nurse will teach her how to prepare meals within the dietary restrictions. What is the *first* step in providing Mrs. Kale with specific instructions?

○ 1. Determine her knowledge level about cholesterol.

○ 2. Ask her to name foods high in fat, cholesterol, and salt.

○ 3. Explain the importance of complying with the diet.

○ 4. Assess the Kales' food preferences.

63. The nurse has been telling Mrs. Kale how to prepare meals that are low in fat, cholesterol, and sodium. Which of these comments indicates that Mrs. Kale needs additional teaching?

○ 1. "I'll use only water-packed tuna."

○ 2. "I'll use a Teflon-coated pan when cooking."

○ 3. "I'll cook more liver with onions."

○ 4. "I'll avoid using steak sauce and catsup."

## THE PATIENT WITH A FEMORAL FRACTURE

Mr. Shawn di Silva, a 28-year-old construction worker, is brought to the hospital emergency room following an accident in which he fell from a beam. He fractured the shaft of his right femur in the fall and has multiple cuts and bruises on his upper body and right arm and hand.

**64.** A booster injection for tetanus is administered in the emergency room when it is determined that Mr. di Silva has not had any immunizations since childhood. Which of the following biologic products will be used to provide Mr. di Silva with passive immunity for tetanus?
- ○ 1. Tetanus toxoid.
- ○ 2. Tetanus antigen.
- ○ 3. Tetanus vaccine.
- ○ 4. Tetanus antitoxin.

**65.** Immunologic protection is provided for Mr. di Silva in order to prevent the pathologic condition called
- ○ 1. tetany.
- ○ 2. lockjaw.
- ○ 3. meningitis.
- ○ 4. gas gangrene.

Mr. di Silva is admitted to the orthopedic unit in balanced skeletal traction using a Thomas splint and Pearson attachment.

**66.** The *major* purpose of traction in this case is to
- ○ 1. improve the patient's comfort.
- ○ 2. separate fracture fragments.
- ○ 3. control internal bleeding.
- ○ 4. maintain skin integrity.

**67.** The nurse is responsible for maintaining effective traction. Which of the following conditions is necessary for effective traction?
- ○ 1. The weights rest securely on the bed frame.
- ○ 2. The ropes are in the wheel grooves of the pulleys.
- ○ 3. The patient is positioned low in the bed.
- ○ 4. The weights are increased by 0.5 pound each shift.

**68.** When a patient is placed in balanced skeletal traction, which of the following actions by the nurse would be appropriate?
- ○ 1. Ensuring that the traction weights hang freely from the bed at all times.
- ○ 2. Gradually increasing the amount of traction weight as the patient's tolerance increases.
- ○ 3. Applying and removing the traction weights at regular intervals throughout the day.
- ○ 4. Removing the weights briefly as needed to reposition the patient in bed.

**69.** What is the purpose of the Pearson attachment on Mr. di Silva's traction setup?
- ○ 1. To support the lower portion of the leg.
- ○ 2. To support the thigh and upper leg.
- ○ 3. To attach the skeletal pin.

- ○ 4. To prevent flexion deformities in the ankle and foot.

**70.** Because of the nature of his fracture, Mr. di Silva is at risk for fat emboli. Which of the following manifestations would the nurse be *most likely* to note if this complication occurs?
- ○ 1. Mental confusion.
- ○ 2. Migrainelike headaches.
- ○ 3. Numbness in the right leg.
- ○ 4. Muscle spasms in the right thigh.

**71.** Which of the following treatments is *most likely* to be used to reduce the surface tension of the fat globules if emboli occur?
- ○ 1. Hypothermia.
- ○ 2. Oxygen therapy.
- ○ 3. Intravenous heparin.
- ○ 4. Anticholesterol drugs.

**72.** Mr. di Silva is quite upset and agitated about his injury and its treatment. He says, "How can I stay like this for weeks? I can't even move!" The nurse should explain that while he is in traction, he
- ○ 1. can turn from side to side in bed and sit up.
- ○ 2. must lie flat in bed and cannot turn at all.
- ○ 3. can sit up straight in bed but cannot turn.
- ○ 4. can turn slightly from side to side and sit up 30° to 40°.

**73.** Because of the use of the Thomas splint, it will be essential for the nurse to assess Mr. di Silva regularly for
- ○ 1. signs of skin pressure in the groin area.
- ○ 2. decreased breath sounds.
- ○ 3. skin breakdown behind the knee.
- ○ 4. urinary retention.

**74.** The nurse plans to teach Mr. di Silva about the traction. What would be the *most appropriate* plan?
- ○ 1. Give cursory explanations for the first few days so as not to overwhelm him.
- ○ 2. Initiate teaching just before the administration of pain medication so that he is alert.
- ○ 3. Use medical terminology exclusively so that he will recognize the terms when the doctors use them.
- ○ 4. Relate the information about the traction to his existing knowledge of construction when possible.

**75.** Mr. di Silva has a nursing diagnosis of "self-care deficit due to the confinement of traction." Which of the following indicates a *successful* outcome for this diagnosis?
- ○ 1. Mr. di Silva assists as much as possible in his care and his participation increases over time.
- ○ 2. Mr. di Silva allows the nurse to complete his care in an efficient manner and does not interfere.

○ 3. Mr. di Silva's wife assumes responsibility for his care and compensates for his deficit.

○ 4. Mr. di Silva allows his wife to complete his care because he knows she needs to feel useful.

76. In order to prevent infection and development of osteomyelitis, the nurse provides pin site care and inspects the site daily for evidence of infection. Which of the following clinical manifestations at the pin site alerts the nurse to infection?

○ 1. Slight serous oozing.

○ 2. Lack of scab formation.

○ 3. Itching.

○ 4. Pain.

77. Mr. di Silva becomes constipated from the decreased mobility imposed by his treatment. Which of the following breakfasts would be most helpful in re-establishing a normal bowel routine?

○ 1. Eggs and bacon, buttered toast, orange juice, and coffee.

○ 2. Corn flakes with sliced banana, milk, English muffin and jelly.

○ 3. Orange juice, breakfast pastries (doughnut and danish), coffee.

○ 4. Orange, raisin bran and milk, wheat toast and butter.

## THE PATIENT WITH A SPINAL CORD INJURY

Ms. Andrea Pulaski, 25, fell during a rock-climbing trip. She is alert and conscious but cannot move her arms or legs on command.

78. The *priority* concern when moving an individual with a possible spinal cord injury is to

○ 1. wrap and support the extremities, which can easily be injured.

○ 2. move the individual gently to help reduce pain.

○ 3. immobilize the head and neck to prevent further injury.

○ 4. cushion the back with pillows to ensure comfort.

79. It is determined that Ms. Pulaski suffered a C7 spinal cord injury. Which of the following would be the *most important* intervention during the acute stage of her care?

○ 1. Turning and positioning every 2 hours.

○ 2. Maintaining proper alignment.

○ 3. Maintaining a patent airway.

○ 4. Monitoring vital signs.

80. The nurse recognizes that spinal shock is likely to persist for the first several weeks after the injury.

Which of the following would be *unexpected* during the period of spinal shock?

○ 1. Tachycardia.

○ 2. Rapid respirations.

○ 3. Hypertension.

○ 4. Dry warm skin.

81. During the period of spinal shock, the nurse should expect that Ms. Pulaski's bladder function will be

○ 1. spastic.

○ 2. normal.

○ 3. atonic.

○ 4. uncontrolled.

82. Passive range-of-motion exercises for the lower extremities and assisted range-of-motion exercises for the upper extremities are part of Ms. Pulaski's care. Which observation by the nurse would indicate a successful outcome of this treatment?

○ 1. Free, easy movement of the joints.

○ 2. Absence of paralytic footdrop.

○ 3. External rotation of hips at rest.

○ 4. Absence of tissue ischemia over bony prominences.

83. Ms. Pulaski's fracture is surgically repaired. Once healing has begun, daily physical therapy sessions are scheduled that include the use of the tilt table. After the therapist places Ms. Pulaski at a 45° angle, the nurse monitors her. What *critical* factor should the nurse assess?

○ 1. Hypertension.

○ 2. Pedal edema.

○ 3. Facial flushing.

○ 4. Dizziness.

84. After a month of therapy, Ms. Pulaski begins to experience muscle spasms in her legs. She calls the nurse in excitement to report the leg movement. Which response by the nurse is *most accurate?*

○ 1. "These movements indicate that the damaged nerves are healing."

○ 2. "These are good signs. Keep trying to move all the affected muscles."

○ 3. "The return of movement means that eventually you should be able to walk again. The damage is not permanent."

○ 4. "The movements occur from muscle reflexes. They can't be initiated or controlled by the brain."

85. Once muscle spasms have started, the nurse realizes that Ms. Pulaski is at risk for autonomic dysreflexia. Which of the following is *not* an expected symptom of this condition?

○ 1. Sudden severe hypertension.
○ 2. Pounding headache.
○ 3. "Goose bumps" over her trunk and arms.
○ 4. Hot dry skin.

**86.** If autonomic dysreflexia occurs, what is the *priority* nursing intervention?
○ 1. Administer nitroprusside sodium (Nipride) intravenously.
○ 2. Place the patient in a modified Trendelenburg position.
○ 3. Place the patient in Fowler's position.
○ 4. Send a urine sample for culture stat.

**87.** The *most common* stimulus for an episode of autonomic dysreflexia is
○ 1. bowel distention.
○ 2. bladder distention.
○ 3. anxiety.
○ 4. rising intracranial pressure.

**88.** The orthotics department makes a custom trunk brace for Ms. Pulaski. When is the *appropriate time* for the nurse to apply this brace?
○ 1. While Ms. Pulaski is sitting in a chair.
○ 2. Before Ms. Pulaski gets out of bed.
○ 3. As soon as Ms. Pulaski becomes fatigued.
○ 4. When Ms. Pulaski is standing on the tilt table.

**89.** Urinary tract infection is a serious problem following spinal cord injury. Which of the following is the *most important* action to prevent its occurrence?
○ 1. Drink a glass of citrus fruit juice at every meal.
○ 2. Drink at least 2,000 ml of fluid daily.
○ 3. Add extra protein to the daily diet.
○ 4. Ensure that the urine remains alkaline.

**90.** Ms. Pulaski asks the nurse why the dietitian has recommended that she decrease her total daily intake of calcium. Which response contains the *most accurate* information?
○ 1. "Excess dairy products make constipation more common."
○ 2. "Immobility causes the ingested calcium to be absorbed from the intestine in greater quantities."
○ 3. "Lack of weight-bearing causes demineralization of the long bones and increases the kidneys' calcium load."
○ 4. "Dairy products are likely to contribute to weight gain."

**91.** As a first step in teaching Ms. Pulaski about her sexual health, the nurse assesses the patient's understanding of the sexual functioning of a quadriplegic. Which of the following statements indicates accurate understanding?
○ 1. "I won't be able to participate in sexual intercourse until the Foley catheter is removed."
○ 2. "I can participate in sexual activity but might not experience orgasm."
○ 3. "I won't be able to participate in sexual intercourse because it causes hypertension, but other sexual activity is allowed."
○ 4. "I will be able to participate in sexual activity but will be infertile."

**92.** Ms. Pulaski had been a very active outdoor person who enjoyed sports and she talks almost obsessively about her past activities. In tears, one day she asks the nurse, "Why can't I stop talking about these things? I know those days are gone forever." Which response by the nurse would provide the best understanding of the patient's behavior?
○ 1. "Be patient. It takes time to adjust to such a massive loss."
○ 2. "Talking about the past is a form of denial. We have to help you focus on today."
○ 3. "Reviewing your losses is a way of working through your grief. Someday soon you'll be able to let go."
○ 4. "It's a simple escape mechanism to go back to and live again in happier times."

# CORRECT ANSWERS AND RATIONALES

Numbers appear in parentheses following the rationales. The numbers identify textbooks listed in the references at the end of Part IV, where correct answers can be verified.

## *The Patient with Rheumatoid Arthritis*

1. 3. Synovial joints are characteristically affected by rheumatoid arthritis. Synovial membranes in the joints secrete fluid that acts as a lubricant and shock absorber in the joints. As the disease progresses, other parts of the joints become involved and eventually deteriorate. (25, 31)

2. 2. Tinnitus (ringing in the ears) is a common symptom of aspirin toxicity. Dysuria, drowsiness, and chest pain are not associated with aspirin toxicity. (12, 16)

3. 4. The proper use of aspirin therapy in rheumatoid arthritis involves continuous ongoing use of the drug to establish and maintain therapeutic blood levels. Aspirin should not be used on a p.r.n. basis. It should always be buffered with food, and patients should be instructed to observe for symptoms of bleeding. (25, 31)

4. 3. Rheumatoid arthritis affects women about three times more frequently than men. The disease characteristically begins during middle life, between the ages of 25 and 35 years. Osteoarthritis affects women about twice as often as it affects men and has its onset primarily late in life. (25, 31)

5. 4. Both osteoarthritis and rheumatoid arthritis cause joint pain, joint stiffness, and limitations in movement. Inflammation, a characteristic feature of rheumatoid arthritis, produces pronounced swelling, which is not a common feature of osteoarthritis. (25, 31)

6. 4. Osteoarthritis is a degenerative joint disease. The weight-bearing joints, such as the knees, hips, and finger joints, are most often involved. The shoulder joints are least likely to be involved when the patient has osteoarthritis. (25, 31)

7. 3. A patient with osteoarthritis has a disease due mostly to "wear and tear," and it probably resulted from excessive and prolonged mechanical stress on the joints. An overweight person adds to the stress on weight-bearing joints. Therefore, the obese person with osteoarthritis should be taught the importance of losing weight. (25, 31)

8. 3. Drugs that cause gastric irritation are best taken after or with a meal, when stomach contents help minimize the local irritation. (12, 16)

9. 4. When a patient compares her therapy with someone else's, it is best for the nurse to explain truthfully and point out that there are various forms of arthritis. What helps one person may not help another. Avoiding the question or suggesting that the patient should not ask a particular question is not helpful. (11, 38)

10. 3. Arthroplasty is a reconstruction of a joint. Sometimes called plastic surgery of the joint, it is the term used to describe the surgical procedure in this item. An osteotomy refers to cutting on a bone. Surgical fixation of a joint is called an arthrodesis. Osteosynthesis is the surgical fastening of the ends of a fractured bone by mechanical means. (25, 31)

11. 4. Proper positioning to prevent flexion deformities of the joints is an ongoing need for patients with rheumatoid arthritis and should be included in the postoperative care plan. Positioning to promote comfort and avoid venous stasis is important but not unique to patients with rheumatoid arthritis. (25, 31)

12. 2. The needed care following total knee replacement is extremely painful. The patient must make a firm commitment to active participation in the rehabilitation process. Scolding or blaming the patient is useless. The nurse should help the patient understand why the care is necessary and should provide reinforcement every step of the way. (5, 23)

13. 2. An exercise program is recommended to strengthen muscles following arthroplasty. Isometric exercises (muscle setting) strengthen muscles but keep the joint stationary during the healing process. Isometric exercises cost little in terms of time and money, and using such exercises may help improve a patient's morale by involving her in her own care, but these are not necessarily primary reasons for using isometric exercises. Isometric exercises will not help prevent joint stiffness because the joint has been replaced in the patient described in this item. Exercises are also helpful in preventing thrombophlebitis. (9, 25)

14. 3. The quadriceps-setting exercises strengthen the quadriceps femoris, the muscles in the leg that are important for proper walking. These muscles can be exercised in bed by pushing the back of the knee into the mattress. (24, 36)

15. 3. Most elderly people require fewer calories than do younger people because of decreasing activity with increasing age. However, a balanced diet in-

cluding all food nutrients remains important throughout life. For patients with arthritis, it is particularly important to watch caloric intake because excess weight causes added strain and discomfort on affected joints. (7, 13)

**16.** 3. Using prescriptions from a patient's physician is the best way to avoid misuse of drugs. Using testimonials and advertisements is a poor way to select drug therapy. The current abuse and misuse of drugs make it important for nurses to teach patients about using only drugs recommended and prescribed by their physician and about the dangers of relying on others' opinions. The patient described in this item has rheumatoid arthritis, and because of its chronicity and discomfort, many such patients unfortunately succumb to so-called cures. The patient should be taught that at present there is no cure for the disease and many advertised "remedies" may be potentially hazardous. (9, 25)

## The Patient with a Hip Fracture

**17.** 4. After a hip fracture, the leg on the affected side is characteristically shorter than the unaffected leg. Typically, it is also abducted and rotated externally. Pain is usually present. (25, 31)

**18.** 1. Crepitation is used to describe the grating sensation produced when broken bone fragments rub against each other. This sound is often audible but may also be heard on auscultation at the site of a fracture. Ossification is the deposition of lime salts and the formation of bone. Proliferation is growth by multiplication of cells. Consolidation is the conversion of a substance into a solid mass. (25, 29)

**19.** 4. There are various advantages in using a pin for the internal fixation of a fractured hip. This procedure is especially favored for older patients because it makes earlier postoperative ambulation possible and offers good fixation at the fracture site. (25, 31)

**20.** 3. The primary reason for applying suction to a wound drainage tube is to prevent fluid from accumulating in the wound. This greatly enhances wound healing and helps prevent abscess formation. (24, 36)

**21.** 3. Nerve damage may be indicated by the presence of any of the following P's: pain, pallor, pulselessness, paresthesia, and paralysis. Bleeding is not indicative of peripheral nerve damage. Peripheral nerve damage can occur as a result of almost any orthopedic surgery. (5, 26)

**22.** 1. It is best to support a patient's leg in its proper anatomic position and to prevent external rotation by supporting the leg with sandbags. A trochanter roll can often also be used effectively. Sandbags should be placed along the length of the thigh and lower leg. A high footboard helps keep bed linens off of a patient's legs and helps prevent footdrop when the feet are properly supported against the board. A rubber air ring and a metal frame bed cradle will not help prevent external rotation of the legs. (24, 36)

**23.** 1. The measure recommended to prevent flexion of the hip for a bedridden patient is to place bedboards under the mattress of the patient's bed. A trapeze helps the patient move herself in bed. An alternating pressure mattress is used primarily to help prevent decubitus ulcers. Using a footboard is most effective in preventing footdrop. (24, 36)

**24.** 2. Before moving a patient, the nurse should place her feet apart to attain a wide base of support and increased stability of the body. Assuming this stance, flexing the knees a bit, coming down close to the patient, and using the weight of the patient's body as a force to reduce the amount of strain on the nurse's body are recommended techniques when moving a patient. (24, 36)

**25.** 3. Following hip surgery for a fractured femur, a pillow is placed between a patient's legs while lying on the side to help prevent adduction of the thigh. This positioning places the hip in proper alignment. Dislocation of the hip can occur if the leg on the affected side is allowed to adduct. (25, 31)

**26.** 3. A high-backed, straight chair with arm rests is recommended for the patient described in this situation. It will help keep the patient in the best possible alignment following surgery for a hip fracture. Soft, low, and swivel chairs do not promote good body alignment or good security. (25, 31)

**27.** 1. Crossing the legs causes adduction of the hips; following hip surgery, this may result in a dislocation of the operated hip. The patient described in this item should not cross her legs. Elevating the legs, flexing the ankles, and extending the knees are not necessarily contraindicated. (25, 31)

**28.** 3. Some elderly people are not good candidates for crutch walking because they are not strong enough to use crutches or are not coordinated enough to make crutch walking safe. Such factors as visual acuity, reaction time, and level of comprehension *may* influence the ability to learn crutch walking but are not as important as motor coordination. (24, 36)

**29.** 2. A patient being prepared for crutch walking should be taught to support her weight with her hands when crutch walking. Supporting weight in the axillae is contraindicated because of possible nerve damage and circulatory obstruction. A patient should be taught to squeeze a ball vigorously to help strengthen the hands in preparation for weight bearing with the hands. Such activities as brushing the hair, flexing and extending the wrists, and doing push-ups may be indicated, but they are not likely to strengthen the hands. (26, 31)

**30.** 2. Scatter rugs have been found to be the greatest source of danger in the home, especially for elderly people who are unsure of their walking. Falls have been found to account for nearly half the accidental deaths that occur in the home. (26, 31)

**31.** 3. Psyllium hydrophilic mucilloid (Metamucil) stimulates peristalsis by increasing the bulk within the intestinal tract. It causes the formation of a soft, gelatinous, water-retaining substance in the bowel to produce bulk. An example of a laxative that lubricates the stool is mineral oil. An example of a laxative that moistens the stool by increasing the water content of the feces is magnesium citrate. An example of a laxative that stimulates peristalsis by irritating nerve endings in the intestinal mucosa is castor oil. (12, 16)

**32.** 3. Bulk-producing laxatives pick up moisture in the gastrointestinal tract. These laxatives may cause a fecal impaction if the person using such laxatives fails to have a generous fluid intake. (12, 16)

## The Patient with a Herniated Disc

**33.** 3. A typical symptom of a herniated lumbar disc is low back pain that is usually relieved by rest and aggravated by activity that causes an increase in fluid pressure in the spine, such as sneezing, coughing, lifting, and bending. Muscle weakness and sensory losses may occur and there is generally a change in tendon reflexes. Pain radiating to the shoulders that often causes a person to believe he is having a heart attack is a typical symptom when a cervical disc herniates. A loss of voluntary muscle control that is likely to cause chorealike movements and a loss of urinary control are not typical early symptoms of lumbar disc disturbances. (25, 31)

**34.** 1. Hyperextension of the spine occurs when a patient lies on her abdomen (that is, in the prone position). Hyperextension of the spine causes discomfort for a patient with a herniated disc, and therefore the prone position is contraindicated for this patient. The patient described in this item will be most comfortable when in the supine, low Fowler's, or left or right Sims' position. (26, 31)

**35.** 4. A radiopaque dye, usually an iodized oil but in some instances a water-soluble compound, is used for a myelogram. Air *may* be used for an air-con-

trast study. Myelography is used to determine the exact location of a herniated disc. (5, 26)

**36.** 3. Nursing care of patient after a myelogram depends in part on the type of dye used. For example, if an oil contrast such as Pantopaque is used, the patient will usually lie prone for 2 to 4 hours, then on her back for 2 to 4 hours. If a water-soluble contrast is used, the head of the bed is elevated 45° for 8 to 24 hours. This position reduces the rate of upward dispersion of the contrast medium. Regardless of the type of dye used for the test, bed rest is necessary for several hours after a myelogram. Fluid intake is encouraged to replace cerebrospinal fluid, to reduce headache, and to facilitate absorption of retained contrast media. Lower extremity neurologic status is assessed frequently. (26, 31)

**37.** 3. To reach the disc, a portion of the vertebra's lamina is removed to explore the involved nerve root and to remove disc fragments. The laminae help form the posterior arches of the vertebrae. (25, 31)

**38.** 1. A spinal fusion uses a bone graft. Usually, bone from the patient's iliac crest is used, but bone from a bone bank may be selected. The bone graft helps cause a permanent area of stiffness, or immobility, over the involved area. (25, 31)

**39.** 2. Trimethobenzamide hydrochloride (Tigan) is a centrally acting antiemetic and helps control nausea and vomiting. It does not control muscle spasms, anxiety, shivering, dizziness, palpitations, or dry mouth. (12, 16)

**40.** 4. Site D in the diagram given in this item is recommended for injecting the deltoid muscle. This site is the thickest part of the deltoid. It is located by forming an imaginary rectangle on the upper arm that is bounded on the top at the lower edge of the acromium. The lower boundary is opposite the axilla. The two side boundaries are lines parallel to the arm, one-third and two-thirds around the outer aspect of the arm. These boundaries can be identified in the diagram in this item. The site of injection is at the center of this rectangle. (24, 36)

**41.** 2. A back brace should be applied before the patient who has had back surgery is out of bed and before weight is placed on the legs and back. The brace should be placed on the bed while the patient is in the side-lying position. The patient should then be rolled onto the brace. Hyperextension of the back following back surgery is contraindicated. (28, 33)

**42.** 2. Experience has shown that it is best to have the patient wear a thin cotton shirt under a brace. This helps protect the skin and helps keep the brace free of skin oils and perspiration. Using padding may increase pressure points. Lubricating and powdering the skin under the brace do not provide the best protection for the skin from irritation by the brace. (9, 28)

**43.** 3. When the patient feels faint while walking with the nurse, the patient should rest on the nurse's hip after the nurse has formed a wide base of support by separating her feet. This maneuver is relatively easy and can be maintained until help is available. Having the patient close her eyes is unlikely to relieve symptoms of fainting. Maneuvering the patient to the floor requires considerable strength and may result in injury to the patient, especially when done quickly. The patient described in this item cannot bend at the waist because of recent back surgery. (24, 36)

**44.** 1. A patient who has had back surgery should place her feet flat on the floor. This ordinarily provides the greatest comfort because it places no strain on the operative area. If the patient is allowed to choose her own position, she may choose one that places strain on the back. The nurse teaches and explains that placing the feet flat on the floor is recommended. (26, 31)

**45.** 4. After a laminectomy, patients should either lie flat in bed in good alignment or should walk. Sitting for long periods is contraindicated, as pressure is increased to the operative area and alignment is compromised. (26, 31)

**46.** 3. Neostigmine bromide (Prostigmin) stimulates peristalsis by its effects on the smooth muscles in the intestinal tract. Psyllium hydrophilic mucilloid (Metamucil) helps relieve constipation, and constipation predisposes to distention. However, the first choice for relatively early relief of distention is to use the neostigmine bromide. Codeine sulfate and diazepam (Valium) may relieve discomfort and worry but will not relieve the condition causing distention. (12, 16)

### The Patient with Peripheral Vascular Disease

**47.** 1. Inadequate arterial circulation produces symptoms of hypoxia. The skin is cool to the touch, pulses are difficult or impossible to palpate, and exercise causes moderate to severe cramping pain. Ankle edema is associated with venous insufficiency and stasis. (25, 31)

**48.** 4. The dorsalis pedis pulse is found on the medial aspect of the dorsal surface of the foot in line with the big toe. The posterior tibial pulse is on the medial surface of the ankle just behind the medial

malleolus. The popliteal pulse is behind the knee. (24, 36)

**49.** 2. Slow steady walking is a recommended activity for patients with peripheral arterial disease because it stimulates the development of collateral circulation. Patients with peripheral arterial disease should not remain inactive. Elevating the legs above the heart and antiembolism stockings are strategies for venous congestion and may worsen peripheral arterial disease. (25, 31)

**50.** 1. Smoking causes direct and diffuse peripheral vasoconstriction, which worsens the effects of arterial insufficiency. (25, 31)

**51.** 4. Coldness is the assessment finding most consistent with *complete* arterial obstruction. Other expected findings would be paralysis and pallor. Aching pain, burning sensations, and numbness and tingling are earlier signs of tissue hypoxia and ischemia and are associated with incomplete obstruction. (5, 26)

**52.** 2. Encouraging the patient undergoing amputation to verbalize his feelings is the most therapeutic nursing intervention. By eliciting information, the nurse may be able to provide information that will help him cope. The nurse should avoid value-laden responses that may make the patient feel guilty or hostile and block further communication. The nurse should not ignore the patient's expressed concern or make him feel that she does not care. She should not reinforce his concern about invalidism and dependency or assume that his wife is willing to care for him. (10, 23)

**53.** 4. The level of amputation often cannot be accurately determined until surgery, when the surgeon can directly assess the adequacy of the circulation of the stump. A longer stump facilitates prosthesis-fitting, and this aspect will be considered in the final decision. (26, 31)

**54.** 2. The nurse should mark the bloodstain and observe it again in 10 minutes. There is no need to notify the physician immediately, since some oozing and bloody drainage are expected. Given the slight amount of drainage, there is no need either to replace the dressing or reinforce it. (5, 26)

**55.** 4. Hemorrhage is an unexpected, but potential, complication of radical surgery such as amputation. A tourniquet should be available at the bedside during the early postoperative period to deal with such a complication. (5, 26)

**56.** 4. Elevating the stump on a pillow for the first 24 hours after surgery helps prevent edema and promotes comfort by increasing venous return. Elevating the stump more than the first 24 hours is contraindicated because of the potential for developing contractures. Adducting the stump on a scheduled basis prevents abduction contracture. When amputation is done for infection, a guillotine-type procedure is performed and the skin is not sutured. Traction is applied to the stump to prevent skin and muscle retraction. (5, 26)

**57.** 1. Preventing joint contractures is essential to physical mobility. Promoting comfort and preventing edema are appropriate immediate postoperative nursing goals, but attaining them does not affect physical mobility in the immediate and extended postoperative periods. Phantom-limb pain begins from 2 weeks to 2 months after amputation. It occurs briefly in about 30% of patients, but only about 2% of patients experience persistent pain. (26, 31)

**58.** 2. Descriptions of sensations, which may or may not be painful, in the amputated part are common and are known as phantom-limb sensations. The patient should be reassured that these sensations are normal and are not a sign of a mental problem. Denial may be present following amputation. Signs of denial include refusal to look at and/or talk about the amputation. Hallucinations indicate a serious, possibly psychotic condition and should be thoroughly assessed. Referral to an appropriate healthcare provider is in order. Body image disturbances can develop after amputation due to fear, grief, loss of locomotion, and decreased self-esteem related to the loss of the body part. (5, 26)

**59.** 4. Washing and thoroughly drying the stump daily are important hygiene measures to prevent infection. Nothing should be applied to the stump after it is bathed. Powder may cause excessive drying and cracking of the skin, and cream softens the skin excessively. The stump should be assessed daily with a mirror to discover any signs of early skin breakdown. To reduce stump swelling, the prosthesis should be removed only at night. (5, 26)

**60.** 4. The use of crutches requires significant strength from the triceps muscles, and efforts should be focused on strengthening these muscles in anticipation of crutch walking. Bed and wheelchair push-ups are excellent exercises targeted at the triceps muscles. (25, 31)

**61.** 2. The proper use of crutches requires that body weight be primarily supported on the forearms. Improper use of crutches can cause nerve damage from excess pressure. Careful instruction and evaluation of the use of crutches is essential. (24, 36)

**62.** 4. Before beginning dietary interventions, it is important to assess the patient's pattern of food intake, life cycle, food preferences, and ethnic, cultural, and financial influences. (5, 26)

**63.** 3. Liver and organ meats are high in cholesterol and saturated fat and should be limited. Water-packed tuna is one of the leanest fish available. Using a Teflon-coated pan when cooking reduces the need for shortening. Steak sauce and catsup are high in sodium. (5, 26)

## The Patient with a Femoral Fracture

**64.** 4. Passive immunity for tetanus is provided in the form of tetanus antitoxin or tetanus immune globulin. An antitoxin is an antibody to the toxin of an organism. Toxoids, antigens, and vaccines all provide active immunity by stimulating the body to produce its own antibodies. (12, 16)

**65.** 2. The antitoxin is specific for the prevention of tetanus, which is also called lockjaw. The etiologic agent is *Clostridium tetani*. Tetany, which is characterized by intermittent tonic spasms, is caused by hypocalcemia. Meningitis, or inflammation of the membranes of the spinal cord or brain, can be caused by bacteria, viruses, or other organisns that reach the meninges. Gas gangrene is caused by the etiologic agent *Clostridium perfringens*. (25, 31)

**66.** 2. The purpose of traction is to separate the bone fragments. This separation facilitates subsequent internal fixation. Traction immobilizes the fracture site and may increase the patient's comfort. Mobilization could result in further damage. Traction does increase circulation to the affected part but does not control internal bleeding. Traction may create, rather than prevent, a problem with skin integrity. (5, 9)

**67.** 2. For the weights to maintain the therapeutic effect of the traction, they must be properly positioned and free-hanging and should be removed only in life-threatening situations. Effective traction depends on the patient's being positioned at the head of the bed. Sufficient weight is applied initially to overcome spasm in affected muscles. As the muscles relax, the weight may be reduced. (5, 9)

**68.** 1. The appropriate pressures and counterpressures are applied to the fracture site when the traction weights hang freely at all times. They are in place continuously and should never be lifted, reduced, or eliminated. Skin traction may be applied intermittently, but balanced skeletal traction is continuous. (25, 31)

**69.** 2. The Pearson attachment supports the upper portion of the leg and allows for more stability in the overall traction setup. Correct alignment is also easier to maintain. (25, 31)

**70.** 1. Fat emboli usually result in cerebral disturbances that cause mental confusion or agitation from hypoxia. If severe, hypoxia can produce delirium and coma. (25, 26)

**71.** 2. Respiratory failure is a common cause of death following fat emboli. Oxygen therapy appears to reduce the surface tension of the fat globules and supports respiratory function by reducing hypoxia. (25, 26)

**72.** 1. Although normal movement is not possible in skeletal traction, the balanced weights ensure that changes in position do not alter or interfere with the traction pull. Therefore, patients can turn and sit up in bed while the traction is in place. (5, 31)

**73.** 1. The Thomas splint is secured by rings that slip over the thigh. They are placed tight up into the groin and may cause discomfort, pressure, or skin irritation. (5, 31)

**74.** 4. Understanding is enhanced when the learner can relate new information to existing knowledge. Linking the common principles of construction and traction is a perfect way to help the patient in this item learn. It is unwise to overload the patient, but complete simple teaching will facilitate relaxation. Teaching is best done when pain is minimal, because discomfort makes it difficult for the patient to concentrate. The patient may not understand medical terminology, and the nurse should always tailor her teaching to the patient's level. (5, 9)

**75.** 1. Self-care minimizes sensory deprivation and allows the patient control. Involving the patient in his care puts him on track for long-term care. Passivity can indicate denial or depression. Family members can assist, but giving them primary responsibility undermines the patient's self-esteem. (9, 26)

**76.** 4. Inflammation, as evidenced by pain, swelling, and redness, is one of the early signs of infection and needs prompt intervention. Slight oozing at the pin site is expected and decreases bacteria in the pin tract. Crusting or scab formation is to be avoided, as it may trap bacteria in the pin tract. Itching at the pin site may be due to dryness or irritation. (5, 9)

**77.** 4. High-fiber foods provide bulk and decrease water absorption in the bowel. Whole grains and fruits (not juices, which often are strained) should be recommended. Processed foods and breads contain little fiber. (37, 41)

## The Patient with a Spinal Cord Injury

**78.** 3. The immediate concern is to immobilize the head and neck to prevent further trauma when the fractured vertebra may be unstable and easily displaced. Pain is usually not a significant consideration with this type of injury. (26, 31)

**79.** 3. Initial care is focused on establishing and maintaining a patent airway and supporting ventilation. Innervation to the intercostals is affected and if spinal edema extends to the C4 level, paralysis of the diaphragm usually occurs. The effects and extent of edema are unpredictable in the first hours and respiratory status must be closely monitored. Suction equipment should be readily available. (26, 31)

**80.** 3. Spinal shock produces massive vasodilatation and subsequent pooling of blood in the periphery. The patient is relatively hypovolemic and exhibits tachycardia, tachypnea, anxiety, and flushed but dry skin. Hypertension would not be expected. (25, 31)

**81.** 3. During the period of spinal shock, the bladder is completely atonic and will continue to fill passively unless the patient is catheterized. No reflex activity occurs during this period, so reflex emptying does not occur. (25, 31)

**82.** 1. Range-of-motion exercises preserve joint motion and stimulate circulation. Contractures develop rapidly in patients with spinal cord injuries, and the absence of this complication indicates treatment success. Footdrop is prevented by using a footboard. External rotation of the hips is prevented by using trochanter rolls. Following a turning schedule prevents local ischemia over bony prominences. (5, 26)

**83.** 4. Lack of vasomotor tone in the lower extremities causes venous pooling, and the patient may become hypotensive and dizzy when placed in an upright position. The tilt table is used to help the patient overcome vasomotor instability and tolerate an upright position. Some pedal edema could occur, but it would develop gradually and would be less problematic than the hypotension. Elastic stockings are sometimes used to facilitate venous return from the legs. Signs and symptoms of insufficient cerebral circulation are pallor, diaphoresis, tachycardia, and nausea. (5, 26)

**84.** 4. After the spinal shock period, the muscles gradually become spastic due to an increased sensitivity of the lower motor neurons. The movement is not voluntary and cannot be brought under voluntary control. It is expected, but does not indicate that healing is taking place. (17, 31)

**85.** 4. With a cervical injury, the patient has sympathetic fibers that can be stimulated to fire reflexively. The firing is cut off from brain control and is both reflexive and massive. It classically produces pounding headache and dangerously elevated blood pressure, "goose bumps," and profuse sweating. Dry, hot skin occurs during spinal shock. (5, 31)

**86.** 3. Autonomic dysreflexia is a medical emergency. The rising blood pressure can cause a cerebrovascular accident, blindness, or even death. Placing the patient in the Fowler's position decreases the blood pressure. Next, the Foley catheter is checked for patency and the rectum is checked for fecal impaction. The most common cause of autonomic dysreflexia is a distended bladder or rectum. Administering nitroprusside sodium (Nipride) intravenously is an appropriate intervention, if the conservative measures are ineffective. A urine sample for culture should be sent if the patient has an elevated temperature and no other cause for the dysreflexia is found. A urinary tract infection may be causing symptoms. A modified Trendelenburg position is indicated for shock. (17, 31)

**87.** 2. The dysreflexia occurs from a sympathetic response to autonomic nervous system stimulation. A distended bladder is the most common cause. Bowel fullness may also trigger the syndrome. (5, 31)

**88.** 2. Braces are designed to be applied while the patient is lying down. They are custom-designed to fit contours of the chest and buttocks and may not fit properly if applied with the patient in other positions. A poor fit could result in pressure areas and/or inadequate support. (17, 31)

**89.** 2. As soon as the patient's vasomotor status is stable, it is essential for her to drink at least 2,000 ml of fluid daily, unless contraindicated. The increased fluid helps flush out bacteria and prevents urinary stasis. Ingesting an acid-ash diet forms acid urine, which helps prevent urinary tract infection. Most citrus fruits are not metabolized as acids in the body. (37, 41)

**90.** 3. Long-bone demineralization is a serious consequence of the loss of weight-bearing. An excess calcium load is therefore brought to the kidneys and precipitation may occur, thus predisposing the patient to stone formation. Absorption is not altered. (5, 26)

**91.** 2. There are no contraindications to sexual activity in a spinal-cord-injured woman, although she may not be able to experience orgasm. A Foley catheter may be left in place during intercourse in both male and female patients. Because a spinal cord injury does not affect fertility, the patient should have access to family planning information so that an unplanned pregnancy can be avoided. (25, 31)

**92.** 3. Spinal cord injury represents a physical loss, and grief is the normal response to the loss. Working through grief entails reviewing memories and eventually letting go of them. The process may take as long as 2 years. (30, 38)

# *test* 10

, *The Patient with Cataracts*

, *The Patient with Glaucoma*

, *The Patient with a Retinal Detachment*

, *The Patient Undergoing Rhinoplasty*

, *The Patient with Ménière's Disease*

, *The Patient with Cancer of the Larynx*

***Correct Answers and Rationales***

*menieres Disease*
*ca of Larynx*
*clt c Burns*
*ct c Hearing Disorders*

Select the one *best* or *correct* answer and indicate your choice by filling in the circle with a pencil in front of the option you have chosen. If the answer you would prefer is not given, select the one you think is *most appropriate*.

## THE PATIENT WITH CATARACTS *Blurred vision*

Mrs. Josephine Trevor, 76, is admitted overnight for a cataract extraction on her right eye. The procedure is to be done under a local anesthetic. Because Mrs. Trevor lives alone in an isolated location, it was decided that an overnight stay would increase her safety since she has no one to help her at home.

1. As a result of her cataract, Mrs. Trevor is *most likely* to complain of which symptoms?
   ○ 1. Halos and rainbows around lights.
   ○ 2. Eye pain and irritation that is worse at night.
   ○ 3. Blurred vision and the hazy appearance of objects.
   ○ 4. Eyestrain and headache when doing close work.
2. Mrs. Trevor asks the nurse, "What causes cataracts in old people?" Which of the following statements should form the basis for the nurse's response?
   ○ 1. Cataracts usually result from chronic systemic diseases.
   ○ 2. Cataracts are thought to be a result of aging.
   ○ 3. Cataracts are believed to result from eye injuries sustained early in life.
   ○ 4. Cataracts usually result from the prolonged use of toxic substances.
3. Mrs. Trevor says, "The doctor told me he'll remove the lens of my eye. What is the lens for, anyway?" The nurse should explain that the lens of the eye
   ○ 1. produces aqueous humor.
   ○ 2. holds the rods and cones.
   ○ 3. focuses light rays onto the retina.
   ○ 4. regulates the amount of light entering the eye.
4. Preoperatively, the nurse is to instill several types of eye drops into Mrs. Trevor's right eye. The accepted abbreviation for the right eye is
   ○ 1. OD.
   ○ 2. OS.
   ○ 3. OU.
   ○ 4. RE.
5. The nurse is to instill drops of phenylephrine hydrochloride (Neo-Synephrine) into Mrs. Trevor's right eye preoperatively. This preparation acts in the eye to produce
   ○ 1. dilatation of the pupil and dilatation of blood vessels.
   ○ 2. dilatation of the pupil and constriction of blood vessels.
   ○ 3. constriction of the pupil and constriction of blood vessels.
   ○ 4. constriction of the pupil and dilatation of the blood vessels.
6. After instilling eye drops in Mrs. Trevor's eye, the nurse should apply slight pressure against the nose at the inner angle of the patient's closed eye. What is the rationale for this action?
   ○ 1. It prevents the medication from entering the tear duct.
   ○ 2. It prevents the drug from running down the face.
   ○ 3. It allows the sensitive cornea to adjust to the medication.
   ○ 4. It facilitates distribution of the medication over the surface of the eye.
7. Mrs. Trevor tells the nurse that she does not like the idea of being awake during the eye surgery. Which of the following responses is the *most appropriate* for the nurse to make?
   ○ 1. "Have you ever had any reactions to local anesthetics in the past?"
   ○ 2. "What is it that disturbs you about the idea of being awake?"
   ○ 3. "By using a local anesthetic, you won't have nausea and vomiting after the surgery."

**483**

4. "There's really nothing to fear about being awake. You'll be given a medication that will help you relax."

8. A short time after surgery, Mrs. Trevor says, "I am sick to my stomach." The *best* course of action for the nurse to take is to
   1. have the patient take a few deep breaths until the nausea subsides.
   2. explain that this is a very common feeling that will pass quickly.
   3. tell the patient to call the nurse promptly if she vomits.
   4. medicate the patient with an antiemetic, as ordered.

9. Mrs. Trevor's postoperative nursing care plan provides for the activities listed below. Which activity is *contraindicated* for this patient?
   1. Turning to the unoperative side.
   2. Coughing every 2 hours.
   3. Ambulating at least twice every 8 hours.
   4. Deep-breathing every 2 hours.

10. Mrs. Trevor becomes disoriented postoperatively. Which of the following nursing measures is *most likely* to help Mrs. Trevor become reoriented?
    1. Reminding her where she is frequently.
    2. Calling her by familiar family names, such as "Granny."
    3. Dimming her room lights.
    4. Asking friends to make more frequent visits.

11. Mrs. Trevor suddenly complains of a sharp pain in the operative eye and becomes restless. When this occurs, the nurse's action should be guided by knowledge that Mrs. Trevor has *very possibly* developed which of the following postoperative complications?
    1. A detached retina.
    2. A prolapse of the iris.
    3. An extracapsular erosion.
    4. An intraocular hemorrhage.

12. The nurse teaches Mrs. Trevor about activities that she can do postoperatively. Which of the following activities is *contraindicated?*
    1. Walking down the hall unassisted.
    2. Lying in bed on the unoperated side.
    3. Performing routines of isometric exercises.
    4. Bending from the hips to pick up a pair of slippers.

13. Mrs. Trevor will be discharged home tomorrow. What information about her vision will be *most* important for the nurse to include in Mrs. Trevor's discharge plan?
    1. She will need to wear glasses or contact lens to correct her vision.
    2. She will need to wear her glasses only until her eye heals.

3. Cataract glasses correct vision by magnifying objects.
4. She will need to relearn to judge distances accurately.

14. Mrs. Trevor is to be discharged with temporary cataract glasses. To help Mrs. Trevor use these glasses most effectively, the nurse should teach her to
    1. practice reading every day to help strengthen eye muscles.
    2. turn her head so that an object is brought into central vision.
    3. hold an object for inspection at a distance of about 2 feet for best focus.
    4. use the unoperative eye when objects appear double until focus begins to improve.

15. According to her health record, Mrs. Trevor has a long history of hypertension. With this knowledge, the nurse *correctly* judges that the patient may experience eye problems, other than cataracts, because chronic hypertension tends to damage the eye's
    1. iris.
    2. sclera.
    3. retina.
    4. cornea.

16. The day after her discharge, Mrs. Trevor calls her physician's office. Which of the following statements would indicate that she did *not* adequately understand the teaching about the surgery?
    1. "I would like to make an appointment now to get my permanent glasses in 3 months."
    2. "I seem to be catching a cold and am coughing a lot. Should I take a prescription cough medicine?"
    3. "I think the doctor had better check my eye. I've been having a lot of pain today."
    4. "Something is terribly wrong with my vision. I keep trying to climb the stairs but they are not where I put my feet."

## ❦ *THE PATIENT WITH GLAUCOMA*

Mr. Wayne Cummings, 74, is admitted to the hospital for diagnostic tests. He has been treated for chronic open-angle glaucoma for 5 years.

17. Changes in the eye that produce glaucoma are primarily the result of
    1. increased production of aqueous humor.
    2. degeneration of the vascular supply to the cornea.

○ 3. obstruction of the outflow of aqueous humor.

○ 4. senile pupillary degeneration.

18. If Mr. Cummings experienced any symptom of glaucoma, it would most likely be

○ 1. eye pain.

○ 2. excessive lacrimation.

○ 3. flashes of colored light.

○ 4. decreasing peripheral vision.

19. The destructive effects of glaucoma on Mr. Cummings' ocular tissues are due to

○ 1. a paralysis of ciliary muscles.

○ 2. a degeneration of aqueous humor.

○ 3. a precipitate of proteins in the retina.

○ 4. an increase in intraocular pressure.

20. Miotics are frequently used in the basic treatment of glaucoma. They work by

○ 1. paralyzing the ciliary muscle.

○ 2. constricting intraocular vessels.

○ 3. constricting the pupil.

○ 4. relaxing the ciliary muscles.

21. Which of the following is an example of a commonly prescribed miotic?

○ 1. Pilocarpine hydrochloride.

○ 2. Atropine sulfate.

○ 3. Scopolamine hydrobromide.

○ 4. Acetazolamide (Diamox).

22. Glaucoma is a progressive disease that can be easily and effectively treated and yet can lead to blindness if unidentified. The *most effective* health-promotion measure for glaucoma is

○ 1. the need for prompt treatment of all eye infections.

○ 2. the avoidance of extended-wear contact lenses by older people.

○ 3. annual intraocular pressure measurements for all individuals over age 40.

○ 4. appropriate blood pressure control.

23. Mr. Cummings' workup includes tonometry. Which of the following information should the nurse tell Mr. Cummings when preparing him for the procedure?

○ 1. Oral pain medication will be given before the procedure.

○ 2. It is a painless procedure with no side effects.

○ 3. Blurred or double vision may occur after the procedure.

○ 4. Medication will be given to dilate the pupils prior to the procedure.

24. The nurse learns that Mr. Cummings uses timolol maleate (Timoptic) eye drops. It is believed that this beta-adrenergic blocker helps control glaucoma by

○ 1. constricting the pupils.

○ 2. dilating the canals of Schlemm.

○ 3. reducing aqueous humor formation.

○ 4. improving ciliary muscle contractability.

25. The nurse observes Mr. Cummings instill eye drops. Mr. Cummings says, "I just try to hit the middle of my eyeball so they don't run out of my eye." The nurse teaches him to instill the eye drops into the lower conjunctival sac and explains that the method Mr. Cummings is using may cause

○ 1. sclera staining.

○ 2. corneal injury.

○ 3. excessive tear formation.

○ 4. systemic absorption of the drug.

26. The nurse reviews the discharge plan with Mr. Cummings. Which of the following measures should the nurse encourage him to implement?

○ 1. Reducing his daily fluid intake.

○ 2. Wearing dark glasses in the bright sun.

○ 3. Minimizing active exercise.

○ 4. Adding extra lighting to his home.

27. Acute narrow-angle glaucoma is a medical emergency that can quickly lead to blindness. Which of the following clinical manifestations should the nurse associate with this condition?

○ 1. Sudden loss of vision in one eye and headache.

○ 2. Acute light sensitivity and blurred vision.

○ 3. Double vision and headache.

○ 4. Sudden eye pain and colored halos around lights.

28. Mr. Cummings is scheduled for a minor surgical procedure. Which of the following orders would require clarification or correction before the nurse would carry it out?

○ 1. Administer morphine sulfate.

○ 2. Administer atropine sulfate.

○ 3. Teach deep-breathing exercises.

○ 4. Teach leg exercises.

29. At midnight on the day of the procedure, the night nurse makes rounds and notes that Mr. Cummings is sleeping. He is experiencing rapid eye movement (REM) sleep. Which of the following statements *most accurately* describes the normal state of the body during the REM stage of sleep?

○ 1. The person is in a stage of dreaming.

○ 2. The person is in a stage of deep sleep.

○ 3. The person's oxygen needs are at the lowest during this stage.

○ 4. The person's blood pressure is at the lowest during this stage.

30. At 3 a.m., Mr. Cummings is awake. He has not received the sedative that had been ordered on a p.r.n. basis, nor does he routinely take sedatives at home. Which of the following nursing measures that promote sleep should receive the *lowest* priority in this situation?

○ 1. Offering him a bedpan.
○ 2. Giving him a backrub.
○ 3. Changing his position in bed.
○ 4. Administering the sedative to him.

**31.** If Mr. Cummings is denied opportunities to dream while sleeping, he will tend to develop signs of
○ 1. anxiety.
○ 2. insomnia.
○ 3. gastric hyperacidity.
○ 4. involuntary muscular contractions.

**32.** Mr. Cummings' primary nurse notes the next morning that her patient had difficulty sleeping. She explores the issue with Mr. Cummings and finds that he rarely sleeps more than 5 hours each night but takes a nap almost every morning and afternoon. The nurse evaluates Mr. Cummings' sleeping habits as being poor. Which of the following statements *most accurately* describes the nurse's evaluation?
○ 1. The evaluation is correct; frequent short periods of sleep interfere with the quality of sleep.
○ 2. The evaluation is correct; the total number of hours the patient is sleeping is insufficient for a person of his age.
○ 3. The evaluation is incorrect; the total number of hours the patient sleeps in each 24-hour period is more important than when he sleeps.
○ 4. The evaluation is incorrect; sleeping for short periods usually is more healthful than sleeping for one long period in each 24-hour cycle.

## THE PATIENT WITH A RETINAL DETACHMENT

Mr. Herbert Cody, a 70-year-old retired carpenter, is admitted through the emergency department with a diagnosis of detached retina involving the right eye. His eyes are patched bilaterally on admission. His is accompanied by his wife and it is apparent that both Mr. and Mrs. Cody are extremely anxious.

**33.** Which of the following clinical manifestations commonly accompanies a retinal detachment?
○ 1. Sudden severe eye pain and colored halos around lights.
○ 2. Inability to move the eye and loss of light accommodation.
○ 3. A tearing sensation and increased lacrimation.
○ 4. Flashing lights and visual field loss.

**34.** As the nurse completes the admission history, Mr. Cody says that before the physician patched his eye, he was aware of many spots or "floaters." The nurse should explain to Mr. Cody that these spots were caused by
○ 1. pieces of the retina floating in the eye.
○ 2. blood cells released into the eye by the detachment.
○ 3. contamination of the aqueous humor.
○ 4. spasms of the retinal blood vessels traumatized by the detachment.

**35.** Mrs. Cody tells the nurse that she does not understand what happened to her husband's eye. Which of the following *most accurately* describes the pathology of a retinal detachment?
○ 1. A tear in the retina permits the escape of vitreous humor from the eye.
○ 2. The optic nerve is damaged when it is exposed to vitreous humor.
○ 3. The two layers of the retina separate, allowing fluid to enter between them.
○ 4. Retinal injury produces inflammation and edema that increases the intraocular pressure.

**36.** Upon admission to the ophthalmology unit, Mr. Cody is placed on flat bed rest. What is the rationale for this position?
○ 1. It helps reduce intraocular pressure.
○ 2. It facilitates drainage from the eye.
○ 3. It will keep the patient safe while confined to bed.
○ 4. It helps prevent further detachment or tearing of the retina.

**37.** Mr. Cody asks the nurse why his eyes have to be patched. He says the enforced blindness is very frightening and rather disorienting. The nurse should base her reply on the knowledge that eye patches serve to
○ 1. reduce rapid eye movements.
○ 2. decrease the irritation of light entering the damaged eye.
○ 3. protect the injured eye from infection.
○ 4. rest the eyes to promote healing.

**38.** In planning Mr. Cody's care prior to surgery, the nurse should be aware that the major problem for a newly visually impaired client is likely to be
○ 1. threats to his self-concept.
○ 2. problems with communication.
○ 3. loss of basic self-care abilities.
○ 4. financial concerns.

**39.** Mr. Cody remains extremely apprehensive. He says, "I'm afraid of going blind. It would be so hard to live that way." What factor should the nurse consider before responding to his statement?
○ 1. Repeat surgery is impossible, so if this procedure fails vision loss is inevitable.
○ 2. The surgery will only delay blindness in the right eye, but vision is preserved in the left eye.

○ 3. More and more services are available to help the newly blind person adapt to daily living.

○ 4. Optimism is justified because surgical treatment is 70% to 90% successful.

**40.** Mr. Cody's physician reviews the treatment options with Mr. and Mrs. Cody. He explains that the detachment is probably too large to be treated successfully with cryosurgery. This intervention uses extreme cold to

○ 1. seal the margins of the tear.

○ 2. stimulate an inflammatory response and scarring.

○ 3. attach the separated layers of the retina.

○ 4. reduce the metabolic demands of the retina.

**41.** Mr. Cody is scheduled for a scleral buckling. The purpose of this procedure is to

○ 1. remove the torn segment of the retina and stitch down the remaining segment.

○ 2. replace the torn segment of the retina with a strip of retina from a donor.

○ 3. stitch the retina firmly to the optic nerve to give it support.

○ 4. create a splint to hold the retina together until a scar can form and seal off the tear.

**42.** In the immediate postoperative period, Mr. Cody's nursing care should include *all* of the following *except*

○ 1. deep-breathing every 2 hours.

○ 2. providing meaningful stimuli.

○ 3. pressure dressings to both eyes.

○ 4. range-of-motion exercises.

**43.** Mr. Cody is allowed out of bed and the nurse initiates plans for discharge. Mr. Cody understands that his activity needs to be restricted initially. Which of the following activities would be *contraindicated* during the early recovery period?

○ 1. Watching television.

○ 2. Reading.

○ 3. Talking on the phone.

○ 4. Walking in the yard.

**44.** As part of the discharge teaching, the nurse should instruct Mr. Cody to

○ 1. avoid abrupt or jarring motions of his head.

○ 2. exercise his eye muscles each day.

○ 3. turn his entire head rather than just his eyes for sight.

○ 4. avoid activities requiring depth perception.

**45.** Which of the following statements provides the *best* activity guide for Mr. Cody during his rehabilitation period?

○ 1. Activity is resumed gradually and he can resume his usual activities in 5 to 6 weeks.

○ 2. Activity level is determined by patient tolerance and he can be as active as he wishes.

○ 3. Activity levels will be restricted for several months, so he should plan on being sedentary.

○ 4. Activity resumption is controlled by a graduated series of "buckle" exercises.

## THE PATIENT UNDERGOING RHINOPLASTY

Mrs. Annette Sullivan, a 27-year-old mother of two young children, is admitted for elective rhinoplasty. During the admission assessment she says, "I always promised myself that when we finally got our college debts paid off, I would do something about this nose."

**46.** Since the surgery is cosmetic in nature, the nurse completes a thorough psychosocial assessment. Which of the following statements should alert the nurse to potential problems?

○ 1. "My family likes my nose fine, but it has always bothered me."

○ 2. "This awful nose has been the cause of most of my problems in life."

○ 3. "I think I'll feel more self-assured when my nose is smaller."

○ 4. "My aunt had this same surgery done and she looks great now."

**47.** Which of the following statements would indicate that Mrs. Sullivan needed further preoperative teaching?

○ 1. "I hope I don't scare the kids after surgery. I guess I'm going to look pretty beat up."

○ 2. "I'm a little worried about not being able to breathe through my nose at first. That always makes me anxious when I have a bad cold."

○ 3. "Thank goodness for general anesthesia. I sure wouldn't want to be awake while they reshape my nose."

○ 4. "This is going to hurt a lot at first, isn't it?"

**48.** Mrs. Sullivan returns from surgery. In what position should the nurse anticipate placing her?

○ 1. Supine.

○ 2. Left side-lying.

○ 3. Mid-Fowler's.

○ 4. Reverse Trendelenburg.

**49.** In addition to the prescribed analgesic, which of the following interventions is likely to be *most effective* in managing the discomfort of rhinoplasty during the first 24 hours after surgery?

○ 1. Applying warm, moist compresses.

○ 2. Lying in the prone position.

○ 3. Blowing the nose gently.

○ 4. Applying ice compresses.

50. Mrs. Sullivan's postoperative orders include monitoring for bleeding. Which of the following would be an important *initial* clue that bleeding was occurring even if the nasal drip pad remains dry and intact?
   ○ 1. Complaints of nausea.
   ○ 2. Repeated swallowing.
   ○ 3. Rapid respiratory rate.
   ○ 4. Anxiety.

51. On the night of surgery, Mrs. Sullivan complains that the nasal packing is uncomfortable and asks when it will be removed. What information should the nurse give her about removal of the packing?
   ○ 1. The nurse can remove it later that evening.
   ○ 2. The physician will remove it the next morning.
   ○ 3. The physician will remove it at her follow-up visit.
   ○ 4. The patient can remove it after it has been in place for a week.

52. Because the packing blocks Mrs. Sullivan's nose, it will be essential for the nurse to include which of the following in her postoperative care?
   ○ 1. Frequent mouth care.
   ○ 2. Frequent auscultation of the lungs.
   ○ 3. Increased frequency of vital signs.
   ○ 4. Accurate intake and output.

53. In order to promote adequate nutrition in the early postoperative period, the nurse would encourage Mrs. Sullivan to
   ○ 1. increase her fluid intake.
   ○ 2. use a drinking straw.
   ○ 3. request an antiemetic before eating.
   ○ 4. limit her intake of high-fiber foods.

54. The nurse teaches Mrs. Sullivan appropriate nasal care measures to be implemented after the nasal packing is removed. Which of the following measures would the nurse teach Mrs. Sullivan?
   ○ 1. Irrigate the nares with normal saline daily.
   ○ 2. Remove the old blood from inside the nose with cotton-tipped applicators.
   ○ 3. Lubricate the membranes for comfort with a water-soluble lubricant.
   ○ 4. Avoid cleaning the nares for at least 2 days.

55. The nurse should include which of the following pieces of information in Mrs. Sullivan's discharge teaching?
   ○ 1. She should expect tarry stools for several days at home.
   ○ 2. Nausea is an expected outcome of surgery and may persist for several days.
   ○ 3. Brief episodes of epistaxis are expected results of the surgery.
   ○ 4. The pain from surgery should be resolved by the time of discharge.

56. Mrs. Sullivan asks when she will be able to judge the results of the surgery. The *most appropriate* response for the nurse would be
   ○ 1. "Are you concerned about the results?"
   ○ 2. "We encourage people to wait at least 6 months."
   ○ 3. "You'll be able to judge the results in 10 to 14 days."
   ○ 4. "How long did your aunt have to wait?"

57. The nurse would include *all* of the following in Mrs. Sullivan's discharge instructions *except*
   ○ 1. avoid the use of aspirin or aspirin-containing products for analgesia.
   ○ 2. use stool softeners and diet modifications to prevent constipation.
   ○ 3. use over-the-counter medications as needed to prevent excessive coughing.
   ○ 4. blow the nose vigorously each day to prevent the accumulation of dried secretions.

58. Mrs. Sullivan tells the nurse that her 6-year-old daughter has severe nosebleeds. She says, "We both get so scared that I'm not sure I do anything right." Which of the following instructions should the nurse give Mrs. Sullivan about the management of nosebleeds?
   ○ 1. Help the child assume a comfortable position with her head tilted backward.
   ○ 2. Tilt the child's head backward and place firm pressure on the nose.
   ○ 3. Help the child lie on her stomach and collect the blood on a clean towel.
   ○ 4. Place the child in a sitting position with her neck bent forward and apply firm pressure on the nasal septum.

59. If bleeding cannot be effectively and quickly controlled with simple pressure, patients can be safely instructed to soak a gauze square in a topical vasoconstrictor, insert in the nose, and apply pressure. In which common medication would it be appropriate to soak the gauze?
   ○ 1. Neomycin sulfate (Otobiotic).
   ○ 2. Vasopressin tannate (Pitressin).
   ○ 3. Phenylephrine hydrochloride (Neo-Synephrine).
   ○ 4. Lidocaine hydrochloride (Xylocaine).

## THE PATIENT WITH MÉNIÈRE'S DISEASE

Mr. Jeremy Lawler, 58, is undergoing workup by an otolaryngologist for a diagnosis of Ménière's disease.

**60.** The classic triad of symptoms associated with Ménière's disease is
○ 1. vertigo, nausea, and headache.
○ 2. vertigo, tinnitus, and hearing loss.
○ 3. headache, vertigo, and double vision.
○ 4. hearing loss, vertigo, and vomiting.

**61.** Mr. Lawler reports that he has noticed problems with his hearing that have progressively worsened over the last 5 years. *All* of the following are characteristics of sensorineural hearing loss *except*
○ 1. greater loss of high-pitched tones.
○ 2. inability to distinguish and understand speech.
○ 3. the ability to hear better in a noisy environment.
○ 4. speaking in a louder tone of voice.

**62.** Although the etiology of Ménière's disease is incompletely understood, the symptoms are believed to result from
○ 1. infection involving the middle ear.
○ 2. obstruction of the eustachian tubes.
○ 3. bony immobilization of the malleus, incus, and stapes.
○ 4. overaccumulation of endolymph in the vestibular system.

**63.** The symptoms of dizziness and vertigo are both subjective experiences. Which of the following would be the *most accurate* description of the experience of vertigo?
○ 1. A feeling that the environment is in motion.
○ 2. An episode of blackout.
○ 3. Light-headedness.
○ 4. Narrowed vision preceding fainting.

**64.** Mr. Lawler would be experiencing typical symptoms of Ménière's disease if, prior to an attack, he experienced
○ 1. a severe headache.
○ 2. nausea.
○ 3. blurred vision.
○ 4. a feeling of intra-ear fullness.

**65.** Diet modification is part of Mr. Lawler's treatment plan. The nurse would explain that the *most frequently* recommended diet is
○ 1. low-sodium.
○ 2. high-protein.
○ 3. low-carbohydrate.
○ 4. low-fat.

**66.** Which of the following statements would indicate that Mr. Lawler understands the expected course of the disease?
○ 1. The process will gradually extend to the eyes.
○ 2. Control of the episodes is usually possible, but a cure is not yet available.
○ 3. Continued treatment with medication will cure the disease.

○ 4. Bilateral deafness is an inevitable outcome of the disease.

**67.** The potential for injury during an attack of Ménière's disease is great. The nurse should instruct Mr. Lawler to take which *immediate* action when experiencing vertigo?
○ 1. Place his head between his knees.
○ 2. Concentrate on rhythmic deep-breathing.
○ 3. Close his eyes tightly.
○ 4. Lie·down in a reclining or flat position.

**68.** Mrs. Lawler is concerned because during the past year, her husband has curtailed family activities and evenings out. Based on this information, which of the following is the *most appropriate* nursing diagnosis?
○ 1. Social isolation related to attacks of vertigo and hearing loss.
○ 2. Anxiety related to concern about progressive hearing loss.
○ 3. Self-care deficit related to labyrinth dysfunction.
○ 4. Altered sensory perception related to labyrinth dysfunction.

**69.** *All* of the following drugs may be used in the attempt to control Mr. Lawler's symptoms *except*
○ 1. antihistamines.
○ 2. anticholinergics.
○ 3. diuretics.
○ 4. glucocorticoids.

**70.** Mr. Lawler finds the chronic tinnitus to be extremely irritating. Which of the following strategies would be *best* for the nurse to suggest?
○ 1. Maintain a quiet, restful environment.
○ 2. Mask the tinnitus with background music.
○ 3. Ensure adequate levels of vitamin $B_6$ in his diet.
○ 4. Explore the use of a hearing aid.

**71.** The *primary* goal of medical management for Mr. Lawler would be to
○ 1. save his hearing.
○ 2. prevent environmental injury.
○ 3. control the symptoms.
○ 4. help him cope with the disease.

**72.** Which of the following *best* describes the effects of a hearing aid for patients with sensorineural hearing losses?
○ 1. It will make sounds louder and clearer.
○ 2. It will have no effect on hearing.
○ 3. It will make sounds louder but not clearer.
○ 4. It improves the individual's ability to separate words from background noises.

**73.** Ototoxicity is a possible side effect of many commonly prescribed medications. Drugs that posses a significant risk of permanent damage include the

○ 1. salicylates.
○ 2. aminoglycoside antibiotics.
○ 3. digitalis preparations.
○ 4. narcotics.

# THE PATIENT WITH CANCER OF THE LARYNX

Mr. William Gordon, a 63-year-old farmer with intrinsic laryngeal cancer, is admitted to the hospital for a total laryngectomy.

74. While taking Mr. Gordon's nursing history, the nurse identifies risk factors that contribute to the incidence of laryngeal cancer. The development of laryngeal cancer is *most clearly* linked to which of the following factors?
    ○ 1. High-fat, low-fiber diet.
    ○ 2. Heavy use of alcohol.
    ○ 3. Low socioeconomic status.
    ○ 4. Overuse of artificial sweeteners.

75. Because the intrinsic laryngeal cancer was identified early, the nurse would anticipate that Mr. Gordon's *primary* symptom was most likely
    ○ 1. difficulty in swallowing.
    ○ 2. persistent mild hoarseness.
    ○ 3. chronic foul breath.
    ○ 4. nagging unproductive cough.

76. Mr. Gordon is scheduled for radical neck surgery and a total laryngectomy. For which of the following postoperative possibilities should the nurse prepare Mr. Gordon preoperatively?
    ○ 1. A temporary tracheostomy.
    ○ 2. Minimal postoperative pain.
    ○ 3. Immediate speech therapy.
    ○ 4. Normal oral and nasal breathing.

77. The *priority* nursing goal for Mr. Gordon in the immediate postoperative period should be to
    ○ 1. maintain a patent airway.
    ○ 2. establish successful nonverbal communication.
    ○ 3. prevent strain on suture lines.
    ○ 4. prevent hemorrhage.

78. Which of the following measures should the nurse perform in relation to suctioning Mr. Gordon's laryngectomy tube?
    ○ 1. Apply suction while inserting the suction catheter into the tube.
    ○ 2. Change the laryngectomy tube after suctioning the patient.
    ○ 3. Select a suction catheter that approximates the diameter of the laryngectomy tube.

○ 4. Administer high concentrations of oxygen prior to suctioning the patient.

79. Mr. Gordon's respiratory secretions are very sticky. To remove the secretions more easily, the nurse liquefies them before suctioning by instilling the laryngectomy tube with 4 to 5 ml of sterile
    ○ 1. water.
    ○ 2. normal saline.
    ○ 3. bacteriostatic water.
    ○ 4. diluted hydrogen peroxide.

80. While suctioning through Mr. Gordon's laryngectomy tube, the nurse should insert the catheter approximately
    ○ 1. 2″ to 4″ (5 to 10 cm).
    ○ 2. 4″ to 8″ (10 to 20 cm).
    ○ 3. 10″ to 12″ (25 to 30 cm).
    ○ 4. 16″ to 20″ (40 to 50 cm).

81. The *longest* period of time the nurse should suction Mr. Gordon at one time is
    ○ 1. 3 to 5 seconds.
    ○ 2. 10 to 15 seconds.
    ○ 3. 20 to 25 seconds.
    ○ 4. 28 to 30 seconds.

82. After suctioning through Mr. Gordon's laryngectomy tube, the nurse waits a few minutes before suctioning again. The nurse uses intermittent suction *primarily* to help prevent
    ○ 1. stimulating the patient's cough reflex.
    ○ 2. depriving the patient of a sufficient supply of oxygen.
    ○ 3. dislocating the patient's laryngectomy tube.
    ○ 4. clogging the suctioning catheter with secretions.

83. When the nurse wants to suction Mr. Gordon's left bronchus, she would ask the patient to help by
    ○ 1. looking toward the ceiling.
    ○ 2. turning his head to the left.
    ○ 3. bringing his chin toward his chest.
    ○ 4. turning his head to the right.

84. In relation to aseptic technique and the catheter used to suction Mr. Gordon's laryngectomy tube, it is recommended that the nurse use a
    ○ 1. sterile catheter with each suctioning and then discard it.
    ○ 2. sterile catheter for all suctioning during an 8-hour period.
    ○ 3. sterile catheter for all suctioning during a 24-hour period.
    ○ 4. clean catheter with each suctioning and disinfect it between uses.

85. Which of the following signs *most accurately* indicates to the nurse that airway suctioning has been effective for Mr. Gordon?

○ 1. Observing that the patient's respirations are not labored.

○ 2. Hearing a hollow sound when the patient's chest is percussed.

○ 3. Observing that the patient is not raising mucus while coughing.

○ 4. Hearing clear breath sounds during auscultation of the patient's chest.

**86.** A nasogastric tube was inserted during surgery and Mr. Gordon receives tube feedings to meet his needs for fluids and nutrition. The *primary* rationale for tube feedings in this situation is to

○ 1. prevent pain associated with swallowing.

○ 2. ensure an adequate intake.

○ 3. prevent the development of a fistula.

○ 4. allow for adequate suture line healing.

**87.** The nurse develops a postoperative teaching plan for Mr. Gordon. Which of the following should the nurse include in this plan?

○ 1. Instructing him to avoid coughing until the sutures are removed.

○ 2. Telling him that he can speak by covering the stoma with a sterile gauze pad.

○ 3. Reassuring him that normal eating will be possible after healing has occurred.

○ 4. Instructing him to control his oral secretions with tissues or by expectorating into an emesis basin.

**88.** Mr. Gordon appears withdrawn and depressed. He keeps the curtain drawn, refuses visitors, and says he wants to be left alone. Which nursing intervention will *most likely* be therapeutic for Mr. Gordon?

○ 1. Discussing his behavior with his wife.

○ 2. Exploring his future plans.

○ 3. Respecting his need for privacy.

○ 4. Encouraging him to express his feelings nonverbally and in writing.

**89.** Mr. Gordon decides that he wants to learn about esophageal speech. The speech therapist comes to discuss this communication technique and explains that it involves

○ 1. holding an electronic instrument against the esophagus.

○ 2. providing an access route from the trachea to the esophagus.

○ 3. filling the esophagus with air.

○ 4. replacing the larynx with scar tissue.

**90.** Discharge teaching for Mr. Gordon must include management of his artificial airway. Which of the following should the nurse include in her teaching?

○ 1. Covering the stoma with a plastic dressing for showering.

○ 2. Sleeping with the head of the bed flat.

○ 3. Blowing the nose gently.

○ 4. Practicing effective diaphragmatic coughing to raise secretions.

# CORRECT ANSWERS AND RATIONALES

Numbers appear in parentheses following the rationales. The numbers identify textbooks listed in the references at the end of Part IV, where correct answers can be verified.

## *The Patient with Cataracts*

1. 3. A patient who has a cataract usually complains of blurred and hazy vision. This vision distortion is due to opacity of the lens, which blocks light rays from reaching the retina. (25, 31)

2. 2. Aging is the most common cause of cataracts; the next most common cause is injury to the eye. Other causes include the ingestion of injurious substances, such as naphthalene, and the presence of systemic diseases, such as diabetes. (25, 31)

3. 3. The lens of the eye focuses light rays onto the retina. The process of bringing light rays into focus from both near and far objects is called accommodation. The ciliary bodies secrete aqueous humor. The retina houses the rods and cones. The iris regulates the amount of light entering the eye. (25, 31)

4. 1. The accepted abbreviation for the right eye is OD, which stands for "oculis dexter." OS ("oculis sinister") refers to the left eye. OU ("oculis uterque") refers to both eyes. RE is not an accepted abbreviation for the right eye. (24, 36)

5. 2. When used in the eye, phenylephrine hydrochloride (Neo-Synephrine) acts as a mydriatic (that is, it causes the pupil to dilate). It also constricts small blood vessels in the eye. (12, 16)

6. 1. Placing pressure against the nose at the inner angle of the closed eye after administering eye drops prevents the medication from entering the lacrimal (tear) duct. If it enters the tear duct, the medication can enter the nose and pharynx, where it may be absorbed and cause toxic symptoms. Eye drops should be placed in the lower conjunctival sac of the eye. (24, 36)

7. 2. The nurse should give a patient who seems fearful of surgery an opportunity to express her feelings. Only after identifying the patient's concern can the nurse intervene appropriately. Premature explanations and clichés do not provided needed assessment data and ignore the patient's feelings. (11, 38)

8. 4. An antiemetic, as prescribed, should be administered as soon as a patient who has had a cataract extracted complains of nausea. Vomiting can in-crease intraocular pressure, which should be avoided after eye surgery because it can cause complications. (25, 31)

9. 2. Coughing is contraindicated in the post-cataract extraction patient because it increases intraocular pressure. Other activities that are contraindicated because they increase intraocular pressure are turning to the operative side, sneezing, crying, and straining. Turning to the unoperative side, ambulating, and deep-breathing do not affect intraocular pressure. (25, 31)

10. 1. Reality orientation means orienting the patient to person, place, and time frequently. Respect for the patient dictates addressing her by name. Frequent visits by friends may be helpful but should not be the primary strategy for reorienting the patient. Keeping the environment dim and very quiet is likely to increase the patient's confusion. (30, 38)

11. 4. Pain and restlessness following eye surgery should suggest to the nurse that the patient may be experiencing intraocular hemorrhage. The physician should be notified promptly. (25, 31)

12. 4. Bending from the hips to pick up slippers is contraindicated after cataract surgery because it increases intraocular pressure. The patient should be taught to flex her knees when picking up something from the floor. Activities such as walking, lying in bed on the unoperated side, and performing isometric exercises are not contraindicated. (25, 31)

13. 4. After cataract surgery, a patient must relearn to judge distances accurately in order to walk safely. The patient will need glasses or contact lenses to restore vision, and cataract glasses do correct vision by magnifying objects; however, these points are not as important in discharge planning as is relearning to judge distance accurately. (25, 31)

14. 2. Thick, biconvex lenses in glasses are used postoperatively for a patient who has had cataract surgery. Because clear vision is possible only through the center of the lens, the patient should be taught to turn her head so that the object she wishes to see is brought into central vision. It is best to begin wearing these glasses while sitting because of the visual distortion they create. The glasses should be worn at all times when awake. Colors may be distorted in the operated eye for a while. (25, 31)

15. 3. The retina of the eye is especially susceptible to damage when a patient suffers from chronic hypertension. The arterioles supplying the retina are damaged. (25, 31)

**16.** 4. After cataract surgery, the patient must relearn how to judge distances accurately. Therefore, she might be expected to have trouble climbing stairs. She should have been appropriately prepared to deal with this problem safely and needs further teaching. Permanent glasses are prescribed within 12 weeks after surgery. The patient should not experience pain in the operative eye. (25, 31)

## The Patient with Glaucoma

**17.** 3. The causes of glaucoma are not completely understood, but a variety of mechanisms appear to interfere with outflow of the aqueous humor. Obstruction in outflow results in backup of fluid and increased intraocular pressure. (25, 31)

**18.** 4. Although chronic open-angle glaucoma is usually completely asymptomatic in the early stages, peripheral vision gradually decreases. (26, 31)

**19.** 4. Chronic increased intraocular pressure destroys optic-nerve function. Late symptoms due to severe and irreversible eye damage include visual-field loss and reduced visual acuity uncorrectable with glasses. Prompt and continuous health care helps many people escape the destructive effects of glaucoma. (25, 31)

**20.** 3. Miotics constrict the pupil and contract ciliary musculature. Pupillary constriction and contraction of ciliary musculature widen the filtration angle and permit increased outflow of aqueous humor. Miotics also cause vasodilation of the intraocular vessels or where intraocular fluids leave the eye, leading to an increase in aqueous humor outflow. Mydriatics cause cycloplegia, or paralysis of the ciliary muscle. (25, 31)

**21.** 1. Pilocarpine hydrochloride is a commonly prescribed miotic that produces negligible systemic effects. Atropine sulfate and scopolamine hydrobromide have mydriatic effects. Acetazolamide (Diamox), a carbonic anhydrase inhibitor, decreases secretion of aqueous humor in the eye, thus lowering intraocular pressure. (12, 16)

**22.** 3. The most effective health-promotion measure for glaucoma is annual intraocular pressure measurements for all persons over age 40. Glaucoma is insidious and basically asymptomatic and must be diagnosed before patients are aware of any vision changes. (26, 31)

**23.** 2. Tonometry is the measurement of intraocular pressure. It is a simple and painless procedure that requires no particular preparation or post-procedure care. There are no test-related side effects. (25, 31)

**24.** 3. Timolol maleate (Timoptic) is commonly used to control glaucoma. The function of the drug is not entirely understood, but it is believed to reduce aqueous humor formation, thereby reducing intraocular pressure. (12, 16)

**25.** 2. The cornea is a very sensitive part of the eye and may be injured when eye drops fall onto it. Eye drops should be instilled into the lower conjunctival sac of the eye to help prevent corneal damage. (24, 36)

**26.** 4. The use of miotics may compromise a patient's ability to adjust safely to night vision. For safety, extra lighting should be added to the home. The patient does not need to curtail fluid intake. Bright lights are not harmful to the eyes, and exercise is permitted, although excessive exertion should be avoided. (12, 16)

**27.** 4. Acute narrow-angle glaucoma causes abrupt changes in the angle of the iris. Clinical manifestations include severe eye pain, colored halos around lights, and rapid loss of vision. (25, 31)

**28.** 2. Atropine sulfate causes dilatation of the pupils. This action is contraindicated for the patient with glaucoma because it increases intraocular pressure. The drug does not have this effect on intraocular pressure on people who do not have glaucoma. (12, 16)

**29.** 1. When people are awakened from rapid eye movement (REM) sleep, almost all report they were dreaming. Because dreaming is an important part of sleep and necessary for well-being, nurses should avoid waking patients who are in REM sleep whenever possible. During certain stages of sleep, when REM is absent, people are in deep sleep; blood pressure and oxygen needs are low. (10, 23)

**30.** 4. The nurse should use such nursing measures as giving a backrub, offering a bedpan, and changing the patient's position in bed to promote sleep before resorting to the use of a sedative. However, when nursing measures fail, the nurse may judge that a sedative is necessary to promote rest and sleep. The indiscriminate use of sedatives is indefensible. (10, 23)

**31.** 1. Symptoms that commonly occur when people are deprived of dreaming include anxiety, irritability, the inability to concentrate, and depression. Insomnia, gastric hyperacidity, and involuntary muscular contractions are not associated with dream deprivation. (10, 23)

**32.** 3. There appears to be no rigid formula as to what is normal in relation to periodicity and duration of sleep. What is important is for each individual to follow a rest pattern that maintains his well-being. (10, 23)

## The Patient with a Retinal Detachment

**33.** 4. Patients with retinal detachment frequently report flashing lights in the affected eye followed by a loss of vision that is often described as a curtain being slowly drawn across the eye. The detachment is painless, does not involve the eye muscles, and does not cause lacrimation. (25, 31)

**34.** 2. The spots or "floaters" reported by patients with retinal detachment are blood cells released into the vitreous humor by the detachment. (25, 31)

**35.** 3. In a detachment, the two layers of the retina separate as a result of a small hole or tear, trauma, or degeneration. Vitreous humor seeps into the tear and separates the retinal layers. Vitreous humor does not leak out of the eye or cause any direct damage to the optic nerve. Increased intraocular pressure is not associated with retinal detachment. (25, 31)

**36.** 4. The patient's position is determined by the location of the retinal tear. The rationale for rest is the hope that the retina will fall back into place as much as possible before surgery and thus will facilitate adherency of the retina to the choroid. Increased intraocular pressure is not a problem in detached retina. There should be no external drainage from the eye. (5, 26)

**37.** 1. Patching the eyes helps decrease random eye movements that could enlarge and worsen the detachment. Patching the eyes minimizes eye movement. (25, 31)

**38.** 3. Patching the eyes creates temporary blindness. The resulting incapacity makes self-care and independence difficult, if not impossible. This need for assistance in basic self-care activities can be extremely frustrating to the patient and reinforces the threat of potential blindness. (25, 31)

**39.** 4. Untreated retinal detachment results in increasing detachment and eventual blindness, but about 70% to 90% of patients can be successfully treated with surgery. The surgical procedure can be repeated about 10 to 14 days after the first procedure. Many more services are available for the newly blind, but ideally this patient will not need them. (5, 26)

**40.** 2. The use of light, heat, and cold are all strategies that stimulate an inflammatory response in the area of the detachment. The eventual scarring reattaches the separated layers of the retina. (25, 31)

**41.** 4. A choroidal scar will form a permanent seal to close the hole or tear in the retina. A scleral buckle serves as a splint to hold the retina and choroid together until that scar can form. Loss of a portion or the whole retina would interfere with sight. Retinal transplants are not performed. The retina is never stitched to the optic nerve. (26, 31)

**42.** 3. Pressure dressings to the eyes are not used following the surgery, although general eye patching may temporarily be used. Elderly patients in particular need planned meaningful stimuli to prevent disorientation. Routine care includes range-of-motion exercises and deep-breathing. Coughing should be avoided. (5, 26)

**43.** 2. Although restful, reading involves too much jerky eye movement and should be avoided during recovery. Watching television, walking outdoors, and visiting with friends are all appropriate activities and can be encouraged. (25, 31)

**44.** 1. During recovery, the patient should be instructed to avoid abrupt or jarring movements of the head. Activities such as shampooing or brushing the hair may be restricted. No specific eye exercises are prescribed and depth perception is not specially affected by the surgery. (25, 31)

**45.** 1. The scarring of the tear needs time to heal completely. Therefore, resumption of activity is gradual, but the patient may resume his usual activities in 5 to 6 weeks. Successful healing should allow the patient to return to his previous level of functioning. (26, 31)

## The Patient Undergoing Rhinoplasty

**46.** 2. Reconstructive surgery will not correct a basic personality problem. People who blame a small defect for all life's failures are sure to be disappointed after surgery. The goal of cosmetic surgery is to help a person feel better. Cosmetic surgery will assist an emotionally stable person to have more self-assurance. The perception of the defect is considered from the patient's point of view, not that of others. Another person's surgical success often encourages an individual to proceed with her own desires. (26, 31)

**47.** 3. Rhinoplasty is generally performed under regional rather than general anesthesia. The patient is quite sedated but should not believe that she will be "asleep" during the procedure. The surgery does cause significant bruising and discomfort and the packing makes mouth-breathing necessary. (25, 31)

**48.** 3. To assist in breathing, promote comfort, and decrease the amount of edema formation after surgery, the patient is most appropriately positioned in a mid-Fowler's position. (25, 31)

**49.** 4. The most effective means of decreasing discomfort is to decrease local edema. Cold applications, such as ice compresses or an ice bag, are very effective. Heat dilates local vessels and increases local congestion. A mid-Fowler's position is the most desirable position to decrease edema and prevent aspiration. Blowing the nose should be avoided as it can disrupt the surgical site and lead to bleeding. Blowing the nose should be avoided for at least 48 hours after the nasal packing is removed. (26, 31)

**50.** 2. Because of the dense packing, it is relatively unusual for bleeding to be apparent through the nasal drip pad. The blood instead runs down the throat and causes the patient to swallow frequently. The back of the throat can be assessed with a flashlight. The accumulation of blood in the stomach may cause the patient to vomit. Increased respiratory rate occurs in shock, but is not an initial clue of bleeding in the post-rhinoplasty patient. (26, 31)

**51.** 2. The purpose of the packing is to maintain hemostasis and prevent bleeding. Removal of the packing is uncomfortable and must be done carefully. The surgeon generally removes the packing the day after surgery. The physician needs to assess the patient before removing the packing and must be present in case of bleeding. (26, 31)

**52.** 1. Mouth-breathing severely dries the mucous membranes of the oral cavity. Frequent mouth care is necessary for comfort and to combat the anorexia associated with the taste of blood and loss of the sense of smell. The other interventions listed are not targeted at the effects of the packing. (25, 31)

**53.** 1. Although foods as tolerated are encouraged, the nurse should encourage the patient with nasal packing to increase fluid intake because fluids are best tolerated at this time. The presence of nasal packing makes eating very difficult and uncomfortable. The packing blocks the passage of air through the nose and a partial vacuum is created during swallowing. A sucking action may occur when the patient attempts to drink with a straw. Antiemetics are needed only if the patient is nauseated or vomiting. Constipation and the Valsalva maneuver should be avoided; the latter can precipitate nasal bleeding. (26, 31)

**54.** 3. A water-soluble lubricant offsets dryness and increases comfort while healing occurs. The lubricant also prevents secretions from drying and crusting in the nose. The patient should be cautioned not to disturb clots either with her fingers or applicators, as bleeding may occur. (26, 31)

**55.** 1. Nasal bleeding causes stools to have a tarry appearance for several days, and patients should be informed of this. Epistaxis and nausea are not expected outcomes and some discomfort can be expected to persist after discharge. (25, 31)

**56.** 2. Ecchymosis and swelling will be present around the eyes and nose for 10 to 14 days. Firm healing develops on about the 10th day. The cosmetic effect from nasal surgery cannot be judged for 6 to 12 months. This allows the tissue to return to normal and the scar to resolve. (26, 31)

**57.** 4. The patient should avoid blowing her nose for 48 hours after the packing is removed. Thereafter, she should blow her nose very gently using the open-mouth technique to minimize bleeding in the surgical area. She should also take measures to prevent coughing and should avoid the use of aspirin. Constipation can cause straining at the stool that can induce bleeding. (26, 31)

**58.** 4. For the initial management of nosebleeds, the individual should sit up and lean forward with the head tipped downward. The soft tissues of the nose should be compressed against the septum with the fingers. The traditional head-back position allows blood to flow down the throat and can trigger vomiting. (25, 31)

**59.** 3. Phenylephrine hydrochloride (Neo-Synephrine) is a topical vasoconstrictor used to control nosebleeds. A nosebleed (epistaxis) is a potentially serious condition and if emergency measures do not control the bleeding, expert medical care should be obtained. Neomycin sulfate (Otobiotic) is an antibiotic used to treat external ear canal infection. Vasopressin tannate (Pitressin) is a posterior pituitary hormone used to treat nonpsychogenic diabetes insipidus. Lidocaine hydrochloride (Xylocaine) is used as a local and topical anesthetic and in some institutions is the drug of choice in the treatment of ventricular dysrhythmia. (26, 31)

## The Patient with Ménière's Disease

**60.** 2. Ménière's disease involves the inner ear and is characterized by episodes of acute vertigo and tinnitus. It can result in progressive and irreversible hearing loss. The severe vertigo can lead to nausea and vomiting. Double vision and headache are not characteristic features of Ménière's disease. (25, 31)

**61.** 3. Sensorineural hearing loss involves the inner ear and is a common degenerative problem for elderly people. The ability to hear high-pitched sounds is decreased, as is the ability to discriminate and understand sounds, especially in a noisy environment. Misinterpretation of voice levels causes these patients to speak in a louder-than-normal voice. (31, 32)

**62.** 4. It is theorized that Ménière's disease is the result of an initial viral infection involving the inner ear. The symptoms are the result of an overaccumulation of endolymph in the vestibular system that interrupts the balance mechanisms. The eustachian tubes are not blocked. Otosclerosis produces bony immobilization of the ear's conduction system. (31, 32)

**63.** 1. Vertigo is a form of hallucination in which the individual perceives the environment to be moving around him or himself to be moving within the environment. Patients are not light-headed and do not faint or black out. (31, 32)

**64.** 4. Many patients are able to identify an incipient attack of Ménière's disease by perceiving a feeling of fullness in the ear that reflects the evolving congestion. Ménière's disease does not affect vision. Nausea may result once the classic symptoms occur. (25, 31)

**65.** 1. A low-sodium diet is frequently an effective mechanism for reducing the frequency and severity of the disease episodes. Approximately three-quarters of patients with Ménière's disease respond to treatment with a low-salt diet. A diuretic may also be ordered. (5, 25)

**66.** 2. There is currently no cure for Ménière's disease, but the wide range of medical and surgical treatments allows for adequate control in many cases. The disease often worsens, but there is no indication that it spreads to the eyes. The hearing loss is usually unilateral. (5, 31)

**67.** 4. The patient needs to be in a safe and comfortable position during the attacks in Ménière's disease, which may last several hours. The patient's location when the attack occurs may dictate the most reasonable position. Ideally, he should lie down immediately in a reclining or flat position to control the vertigo. The danger of a serious fall is very real. (5, 31)

**68.** 1. Patients with Ménière's disease often curtail social activity because of the embarrassment of having a dizzy spell in public. This seems likely in this situation, based on the wife's information, but would need to be validated by the patient. However, the wife may be a more reliable source of information about social isolation than the patient. The other three diagnoses are appropriate in Ménière's disease but are less directly related to social activity. (5, 31)

**69.** 4. A wide variety of medications are used in the attempt to control Ménière's disease, including antihistamines, anticholinergics, and diuretics. Glu-cocorticoids play no significant role in disease treatment. (25, 31)

**70.** 2. The chronic tinnitus associated with Ménière's disease can be extremely intrusive and frustrating for patients. Quiet environments appear to worsen the patient's perception of the problem, and attempting to mask it with a low-level competing sound such as music is often recommended. (25, 31)

**71.** 1. Uncontrolled Ménière's disease can lead to irreversible hearing loss. Preventing this is the primary goal of medical treatment. All the other goals are important goals for both physicians and nurses during the patient's care. (25, 31)

**72.** 3. Hearing aids have limited use for patients with sensorineural hearing loss because these patients experience problems with sound discrimination as well as volume. A hearing aid can make sounds louder but not necessarily clearer. (25, 31)

**73.** 2. Numerous drugs may cause ototoxicity. Permanent damage to the ear is a possible consequence of the use of aminoglycoside antibiotics, and nurses should monitor patients frequently for these effects. High doses of salicylates do cause hearing impairment, but it is promptly reversible with a simple reduction in total daily dose. (12, 16)

## The Patient with Cancer of the Larynx

**74.** 2. Predisposing factors for laryngeal cancer include chronic irritants such as alcohol, cigarette smoke, and other noxious fumes. Three of four people who develop laryngeal cancer are smokers. The combination of smoking and heavy alcohol intake is even more strongly implicated as a causative agent in laryngeal cancer. Epidemiologic studies indicate that a high-fat diet may be a major factor in the development of cancer of the breast, prostate, and colon. Low socioeconomic status is a predisposing factor in cervical cancer but is not a laryngeal cancer risk factor. Artificial sweeteners have been related to the incidence of bladder cancer. (25, 26)

**75.** 2. Hoarseness occurs early in the development of most intrinsic laryngeal cancers because the tumor presence and growth prevents accurate approximation of the vocal cords during phonation. Foul breath and expectoration of blood are late symptoms. Large extrinsic tumors eventually produce difficulty and pain in swallowing. A nagging cough has no direct relationship to laryngeal cancer. (26, 31)

**76.** 2. Postoperative pain is minimal because the sensory nerves that convey pain are no longer present.

Patients may have a temporary laryngectomy tube, which remains in place until the wound is healed and a permanent fistula has formed, usually in 2 or 3 weeks. Speech therapy is delayed until healing occurs. Surgery permanently alters the airway and necessitates breathing through the permanent tracheal opening. (14, 25)

**77.** 1. Maintaining a patent airway is *the* priority nursing goal in the immediate postoperative period. The patient's ability to cough and breathe deeply is impaired because the glottis is removed. Nonverbal communication is important but is not the priority postoperative nursing goal. Promoting comfort, reducing strain on suture lines, and preventing hemorrhage are important nursing goals, but patent airway is *the* priority. (26, 31)

**78.** 4. Patients are hyperoxygenated prior to suctioning to prevent hypoxia. Suction is never applied while inserting the catheter into the airway. The suction catheter should be about half the diameter of the tube; a larger-diameter suction catheter would interfere with airflow during the procedure. Laryngectomy tubes are not changed after suctioning the patient. (26, 31)

**79.** 2. Sterile normal saline is the solution of choice for instilling into a laryngectomy tube cannula to help liquefy sticky secretions. Normal saline is less irritating to mucous membranes than plain water, diluted hydrogen peroxide, and bacteriostatic water. The area around a laryngectomy stoma may be cleansed with an applicator moistened with diluted hydrogen peroxide, but the nurse should be careful that none enters the stoma because of its irritating effects on respiratory mucosa. Furthermore, it is important to prevent aspiration. (5, 31)

**80.** 3. To be effective, the catheter should be inserted about 10″ to 12″ (25 to 30 cm) when suctioning through a laryngectomy tube. Inserting it further may damage respiratory tissues. Inserting it less than the recommended distance is unlikely to make suctioning effective, although some texts recommend inserting the catheter 8″ to 12″ (20 to 30 cm). (5, 26)

**81.** 2. The patient should *not* be suctioned longer than 10 to 15 seconds at a time. Sectioning longer than 15 seconds at a time is likely to remove so much oxygen from the patient's respiratory tract that he may become hypoxic. (5, 26)

**82.** 2. After being suctioned, the patient should rest 3 minutes before being suctioned again, unless secretions interfere with breathing. Intermittent suctioning prevents depriving the patient of oxygen. Hypoxia can lead to cardiac dysrhythmias and car-

diac arrest. One hundred percent oxygen should be administered between suctioning. (5, 26)

**83.** 4. Having the patient turn his head to the right may help the catheter enter the left bronchus. Conversely, having the patient turn his head to the left may help the catheter enter the right bronchus. (26, 36)

**84.** 1. The recommended technique is to use a sterile catheter for each suctioning when the patient has a laryngectomy or tracheostomy tube. There is danger of introducing organisms into the respiratory tract when strict aseptic technique, including a change of catheter for each suctioning, is not used. (5, 36)

**85.** 4. Hearing clear breath sounds during auscultation of the patient's chest is the most accurate method for evaluating the effectiveness of tracheobronchial suctioning. Auscultation should also be used to determine whether the patient needs suctioning. Assessment techniques such as observing whether the patient's respirations are labored, observing whether he raises mucus while coughing, and hearing a hollow sound when his chest is percussed are not the most accurate methods for evaluating the effectiveness of tracheobronchial suctioning. (5, 36)

**86.** 4. A nasogastric tube is usually inserted during surgery to instill food and fluids postoperatively. The tube allows the suture line to heal adequately, minimizes contamination of the pharyngeal and esophageal suture lines, and prevents fluid from leaking through the wound into the trachea before healing occurs. Normal oral feedings are resumed as soon as the nasogastric tube is removed, usually within 10 days after surgery. A tracheoesophageal fistula is a rare potential complication of total laryngectomy and may occur if radiation therapy has compromised wound healing. (25, 31)

**87.** 3. Normal eating is possible once the suture line has healed. Coughing is essential to keep the airway patent. Since the larynx has been removed, the patient cannot speak. Swallowing is unaffected and the patient should have no problem controlling oral secretions. (25, 31)

**88.** 4. The laryngectomy patient has undergone body changes and permanent loss of verbal communication. He may feel isolated and insecure. The nurse can encourage his expression of feelings and use this information to develop an appropriate care plan. Discussing the patient's behavior with his wife may not reveal the patient's feelings. Exploring future plans is not appropriate at this time because more information about the patient's behavior is needed before proceeding on this level. The nurse can respect the patient's need for privacy while encouraging him to express his feelings. (26, 31)

**89.** 3. Esophageal speech requires filling the esophagus with air and allowing it to vibrate out. An artificial larynx (electrolarynx) is a hand-held speech aid placed against the neck. An access route from the trachea to the esophagus is required for tracheoesophageal shunting. This provides pulmonary power to the pharyngeal sphincter, which provides vibrations for a pseudovoice. Replacing the larynx with scar tissue would not facilitate speech. (26, 31)

**90.** 4. Coughing maintains a patent airway because it removes secretions. Plastic should never be placed over the stoma because breathing is impossible through plastic. Elevating the head of the bed promotes drainage of secretions and prevents strain on suture lines. Blowing the nose is impossible because there is no longer a connection between the lower airway and nose. (26, 31)

# test 11

The Patient in Pain

The Patient with Pernicious Anemia

The Patient with Hodgkin's Disease

The Patient Requiring Cardiopulmonary Resuscitation

The Patient with Burns

The Patient in Shock

Correct Answers and Rationales

Select the one *best* or *correct* answer and indicate your choice by filling in the circle with a pencil in front of the option you have chosen. If the answer you would prefer is not given, select the one you think is *most appropriate*.

## THE PATIENT IN PAIN

Mr. Lee Fong, 34, is admitted to the hospital after experiencing multiple trauma as a result of an automobile accident. He has three fractured ribs, a hairline fracture of the pelvis, and a compound fracture of his right tibia and fibula, in addition to soft-tissue injuries. He is in severe pain when he arrives on the unit after emergency surgery.

1. The nurse's first action after a careful assessment is to administer Mr. Fong's prescribed narcotic of 100 mg of meperidine hydrochloride (Demerol). This medication will be effective in relieving Mr. Fong's pain because of the drug's ability to
   ○ 1. reduce the perception of pain.
   ○ 2. decrease the sensitivity of pain receptors.
   ○ 3. interfere with pain impulses traveling along sensory nerve fibers.
   ○ 4. block the conduction of pain impulses along the central nervous system.

2. Mr. Fong continues to experience severe pain and requires frequent medication. A nursing assistant expresses her surprise, saying, "I thought Oriental people were very stoic about pain." Which of the following statements about pain is *correct?*
   ○ 1. The level of pain perception varies widely from person to person.
   ○ 2. The level of pain tolerance is about the same in all people.
   ○ 3. The level of pain tolerance is determined by an individual's genetic makeup.
   ○ 4. The level of pain perception is about the same in all people.

3. The nurse decides to call a conference to review and discuss the physiology and management of pain. The nurses discuss the gate-control theory of pain. This theory holds that there is a regulatory process that controls impulses reaching the brain. This regulatory process is believed to be located in the
   ○ 1. brain stem.
   ○ 2. cerebellum.
   ○ 3. spinal cord.
   ○ 4. hypothalamus.

4. Various nursing measures to help promote comfort for patients in pain are discussed. Which of the following nursing measures should be selected for use in caring for a patient in pain if the gate-control theory is used to guide intervention?
   ○ 1. Giving the patient a backrub.
   ○ 2. Repositioning the patient in bed.
   ○ 3. Giving the patient a prescribed analgesic.
   ○ 4. Loosening a tight abdominal binder.

5. Common behavioral responses to pain are discussed. The body typically and automatically responds to pain *first* by attempts to improve its ability to
   ○ 1. tolerate the pain.
   ○ 2. decrease the perception of pain.
   ○ 3. escape the source of pain.
   ○ 4. divert attention from the source of pain.

6. The nurses caring for Mr. Fong find it difficult to satisfactorily relieve his pain. Which of the following measures should they take into consideration as they continue their efforts to promote Mr. Fong's comfort?
   ○ 1. Improving the nurse–patient relationship.
   ○ 2. Enlisting the help of the patient's family.
   ○ 3. Allowing the patient additional time for privacy to work through his responses to pain.
   ○ 4. Arranging to have the patient share a room with a patient who has little pain.

7. After 5 days of hospitalization, Mr. Fong is noted to be asking for pain medication with increasing

frequency and exhibiting increased anxiety and restlessness. What is the probable cause of his behavior?

○ 1. His physical condition is deteriorating.
○ 2. He is becoming addicted to the narcotic.
○ 3. His coping mechanisms are exhausted.
○ 4. He has developed tolerance to his narcotic dosage.

8. Mr. Fong tells the nurse, "If I could be among my people, I could have acupuncture for this pain." The nurse should understand that the use of acupuncture in the Oriental culture is based on the theory that it

○ 1. eliminates evil spirits.
○ 2. promotes tranquility with God.
○ 3. restores the balance of energy.
○ 4. blocks nerve pathways to the brain.

9. When Mr. Fong complains of pain at the site of his surgical incision, where in the brain is he perceiving the pain?

○ 1. In the thalamus.
○ 2. In the brain stem.
○ 3. In the cerebellum.
○ 4. In the cerebral cortex.

10. Mr. Fong experiences acute pain during his elaborate dressing changes. He is encouraged to watch television during the procedure. This strategy helps a patient cope with the pain by

○ 1. relieving the source of the pain.
○ 2. dissipating the stimulus for pain.
○ 3. decreasing the perception of pain.
○ 4. interfering with the pathway along which the pain impulse travels.

11. Mr. Fong's physician decides to switch him to oral meperidine hydrochloride (Demerol). His current dose is 75 mg IM q 4h p.r.n. What dosage of oral meperidine hydrochloride will be required to provide an equivalent analgesic dose?

○ 1. 50 to 75 mg.
○ 2. 75 to 100 mg.
○ 3. 100 to 150 mg.
○ 4. 250 to 300 mg.

12. One day, Mr. Fong states that he is about to have a migraine headache. He states that he has suffered frequent migraines for several years. Ergotamine tartrate (Gynergen) is prescribed. The nurse judges *correctly* that the desired effect of the drug is being accomplished when the patient reports that it

○ 1. aborts the attack of migraine.
○ 2. lengthens the intervals between attacks of migraine.
○ 3. relieves the sleeplessness he experienced in the past after an attack of migraine.

○ 4. decreases the visual problems he experienced in the past after an attack of migraine.

13. The pain associated with Mr. Fong's migraine headaches is believed to be due to

○ 1. dilatation of the cranial arteries.
○ 2. a temporary decrease in intracranial pressure.
○ 3. irritation and inflammation of the openings of the sinuses.
○ 4. sustained contraction of muscles around the scalp and face.

14. Mr. Fong is evaluated at the pain center and biofeedback theory is suggested. The purpose of biofeedback is to enable Mr. Fong to exert control over his physiologic processes by

○ 1. regulating his body processes by electrical control.
○ 2. shocking himself when an undesirable response is elicited.
○ 3. monitoring his body processes for the therapist to interpret.
○ 4. translating signals of his body processes into observable forms.

15. One of the *most important* prerequisites for Mr. Fong's biofeedback training is that he must

○ 1. have no physiologic deficits.
○ 2. have exhausted all other means of treatment.
○ 3. be passive and relaxed at the therapist's directions.
○ 4. take an active and responsible part in the training.

16. What will Mr. Fong be taught to observe as a sign that biofeedback is having its desired effects in terms of helping him relieve the discomfort of migraine headaches?

○ 1. Decreasing baseline respiratory rate.
○ 2. Increasing temperature of the hands.
○ 3. Decreasing heart rate and blood pressure.
○ 4. Increasing frequency and amplitude of the brain's alpha waves.

# THE PATIENT WITH PERNICIOUS ANEMIA

Mrs. Bernice Lory, 75, comes to a clinic for health care. Because of the symptoms she reports, it is suspected that she may have pernicious anemia. Mrs. Lory is accompanied by her husband, an alert, 69-year-old retired teacher.

17. If Mrs. Lory has pernicious anemia, the nurse can anticipate that a clinical manifestation she will no doubt present is

○ 1. incontinence.
○ 2. a sore tongue.
○ 3. impaired vision.
○ 4. itchy skin.

18. The nurse prepares Mrs. Lory for a gastric analysis as part of her initial assessment. A *typical* laboratory finding when gastric samples from a person with pernicious anemia are analyzed is
○ 1. a high bile concentration.
○ 2. an absence of hydrochloric acid.
○ 3. a low bicarbonate concentration.
○ 4. the presence of immature red blood cells.

19. Mrs. Lory is given radioactive $B_{12}$ in water for a Shilling test. The *primary* purpose of this test is to measure the patient's ability to
○ 1. store vitamin $B_{12}$.
○ 2. digest vitamin $B_{12}$.
○ 3. absorb vitamin $B_{12}$.
○ 4. produce vitamin $B_{12}$.

20. Mrs. Lory is likely to suffer from the symptoms of vitamin $B_{12}$ deficiency, even though she consumes normal amounts of food containing this vitamin. What is the reason for this vitamin deficiency?
○ 1. The inability to absorb the vitamin because the stomach is not producing enough acid.
○ 2. The inability to absorb the vitamin because the stomach is not producing enough intrinsic factor.
○ 3. The excessive excretion of the vitamin because of kidney dysfunction.
○ 4. The increased requirement for the vitamin because of rapid red blood cell production.

21. When the nurse plans a teaching program for the Lorys in relation to Mrs. Lory's illness, their ages are taken into consideration. A common behavioral characteristic of the elderly person that should influence the nurse's teaching program is that, when compared with a younger adult, the elderly person tends to
○ 1. adjust more slowly to change.
○ 2. show less interest in hygiene habits.
○ 3. resent needing health care more strenuously.
○ 4. be less concerned about having a physical illness.

22. Vitamin $B_{12}$ is prescribed for Mrs. Lory. The nurse should understand that the unit of measure used for prescribing dosages of vitamin $B_{12}$ is a
○ 1. unit.
○ 2. milliliter.
○ 3. milligram.
○ 4. microgram.

23. After starting therapy for pernicious anemia, Mrs. Lory asks the nurse how long it will be before she feels better. The nurse should explain that after treatment is started, relief of symptoms for *most* people with pernicious anemia who are free of complications can be measured in terms of
○ 1. hours.
○ 2. days.
○ 3. weeks.
○ 4. months.

24. Mrs. Lory asks why she cannot take vitamin $B_{12}$ orally. The nurse should explain that oral administration is *unsatisfactory* because
○ 1. gastric juices destroy oral preparations of vitamin $B_{12}$.
○ 2. oral preparations of vitamin $B_{12}$ are rapidly excreted from the body.
○ 3. a lack of intrinsic factor prevents the absorption of vitamin $B_{12}$.
○ 4. intestinal secretions impede the absorption of oral preparations of vitamin $B_{12}$.

25. Mr. Lory asks to be taught to administer vitamin $B_{12}$ to his wife. He will use the ventrogluteal site. Which of the following positions will help *most* to decrease Mrs. Lory's discomfort when Mr. Lory injects the vitamin $B_{12}$?
○ 1. Having her lie on her side with her legs extended.
○ 2. Having her lie on her abdomen with her toes pointing inward.
○ 3. Having her lean over the edge of a low table with her hips well flexed.
○ 4. Having her stand in the upright position with her feet comfortably apart.

26. The nurse teaches Mr. Lory to leave a small air bubble in the syringe before injecting the vitamin. The *primary* purpose of the bubble is that it helps
○ 1. relieve excessive pressure in the tissue.
○ 2. prevent medication from escaping from the tissue.
○ 3. disperse medication in the tissue more extensively.
○ 4. push the medication remaining in the needle into the tissue.

27. When Mr. Lory is locating the ventrogluteal site before giving the intramuscular injection, the palm of his hand should be placed on Mrs. Lory's
○ 1. iliac crest.
○ 2. greater trochanter.
○ 3. anterior superior iliac spine.
○ 4. posterior superior iliac spine.

28. The nurse teaches Mr. Lory to hold the gauze pledget against the site of the injection while he removes the needle from Mrs. Lory's muscle. This technique helps

○ 1. seal off the track left by the needle in the tissue.
○ 2. hasten the spread of the medication in the tissue.
○ 3. avoid the discomfort of the needle pulling on the skin.
○ 4. prevent organisms from entering the body through the skin puncture.

29. Mr. Lory uses disposable needles and syringes. The nurse should teach him to break the needle at the hilt before disposing of it in order to
○ 1. destroy equipment that cannot be safely sterilized.
○ 2. prevent injury to the people who handle the garbage.
○ 3. prevent its reuse by people who abuse injectable drugs.
○ 4. discard any medication that may remain in the needle or syringe.

30. Mr. Lory asks why he should not give the intramuscular injection into his wife's upper arm. The nurse should explain that the deltoid muscle is rarely used because the muscle
○ 1. is small.
○ 2. is difficult to locate.
○ 3. has many pain receptors.
○ 4. has a poor blood supply.

31. In relation to the toxic effects of vitamin $B_{12}$, the nurse should teach Mrs. Lory that
○ 1. this vitamin is remarkably free of toxicity.
○ 2. ringing in the ears is a common symptom of toxicity.
○ 3. nausea and vomiting are common symptoms of toxicity.
○ 4. skin rashes and itching are common symptoms of toxicity.

32. If Mrs. Lory did not have pernicious anemia, from which of the following foods would her body normally obtain its best supply of vitamin $B_{12}$?
○ 1. Fresh fruits.
○ 2. Green leafy vegetables.
○ 3. Meats and dairy products.
○ 4. Whole-wheat breads and cereals.

## THE PATIENT WITH HODGKIN'S DISEASE

Mr. John Ketter has Hodgkin's disease and is admitted to the hospital for staging. He is to have a bone-marrow biopsy.

33. Mr. Ketter's illness was diagnosed early in its course. Which of the following symptoms *most likely* first brought Mr. Ketter to seek health care?

○ 1. Difficulty swallowing.
○ 2. Swollen cervical lymph nodes.
○ 3. Difficulty breathing.
○ 4. A feeling of fullness over the area of his liver.

34. Hodgkin's disease typically affects individuals in which of the following age groups?
○ 1. Children (6 to 12 years of age).
○ 2. Teenagers (12 to 20 years of age).
○ 3. Young adults (20 to 40 years of age).
○ 4. Older adults (40 to 50 years of age).

35. The process of staging Mr. Ketter's illness will provide health-care personnel with information useful for *all* of the following purposes *except* that of
○ 1. prescribing the patient's therapy.
○ 2. determining the extent of the patient's disease.
○ 3. estimating the activity of the patient's disease.
○ 4. identifying the cell causing the patient's disease.

36. The nurse can anticipate that a bone-marrow specimen is *most likely* to be obtained from Mr. Ketter's sternum or
○ 1. rib.
○ 2. femur.
○ 3. vertebra.
○ 4. iliac crest.

37. Mr. Ketter's nutritional state is noted to be below par. Which of the following blood examinations is *most helpful* in determining whether Mr. Ketter's diet contains inadequate protein?
○ 1. Red blood cell count.
○ 2. Bilirubin level.
○ 3. Reticulocyte count.
○ 4. Serum albumin level.

38. Mr. Ketter undergoes radiation therapy. After he receives therapy, his skin is red and moist. Which of the following nursing measures is generally recommended for the care of affected skin areas?
○ 1. Wash the area with water and pat dry.
○ 2. Apply a mild emollient to the area and massage dry.
○ 3. Cover the area with an antiseptic ointment and sterile gauze.
○ 4. Cover the area with a light dressing or gauze bandage.

39. Mr. Ketter's treatment plan also includes a multiple chemotherapy protocol. While caring for Mr. Ketter during chemotherapy, the nurse should recognize that a *disadvantage* in the use of antineoplastic drugs is that they
○ 1. fail to distinguish between tumor cells and normal cells.
○ 2. predispose to focal infections in tumor cells and normal cells.

3. tend to accumulate, resulting in dangerously high blood levels of the drug.

4. occupy normal defenses that would normally help control the growth of tumor cells.

**40.** The chemotherapy is extremely toxic to the bone marrow. Mr. Ketter develops thrombocytopenia (low platelet count). The nurse should therefore take precautions to help control

○ 1. bleeding.
○ 2. diarrhea.
○ 3. infection.
○ 4. hypotension.

**41.** Mr. Ketter is placed in reverse (protective) isolation. Which of the following statements *best* describes the primary purpose of reverse isolation?

○ 1. Reverse isolation helps prevent the spread of organisms to the patient from sources outside his environment.

○ 2. Reverse isolation helps prevent the spread of organisms from the patient to health-care personnel, visitors, and other patients.

○ 3. Reverse isolation helps prevent the spread of organisms by using special techniques to destroy discharges from the patient's body.

○ 4. Reverse isolation helps prevent the spread of organisms by using special techniques to handle the patient's linen and personal items.

**42.** Mr. Ketter is discharged home but is readmitted frequently with exacerbations that prove to be resistant to the aggressive treatment protocol. He is finally readmitted as death appears imminent. The nurse should be aware that one of the *greatest* emotional problems hospitalized terminally ill patients face is

○ 1. fear of pain.
○ 2. fear of further therapy.
○ 3. feelings of being isolated.
○ 4. feelings of social inadequacy.

**43.** Which of the following statements *best* explains the common observation that health-care personnel avoid the terminally ill patient?

○ 1. The family members who are present are able to provide essential care.

○ 2. Staff members have failed to understand their own feelings about death and dying.

○ 3. The dying patient requires a minimal amount of physical care to be comfortable.

○ 4. It is best to avoid interrupting the patient so as to protect his right to die with dignity.

**44.** The nurse caring for Mr. Ketter concludes that he has accepted his impending death when Mr. Ketter says,

○ 1. "I have done all the talking that needs to be done."

○ 2. "I really don't think you're trying to help me anymore."

○ 3. "I'm too young to die, but I guess I have no choice in the matter."

○ 4. "I wish I were well enough to spend one more night with my friends."

**45.** Mr. Ketter slips into a coma. The nurse offers sound advice to his family when she explains that the last body sense to lapse into unconsciousness is the sense of

○ 1. smell.
○ 2. sight.
○ 3. touch.
○ 4. hearing.

**46.** When Mr. Ketter dies, Mrs. Ketter cries angrily, "Why him? Why couldn't you help him?" Authorities describe such an angry emotional outburst as typical when the bereaved relative is

○ 1. fearful of death.
○ 2. in an early stage of grief.
○ 3. covering up true feelings.
○ 4. experiencing feelings of paranoia.

**47.** When Mrs. Ketter expresses her anger, it would be *best* for the nurse to

○ 1. offer to call a relative or friend to be with her.
○ 2. remain with her and listen to what she is saying.
○ 3. leave her alone so that she can work through her emotions in private.
○ 4. explain that everything possible was done for her husband.

## THE PATIENT REQUIRING CARDIOPULMONARY RESUSCITATION

A nurse is called to her neighbor's home when 56-year-old Mr. Ben Chavez collapses. After a quick assessment of the victim, the nurse knows that cardiopulmonary resuscitation (CPR) is necessary. The nurse instructs Mrs. Chavez to call the rescue squad.

**48.** Mr. Chavez is lying in an upholstered reclining chair when the nurse arrives. Where should the victim be positioned for cardiopulmonary resuscitation (CPR)?

○ 1. On the sofa.
○ 2. On the floor.
○ 3. On the tipped-back reclining chair.
○ 4. On a mattress pulled onto the floor.

**49.** After positioning Mr. Chavez, the nurse's *next* course of action should be to

○ 1. open the victim's airway.
○ 2. elevate the victim's head slightly.

3. give the victim four quick breaths.

4. administer 15 quick cardiac compressions.

**50.** Mr. Chavez's teenaged son steps forward and tells the nurse that he knows CPR and can help. The nurse initiates external cardiac compressions while the son administers artificial ventilations. The rate at which the nurse should administer cardiac compressions should be

1. 40 to 60 per minute.

2. 50 to 70 per minute.

3. 60 to 80 per minute.

4. 80 to 100 per minute.

**51.** What is the compression-ventilation ratio for two-rescuer CPR?

1. 4:1.

2. 5:1.

3. 5:2.

4. 6:3.

**52.** The xiphoid process at the lower end of Mr. Chavez's sternum should *not* be deeply compressed when performing external cardiac compression because of the danger of lacerating the victim's

1. lung.

2. liver.

3. stomach.

4. diaphragm.

**53.** When performing external chest compressions on an adult, the nurse should depress the sternum

1. $1/2"$ to $1"$.

2. $1"$ to $1 1/2"$.

3. $1 1/2"$ to $2"$.

4. $2"$ to $2 1/2"$.

**54.** During CPR, Mr. Chavez's pulse should be checked at regular intervals using the

1. radial artery.

2. celiac artery.

3. carotid artery.

4. brachial artery.

**55.** If Mr. Chavez's chest wall fails to rise with each inflation when the rescue breathing is administered, the *most likely* reason is that the

1. airway is not clear.

2. victim is beyond resuscitating.

3. inflations are being given at too rapid a rate.

4. rescuer is using inadequate force for cardiac massage.

**56.** As Mr. Chavez's son provides rescue breathing, Mr. Chavez will exhale by

1. normal relaxation of the chest.

2. gentle pressure of the rescuer's hand on the upper chest.

3. the pressure of the cardiac compressions.

4. turning his head to the side.

**57.** Mr. Chavez is transported by ambulance to the hospital's emergency room, where the admitting nurse quickly assesses the patient's condition. Of the following observations, the one *most often* recommended for determining the effectiveness of CPR is noting whether the victim's

1. pulse rate is normal.

2. pupils are reacting to light.

3. mucous membranes are pink.

4. systolic blood pressure is at least 80 mm Hg.

**58.** Mr. Chavez receives epinephrine (Adrenalin) in the emergency room. This drug is administered *primarily* because of its ability to

1. dilate bronchioles.

2. constrict arterioles.

3. free glycogen from the liver.

4. enhance myocardial contractility.

**59.** Mr. Chavez regains consciousness and is breathing spontaneously. He is confused and very anxious. Which of the following courses of action is likely to give this patient the *most* support while life-saving measures are being performed?

1. Occasionally hold his hand firmly.

2. Ask him if he knows why he is afraid.

3. Remind him that his wife is in the waiting room.

4. Tell him that he can help most by trying to relax.

**60.** It is estimated that the maximum amount of time Mr. Chavez could have been without cardiopulmonary functioning and still *not* experience permanent brain damage is between

1. 1 and 2 minutes.

2. 4 and 6 minutes.

3. 8 and 10 minutes.

4. 12 and 15 minutes.

**61.** If the nurse had been summoned because Mr. Chavez was choking on a piece of food such as meat, she would most probably use the Heimlich maneuver (subdiaphragmatic abdominal thrusts) to dislodge the food from the victim's airway. If the nurse uses the following techniques when performing the Heimlich maneuver, which is in *error*?

1. The nurse stands behind the victim.

2. The nurse places the palms of her hands flat against the victim's abdomen.

3. The nurse allows the victim to fall over her arms as they encircle him.

4. The nurse uses pressure to produce an upward thrust on the victim's abdomen.

**62.** What is being used to force debris from Mr. Chavez's airway if he is choking on a piece of food and the nurse uses the Heimlich maneuver?

1. The victim's glottis.

2. The victim's stomach contents.

3. Residual air in the victim's lungs.

4. Pressure applied to the victim's sternum.

# THE PATIENT WITH BURNS

Mr. Arnold Paul, 25, is admitted to the hospital after sustaining burns to his chest, abdomen, right arm, and right leg. The accident occurred when gasoline ignited while he was cleaning the engine of his motorcycle.

63. Mr. Paul tells the emergency-room nurse that when he realized his clothes were on fire, he ran into his house to telephone for help. If the following courses of action had been available to Mr. Paul, it would have been *best* for him to
    ○ 1. fall to the ground and roll.
    ○ 2. take off the clothing immediately.
    ○ 3. stand still and call for help.
    ○ 4. spray the clothing with fire extinguisher liquid.

64. Which of the following would have provided the *best* emergency care for Mr. Paul at the site of the accident?
    ○ 1. Pouring cool water over the areas.
    ○ 2. Applying clean dry dressings to the areas.
    ○ 3. Rinsing the areas with a warm mild soap solution.
    ○ 4. Applying a mild antiseptic ointment to the areas.

65. The shaded areas in the diagram below indicate the burned areas on Mr. Paul's body. The nurse uses the "rule of nines" to approximate the percentage of Mr. Paul's body that is burned, which is about

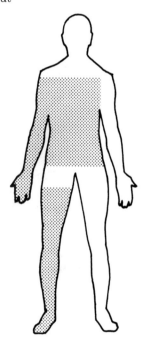

    ○ 1. 18%.    ○ 3. 45%.
    ○ 2. 27%.    ○ 4. 64%.

66. By which of the following *physical* processes is Mr. Paul losing significant amounts of fluid from the burned areas?
    ○ 1. Diffusion.
    ○ 2. Dispersion.
    ○ 3. Evaporation.
    ○ 4. Condensation.

67. Mr. Paul can be expected to have a fluid derangement during the first 2 days following his accident. The nurse should recognize that the fluid derangement is due to a fluid shift that results from an increase in the
    ○ 1. permeability of capillary walls.
    ○ 2. total volume of intravascular plasma.
    ○ 3. total volume of circulating whole blood.
    ○ 4. permeability of the tubules in the kidneys.

68. During the first 48 to 72 hours of fluid resuscitation, it would be *best* for the nurse to adjust Mr. Paul's intravenous fluid rate by evaluating his
    ○ 1. daily body weight.
    ○ 2. hourly body temperature.
    ○ 3. hourly urinary output.
    ○ 4. hourly urine specific gravity.

69. An open method is used to care for Mr. Paul's burned chest and abdomen while a closed method is used for his burned extremities. Which of the following actions should the nurse take to help prevent discomfort caused by air currents over Mr. Paul's chest and abdomen?
    ○ 1. Keeping the patient well sedated.
    ○ 2. Adding humidity to the patient's room air.
    ○ 3. Supporting the patient's upper bed linens on a cradle.
    ○ 4. Keeping the door and windows closed in the patient's room.

70. Which of the following techniques should the nurse use when bandaging Mr. Paul's hand to maintain its functional alignment?
    ○ 1. Wrap the thumb separately from the fingers.
    ○ 2. Wrap an extended fist with recurrent bandages.
    ○ 3. Curve the fingers and thumb over a roll of gauze.
    ○ 4. Secure the fingers to a flat, well-padded handboard.

71. Another precaution the nurse should take when bandaging Mr. Paul's hand is to make certain that
    ○ 1. the patient's hand and finger surfaces do not touch.
    ○ 2. the material used for bandaging is free of elastic.
    ○ 3. the patient's hand and fingers are not elevated above the level of the heart.
    ○ 4. the material used for bandaging is moistened with sterile water or normal saline solution.

72. Mr. Paul is to have whirlpool baths with dressing changes. Which of the following activities should the nurse include on Mr. Paul's care plan, to be carried out about a half-hour prior to his daily whirlpool bath and dressing changes?
    - ○ 1. Soak the dressing.
    - ○ 2. Remove the dressings.
    - ○ 3. Administer an analgesic.
    - ○ 4. Slit the dressing with blunt scissors.

73. Mr. Paul receives total parenteral nutrition (TPN) beginning on the 4th day of hospitalization. The *primary* reason for this therapy is to help
    - ○ 1. correct water and electrolyte imbalances.
    - ○ 2. facilitate rest for the gastrointestinal tract.
    - ○ 3. provide supplemental vitamins and minerals.
    - ○ 4. ensure an adequate intake of calories and proteins.

74. Mr. Paul hears physicians using the term "eschar" when speaking about his burn wounds and asks the nurse what the word means. Which of the following descriptions *best* defines eschar?
    - ○ 1. Scar tissue in a developmental stage.
    - ○ 2. Crust formation without a blood supply.
    - ○ 3. Burned tissue that has become infected.
    - ○ 4. Viable living tissue with a rich blood supply.

75. Mr. Paul is prepared for skin-graft procedures that will begin with porcine (pigskin) grafts. An advantage of using biologic grafts on burns, such as the porcine graft Mr. Paul receives, is that they appear to help
    - ○ 1. encourage formation of tough skin.
    - ○ 2. promote the growth of epithelial tissue.
    - ○ 3. provide for permanent wound closure.
    - ○ 4. facilitate development of subcutaneous tissue.

76. Which of the following conditions will have the *least* influence on the survival and effectiveness of Mr. Paul's skin grafts?
    - ○ 1. The absence of infection in the wounds.
    - ○ 2. An adequate vascularization in the grafted area.
    - ○ 3. Immobilization of the area being grafted.
    - ○ 4. The use of analgesics as necessary for the relief of pain.

77. Mr. Paul has a pedicle-flap skin graft in one area of his body. The nurse should recognize that a characteristic of this type of graft is that it
    - ○ 1. carries its own blood supply.
    - ○ 2. is made of a polyurethane film.
    - ○ 3. is derived from the skin of a cadaver.
    - ○ 4. consists of a layer of full-thickness skin.

78. While caring for Mr. Paul, the nurse observes him for signs and symptoms of a complication believed to be due primarily to stress. This stress-related complication is
    - ○ 1. infection.
    - ○ 2. gastric dilatation.
    - ○ 3. nitrogen imbalance.
    - ○ 4. gastrointestinal ulceration.

## THE PATIENT IN SHOCK

Ms. Georgeanna Bilosky, 47, has had a gastric ulcer for years. Today, when she started vomiting blood, her neighbor drove her to the emergency room.

79. Ms. Bilosky is presumed to be in the early stages of hypovolemic shock. *All* of the following assessment data indicate early shock *except*
    - ○ 1. bradycardia.
    - ○ 2. tachypnea.
    - ○ 3. restlessness.
    - ○ 4. cool clammy skin.

80. *All* of the following major pathophysiologic changes occur during the early stage of shock *except* increased
    - ○ 1. levels of glucocorticoids.
    - ○ 2. capillary fluid pressure.
    - ○ 3. secretion of epinephrine.
    - ○ 4. levels of ADH.

81. If Ms. Bilosky had blood gases drawn while still in the early stage of shock, what would the nurse expect the results to indicate?
    - ○ 1. Respiratory alkalosis.
    - ○ 2. Respiratory acidosis.
    - ○ 3. Metabolic alkalosis.
    - ○ 4. Metabolic acidosis.

82. One of the body's compensatory mechanisms in early hypovolemic shock is a shift of fluid from the interstitial to the vascular compartment. What clinical manifestation could the nurse anticipate because of this compensatory mechanism?
    - ○ 1. Confusion.
    - ○ 2. Lethargy.
    - ○ 3. Nausea.
    - ○ 4. Thirst.

83. If none of the following bed positions is contraindicated for Ms. Bilosky, which position is preferred?
    - ○ 1. Flat in bed.
    - ○ 2. Head of the bed elevated 45°.
    - ○ 3. Flat with lower extremities elevated.
    - ○ 4. Flat with feet elevated and head below the level of the heart.

84. Ms. Bilosky is receiving oxygen via nasal cannula at 4 liters per minute. Her respiratory rate is between 20 and 24 per minute. The nurse would correctly interpret this respiratory rate to indicate

1. effective fluid and oxygen therapy.
2. inadequate oxygen therapy.
3. progression into late or noncompensatory shock.
4. deterioration of the acid-base balance.

85. Fluid resuscitation is ordered for Ms. Bilosky. Dextran 70 (Expandex) is started while blood is being typed and matched. A characteristic of this plasma substitute is that it
    1. can be administered only once.
    2. has no ability to carry oxygen.
    3. must be stored in a refrigerator.
    4. does not interfere with normal blood clotting.

86. Ms. Bilosky receives an intravenous infusion of packed red blood cells and normal saline. Which of the following factors may complicate the transfusion of packed red blood cells, compared to the transfusion of stored whole blood?
    1. Decreased $O_2$ carrying capacity.
    2. Viscosity of the product.
    3. Pain at the intravenous site.
    4. Increased metabolic complications.

87. Ms. Bilosky is not responding adequately to fluid replacement. An intravenous infusion of dopamine hydrochloride (Intropin) is started. Dopamine hydrochloride is frequently the drug of choice in the treatment of shock primarily because it
    1. is a potent vasodilator.
    2. does not stress the heart.
    3. supports renal perfusion.
    4. is free of serious side effects.

88. Which of the following urinary symptoms would suggest to the nurse that Ms. Bilosky's glomerular filtration has *most likely* been impaired by the shock state?
    1. A decreased urinary pH.
    2. A decreased urinary output.
    3. An increased urinary pH.
    4. An increased urinary output.

89. Which of the following would be the *best* indication that Ms. Bilosky's fluid replacement is adequate?
    1. Urine output greater than 35 ml per hour.
    2. Systolic blood pressure above 110 mm Hg.
    3. Diastolic blood pressure above 90 mm Hg.
    4. Urine output of 20 to 30 ml per hour.

90. Ms. Bilosky's condition stabilizes, but medical intervention fails to stop the gastric bleeding. She is scheduled for surgery within the next 6 hours. Ms. Bilosky is resting quietly. The nurse ensures that Ms. Bilosky is warm but not overheated and that the light in the room is lowered. The nurse gives Ms. Bilosky and her family calm, simple answers to their questions about the surgery. Which is the *major* goal behind these interventions?
    1. Stabilize fluid and electrolyte balance.
    2. Minimize oxygen consumption.
    3. Increase patient and family comfort.
    4. Prevent infection.

# CORRECT ANSWERS AND RATIONALES

Numbers appear in parentheses following the rationales. The numbers identify textbooks listed in the references at the end of Part IV, where correct answers can be verified.

## *The Patient in Pain*

**1.** 1. Narcotic analgesics relieve pain by reducing or altering the perception of pain. They do not decrease the sensitivity of pain receptors, interfere with pain impulses traveling along sensory nerve fibers, or block the conduction of pain impulses in the central nervous system. (25, 31)

**2.** 4. Nurses typically have multiple misconceptions about patients and pain, which is a highly individual experience. Research indicates that although pain tolerance varies widely among people due to individual and cultural factors, most people *perceive* a painful stimulus at about the same point. (25, 31)

**3.** 3. According to the gate-control theory, the regulatory process that controls pain impulses reaching the brain most probably takes place in the spinal cord. (25, 31)

**4.** 1. According to the gate-control theory of pain, stimulating large-diameter cutaneous fibers in the skin appears to close the gate, and as a result pain impulses cannot travel from the spinal cord to the brain. Giving a backrub to a patient in pain reflects the gate-control theory because rubbing the back acts to stimulate cutaneous fibers in the skin. (25, 31)

**5.** 3. Responses to pain are directed initially toward the body's ability to escape or flee the source of pain. The response is typical of the fight-or-flight phenomenon, which was first described by Walter B. Cannon when he worked on theories of homeostasis and fear. (26, 31)

**6.** 1. Sometimes, all measures seem doomed to failure when a nurse is caring for patients with severe pain. Experience has demonstrated that patients who feel confidence in personnel caring for them do not require as much therapy for pain relief as those who have less confidence. Without the confidence developed in a good nurse-patient relationship, nothing seems to work; with it, often amazing results have been obtained by measures that ordinarily are only modestly effective. Other measures that help strengthen the nurse-patient relationship and promote pain relief include discussing pain with the patient, allowing the patient to help decide on a method of relief, and visiting and remaining with the patient in pain. (25, 26)

**7.** 4. Physical tolerance to an existing narcotic dose develops rapidly with frequent use. Patients then experience increased discomfort, ask for medication frequently, and exhibit anxious and restless behavior, which is often misinterpreted as indicative of developing dependence or addiction. (25, 26)

**8.** 3. Acupuncture, like acumassage and acupressure, is believed by people in the Oriental culture to help restore the energy balance within the body. Pressure, massage, and fine needles are used on energy pathways to help restore the body's balance, according to folk medicine of the Orientals. In the Western world, it is thought that the gate-control theory may be applicable to an understanding of acupuncture, acumassage, and acupressure. (5, 23)

**9.** 4. Pain is perceived in the cerebral cortex. (25, 31)

**10.** 3. Distraction cannot alter the physical transmission of the pain impulse, but it can help alter the patient's awareness of the pain experience. (25, 31)

**11.** 4. The equianalgesic dose of oral meperidine hydrochloride (Demerol) is up to 4 times that of the intramuscular dose. Although meperidine hydrochloride can be given orally, it is more effective when given intramuscularly. (12, 16)

**12.** 1. Ergotamine tartrate (Gynergen) is used to help abort an attack of migraine headache. The drug acts as a vasoconstrictor. It should be taken as soon as the patient recognizes that he is about to have a migraine headache. The drug is not used to lengthen intervals between headaches, relieve sleeplessness after an attack, or decrease visual problems after an attack. It is useless to administer ergotamine tartrate after a migraine headache has started. (12, 16)

**13.** 1. A vascular disturbance involving branches of the carotid artery is believed to cause migraine headaches. Vasoconstriction of blood vessels appears to occur first. The extra- and intracranial arteries then dilate, causing the headaches. It has been noted that a family history of migraine is present in more than half the patients with migraine headaches. (25, 31)

**14.** 4. The purpose of biofeedback is to translate body processes into observable signs and help the person using it to exercise at least some control over certain body processes. For example, the patient uses a biofeedback machine that measures his pulse rate and displays the information. He is then instructed to try to lower his pulse rate, using such techniques as listening to relaxing music or thinking of a pleasant scene. If any action he performs lowers his pulse rate, he learns to continue to do whatever it was that decreased his pulse rate. The reinforcement of learning is immediate because the person can see the results of his actions. (25, 31)

**15.** 4. Patients are taught to carry out biofeedback procedures themselves. This requires the patient to take an active and responsible part in the program. (25, 31)

**16.** 2. It has been observed that migraine headaches are relieved by a regulation of blood flow from the head to the hands. This transfer of blood to the hands increases the skin temperature of the hands because of the influx of blood. (25, 31)

## The Patient with Pernicious Anemia

**17.** 2. Patients with pernicious anemia almost always complain of having a sore tongue. The tongue appears smooth and red. (25, 31)

**18.** 2. Patients with pernicious anemia demonstrate a lack of hydrochloric acid in gastric secretions. (25, 31)

**19.** 3. Pernicious anemia is caused by the body's inability to absorb vitamin $B_{12}$. This is caused by a lack of the intrinsic factor in the gastric juices. The Shilling test helps diagnose pernicious anemia by determining the patient's ability to absorb vitamin $B_{12}$. (25, 31)

**20.** 2. Most patients with pernicious anemia have a defective production of intrinsic factor in the stomach. Intrinsic factor attaches to the vitamin in the stomach and forms a complex that allows the vitamin to be absorbed in the small intestine. (13, 40)

**21.** 1. The elderly person tends to adjust more slowly to change than does a younger person. The elderly person does not necessarily lose intellectual capacity. It has not been shown that elderly people, when compared with younger adults, are less interested in habits of hygiene, less concerned about having illness, or resentful of needing health care. (23, 34)

**22.** 4. Vitamin $B_{12}$ is measured in micrograms. One microgram is a millionth of a gram. (25, 31)

**23.** 2. Dramatically quick recovery from symptoms has been observed in people with pernicious anemia, even those who are very ill, after treatment is initiated. However, symptoms due to permanently damaged tissues will not be relieved. (26, 31)

**24.** 3. Pernicious anemia is caused by the absence of intrinsic factor, which is necessary for the absorption of vitamin $B_{12}$ in the gastrointestinal tract. In the absence of intrinsic factor, orally administered vitamin $B_{12}$ cannot be absorbed in the body. (25, 31)

**25.** 2. The position of choice to promote comfort when injecting at the ventrogluteal site is to have the patient lie on the abdomen with the toes pointing inward. This positioning promotes muscle relaxation, which, in turn, decreases the discomfort of having a tense muscle injected. (24, 36)

**26.** 4. Injecting a small air bubble after the medication when giving an intramuscular injection pushes any medication remaining in the needle into muscle tissue. (24, 36)

**27.** 2. The palm of the hand should be placed on the patient's greater trochanter when the ventrogluteal site is being located. The index finger is placed on the anterior superior iliac spine. The posterior iliac spine is a landmark for locating the dorsogluteal site. The site should be *carefully* and *correctly* identified to avoid tissue or nerve damage. (24, 36)

**28.** 3. Holding a pledget against an injection site while removing the needle helps prevent the needle from pulling on the skin. The technique makes any injection less uncomfortable. (24, 36)

**29.** 3. The primary reason for breaking a disposable needle at its hilt is to prevent it from being used by people who abuse injectable drugs. Drug abusers have been known to use discarded needles when they were not broken at the hilt before being discarded. (24, 36)

**30.** 1. Because the deltoid muscle is small, it is relatively uncomfortable to have this muscle injected. It is very easy to locate. It has pain receptors and a good blood supply, just as other muscles in the body. (24, 36)

**31.** 1. Vitamin $B_{12}$ is remarkably free of toxicity. When allergic reactions have occurred, it is believed that they were the result of impurities or the preservative in the $B_{12}$ preparation. (12, 16)

**32.** 3. Good sources of vitamin $B_{12}$ include meats and dairy products. Many fresh fruits are good sources of vitamin C. Green leafy vegetables are good sources of vitamin A, vitamin $B_2$, and vitamin $B_9$ (folic acid). Whole-wheat breads and cereals are good sources of vitamin $B_1$, vitamin $B_2$, vitamin $B_3$, vitamin $B_6$, and vitamin E. (13, 40)

## The Patient with Hodgkin's Disease

**33.** 2. A characteristic early sign of Hodgkin's disease is the presence of swollen cervical lymph nodes. The disease originates in the lymphatic system but its cause is unknown. (25, 31)

**34.** 3. Hodgkin's disease most often strikes the young adult, usually between the ages of 20 and 40 years. A resurgence in incidence is noted after age 50. The disease is seen somewhat more often in men than in women. (25, 31)

**35.** 4. Staging of Hodgkin's disease is done to determine the extent and activity of the disease in order to prescribe the patient's therapy appropriately. The nature of the cell causing the disease is studied microscopically, not by staging. (14, 25)

**36.** 4. The iliac crest and the sternum are the most common sites for obtaining bone-marrow specimens in adults. These sites are usually selected because they are easily accessible and removed from major organs, but other sites may be used also. (14, 25)

**37.** 4. Serum albumin levels help determine whether protein intake is sufficient. Proteins are broken down into amino acids during digestion. Amino acids are absorbed in the small intestine, and albumin is built from amino acids. (6, 41)

**38.** 1. Washing the area with water and patting it dry is most often recommended for the patient receiving radiation therapy. It is least irritating and most comfortable. Emollients, ointments, and coverings should not be placed over irradiated skin. (14, 25)

**39.** 1. Chemotherapy agents attack both normal and cancerous cells. Rapidly replicating cells such as bone marrow, mucous membranes, and hair follicles are at particular risk. This characteristic of chemotherapy is responsible for the multiple negative side effects associated with its use. (14, 25)

**40.** 1. Thrombocytopenia is a low platelet count that leaves the patient at a potentially life-threatening risk for spontaneous hemorrhage. (25, 31)

**41.** 1. The primary purpose of reverse (protective) isolation is to reduce the spread of organisms from sources outside the environment to the patient. (25, 36)

**42.** 3. Terminally ill patients most often describe feelings of isolation because they tend to be ignored, are often left out of conversations, especially those dealing with the future, and sense the attitudes of discomfort that many people feel in their presence. Helpful nursing measures to overcome these feelings include taking the time to be with the patient, offering him opportunities to talk about his feelings, and answering his questions honestly. (30, 38)

**43.** 2. Health-care personnel may avoid the terminally ill patient because they are uncomfortable about death and do not understand their own feelings about dying. Family members should not be expected to assume responsibility for patient care, but they should be involved in the patient's care to the extent they desire. Skilled and knowledgeable nursing care is required to make a dying patient comfortable. Interrupting the patient does not nec-

essarily interfere with his right to die with dignity. (30, 38)

**44.** 1. According to Kübler-Ross, a terminally ill patient is generally in a stage of having accepted his finiteness when he shows that he wishes privacy and that he has said everything that needs saying. It is a period of peace and tranquility. However, the patient still needs attention, and the nurse should be alert to comments that may reflect defeat rather than acceptance during this time. Being critical of caretakers typically occurs when a patient is in a stage of anger and is asking, "Why me?" The stage of depression is one of sadness, often with crying. The patient has not accepted death even though he is dying. There is an expression of "Yes, me, unfortunately." A stage of bargaining for time to do one more thing before dying occurs before the acceptance stage. The patient may appear to be at peace with death but really is not. (30, 38)

**45.** 4. Hearing is thought to be the last sense to leave the body. Although the patient is unconscious, he may still be able to hear. (25, 31)

**46.** 2. The stages of grief are fairly predictable. Anger is an early sign of grief. The characteristic expression of anger is, "Why him?" Following a stage of anger, bereaved people normally work through grief until they accept the death. (30, 38)

**47.** 2. When a person expresses anger, it is best for the nurse to allow her time to do so and to listen quietly. The angry behavior acts to relieve a charged emotional situation. Offering to call a relative or friend for the bereaved person turns a nursing responsibility over to others. Allowing the person to remain alone and explaining that everything possible was done for the loved one are of little value in an emotional situation. (30, 38)

## The Patient Requiring Cardiopulmonary Resuscitation

**48.** 2. A victim requiring CPR should be placed flat on his back on a *firm* surface. If he is placed on a surface with "give," such as a mattress, sofa, or upholstered piece of furniture, the nurse's efforts to apply sufficient pressure to compress the heart will be ineffective. In a hospital, it is usual to slip a board under a patient who is in bed before administering CPR. (25, 31)

**49.** 1. The ABCs of CPR are carried out in sequence. The "A" stands for airway, which should be opened *first* by lifting the jaw forward. Any obvious debris in the mouth, such as loosened dentures, should be removed. CPR cannot help unless the airway is open for the victim to receive air. The "B" stands for breathing and the "C" stands for circulation. Rescue breathing and cardiac compression follow immediately after the airway is open, if necessary. (25, 31)

**50.** 4. The external cardiac compression rate for two-rescuer CPR is 80 to 100 per minute so as to ensure adequate oxygenation. (25, 31)

**51.** 2. With two-rescuer CPR, the compression-ventilation ratio is 5:1, with a 1 to 1½ second pause for ventilation. (25, 31)

**52.** 2. The liver, because of its location near the xiphoid process, is the organ most easily damaged when pressure is exerted over the xiphoid process during resuscitation. The pressure on the victim's chest wall should be great enough to compress the heart but not so great that it will damage internal organs. (25, 31)

**53.** 3. An adult's sternum must be depressed 1½″ to 2″ with each compression to ensure adequate pumping. (25, 31)

**54.** 3. The carotid artery is used to check the effects of CPR. It is the nearest the rescuer, ordinarily is easily accessible, and will usually have a pulse when more peripheral pulses have diminished and are no longer palpable. (25, 31)

**55.** 1. When the airway is not clear, it is impossible to inflate the lungs during CPR. A common sign of an obstructed airway is present when a victim's chest wall fails to rise with each inflation. (25, 31)

**56.** 1. The exhalation phase of ventilation is a passive activity and will occur during CPR as part of the normal relaxation of the chest. No action on the part of the rescuer is necessary. (25, 31)

**57.** 2. The reaction of the pupils is the best indication of whether oxygenated blood is reaching the patient's brain. If the pupils remain widely dilated and do not react to light, it is likely that serious brain damage has occurred. (25, 31)

**58.** 4. Epinephrine is administered during resuscitation primarily for its ability to improve cardiac activity. Epinephrine has great affinity for adrenergic receptors in cardiac tissue and acts to strengthen and speed the heart rate, as well as to increase impulse conduction from atria to ventricles. Epinephrine will constrict arterioles, but this is not the primary reason for administering it during CPR. (12, 25)

**59.** 1. Communicating by touch, such as holding the patient's hand firmly, is often an effective way to offer the patient emotional support. Such measures as asking the patient why he is fearful and telling him a family member is nearby and to relax offer little if any emotional support to the patient in distress. (11, 38)

**60.** 2. It has been estimated that a person can be without cardiopulmonary function for a maximum of 4 to 6 minutes. After that, permanent brain damage is almost certain. To prevent permanent brain damage, it is important to begin CPR *promptly* without wasting time when a victim suffers cardiopulmonary failure. (25, 31)

**61.** 2. The nurse stands behind the victim and wraps her arms around the victim's waist. She forms a fist with one hand and places the thumb side of the fist against the victim's abdomen in the midline slightly above the navel and well below the xiphoid process. She grasps the fist with the other hand and presses the fist into the victim's abdomen with a quick upward thrust. (25, 31)

**62.** 3. Residual air in the victim's lungs is used to force debris from the airway when the Heimlich maneuver (subdiaphragmatic abdominal thrusts) is used. (25, 31)

## The Patient with Burns

**63.** 1. The priority action is to stop the burning. If the victim's clothing is on fire, the victim should drop to the ground and roll to extinguish the flames. Running is a natural response, but it only fans the flames. Standing still causes the flames and smoke to engulf the face, possibly igniting the hair and causing an inhalation injury. Falling to the ground and rolling would take less time than trying to use a fire extinguisher. (5, 31)

**64.** 1. The recommended emergency treatment of a heat burn is immersion in cool water or application of clean, cool wet packs. This helps relieve pain and diminishes tissue damage by cooling the tissue. Ice is not recommended because it may cause the patient to become hypothermic and may further damage burn lesions. Clothing should not be removed, nor should ointments be applied. Applying antiseptics or ointments are contraindicated because they may lead to further tissue damage. (5, 31)

**65.** 3. According to the "rule of nines," the patient described in this item has sustained burns on approximately 45% of his body. His right arm is calculated as being 9%; his right leg is 18%; and his anterior trunk is 18%. The total is about 45%. (25, 31)

**66.** 3. A burn victim loses much body fluid by the process of evaporation. The capillaries dilate and there is increased capillary permeability at the site of the burn. Plasma seeps out into the burned tissue and evaporation causes fluid loss. The physical processes of diffusion, dispersion, and condensation do not account for fluid loss from the site of burns. (25, 31)

**67.** 1. When a burn occurs, the capillaries and small vessels dilate, and the damage to cells causes a release of a histaminelike substance. This substance causes the capillary walls to become more permeable, and significant quantities of fluid are lost. The initial fluid derangement following a burn is a plasma-to-interstitial fluid shift. (25, 31)

**68.** 3. During the first 48 to 72 hours of fluid resuscitation, hourly urine output is the most accessible and generally reliable index of adequate fluid replacement. The adequacy of fluid volume is also assessed by monitoring mental status, vital signs, peripheral perfusion, and body weight. Pulmonary artery end-diastolic pressure (PAEDP) and even central venous pressure (CVP) are preferred guides to fluid administration, but urinary output is best when PAEDP or CVP is not used. After the first 48 to 72 hours, the urinary output is no longer a reliable guide to fluid needs. The patient enters the diuretic phase as edema reabsorption occurs, and urinary output increases dramatically. (25, 31)

**69.** 3. Bed linens should be kept off a burn wound when the open method of wound care is used. To prevent drafts over the burn areas, it is best to place a cradle on the bed and drape bed linens over the cradle. Adding humidity to inspired air, keeping the patient well sedated, and keeping doors and windows closed do not help prevent discomfort due to air currents passing over a patient's burned chest and abdomen. (5, 26)

**70.** 3. It is important to bandage a body part so that it is held in a normal anatomic alignment to prevent contractures and deformities. When bandaging a hand, this is best accomplished by curving the fingers and thumb over a roll of gauze or a commercial hand holder. See also the next item on techniques for bandaging a hand. (3, 39)

**71.** 1. When bandaging the fingers and hands, it is important that skin surfaces not touch. Allowing skin surfaces to touch interferes with normal healing and is likely to be irritating to the surfaces. Bandages on burns may be elasticized and often are used to form an occlusive pressure dressing. The bandages may be impregnated with antimicrobial agents but are not ordinarily kept moist with water or normal saline. A bandaged hand is ordinarily elevated to prevent edema. (3, 39)

**72.** 3. Removing dressings from a patient who has severe burns will expose sensitive nerve endings to the air. This is very painful. It is recommended that a patient receive a prescribed analgesic about a half-hour before the dressing change to promote comfort. (3, 25)

**73.** 4. Nutritional support with sufficient calories and protein is extremely important following severe burns because of the loss of plasma protein through injured capillaries and an increased metabolic rate. Gastric dilatation and paralytic ileus commonly occur when a patient is severely burned. Oral fluids and foods are then contraindicated. Parenteral nutrition is also used if the patient is unable to take sufficient nourishment orally or by gastric gavage. Parenteral nutrition then becomes an effective method for supplying the body with nutrients, and especially with protein, which the burn victim needs in larger-than-average amounts. (3, 25)

**74.** 2. Eschar is dead tissue, heavily contaminated with bacteria and without a blood supply. It is tissue that sloughs. Eschar has also been defined as devitalized skin. When eschar sloughs, an open wound that is almost always infected results. (3, 25)

**75.** 2. Biologic dressings, such as a porcine graft, serve many purposes for a patient with severe burns: they enhance the growth of epithelial tissues and minimize the overgrowth of granulation tissue, prevent loss of water and protein, decrease pain, increase mobility, and help prevent infection. (3, 39)

**76.** 4. The use of analgesics to keep a burn victim comfortable is important but is unlikely to influence graft survival and effectiveness. Such factors as the absence of infection, adequate vascularization, and immobilization of the grafted area promote an effective graft. (3, 39)

**77.** 1. A pedicle-flap skin graft has its own blood supply and does not depend on the recipient site for its blood supply. Examples of free grafts (that is, grafts completely separated from a donor site and without their own blood supply) include grafts of split-thickness and full-thickness skin, skin from animals and cadavers, and polyurethane film. (25, 39)

**78.** 4. Gastrointestinal ulceration is observed in about 50% of patients suffering from severe burns. The incidence of ulceration seems proportional to the extent of the burns. The ulcers are referred to as Curling's or stress ulcers. Such complications as infection, gastric dilatation, and nitrogen imbalance may occur following burns, but they are not attributed to stress. (25, 39)

## The Patient in Shock

**79.** 1. The body responds to the challenge of early hypovolemic shock by adrenergic stimulation. Widespread vasoconstriction conserves fluid, supporting blood pressure and producing the classic cool and clammy skin. Patients are typically anxious, and adrenergic stimulation causes both heart and respiratory rates to increase. Bradycardia would be unexpected. (25, 31)

**80.** 2. In the early compensatory stage of shock, the precapillary arteriole sphincters contract. This causes a decrease in capillary fluid pressure, which allows fluid to shift from the interstitial to the intravascular space in order to increase vascular volume. Epinephrine and norepinephrine are increased, resulting in increased cardiac output. Glucocorticoids and mineralocorticoids are increased. This results in sodium and fluid retention, which also increases intravascular volume. Decreased blood flow to the heart occurs in the late or noncompensatory stage of shock. (21, 31)

**81.** 1. As a compensatory measure in the early stage of shock, the patient hyperventilates in response to hypoxemia. Hyperventilation is an attempt to provide more oxygen to the tissues in the face of a decreased circulating volume. Hyperventilation increases minute volume and results in a decreased $PaCO_2$, while the $PaO_2$ remains normal. This is the classic picture of respiratory alkalosis. Metabolic acidosis and respiratory acidosis occur in the advanced stage of shock. (21, 31)

**82.** 4. The body is very sensitive to fluid balance. The fluid shift to the vascular compartment causes tissue dehydration, which stimulates the thirst center in the hypothalamus. Thirst alerts the body to the need to increase fluid intake. Since the patient in hypovolemic shock due to a gastric bleed is likely to be n.p.o., mouth care may help relieve the symptom. Nausea is not a common symptom in shock. Lethargy and confusion are signs of late shock. (21, 31)

**83.** 3. A patient in shock is best positioned flat in bed with the feet elevated to bring peripheral blood into the central circulation. The Trendelenburg position with the head lower than the heart was formerly recommended but has been found to inhibit respiratory expansion and possibly to cause congestion in the head, increasing intracranial pressure. (25, 31)

**84.** 1. Patients in early shock typically hyperventilate. A return to a normal respiratory rate with the administration of fluid and oxygen therapy indicates improvement and stabilization. In late shock, the respiratory rate is increased and the respirations are shallow. In metabolic acidosis, respiratory rate and depth are increased. (21, 31)

**85.** 2. A plasma expander such as Dextran 70 (Expandex) cannot carry oxygen. It can be stored without refrigeration and used repeatedly as needed. It can coat blood platelets and interfere with normal blood clotting. Dextran 40 has a lower molecular weight. It does not interfere with blood

clotting but is less effective as a volume expander. (25, 31)

**86.** 2. The increased viscosity of packed red blood cells requires a slow infusion rate. Administering the packed cells via a Y-connector tubing with normal saline allows the infusion rate to be increased. Stored whole blood and packed red blood cells increase the $O_2$ carrying capacity of the blood, but packed cells do so with less volume loading. The patient should not experience pain at the intravenous site. Packed red blood cells cause fewer metabolic problems than stored whole blood because the former contains a decreased amount of transfused antibodies and electrolytes. (21, 31)

**87.** 3. Dopamine hydrochloride (Intropin) is a potent vasoconstrictor. It is ideally suited for use in the treatment of shock because while it constricts the peripheral vessels, it dilates the renal and mesenteric arteries, supporting perfusion to the kidney. (25, 31)

**88.** 2. A decreased urinary output is a typical sign of impaired glomerular filtration. The pH level of the urine is not necessarily affected by shock, although the falling output is usually accompanied by an increase in urine specific gravity. (25, 31)

**89.** 1. The urinary output provides the most sensitive indication of the patient's response to shock therapy. The patient's blood pressure is a more accurate reflection of the adequacy of the vasoconstriction than of tissue perfusion. Hourly urine output should be consistently above the obligatory levels of 30 to 35 ml per hour. (25, 31)

**90.** 2. Bed rest decreases the body's need for oxygen and nutrients, substances already deficient in the patient in shock. These interventions are not directly related to fluid and electrolyte balance or to the prevention of infection. These interventions may increase the comfort of the patient and the family, but this is not the major goal. (21, 31)

## REFERENCES FOR PART IV
### The Nursing Care of Adults with Medical/Surgical Disorders

1. Andreoli KG, Zipes DP, Heger JJ, Faust S. Comprehensive Cardiac Care. 6th ed. St. Louis: CV Mosby, 1987.
2. Bates B. A Guide to Physical Assessment. 4th ed. Philadelphia: JB Lippincott, 1987.
3. Bernstein NR, Robson MC. Comprehensive Approaches to the Burned Person. Garden City, NY: Medical Examination, 1983.
4. Billings DM, Stokes LG. Medical-Surgical Nursing. St. Louis: CV Mosby, 1987.

5. Brunner LS, Suddarth DS. Textbook of Medical-Surgical Nursing. 6th ed. Philadelphia: JB Lippincott, 1988.
6. Burtis G, Davis J, Martin S. Applied Nutrition and Diet Therapy. Philadelphia: WB Saunders, 1988.
7. Christian JL, Gregor JL. Nutrition for Living. 2nd ed. Menlo Park, CA: Benjamin/Cummings, 1988.
8. Conway-Rutowski B. Carini and Owen's Neurological and Neurosurgical Nursing. St. Louis: CV Mosby, 1982.
9. Farrell, J. Illustrated Guide to Orthopedic Nursing. 2nd ed. Philadelphia: JB Lippincott, 1982.
10. Flynn JBM, Heffron PB. Nursing—From Concept to Practice. 2nd ed. Norwalk, CT: Appleton & Lange, 1988.
11. Gerrard BA, Boniface WJ, Love BH. Interpersonal Skills for Health Professionals. 2nd ed. Reston, VA: Reston Publishing, 1985.
12. Govoni LE, Hayes JE. Drugs and Nursing Implications. 5th ed. New York: Appleton-Century-Crofts, 1985.
13. Green M, Harry J. Nutrition in Contemporary Nursing Practice. 2nd ed. New York: John Wiley & Sons, 1987.
14. Groenwald SL. Cancer Nursing: Principles and Practice. Boston: Jones & Bartlett, 1987.
15. Guzzetta CE, Dossey BM. Cardiovascular Nursing: Bodymind Tapestry. St. Louis: CV Mosby, 1984.
16. Hahn AB, Oestreich SJK, Barkin RL. Mosby's Pharmacology in Nursing. 17th ed. St. Louis: CV Mosby, 1986.
17. Hickey J. The Clinical Practice of Neurological and Neurosurgical Nursing. Philadelphia: JB Lippincott, 1986.
18. Hogan R. Human Sexuality—A Nursing Perspective. 2nd ed. Norwalk: Appleton-Century-Crofts, 1986.
19. Horvath PT, ed. Care of the Adult Cardiac Surgery Patient. New York: John Wiley & Sons, 1984.
20. Kee J. Laboratory and Diagnostic Tests with Nursing Implications. 2nd ed. Norwalk: Appleton & Lange, 1986.
21. Kenner CV, Guzzetta CE, Dossey BM. Critical Care Nursing: Body, Mind and Spirit. Boston: Little, Brown, 1986.
22. Kneisel CR, Ames SW. Adult Health Nursing: A Biopsychosocial Approach. Reading, MA: Addison-Wesley, 1986.
23. Kozier B, Erb G. Fundamentals of Nursing. 3rd ed. Reading, MA: Addison-Wesley, 1987.
24. Kozier B, Erb G. Techniques in Clinical Nursing. 2nd ed. Reading, MA: Addison-Wesley, 1987.
25. Lewis SM, Collier IC. Medical Surgical Nursing: Assessment and Management of Clinical Problems. 2nd ed. New York: McGraw-Hill, 1987.
26. Luckmann J, Sorensen K. Medical-Surgical Nursing: A Psychophysiologic Approach. 3rd ed. Philadelphia: WB Saunders, 1987.
27. Malasanos L, Barkauskas V, Stoltenberg-Allen K. Health Assessment. 3rd ed. St. Louis: CV Mosby, 1986.
28. Martin N, et al. Comprehensive Rehabilitation Nursing. New York: McGraw-Hill, 1980.
29. Mosby's Medical and Nursing Dictionary. St. Louis: CV Mosby, 1986.
30. Pasquali E, Arnold H, DeBasio H, Alesi E. Mental Health Nursing: A Holistic Approach. St. Louis: CV Mosby, 1985.
31. Phipps WJ, Long BC, Woods NF. Medical-Surgical Nursing Concepts and Clinical Practice. 3rd ed. St. Louis: CV Mosby, 1987.
32. Porth CM. Pathophysiology. 2nd ed. Philadelphia: JB Lippincott, 1986.
33. Rehabilitation Nursing: Concepts and Practice—A Core Curriculum. 3rd ed. Evanston, IL: The Rehabilitation Nursing Foundation, 1987.
34. Rorden JW. Nurses as Health Teachers. Philadelphia: WB Saunders, 1987.
35. Rudy E. Advanced Neurological and Neurosurgical Nursing. St. Louis: CV Mosby, 1985.
36. Smith S, Duell D. Clinical Nursing Skills. 2nd ed. Los Altos, CA: National Nursing Review, 1988.
37. Suitor CW, Crowley MF. Nutrition: Principles and Application in Health Promotion. 2nd ed. Philadelphia: JB Lippincott, 1984.
38. Sundeen S, Stuart G, Rankin E, Cohen S. Nurse-Client Interaction: Implementing the Nursing Process. St. Louis: CV Mosby, 1985.
39. Wachtel TL, Kah V, Frank HA. Current Topics in Burn Care. Rockville: Aspen Publishers, 1983.
40. Whitney EN, Cataldo CB, Rolfes SR. Understanding Normal and Clinical Nutrition. 2nd ed. St. Paul: West Publishing Company, 1987.
41. Zeman FJ, Ney DM. Applications of Clinical Nutrition. Englewood Cliffs, NJ: Prentice-Hall, 1988.

# PART V

## Postreview Comprehensive Tests

These four tests resemble the National Council Examination for Registered Nurses (NCLEX-RN). Just as the examination is comprehensive, so are these tests. The licensure examination is timed, and you will be given 90 minutes to complete each of its four parts. Therefore, completing these four comprehensive tests in this section within 90 minutes each will enable you to simulate the state board examination.

After you have completed the four comprehensive tests, refer to the sections entitled "Correct Answers and Rationales" to reinforce or increase your knowledge and to evaluate your success. Study the rationale for each item carefully. Reading the rationales for items that you answered correctly reinforces your knowledge, while reading the rationales for items that you answered incorrectly clarifies misconceptions and expands your knowledge.

To evaluate your success on a comprehensive test, make a check mark next to the items you answered incorrectly and then determine the percentage of items you answered correctly. To do so, divided the number of your correct responses by the total number of questions in the test and multiply by 100. For example, if you answered 80 of 90 questions correctly, divide 80 by 90 and multiply by 100. The result is 89%. If you answered more than 75% of the items correctly, you are most likely prepared to write NCLEX-RN. If, however, you answered less than 75% of the items correctly, carefully examine the items that you answered incorrectly. Did you answer incorrectly because of lack of content knowledge or because you did not read carefully? Errors attributable to not reading the question carefully indicate the need to revise your test-taking strategies (see the introduction to this book). Lack of knowledge indicates the need for further review in that content area. If you identify areas in which you need more concentrated review, you can complete the questions in the section of this book devoted to that clinical area. More information about NCLEX-RN and the format and use of this review is contained in the introduction to this book.

# *comprehensive* *test* 1

Select the one *best* or *correct* answer and indicate your choice by filling in the circle with a pencil in front of the option you have chosen. If the answer you would prefer is not given, select the one you think is *most appropriate*.

A school nurse assesses 15-year-old Joan King prior to Joan's participating in an active sports program in her high school.

**1.** During an interview, Joan tells the nurse that she likes being with her friends more than with her family at home. She belongs to several clubs, talks on the telephone "a lot," likes dancing and movies, has started to date, and does volunteer work. Her many activities with her peers are likely to help Joan *most* eventually to answer the question
- ○ 1. Who am I?
- ○ 2. Can I succeed?
- ○ 3. Who can I trust?
- ○ 4. What work shall I choose?

**2.** Joan has been volunteering with some of her friends in areas considered the "slums" of the city in which they live. Which of the following measures related to disease prevention/detection should the nurse suggest Joan have done if she has not already done so?
- ○ 1. Have pertussis vaccine.
- ○ 2. Have tuberculin testing.
- ○ 3. Have typhoid fever vaccine.
- ○ 4. Have a smallpox vaccination.

**3.** When assessing Joan's physical status, the nurse measures skin-fold thicknesses. These data enable the nurse to estimate the
- ○ 1. quantity of body fat.
- ○ 2. tonus of body musculature.
- ○ 3. amount of body surface area.
- ○ 4. status of the integumentary system.

**4.** Joan says to the nurse, "Occasionally I masturbate. Is anything wrong with that?" The nurse's *best* response to Joan's question is,
- ○ 1. "No, not if you find that it relieves tensions that are sexual in nature."
- ○ 2. "Yes, because masturbation may interfere with the normal development of your sex organs."

- ○ 3. "Maybe, because masturbation could cause a disturbance in the development of your sexual identity."
- ○ 4. "We don't know. Some say masturbation may lead to a lack of interest in sexual intimacy later, but we're not sure."

**5.** After analyzing Joan's typical daily diet, the nurse determines that Joan is eating many snack foods that predispose to caries. The nurse develops a plan for helping Joan minimize her intake of cariogenic snacks. The plan should include explaining that which of the following snack foods is a good alternative to cariogenic snacks?
- ○ 1. Granola bars.
- ○ 2. Popcorn.
- ○ 3. Vanilla ice cream.
- ○ 4. Caffeine-free soft drinks.

**6.** The nurse learns that Joan's mother took diethylstilbestrol (DES) when she was pregnant with Joan. Which of the following suggestions is *most appropriate* for the nurse to make in this situation?
- ○ 1. "Don't use 'the pill' for contraception."
- ○ 2. "Let me take a Pap smear for laboratory study."
- ○ 3. "Avoid using tampons for protection during menstruation."
- ○ 4. "Please see a gynecologist of your choice as soon as you can."

**7.** Joan wears soft contact lenses. They are not the extended-wear type. She says to the nurse, "They're great. I forget about them because they're so comfortable." The nurse cautions Joan not to sleep with her contacts in place because overuse of the lenses predisposes the patient to damage of the
- ○ 1. pupil.
- ○ 2. sclera.
- ○ 3. cornea.
- ○ 4. optic nerve.

A nurse helps care for patients admitted to a hospital's emergency department.

**8.** Mr. Kevin Long suffered a cardiac arrest and is receiving cardiopulmonary resuscitation in the emergency room after being brought in by the rescue squad. On assessment the nurse notes that Mr. Long's pupils constrict when exposed to light. This finding indicates that the oxygen supply is *adequate* to Mr. Long's
- ○ 1. lungs.
- ○ 2. heart.
- ○ 3. brain.
- ○ 4. kidneys.

**9.** Mr. Joshua North comes to the emergency room with severe epistaxis (nosebleed) that he has been unable to control. The nurse should anticipate that his treatment is *most likely* to include swabbing the bleeding nostril with a cotton applicator moistened with
- ○ 1. vitamin K (AquaMEPHYTON).
- ○ 2. protamine sulfate.
- ○ 3. diphenhydramine hydrochloride (Benadryl).
- ○ 4. phenylephrine hydrochloride (Neo-Synephrine).

**10.** Ms. Edith Carrigan comes to the emergency room because of vertigo and tinnitus. During the physical assessment, the nurse will need to be particularly alert to identify supporting signs involving the
- ○ 1. eyes.
- ○ 2. ears.
- ○ 3. nose and sinuses.
- ○ 4. throat and mouth.

**11.** Ms. Karen Compton comes to the emergency room because she has been stung by a bee. The nurse observes the bee sting for initial signs and symptoms of acute inflammation, one of which *typically* is
- ○ 1. numbness.
- ○ 2. swelling.
- ○ 3. blanching of the skin.
- ○ 4. the presence of an exudate.

**12.** Mr. and Mrs. Worth bring their 4-year-old daughter to the emergency room because she has an acute ear infection. During the admission history, the nurse learns that the Worths live in a rural area where the drinking water is not fluoridated. Health teaching for the family should include informing them that a significant amount of fluoride can be obtained in
- ○ 1. tea.
- ○ 2. yogurt.

- ○ 3. citrus juices.
- ○ 4. natural cheeses.

Mr. John Carson, 64, is admitted to an emergency room of a hospital with what he believes is a heart attack. Mr. Carson describes having palpitations, a choking sensation, and tightness in the chest. He is noted to be hyperventilating and says during an initial interview, "My wife left me with all the chores and I don't know what to do. Now this. Not until she died about 6 months ago did I realize how much I need her." A physical examination is essentially negative.

**13.** The nurse analyzes the results of Mr. Carson's blood gas studies. In this situation, the blood gas studies would evidence an excessive loss from the body of
- ○ 1. sodium.
- ○ 2. oxygen.
- ○ 3. potassium.
- ○ 4. carbon dioxide.

**14.** Mr. Carson's medical diagnosis is acute anxiety attack. While planning nursing care for Mr. Carson, an important ingredient the nurse should prepare to display in her behavior is
- ○ 1. calmness.
- ○ 2. sympathy.
- ○ 3. cheerfulness.
- ○ 4. friendliness.

**15.** Mr. Carson is referred to a psychiatric clinic for help and is scheduled for counseling. He describes attacks of anxiety that usually occur shortly after work when he is preparing his evening meal. Which of the following questions is *most appropriate* for the admitting nurse to ask the patient *first* in an effort to learn how the patient can be helped?
- ○ 1. "When during the day do you most often think of your wife?"
- ○ 2. "Where do you feel most uncomfortable when you are anxious?"
- ○ 3. "Why do you think you feel anxious when returning from work?"
- ○ 4. "What do you do when you are anxious to help yourself feel better?"

**16.** During an early counseling session, the patient says, "I guess I can't make it without my wife. I can't even sleep without her." Of the following possible responses the nurse could make, the *most therapeutic* is
- ○ 1. "Things always look worse before they get better."

2. "I'd say that you're not giving yourself a fair chance."

3. "I'd bet on you to make it, given a little more time. Don't hurry yourself."

4. "I'd be interested in knowing more about what you mean when you say you can't make it without your wife."

17. During Mr. Carson's final counseling session with the nurse, he makes the comments given below. Which comment is *least reflective* of having attained success with counseling techniques?

1. "I am beginning to think I enjoy sack time (sleep) too much."

2. "Did I tell you that I met a lady and we enjoy watching TV together?"

3. "I would like to go on with these sessions. They are most interesting."

4. "It has become a game of fun to see how many different things I can do to feel better."

18. During a follow-up session with Mr. Carson some time later, the nurse judges that he is beginning to accomplish a developmental task of the elderly person when she observes that he is showing evidence of

1. trust.

2. generativity.

3. self-identity.

4. personal integrity.

A nurse is helping care for Ms. Georgia Abbott, who is pregnant with her first baby. She is in the first trimester of pregnancy.

19. Ms. Abbott's last menstrual period began on April 10. According to Näegele's rule, her estimated date of delivery is

1. December 17.

2. January 10.

3. January 17.

4. February 10.

20. Ms. Abbott complains of morning sickness. The nurse should suggest that to help relieve the discomfort, the patient should eat a diet low in

1. fat.

2. protein.

3. roughage.

4. carbohydrates.

21. Iron supplements are prescribed for Ms. Abbott. It is important for the nurse to plan to teach her that absorption of the iron is improved if iron supplements are taken with

1. milk.

2. yogurt.

3. orange juice.

4. cranberry juice.

22. Ms. Abbott says she read a magazine article about nutrition in which trace minerals were mentioned but not defined. She asks the nurse what trace minerals are. The nurse explains correctly when she points out that these minerals are important for health but are so named because they are

1. needed by the body only during childhood.

2. needed by the body in relatively small amounts.

3. easily obtained by the body when milk intake is adequate.

4. easily obtained by the body when major minerals are consumed in adequate amounts.

23. Ms. Abbott says to the nurse, "I have several beers or highballs every day. Is that O.K.?" Which of the following statements offers the nurse the *best* guide when she responds to Ms. Abbott's question?

1. There is probably no safe level of daily alcohol intake during pregnancy.

2. Drinking alcohol is probably safe during pregnancy if drinking is limited to several beers per day.

3. Drinking alcohol is probably safe during pregnancy if drinking is limited to several servings of wine per day.

4. Drinking alcohol is probably safe during pregnancy if drinking is limited to several ounces of liquor per day.

24. When Ms. Abbott is about 7 months pregnant, she and the nurse discuss her concerns about having sexual intercourse. "At times, I don't want intercourse. I don't know why. I try to remain distant from my husband at those times," she says. In response to the patient's statement, the nurse should explain that

1. sexual drives normally tend to fluctuate during pregnancy.

2. a low sexual drive is often a sign of impending labor.

3. a low sexual drive serves as nature's signal to discontinue sexual intimacies and intercourse until after delivery.

4. sexual drives normally are stronger during pregnancy and the problem should be discussed with her physician.

25. When Ms. Abbott says she tries to control her weight by omitting breakfast, the nurse should caution her against this practice because the patient may develop

1. uremia.

2. ketosis.

○ 3. hypertension.

○ 4. hyperglycemia.

**26.** Ms. Abbott asks how blood reaches her baby and why newborns sometimes need heart surgery. The nurse explains fetal circulation and includes a description of the functioning of the foramen ovale, which allows blood in the fetal circulatory system to pass directly from the right atrium to the

○ 1. aorta.

○ 2. left atrium.

○ 3. left ventricle.

○ 4. right ventricle.

Mr. John Korrick, 48, is admitted to the hospital with congestive heart failure. He presents with signs of edema and severe lethargy.

**27.** When planning care for Mr. Korrick, the nurse should keep in mind that the *primary* pathophysiology underlying the patient's illness is failure of the heart's muscles to

○ 1. contract effectively.

○ 2. maintain a regular rhythm.

○ 3. experience full refractory periods.

○ 4. initiate electrical currents properly.

**28.** Digoxin (Lanoxin) is prescribed for Mr. Korrick. While observing the patient for evidence of toxicity, the nurse should be *especially* careful to monitor the patient's

○ 1. pulse rate.

○ 2. fluid intake.

○ 3. blood pressure.

○ 4. respiratory rate.

**29.** Diuretic therapy with furosemide (Lasix) is started for Mr. Korrick. The nurse judges that the therapy is proving effective when she observes that compared with admission data obtained 3 days previously, the patient now

○ 1. eats better.

○ 2. weighs less.

○ 3. is less thirsty.

○ 4. has clearer urine.

**30.** Dietary measures need to be taken to help prevent Mr. Korrick from developing hypokalemia from diuretic therapy. Which of the following foods is the *poorest* source of potassium?

○ 1. Rice.

○ 2. Cantaloupe.

○ 3. Dried prunes.

○ 4. Grapefruit juice.

**31.** Because Mr. Korrick is on a sodium-restricted diet, the nurse teaches him to avoid certain over-the-counter preparations. Mr. Korrick's selection of which of the following items indicates that he has understood the teaching?

○ 1. Throat lozenges, such as Sucrets.

○ 2. Analgesics, such as aspirin and acetaminophen (Tylenol).

○ 3. Alkalizers, products such as Rolaids and Alka-Seltzer.

○ 4. Nasal decongestants, such as Neo-Synephrine.

**32.** Mr. Korrick's care plan states that he is to be up in a chair three times daily for 1 hour. The *primary* purpose of this order is to help

○ 1. strengthen heart muscles.

○ 2. improve arterial blood pressure.

○ 3. limit the volume of circulating blood.

○ 4. decrease the return of venous blood to the heart.

**33.** Mr. Korrick is at risk for developing a decubitus ulcer. The nursing measure that will help *most* to prevent decubitus ulcer formation is to

○ 1. reposition the patient every few hours.

○ 2. be sure the patient eats a balanced diet.

○ 3. ensure that the patient has a generous fluid intake.

○ 4. perform passive range-of-motion exercises with the patient twice a day.

**34.** Mr. Korrick's primary nurse reviews comments that Mr. Korrick made during conversations with her. Which of the following statements *best* reflects Mr. Korrick's developmental concerns at this time in his life?

○ 1. It is time to reevaluate life's goals.

○ 2. The selection of a career is important.

○ 3. Leisure-time activities are a center of focus.

○ 4. Stress associated with illness precipitates a need to settle down.

A nurse is caring for Roy Donald, who was born with a cleft lip and palate.

**35.** Baby Donald's nursing-care plan should indicate that when feeding the infant his formula, the nurse should be *sure* to

○ 1. bubble the infant often.

○ 2. hold the infant in a supine position.

○ 3. give the infant a little water before giving the formula.

○ 4. limit feeding time to no more than 5 to 10 minutes.

36. Baby Donald's lip is repaired soon after birth. It is *best* for the nurse to cleanse the suture line postoperatively with
   ○ 1. plain water.
   ○ 2. normal saline.
   ○ 3. baking soda solution.
   ○ 4. half-strength hydrogen peroxide.

37. In restraining Baby Donald postoperatively, the nurse would be considered in error *unless* she uses
   ○ 1. a vest restraint.
   ○ 2. elbow restraints.
   ○ 3. mitten restraints.
   ○ 4. a mummy restraint.

38. Roy's palate is repaired when he is 3½ years old. During the postoperative period, the nurse observes Roy closely for signs of excessive bleeding. Which of the following signs is a common *early* sign of hemorrhage after a palate repair?
   ○ 1. Excessive crying.
   ○ 2. Frequent swallowing.
   ○ 3. Refusal to take fluids.
   ○ 4. An expiratory grunt.

39. If Roy's dentition is normal, he has all his primary teeth at his age of 3½ years. What is the total number of primary teeth that Roy should have?
   ○ 1. 14.
   ○ 2. 16.
   ○ 3. 20.
   ○ 4. 24.

40. The nurse assesses Roy's motor behaviors. She is *unrealistic* if she expects Roy, at 3½ years old, to be able to
   ○ 1. feed himself.
   ○ 2. tie his shoelaces.
   ○ 3. button his clothes.
   ○ 4. control his bowels.

41. The nurse plans to discuss long-term rehabilitation for Roy with his parents. She should know that after repair of his palate, Roy will *most likely* require the help of a
   ○ 1. speech therapist.
   ○ 2. physical therapist.
   ○ 3. respiratory therapist.
   ○ 4. psychological counselor.

A nurse is caring for Ms. Gloria Smith, who is in active labor in a hospital's labor suite. It is determined that the fetal head is presenting.

42. The nurse should be prepared to help Ms. Smith throughout labor and especially when discomfort is likely to be intense. During which stage of labor do patients usually require the *most* encouragement and support because of the intensity of discomfort?
   ○ 1. During the early part of stage 1.
   ○ 2. During the transition part of stage 1.
   ○ 3. During stage 2.
   ○ 4. During stage 3.

43. About midway between Ms. Smith's contractions, the nurse notes that the fetal heart rate is between 140 and 150 beats per minute. The nurse should interpret this rate to be
   ○ 1. within normal range.
   ○ 2. below normal range.
   ○ 3. slightly above normal range.
   ○ 4. markedly above normal range.

44. Ms. Smith is moved to the delivery room. In relation to uterine contractions, at what time is it considered *best* to deliver the head of Ms. Smith's baby?
   ○ 1. Midway between contractions.
   ○ 2. As soon as a contraction begins.
   ○ 3. During the last part of a contraction.
   ○ 4. Immediately before a contraction.

45. During Ms. Smith's delivery, the umbilical cord is noted to encircle the infant's neck. If pressure is allowed to persist on the cord, a *primary* danger is that the
   ○ 1. umbilical cord is likely to tear.
   ○ 2. placenta is likely to separate prematurely.
   ○ 3. infant will fail to move through the normal delivery process.
   ○ 4. infant will fail to receive adequate oxygen.

46. After the infant is delivered, the oxytocic agent ergonovine is prescribed for Ms. Smith. The nurse judges that the medication has accomplished its *primary* purpose when the patient's
   ○ 1. uterus relaxes.
   ○ 2. blood pressure rises.
   ○ 3. uterine contractions increase.
   ○ 4. umbilical cord ceases to pulsate.

47. Shortly after the birth of Ms. Smith's baby, the nurse judges that the placenta is about to be delivered. A common sign of placental separation is present when the
   ○ 1. uterus begins to feel soft.
   ○ 2. vaginal bleeding temporarily stops.
   ○ 3. mother begins to bear down of her own accord.
   ○ 4. umbilical cord lengthens outside the vagina.

48. When Ms. Smith is ready to be moved from the delivery table, the nurse removes her legs slowly and simultaneously from the stirrups. The nurse's action is correct because this technique helps prevent

○ 1. inverting the uterus.
○ 2. cramping in the leg muscles.
○ 3. damaging nerves in the popliteal spaces.
○ 4. overstretching blood vessels in the legs.

**49.** Several hours after delivery, Ms. Smith begins to cry. She says, "I don't know why I feel this way." Of the following comments the nurse could make, the *most* therapeutic is
○ 1. "You have a lovely baby. There's no need to cry."
○ 2. "You're saying you don't know why you're crying?"
○ 3. "Shall I call your doctor for a medication to help you?"
○ 4. "Many mothers cry after the birth of a baby. You'll soon feel better."

**50.** About 6 hours after delivery, the nurse helps Ms. Smith ambulate. The *primary* purpose of walking is to prevent
○ 1. afterpains.
○ 2. endometritis.
○ 3. vulvar edema.
○ 4. thrombophlebitis.

A nurse works in a clinic for both well and ill children.

**51.** Ten-month-old Sharon Celoni is brought to the clinic by her mother because she has a cold. When examining the infant, the nurse notes that Sharon's nasal secretions are thick and sticky. To help relieve nasal stuffiness, the nurse should teach the mother to suction the nasal passages with a bulb syringe after first instilling into each nostril a drop or two of warm
○ 1. normal saline.
○ 2. baking soda solution.
○ 3. half-strength hydrogen peroxide.
○ 4. phenylephrine hydrochloride (Neo-Synephrine).

**52.** One-month-old Gregory Morris is brought to the clinic. Gregory's parents describe *typical* signs of pyloric stenosis, one of which is persistent
○ 1. cyanosis.
○ 2. vomiting.
○ 3. diarrhea.
○ 4. refusal to eat.

**53.** Brian Kelly, a well 2-month-old infant, is brought to the clinic by his mother to start immunizations. Which of the following immunizations should the mother be advised to have for her infant at this time?
○ 1. Trivalent oral polio (TOP) and diphtheria, pertussis, and tetanus.

○ 2. Trivalent oral polio (TOP) only.
○ 3. Diphtheria, pertussis, and tetanus.
○ 4. Measles, mumps, and rubella (MMR).

**54.** Ms. Peplau is disturbed because her 4-year-old child, Janice, sucks her thumb. The mother and the nurse decide on a strategy to change the child's behavior by using techniques of behavior modification. These techniques are based on the principle that the child's behavior is *best* changed by
○ 1. wrapping her thumb so that she is reminded not to suck.
○ 2. punishing the child with brief periods of isolation when she sucks her thumb.
○ 3. explaining to the child in language she understands why thumb-sucking is undesirable.
○ 4. rewarding the child if she is in situations when she ordinarily would suck her thumb but does not do so.

**55.** Bobby Sing, 11, has ringworm (tinea). Griseofulvin (Fulvicin) is prescribed for him. To enhance the drug's rate of absorption, the nurse should teach Bobby's mother that griseofulvin is *best* taken with a meal that is high in
○ 1. fat.
○ 2. protein.
○ 3. roughage.
○ 4. carbohydrates.

**56.** Two-year-old George Vasquez, the child of migrant workers, has roundworms. During clinic visits, the nurse teaches George's mother the importance of providing George with a nourishing diet and of having safe milk and water supplies and teaches her how to carry out sanitary measures in the child's environment. If, after treatment for roundworms, the child becomes reinfected, the nurse should *most certainly* determine whether the mother understands instructions in relation to the importance of
○ 1. preparing a nourishing diet for the child.
○ 2. ensuring that the child's milk supply is safe.
○ 3. observing sanitary measures in the child's environment.
○ 4. boiling the child's drinking water when the water supply is believed unsafe.

**57.** Three-year-old Sandy Korkian has cystic fibrosis. Which of the following systems of the body should the nurse assess with special care because it is the system *most frequently* involved in the morbidity and mortality of cystic fibrosis?
○ 1. The digestive system.
○ 2. The respiratory system.
○ 3. The cardiovascular system.
○ 4. The musculoskeletal system.

A nurse working in a crisis center answers a telephone hotline and sees walk-in patients also.

**58.** Ms. Betty Astry comes to the crisis center because, she says, "I feel terrible, so down. I don't know why I feel this way. I was walking by and thought you might help me." One part of the nurse's assessment of this patient includes using the Holmes and Rahe Social Readjustment Rating Scale to analyze data. If the following changes had occurred in Ms. Astry's life during about the last year, which has the *highest* Life Change Unit (LCU) value and therefore adds *most* to the risk of the patient's developing health problems?
  ○ 1. The patient was divorced.
  ○ 2. The patient's sister died.
  ○ 3. The patient was fired from her job.
  ○ 4. The patient moved to a smaller apartment.

**59.** The crisis-center nurse is helping people who have suffered from the effects of a severe flood. She interviews Mr. Wilson, whose pregnant wife is missing and whose home has been destroyed. The patient keeps talking rapidly about his experience and says, "I can't see how I can ever rebuild my life." When the nurse has the opportunity to comment, it would be *best* for her to say
  ○ 1. "If you start organizing your life now, I'm sure all will be fine."
  ○ 2. "This has been a bad experience, but go on. Tell me more about how you feel."
  ○ 3. "Let me note a few of the things you said before you continue with your story."
  ○ 4. "Think some more of what happened tonight, so that we can continue with this tomorrow. For now, let's discuss how you might rebuild your life."

**60.** Several days later, shortly after Mr. Wilson's wife has been found dead, Mr. Wilson returns to the crisis center and says he thinks it would be better to "end it all right now and join my wife and kid, wherever they are." The nurse has already determined that he has no history of major psychological problems. In terms of the seriousness of the patient's suicide threat, this patient's risk should be considered as *most probably*
  ○ 1. very low; as long as the patient speaks of suicide, he is unlikely to carry out the act.
  ○ 2. low; a person who has not had psychological problems in the past rarely carries out a first suicide threat.
  ○ 3. moderate; the patient appears to be making an effort to gain attention and extra support.
  ○ 4. high; the patient's suicide threat can be considered a call for help and should be taken seriously.

**61.** The nurse at the crisis center helps Mr. Wilson obtain psychological counseling with a nurse who makes plans to begin a one-to-one relationship with the patient. Her care plan for Mr. Wilson should indicate that she will begin the relationship by
  ○ 1. having the patient confirm her nursing diagnosis.
  ○ 2. setting goals that she hopes to attain in the relationship.
  ○ 3. defining the relationship to be developed between the nurse and the patient.
  ○ 4. planning a schedule of meetings mutually convenient for the nurse and the patient.

**62.** During one meeting, Mr. Wilson says, "I could hate God for that flood." The nurse responds, "Oh, don't feel that way. We're making progress in these sessions." When the nurse evaluates her statement, she concludes that she has *most clearly* demonstrated a failure to
  ○ 1. look for meaning in what the patient says.
  ○ 2. explain to the patient why he may think as he does.
  ○ 3. add to the strength of the patient's support system.
  ○ 4. give the patient credit for being able to solve his own problems.

**63.** One evening, the nurse answers the telephone hotline. The man speaking is Mr. Charles Johnson, who has been at the crisis center once in the past when he made a suicide threat. Mr. Johnson says, "Don't try to help me anymore. This is it. I've had enough and I have a gun in front of me now." He then hangs up the telephone. The nurse's *best* course of action in this situation is *first* to call
  ○ 1. the patient back to calm him.
  ○ 2. the police to request their intervention.
  ○ 3. his wife at work to suggest she hurry home.
  ○ 4. a neighbor to ask him to go to the patient's home immediately.

**64.** Two boys in their early teens come to the crisis center. One says, "Can you help? Our friend Jake is sick in the car. We don't know what's wrong but he uses lots of stuff to feel better." After bringing Jake into the center, the nurse judges that Jake has *most probably* been using marijuana because his eyes
  ○ 1. are bloodshot.
  ○ 2. have dilated pupils.
  ○ 3. have pinpoint pupils.
  ○ 4. show rapid movement.

**65.** In planning Jake's care, the nurse takes into consideration that his *priority* need at this time is for
○ 1. physical activity.
○ 2. large amounts of fluid.
○ 3. reassurance in a calm environment.
○ 4. close contact with his friends.

**66.** Jake also admits to using cocaine and says, "When I stop using, I feel bad." The nurse asks him to tell her more about what happens when he stops using cocaine. Which of the following effects is Jake *most likely* to describe as occurring after he stops using cocaine?
○ 1. Depression.
○ 2. Palpitations.
○ 3. Hallucinations.
○ 4. Double vision.

**67.** The nurse talks with Jake on and off for several hours. She listens closely to his comments and analyzes her findings in terms of the psychodynamics that appear to be most clearly related to the personality of someone who abuses various substances. Chemical abusers generally have feelings of
○ 1. depression.
○ 2. superiority.
○ 3. low self-esteem.
○ 4. exaggerated well-being.

**68.** The nurse has conducted classes about substance abuse and evaluates the success of her classes. Data indicate that the class to help decrease marijuana use has not been successful. The nurse attributes this *primarily* to the fact that there is
○ 1. no evidence that marijuana is harmful.
○ 2. no known cure at present for marijuana addiction.
○ 3. little social stigma attached to the use of marijuana.
○ 4. very little known about the active ingredient in marijuana.

A nurse working in a community center cares for battered children and counsels their parents. The nurse counsels Mr. and Mrs. Warner, who were referred to the center because of suspected child abuse. It is established that the child being abused is Amy, age 3. Amy has three older sisters.

**69.** During counseling, the nurse should recognize that Amy's parents give a *typical* description of the abused child when they say Amy
○ 1. tends to lie and cheat frequently.
○ 2. always keeps running away from home.

○ 3. does not show respect for authority.
○ 4. always has been different from her sisters.

**70.** The nurse also notes that the Warners present a common finding of parents who abuse children when she learns that they
○ 1. were abused children also.
○ 2. married at a very early age.
○ 3. did not want more than two children.
○ 4. were disappointed when all the children were female.

Ms. Mary Ortez, 34, recently came to this country from Puerto Rico and is hospitalized with rheumatoid arthritis.

**71.** The nurse assesses Ms. Ortez's musculoskeletal system and notes the presence of crepitation. The term crepitation refers to
○ 1. swelling in an affected joint.
○ 2. irregularity in the shape of an affected joint.
○ 3. elevated skin temperature over an affected joint.
○ 4. grating sounds when an affected joint is moved.

**72.** After assessing Ms. Ortez, the nurse establishes four broad goals of nursing care. Assuming that the goals are legitimate and based on accurate data, which should have the *highest* priority at this time for the patient?
○ 1. To teach the patient how to use correct body mechanics.
○ 2. To teach the patient to avoid rushing through activities of daily living.
○ 3. To teach the patient how to reduce her daily food intake for weight control.
○ 4. To teach the patient how to arrange her kitchen so that utensils are easy to reach.

**73.** While teaching Ms. Ortez about her illness, the nurse notes that the patient appears uninterested. The nurse changes her course of action because she realizes that a common characteristic of people from Spanish-speaking cultures is that most believe that what happens, including illness, is *most often* controlled by
○ 1. God.
○ 2. phases of the sun and moon.
○ 3. a person capable of casting spells.
○ 4. improperly balanced fluid and food intake.

**74.** The nurse establishes priorities in terms of nursing interventions planned for Ms. Ortez. When following Abraham Maslow's hierarchy of human needs, which of the following nursing measures should have *highest* priority?

○ 1. Helping the patient develop a positive self-concept.

○ 2. Encouraging family members and friends to visit the patient.

○ 3. Administering a prescribed medication for the relief of pain.

○ 4. Assisting the patient with a bath before she has physical therapy.

**75.** The nurse also uses the concept of the wellness-illness continuum while planning Ms. Ortez's care. The continuum will *best* serve to guide the nurse when she uses it to teach the patient how to

○ 1. avoid the crippling effects of her disease.

○ 2. delay the progression of disease in her body.

○ 3. select an appropriate diet so that she will not gain weight.

○ 4. use health strengths so that she can function as effectively as possible.

**76.** Ms. Ortez has been taking prescribed aspirin in large doses prior to her admission to the hospital. She complains of stomach irritation, sometimes with vomiting, from the aspirin. If her typical daily intake includes the following, the one *most likely* contributing to her gastrointestinal irritation is

○ 1. dry toast several times a day.

○ 2. a hard-boiled egg at least once a day.

○ 3. sweetened tea with each meal.

○ 4. several ounces of wine before her evening meal.

**77.** Ms. Ortez is being helped out of bed and into a chair. Which type of chair is *most suitable* for her?

○ 1. A rocking chair.

○ 2. An upholstered chair.

○ 3. A straight-back chair.

○ 4. A stool with a low back support.

**78.** To help prevent hip-flexion deformities, which of the following positions in bed should Ms. Ortez be helped to assume several times a day?

○ 1. A prone position.

○ 2. A very low Fowler's position.

○ 3. A modified Trendelenburg position.

○ 4. A right or left side-lying position.

**79.** Ms. Ortez tells the nurse, "I have so much pain right now. I tried a pill with aspirin and codeine that my neighbor gave me in Puerto Rico and it helped so much. Can't I have a pill like that here?" Which of the following statements should guide the nurse when she teaches Ms. Ortez why codeine and aspirin are contraindicated for her?

○ 1. Codeine used over a period of time is habit-forming.

○ 2. Codeine becomes a serious respiratory depressant in time.

○ 3. Codeine for the control of pain is relatively ineffective unless administered subcutaneously.

○ 4. Codeine combined with aspirin acts to potentiate the irritating effects of aspirin on gastrointestinal mucosa.

**80.** If Ms. Ortez suffered from degenerative joint disease (osteoarthritis) instead of rheumatoid arthritis, one goal the nurse should certainly strive to attain is to

○ 1. relieve discomfort.

○ 2. prevent dehydration.

○ 3. prevent decubitus ulcers.

○ 4. increase vitamin C intake.

Ms. Sonia Torry, who has signs of preeclampsia, is admitted to the hospital.

**81.** Of the following signs, the one that Ms. Torry most likely developed *earliest* and is *most characteristic* of preeclampsia is

○ 1. vaginal bleeding.

○ 2. dizziness with tinnitus.

○ 3. a sudden rise in blood pressure.

○ 4. a sharp pain in the epigastric area.

**82.** If the following orders appear on Ms. Torry's care plan, which should the nurse question as possibly being in *error*?

○ 1. Weigh the patient weekly.

○ 2. Record the patient's intake and output.

○ 3. Keep a padded mouth gag at the patient's bedside.

○ 4. Send a specimen of the patient's urine daily to the laboratory to check for proteinuria.

**83.** Ms. Torry's condition worsens. The nurse should recognize that the patient has eclampsia when she

○ 1. develops anuria.

○ 2. has a convulsion.

○ 3. goes into premature labor.

○ 4. becomes hypotensive suddenly.

**84.** Magnesium sulfate is prescribed for Ms. Torry. Which of the following should the nurse have ready in case the patient develops magnesium toxicity?

○ 1. Atropine sulfate.

○ 2. Protamine sulfate.

○ 3. Naloxone (Narcan).

○ 4. Calcium gluconate.

Mr. David Ury, 67, is admitted to the hospital. A partial gastrectomy is to be performed for recurrent peptic ulcers.

**85.** While preparing Mr. Ury for surgery, the nurse assesses him for psychosocial problems that may cause preoperative anxiety. It is believed that the *most* devastating fear a preoperative patient is likely to experience is a fear of

○ 1. the unknown.
○ 2. changes in body image.
○ 3. the effects of anesthesia.
○ 4. being separated from family members.

**86.** When Mr. Ury returns to his room from the post-anesthesia recovery room, he is alert and oriented to person, place, and time. To minimize tension on his abdominal incision and to allow his cardiovascular and respiratory systems to function optimally, the nurse should position him in bed in which position?

○ 1. Prone.
○ 2. Supine.
○ 3. Low Fowler's.
○ 4. Right or left Sims'.

**87.** Mr. Ury is to use an incentive spirometer postoperatively, *primarily* to help

○ 1. promote gastric drainage.
○ 2. decrease cardiac irritation.
○ 3. stimulate deep respirations.
○ 4. prevent metabolic alkalosis.

Mr. Arnold Kosta, a 25-year-old construction worker, comes to the emergency department complaining of back and left flank pain. Initially the pain was dull and constant, but now Mr. Kosta reports that he has periods of complete comfort alternating with periods of excruciating pain. A tentative diagnosis of renal calculi is made.

**88.** Which of the following associated signs and symptoms is *inconsistent* with a diagnosis of renal calculi?

○ 1. Pain radiating to the external genitalia.
○ 2. Uncontrolled diarrhea.
○ 3. Microhematuria.
○ 4. Nausea and vomiting.

**89.** Mr. Kosta is scheduled for an intravenous pyelogram (IVP). The nurse teaches him what to expect when the dye is injected. Mr. Kosta has correctly understood the teaching when he tells the nurse that when the dye is injected he may experience

○ 1. a metallic taste.
○ 2. flushing of the face.
○ 3. cold chills.
○ 4. chest pain.

**90.** Mr. Kosta's stone does not pass. He is scheduled for a ureterolithotomy via a flank incision. Given the specific surgical procedure, the nurse would plan to monitor Mr. Kosta postoperatively for the development of

○ 1. parotitis.
○ 2. infection.
○ 3. deep vein thrombosis.
○ 4. respiratory alkalosis.

# CORRECT ANSWERS AND RATIONALES

Numbers appear in parentheses following the rationales. The numbers identify textbooks listed in the references at the end of Part V, where correct answers can be verified.

**1.** 1. Adolescents are especially concerned with the normal psychosocial process of developing a sense of identity. They want most to know who they are. The teen years are also a time when an adolescent is learning to be comfortable with her own body, which also fosters self-identity. Teenagers prefer spending time with their peers so that ideas can be exchanged without fear of criticism from figures of authority while self-identity develops. (26, 40)

**2.** 2. Tuberculosis is found most often in the so-called slums of urban areas where unhealthy and crowded conditions prevail and where there is poor sanitation and inadequate health care. A person working in such an area should have tuberculin testing to detect a possible tuberculous infection. If the test is positive, preventive measures are started. If the person has already contracted tuberculosis, a therapeutic regimen is begun. Smallpox vaccinations are no longer used in this country, but may be advised for people traveling in certain parts of Asia and Africa. Typhoid fever vaccine is used during epidemics, in certain rural areas, or prior to traveling to certain foreign countries. Pertussis vaccine is used only for children under about 6 years of age. (26, 40)

**3.** 1. Part of an adolescent's nutritional assessment may include a study of skin-fold thicknesses, which reveals the quantity of body fat. Measurements are ordinarily taken of the triceps, scapular, suprailiac, midaxillary, and medial calf skin-folds. These measurements are compared with each other as well as with those of other adolescents. Certain conclusions can then be drawn about the adolescent's nutritional status and obesity. (26)

**4.** 1. Masturbation, which is sexual self-stimulation, releases sexual tension and helps the individual learn about her sex organs and their function. Masturbation is not considered a disease, nor has it been found to interfere with normal physical sexual development, sexual self-identity, or interest in sexual intimacy later in life. (26, 40)

**5.** 2. Popcorn is an example of a minimally cariogenic snack. Other snacks that help prevent caries include raw vegetables, fresh fruits, whole-grain cereals and breads, sunflower seeds, plain yogurt, and natural cheeses. Vanilla ice cream, granola bars, and soft drinks, including those that are caffeine free, are examples of cariogenic nutrients. (26, 40)

**6.** 4. Diethylstilbestrol (DES) is contraindicated during pregnancy. Studies have shown that daughters of women who used DES during pregnancy may have an increased risk of developing vaginal or cervical adenocarcinoma. The nurse should refer the adolescent female described in this item to a gynecologist for examination because of her perinatal history. (33)

**7.** 3. Soft contact lenses that are not of the extended-wear type and hard contact lenses should be removed daily and should not be kept in place while sleeping. Overuse is likely to lead to corneal ulceration and abrasions. Contact lenses do not damage the pupils, sclera, or optic nerve. (28, 40)

**8.** 3. When pupils constrict in the presence of light while the patient is receiving cardiopulmonary resuscitation, it is safe to judge that the brain is receiving an adequate flow of oxygenated blood. A sufficient flow of oxygen to the brain is vital to sustain life. (6, 34)

**9.** 4. Phenylephrine hydrochloride (Neo-Synephrine) is an adrenergic agent and, when placed on the nasal mucosa, acts as a vasoconstrictor. Therefore, a cotton applicator moistened with the solution is often used to help control a nosebleed. Additional treatment includes having the patient sit upright, having him breathe through his mouth and refrain from talking, and compressing the outer part of his nose against the septum. Vitamin K is essential for prothrombin production in the body but is not used when hemorrhage is caused by a deficiency of the vitamin. Protamine sulfate is a heparin antidote and acts to prolong clotting time. Diphenhydramine hydrochloride (Benadryl) is an antihistamine often used to relieve the symptoms of a cold. (6, 17)

**10.** 2. Vertigo (dizziness) and tinnitus (ringing in the ears) are abnormal findings ordinarily associated with a disturbance in the proper functioning of the ears. (6, 28)

**11.** 2. Cardinal signs of an acute inflammation include swelling, warmth, pain (not numbness), redness (not blanching of the skin), and a loss of function in the part involved. An exudate is not typical of an acute inflammation but often occurs when an inflammation becomes chronic. (6, 28)

**12.** 1. Tea contains a significant amount of fluoride. Foods in general contain very limited amounts. In most communities water is fluoridated, an effective and safe practice that helps prevent dental caries. Fluoride drops or tablets may also be used to provide fluorine, but the nurse should observe careful safety measures while using them because children accidentally may take them in sufficient quantities to result in serious toxicity. (36, 42)

**13.** 4. Hyperventilation causes the loss of an excessive amount of carbon dioxide through the respiratory process. This results in a decrease in the carbonic acid content of the blood. The kidneys will try to compensate by eliminating bicarbonate to maintain normal carbonic acid-bicarbonate ratios. If compensatory efforts are insufficient, the patient will develop respiratory alkalosis. (6, 23, 28)

**14.** 1. Nurses caring for a very anxious patient should be calm and sufficiently authoritative to help the patient understand that they can provide controls for the patient when he cannot do so on his own. If possible, the patient should be kept in a quiet, relatively small room, because he is already overwhelmed by external stimuli. (16, 36)

**15.** 4. The nurse should first assess the patient who is subject to anxiety attacks by determining what behavior ordinarily relieves his anxiety. However, nursing care of an anxious patient must ultimately take into account all parts of the patient's anxiety, including what leads to attacks and what happens during an attack. Then the nurse can help the patient understand his anxiety, what personal needs may be unmet, and how to cope with his problem with behavior that is more satisfactory than having an anxiety attack. (3, 36)

**16.** 4. The nurse is using a technique of communication to help the patient explore his feelings when she says she is interested in knowing more about his problem. Clichés and statements that make unwarranted judgments about the patient are rarely, if ever, helpful. (36)

**17.** 3. Interventions have been effective when the patient has learned various ways to help himself feel and sleep better and is finding interests outside himself and his own activities of daily living. The patient is expressing uncertainty and continued dependence on the nurse when he says he would like to continue with the sessions. The nurse will wish to explore these feelings of dependence to determine whether further counseling is indicated or whether the patient's strengths in handling and preventing anxiety are sufficiently strong that he can cope with problems effectively on his own. (36)

**18.** 4. Erik Erikson is credited with a theory that describes typical developmental tasks during various ages of life. The elderly person experiences positive resolution of a central task by developing integrity rather than falling into a state of despair. Typical signs of personal integrity include finding meaningfulness in life and finding new interests and

relationships. Developing trust rather than suffering with mistrust typically occurs during infancy; self-identity is an important developmental task of teenagers; and generativity is a task typical of people during middle adulthood. (36)

**19.** 3. According to Näegele's rule, the estimated date of confinement is determined as follows: First day of the last menstrual period minus 3 calendar months plus 7 days plus 1 year. The patient's last menstrual period began on April 10; April 10 minus 3 calendar months is January 10; add 7 days. The patient's estimated date of confinement is January 17 of the following year. (27)

**20.** 1. Small, frequent low-fat meals are recommended to help relieve morning sickness. Other remedies include eating a dry starchy food, such as crackers or melba toast, before arising in the morning, limiting fluid intake with meals, eating high-protein or high-carbohydrate meals, and eating small meals five or six times a day. (27)

**21.** 3. Taking iron with citrus fruit or its juice, such as orange juice, improves the absorption of the mineral. Ferric iron is poorly absorbed (that is, it has low bioavailability within the intestinal tract). However, absorption is improved in the presence of an acidic medium. Vitamin C (ascorbic acid) has been found to be particularly helpful in reducing $Fe^{+++}$ to $Fe^{++}$ for better absorption of supplemental iron as well as of dietary iron. (1, 22, 27, 42)

**22.** 2. Trace minerals are also sometimes called micronutrients. They are so named because the body needs relatively small amounts of them for health. Examples of trace minerals include iron, iodine, fluorine, zinc, copper, and chromium. They are usually obtained in adequate amounts when a wellbalanced, nutritious diet is eaten. Milk is very poor in iron and copper, two trace minerals required by the body for health. Micronutrients are required throughout life. They do not derive from major minerals. (27)

**23.** 1. There is no safe level of alcohol consumption during pregnancy. It has been demonstrated that alcohol crosses the placenta, although it is not known whether it is the ethanol or the result of alcohol breakdown, acetaldehyde, that causes problems. Outright alcoholism is not required to place a fetus at risk. The use of alcohol during pregnancy includes these risks: changes in the development and growth of the fetus, low birth weight, short stature, small head, and various joint and heart defects, mental retardation, motor dysfunction, and spontaneous abortion. (27)

**24.** 1. Sexual drives during pregnancy tend to fluctuate. A pregnant woman may not wish to have sexual intercourse, for no specific reason. Communication between the expectant parents is essential and both should understand that sexual drives normally fluctuate during pregnancy. A man may also experience emotional instability from time to time during his partner's pregnancy. (27)

**25.** 2. A condition sometimes called accelerated starvation may occur if a pregnant woman does not eat for 12 hours or more. Blood glucose and alanine levels tend to fall below normal and plasma-free fatty acids increase. The resulting condition, ketosis, places the normal intellectual development of the fetus at risk. Everyone, and especially pregnant women, should eat regularly and control their weight, if it becomes necessary, by means other than skipping meals. (27)

**26.** 2. The blood enters the fetal heart from the inferior vena cava and empties into the right atrium. From there, most blood goes directly into the left atrium through the foramen ovale. Blood then flows to the left ventricle and from there to the aorta. The foramen ovale is a special fetal structure that helps much blood to bypass pulmonary circulation. Normally, the foramen ovale closes at birth. (27)

**27.** 1. The primary pathophysiology underlying cardiac failure involves impaired contractural properties of heart muscles. A variety of causes can impair heart muscle function, such as atherosclerosis, hypertension, and inflammatory or degenerative muscle disease. The heart muscles would be in a state of sustained contraction if they failed to have periods of refraction. This is not part of the pathophysiology of congestive heart failure. The heartbeat is initiated in the SA node, which consists of specialized cells controlled by the sympathetic and parasympathetic nervous system. These cells start an impulse that sweeps through the heart's musculature. (6, 23)

**28.** 1. Common signs and symptoms of digitalis toxicity include bradycardia, anorexia, nausea, vomiting, headaches, and general malaise. Urinary output should also be carefully monitored for patients taking digitalis preparations when they have poor renal function and electrolyte depletion. (6, 17)

**29.** 2. The primary purpose of a diuretic for patients with congestive heart failure is to promote the excretion of sodium and water through the kidneys. As a result, excessive body water that tends to accumulate in patients with congestive heart failure is eliminated, and this loss of water will cause the patient to lose weight. Monitoring the patient's weight daily helps evaluate the effectiveness of diuretic therapy. (6, 17)

**30.** 1. Practically all foods contain at least some potassium. However, rice is very low in potassium.

Bananas, grapefruit and orange juice, cantaloupe, nectarines, dried prunes and figs, potatoes, and tomato juice are examples of foods especially rich in potassium. (37, 42)

**31.** 3. Alkalizers, such as Rolaids and Alka-Seltzer, have a high sodium content and should be avoided by patients on a sodium-restricted diet. Patients should be taught to read labels carefully. Other preparations that may contain sodium include cough syrups, laxatives, and sedatives. A patient on a sodium-restricted diet should consult a physician when there is a question about any over-the-counter preparation. (6, 13)

**32.** 4. Having the patient sit in a chair and keeping the head of his bed elevated while he is in bed help decrease the return of venous blood to the heart and lungs. This relieves pulmonary congestion and gives the diaphragm maximum space to function. Sitting in a chair does not limit the volume of circulating blood, improve arterial blood pressure, or increase the strength of heart muscles. (6, 23)

**33.** 1. The most important measure to help prevent decubitus ulcer formation is to be sure the patient whose activity is limited is repositioned frequently, as often as every 1 to 2 hours. A decubitus ulcer is an area of cellular necrosis caused by the lack of blood circulation to the involved area. Blood circulation is impeded by pressure on the site, usually over bony prominences, causing collapse of blood vessels, especially the arterioles and capillaries. As a result of the poor circulation, the cells are inadequately nourished and eventually die. Adequate hydration and nutrition are also important because healthy cells are less likely to deteriorate. However, unless pressure over an at-risk area is relieved, the cells will die. (20, 34)

**34.** 1. During middle adulthood (45 to 55 years of age), most people go through a process of taking stock. They become very aware of time left to live. This appears to be especially true of men. Death now becomes more of a reality instead of something that happens only to others. Selecting career goals and leisure-time activities and settling down are more typical concerns of younger adults. (6, 19)

**35.** 1. When feeding an infant with a cleft lip and palate, the nurse should bubble the infant often because he swallows large amounts of air due to his open lip and palate. To prevent aspiration, the infant should be held in an upright position and fed slowly. A little water is ordinarily offered after a formula feeding to help wash away formula that may have adhered to the clefts. (25, 40)

**36.** 4. A half-strength hydrogen peroxide solution is recommended to clean the suture line after the repair of a cleft lip. The foaming action created by the release of oxygen from the solution helps break up and remove debris from the suture line. (25, 32)

**37.** 2. To help prevent injury to the operative area following surgery for the repair of a cleft lip, the nurse should use elbow restraints or a clove-hitch restraint on the infant. Mitten restraints and a vest restraint still allow the infant to touch the operative site. A mummy restraint is inappropriate because it does not allow for movement, and the infant needs some activity. Mummies are used for a procedure such as insertion of a needle into a scalp vein or a jugular vein. (25, 40)

**38.** 2. Frequent swallowing is a common early sign of excessive bleeding following the repair of a cleft palate. The youngster may be fussy and cry and may not be interested in taking fluids, but these behaviors do not necessarily indicate hemorrhage. An expiratory grunt is abnormal but unrelated to excessive bleeding. (25)

**39.** 3. At about 3 to 4 years of age, a child normally has all of his primary teeth, which total 20 in number. By about 5 years of age, the child normally has 24 teeth (that is, the 20 primary teeth and 4 permanent molars). (25, 40)

**40.** 2. It is unrealistic to expect a 3½-year-old child to be able to tie his shoelaces. This fine motor skill is usually not accomplished until a child is about 5 years old. A 3½-year-old can be expected to be able to button clothes and feed himself. He also can control his bowel movements but may still occasionally have accidents. (25, 40)

**41.** 1. Difficulties with speech and hearing are common following the repair of a cleft palate. For some children, speech therapy may be required for years. (32, 40)

**42.** 2. The transition part of stage 1 is ordinarily the most difficult period of labor. It is the time when patients are most likely to lose control. The mother also usually suffers from fatigue during transition, may be nauseated, and has very forceful contractions. (27)

**43.** 1. The normal range for the fetal heart rate about midway between contractions is between 120 and 160 beats per minute. During and immediately after a contraction, the rate is normally lower; this lower rate tends to be greater for primigravidas than for multigravidas. (27)

**44.** 1. It is best to deliver an infant's head slowly about midway between uterine contractions. Ritgen's technique is one maneuver that is often used. When the infant's head causes distention of the perineum as it delivers, downward pressure is placed on the occiput while forward pressure is placed on the

baby's chin. This technique allows control of the head and facilitates extension of the head to help prevent perineal lacerations. (27)

**45.** 4. If the umbilical cord encircles the infant's neck, the pressure of the infant on the cord will interfere with the infant's oxygen supply. If the cord is too tightly encircled to be slipped over the head, it is ordinarily clamped and cut and the infant is delivered quickly before asphyxiation results. (27)

**46.** 3. Oxytocic agents are sometimes used after the delivery of an infant to stimulate uterine contractions and to minimize blood loss. Ergonovine causes a rise in blood pressure, but it is not used for this purpose after delivery. A derivative of ergonovine, methylergonovine maleate (Methergine), is sometimes used because it is believed to cause less of an increase in blood pressure than does ergonovine. (27)

**47.** 4. Common signs of placental separation include a lengthening of the umbilical cord outside of the vagina; a firming of the uterus; sudden vaginal bleeding (usually a spurt or a trickle); an elevation of the uterus into the abdomen; and a change in the shape of the uterus from a disclike to a globular shape. The patient is asked to bear down to help expel the placenta because the urge to do so does not ordinarily occur spontaneously. (27)

**48.** 2. Cramping and an uncomfortable twitching of leg muscles are prevented when a patient's legs are removed from stirrups slowly and simultaneously. The technique is not used to prevent stretching of blood vessels, damage to nerves in the popliteal spaces, or inversion of the uterus. (27)

**49.** 2. When a mother cries soon after the delivery of her baby and says she does not know why she is crying, the nurse should encourage the patient to talk about her feelings. By validating the patient's statements, the nurse provides an open channel of communication. Various emotional reactions shortly after delivery are not uncommon and help relieve tension. The nurse ignores the mother's feelings when she tells her there is no need to cry, asks if she should obtain medications, or explains that her reactions are normal. (27)

**50.** 4. Early ambulation is credited with helping prevent thrombophlebitis and pulmonary embolus. Early ambulation also helps prevent subinvolution of the uterus and complications related to urinary and intestinal elimination. Most women feel less weak and psychologically better with early activity after delivery. (27)

**51.** 1. Instilling a few drops of normal saline into each nostril helps loosen nasal secretions, making it easier to suction them with a bulb syringe. Hydrogen peroxide and baking soda are not recommended for this procedure. Phenylephrine hydrochloride (Neo-Synephrine) relieves a stuffy nose because it acts as a nasal decongestant. It is not used to loosen nasal secretions. (40)

**52.** 2. The most typical sign of pyloric stenosis is persistent vomiting, which is often projectile. Other signs include small, constipated stools, failure to gain weight, hunger, a hard mass in the abdomen, and peristalsis visible on the wall of the abdomen. Signs are due to a constricture at the pyloric sphincter that prevents food from entering the duodenum properly. The vomitus may contain blood but does not contain bile. Usual therapy is a surgical procedure to enlarge the opening at the site of the obstruction. (25, 40)

**53.** 1. For a healthy infant, trivalent oral polio (TOP) and diphtheria, pertussis, and tetanus (DPT) should be given when the infant is about 2 months old. Boosters are recommended when the infant is 4 and 6 months old. Immunization for measles, mumps, and rubella (MMR) usually should be given when the child is about 15 months old. (25, 40)

**54.** 4. Behavior modification is based on the principle that rewarded behavior is reinforced and promotes change from undesirable behavior. Explaining, punishing, and using a technique to remind a child of thumb-sucking are not related to change when techniques of behavior modification are used. (32, 40)

**55.** 1. In most instances, taking food with a drug tends to decrease the rate of absorption of the drug. One exception is griseofulvin (Fulvicin), an antifungal agent. For reasons not entirely clear, the drug is absorbed more quickly when it is given with a high-fat meal. (33)

**56.** 3. Roundworms (*Ascaris lumbricoides*) are spread when sanitary conditions in the environment are poor. The eggs of the roundworm are ingested, either directly or indirectly. Reinfestation is believed to recur most often when playing areas are contaminated, hands are not washed, and disposal of human feces is poor. (32, 40)

**57.** 2. Complications involving the respiratory system most often cause morbidity and mortality in the child with cystic fibrosis. Many pathologic changes occur in the respiratory system as a result of the disease, such as loss of cilia, an increase in mucus-secreting cells with the production of copious amounts of sticky secretions, bronchiectasis, bronchiolitis, and atelectasis. (32, 40)

**58.** 1. A change in marital status carries the highest score in terms of risk of developing health problems, according to the Holmes and Rahe Social Readjustment Scale. The death of a spouse has a 100-point value; divorce, 73 points; marital separation, 65 points; the death of a family member, 63 points; being fired from a job, 47 points; changing residence, 20 points. If the patient described in this situation has a total score of 203, she is going through a moderate life crisis. A score of 300 or more suggests a major life crisis. (3, 36)

**59.** 2. At the time of a major crisis, such the flood described in this item, the person suffering great loss is best helped by being allowed time to talk out his experience and describe his feelings. Telling the patient to think more about what happened for further discussion the next day and suggesting he start to rebuild his life is nurse-centered rather than patient-centered and is unlikely to help the patient. Asking the patient to stop talking so that the nurse can write notes places more emphasis on her needs than on those of the patient. Clichés such as "Everything will be fine" are not helpful. (3, 36)

**60.** 4. The patient who threatens suicide should be considered at high risk, and his threat should be taken seriously as a call for help. It is untrue that a suicide threat is only a bid for attention, that people who talk about suicide will not do it, and that without a history of psychological problems a first threat is very unlikely to be carried out. (3, 36)

**61.** 3. After determining that a nurse and a patient will collaborate in a one-to-one relationship, the relationship should be defined so that the patient and nurse become committed to a relationship that each can maintain. After the relationship is defined, other actions, such as scheduling meetings, setting goals, and developing nursing diagnoses, can be performed. Defining the relationship is described as the first phase of a working relationship, which is the orientation phase. This phase is followed by the working phase and ends with a resolution phase. (3, 36)

**62.** 1. Behavior is caused, and therefore people handle problems and situations in terms of what they consider important to them, not necessarily in terms of what others may think is important. Such clichés as "Don't feel that way" are rarely helpful because they ignore the patient's feelings and his interpretation of the situation in which he finds himself. They fail to focus on the patient and what he feels. (3, 36)

**63.** 2. The nurse's first responsibility when a patient threatens suicide is to do whatever can most quickly be done to protect the patient from himself. When the nurse is in a crisis center and the patient is at home, it is best to call the police to intervene. They are able to reach the patient quickly and are familiar with handling a person threatening to destroy himself. Outsiders, such as a neighbor or even the patient's wife, may be hurt, especially when the patient has a weapon. It is appropriate to err on the side of safety rather than to assume the patient is not serious about a suicide threat. (3, 36)

**64.** 1. Marijuana causes dilatation of arterioles, and this causes a marked redness of the eyes; they become bloodshot. Heroin characteristically causes pinpoint pupils, cocaine causes dilatation of the pupils, and phencyclidine (PCP) causes rapid eye movements. (32, 36)

**65.** 3. A person suffering from the ill effects of chemical abuse needs reassurance, acceptance, and a calm, quiet environment. Various stimuli, physical activities, and fluids are less likely to provide the kind of environment the patient needs at this time. (36)

**66.** 1. Depression typically occurs after a person stops using cocaine. Some people experience "cocaine bugs" and describe bugs crawling under their skin. Hallucinations, double vision, and palpitations are not associated with cocaine withdrawal. (36)

**67.** 3. People who abuse chemicals most often reveal feelings of self-failure, poor self-esteem, dependency, and passivity. They tend to be seeking experiences that will alter these feelings and often turn to chemicals to accomplish their goal. These feelings often make substance abuse a difficult problem with which to deal because the chemicals meet an important need in the mind of the abuser. (36)

**68.** 3. It is estimated that millions of Americans use marijuana regularly, and many people believe it should be legalized. Punitive measures and educational efforts to decrease its use have not fared well, most probably because little social stigma is attached to its use. Marijuana is not generally considered addictive, but it may cause psychological dependency. The active ingredient in marijuana has been well studied and its effects have been documented. Marijuana is not without harmful effects. (36)

**69.** 4. A very typical finding when the parents of abused children are interviewed is that they describe the abused child as being different from other children, including her siblings. They will frequently say the child whines a lot, cries, and is sullen. When a child is being abused, very often the nurse will find other crisis or near-crisis situations in the home, such as unemployment, financial strains, alcoholism, and the like. If one child in a family is being abused, the siblings are at risk for being abused also. (32, 36)

**70.** 1. Child abuse can be a vicious cycle because abused children very often become abusive par-

ents. Marrying at an early age, disappointment on the part of parents at the sex of their children, and having unwanted children are not necessarily associated with child abuse. (32, 36)

**71.** 4. Crepitation, or crepitus, is used to describe various abnormal sounds or noises. In patients with rheumatoid arthritis, a characteristic grating sound is heard when an affected joint is moved. The sound is caused by the rubbing together of dry synovial surfaces in the joint. Affected joints in patients with rheumatoid arthritis also present such typical signs as tenderness, warmth of the skin, and irregularities in the shape of joints. (6, 24)

**72.** 3. All the goals described in this item are typical and appropriate for a patient with rheumatoid arthritis. However, for overweight patients with rheumatoid arthritis, it is especially important to help them lose weight, because obesity causes such stress on weight-bearing joints that further damage is likely to occur. (6, 23)

**73.** 1. Most people of Spanish-speaking cultures accept religion as a fundamental part of their lives. They tend to believe that God gives health and allows illness for a reason. Illness may be considered a punishment or a cross to bear. This aspect of the culture could cause a patient to show little interest in learning about illness. (12, 19)

**74.** 3. Abraham Maslow's theory about the hierarchy of human needs is often helpful in establishing priorities in nursing care. Maslow ranks physical needs—the need for oxygen, food, water, elimination, rest, sleep, and freedom from pain—as having the highest priority. The needs for safety, security, belonging, affection, esteem, and self-actualization, according to Maslow, are met only after physical needs are first met. (6, 23)

**75.** 4. It is important for the nurse to plan care for a patient with rheumatoid arthritis that emphasizes how the patient can avoid the crippling effects of the disease, delay the progression of the disease, and select an appropriate diet to avoid weight gain. But the concept of the wellness-illness continuum emphasizes teaching how a patient can use remaining health strengths so that, despite limitations due to a disease, the patient can still function as effectively as possible. (6, 23)

**76.** 4. Gastrointestinal irritation is a common side effect of many drugs, including aspirin, especially when aspirin is taken in large doses. Such signs as anorexia, nausea, vomiting, diarrhea, and constipation are also common. A few drugs, when taken with other chemicals, are especially likely to cause gastrointestinal irritation, to the point of doing direct damage to gastric mucosa. One such combination is aspirin and alcoholic beverages. (37, 42)

**77.** 3. To help prevent flexion deformities, a straight-back chair with a seat that allows the feet to rest flat on the floor is recommended. Upholstered chairs, rocking chairs, and stools with back supports do not support the body in proper alignment as well as a straight-back chair does. (6, 34)

**78.** 1. To help prevent flexion deformities, patients with rheumatoid arthritis should lie in a prone position in bed several times a day for about a half-hour. This positioning helps keep the hips and the knees in an extended position and prevents joint flexion. (6, 23)

**79.** 1. For patients with chronic diseases who are very likely to require medications for pain control over a period of time, narcotic analgesics, such as codeine, are contraindicated because of their habit-forming characteristics. Codeine is an effective analgesic and is well absorbed from the gastrointestinal tract when administered orally. Codeine has not been found to potentiate the irritating effects of aspirin on gastrointestinal mucosa, although some patients experience epigastric distress after taking it orally. When the patient in this item mentions using a neighbor's medication, the nurse should plan to teach her about the dangers of using medications prescribed for others. (6, 17)

**80.** 1. The most common symptom of degenerative joint disease (osteoarthritis) is pain. Discomfort generally decreases with rest. In contrast, patients with rheumatoid arthritis usually feel more comfortable if they are active. The pain associated with osteoarthritis is related to joint degeneration and muscle spasms. Analgesics are almost always required to control pain and discomfort. (6, 23)

**81.** 3. The three classic signs of preeclampsia are sudden hypertension (usually the earliest sign), albuminuria, and edema. Pain in the epigastric area is typically a late sign. Because preeclampsia is a serious complication of pregnancy, it is very important for every pregnant woman to have her blood pressure checked regularly and frequently during pregnancy so that the complication can be discovered and treated early. (30)

**82.** 1. Because a preeclamptic patient should be observed carefully for water retention and edema, she should be weighed daily. Typical orders when preeclampsia is present include keeping a padded mouth gag at the patient's bedside in case of a convulsion, recording the patient's intake and output, and performing a daily urinalysis for proteinuria. (30)

**83.** 2. A patient is considered to have eclampsia when she has a convulsion. Eclampsia is almost always preceded by preeclampsia. (30)

**84.** 4. The antidote for magnesium sulfate is calcium gluconate. The antidote should be kept ready whenever a patient receives magnesium sulfate. Symptoms of magnesium excess include lethargy, impaired respirations, and coma. Protamine sulfate is an antidote for heparin. Naloxone (Narcan) is an antidote for opiates. (22, 30)

**85.** 1. Anxieties in preoperative patients may be caused by many different fears, such as fear of the effects of anesthesia, the effects of surgery on body image, being separated from family and friends, job loss and disabilities, pain, and death. But the fear of the unknown most probably looms as the greatest because the patient feels helpless and doomed. Therefore, an important part of preoperative nursing is to assess the patient for anxieties and explore possible causes. Interventions can then be used to help the patient and to offer him emotional support so that he is in the best possible psychological condition for surgery. (6, 19)

**86.** 3. A patient who has had abdominal surgery is best placed in a low Fowler's position postoperatively. This positioning relaxes abdominal muscles and provides for maximum respiratory and cardiovascular function. (6, 19)

**87.** 3. Incentive spirometry is used postoperatively to promote lung expansion. The machine is set at a preselected target, and the patient is taught proper breathing techniques preoperatively so that he can reach the target. (6, 19)

**88.** 2. Uncontrolled diarrhea is not consistent with a diagnosis of renal calculi. Pain (renal colic), the major symptom in an acute episode of renal calculi, radiates to the external genitalia. Microhematuria is nearly always present. Nausea and vomiting often accompany the renal colic. (6, 28)

**89.** 2. As the dye is injected, the patient may experience a feeling of warmth, a flushing of the face, and a salty taste in the mouth. The patient should not experience chest pain. (6, 28)

**90.** 2. The patient is at risk for infection. The flank incision, which makes it difficult to take deep breaths, predisposes the patient to atelectasis and respiratory acidosis. Urinary tubes predispose him to urinary tract infection. Parotitis, or "surgical mumps," is a secondary staphylococcal infection that develops in the parotid glands due to debilitation and poor oral hygiene. The lithotomy position, not the lateral position in which the patient will be positioned intraoperatively, is associated with deep vein thrombosis. (6, 28)

*asmatic pt = lots of fl*
*have fear pos. high fra*
*tolerate swimming*
*epinephrine release*
*bronchial muscles*
*The tip of the pacemaker*
*placed in R ventricle*

Select the one *best* or *correct* answer and indicate your choice by filling in the circle with a pencil in front of the option you have chosen. If the answer you would prefer is not given, select the one you think is *most appropriate*.

Jerry Fein, 9, is admitted to the emergency room because of an attack of bronchial asthma. His respirations are very labored.

**91.** Jerry is reacting emotionally to dyspnea in a way typical of patients with asthma. Therefore, the nurse should work toward the goal of helping him overcome feelings of
○ 1. fear.
○ 2. depression.
○ 3. exhilaration.
○ 4. irritability.

**92.** Subcutaneous epinephrine is prescribed for Jerry and is observed to relieve his dyspnea after being administered a second time. Epinephrine acts to relieve dyspnea by helping to
○ 1. relax bronchial smooth musculature.
○ 2. inflate collapsed alveoli in the lungs.
○ 3. inhibit the body's release of histamine.
○ 4. decrease the viscosity of mucous secretions.

**93.** In which of the following positions is Jerry likely to be *most* comfortable upon admission?
○ 1. The prone position.
○ 2. The supine position.
○ 3. A high Fowler's position.
○ 4. Either side-lying position.

**94.** After Jerry's condition stabilizes, the nurse learns that Jerry had not been complying with prescribed drug therapy. Which of the following drugs is *most likely* to be prescribed for Jerry, *primarily* as a prophylactic agent?
○ 1. Ephedrine.
○ 2. Ammonium chloride.
○ 3. Cromolyn sodium (Intal).
○ 4. Isoproterenol hydrochloride (Isuprel).

**95.** The nurse should also determine whether Jerry is complying with other prescribed therapy. She should try to learn whether Jerry's daily intake of nutrients includes larger-than-average amounts of

○ 1. fruits.
○ 2. fluids.
○ 3. foods high in vitamin C.
○ 4. foods high in potassium.

**96.** To promote Jerry's physical and psychosocial development, the nurse encourages him to participate in various activities with his peers. Jerry asks, "But what can I do?" If Jerry expresses interest in the following activities, which is *best* for him to pursue?
○ 1. Swimming.
○ 2. Wrestling.
○ 3. Playing basketball.
○ 4. Playing ice hockey.

Mr. Jack Kemps, 72, is admitted to the hospital for a pacemaker insertion.

**97.** Mr. Kemps has the equipment listed below in his home. The item *most likely* to present a hazard, even when the pacemaker and the item are in good working order, is the
○ 1. dehumidifier.
○ 2. electric razor.
○ 3. microwave oven.
○ 4. high-fidelity record player.

**98.** Mr. Kemps asks the nurse, "Where did they put the tip of my pacemaker? Is it in my heart?" The nurse should base her response on knowledge that most often, the tip of the catheter on the pacemaker is placed in the
○ 1. left atrium.
○ 2. right atrium.
○ 3. left ventricle.
○ 4. right ventricle.

**99.** Which of the following electrocardiograms would indicate to the nurse that a patient has a pacemaker?

○ 1.

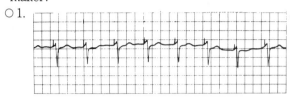

○ 2.

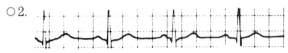

○ 3.

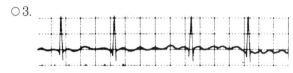

○ 4.

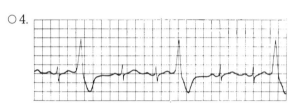

**100.** Mr. Kemps has a *demand* pacemaker. The nurse explains that this pacemaker functions by providing

○ 1. stimuli to the heart muscle only when the heart begins to beat irregularly.

○ 2. continuous stimuli to the heart muscle, resulting in a predetermined heart rate.

○ 3. stimuli to the heart muscle only when the heart rate falls below a specified level.

○ 4. continuous stimuli to the heart muscle whenever ventricular fibrillation is present.

**101.** Mr. Kemps says he is afraid of his pacemaker. Which of the following responses would be *most appropriate* for the nurse to make?

○ 1. "All patients are scared at first, but you have nothing to fear."

○ 2. "Tell me more about what frightens you about your pacemaker."

○ 3. "There is no need to worry if you see your doctor as regularly as he suggests."

○ 4. "Here is a manual for you to read before I begin to teach you about your pacemaker."

**102.** The nurse teaches Mr. Kemps what to expect when his pacemaker begins to fail. Which of the following statements is *correct*?

○ 1. "You will have nausea."

○ 2. "You will have tremors."

○ 3. "You will have headaches."

○ 4. "You will be dizzy."

**103.** Mr. Kemps says, "It's harder every day to be someone. Everyone is in such a hurry to get things done, and *their* way." After analyzing the patient's comment, the nurse judges that Mr. Kemps has described a common problem experienced by the elderly patient when his life-style threatens the need for

○ 1. feeling self-esteem.

○ 2. being able to communicate effectively.

○ 3. being able to express hostility openly.

○ 4. feeling secure about having adequate health care.

**104.** Which of the following comments that a person of Mr. Kemps' age could make *best* illustrates that the person is *failing* to come to terms with his life?

○ 1. "Life ends for all."

○ 2. "Life has little meaning any more."

○ 3. "Life on earth is short, but I did a lot in my time."

○ 4. "Life has not always been easy, but we learn from hardships."

Ms. Betty Stein, 24, is about 7 months pregnant.

**105.** Ms. Stein has received permission from her physician to make an 8-hour auto trip. The nurse discusses the trip with Ms. Stein to determine whether the patient understands precautions she should take while traveling. The nurse is justified in deciding that the patient understands instructions when Ms. Stein says that during the trip she plans to

○ 1. drink fluids every 1 to 2 hours.

○ 2. have a snack approximately every 2 hours.

○ 3. sleep for about 1 hour at the halfway mark.

○ 4. take a 10- to 15-minute rest period every few hours.

**106.** Ms. Stein complains of low backaches. If the patient wears the following articles of clothing, which item is *most probably* contributing to her backaches?

○ 1. Pull-on slacks.

○ 2. Knee-high stockings.

○ 3. An elasticized girdle.

○ 4. Sandals with flat insteps.

**107.** Ms. Stein is admitted to the hospital, but she thinks she is in false labor. The nurse judges *correctly* that Ms. Stein is in true labor because contractions are occurring regularly and the patient's

○ 1. cervix is dilating.

○ 2. fetus is in the pelvis.

○ 3. membranes have ruptured.

○ 4. mucus plug in the cervical canal is expelled.

108. If Ms. Stein's cord prolapses when her membranes rupture, what position should the nurse help the patient assume in bed?

○ 1. A supine position.

○ 2. A knee-chest position.

○ 3. A low Fowler's position.

○ 4. Flat in bed on either side.

109. After delivering a 6-pound, 12-ounce infant, Ms. Stein says, "It was really a wonderful experience to participate in my labor and deliver while wide awake." The nurse is justified in her evaluation when she gives *most* credit for the mother's feelings of satisfaction to the fact that Ms. Stein

○ 1. is at an ideal age for childbirth.

○ 2. has attended prepared childbirth classes.

○ 3. has had no complications during pregnancy.

○ 4. has delivered an infant of lower-than-average birth weight.

110. After the birth of Ms. Stein's infant, the nurse helps promote maternal-infant bonding. It is generally believed that this is *best* initiated when the mother is allowed to

○ 1. nurse her infant.

○ 2. hear her infant cry.

○ 3. wrap her infant in a receiving blanket.

○ 4. experience eye-to-eye contact with her infant.

111. Which of the following pharmaceutical preparations should the nurse have ready for immediate administration if Ms. Smith is at risk for postpartum hemorrhage?

○ 1. An oxytocic preparation.

○ 2. A cortisone preparation.

○ 3. A prostaglandin preparation.

○ 4. A magnesium sulfate preparation.

112. After Ms. Stein is moved from the delivery room to her room, the nurse recommends that during rest periods Ms. Stein use the prone position from time to time. If the patient uses the following techniques when lying on her abdomen, which is in *error*?

○ 1. Her head rests on the mattress.

○ 2. Her feet rest on the mattress.

○ 3. Her face is turned to one side.

○ 4. Her forearms are alongside her head with the elbows flexed.

113. Ms. Stein complains of afterpains on her 3rd postpartum day. The nurse explains *correctly* that afterpains are *most* common when the mother

○ 1. is nursing her baby.

○ 2. is experiencing urinary retention.

○ 3. has inhalation analgesia during labor.

○ 4. had an episiotomy at the time of delivery.

A graduate engineering student, Mr. John Henderson, 24, has noticed some itchiness on his skin over the past month. Now he notices an enlargement on his neck and checks in at the student health center. He is admitted to the hospital and is diagnosed as having stage I Hodgkin's disease. He is discharged and started on a 4-week course of local nodal radiotherapy as an outpatient.

114. Mr. Henderson spends a lot of time talking about his fate. Which of the following statements indicates that he understands his prognosis?

○ 1. "I'm going to pack a lot of living into the 4 or 5 years that I have left."

○ 2. "I hate never having the chance to use all the education I've received."

○ 3. "If I had caught this in an early stage, it might have been better."

○ 4. "I'm very fortunate to have a cancer that has such a good chance for a cure."

115. Radiation therapy is instituted, and after 1 week the radiation site becomes red and irritated. Which of the following statements indicates that Mr. Henderson treated the area appropriately at home?

○ 1. "I applied aloe vera lotion to the area."

○ 2. "I applied moist cool soaks to the area."

○ 3. "I applied nothing to the area, just kept it dry."

○ 4. "I applied a hot-water bottle to the area."

116. After 2 weeks of therapy, Mr. Henderson becomes discouraged. He tells the nurse that he is so tired he can barely keep up with this studies. What information would the nurse use in planning her response?

○ 1. Fatigue is one of the most common problems associated with radiotherapy and will continue throughout therapy.

○ 2. Fatigue is a transient problem that will resolve as radiotherapy continues.

○ 3. Fatigue is unrelated to the radiotherapy and another possible cause should be sought.

○ 4. Fatigue indicates that the disease is eradicated and that radiotherapy is not needed.

117. Mr. Henderson explains to the nurse the monitoring he will be doing at home between treatments. Which of the following statements indicates that he knows how to detect a *major* complication?

○ 1. "I'll measure the circumference of my neck every day."

○ 2. "I'll take my temperature every day."

○ 3. "I'll monitor the loss of my body hair every week."

○ 4. "I'll check the circulation in my arms every day."

Mr. William Story, a 59-year-old construction worker, makes an appointment to see his physician. The office nurse obtains Mr. Story's initial health history. When the physician reads the history, he tells the nurse that he suspects that Mr. Story may have non-insulin-dependent diabetes mellitus.

**118.** While obtaining the health history, Mr. Story says he is not feeling right and makes the statements given below. Which is *most probably unrelated* to diabetes mellitus, if it is established that the patient has the disease?
- ○ 1. "I have this cut on my hand that doesn't want to heal."
- ○ 2. "No matter how much I drink, I still seem to be thirsty all the time."
- ○ 3. "I seem to be unable to get an erection. I've never been impotent before."
- ○ 4. "In the past couple of weeks, I've been having a great deal of trouble starting to urinate."

**119.** It is established that Mr. Story has diabetes mellitus and the sulfonylurea tolbutamide (Orinase) is prescribed for him. The sulfonylureas function in the body by
- ○ 1. decreasing gluconeogenesis in the liver.
- ○ 2. potentiating the action of insulin in body cells.
- ○ 3. promoting the excretion of excess glucose through the kidneys.
- ○ 4. stimulating the beta cells in the pancreas to secrete more insulin.

**120.** When Mr. Story's blood glucose levels begin to fluctuate widely, tolbutamide therapy is discontinued and he is admitted to the hospital to begin insulin therapy. The nurse learns that the patient smokes one to two packs of cigarettes daily, has "two or three drinks" on social occasions, is obese, and works in an occupation that requires him to be outdoors all year. All of the following goals are important, but to help control his diabetes it will be *most important* for the nurse to help Mr. Story
- ○ 1. lose weight.
- ○ 2. stop smoking.
- ○ 3. limit exposure to the cold.
- ○ 4. avoid drinking alcoholic beverages.

**121.** Mr. Story is taught how to give himself NPH insulin. If the nurse notes that the patient is using the following techniques when administering insulin to himself, which technique is in *error*?
- ○ 1. The patient shakes the insulin vial before withdrawing insulin.
- ○ 2. The patient introduces the needle into subcutaneous tissue with a dartlike action.

- ○ 3. The patient pulls back on the syringe plunger as soon as the needle is in place in subcutaneous tissue.
- ○ 4. The patient holds an antiseptic sponge against the needle when removing it from subcutaneous tissue.

**122.** Mr. Story is being taught dietary management. He is of Italian ancestry and says, "How will I ever live without my pasta!" Which of the following responses would be *best* for the nurse to make in this situation?
- ○ 1. "After you are well regulated on insulin, maybe you can eat some pasta."
- ○ 2. "Many people have given up pasta, and I'm sure you'll be able to, also."
- ○ 3. "I think this is something to discuss with your doctor. He may allow you to eat pasta."
- ○ 4. "You don't need to give up pasta, but the amount will need to be regulated in your diet."

**123.** After Mr. Story has been on insulin therapy for some time, laboratory findings demonstrate high fasting blood sugars each morning. He is believed to be suffering from the Somogyi, or dawn, phenomenon. The nurse should understand that this condition has *most often* been found to be due to
- ○ 1. dietary noncompliance.
- ○ 2. excessive dosages of insulin.
- ○ 3. beginning atherosclerotic changes in large arteries.
- ○ 4. pathologic changes in the autonomic nervous system.

A nurse helps care for Baby Boy Duggan, a newborn, and assesses his physical condition.

**124.** Immediately after the birth of Baby Duggan, the nurse should plan that her *first* efforts should be directed toward helping with
- ○ 1. cutting the umbilical cord to prevent blood loss.
- ○ 2. wrapping the infant in a receiving blanket to prevent hypothermia.
- ○ 3. using prophylaxis to protect the infant's eyes from ophthalmia neonatorum.
- ○ 4. ensuring that the infant's airway is open to promote pulmonary function.

**125.** The nurse determines Baby Duggan's Apgar score. What is the *highest* score the infant can receive when his reflex irritability is assessed?
- ○ 1. 1.
- ○ 2. 2.
- ○ 3. 5.
- ○ 4. 10.

**126.** The nurse includes assessing Baby Duggan's eyes in her plans. To facilitate her task, in which of the following positions should she plan to place the infant so that his eyes are likely to open spontaneously?

○ 1. On his abdomen.

○ 2. On either side.

○ 3. On his back with his head lowered.

○ 4. On his back with his head elevated.

**127.** Baby Duggan's rooting reflex is *best* tested during assessment when the nurse

○ 1. strokes the infant's cheek.

○ 2. places her finger in the infant's hand.

○ 3. holds the infant upright, then allows his feet to touch a firm surface.

○ 4. supports the infant's head, then allows it to drop back a short distance.

Ethel North, 5, is to be admitted to a hospital. She is acutely ill with meningitis.

**128.** When the nurse is notified that Ethel is to be admitted, the type of isolation she should plan to use for the patient is

○ 1. strict.

○ 2. enteric.

○ 3. protective. *or reverse*

○ 4. respiratory.

**129.** The nurse obtains Ethel's nursing history from the child's mother. If the child has had the following illnesses relatively recently, which *most likely* predisposed her to meningitis?

○ 1. Otitis media. *middle ear*

○ 2. A broken arm.

○ 3. Pinworms, for which she was treated.

○ 4. Diarrhea following food poisoning.

**130.** The nurse assesses Ethel to determine whether the patient has pain and stiffness in her neck. The nurse's technique is in error *unless* she carries out this assessment while Ethel is in the

○ 1. prone position.

○ 2. supine position.

○ 3. high Fowler's position.

○ 4. right or left side-lying position.

**131.** Ethel undergoes a lumbar puncture. The nurse judges that Ethel is *not* experiencing a headache following the lumbar puncture *primarily* because nursing care following the procedure included

○ 1. darkening the child's room.

○ 2. positioning the child in bed in the supine position.

○ 3. offering the child a high-carbohydrate snack.

○ 4. encouraging the child to take generous amounts of fluid.

**132.** Ampicillin is prescribed for Ethel. By which route should the nurse be prepared to administer the medication?

○ 1. The oral route.

○ 2. The intravenous route.

○ 3. The intramuscular route.

○ 4. The subcutaneous route.

**133.** Mannitol is prescribed for Ethel when she presents signs and symptoms typical of cerebral edema. The nurse is justified in judging that mannitol is accomplishing its *primary* purpose when Ethel says which of the following?

○ 1. "I'm so tired."

○ 2. "I can turn my neck a little."

○ 3. "I don't feel so hot anymore."

○ 4. "I keep having to go to the toilet."

**134.** During Ethel's convalescence, the nurse should be *especially* mindful to help Ethel deal with feelings about her illness. A feeling typical for her age is

○ 1. pity.

○ 2. anger.

○ 3. guilt.

○ 4. sorrow.

Mrs. Tanya Bloom is admitted to the emergency room. She has cut her finger and the wound is bleeding profusely. She says, "Just let me alone. I'll be fine just as soon as you fix my finger." She displays signs of intoxication and a blood test confirms it.

**135.** After Mrs. Bloom's wound is sutured but before she leaves the emergency room, it would be *best* for the nurse to see to it that the patient

○ 1. takes a nap.

○ 2. does some exercising.

○ 3. restricts fluid intake.

○ 4. drinks generous amounts of black coffee.

**136.** Mr. Bloom is notified of his wife's admission to the emergency room. If he makes the following statements about his wife, which is *least typical* of a person who is abusing alcohol?

○ 1. "She uses alcohol and tranquilizers to steady her nerves."

○ 2. "Whenever she has a problem, she seems to hit the bottle."

○ 3. "Her drinking certainly hasn't interfered with her eating."

○ 4. "She has stopped drinking several times, sometimes for as long as 4 months."

**137.** Mrs. Bloom mumbles with some uncertainty when asked how she cut her finger and then says, "While cutting flowers in our garden." Mr. Bloom says they do not have a flower garden. Filling in gaps of memory, as Mrs. Bloom has done, is called

○ 1. displacement.
○ 2. confabulation.
○ 3. disorientation.
○ 4. flight of ideas.

**138.** About 2 weeks after receiving care in the emergency room, Mrs. Bloom admits to her husband that she has a drinking problem and decides to do something about it. Of *critical* importance for her successful rehabilitation is

○ 1. her emotional support system.
○ 2. her motivation to change her behavior.
○ 3. the presence of self-help groups in the community.
○ 4. the presence of local health centers for alcoholics.

**139.** Mrs. Bloom admits herself to a rehabilitation program for alcoholics. Plans are made to care for her if she begins to have delirium tremens (DTs). An appropriate intervention for the nurse to take when DTs occur is to

○ 1. help the patient remain awake.
○ 2. place the patient in restraints.
○ 3. keep the patient's room well lighted.
○ 4. agree with the patient's visual misinterpretations.

**140.** The nurse judges that Mrs. Bloom is possibly developing Wernicke-Korsakoff syndrome when she shows signs of

○ 1. fear and paranoia.
○ 2. aggression and hostility.
○ 3. memory loss and disorientation.
○ 4. depression and suicidal tendencies.

**141.** Mrs. Bloom agrees to undergo disulfiram (Antabuse) therapy. The nurse is justified in believing that Mrs. Bloom *most probably* has drunk alcohol while taking disulfiram when the patient has

○ 1. vertigo.
○ 2. hallucinations.
○ 3. diarrhea and fever.
○ 4. nausea and vomiting.

**142.** The nurse tells Mrs. Bloom about Alcoholics Anonymous (AA), and when the patient is ready for discharge she decides to attend an AA meeting. AA has helped in the rehabilitation of many alcoholics, *most probably* because many people find it easier to change their behavior when they

○ 1. have the support of rehabilitated alcoholics.

○ 2. know rehabilitated alcoholics will sympathize with them.
○ 3. can depend on rehabilitated alcoholics to help them identify personal problems related to alcoholism.
○ 4. realize rehabilitated alcoholics will help them develop mechanisms to cope with their alcoholism.

George Dural, 61, is admitted to the hospital. He has been suffering from emphysema for about 5 years.

**143.** Mr. Dural is ordered to receive a loading dose of 400 mg of aminophylline intravenously. Each ampule of aminophylline contains 250 mg of the drug in 10 ml of solution. How many milliliters of the solution should Mr. Dural receive?

○ 1. 12 ml.
○ 2. 15 ml.
○ 3. 16 ml.
○ 4. 18 ml.

**144.** The *primary* purpose of administering aminophylline to Mr. Dural is that the drug acts to

○ 1. relieve diaphragmatic spasms.
○ 2. relax smooth muscles in the bronchioles.
○ 3. promote efficient pulmonary circulation.
○ 4. stimulate chemoreceptors in the medullary respiratory center.

**145.** Mr. Dural is receiving continuous oxygen therapy. Depression of ventilation is likely to occur unless the nurse ensures that the patient receives oxygen that is administered

○ 1. warmed.
○ 2. humidified.
○ 3. at a low flow rate.
○ 4. through a nasal cannula.

**146.** Mr. Dural's blood gases are monitored closely while he receives oxygen therapy. A *normal* range of $PaO_2$ for a healthy patient of Mr. Dural's age is between about

○ 1. 50 and 60 mm Hg.
○ 2. 60 and 70 mm Hg.
○ 3. 70 and 80 mm Hg.
○ 4. 80 and 90 mm Hg.

**147.** The nurse examines Mr. Dural to determine whether his neck veins are distended. If they are, the nurse is justified in concluding that his disease has advanced beyond lung pathology. Accordingly, the nurse should continue her assessment for signs that would indicate the patient is likely to be developing

○ 1. empyema.
○ 2. renal failure.
○ 3. hepatic insufficiency.
○ 4. right-sided heart failure.

**148.** Mr. Dural's sputum is very thick and tenacious. In addition to a high fluid intake, which of the following measures should be included in the patient's nursing care plan to help reduce the tenacity of respiratory secretions?
○ 1. Having the patient use postural drainage.
○ 2. Humidifying the air the patient inspires.
○ 3. Giving the patient low concentrations of oxygen.
○ 4. Instructing the patient to use diaphragmatic breathing.

**149.** The nurse teaches Mr. Dural to use pursed-lip breathing. The *primary* purpose of this type of breathing is to help
○ 1. increase intrapulmonic pressure.
○ 2. promote a regular breathing pattern.
○ 3. prevent collapse of alveolar tissues.
○ 4. sensitize central chemoreceptors in the medulla.

Anne Simon, 16, is pregnant and is being seen by a nurse in a maternity clinic.

**150.** When the nurse inquires about Anne's marital status while interviewing her, the patient appears uneasy and says, "Do I have to discuss that with you?" The nurse's *best* answer would be
○ 1. "Yes, if you want me to care for you."
○ 2. "Yes, because I need to know to complete your records."
○ 3. "No, but it would be helpful in planning your care."
○ 4. "No, but I do want you to know I'm sorry for you."

**151.** An admission interview indicates that Anne's lifestyle is typical of a low socioeconomic status. As a result, the nurse should be *especially* alert during Anne's pregnancy to determine whether she is likely to develop a problem related to
○ 1. activity.
○ 2. nutrition.
○ 3. rest and sleep.
○ 4. personal cleanliness.

**152.** Anne tells the nurse, "My grandmom says I'll lose a tooth because I'm pregnant. Is that true?" The nurse should explain that eating a proper diet will prevent tooth loss and teaches the importance of an adequate intake of the mineral

○ 1. iron.
○ 2. zinc.
○ 3. calcium.
○ 4. potassium.

**153.** Anne is admitted to the hospital and delivers a baby girl. Baby Simon is given vitamin K shortly after birth *primarily* to help
○ 1. stimulate respirations.
○ 2. improve blood clotting.
○ 3. increase calcium absorption.
○ 4. start peristaltic movements.

**154.** When the nurse is giving Baby Simon an intramuscular injection of vitamin K, her technique is *correct* when the muscle she injects is the
○ 1. biceps brachii muscle.
○ 2. biceps femoris muscle.
○ 3. rectus femoris muscle.
○ 4. gluteus maximus muscle.

**155.** Anne asks if she should clean her nipples before nursing her baby. The nurse should recommend that before nursing, Ann should clean her nipples with
○ 1. alcohol.
○ 2. plain water.
○ 3. soap and water.
○ 4. a diluted antiseptic solution.

A nurse discusses the care of 6-week-old Gretchen Small with the infant's mother. The infant has colic, and Mrs. Small says Gretchen cries lustily for long periods of time.

**156.** The nurse assesses Gretchen and finds her essentially healthy. She should teach the mother that a technique that sometimes helps prevent colic is to
○ 1. position the infant on either side for sleeping.
○ 2. bubble the infant several times while feeding her.
○ 3. feed the infant small amounts of formula at frequent intervals.
○ 4. offer the infant a little water immediately before feeding her.

**157.** Which of the following behaviors should the nurse expect of a healthy 6-week-old infant?
○ 1. The infant can roll over.
○ 2. The infant demonstrates fear of strangers.
○ 3. The infant holds a nursing bottle fairly well.
○ 4. The infant can hold up her head when lying on her abdomen.

Mr. Morris is admitted to a hospital for the mentally ill because of an obsessive-compulsive disorder. He washes his feet endlessly because he thinks they are so dirty that he cannot put on his socks and shoes.

**158.** Mr. Morris is using ritualistic behavior because of his obsessive-compulsive disorder *primarily* to relieve discomfort associated with feelings of
- ○ 1. depression.
- ○ 2. ambivalence.
- ○ 3. irrational fear.
- ○ 4. intolerable anxiety.

**159.** As he busily scrubs his feet, Mr. Morris tells the nurse, "Never mind if I look silly to you. I must finish before I can put on my socks and shoes and go to lunch." When analyzing the patient's statement, the nurse should be guided by knowledge that patients with obsessive-compulsive disorders tend to
- ○ 1. be unaware of the disruptive nature of their ritualistic behavior.
- ○ 2. be aware of the unreasonableness of their ritualistic behavior.
- ○ 3. expect health professionals to stop them from performing their ritualistic behavior.
- ○ 4. make frequent attempts to test the skill of those helping them overcome their ritualistic behavior.

**160.** As a result of Mr. Morris's frequent foot-washing, he is usually late for meals, group activities, therapy sessions, and other occasions. It is *most probably best* for the nurse to help overcome this habitual tardiness by planning to
- ○ 1. explain to the patient how his tardiness for scheduled activities interferes with his getting well.
- ○ 2. help the patient stop his ritualistic behavior when it is time for him to leave for scheduled activities.
- ○ 3. allow the patient to decide whether he wishes to attend scheduled activities or do his ritualistic behavior.
- ○ 4. remind the patient early enough that he can carry out his ritualistic behavior in time to arrive for scheduled activities.

Ms. Janet Farrell is admitted to the hospital. She has a malignant growth on the larynx and will have a laryngectomy.

**161.** The nurse obtains Ms. Farrell's health history upon admission to the hospital. The patient is *most likely* to state that the *earliest* symptom that made her realize she may have a health problem occurred when she noted having
- ○ 1. a sore throat.
- ○ 2. chronic hoarseness.
- ○ 3. pain radiating to her ear.
- ○ 4. difficulty swallowing.

**162.** The nurse learns from the patient's sister that it was 3 months before Ms. Farrell sought health care after she first had symptoms of a tumorous growth on her larynx. "I'll be O.K.," she said. "Just give me a little time." The common emotional response Ms. Farrell was *most probably* demonstrating during the first stage of her illness is
- ○ 1. anger.
- ○ 2. denial.
- ○ 3. dependency.
- ○ 4. aggression.

**163.** Ms. Farrell is prepared for a total laryngectomy. Of the following nursing measures, the one that should have *highest* priority in preparing Ms. Farrell for surgery is ensuring that she has
- ○ 1. adequate nourishment.
- ○ 2. thorough oral hygiene.
- ○ 3. proper bowel elimination.
- ○ 4. a high level of fluid intake.

**164.** Following the laryngectomy, the nurse carefully observes Ms. Farrell for signs of rupture of the carotid artery. If any such signs occur, immediate emergency care includes calling for help while simultaneously
- ○ 1. raising the head of the patient's bed.
- ○ 2. suctioning the patient's laryngectomy tube.
- ○ 3. applying a clamp to the patient's bleeding artery.
- ○ 4. applying pressure over the patient's bleeding artery.

**165.** Ms. Farrell begins oral feedings 9 days postoperatively. After the patient starts oral feedings, it is important for the nurse to help the patient develop the ability to
- ○ 1. cough.
- ○ 2. belch.
- ○ 3. hiccup.
- ○ 4. sneeze.

**166.** Ms. Farrell convalesces without problems. If she says she enjoys the following leisure-time activities, the one the nurse should teach her to *avoid* is
- ○ 1. bowling.
- ○ 2. swimming.
- ○ 3. attending sports events.
- ○ 4. tending a flower garden.

Melissa Younger, 9, is admitted to the pediatric unit of a hospital after an emergency appendectomy. The appendix had not ruptured and the surgical procedure was uncomplicated.

167. When Melissa wakes from the anesthesia following surgery, she asks the nurse if she is going to die. When responding to Melissa's question, the nurse should recognize that, at Melissa's age, it is *most* common for her to think of death as being
    ○ 1. a happy event.
    ○ 2. a reversible event.
    ○ 3. an event of fantasy.
    ○ 4. an irreversible event.

168. Following the appendectomy, which of the following measures should the nurse use to help determine whether Melissa is ready to take oral fluids?
    ○ 1. Asking her if she is thirsty.
    ○ 2. Determining that she is fully conscious.
    ○ 3. Auscultating her abdomen for evidence of bowel sounds.
    ○ 4. Palpating her epigastric area for evidence of discomfort.

169. The nurse should assess for pediculosis capitis (head lice) when she notes that Melissa
    ○ 1. has spotty baldness.
    ○ 2. scratches her scalp frequently.
    ○ 3. twirls strands of hair frequently.
    ○ 4. has wheals with blistering on the scalp.

170. The nurse assesses Melissa's typical at-home diet after interviewing the child's mother. The nurse judges that Melissa's protein intake falls short of recommended standards. If Melissa likes the following foods, which should the nurse recommend that the mother use to improve Melissa's protein intake?
    ○ 1. Raw apple.
    ○ 2. Carrot sticks.
    ○ 3. Peanut butter.
    ○ 4. Graham crackers.

171. At Melissa's age (9 years), the child's dominant influence as she develops social skills and industry typically is/are her
    ○ 1. peers.
    ○ 2. mother.
    ○ 3. father.
    ○ 4. siblings.

172. The hospital has a television in each child's room. A group of nurses are discussing the possible influence of television programs on personality development in children of Melissa's age. Which of the following statements *most accurately* reflects present knowledge concerning television and its effects on children?

○ 1. Research clearly shows that television has a negligible influence on the behavior of school-age children.
○ 2. Research clearly shows that television has a marked influence on the behavior of school-age children.
○ 3. Research clearly shows that a child's intelligence is the deciding factor in determining how much television influences the behavior of school-age children.
○ 4. Research has not yet clearly established the nature of the influence television has on the behavior of school-age children.

Gloria Young, 16, is admitted to the hospital with acute glomerulonephritis.

173. It is *most likely* that the nurse will learn that Gloria recently suffered from an infection in which the causative organisms were
    ○ 1. Group A streptococci.
    ○ 2. *Diplococcus pneumoniae.*
    ○ 3. *Pseudomonas aeruginosa.*
    ○ 4. *Haemophilus influenzae.*

174. When planning Gloria's care, which of the following orders should the nurse *most certainly* include?
    ○ 1. Record the patient's intake and output.
    ○ 2. Observe respiratory isolation techniques for the patient.
    ○ 3. Obtain arterial blood for daily evaluation of blood serum gases.
    ○ 4. Offer nourishment of the patient's choice at midmorning, midafternoon, and midevening.

175. Gloria tells the nurse she dislikes bedtime because she has insomnia and has been bothered with it for a long time. If none of the following bedtime snacks is contraindicated for Gloria, which is *most likely* to help promote sleep?
    ○ 1. An apple.
    ○ 2. Dried figs.
    ○ 3. Cheese cubes.
    ○ 4. Toast and jelly.

Mrs. Agnes Hanson, a 64-year-old high-school librarian, goes to her ophthalmologist for a routine visit. She complains of some difficulty seeing. Glaucoma is suspected.

**176.** Which of the following is an *early* symptom of glaucoma?
- ○ 1. Hazy vision.
- ○ 2. Loss of central vision.
- ○ 3. Impaired peripheral vision.
- ○ 4. Blurred or "sooty" vision.

**177.** Timolol maleate (Timoptic) eye drops, a beta-adrenergic receptor blocking agent, are ordered because they do not interfere with vision. Of what common side effect would the nurse tell Mrs. Hanson to be aware?
- ○ 1. Slight bradycardia at rest.
- ○ 2. Nausea and vomiting.
- ○ 3. Vivid dreams.
- ○ 4. Migraine headaches.

**178.** Mrs. Hanson asks about the seriousness of glaucoma. On which of the following statements about glaucoma should the nurse base her answer?
- ○ 1. Glaucoma is a serious disease that if untreated leads to blindness.
- ○ 2. Glaucoma can be annoying, but it has no serious long-term effects.
- ○ 3. Glaucoma is a common disease that can be cured with either medical or surgical intervention.
- ○ 4. Glaucoma is a serious disease that eventually leads to blindness, despite treatment.

**179.** The nurse teaches Mrs. Hanson to avoid activities that increase intraocular pressure, such as
- ○ 1. watching television.
- ○ 2. knitting with fine yarn.
- ○ 3. eating a high-fat diet.
- ○ 4. shoveling snow.

**180.** Because of continuing problems, Mrs. Hanson underwent laser trabeculoplasty. She has returned for a regularly scheduled follow-up visit. Which of the following indicates that the nurse's medication teaching for Mrs. Hanson's postoperative period was successful?
- ○ 1. The patient began tapering her regular eye drops 1 week postoperatively.
- ○ 2. The patient continued to use her regular eye drops until this visit.
- ○ 3. The patient stopped using her regular eye drops the day of surgery.
- ○ 4. The patient replaced her regular eye drops with steroid eye drops.

# CORRECT ANSWERS AND RATIONALES

Numbers appear in parentheses following the rationales. The numbers identify textbooks listed in the references at the end of Part V, where correct answers can be verified.

**91.** 1. A person who has trouble breathing typically exhibits signs and symptoms of fear and anxiety. The experience of not being able to breathe can be devastating, and fear and anxiety tend to intensify the dyspnea. Therefore, the nurse should work calmly as she offers reassurance, emotional support, and explanations of procedures to the extent that the patient can understand. The environment should be comfortable and quiet. The child's parents, who are also usually fearful and anxious, should be offered similar care. Depression, exhilaration, and irritability are not ordinarily associated with dyspnea. (32, 40)

**92.** 1. Epinephrine's main effect is to relax bronchial muscles. The adrenergic drug also increases the vital capacity of the lungs by relieving the congestion of mucosa in the bronchial passages. The drug's action is rapid but of short duration, and therefore it may be administered a second time when the first administration is not sufficiently effective. Cromolyn sodium (Intal) inhibits the body's release of histamine. Expectorants are used to decrease the viscosity of mucous secretions. In asthma, the alveoli in the lungs are already hyperinflated because of the gases trapped in the lungs. Typically, expiratory efforts cannot rid the lungs of air because the lumen of the patient's airway narrows during an asthma attack. (32, 33)

**93.** 3. A dyspneic patient is almost always most comfortable in a high Fowler's position, or he may be comfortable when leaning over an overbed table. These positions maximize the lungs' capacity to ventilate. (25, 40)

**94.** 3. Cromolyn sodium (Intal) is a prophylactic agent for bronchial asthma that inhibits the body's release of histamine. Ephedrine is a sympathomimetic bronchodilator but is best suited to prevent a severe asthma attack when early signs and symptoms have already appeared. Ammonium chloride is an expectorant; it increases secretory action and thereby decreases the viscosity of respiratory secretions. Isoproterenol hydrochloride (Isuprel) is a bronchodilator and may be used for an asthma attack or *status asthmaticus*. (33, 40)

**95.** 2. Patients with asthma are encouraged to drink as much as two to three times the daily normal intake. A large fluid intake helps prevent dehydration and serves as an excellent diluent of respiratory mucus for easier expectoration. (32, 40)

**96.** 1. Children with asthma tolerate swimming very well, probably because the sport requires rhythmic deep-breathing with prolonged expiration. Other sports in which many asthmatics learn to participate include skiing, baseball, and soccer, because these sports have periods of rest following activity. Activities requiring long periods of endurance, such as wrestling, ice hockey, basketball, and running, are less well tolerated. Playing a wind instrument is recommended because it requires pursed-lip breathing, which helps rid the lungs of wastes. (40)

**97.** 3. The microwave oven *may* interfere with proper pacemaker functioning. Microwave ovens have a particular frequency and wave length of electromagnetic energy that may be picked up by the pacemaker and may cause heart stimulation. Some microwave ovens are advertised as safe for patients with pacemakers, and they probably are. But for years, patients with pacemakers were warned to avoid microwave ovens, and they should be taught that there appear to be few, if any, electrical hazards with pacemakers and ovens now being manufactured. (6, 23)

**98.** 4. The tip of the catheter is placed in the apex of the right ventricle, which is muscular and thicker than the atrial wall; there is less tendency for the lead to become dislodged or rupture through the wall in this location. If there *may* be danger of perforating the right ventricle wall, the tip of the catheter may be placed in the pulmonary outflow path in the right ventricle. (15, 21)

**99.** 1. The electrical stimulus of an artificial pacemaker appears on an EKG as a small vertical line, or a spike, just before the QRS complex. (15, 21)

**100.** 3. In contrast to a fixed-rate pacemaker, a demand pacemaker functions only when the heart rate falls below a certain level. Fixed-rate pacemakers stimulate heart contractions at a constant rate independent of the patient's heart rate. They are much less common than demand pacemakers. (15, 21)

**101.** 2. The nurse should give the frightened patient an opportunity to express his fears rather than suggesting that there is no need for concern or handing him a manual to read. Listening to the patient's fears gives the nurse a chance to select appropriate nursing interventions that may help alleviate his fears. (6, 19)

**102.** 4. Symptoms of a failing pacemaker result from poor perfusion of blood in the brain, heart, and skeletal muscles. The patient will report such symptoms as feeling dizzy and faint, having chest pain, palpitations, or shortness of breath, and being overly tired. Fluids may be retained also, causing the patient to report symptoms of edema such as swollen ankles and fingers. (15, 21)

**103.** 1. A developmental task of the elderly person is to build and maintain self-esteem and feelings of worth. The patient who says he finds it difficult "to be someone" displays problems with the task of developing self-esteem. His statement less clearly demonstrates that he finds it difficult to communicate effectively, feels insecure about having inadequate health care, or finds it difficult to express hostility, although these problems may also arise in the elderly person. (6, 19)

**104.** 2. As life reaches its end, the older person often has problems finding meaning and value in what remains of life. Failing to find meaning and value often leads to bitterness and depression. For successful development in old age, the elderly person needs to accept his finiteness and come to terms with the knowledge that life ends for all. Such comments as "Life has not always been easy but we learn from hardships" and "Life on earth is short but I did a lot in my time" suggest that he has come to terms with the past, present, and most probably the future and has maintained his integrity and self-worth. (6, 19)

**105.** 4. There are few travel restrictions when a pregnant woman is free of complications and when she avoids undue fatigue. She should plan to take 10- to 15-minute rest periods every few hours when traveling by car. This schedule helps prevent fatigue and, when the breaks include walking and stretching, improves circulation. Pregnant women should use seat belts and shoulder belts. The seat belts should be worn below the level of the abdomen. (27)

**106.** 4. Shoes with little or no arch support are likely to contribute to backaches, aching legs, poor posture, and general fatigue for the pregnant woman. Flat- or low-heeled shoes with a good arch support are recommended. Knee-high stockings are not recommended because the elastic at the top is likely to constrict circulation in the legs. However, they do not necessarily cause low back pain. A loosely elasticized girdle helps support the abdomen and may relieve backaches. Pull-on slacks are satisfactory if they are comfortable. (27)

**107.** 1. A sign of true labor is that the cervix gradually dilates when contractions are regular. In false labor, no change in the cervix is noted and contractions are usually irregular. The patient's membranes may rupture before true labor starts. The presence of the fetus in the pelvis is not a sign of true labor. The

mucus plug in the cervical canal and the presence of show are signs of impending labor. (27)

**108.** 2. To help the presenting part of the fetus move off a prolapsed cord, the patient should be helped into the knee-chest position. If this is impossible, the head of the bed should be lowered. A prolapsed cord should be treated as an emergency because the fetus' life is at risk due to possible asphyxiation. Pressure must be relieved from the cord. (27)

**109.** 2. The current opinion is that prepared childbirth classes are critically important in helping a mother cope and find satisfaction with the birthing experience. The goal of these classes is to help a mother help herself during labor and delivery. Although every person responds differently to the birthing process and requires individualized care, proper prenatal education appears to help lead to a satisfying outcome. Prepared childbirth classes typically include fathers, which also has been found to enhance the birthing experience for both parents. (27)

**110.** 4. Maternal-infant bonding is best initiated when the mother has eye-to-eye contact with the newborn as soon after birth as possible. This is best accomplished by allowing the mother to assume a position so that when holding her baby, she is face-to-face with the infant. Typically, the mother then touches the baby with her fingers and then with her hands in an exploring manner. (27)

**111.** 1. The nurse should have an oxytocic preparation of the physician's choice ready for immediate administration if the patient is at risk for postpartum hemorrhaging. Oxytocics cause the uterus to contract. A relaxed uterus is a primary cause of postpartum hemorrhage. Magnesium sulfate relaxes uterine muscles and may be used to overcome uterine tetany. Prostaglandin preparations are sometimes used in obstetrics to induce labor. Cortisone preparations are sometimes used to help overcome certain problems associated with infertility. (27)

**112.** 2. Lying on the abdomen following delivery is believed to help the uterus return to its normal position. When the patient is in the prone position, the feet are of primary concern. They should rest over a pillow or over the end of the mattress to prevent being forced into the uncomfortable position of footdrop. The forearms are placed alongside the head while the elbows are flexed, or they may be placed comfortably at the patient's sides. The patient's head may be allowed to lie flat on the mattress or may rest on a very small pillow. This positioning of the head prevents hyperflexion of the neck. The face is turned to either side for comfort. (29)

**113.** 1. Afterpains are common when a mother breast-feeds her infant. Suckling releases oxytocin from the mother's pituitary gland, causing the uterus to contract. Other factors that contribute to after-pains are retention of material in the uterus and a greatly distended uterus during pregnancy. (27)

**114.** 4. Patients with stage I Hodgkin's disease treated with radiotherapy currently have a 95% 5-year survival rate and are considered cured. In stage I, the earliest stage, the disease is limited to a single node and contiguous structure, or a single extralymphatic organ or site. (6, 28)

**115.** 3. Lotions, creams, and powders may increase irritation and should be avoided. The area should be kept dry and open to the air. Radiated skin is temperature-sensitive, and a hot-water bottle could cause a burn. (6, 28)

**116.** 1. Fatigue or lethargy is one of the most common problems associated with radiotherapy. It lasts during therapy and for varying periods after the end of therapy. Extra rest and a reduction in normal activity are often necessary to maintain a reasonable energy level. Informing the patient about the fatigue before treatment enables him to schedule his activities accordingly. (6, 28)

**117.** 2. Patients with Hodgkin's disease are extremely vulnerable to infection because of the defective immune responses caused by the tumor, as well as the bone-marrow depression and low white blood count caused by the radiation. Fever is the most sensitive indicator of infection and should be reported immediately so that treatment can be initiated. Loss of hair is unusual in radiation to the neck. Neck circumference and upper-extremity circulation are not related to major complications. (6, 28)

**118.** 4. It is unlikely that having trouble starting urination is related to having diabetes. Common signs and symptoms of diabetes mellitus include wounds that heal slowly or not at all, impotence, thirst, hunger, and frequent voiding. Additional signs and symptoms include fatigue, itching of the skin, blurred vision, irritability, and muscle cramps, especially in the legs. (6, 23)

**119.** 4. The primary action of oral hypoglycemic agents is to stimulate the secretion of insulin by the beta cells in the pancreas' islets of Langerhans. The sulfonylureas may also alter cell-receptor sensitivity to insulin. Oral hypoglycemics can be used only when some function of the beta cells remains. They cannot be used when beta cells no longer function. The sulfonylureas do not influence urinary excretion of glucose, gluconeogenesis in the liver, or the action of insulin in body cells. (6, 17)

**120.** 1. The etiology of diabetes mellitus is not clearly understood, but obesity appears to be a contributing factor, especially in patients with non-insulin-dependent diabetes. Because weight reduction is critically important, one of the nurse's goals should be to help the patient plan a program to lose weight. Smoking and exposure to cold do not appear to predispose to diabetes, but smoking is unhealthful for everyone. This is especially true for diabetics because of their susceptibility to vascular complications. Diabetics who drink alcohol must learn to take into account the caloric intake of the beverage when planning dietary management. Drinking alcohol may make it difficult to lose weight, because alcohol is high in calories. (6, 7)

**121.** 1. The patient should be instructed to mix the sediment that accumulates in a vial of NPH insulin by rolling the vial gently between the palms of the hands or by turning the vial upside down several times. Shaking the vial is *not* recommended because it produces bubbles that make it difficult to withdraw accurate doses of insulin. Proper techniques of self-administering insulin include introducing the needle with a dartlike action, pulling back on the plunger as soon as the needle is in place to determine whether the needle is in a vein, and holding an antiseptic sponge against the needle when removing it from tissue to prevent the discomfort of the needle pulling on the skin. (23, 28)

**122.** 4. When teaching dietary alterations to a patient with diabetes mellitus, the nurse should take into account his food preferences and cultural background. Neglecting to do so often results in dietary noncompliance. In exchange lists, which most diabetics are taught to use, pastas are classified as a cereal. (9, 19)

**123.** 2. The Somogyi, or dawn, phenomenon is due to excessive insulin administration. The patient has high fasting blood sugars each morning when dietary noncompliance is not a factor. Some patients describe middle-of-the-night symptoms resembling symptoms of hypoglycemia. It is believed that when hypoglycemia occurs, the body demonstrates a rebound hyperglycemic action that causes the high fasting blood sugars in the morning. Usually, insulin dosages are reduced for patients suffering from the Somogyi effect. (9, 19)

**124.** 4. The first order of business after the birth of a baby is to ensure that the infant's airway is clear. Clearing the airway is started immediately after the delivery of the infant's head, when debris is cleared from the nose and mouth. The infant is often kept in the face-down position immediately after delivery to promote drainage from the respiratory passages. Suctioning the respiratory passages is also sometimes used. *After* the infant's respiratory system is functioning satisfactorily, other procedures can be carried out, such as cutting the cord, wrapping the infant, and instilling eye drops. (6, 40)

**125.** 2. Apgar scoring takes into account five aspects of the infant's condition: heart rate, respiratory effort, muscle tone, reflex irritability, and color. The highest possible score on each of these five items is 2, so 10 is the highest possible total Apgar score. (6, 32, 40)

**126.** 4. A newborn's eyes are closed most of the time. To facilitate an examination of the eyes, the infant's head should be lifted. He will then tend to open his eyes spontaneously. The infant is also likely to open his eyes when rocked. (6, 32, 40)

**127.** 1. The rooting reflex is best tested by stroking a newborn's cheek or the corner of his mouth. The normal newborn will turn to the stimulus and open his mouth. The grasp reflex is tested by placing a finger in the infant's hand. He will normally grasp the finger securely. The Moro reflex is best tested by supporting the infant's head, then allowing it to drop back a short distance. Normally, the arms will extend laterally and the hands will open; the infant then flexes his arms and brings them together as though embracing. The stepping or dancing reflex is tested by holding the infant upright while allowing his feet to touch a firm surface. He will normally move his feet in stepping or dancing movements. (6, 32, 40)

**128.** 4. The recommended type of isolation used for a child with meningitis is respiratory isolation. This requires a private room with a door that must be kept closed. Gowns and gloves are not necessary, but a mask should be worn by people entering the room. These techniques are used until 24 hours after successful therapy has been started. (26, 40)

**129.** 1. Meningitis is almost always preceded by an infection elsewhere in the body. Such infections include otitis media, nasopharyngitis, mastoiditis, and infections of the bone, lungs, heart, and skin. It is unlikely that a broken bone, food poisoning, and pinworms predisposed this child to meningitis. (25, 40)

**130.** 2. Neck rigidity and pain are assessed by having the child lie in the supine position. The examiner lifts the child's head and moves the neck in all directions. During this exam, a child with meningitis typically demonstrates pain and rigidity of the neck. If the child has involuntary bending of the hips and knees during passive flexion of the neck, Brudzinski's sign is positive, suggesting meningeal inflammation. (26, 32)

**131.** 2. After a lumbar puncture, a child should be placed in the supine position in bed to help prevent headaches. The supine position helps prevent cerebrospinal fluid from leaking through the puncture in the dura into the arachnoid spaces; such leakage is believed to cause headaches. Fluids, high-carbohydrate snacks, and a darkened room are unlikely to prevent headaches following a lumbar puncture. (26, 32)

**132.** 2. Typically, antibiotic therapy is used for children with meningitis. The drug is almost always given by the intravenous route through the intravenous line used to infuse fluids. (26, 32)

**133.** 4. Mannitol is an osmotic diuretic. It is used for its diuretic effect to help relieve cerebral edema by increasing the output of fluids through the kidneys. (22, 33)

**134.** 3. Many preschoolers have great feelings of guilt about hospitalization because they associate being ill with bad behavior. Anger, pity, and sorrow are not necessarily associated with illness, but occasionally a nurse may become aware that a patient has such feelings. The nurse's primary role is to allow the child to express her feelings and correct any misperceptions. (25, 32)

**135.** 1. It is best to overcome the effects of excessive alcohol intake by "sleeping it off." Alcohol is not used directly by muscle cells, and therefore physical activity does not affect the rate at which alcohol is removed from the patient's bloodstream. Restricting fluids or drinking black coffee does not hasten removal of alcohol from the body. (5, 6)

**136.** 3. There is no precise profile of a person suffering from alcoholism, but common behavioral traits include a history of refraining from drinking for periods of time only to return to excessive drinking, using alcohol as a solution for personal problems, and demonstrating multiple substance abuse. An inadequate diet is common, and many chronic alcoholics suffer from malnutrition. A magnesium deficit is often noted, and Wernicke-Korsakoff syndrome, caused by a vitamin B deficiency, is noted in some alcoholics. Poor digestion and absorption of food constituents also seriously compromise the utilization of food in the alcoholic due to the damaging effect of alcohol on the stomach and small intestine and subsequently on the liver and pancreas. (16)

**137.** 2. Making up stories to fill in memory gaps is called confabulation. Displacement is a defense mechanism that refers ideas and feelings to something or someone not responsible for them. Disorientation is a loss of understanding in relation to place, time, or identity. Flight of ideas is a rapid shift of thoughts from one subject to another before any idea has been finished. (16)

**138.** 2. The patient with an alcohol problem must be motivated to change her behavior before rehabilitation can be expected to succeed. Such other factors as a support system in the home, a community health center for alcoholics, and self-help groups can play an important role, but they cannot be expected to help unless the patient wants to solve her alcohol-abuse problem. (16, 36)

**139.** 3. Delirium tremens often occurs after the patient who has been abusing alcohol does not drink alcohol for about 24 to 72 hours. It is a serious complication and can be life-threatening. The patient should be kept in a private room, which should be well lighted to reduce shadows and visual hallucinations. A calm, nonstressful environment is recommended and the patient should be given prescribed sedation. Restraints are used only as a last resort; it is preferable to stay with the patient and calm her with touch, reassurance, and the nurse's presence. The nurse's attitude of acceptance and support is important. One method to help strengthen the patient's link with reality is to explain her visual misinterpretations, rather than to agree with them. (5)

**140.** 3. Memory loss and disorientation are typical signs of Wernicke-Korsakoff syndrome; so also is confabulation. The syndrome is believed to be due to a vitamin B deficiency and usually occurs in patients with long-standing alcoholism who have neglected their diets. (16)

**141.** 4. Disulfiram (Antabuse) is used for patients suffering from alcohol abuse because the drug sensitizes them to alcohol. When a patient drinks alcohol while taking the drug, the adverse effects that result include flushing of the face, neck, and upper trunk, hyperventilation, and a rapid pulse rate. Nausea and severe vomiting then typically follow. These symptoms are often accompanied by pallor, hypotension, headaches, palpitations, dyspnea, and faintness. (17)

**142.** 1. Membership in Alcoholics Anonymous (AA) is voluntary. Its rehabilitated members are available to support alcoholics, and the understanding and influence of these rehabilitated members often enable alcoholics to change their own behavior. The role of rehabilitated members does not include helping people abusing alcohol to identify personal problems, sympathizing with them, or helping them develop defense mechanisms to cope with alcoholism. AA is not entirely unlike other groups of people who organize to help those with disorders similar to their own. For example, ostomy clubs have helped many people with new ostomies learn to adjust to a change in their bodies and to live useful and fulfilling lives. (36)

**143.** 3. One formula that can be used to determine liquid dosage is by proportion:

$$250 \text{ mg} : 10 \text{ ml} :: 400 \text{ mg} : x$$

$$250\,x = 4{,}000$$

$$4{,}000 \div 250 = 16 \text{ ml}$$

Another method is:

$$\frac{\text{Dose desired}}{\text{Dose on hand}} \times \text{Quantity} = x$$

$$\frac{400 \text{ mg}}{250 \text{ mg}} \times 10 \text{ ml} = x$$

$$4{,}000 \div 250 = 16 \text{ ml}$$

A typical loading dose for aminophylline is about 6 mg/kg of body weight administered over 20 to 30 minutes. Assume the patient weighs 154 pounds (70 kg). 6 mg/kg × 70 kg = 420 mg. The loading dose of 400 mg when the patient weighs 70 kg is within normal range. (13, 17)

**144.** 2. Aminophylline is a bronchodilator that relaxes smooth muscles in the bronchioles. It is used in patients with emphysema to improve ventilation by dilating the bronchioles. (6, 17)

**145.** 3. The patient with emphysema has a chronic retention of excessive carbon dioxide; as a result, the normal stimulus for respirations in centers in the medulla becomes ineffective. Instead, peripheral pressoreceptors in the aortic arch and carotid arteries, which are sensitive to oxygen blood levels, stimulate respirations. If the emphysemic patient receives high concentrations of oxygen, the blood level of oxygen will rise excessively, the stimulus for respiration will decrease, and the patient is likely eventually to have respiratory failure. (23, 28)

**146.** 3. Authorities differ slightly about normal $PaO_2$ ranges for people of about 60 years of age, but a range of 70 to 80 mm Hg is common. Because of poor gas exchanges in the diseased lungs, the patient with emphysema typically has a lower-than-average $PaO_2$ and a higher-than-average $PaCO_2$. (21, 28)

**147.** 4. Right-sided heart failure, or cor pulmonale, is a complication of emphysema. Typical signs of the disorder include distended neck veins, dependent edema, and pain in the upper right abdomen. Emphysema results in poor arterial oxygen saturation and poor excretion of carbon dioxide. These pathologic conditions result in vasoconstriction of pulmonary arteries, which in turn causes increased resistance to blood circulation in the pulmonary system. This leads to increased work for the right ventricle of the heart, and eventually to right-sided heart failure. (6, 23)

**148.** 2. Measures to reduce the tenacity of respiratory secretions include humidifying inspired air and encouraging a high level of fluid intake. In postural drainage, the force of gravity is used to help promote drainage of secretions. Diaphragmatic breathing helps strengthen and increase the use of the diaphragm in breathing but does not reduce the tenacity of sputum. Oxygen does not reduce the tenacity of respiratory secretions. (6, 23)

**149.** 3. Pursed-lip breathing helps prevent collapse of alveolar tissues in the lungs. In the presence of emphysema, a chronic state of hyperinflation results because of obstruction of bronchioles and a loss of elasticity in the lower pulmonary system, causing alveolar lung tissues to collapse. Hyperinflation can be somewhat relieved when accumulated air is forcefully exhaled through pursed-lip breathing to reduce intrapulmonary pressure. When alveoli function effectively, the exchange of gases in the lungs occurs properly. Pursed-lip breathing is not used primarily to promote a regular breathing pattern, although more regular breathing may result. Pursed-lip breathing is not used to sensitize central chemoreceptors in the medulla. (6, 21)

**150.** 3. Because of problems associated with pregnant, unmarried teenagers, it is important for the nurse to learn about psychosocial factors in the patient's life. When psychosocial problems exist, as they often do for these young women, the nurse can plan to do whatever is possible to make the patient's pregnancy a healthful experience, in cooperation with other health-team members. To help a reluctant patient, the nurse should be nonjudgmental and accepting and should provide open channels of communication. Threatening to withhold care if certain information is not given, saying that information is necessary for the record, and offering sympathy are unlikely to gain the patient's trust and cooperation. (27)

**151.** 2. All the factors in this item (activity, exercise, nutrition, fluid intake, rest and sleep, and personal cleanliness) influence a patient's pregnancy. However, probably the most common and important problem associated with a low socioeconomic status is inadequate or poor nutrition. Especially common problems include iron-deficiency anemia and inadequate intakes of vitamins A and C, and riboflavin. (27)

**152.** 3. An adequate calcium intake will help prevent tooth loss in the pregnant woman. When calcium intake is low, the fetus receives calcium from the mother, often indirectly from her teeth and bones. (27)

**153.** 2. The newborn's lower gastrointestinal tract does not contain the bacteria necessary to produce vitamin K. As a result, poor blood clotting is present. The deficiency is overcome when vitamin K is given to the newborn. (27)

**154.** 3. Intramuscular injections should be given to a newborn in the rectus femoris muscle on the anterior of the thigh. It is a relatively large muscle, convenient to use, and free of nerves that could be injured. Gluteus muscles should *not* be used, because of the danger of injuring the sciatic nerve. The biceps brachii muscle, located in the arm, and the biceps femoris muscle, located in the back of the leg, are unsuitable sites. (27)

**155.** 2. Before nursing, the mother should cleanse her nipples with plain water. Water will not wash off the nipples' normal antiseptic lubricant, lysozyme. Soap, antiseptics, and alcohol tend to dry the nipples and predispose to cracking. (27)

**156.** 2. The cause of colic is not understood, but it is believed to result from an accumulation of air in the intestines. Allergies, over- and underfeeding, and parental tensions may also be causative factors. To help prevent the accumulation of air in the gastrointestinal tract, the infant should be bubbled frequently during feedings, fed slowly, and held upright for a half-hour or so after feedings. The mother should be helped to relax if tension appears to have a role in the colic. The problem usually disappears on its own when the infant reaches about 3 months of age. Colic does not appear to interfere with the normal growth and development of an otherwise healthy infant. (26, 36)

**157.** 4. Beginning at about 1 month to 6 weeks, a healthy infant can hold up his head when lying on his abdomen. An infant starts holding a bottle fairly well beginning at about 6 months of age. An infant can roll over at about 4 to 5 months of age. An infant normally begins to show fear of strangers at about 6 to 7 months of age. (26, 40)

**158.** 4. The person suffering from an obsessive-compulsive disorder has an uncontrollable and persistent need to carry out behavior that helps relieve intolerable anxiety. An irrational fear is called a phobia. Ambivalence refers to two simultaneous opposing feelings. In depression, the patient feels extreme sadness. (3, 36)

**159.** 2. A common characteristic of the person with an obsessive-compulsive disorder is that he recognizes that his behavior is irrational but cannot change it. (3, 36)

**160.** 4. Coping with compulsive behavior can be very frustrating. Interfering with the patient's behavior is ordinarily not helpful and may cause the patient to become negative and more firmly committed to the behavior. Nor does it help to explain how his behavior may interfere with getting well. Allowing the patient to decide whether he will carry out his behavior or attend meals, group activities, therapy sessions, and the like usually means the patient will favor his abnormal behavior over activities that he requires for healthful living. Therefore, in the situation described, it would be best for the nurse to remind the patient in sufficient time so that he can carry out his ritualistic behavior and arrive on time for scheduled activities. (3, 36)

**161.** 2. Hoarseness that fails to subside with conservative care is an early sign of cancer of the larynx. Difficulty with swallowing is a later symptom and occurs as the tumor enlarges to the point that it obstructs swallowing. A sore throat is not an early symptom of laryngeal cancer. Pain that radiates to the ear is a likely indication that the tumor is metastasizing. (6)

**162.** 2. People react to illnesses in their own unique way. However, a common emotional response during the first stage of an illness, especially when the illness is not a sudden one of catastrophic proportion, is denial, which the patient described in this item appears to be demonstrating. Other early emotional responses to illness include anxiety, shame, and guilt. Patients are less likely to demonstrate dependence, aggression, or anger during the first stage of an illness. (6)

**163.** 2. Preparing a patient for surgery includes attending to oral hygiene, giving adequate nourishment and fluid, and providing for proper bowel elimination. However, before a laryngectomy, the highest priority is ensuring thorough and regular oral hygiene. This measure is especially significant in helping to prevent postoperative infection. An antibiotic may be prescribed preoperatively, also with the intent of reducing the possibility of postoperative infection. Oral hygiene is also important postoperatively to help prevent infection. In addition, because the patient's exhaled air does not pass through his mouth following a total laryngectomy, the patient may be unaware of halitosis. The nurse should help prevent it by ensuring that oral hygiene is performed. (5, 6)

**164.** 4. Rupture of the carotid artery is a serious complication after a laryngectomy. It is more likely to occur if the patient has a wound infection at the site of surgery. While calling for help, the nurse should apply pressure over the bleeding artery and reassure the patient. Neither suctioning the laryngectomy tube nor raising the head of the bed will stop the bleeding. It is neither practical nor safe to try to clamp the bleeding artery. (6)

**165.** 2. Patients with a total laryngectomy can eventually learn to produce sounds by ejecting air under pressure from the esophagus. At first, they must do this by using the air of a belch. Therefore, a patient should begin learning how to belch when starting to take oral feedings following a total laryngectomy. Coughing, sneezing, and hiccuping will not help the patient during speech rehabilitation. (6, 28)

**166.** 2. A patient who has had a total laryngectomy will drown if water enters the stoma; therefore, swimming is contraindicated. A plastic bib or a hand held over the stoma is recommended during showering. The patient should be encouraged to exercise but not to the point of fatigue. Bowling, tending a flower garden, and attending sports events are not contraindicated. (6, 19)

**167.** 4. By the time a child reaches the age of about 8 to 10 years, he will normally view death as irreversible and will fear it. The nurse should be aware of this and should answer questions about death accordingly. For the child described in this item, death is not a threat; therefore, the nurse should reassure her and allow her to express her fears freely. Children under about 6 or 7 years of age often view death as reversible. (32, 40)

**168.** 3. After an uncomplicated appendectomy, fluid intake is started early in the postoperative period. But before doing so, the nurse should auscultate the patient's abdomen to determine whether bowel sounds are present. If they are not, fluids should be withheld until bowel sounds are heard. Asking the patient whether he is thirsty, making sure he is fully conscious, and palpating the abdomen for pain will not help determine whether he has bowel sounds and is ready to take oral fluids. (32, 40)

**169.** 2. A typical sign of pediculosis capitis (head lice) is frequent scratching of the scalp, because the condition causes severe itching. Scratch marks are usually easily visible. Several pharmaceutical preparations are available that destroy the lice and nits. Since head lice are easily transmitted to others, members of the child's family and her peers should be examined for infestation also. Spotty baldness often occurs when a patient has tinea capitis (scalp ringworm). Wheals, smooth elevated areas that often itch, are common when an allergy is present. Wheals with blistering are often present when a child has mosquito bites. (32, 40)

**170.** 3. Peanut butter is rich in protein, as are milk, eggs, cheese, meat, fish, legumes, and nuts. Carrot sticks, graham crackers, and raw apples are low in protein. (7, 25)

**171.** 1. A child normally develops social skills between the preschool and the adolescent years. The dominant influence during the middle childhood years comes characteristically from peers and people such as teachers and peers' parents. The child normally works on developing a sense of industry and competency. These developmental tasks can be seen as the child accepts work for the sake of work and play for the sake of play, and recognizes the difference between work and play. (25, 40)

**172.** 4. Most authorities agree more research is needed to determine the amount of influence television has on the behavior of school-age children. One limiting feature of present research is that the studies have been carried out mostly in contrived settings. Also, it has been shown that individual personality variables play an important part in the extent of influence television has on a child. Some authors point out that excessive television interferes with a child's opportunities to interact with people, objects, and the environment. Nurses should keep up-to-date on such research, because television is popular with children. (32, 40)

**173.** 1. A history of a throat infection with Group A streptococci is present in most cases of acute glomerulonephritis. Ordinarily, the infection occurs 2 to 3 weeks before the onset of nephritis. Glomerulonephritis typically strikes young people. (32, 40)

**174.** 1. A patient with acute glomerulonephritis typically has scanty urinary output; some patients may produce no urine (anuria). Urinary output increases as the patient's condition improves. Fluids are administered to the patient according to clinical findings. It is very important to keep accurate records of the patient's intake and output to make accurate judgments about the nursing and medical management of the patient. (32, 40)

**175.** 3. A high-protein snack before bedtime is recommended for people with insomnia because an amino acid derived from protein is believed to help induce sleep. Of the snacks described in this item, only cheese cubes are high in protein; apples, jellied toast, and dried figs have a low protein content. (7, 29)

**176.** 3. In glaucoma, peripheral vision is impaired long before central vision is impaired. Hazy, blurred, or distorted vision is consistent with a diagnosis of cataracts. Loss of central vision is consistent with senile macular degeneration but occurs late in glaucoma. Blurred or "sooty" vision is consistent with a diagnosis of detached retina. (6, 21)

**177.** 1. Timolol maleate (Timoptic) eye drops reduce elevated, as well as normal, intraocular pressure and help prevent visual field loss. As with other topically applied ophthalmic drugs, this drug is absorbed systemically; its major side effects are slight bradycardia at rest, anorexia, and headache. Nausea and vomiting and vivid dreams are side effects of timolol maleate (Blocadren), an antihypertensive agent. (13, 17)

**178.** 1. Glaucoma is caused by obstruction in any of the outflow channels in the eye, resulting in increased intraocular pressure. If untreated, increased intraocular pressure can damage the optic nerve and can lead to blindness. Although glaucoma cannot be cured, it can usually be controlled. (6, 21)

**179.** 4. Excessive exertion, such as shoveling snow and heavy lifting, increases intraocular pressure, as does any activity that causes a person to perform the Valsalva maneuver. Watching television and knitting do not increase intraocular pressure. Dietary fat does not affect intraocular pressure. (6, 21)

**180.** 2. Laser trabeculoplasty produces a nonpenetrating thermal burn that changes the configuration of the trabecular meshwork and leads to an increased outflow of aqueous humor. Because 4 to 8 weeks are required to determine if the procedure is successful, medications prescribed preoperatively to decrease intraocular pressure are continued postoperatively. In addition to these glaucoma medications, a steroid or combination antibiotic/steroid may be prescribed to reduce inflammation or prevent infection. (6, 28)

# comprehensive test 3

Select the one *best* or *correct* answer and indicate your choice by filling in the circle with a pencil in front of the option you have chosen. If the answer you would prefer is not given, select the one you think is *most appropriate*.

Mr. Jacob Pinsky, 80, has an indirect inguinal hernia on the right side. A herniorrhaphy is scheduled.

**181.** While admitting Mr. Pinsky, the nurse notes that he is wearing a hearing aid. Which of the following courses of action would be *best* for the nurse to take in relation to the hearing aid?
- ○ 1. Send it home with his daughter for safekeeping.
- ○ 2. Label it and place it in a locked cupboard for safekeeping.
- ○ 3. Encourage the patient to wear it as he ordinarily does at home.
- ○ 4. Instruct the patient to keep it in the drawer of his bedside stand.

**182.** Which of the following positions permits the *best* assessment of Mr. Pinsky's inguinal hernia?
- ○ 1. The upright position.
- ○ 2. The sitting position.
- ○ 3. The left side-lying position.
- ○ 4. The right side-lying position.

**183.** Which of the following adjustments in the average adult dosage of preoperative medications should the nurse expect for Mr. Pinsky?
- ○ 1. A larger-than-average dosage; elderly patients tend to have a decreased ability to absorb drugs.
- ○ 2. A larger-than-average dosage; elderly patients tend to have a decreased ability to maintain adequate blood levels of most drugs.
- ○ 3. A smaller-than-average dosage; elderly patients tend to have an increased sensitivity to most drugs.
- ○ 4. A smaller-than-average dosage; elderly patients tend to have an increased susceptibility to allergic reactions to most drugs.

**184.** Atropine sulfate is prescribed for Mr. Pinsky preoperatively. The nurse should explain to the patient that the medication will *most probably* cause him to feel

- ○ 1. numb.
- ○ 2. dizzy.
- ○ 3. hungry.
- ○ 4. thirsty.

**185.** The nurse in the surgical reception area prepares Mr. Pinsky's skin for surgery. The *primary* goal of preoperative skin preparation is to
- ○ 1. render the operative area free of organisms.
- ○ 2. improve the field of vision for the physician.
- ○ 3. decrease the number of organisms on the surface of the skin.
- ○ 4. enhance the skin's natural defenses against organisms.

**186.** A depilatory is used to remove body hair from Mr. Pinsky's operative site rather than a razor. The *primary* reason for using a depilatory is that, in contrast to a razor, a depilatory
- ○ 1. leaves the skin cleaner.
- ○ 2. removes body hair more quickly.
- ○ 3. tends to irritate the skin less.
- ○ 4. is more effective in removing fine body hair.

**187.** Mr. Pinsky receives spinal anesthesia. The position of choice for administering spinal anesthesia is to have the patient lie on his
- ○ 1. side with his legs well flexed.
- ○ 2. side with his legs well extended.
- ○ 3. abdomen with his arms at his side.
- ○ 4. abdomen with his arms folded under his head.

**188.** Which of the following assessments should the nurse perform and document in the patient's record to indicate that Mr. Pinsky is recovering from anesthesia?
- ○ 1. The level of consciousness.
- ○ 2. The rate and depth of respirations.
- ○ 3. The rate of capillary refill in the toes.
- ○ 4. The degree of response to pin pricks in the legs and toes.

**189.** Mr. Pinsky's scrotum is swollen and painful 2 days postoperatively. A nursing measure *most likely* to promote comfort for Mr. Pinsky is to

○ 1. apply a snug binder on the patient's abdomen.
○ 2. have the patient wear a truss to support the scrotum.
○ 3. elevate the scrotum and place ice bags on the area intermittently.
○ 4. have the patient lie on his side and place a pillow between his legs.

Ms. Kim Ling visits her physician when she thinks she is pregnant.

**190.** If the nurse gathers the following information about Ms. Ling, which finding should she interpret as a *probable* sign of pregnancy?
○ 1. The patient has morning sickness.
○ 2. The patient's pregnancy test is positive.
○ 3. The patient is having menstrual suppression.
○ 4. The patient complains of a frequent need to void.

**191.** On a subsequent visit, Ms. Ling says she is "feeling life," an expression synonymous with the term
○ 1. quickening.
○ 2. lightening.
○ 3. ballottement.
○ 4. Chadwick's sign.

**192.** Later in Ms. Ling's pregnancy, the nurse learns that she is using Alka-Seltzer and baking soda to relieve heartburn. The nurse is justified in suggesting that the patient avoid these two remedies for heartburn when the patient complains of
○ 1. diarrhea.
○ 2. flatulence.
○ 3. symptoms associated with water retention.
○ 4. frequent urination.

**193.** The nurse notes that on Ms. Ling's previous visit, the examiner documented hearing funic souffles when the patient's abdomen was auscultated. This means the examiner heard a sound that is considered
○ 1. abnormal; it is the sound of blood passing through a defective placenta.
○ 2. abnormal; it is the sound of blood passing through a defective valve in the fetal heart.
○ 3. normal; it is the sound of blood passing through uterine vessels.
○ 4. normal; it is the sound of blood passing through the umbilical cord.

**194.** When Ms. Ling complains of a common discomfort of pregnancy, the nurse teaches her to use the tailor-sitting position. On her next visit, the nurse judges that the position has been effective when Ms. Ling says she is now less bothered by

○ 1. hemorrhoids.
○ 2. leaking urine.
○ 3. low backaches.
○ 4. leg varicosities.

Ms. Roberta Thomas, a 64-year-old college professor, is admitted to the hospital with peptic (duodenal) ulcers.

**195.** The discomfort that *most probably* brought Ms. Thomas to seek health care is pain that is
○ 1. relieved by eating.
○ 2. relieved by resting.
○ 3. increased by physical activity.
○ 4. increased by excretory efforts.

**196.** Ms. Thomas tells the nurse that she has been using bicarbonate of soda frequently to relieve heartburn and indigestion. By so doing, the patient increases her risk of developing
○ 1. constipation.
○ 2. dehydration.
○ 3. metabolic alkalosis.
○ 4. iron-deficiency anemia.

**197.** The heartburn for which Ms. Thomas has been using bicarbonate of soda *usually* occurs as a result of
○ 1. eating too much food at one time.
○ 2. regurgitating stomach contents into the esophagus.
○ 3. having an allergy to something that is being eaten.
○ 4. placing undue work on the heart because of a stressful environment.

**198.** Ms. Thomas has an x-ray examination of her upper gastrointestinal tract (a GI series). The nurse should anticipate that following Ms. Thomas's GI series, measures are *usually* taken to guard against the patient's developing
○ 1. diarrhea.
○ 2. heartburn.
○ 3. constipation.
○ 4. nausea and vomiting.

**199.** If Ms. Thomas says she uses the following medications at home, which should the nurse teach her to *avoid* because of her peptic ulcers?
○ 1. Aspirin for occasional headaches.
○ 2. Scopolamine to prevent seasickness when boating.
○ 3. Psyllium hydrophilic mucilloid (Metamucil) for occasional constipation.
○ 4. Phenylephrine (Neo-Synephrine) for an upper respiratory infection.

**554**

A nurse is caring for Baby Boy Cranston, a preterm infant.

**200.** Which of the following criteria is *least likely* to be used to establish Baby Cranston's prematurity?
○ 1. His birth weight.
○ 2. His gestational age.
○ 3. The status of his muscle tonus.
○ 4. The status of his pupillary reactions to light.

**201.** Baby Cranston is fed by gastric gavage with a tube that enters his nostril. The distance the nurse should insert the tube so that it reaches the stomach should be equivalent to the distance from the
○ 1. infant's mouth to the bottom of the stomach.
○ 2. bridge of the infant's nose to the xiphoid process.
○ 3. tip of the infant's nose, to an earlobe, to the xiphoid process.
○ 4. middle of the infant's forehead, to an earlobe, to the bottom of the rib cage.

**202.** Sodium bicarbonate is prescribed for Baby Cranston when laboratory studies reveal that he suffers from hyponatremia. The nurse is justified in judging that too much sodium bicarbonate is being administered when the infant has signs of
○ 1. diarrhea.
○ 2. fluid retention.
○ 3. increased irritability.
○ 4. spasms of the feet and hands.

**203.** The nurse closely monitors Baby Cranston's vital signs. It is *most often* recommended that the pulse rate should be obtained over
○ 1. a femoral artery.
○ 2. a carotid artery.
○ 3. the ascending aorta.
○ 4. the apex of the heart.

**204.** Baby Cranston receives supplemental oxygen. Oxygen toxicity due to high elevations in his blood $PaO_2$ predisposes him to
○ 1. deafness.
○ 2. blindness.
○ 3. mental retardation.
○ 4. respiratory distress syndrome.

Ms. Rena Jackson, 70, participates in a screening test for carcinoma of the lower intestine. The test is positive. Ms. Jackson seeks health care and learns that she has carcinoma of the colon. She is admitted to the hospital and will have surgery to perform a colostomy.

**205.** The screening test Ms. Jackson *most likely* had was one that examined the stool for evidence of

○ 1. pus.
○ 2. mucus.
○ 3. occult blood.
○ 4. malignant cells.

**206.** The nurse notes that Ms. Jackson's skin is dry and flaky and feels warm to the touch. Her oral mucous membrane is cracked. The nurse judges that Ms. Jackson is dehydrated. To validate this observation, the nurse should check the patient's
○ 1. skin turgor.
○ 2. eye grounds.
○ 3. respiratory rate.
○ 4. urine specific gravity.

**207.** Kanamycin sulfate (Kantrex) is prescribed preoperatively for Ms. Jackson. This drug is prescribed *primarily* because it helps
○ 1. inhibit spasticity of the colon.
○ 2. coat irritated walls in the colon.
○ 3. reduce the bacterial count in the colon.
○ 4. slow metastatic growth of the malignant tumor.

**208.** Ms. Jackson is being taught deep-breathing exercises preoperatively. After taking a deep inhalation, the patient should be taught *next* to
○ 1. close the glottis tightly.
○ 2. make a short, hacking cough.
○ 3. exhale slowly but thoroughly.
○ 4. hold the breath for a few seconds.

**209.** The nurse teaches Ms. Jackson to perform leg exercises. The *primary* purpose for having Ms. Jackson use leg exercises postoperatively is to help prevent
○ 1. venous stasis.
○ 2. paralytic ileus.
○ 3. decubitus ulcers.
○ 4. urinary retention.

**210.** Ms. Jackson expresses concern over how she will look after her surgery and says she feels "disgusted already." The nurse works to help Ms. Jackson accept a change in body image. The nurse should keep in mind that the groundwork for the development of the basic body image is *most probably* started during which stage of life?
○ 1. Childhood.
○ 2. Adolescence.
○ 3. Early adulthood.
○ 4. Middle adulthood.

**211.** The recovery-room nurse observes Ms. Jackson for signs of postoperative shock. Of the following conditions, which is the *most common* cause of postoperative shock?
○ 1. Adrenal failure.
○ 2. Excessive bleeding.
○ 3. A transfusion reaction.
○ 4. An untoward drug reaction.

**212.** The nurse assesses Ms. Jackson for cyanosis. Because the patient is black, it would be *best* for the nurse to assess for cyanosis by examining
○ 1. her retinas.
○ 2. her nail beds.
○ 3. her oral mucous membranes.
○ 4. the skin on the inner aspects of her wrists.

**213.** Before Ms. Jackson is helped to ambulate, she is first prepared for dangling on the side of her bed. Which of the following measures should the nurse plan to carry out before helping Ms. Jackson dangle?
○ 1. Administer a prescribed analgesic.
○ 2. Encourage the patient to take a short nap.
○ 3. Have the patient carry out leg exercises for a few minutes.
○ 4. Help the patient assume a high Fowler's position for a few minutes.

**214.** Ms. Jackson develops an incisional abscess. A debridement is done and a small drain is left in the wound. The drain is accomplishing its intended purpose when it
○ 1. is used to irrigate the wound.
○ 2. permits the escape of wound drainage.
○ 3. decreases the discomfort in the surrounding tissues.
○ 4. allows for the introduction of antibiotics into the wound.

**215.** In contrast to younger mature adults, Ms. Jackson has a higher risk of a postoperative infection *primarily* because elderly people have
○ 1. atrophy of lymph nodes.
○ 2. considerable loss of neurons in the body.
○ 3. reduced ability to maintain physiologic homeostasis.
○ 4. decreased interest in healthful habits of daily living.

**216.** The nurse irrigates Ms. Jackson's colostomy. When Ms. Jackson complains of abdominal cramping while fluid is being introduced through the stoma, the nurse's *best* course of action is to
○ 1. help the patient turn onto her side.
○ 2. remove the irrigating cone from the stoma.
○ 3. have the patient take several deep breaths.
○ 4. slow the flow of irrigating solution temporarily.

Ms. Grace Martin is admitted to the hospital in the first stage of labor.

**217.** The nurse times the frequency of Ms. Martin's contractions *correctly* when she determines the time interval between the

○ 1. beginning and the end of one contraction.
○ 2. end of one contraction and the beginning of the next contraction.
○ 3. end of one contraction and the end of the next contraction.
○ 4. beginning of one contraction and the beginning of the next contraction.

**218.** The position of choice during the first stage of labor is
○ 1. a sitting position.
○ 2. a low Fowler's position.
○ 3. either side-lying position.
○ 4. any position of comfort.

**219.** A vaginal examination is to be performed on Ms. Martin. In addition to a lubricating agent, which of the following should the nurse have ready?
○ 1. A speculum.
○ 2. Waterproof gloves.
○ 3. Nitrazine paper.
○ 4. A fetal heart stethoscope.

**220.** Ms. Martin is offered a bedpan or helped to the bathroom by the nurse every few hours *primarily* because a full bladder during labor
○ 1. increases the risk of urinary incontinence.
○ 2. predisposes to a prolapse of the umbilical cord.
○ 3. causes a decrease in the frequency of uterine contractions.
○ 4. interferes with the descent of the infant in the birth canal.

**221.** Immediately after Ms. Martin's membranes rupture, the nurse should listen to the fetal heartbeat for signs of a prolapsed cord. The *most typical* sign of fetal distress due to pressure on the cord is
○ 1. an increasingly arrhythmic fetal heartbeat before contractions.
○ 2. a persistently slow fetal heartbeat after contractions.
○ 3. a steadily increasing fetal heartbeat during contractions.
○ 4. an intermittently rapid and slow fetal heartbeat between contractions.

**222.** In keeping with the gate-control theory for the relief of pain, the nurse suggests to Ms. Martin that she use her hands to make circular, massagelike movements over her abdomen when she feels discomfort. An anatomic characteristic of the skin believed important for closing the gating mechanism and halting the transmission of pain impulses is that the skin
○ 1. is well supplied with blood vessels.
○ 2. is normally well lubricated with oily sebum.
○ 3. has many large-diameter sensory nerve fibers.
○ 4. has many receptors that are responsive to pressure changes.

Stacey Johnson, 10, is admitted to the hospital acutely ill with rheumatic fever. Her mother accompanies her.

**223.** When planning Stacey's nursing care, the goal of *highest priority* during the patient's acute illness should be helping Stacey to
○ 1. maintain bed rest.
○ 2. obtain sufficient nourishment.
○ 3. take generous amounts of liquids.
○ 4. carry out range-of-motion exercises.

**224.** When the nurse obtains Stacey's health history from the mother, Mrs. Johnson says that Stacey was ill a short time ago. It is *most probable* that the child was ill with
○ 1. cystitis.
○ 2. chicken pox.
○ 3. a sore throat.
○ 4. a gastrointestinal upset.

**225.** Stacey complains of pain in her joints. Nursing measures to help minimize joint discomfort include positioning the patient in proper body alignment and
○ 1. massaging the affected joints.
○ 2. passively exercising the affected joints.
○ 3. applying warmth to affected joints.
○ 4. moving the affected joints as little as possible.

Ms. Terry Wolcox comes to the emergency room complaining of a fever and a sore throat. While examining the patient, the nurse notes that Ms. Wolcox has many bruises in various stages of healing. She suspects the patient may be the victim of abuse.

**226.** When Ms. Wolcox notes that the nurse observes her bruises, she says her fever caused her to become confused and clumsy and that she fell several times and bruised herself. If Ms. Wolcox is being abused and denying it, this behavior by the patient is *most probably* due to
○ 1. gaining pleasure from being abused.
○ 2. fearing that she will be blamed for her plight.
○ 3. believing that because she is ill, the abuse will now end.
○ 4. thinking that she can handle the problem as soon as she is well.

**227.** Which of the following statements that the nurse could make to Ms. Wolcox is *most likely* to help facilitate the patient's admitting and describing her abuse?
○ 1. "How did you hurt yourself?"
○ 2. "When were you in an accident?"

○ 3. "Is there someone doing this to you?"
○ 4. "How long have you had these bruises?"

**228.** When the nurse documents Ms. Wolcox's initial care, which of the following statements is *least helpful* in assisting others giving her health care?
○ 1. "Requests that her bruises not be described to a doctor."
○ 2. "Seems fearful to discuss how bruises on her body had been caused."
○ 3. "Asks that her husband not be called at work because she says she knows he is very busy."
○ 4. "Refuses a follow-up appointment because she states that she has a child at home who needs her care."

**229.** A few days later, Ms. Wolcox returns to the emergency room and, sobbing, tells the nurse, "I guess you really know that my husband beats me and that's why I have bruises all over my body. I don't know what to do. I'm afraid he'll kill me one of these times." Which of the following responses *best* shows that the nurse recognizes the patient's needs at this time?
○ 1. "The fear that your husband will kill you is unfounded."
○ 2. "We can begin by discussing various options open to you."
○ 3. "You can legally leave your husband because he has no right to hurt you."
○ 4. "We can begin by listing ways to avoid making your husband angry with you."

**230.** Some nurses find working with battered women, such as Ms. Wolcox, frustrating *primarily* because
○ 1. the legal system in this country lacks procedures to protect battered women.
○ 2. crisis intervention is rarely useful as a therapeutic strategy.
○ 3. society in general has supported beating of women by men as part of the male machismo.
○ 4. the incidence of women being battered is so small that few people are interested in helping to solve the problem.

Ms. Georgia Small is to be admitted to the emergency room with extensive burns over a large part of her body that occurred when she fell asleep in bed with a lighted cigarette.

**231.** How is the extent of the burn quickly estimated in the emergency room?
○ 1. The percentage of the burned area is correlated with the patient's admission weight.

○2. The body is divided into areas equal to multiples of nine, and the calculation is based on areas affected.

○3. The circumference of the body is calculated and unburned areas are measured and subtracted from the total.

○4. The area burned is measured in square inches; that total is multiplied by a factor of 0.862.

**232.** What would be the *priority* intervention for Ms. Small in the emergency room?

○1. Inserting a large-caliber intravenous line.

○2. Administering intramuscular morphine.

○3. Initiating endotracheal intubation.

○4. Administering tetanus toxoid.

**233.** Fluid resuscitation is quickly initiated. Lactated Ringer's is used with the consensus resuscitation formula as a base. Which of the following indicates adequate resuscitation?

○1. Urine output of more than 30 ml per hour.

○2. Pulse rate more than 120 beats per minute.

○3. Systolic blood pressure greater than 130 mm Hg.

○4. A 5% weight gain in the first 72 hours.

**234.** The nurse on the burn unit cleanses Ms. Small's burn with a dilute solution of povidone-iodine. At the same time, the body hair in and around the wound is closely clipped. What is the rationale for this intervention?

○1. To decrease the risk of infection.

○2. To promote comfort during dressing changes.

○3. To maximize visibility of the burn wound.

○4. To promote healing by increasing circulation.

**235.** A cream containing mafenide acetate (Sulfamylon Acetate) is applied over one area of Ms. Small's body. Before applying the cream, the nurse should plan to prepare the patient by explaining that the cream is *likely* to cause

○1. nausea.

○2. a strange taste in the mouth.

○3. a burning sensation on the body.

○4. a stain on skin surrounding the burn area.

**236.** Ms. Small is judged to have a negative nitrogen balance. Because of this, it is *particularly* important that she receive a generous intake of which of the following nutrients?

○1. Fats.

○2. Proteins.

○3. Minerals.

○4. Carbohydrates.

**237.** The nurse should ensure that Ms. Small's diet is also especially rich in vitamin

○1. A.

○2. B.

○3. C.

○4. D.

**238.** Ms. Small is friendly and cooperates with the nurses, but whenever the nurse discusses her injury, she changes the subject. She repeatedly says she is fine and seems almost euphoric. Ms. Small's behavior is indicative of

○1. regression.

○2. denial.

○3. depression.

○4. flood reaction.

Mrs. Monica Baker, 68, is believed to have pernicious anemia.

**239.** If Mrs. Baker has pernicious anemia, the sign or symptom that *most probably* caused her to seek health care is

○1. dark stools.

○2. a tendency to bleed.

○3. sudden weight loss.

○4. feelings of unusual fatigue.

**240.** It is determined that Mrs. Baker has pernicious anemia, and intramuscular vitamin $B_{12}$ therapy is prescribed. Mrs. Baker asks when she can stop taking the injections. Which of the following statements should guide the nurse's response?

○1. Injections will be necessary for the rest of the patient's life.

○2. Injections will be necessary between remissions in the patient's disease.

○3. Injections will be necessary until the patient's disease process has been successfully controlled.

○4. Injections will be necessary until the patient's dietary regimen has been successfully established.

**241.** If Mrs. Baker's pernicious anemia is allowed to progress without treatment, degenerative changes are *most likely* to occur in the

○1. nervous system.

○2. endocrine system.

○3. musculoskeletal system.

○4. gastrointestinal system.

Larry Heller, 9, is admitted to the emergency room in a state of ketoacidosis due to uncontrolled diabetes mellitus. He is accompanied by his father.

**242.** The nurse monitors Larry's respirations and notes a *typical* finding in the presence of ketoacidosis, which is
○ 1. dyspnea.
○ 2. orthopnea.
○ 3. Kussmaul respirations.
○ 4. Cheyne-Stokes respirations.

**243.** Intravenous insulin is prescribed for Larry. The nurse should question the order *unless* the type of insulin prescribed for Larry is
○ 1. globulin zinc insulin (ILETIN).
○ 2. protamine zinc insulin (PZI).
○ 3. regular crystalline insulin.
○ 4. isophane insulin suspension (NPH).

**244.** Larry and his parents did not know he had diabetes until his admission to the hospital. If his father makes the following comments about Larry, which one is *least typical* of insulin-dependent diabetes mellitus?
○ 1. "He has been drinking a lot of water lately."
○ 2. "It happened so fast. Almost overnight, he became very sick."
○ 3. "He eats well but hasn't gained weight lately."
○ 4. "He sleeps soundly and sometimes wakes up with nightmares."

**245.** While Larry is hospitalized, the nurse plans a teaching program with Larry and his father. U-100 insulin is prescribed for Larry. To understand how to determine a proper dosage, the plan should include teaching Larry and his father that U-100 means Larry's
○ 1. insulin contains 100 units per milliliter.
○ 2. proper dosage is 100 units of insulin daily.
○ 3. vial of insulin contains 100 units of insulin.
○ 4. insulin is compatible with other types of insulin.

**246.** The nurse teaches Larry and his father how to give insulin injections and explains how to rotate the injection site. Larry says, "It's easier to give the shot in my leg. Do I have to switch around to different spots all the time?" In words he can understand, the nurse should explain that rotating the site of injection is important in helping to prevent
○ 1. development of resistance to insulin.
○ 2. atrophy of fat in subcutaneous tissues.
○ 3. exceedingly rapid absorption of insulin.
○ 4. damage to nerves in the area of injection.

**247.** The nurse teaches Larry and his father the signs of hypoglycemia and explains what items help relieve the problem. Larry says, "Oh good! Candy! I'll use my favorite—a chocolate bar." The nurse should suggest using hard candies instead, *primarily* because chocolate candy

○ 1. is absorbed slowly in the body.
○ 2. depresses the appetite in the presence of hypoglycemia.
○ 3. may cause an allergic reaction to insulin.
○ 4. predisposes to nausea and vomiting in the presence of hypoglycemia.

**248.** Larry's father says, "The symptoms of too much and too little insulin are confusing. If we don't know which it is, what do we do?" What is the nurse's *best* advice?
○ 1. "Call Larry's physician immediately."
○ 2. "Assume Larry has had too much insulin."
○ 3. "Assume Larry has had too little insulin."
○ 4. "Take Larry to the nearest emergency room."

**249.** The nurse learns from Larry's father that Larry likes to swim. What advice should the nurse plan to give Larry about swimming?
○ 1. Swimming is too strenuous for most diabetics.
○ 2. He should have a snack before swimming.
○ 3. He should increase his insulin dosage before swimming.
○ 4. Swimming is appropriate if limited to no more than 15 or 20 minutes.

**250.** Because Larry is overweight for his age, he should be taught the value of a balanced diet and how properly to decrease his intake of
○ 1. fats.
○ 2. fluids.
○ 3. calories.
○ 4. carbohydrates.

A nurse works in a hospital's emergency room.

**251.** Ms. Gunderson fell and suffered a laceration of her lower leg. Arterial bleeding is profuse at the site of the wound. After exposing the leg, the nurse should *next*
○ 1. apply a tourniquet to the patient's leg.
○ 2. place a pressure dressing over the patient's wound.
○ 3. place the patient in a modified Trendelenburg position.
○ 4. apply pressure with her hand on the patient's femoral artery.

**252.** Mr. Welch has a sucking stab wound in the chest wall. Of the following courses of action, the nurse should *first*
○ 1. start to administer oxygen.
○ 2. prepare to do a tracheostomy.
○ 3. prepare for endotracheal intubation.
○ 4. cover the wound with a petroleum-impregnated gauze dressing.

**253.** Mr. Wendell is admitted to the emergency room in acute respiratory distress. When managing an acute respiratory emergency, the nurse should *first*

○ 1. start oxygen therapy.
○ 2. provide an open airway.
○ 3. give mouth-to-mouth resuscitation.
○ 4. start giving sodium bicarbonate intravenously.

**254.** Mr. Cocker was hurt while diving into shallow water, and a spinal-cord injury is suspected. The nurse should judge that Mr. Cocker's friends transported him to the hospital correctly when they moved the victim by placing him

○ 1. on his back on a board.
○ 2. in a sitting position on a straight-back chair.
○ 3. on their chests while using a three-carrier lift.
○ 4. on a stretcher made with a blanket and poles.

Mr. Ron Wagner is admitted to a hospital for the mentally ill. He is accompanied by his wife, who reports that her husband has been "on a spending spree; he sent roses to everyone we know. He's playing the seductive game with women he meets, and he says he's next in line for the throne in some country in Europe."

**255.** While being admitted to the hospital, Mr. Wagner becomes very active, moves about, and then puts his arm around the nurse in a show of affection and says to her, "I sure like you a lot, honey. I can do a lot for you in the real world out there." In this situation, what would be the nurse's *best* response?

○ 1. "Let's get some popcorn and a soda."
○ 2. "I'll have to tell my supervisor if you don't stop this minute."
○ 3. "You know you shouldn't do this. It's against the rules of the hospital."
○ 4. "Please stop. I'm very uncomfortable with your display of affection."

**256.** An important goal of nursing care for Mr. Wagner is to help him

○ 1. join in group activities.
○ 2. get enough rest.
○ 3. select leisure-time activities.
○ 4. find ways to promote cardiopulmonary stimulation.

**257.** Mr. Wagner uses the telephone as often as several times an hour. The behavior is judged to be inappropriate but in keeping with his hyperactive behavior. In a nursing-team conference, the team considers various ways to handle the problem.

The *best* course of action for the nurses to follow is to

○ 1. take the patient back to his room each time he goes to the telephone.
○ 2. explain that because he abused telephone privileges, he can no longer use it.
○ 3. work out a plan with the patient about the number of telephone calls he can make each day.
○ 4. allow the patient to use the telephone when he likes until he begins to show improvement from therapy.

**258.** Lithium carbonate (Lithane) is prescribed for Mr. Wagner. The patient will be monitored to determine a maintenance dosage. An appropriate directive on Mr. Wagner's nursing care plan should stipulate that, twice a week, which of the following specimens should be obtained?

○ 1. Urine.
○ 2. Stool.
○ 3. Blood.
○ 4. Saliva.

**259.** After Mr. Wagner receives lithium carbonate (Lithane) for a while, the nurse judges *correctly* that the patient is exhibiting a typical sign of lithium toxicity when he demonstrates

○ 1. insomnia.
○ 2. disorientation.
○ 3. excessive perspiration.
○ 4. lack of muscle coordination.

**260.** Mr. Wagner is ready to go home. Because he will continue to take lithium carbonate (Lithane) at home, the nurse should plan to teach Mr. Wagner and his wife that his diet should *most certainly not* be low in

○ 1. fats.
○ 2. salt.
○ 3. eggs.
○ 4. sugar.

Jerry Sanders is born at 30 weeks gestation and weighs 3 pounds (1,250 g). He remains in the neonatal intensive care unit until his weight increases to 5 pounds (2,250 g). He is then discharged home in the care of his parents. Jerry needs an apnea monitor and has a tracheostomy.

**261.** Which of the following statements made by Mrs. Sanders indicates to the nurse that more teaching is needed about tracheostomy care in the home?

○ 1. "I won't use hair spray in the room with Jerry."
○ 2. "I'll call the doctor if yellow-green mucus drains from the ostomy."

○ 3. "I'll keep Jerry inside on windy days."

○ 4. "I can use gauze pads around the tracheostomy if I don't cut them."

262. The nurse teaches Mr. and Mrs. Sanders the correct use of the apnea monitor. What is the *first* step the parents should take if the monitor alarm rings and the child is not breathing?

○ 1. Call the rescue squad.

○ 2. Begin mouth-to-mouth resuscitation.

○ 3. Palpate the brachial pulse.

○ 4. Shake the child gently.

263. The visiting nurse notes that sensory stimulation for Jerry's optimal growth and development is limited in the home. What advice should the nurse give the parents to improve auditory stimulation for the infant?

○ 1. Play classical music for the infant.

○ 2. Play jazz music for the infant.

○ 3. Play rock music for the infant.

○ 4. Speak to the infant in a monotone voice.

Mrs. Faye Morris is a 25-year-old gravida 2, TPAL 1001, who had a previous cesarean delivery for breech presentation. She comes to the prenatal clinic for a routine visit.

264. The nurse tells Mrs. Morris about laboratory tests that can be performed during the second trimester. The nurse correctly advises Mrs. Morris that for the procedure of alpha-fetoprotein testing

○ 1. her abdomen will be shaved and a sample of amniotic fluid will be withdrawn.

○ 2. she will have to drink six glasses of water and an ultrasonic examination will be performed.

○ 3. a venipuncture will be performed and a sample of her blood sent to the laboratory for analysis.

○ 4. an electronic fetal monitor will be attached and her baby's activity assessed.

265. Mrs. Morris discusses vaginal birth after cesarean section (VBAC) with the nurse. Which statement made by Mrs. Morris indicates that she needs more teaching?

○ 1. "I can have only minimal, if any, analgesia or anesthesia if I have a VBAC."

○ 2. "I'll have to have a cesarean section if this baby is in a breech presentation."

○ 3. "I can use the birthing suite during labor."

○ 4. "I might need continuous electronic monitoring during labor."

266. The nurse would advise Mrs. Morris to report which of the following occurrences, which will help confirm the gestational age of the fetus?

○ 1. Increased fetal movement after meals.

○ 2. Date of quickening.

○ 3. Appearance of abdominal striae.

○ 4. Decrease in urinary frequency.

267. Mrs. Morris is admitted in labor and vaginally delivers a 7.5-pound (3,200-g) baby boy. She is a candidate for early postpartal discharge (12 hours after delivery). What assessment is *essential* for the nurse to make *before* Mrs. Morris is discharged?

○ 1. Establishment of lactation.

○ 2. Return of normal bowel function.

○ 3. Development of lochia serosa.

○ 4. Firmness of fundus.

268. On Mrs. Morris' 3rd postpartal day, the nurse makes a home visit. In assessing light-skinned Baby Morris for jaundice, the nurse should

○ 1. press the skin over the infant's forehead.

○ 2. assess the color of the infant's gums.

○ 3. check the color of the infant's stool.

○ 4. assess the color of the infant's urine.

269. Baby Morris is admitted to the hospital with a diagnosis of physiologic jaundice. He is placed under bilirubin lights for phototherapy. Nursing care for Baby Morris while receiving phototherapy should include

○ 1. covering the infant with a blanket.

○ 2. keeping the infant under the lights continuously.

○ 3. applying eye patches during therapy.

○ 4. covering the infant's head with a stockinette cap.

270. When Mrs. Morris visits her son in the hospital, she becomes alarmed and exclaims, "My baby is changing color!" The nurse can *best* allay Mrs. Morris' anxiety by telling her that "tanning" sometimes occurs and that

○ 1. the tanning should disappear in about 3 weeks.

○ 2. the darkened skin color will lighten to normal during the school-age years.

○ 3. the alternative to the permanent tanning is brain damage from an accumulation of bilirubin in the blood.

○ 4. the apparent color change is due to the type of room lights used in the nursery.

# *CORRECT ANSWERS AND RATIONALES*

Numbers appear in parentheses following the rationales. The numbers identify textbooks listed in the references at the end of Part V, where correct answers can be verified.

**181.** 3. It is best to advise a patient who has a hearing aid to use it during hospitalization just as he does at home so that there will be no increase in sensory loss. There is no need to remove it, and he would probably be uncomfortable without it. (6, 24, 28)

**182.** 1. For best assessment of an inguinal hernia, the patient should be in a standing, or upright, position. The sitting and side-lying positions do not help the examiner palpate for the inguinal ring. The patient may be asked to lie down after being examined in the standing position to determine whether the hernia can be reduced and its sac contents returned to the abdominal cavity. (6, 23)

**183.** 3. A nurse can expect a smaller-than-average drug dosage for an elderly patient because the elderly patient tends to have an increased sensitivity to most drugs. Smaller-than-average doses of pharmaceutical agents are not prescribed for the elderly because of increased susceptibility to allergic reactions, although, like younger adults, the elderly may be allergic to certain medications. (6, 19)

**184.** 4. Atropine sulfate is a cholinergic blocking substance whose actions include decreasing secretions from the salivary glands. The patient should be told that he is likely to be thirsty after receiving the drug. Such symptoms as hunger, dizziness, and numbness are not associated with atropine sulfate. (17, 28)

**185.** 3. Preoperative skin preparation is done primarily to reduce the number of organisms in the operative area. The skin cannot be rendered free of organisms. Skin preparation does not improve the field of vision for the physician. The skin's defenses are not necessarily improved, but when fewer organisms are present, there is less likelihood of a postoperative infection. (6, 23)

**186.** 3. Depilatories are becoming more popular for preparing the skin at and near an operative site primarily because they are less irritating to the skin than a razor. Shaven, irritated skin becomes a portal of entry for organisms. Studies have shown that well-cleaned but unshaven skin at the site of surgery is less often implicated in postoperative wound infections than shaven skin. If a razor is used to prepare the skin, it should be used with the greatest care possible to minimize skin irritation. (6, 23)

**187.** 1. For the convenience of the anesthesiologist and in order to open the spaces between the vertebrae to the greatest extent, the patient should be on his side with his legs well flexed when receiving spinal anesthesia. Other positions will interfere with a convenient and safe procedure. (23, 28)

**188.** 4. Because the patient's legs will be anesthetized, when the patient starts feeling sensations in his toes and legs it can be assumed that he is recovering from spinal anesthesia. The anesthesia should not alter skin color. Because the patient receiving spinal anesthesia is conscious, he will not ordinarily be disoriented, nor will his respiratory rate be affected unless a complication is present. (6, 23)

**189.** 3. A swollen, painful scrotum following a herniorrhaphy is relatively common. Elevating the scrotum, as on a rolled towel, and placing ice bags on the area intermittently are helpful. Applying a binder or a truss and having the patient lie on his side with a pillow between his legs are unlikely to promote comfort when the scrotum is swollen. (6, 23)

**190.** 2. Probable signs of pregnancy include a positive pregnancy test, an enlarged uterus, Hegar's sign, and Braxton-Hicks contractions. A fetal outline can be distinguished. Presumptive signs of pregnancy include amenorrhea, morning sickness, frequency of voiding, breast tenderness, pigmentation of the skin, and quickening. Positive signs of pregnancy include fetal heart sounds, fetal movements, and a fetal outline visible by an x-ray examination or by ultrasonography. (30)

**191.** 1. The term "quickening" is synonymous with "feeling life." It is a probable sign of pregnancy, rather than a positive sign, because the sensation of feeling life can be confused with the feeling associated with the movement of flatus in the intestines. Chadwick's sign, a dark discoloration of the patient's vaginal tissues, is a presumptive sign of pregnancy. Ballottement is present when, upon examination, the fetus can be moved about in the uterus; it is a probable sign of pregnancy. Lightening occurs when the uterus descends into the pelvis; it usually occurs about 2 to 3 weeks before labor in primiparas and at or near the onset of labor in multiparas. (30)

**192.** 3. Baking soda and many over-the-counter preparations, including Alka-Seltzer, contain sodium, which tends to cause water retention. Products better for relieving heartburn include antacids that contain a magnesium or aluminum base. Alternately, the discomfort may be relieved by drinking milk or carbonated beverages or sipping water. Sitting up, trying to relax, and deep-breathing are also often helpful. Suggestions for helping to prevent heartburn include eating small but more frequent meals, wearing clothes loose at the waist, and staying in an upright position after meals. (27)

**193.** 4. Funic and uterine souffles are normal sounds heard over a pregnant uterus. Funic souffles, the soft, murmuring sounds of blood passing through the umbilical cord, are a positive sign of pregnancy because they can be heard at approximately the same rate as the fetal heartbeat. The sounds of blood passing through uterine vessels are called uterine souffles. They are caused by maternal blood and are heard at approximately the same rate as the mother's heartbeat. (30)

**194.** 3. Tailor-sitting is often recommended for pregnant women with low backaches. The knee-chest position also sometimes helps relieve backaches. Exercises that help relieve backaches include pelvic tilts and knee-chest twists. The knee-chest position often helps relieve discomforts associated with hemorrhoids. Leg elevations are recommended for leg varicosities. Pelvic-floor contractions are used when leaking urine is a problem. (30)

**195.** 1. The pain of a duodenal peptic ulcer is ordinarily relieved by eating or by taking alkalis. The food and alkalis help to neutralize excess acids that irritate gastrointestinal mucosa. The pain will gradually go away when the secretion of acid in the stomach eventually stops. (6)

**196.** 3. The indiscriminate use of bicarbonate of soda may result in metabolic alkalosis. The product is emptied from the stomach very quickly. Using bicarbonate of soda is unrelated to the development of constipation, dehydration, and iron-deficiency anemia. Renal calculi, hypernatremia, and hyperkalemia can occur with the excessive use of bicarbonate of soda. (6, 19, 27)

**197.** 2. The sensation most people refer to as heartburn is caused by the regurgitation of stomach contents into the esophagus. It has nothing to do with the functioning of the heart. (23)

**198.** 3. The barium sulfate used for x-ray examination of the upper and lower gastrointestinal tract is likely to produce constipation and fecal impaction because the barium dries into a chalky, hard substance. A prescribed laxative should be administered after the procedure to prevent constipation and fecal impaction. (6, 19, 27)

**199.** 1. Aspirin is a medication people with peptic ulcers should be taught to avoid because it irritates the gastrointestinal mucosa. A nonaspirin analgesic should be used. Phenylephrine (Neo-Synephrine) for relieving cold symptoms, psyllium hydrophilic

mucilloid (Metamucil) for occasional constipation, and scopolamine for seasickness are not necessarily contraindicated for the person with peptic ulcers. (6, 17)

**200.** 4. An infant that weighs 2,500 g or less at the time of birth is called a low-birth-weight baby. A premature baby is one whose birth weight is low and whose gestational age, estimated on the basis of the mother's last menstrual period, is less than 37 weeks. Various criteria are used to help confirm gestational age, including a study of the status of the infant's muscle tonus. The ability of an infant's pupils to react to light is not used to help establish prematurity. (32, 40)

**201.** 3. A tube used for gastric gavage for an infant should be inserted a distance equivalent to the distance from the tip of the infant's nose, to an earlobe, to the xiphoid process. If the tube is inserted through the mouth, the distance to insert the tube should be equivalent to the distance from the bridge of the nose to the xiphoid process. These distances ensure that the tube reaches the infant's stomach. (25, 40)

**202.** 2. The immaturity of the kidneys of premature babies often causes a greater-than-average amount of sodium to escape from the urinary tract. Sodium bicarbonate is used to correct the sodium imbalance. However, if too much is administered, fluid retention with edema, water intoxication, and hemorrhage may result. (27, 32, 40)

**203.** 4. The most frequently recommended procedure is to take an infant's pulse rate by auscultating over the apex of the heart. This technique gives the most accurate data. (27, 32, 40)

**204.** 2. Careful monitoring of blood levels of $PaO_2$ are essential when oxygen is being administered to a premature infant. Levels that are too high are likely to cause vasoconstriction of vessels in the infant's retinas, a condition likely to result in retrolental fibroplasia and irreversible blindness. Respiratory distress syndrome is caused by a deficiency of surfactant. (25, 40)

**205.** 3. An important technique for diagnosing carcinoma of the colon is to examine the stool for the presence of occult blood. Three commonly used tests to detect occult blood are the orthotoluidine (Occultest), the benzidine, and the guaiac (Hemoccult) tests. Positive results indicate the presence of blood in the stool, a common symptom of carcinoma of the colon. If bleeding occurs in the colon or higher in the gastrointestinal tract, blood causes the stool to become dark and to have a very unpleasant odor. If bleeding occurs in the rectum, gross blood appears in the stool. Tests of the stool for the presence of occult blood are simple to perform and help diagnose colon carcinoma early in many patients. The test is recommended as part of a routine examination for all people over 40 years of age. (11, 21, 28)

**206.** 4. A high urine specific gravity is often the result of dehydration. Skin turgor does not accurately indicate an elderly person's hydrational status because skin in the elderly becomes dry and inelastic. In a younger person skin turgor accurately reflects dehydration. When a patient is dehydrated, skin loses its elasticity, remaining puckered when the nurse compresses a fold of skin between her fingers. Assessing eye grounds and respiratory rate will not help the nurse validate dehydration in a patient. (23, 28)

**207.** 3. Kanamycin sulfate (Kantrex) is an antimicrobial agent frequently used before bowel surgery to reduce the bacterial count in the colon. The procedure helps make the surgical site as clean as possible and helps prevent postoperative infections at the site of surgery. (17, 28)

**208.** 4. After taking a deep breath while inhaling slowly, a patient should be instructed to hold the breath for 3 to 5 seconds before exhaling. This technique of holding the breath after inhalation allows for maximum oxygen absorption. Teaching a patient how to cough properly is ordinarily carried out preoperatively, but the technique is used postoperatively only if a patient has accumulated secretions in the airway. The patient should be relaxed while deep-breathing and should not be told to close the glottis tightly because this defeats relaxation. (6, 23)

**209.** 1. Postoperative leg exercises are performed primarily to promote circulation and to prevent venous stasis, which is believed to play a very significant role in the development of venous thrombosis, thrombophlebitis, and deep vein thrombosis. (6, 19)

**210.** 1. A knowledge of the concept of body image is important in helping patients adjust to a change in their body. The body image is developed over a period of time, but it is believed that the formative years of childhood are especially important in terms of integrating experiences that result in the development of a basic body image. It can be assumed that because the patient described in this item is 65 years old, feelings about her body image are likely to be well established, and it will take time and patience on the nurse's part to help the patient accept a change in her body image. (6, 23)

**211.** 2. Postoperative shock is most commonly caused by excessive bleeding. This type of shock is called hypovolemic shock. Adrenal failure, a transfusion reaction, and an untoward drug reaction are not typical postoperative conditions that lead to shock. (6, 23)

**212.** 3. In black people, cyanosis can best be detected by examining the conjunctiva, lips, and oral mucous membranes. (2, 24, 28)

**213.** 4. Many patients feel faint and weak when helped to ambulate for the first time postoperatively. It is helpful to prevent these feelings by giving the circulatory system time to adjust before patients plan to assume a standing position. This is best done by helping patients into a high Fowler's position in bed for a few minutes. After becoming accustomed to a sitting position, the patient can then be helped to dangle at the edge of the bed before ambulating. Preparations for ambulating help give the circulatory system time to adjust to the patient's upright position. (19, 34)

**214.** 2. A drain in a patient's wound allows drainage of blood, lymph, and other debris from the wound. Most drains are not used to introduce antibiotics into the wound or to irrigate the wound. When drainage occurs from the wound, some discomfort may be relieved, but a drain is not used primarily to relieve discomfort. (21, 23)

**215.** 3. Postoperative infections tend to occur more frequently among elderly patients than among younger mature adults for several reasons. Physiologic homeostasis is less efficiently maintained in the elderly. When an infection or trauma occurs, such as a surgical procedure, the elderly patient has little reserve power to combat stress placed on the body. Arteriosclerosis and poor circulatory efforts, often present in the elderly, tend to increase the risk of infection. It is true that there is a loss of neurons as the body ages, but this fact does not explain the increased incidence of postoperative infections. It has not been demonstrated that the elderly have a decreased interest in healthful habits of daily living or that atrophy of lymph nodes occurs to decrease resistance to infection. (6, 23)

**216.** 4. The amount of irrigating solution and the pressure at which it is given distend the bowel and promote peristalsis. Feces are then excreted through the stoma. If, while administering the irrigating solution, the patient complains of cramping, it is best to continue with the irrigation but to slow the flow rate temporarily. If cramping continues and becomes severe, it is best to halt the flow of solution for a minute or two. Deep-breathing or lying on the side will not help relieve cramping during a colostomy irrigation. Cramping will usually subside when proper measures are used without removing the irrigating cone from the stoma. (6, 19)

**217.** 4. The frequency of contractions is the interval between the beginning of one contraction and the beginning of the next. The duration of a contraction is the interval between the beginning and the end of one contraction. The intensity of contractions is estimated and categorized as mild when uterine muscles become somewhat tense, moderate when uterine muscles become moderately strong, and strong when the uterine muscles are so firm they feel wooden. (27, 30)

**218.** 4. If the patient is not being monitored, she should be encouraged to assume any position of comfort. There is no need to keep her in one position, especially on her back, which tends to predispose to hypotension. (27, 30)

**219.** 2. Vaginal, as well as rectal, examinations may be done to evaluate the progress of labor. A lubricating agent and waterproof gloves are necessary for these examinations. The gloves and agent should be sterile for the vaginal examination; they should be clean but not necessarily sterile for the rectal examination. A fetal heart stethoscope is required for obtaining the fetal heart rate. A speculum is used to examine the vagina. Nitrazine test paper is used to help determine whether vaginal secretions contain amniotic fluid. (27, 30)

**220.** 4. A full bladder during labor may impede labor primarily by interfering with the descent of the infant in the birth canal. In addition, a full bladder adds to the discomfort of the mother and predisposes to urinary retention after delivery. A full bladder *may* influence the intensity of uterine contractions. If the patient is unable to void, consideration may have to be given to catheterizing her. However, efforts should first be used to promote normal voiding. (27, 30)

**221.** 2. It is imperative that the fetal heartbeat be assessed after the membranes rupture, and again in a few minutes, to determine whether there is pressure on the cord. A sign of fetal distress is a persistently slow fetal heartbeat after contractions, as well as early during a contraction. The physician should be notified promptly of bradycardia. (27, 30)

**222.** 3. According to the gate-control theory, stimulation of large-diameter sensory nerve fibers closes the gating mechanism to prevent the transmission of pain impulses from reaching the brain. The skin has many large-diameter nerve fibers, and therefore cutaneous stimulation is a common method for relieving discomfort. (27, 30)

**223.** 1. The highest priority when caring for a patient who is acutely ill with rheumatic fever is to help the patient maintain bed rest. In most cases, the patient should not be out of bed, and nursing care should include measures to ensure personal hygiene, proper nutrition, and proper elimination. The heart needs maximum rest to prevent complications, which can be very serious. (25, 40)

**224.** 3. It has been said that if children with sore throats were cared for properly, rheumatic fever could be eliminated. An untreated streptococcal throat infection most frequently precedes rheumatic fever. School nurses in particular play an important role in the prevention of rheumatic fever and often screen for sore throats among school-age children. (25, 40)

**225.** 4. Patients acutely ill with rheumatic fever may complain of arthralgia, which may at times be severe. Nursing measures to help minimize the discomfort include moving the affected joints as little as possible, positioning the patient in proper body alignment, and using a bed cradle to prevent bed linens from resting on the patient. Massaging the joints, applying heat or cold, and exercising the affected joints are likely to make matters worse. (25, 40)

**226.** 2. A common reason why battered women deny being abused is that they are afraid they will be blamed for their plight. It is mostly a myth that battered women are masochistic and gain pleasure from abuse. Most abused women realize that the abuse is unlikely to stop, and they suffer from fear, shame, hopelessness, and helplessness. (16)

**227.** 3. A question from the nurse that helps the patient describe her health problem is most helpful when abuse is suspected. Statements that help the patient avoid the issue are least helpful. Even if the patient does not want to discuss possible causes of bruises due to abuse, helping her to express her thoughts in a supportive atmosphere often helps open channels of communication. (16, 19)

**228.** 2. Information documented on a patient's record should be as objective as possible so that other health personnel can verify findings as necessary. Stating that a patient seems fearful to discuss how bruises on her body had been caused is subjective and expresses the nurse's opinion. Rather than stating her opinion, the nurse should state exactly what the patient said. (16, 19)

**229.** 2. The patient in this situation is asking for help when she says she does not know what to do about being abused by her husband. The nurse's best course of action is to explain various options that are open to her. This technique helps the patient make decisions based on appropriate knowledge. (16, 36)

**230.** 3. Battering of women, until the last decade or two, was often looked upon as part of a male mystique that supports a macho image. Although society's viewpoints are changing, this attitude has often made trying to stop battering of women a frustrating experience. The incidence of battering is unknown, but it is believed to be more common than generally thought. Many more people than in the past are working to solve the problem. Crisis intervention is useful and is often believed to halt battering that could lead to more violence, even to murder. The legal system in this country has procedures to help battered women, although the procedures may be poorly used. (3, 16, 36)

**231.** 2. The rule of nines is used to determine the extent of burns quickly. A chart with the body areas divided into areas equal to multiples of nine is used. Affected areas are shaded and the total shaded areas calculated. Other, more detailed charts can be used later for more specific calculation. It is impractical to measure the body when more critical care is indicated. Weight is not a reliable measure of the extent of burns. (21, 28)

**232.** 3. Establishing an airway is the priority intervention in trauma cases. Prophylactic intubation is initiated if heat has been inhaled or if the neck, head, or face is involved. Swelling of the upper airways can progress to obstruction. After the airway has been established, circulating support is the next priority. Fluid is best replaced via two large-caliber peripheral catheters. However, one peripheral line and one central line are preferable if the burn is large or complicated by inhalation injuries. Partial-thickness burns are painful, but morphine sulfate, the analgesic of choice, would not be administered until the patient was stable; furthermore, the intravenous route would be used. Tetanus prophylaxis is begun in the emergency room but is not the priority intervention. (21, 28)

**233.** 1. Hourly urine output is the most accessible and generally reliable index of adequate fluid replacement because of the kidney's sensitivity to circulating volume. A pulse rate of 120 or less indicates successful resuscitation. A higher rate indicates stress on the cardiovascular system. A systolic blood pressure more than 130 mm Hg is unrealistic because the loss of skin integrity causes severe fluid loss; a systolic blood pressure around 100 is more realistic. A weight gain of 15% to 20% is expected during the first 72 hours of fluid resuscitation. (6, 28)

**234.** 1. Hair attracts and shelters bacteria. The skin is the major barrier to infection and its disruption increases the risk of infection. Clipping hair in and around the burn decreases the risk of contamination. (21, 28)

**235.** 3. Mafenide acetate (Sulfamylon acetate) causes a burning pain after it is applied to a burn area. The discomfort is sometimes severe enough that the nurse should consider administering a prescribed analgesic before applying the cream. (6, 21, 28)

**236.** 2. Nutritionists often speak of protein nutrition in terms of nitrogen balance because nitrogen is the element that makes proteins different from carbohydrates and fats. Large amounts of protein are lost with exudates from burn wounds, and therefore a patient in a state of negative nitrogen balance needs proteins to return to nitrogen balance. (21, 42)

**237.** 3. Collagen is protein found between cells, and it forms a major structural protein in the body. Collagen is a key element in wound healing and is necessary to restore skin. All nutrients are important in one way or another for good wound healing, but an adequate intake of vitamin C and the mineral zinc are especially important for collagen formation. (7, 21, 42)

**238.** 2. Denial is a coping mechanism used when a patient is unable to accept the present condition. It buffers the patient from the impact of overwhelming crisis. The behavior indicates a distorted comprehension of the burn. Regression produces infantile, demanding behavior. Depression results in lethargic, apathetic behavior. Flood reaction causes the patient to try urgently to settle family and financial problems. (6, 19)

**239.** 4. A patient with pernicious anemia characteristically seeks health care because of unusual fatigue and listlessness. Energy is poor because the drop in red blood cells causes the body to be poorly oxygenated. The onset of pernicious anemia is usually rapid. Pernicious anemia is sometimes referred to as a vitamin $B_{12}$ deficiency when there is an absence of the intrinsic factor being secreted by the cells of the stomach. (6, 23)

**240.** 1. Vitamin $B_{12}$ therapy for pernicious anemia must continue for life to prevent recurrence of symptoms because the intrinsic factor does not return to gastric secretions, even with therapy. (6, 23)

**241.** 1. Patients who do not have therapy for pernicious anemia will eventually develop neurologic problems due to irreversible neural damage. (23, 28)

**242.** 3. Kussmaul respirations, which are deep and rapid, are typical of the patient with ketoacidosis. They are not necessarily labored or difficult, although accessory muscles may be used to help improve ventilation. The body is attempting to compensate for acidosis with Kussmaul respirations by increasing respiratory efforts to "blow off" carbon dioxide and thereby to decrease the carbonic acid content of the blood and reduce its pH. (32, 40)

**243.** 3. Regular crystalline insulin is used for intravenous administration. Globulin zinc insulin

(ILETIN), protamine zinc insulin (PZI), and iso-phane insulin suspension (NPH) are not appropriate for intravenous use. (32, 40)

**244.** 4. The three classical signs of diabetes mellitus are eating well without gaining weight (polyphagia), excessive thirst (polydipsia), and frequent voiding (polyuria). Insulin-dependent diabetes mellitus, also known as juvenile-onset diabetes, characteristically has a rapid onset, in contrast to non-insulin-dependent (adult-onset) diabetes mellitus, which has a slow onset. Tiredness is often described, but not necessarily nightmares. (32, 40)

**245.** 1. U-100 describes the concentration of insulin in the vial and means there are 100 units of insulin in each milliliter of solution. In the past, other concentrations of insulin were available, but concentrations now are standardized as U-100 to help avoid errors. (25, 32)

**246.** 2. Atrophy of fat in subcutaneous tissues and scarring result when the same site is injected repeatedly with insulin. In addition to tissue damage, poor absorption of insulin also results. Although many patients say it is less uncomfortable when the same site is injected, this practice should be avoided to prevent insulin-induced atrophy at the site. (32, 40)

**247.** 1. Because of its high fat content, chocolate candy is absorbed slowly in the body. In the presence of hypoglycemia, a carbohydrate that is absorbed very rapidly, such as hard candy, sugar, and orange juice, should be used. There are also quick-acting commercial products to help overcome hypoglycemia. Glucagon is available by prescription for subcutaneous injection for treating hypoglycemia. (25, 26)

**248.** 2. Patients should be taught how to manage hypoglycemia and hyperglycemia when they occur, although the patient still may need medical care after treatment is initiated. However, when there is doubt as to whether the patient has hyperglycemia or hypoglycemia, it should be assumed that the condition is hypoglycemia and the patient should be given a simple carbohydrate. It is better to give the patient something to combat hypoglycemia than to aggravate the situation by causing an even more profound state of hypoglycemia if the problem turns out to be too much insulin. (25, 40)

**249.** 2. The patient with diabetes mellitus should be encouraged to exercise regularly, and swimming is one of many satisfactory sports. Swimming does not necessarily need to be limited, but it should be in keeping with the patient's ability. However, exercise reduces the body's need for insulin, and therefore the patient should eat a snack about an hour before exercising or should reduce his insulin intake somewhat. He should also be prepared to manage hypoglycemia, should it occur. Increasing insulin dosage before exercising is contraindicated. (25, 40)

**250.** 3. The overweight individual should be taught to eat a balanced diet as prescribed for him in terms of percentages of nutrients to eat each day, but he also should be taught to decrease his total caloric intake. Decreasing the intake of fats or carbohydrates *only* is likely to lead to an unbalanced diet. Insulin dosages may have to be lowered and the patient should be taught to be especially alert to signs of hypoglycemia when caloric intake is decreased. (7, 40)

**251.** 4. Initial emergency care for profuse bleeding is to apply pressure over the artery involved, in this situation the femoral artery. A pressure dressing should then be applied. A tourniquet should be used only as a last resort to control bleeding. The modified Trendelenburg position *may* be used later if the patient develops signs of shock due to excessive bleeding. (6, 23)

**252.** 4. The first course of action when a patient has a sucking chest wound is to take steps to stop air from entering the chest cavity, which will cause the lung to collapse. This is best done in an emergency situation by applying an air-occlusive dressing over the wound. Such measures as starting oxygen therapy, preparing for a tracheostomy, and preparing for endotracheal intubation *may* become necessary but do not have the same priority upon admission as closing the wound. (6, 23)

**253.** 2. Unless the airway is open for the entry of air or oxygen, such measures as starting oxygen therapy, giving mouth-to-mouth resuscitation, and giving sodium bicarbonate will not be of value. The airway first must be open. Ensuring that a patient's airway is open is an important first step in emergency care. (6, 23)

**254.** 1. A patient with a possible spinal-cord injury should be transported in such a way as to minimize movement, twisting, turning, and bending of the spine. Injury to the cord may be increased if the spine is not held straight. The best way to transport a potentially spinal-cord-injured patient is to place him on a flat board while he lies flat on his back. (6, 23)

**255.** 4. The overactive patient needs to have limits set, especially when his behavior is demanding or seductive. The patient should be told to stop his behavior and the nurse should explain her intolerance for it. Telling a seductive patient that it is against the rules for patients and nurses to display affection toward each other does not tell the patient that his behavior is unacceptable, nor will it help to threaten him by saying the supervisor will be notified. It may become appropriate to divert the patient's attention, for example by suggesting something to eat and drink, but first limits should be set and explained to the patient. (6, 16)

**256.** 2. Patients displaying hyperactive behavior are on the go almost constantly, very often to the point of jeopardizing their health for lack of rest and sleep. Therefore, the nurse should make concerted efforts to ensure that these patients have sufficient rest. Most often, hyperactive patients do not need assistance in joining groups, finding things to do, and promoting cardiopulmonary activity; in fact, almost the opposite is true. (6, 16)

**257.** 3. A hyperactive patient needs help in setting limits on his behavior. The best course of action when the patient described in this item abuses telephone privileges is to work out a plan with him about the number of calls he can make each day. The agreed-upon plan should then be followed. (6, 16)

**258.** 3. Serum blood levels are ordinarily monitored when a patient is receiving lithium carbonate (Lithane). Lithium carbonate may be found in a patient's saliva, but it is not typical to monitor the drug by examining saliva. (13, 17)

**259.** 4. Lack of muscle coordination and weakness are typical signs of lithium toxicity; so, also, are drowsiness and dehydration with dry skin and mucous membranes. Additional untoward reactions to the drug may affect the central nervous system, cardiovascular system, gastrointestinal system, genitourinary system, and autonomic nervous system. (13, 17)

**260.** 2. Lithium carbonate (Lithane) affects the renal tubules by decreasing sodium resorption. As a result, the patient may suffer from sodium depletion. A patient taking this drug should have essentially a normal diet, but one that includes salt. If the body has insufficient sodium, the patient is likely to have a decreased tolerance for lithium carbonate. (13, 17)

**261.** 3. A patient with a tracheostomy can be taken outside on windy or hot dry days if the tracheostomy is covered with a scarf or handkerchief. If gauze sponges are used around the tracheostomy site, they should not be cut to avoid getting loose strings in the ostomy. Aerosol sprays can get into the tracheostomy and cause lung irritation. Yellow-green mucus may be a sign of infection and should be reported to the physician. (40)

**262.** 4. When the apnea monitor alarm rings and the child is not breathing, the first action is to shake the child gently and wait 10 seconds for breathing to resume. If the child does not begin to breathe spontaneously, cardiopulmonary resuscitation should begin immediately. Shaking usually stimulates breathing and no further action is needed. (40)

**263.** 1. Stimulation should be offered only when the infant is alert, and then only for short periods. Auditory stimulation includes playing classical music for the infant (jazz and rock are less effective), calling the infant by name at each interaction, speaking with a variety of voice inflections, and alternating adult with baby talk. (40)

**264.** 3. Maternal serum is assessed for alpha-fetoprotein (AFP) between 15 and 20 weeks gestation. If the value is elevated, a second sample is drawn. If follow-up is needed, an amniocentesis is performed and a small amount of amniotic fluid removed for analysis. A sonogram may detect serious fetal defects but does not provide AFP levels. An electronic fetal monitor is used antepartally for stress and nonstress testing. (27)

**265.** 1. Analgesia or anesthesia is allowed in vaginal birth after cesarean section. VBAC may be considered if no contraindications exist for vaginal delivery. Electronic monitoring is available and facilities should be ready if a cesarean section is necessary. Breech presentation is a criterion for a cesarean section according to accepted guidelines. A VBAC patient can use the birthing suite if she meets the criteria for good labor assessment. (27)

**266.** 2. Quickening, or the first maternal perception of fetal movement, occurs between 18 and 20 weeks gestation. Adding 20 weeks to the date of quickening can help determine the date of confinement; this date should be compared to the date of the last normal menstrual period. Fetal movement normally increases after meals. Maternal striae appear as the abdomen stretches but not at any certain gestational age. Urinary frequency, which usually disappears as the fetus rises in the pelvis and reappears after the baby has dropped, is an unreliable indicator of gestational age. (27)

**267.** 4. The mother may be discharged as soon as 6 hours after a vaginal delivery. Criteria for early discharge include a firm uterine fundus. Lactation is not expected to be established within the first 24 hours after delivery. Lochia will be rubra for about 3 days, and the patient will not be expected to have a bowel movement until the 2nd or 3rd day after delivery. (27)

**268.** 1. Newborns are routinely assessed for evidence of jaundice. Applying pressure to the skin, especially over bony prominences such as the nose and sternum, causes blanching and allows the yellow skin to be more noticeable. In dark-skinned infants, the color of the gums is the most reliable indicator of jaundice. (27)

**269.** 3. During phototherapy, the infant's eyes are covered to prevent exposure to the light. Phototherapy can damage the photoreceptors in the retina. Once each nursing shift, the infant is removed from the lights and the eyes assessed for discharge. The infant is placed under the fluorescent light nude, expect for minimal covering over the genitals, and is turned frequently because in order for phototherapy to be effective, the light must come in

contact with the skin surface. Light in the blue range is believed to decompose bilirubin by the process of photo-oxidation. Stockinette caps may be used to cover the heads of premature infants 37 gestational weeks or younger to prevent phototherapy-induced hypocalcemia. The infant in this item is not premature. (25, 40)

**270.** 1. Newborns receiving phototherapy sometimes tan. This is not a permanent condition and disappears in about 3 weeks. Understanding the process involved in phototherapy can help alleviate the mother's anxiety. (25, 40)

# comprehensive test 4

Select the one *best* or *correct* answer and indicate your choice by filling in the circle with a pencil in front of the option you have chosen. If the answer you would prefer is not given, select the one you think is *most appropriate*.

Josh Dretakis was born prematurely at 34 weeks gestation and is immediately admitted to the neonatal intensive care unit. He is 5 days old and is being weaned from respiratory support. Recurrent apnea and increased $PaCO_2$ suggest possible patent ductus arteriosus.

**271.** Given a tentative diagnosis of patent ductus, what other early clinical manifestations would the nurse expect to find?
- ○ 1. Bounding peripheral pulses.
- ○ 2. Pericardial hypoactivity.
- ○ 3. Intermittent murmur.
- ○ 4. Narrowing pulse pressure.

**272.** In fetal circulation, the ductus arteriosus carries blood from the
- ○ 1. pulmonary vein to the coronary artery.
- ○ 2. pulmonary artery to the coronary artery.
- ○ 3. pulmonary vein to the descending aorta.
- ○ 4. pulmonary artery to the descending aorta.

**273.** In a full-term infant, the ductus arteriosus functionally closes within
- ○ 1. the first 3 days of life.
- ○ 2. 1 week of birth.
- ○ 3. 2 weeks of birth.
- ○ 4. 3 weeks of birth.

**274.** Mrs. Dretakis asks the nurse about tests that will be used to confirm the diagnosis of patent ductus arteriosus. The nurse should be aware that the test *least likely* to be helpful in confirming the diagnosis in preterm infants is
- ○ 1. a cardiac catheterization.
- ○ 2. a chest x-ray.
- ○ 3. an echocardiogram.
- ○ 4. an electrocardiogram.

**275.** Diagnostic studies confirm the diagnosis of patent ductus arteriosus. In discussing the diagnosis with Josh's parents, the nurse would explain that patent ductus arteriosus is
- ○ 1. nearly twice as common in males as in females.

- ○ 2. one of the rarest cardiac anomalies.
- ○ 3. a contributing factor in respiratory distress.
- ○ 4. found in almost one third of premature infants.

**276.** A decision is made to try to close the patent ductus arteriosus pharmacologically, and Josh is given indomethacin (Indocin). Mr. Dretakis asks the nurse how the drug works. Which of the following facts should be the basis for the nurse's response?
- ○ 1. Indomethacin binds with opiate receptors.
- ○ 2. Indomethacin inhibits prostaglandin synthesis.
- ○ 3. Indomethacin decreases smooth muscle relaxation.
- ○ 4. Indomethacin inhibits the effect of acetylcholine.

**277.** Josh develops congestive heart failure. Digoxin and furosemide (Lasix) are ordered in addition to the indomethacin (Indocin). Which of the following electrolyte values should the nurse monitor *most closely* while Josh is receiving these medications?
- ○ 1. Sodium and potassium.
- ○ 2. Sodium and chloride.
- ○ 3. Potassium and chloride.
- ○ 4. Potassium and calcium.

**278.** Josh is now 6 weeks old. The patent ductus arteriosus has closed, and his respiratory and cardiac problems have resolved. He is to be discharged home soon without medication, and the nurse prepares his parents for his discharge. Which of the following statements indicates that Mrs. Dretakis has understood the teaching?
- ○ 1. "I'll count his pulse for a full minute every morning."
- ○ 2. "I'll be alert to any signs of decreasing appetite or vomiting."
- ○ 3. "I'll carefully limit the amount of fluid that he drinks."
- ○ 4. "I'll place his cradle gym within his sight."

Mrs. Kimberly Erikson, 32, is experiencing increasing fatigue and weakness that interfere with her activities of daily living. A Tensilon test and electromyography (EMG) confirm a diagnosis of myasthenia gravis.

**279.** The nurse's assessment of Mrs. Erikson *most likely* would disclose
- ○ 1. paresthesias in the extremities.
- ○ 2. depressed deep tendon reflexes.
- ○ 3. atrophy of the arm and leg muscles.
- ○ 4. bilateral ptosis of the eyelids.

**280.** The *primary* nursing goals for the care of a patient with myasthenia gravis are to conserve the patient's energy and to
- ○ 1. provide a safe environment.
- ○ 2. maintain respiratory function.
- ○ 3. provide psychological support and reassurance.
- ○ 4. promote comfort and relieve pain.

**281.** Pyridostigmine bromide (Mestinon) timespan tablets are ordered b.i.d. The nurse must be able to distinguish cholinergic crisis (too much medication) from myasthenic crisis (too little medication) in a patient on anticholinesterase therapy. *All* of the following are present in cholinergic crisis *except*
- ○ 1. improved muscle strength after IV edrophonium chloride (Tensilon).
- ○ 2. increased weakness of skeletal muscles.
- ○ 3. respiratory embarrassment.
- ○ 4. abdominal cramps and increased salivation.

**282.** The nurse teaches Mrs. Erikson about myasthenia gravis. Mrs. Erikson has formed a realistic concept of her condition when she says that by taking her medication and pacing her activities
- ○ 1. she will live longer, but ultimately the disease will cause her death.
- ○ 2. her symptoms will be controlled, and eventually the disease will be cured.
- ○ 3. she should be able to control the disease and have a healthy life-style.
- ○ 4. her fatigue will be relieved, but she should expect occasional periods of muscle weakness.

Mr. George Holmen, 77, is admitted to the hospital for elective surgery to repair an abdominal aortic aneurysm. In taking his health history, the nurse learns that he has been taking medication because of the aneurysm.

**283.** Which of the following categories of medications has Mr. Holmen *most likely* been taking?

- ○ 1. Anticoagulants.
- ○ 2. Antihypertensives.
- ○ 3. Diuretics.
- ○ 4. Corticosteroids.

**284.** Mr. Holmen may experience some loss of environmental control because of the hospitalization. Which of the following nursing interventions should the nurse include in Mr. Holmen's nursing care plan to minimize this experience?
- ○ 1. Orient the patient to his hospital room.
- ○ 2. Ask the patient where he would like to put his personal belongings.
- ○ 3. Ensure the patient that he will have continuity of nursing care.
- ○ 4. Ask the psychiatric clinical nurse specialist to see the patient.

**285.** The surgeon explains the surgical procedure to Mr. and Mrs. Holmen, and later they discuss what they were told with the nurse. Which of the following statements indicates that they have understood the surgical procedure correctly?
- ○ 1. "The aneurysm will be replaced by a saphenous vein graft."
- ○ 2. "The aneurysm will be removed and the aorta anastomosed."
- ○ 3. "The aneurysm will be removed and a donor aorta inserted."
- ○ 4. "The aneurysm will be replaced with a Teflon graft."

**286.** When the nurse prepares Mr. Holmen for surgery, he displays nervous behavior and says, "I hope I'm doing the right thing by having surgery." What would the nurse's *most therapeutic* response be?
- ○ 1. "Your doctor has done this type of surgery many times."
- ○ 2. "You seem anxious about the surgery."
- ○ 3. "Everybody feels anxious the morning of surgery."
- ○ 4. "You can always cancel surgery, if you want."

**287.** The surgery is successful and Mr. Holmen will be discharged in a few days. The nurse prepares him for discharge by suggesting dietary modifications to reduce the risk of atherosclerosis. Selecting which of the following menus indicates that Mr. Holmen will *not* need additional dietary instruction?
- ○ 1. Veal, broccoli, and a slice of whole-wheat bread.
- ○ 2. Scrambled eggs, bacon, and an English muffin.
- ○ 3. Cheese fettucine, spinach, and strawberries.
- ○ 4. Chicken, French bread, and chocolate ice cream.

Allan Cook, 6, comes to the clinic for a follow-up visit. Two months ago, Allan had bilateral otitis media and an upper respiratory infection. He was treated successfully with a course of antibiotics, but his mother reports that since then he has been pale, listless, and anorexic. Upon physical examination, the nurse notes a low-grade fever, weight loss of 2 pounds in the last 2 months, and several unexplained bruises. Leukemia is suspected and diagnostic tests are ordered.

**288.** Which of the following is a *definitive* diagnostic test for leukemia?
- ○ 1. Bone-marrow aspiration.
- ○ 2. Complete blood count.
- ○ 3. Lumbar puncture.
- ○ 4. Chest x-ray.

**289.** The diagnosis of acute lymphoid leukemia (ALL) is confirmed and Allan is admitted to the hospital to begin chemotherapy immediately. While taking a nursing history, the nurse discovers that Allan's immunizations are current *except* for the measles-mumps-rubella (MMR), which he never received. What would be the appropriate course of action regarding the administration of the MMR immunization to Allan?
- ○ 1. It should be given immediately because his susceptibility to these diseases is increased.
- ○ 2. It should not be given until 3 months after the termination of chemotherapy.
- ○ 3. Only the mumps-rubella vaccines should be given now because they are inactivated viruses.
- ○ 4. It should be given now, but in two divided doses so as not to overwhelm the immune system.

**290.** Mrs. Cook asks the nurse about Allan's prognosis. The nurse should base her answer on knowledge that the *most important* prognostic factors in determining long-term survival for children with acute lymphoid leukemia (ALL) are the initial white blood count and
- ○ 1. sex.
- ○ 2. histologic type of disease.
- ○ 3. red blood count.
- ○ 4. patient's age at diagnosis.

**291.** Allan's induction chemotherapy begins immediately. He receives prednisone, vincristine sulfate (Oncovin), and L-asparaginase (Elspar). Because Allan is receiving vincristine sulfate, which of the following side effects should the nurse report to the physician *immediately*?
- ○ 1. Jaw pain.
- ○ 2. Fever.
- ○ 3. Urinary retention.
- ○ 4. Anorexia.

**292.** Maintaining Allan's nutritional status at an optimal level is an important nursing goal. To attain this goal the nurse would

- ○ 1. encourage Allan to select his meals from the hospital menu.
- ○ 2. suggest that Allan eat three meals a day and avoid between-meal snacks.
- ○ 3. discourage Allan's mother from bringing food from home that might be incompatible with Allan's diet.
- ○ 4. close the curtains around Allan's bed at meal time so that he is not distracted.

**293.** Allan begins to experience nausea and vomiting as a side effect of the chemotherapy. He has a p.r.n. antiemetic order. Based on knowledge of nausea control, the nurse administers the antiemetic
- ○ 1. as soon as Allan says he feels nauseated.
- ○ 2. as needed during therapy; the chemotherapeutic agents are administered in the morning before Allan eats.
- ○ 3. 1 hour before beginning Allan's chemotherapy and every 2 to 6 hours for the next 24 hours.
- ○ 4. concurrently with the chemotherapeutic agents, but only after Allan has been n.p.o. for 6 hours.

During an office visit, Mr. Richard Pfeifer, 72, reports he has generalized crampy abdominal discomfort and alternating bouts of constipation and diarrhea. Physical examination reveals left lower quadrant abdominal tenderness on palpation. A barium enema shows multiple diverticula in the sigmoid colon. The diagnosis is diverticulitis.

**294.** Propantheline bromide (Pro-Banthine) is ordered to relieve the crampy abdominal pain. The nurse tells Mr. Pfeifer that in addition to the pain relief, he may experience dryness of the mouth and
- ○ 1. urinary frequency.
- ○ 2. bradycardia.
- ○ 3. diarrhea.
- ○ 4. blurred vision.

**295.** Treatment of diverticulitis is important to prevent the development of peritonitis from a perforated diverticulum. Care of Mr. Pfeifer would include assessment for which symptom of peritonitis?
- ○ 1. Hyperactive bowel sounds.
- ○ 2. Rigid abdominal wall.
- ○ 3. Explosive diarrhea.
- ○ 4. Excessive flatulence.

**296.** The nurse teaches Mr. Pfeifer about dietary management during the acute stage of diverticulitis. Mr. Pfeifer's selection of which of the following foods indicates that he needs additional teaching?

○ 1. Bran cereals and unpeeled apples.
○ 2. Cookies and candy.
○ 3. Pasta and white bread.
○ 4. Beef and pork.

**297.** Mr. Pfeifer responds to conservative therapy and his symptoms subside. Which of the following maintenance therapeutic diets would the nurse anticipate being ordered for Mr. Pfeifer?
○ 1. Low-residue.
○ 2. Low-fat.
○ 3. High-fiber.
○ 4. Bland.

**298.** Mr. Pfeifer has presbycusis. When instructing him about his therapeutic diet, the nurse can facilitate communication by
○ 1. accentuating vowels.
○ 2. raising the tone of her voice.
○ 3. overarticulating her words.
○ 4. talking at a moderate rate.

Mrs. Odom is a 21-year-old gravida 1, TPAL 000, admitted to the labor and delivery suite. On admission she is 4 centimeters dilated, 95% effaced, and at station minus-1, with a vertex presentation.

**299.** Upon Mrs. Odom's admission, the nurse applies an external electronic monitor, or tocodynamometer. An external electronic monitor enables the nurse to assess
○ 1. contraction compensation.
○ 2. contraction quality.
○ 3. periodic changes in fetal heart rate.
○ 4. fetal heart baseline variability.

**300.** The physician orders 1 mg butorphanol tartrate (Stadol) IV push for Mrs. Odom. The nurse would administer this medication correctly by giving it
○ 1. between contractions.
○ 2. during three to five contractions.
○ 3. in a bolus with one contraction.
○ 4. in 100 ml of normal saline.

**301.** Over the next 3 hours, Mrs. Odom dilates 1 additional centimeter. Which Friedman labor pattern is she exhibiting?
○ 1. Prolonged latent-phase labor.
○ 2. Protracted active-phase labor.
○ 3. Prolonged deceleration-phase labor.
○ 4. Secondary arrest of dilatation.

**302.** The physician ruptures Mrs. Odom's membranes and applies an internal scalp electrode to the fetus. The nurse observes that the monitor tracing is exhibiting moderate variable decelerations. The nurse's *first* action should be to

○ 1. turn the patient onto her side.
○ 2. administer oxygen at 6 L/minute per protocol.
○ 3. chart the observation on the labor record.
○ 4. notify the physician of the decelerations.

**303.** Mrs. Odom remains 8 centimeters dilated for 2 hours, and the physician decides to perform a cesarean section for cephalopelvic disproportion. A newborn problem the nurse should anticipate following a cesarean delivery is
○ 1. increased muscle tone.
○ 2. high-pitched cry.
○ 3. increased nasopharyngeal secretions.
○ 4. difficulty with nipple grasping.

**304.** Even though Mr. Odom was with his wife during labor, he decides not to stay with her during the cesarean section. Which of the following nursing interventions would be *least* effective in promoting Mr. Odom's attachment to the newborn?
○ 1. Encouraging Mr. Odom to carry the baby to the nursery.
○ 2. Having Mr. Odom hear the baby's first cry.
○ 3. Having Mr. Odom accompany the nurse as she transports the infant to the nursery.
○ 4. Encouraging Mr. Odom to hold the baby after discharge.

While playing in the kitchen, 18-month-old Jennifer Gulino pulls a pan of boiling water from the stove onto herself.

**305.** *Immediate* care for Jennifer should include
○ 1. immersing the burned areas in cool water.
○ 2. applying a topical ointment.
○ 3. covering the burned clothing with a clean, dry cloth.
○ 4. covering the burned areas with clean, dry linens.

**306.** Mrs. Gulino calls an ambulance, and she and Jennifer are taken to the nearest emergency center. Jennifer is taken into a treatment room and her mother starts to go with her. Which of the following statements would be *best* for the nurse to make to Mrs. Gulino?
○ 1. "It would be best if you would wait here. I'll keep you informed of what's happening."
○ 2. "I can see that you're upset. Why don't I wait in the waiting room with you?"
○ 3. "You may stay with Jennifer, but children usually do better if their parents stay in the waiting room."
○ 4. "Staying with Jennifer may be difficult for you, but you may be able to help keep her calm."

**307.** Jennifer's burns are classified as partial- and full-thickness, involving 25% of her body surface. They involve the chest, thighs, and face. Which of the following systemic responses would be expected?
○ 1. Decreased metabolic rate.
○ 2. Decreased oxygen consumption.
○ 3. Decreased cardiac output.
○ 4. Decreased hematocrit.

**308.** The nurse anticipates that Jennifer's *immediate* treatment should include
○ 1. fluid replacement with a hypertonic solution.
○ 2. insertion of a Foley catheter.
○ 3. placement on a cooling blanket.
○ 4. administration of intramuscular analgesics.

**309.** Which of the following outcomes indicates that the goal of nursing care during the acute phase of burn care has been attained?
○ 1. Burn shock is prevented.
○ 2. Baseline information is obtained.
○ 3. Bacterial growth in the wound is controlled.
○ 4. The burn wound is assessed.

**310.** Jennifer's condition stabilizes after 3 days. She is now in the management phase of a burn. The nurse judges that the primary danger in this phase has been avoided when Jennifer does *not* develop
○ 1. contractures.
○ 2. an infection.
○ 3. Curling ulcer.
○ 4. shock.

**311.** Before dressing the wound, the nurse notes the areas likely to be full-thickness burns. Which of the following characteristics describes full-thickness burns?
○ 1. They have the most blisters.
○ 2. They cause little pain.
○ 3. They blanch to the touch.
○ 4. They bleed excessively.

**312.** Given Jennifer's age and stage of development, which of the following interventions would the nurse include on Jennifer's nursing care plan?
○ 1. Keep her slightly sedated.
○ 2. Allow her to help with her care.
○ 3. Disturb her as little as possible.
○ 4. Discourage movement that is painful.

**313.** The nurse applies silver sulfadiazine (Silvadene cream) to Jennifer's burns. Which of the following statements is *most accurate* about this preparation?
○ 1. It is difficult to apply.
○ 2. It absorbs very quickly.
○ 3. It is bactericidal for up to 48 hours.
○ 4. It is painful when first applied.

**314.** The nurse prepares to change Jennifer's dressing. What should the nurse do *immediately before* beginning the dressing change?
○ 1. Give Jennifer an injection of morphine sulfate.
○ 2. Make sure all the necessary supplies are in Jennifer's room.
○ 3. Ask Jennifer's parents to assist with the dressing change.
○ 4. Encourage Jennifer to remain very quiet during the dressing change.

**315.** Jennifer receives nasogastric feedings to provide her with needed nutrition because her oral intake is minimal. The nurse develops a plan to increase Jennifer's oral intake. The *most important* nursing intervention in attaining this goal is to
○ 1. schedule her meals long after dressing changes.
○ 2. encourage her parents to bring her favorite foods from home.
○ 3. have her feed herself while sitting in a highchair.
○ 4. provide nourishing snacks between meals.

**316.** Jennifer progresses to the rehabilitative phase of burn care and is scheduled for skin grafting on her upper thighs. The nurse anticipates that when Jennifer returns from the grafting procedure, the mesh grafts may be covered with
○ 1. moist saline dressings covered with dry gauze.
○ 2. a thin layer of plastic wrap covered with elasticized gauze.
○ 3. dry sterile gauze covered with elasticized netting.
○ 4. antibiotic-impregnated gauze covered with a plastic wrap.

**317.** Jennifer's burns, graft sites, and donor sites heal and she is to be discharged home within a few days. The nurse teaches Jennifer's mother about Jennifer's post-discharge skin care. Which of the following statements would indicate that Jennifer's mother has understood the teaching?
○ 1. "I will bathe her twice a week."
○ 2. "I will not take her swimming."
○ 3. "I will avoid using sunscreen on her thighs."
○ 4. "I will apply lubricating cream daily."

Mrs. Jane Kramer, 32, comes to the emergency department with a neighbor. Mrs. Kramer has multiple bruises on her face and arms, a black eye, and a broken nose. She says that these injuries occurred when she "fell down the stairs." The nurse suspects that Mrs. Kramer may have been physically assaulted.

**318.** During the admission interview, it would be *best* for the nurse to

○ 1. ask the patient specifically about the possibility of physical abuse.

○ 2. tell the patient that it is difficult to believe that such injuries are the result of a fall.

○ 3. tell the patient that social services must be notified of the situation.

○ 4. use sensitive questioning to ask the patient if she has been battered.

**319.** After talking with the nurse, Mrs. Kramer admits to being physically abused by her husband. She says that she has never called the police because her husband has threatened to kill her if she does. She says, "I don't want to get him into trouble because he's the father of my children. I don't know what to do!" Which of the following nursing interventions would be *most therapeutic* at this time?

○ 1. Express concern for the patient's safety.

○ 2. Help the patient identify the behaviors that provoke the abuse.

○ 3. Teach the patient ways to reduce the stress within her family.

○ 4. Tell the patient that she should leave her husband.

**320.** During the conversation with the nurse, Mrs. Kramer says, "Let me try to explain why I stay with my husband." Which of the following reasons would Mrs. Kramer be *least likely* to mention?

○ 1. "I'm responsible for keeping my family together."

○ 2. "When it's not too bad, the abuse adds spice to our relationship."

○ 3. "I have only a sixth-grade education."

○ 4. "I'm not sure I could get a job that paid even minimum wage."

**321.** Assessing Mrs. Kramer's family system is likely to reveal the existence of which of the following situations?

○ 1. A balance of power.

○ 2. An emphasis on egalitarian roles.

○ 3. Strong support systems.

○ 4. Lack of religious affiliation.

**322.** The nurse planning interventions for Mrs. Kramer bases the plan on knowledge that

○ 1. a woman in crisis in unlikely to be receptive to professional help.

○ 2. the patient can control the batterer.

○ 3. assessment of the patient's level of danger is a prerequisite to intervention.

○ 4. success is least likely with a multidisciplinary approach.

**323.** A nurse prepares to present a community program about women who are victims of physical abuse. Which of the following facts could the nurse present about the incidence of battering?

○ 1. Battering rarely results in death.

○ 2. Battering is a major cause of injury to women.

○ 3. Battering occurs primarily in lower socioeconomic groups.

○ 4. Battering rarely occurs when women are pregnant.

Ms. Janice Chanute, a 20-year-old single parent, brings her 3-year-old son Tyler into the emergency department because "he fell." He has bruises on his face, arms, and legs, and his mother says that she did not witness the fall. Because the reported cause of injury is vague, the nurse suspects child abuse. While the nurse is examining Tyler, Ms. Chanute says, "Sometimes I guess I'm pretty rough with Tyler. He's so demanding! I'm alone and I try to do my best, but I just don't know how to manage him."

**324.** Referral to which type of program would be *most appropriate* for Ms. Chanute at this time?

○ 1. An assertiveness-training program.

○ 2. A program for single parents.

○ 3. A parenting education program.

○ 4. A women's support group.

**325.** Tyler is admitted overnight for observation. To decrease the child's anxiety, the nurse does which of the following when caring for him?

○ 1. Moves quickly around the child.

○ 2. Keeps the child away from the center of activity.

○ 3. Avoids the use of night lights.

○ 4. Avoids making loud noises.

Mr. Doug Shaller, a 52-year-old journalist, comes to the emergency department after experiencing a sudden onset of severe "ripping" abdominal pain. He is pale, diaphoretic, and tachycardic. After being examined by a physician, Mr. Shaller is rushed to x-ray for an abdominal computed tomography (CT) scan. Abdominal aortic aneurysm is suspected.

**326.** The nurse accompanies Mr. Shaller to the procedure and while en route briefly explains the CT scan. She judges that he has understood the teaching when he says that the examination will involve

○ 1. the injection of air into the lumbar space.

○ 2. the use of x-rays.

○ 3. high-frequency sound waves.

○ 4. the injection of radioactive dye.

**327.** Results of the CT scan show that Mr. Schaller has a dissecting abdominal aortic aneurysm. Mr. Schaller asks what this means. The nurse bases her answer on knowledge that the aneurysm is

○ 1. a pulsating hematoma resulting from a clot on the outside of the vessel.

○ 2. a ballooning of the entire circumference of the aorta.

○ 3. a saclike dilatation on one side of the vessel.

○ 4. a hematoma accumulating between the intimal and medial layers of the vessel.

**328.** Mr. Schaller loses consciousness and is prepared for emergency surgery. His family is summoned, and his wife and two teenaged children arrive just as he is wheeled into the operating room. The nurse explains that they can wait in the critical-care unit family room and shows them where it is. Mrs. Schaller asks many questions and repeatedly says, "What will I do without my husband?" Which of the following would be the nurse's *best initial* response?

○ 1. "Tell me more about your fears."

○ 2. "Are you afraid your husband is going to die?"

○ 3. "Try not to worry; your husband's surgeon is the best."

○ 4. "Would you like me to telephone your priest or minister?"

**329.** Mr. Schaller returns to the critical-care unit on a ventilator. He has an altered level of consciousness and his condition is unstable. A collaborative problem identified is "potential complication: hemorrhage." To detect hemorrhage as soon as possible, the nurse would plan to

○ 1. check the patient's blood pressure every hour.

○ 2. measure the patient's abdominal girth every 8 hours.

○ 3. measure the patient's urinary output every 2 hours.

○ 4. check the operative site for bleeding every 15 minutes.

**330.** Mr. Schaller exhibits signs and symptoms of hemorrhage, and hypovolemic shock develops. The nurse notifies the surgeon, but the hemorrhaging continues and Mr. Schaller dies. After learning that Mr. Schaller has died, his family says they want to see him. In response to their request, the nurse plans *first* to wash Mr. Schaller and then to

○ 1. accompany his family into the room.

○ 2. allow them to be alone with him.

○ 3. suggest that they wait until the priest arrives.

○ 4. ask them if they want the physician to be with them.

Mrs. Jenny Twining, 34, has chronic schizophrenia and is admitted for the third time to a state mental institution under a 72-hour involuntary commitment for evaluation. When she is admitted, Mrs. Twining tells the nurse, "I didn't do anything wrong. I was just carrying out the orders God gave me to paint an 'X' upon the door of all sinners."

**331.** Several hours after being admitted, Mrs. Twining wants to leave the hospital. In addition to explaining that the staff is concerned about her health and safety, the nurse would also tell Mrs. Twining that

○ 1. it will take about 3 days to complete the evaluation.

○ 2. she must stay at least 2 days but then may be able to leave.

○ 3. the court has mandated a 72-hour evaluation.

○ 4. the court has mandated that she stay until she is well.

**332.** Mrs. Twining tells the nurse, "I'm gonna divorce my no-good husband. I hope he rots in hell. But I miss him so bad. I love him. When's he gonna come get me out of here?" Mrs. Twining is displaying

○ 1. ambivalence.

○ 2. autistic thinking.

○ 3. associative looseness.

○ 4. auditory hallucinations.

**333.** Mrs. Twining tells the nurse, "Everybody smiles at me because they know that I was chosen by God for this mission." This statement reflects

○ 1. an idea of reference.

○ 2. a thought insertion.

○ 3. a visual hallucination.

○ 4. a neologism.

**334.** Mrs. Twining's belief in her mission from God can be referred to as a religious delusion of grandeur. A *primary* purpose of such delusions is to provide

○ 1. a sexual outlet.

○ 2. comfort.

○ 3. safety.

○ 4. self-esteem.

**335.** The treatment team persuades Mrs. Twining to sign herself in as a voluntary patient. Haloperidol (Haldol) 10 mg b.i.d. is ordered for Mrs. Twining, and she improves. She is not considered dangerous to herself or others but remains delusional. One morning during the second week of her hospitalization, she refuses to take the haloperidol. Which of the following interventions should the nurse plan to take?

○ 1. Summon another nurse to help her ensure that the patient takes her medication.

 2. Tell the patient that she can take the medication either orally or via injection.

 3. Withhold the medication until she determines why the patient is refusing to take it.

 4. Tell the patient that she needs to take her "vitamin" to stay healthy.

**336.** Because Mrs. Twining is receiving haloperidol (Haldol), the nurse plans to assess her for the development of

 1. hypertensive episodes.

 2. extrapyramidal symptoms.

 3. euphoria.

 4. lithium toxicity.

**337.** Mrs. Twining is no longer delusional and is being considered for discharge soon. Determining her readiness for discharge *must* include an assessment of her

 1. medication knowledge.

 2. activity level.

 3. ability to be employed.

 4. understanding of her disease.

**338.** Mrs. Twining is discharged and referred to a nurse at the comprehensive care center in her home town. During their initial session, the nurse asks Mrs. Twining about her current living situation, daily activities, and the recurrence of psychotic symptoms. The nurse would judge the initial session a success, in terms of data-gathering, if she also could obtain information about the

 1. history and course of the patient's illness.

 2. patient's financial status.

 3. patient's recollections of childhood.

 4. patient's goals for the future.

Mrs. Twining has no children, is separated from her husband, and receives Supplemental Security Income. Although she lives with her mother and older sister, she manages her own medication. Mrs. Twining's mother is in poor health and receives Social Security benefits; Mrs. Twining's sister works outside the home. Mrs. Twining's father is dead; she says he died in a mental institution in a neighboring state. She does not know his diagnosis and has little recollection of him.

**339.** Which of the following areas should the nurse address *first* in Mrs. Twining's care?

 1. Family issues.

 2. Marital issues.

 3. Financial issues.

 4. Medication issues.

**340.** About 6 months after stabilization, Mrs. Twining begins to skip her medication and her counseling

sessions. She tells the nurse that she just forgets to take the medication when things are going well. The nurse develops a plan to help Mrs. Twining continue to take her medication. Which of the following interventions would the nurse include in this plan?

 1. Explain the negative effects that skipping the medication have on the patient's condition.

 2. Consult with the staff psychiatrist about changing the medication to fluphenazine decanoate (Prolixin Decanoate) injections administered by the nurse.

 3. Have the patient's family begin long-term commitment procedures so that the patient's medication regimen can be more closely supervised.

 4. Refer the patient to a partial hospitalization program so that she can participate regularly in group therapy sessions.

**341.** Mr. Twining telephones the nurse to ask for information about his wife's condition. Which of the following responses by Mr. Twining shows that he has understood her explanation about her ability to provide such information?

 1. "I'll meet you in the conference room so that we can discuss her progress."

 2. "I'll ask her physician for permission to read her medical record."

 3. "I'll ask my wife to give you permission to discuss her care with me."

 4. "I'll try to attend my wife's next team treatment case conference."

Mrs. Lorraine Shelby, a 37-year-old music teacher, is admitted to a medical unit for neurologic evaluation.

**342.** While taking the admitting history, the nurse learns that Mrs. Shelby has experienced weakness and fatigue, incoordination, and paresthesias for the past 2 months. These are hallmark clinical manifestations of

 1. multiple sclerosis.

 2. myasthenia gravis.

 3. Parkinson's disease.

 4. amyotrophic lateral sclerosis.

**343.** As part of the neurologic examination, the nurse asks Mrs. Shelby to walk across the room and then back to the bed. Mrs. Shelby lacks coordination and is unsteady. The nurse correctly interprets this gait to be

 1. spastic.

 2. waddling.

○ 3. ataxic.

○ 4. hemiplegic.

**344.** Upon further questioning, Mrs. Shelby says that she has had difficulty walking for the past 2 months and has had numerous falls. She has also had a problem with grip strength and has spilled coffee and often dropped things. Based on this additional assessment data, the nurse would plan interventions related to which of the following nursing diagnoses?

○ 1. Impaired physical mobility related to muscle dysfunction.

○ 2. Disturbance in self-concept related to debilitating condition.

○ 3. Potential for injury related to weakness and muscle dysfunction.

○ 4. Activity intolerance related to fatigue.

**345.** The nurse teaches Mrs. Shelby techniques that will enable her to walk with less difficulty and that will help prevent falls. Which of Mrs. Shelby's behaviors indicate that she has understood the teaching?

○ 1. She takes short, shuffling steps.

○ 2. She walks with her feet wide apart.

○ 3. She uses a walker correctly.

○ 4. She uses a heel-toe, heel-toe gait.

**346.** Mrs. Shelby's physician explains the medications used in the treatment of her disease. Later, she discusses with the nurse what the physician told her. The nurse judges that Mrs. Shelby understood the explanation when she says that a course of which of the following medications is *most likely* to relieve her symptoms?

○ 1. Diphenhydramine hydrochloride (Benadryl).

○ 2. Neostigmine bromide (Prostigmin).

○ 3. Levodopa.

○ 4. Adrenocorticotrophic hormone (ACTH).

**347.** The nurse assesses Mrs. Shelby for euphoria. Which of the following clinical manifestations is characteristic of euphoria?

○ 1. Inappropriate laughter and giddiness.

○ 2. Mood elevation with an exaggerated sense of well-being.

○ 3. Slurring of words when excited.

○ 4. Visual hallucinations and giddiness.

**348.** Mrs. Shelby experiences bladder control problems. She and the nurse identify several interventions to promote urinary continence, such as having the bedpan within easy reach and developing a drinking and voiding schedule. Which of the following patient outcomes indicates the success of these interventions?

○ 1. The patient is continent 24 hours a day.

○ 2. The patient states that her bladder control is improved.

○ 3. The patient monitors herself for urinary retention.

○ 4. The patient complies with the drinking and voiding schedule.

**349.** In preparing Mrs. Shelby for discharge, the nurse discusses activities of daily living and their relationship to her disease. Which of the following suggestions should the nurse emphasize?

○ 1. Accept the need for quiet living and a sedentary life-style.

○ 2. Remain active while avoiding emotional upset, fatigue, and infection.

○ 3. Adhere to good health habits so as to alter the course of the disease.

○ 4. Practice using mechanical aids that will be needed in the future.

**350.** Mrs. Shelby asks the nurse about the effect of her disease on sexual function, and the nurse teaches her how to combat problems that interfere with sexual activity. Which of the following statements made by Mrs. Shelby indicates that she has understood the teaching?

○ 1. "I will use lubricants and stimulants."

○ 2. "I will do perineal tightening exercises every day."

○ 3. "I will take a hot bath before having intercourse."

○ 4. "I will rest before having intercourse."

**351.** During the community health nurse's second visit to Mrs. Shelby, she observes that Mrs. Shelby looks unkempt and sad. Mrs. Shelby suddenly says, "I can't even find the strength to comb my hair" and bursts into tears. Which of the following statements would be *best* for the nurse to make?

○ 1. "It must be frustrating not to be able to care for yourself."

○ 2. "How many days have you been unable to comb your hair?"

○ 3. "Why hasn't your husband been helping you?"

○ 4. "Tell me more about how you're feeling."

Mrs. Ruby Langford, a 20-year-old student, is pregnant. Due to a history of rheumatic heart disease as a child, she is classified as a class II cardiac patient with her pregnancy.

**352.** The nurse counsels Mrs. Langford about her activity during pregnancy. The nurse judges that Mrs. Langford has understood the teaching when she makes which of the following statements?

○ 1. "I won't perform any physical activity during the third trimester."

○ 2. "I'll continue my usual daily activities and rest for 30 minutes each day."

○ 3. "I'll remain on bed rest throughout my pregnancy."

○ 4. "I'll walk more to increase circulation to the growing fetus."

**353.** Mrs. Langford goes into labor. Her physician advises her to have a continuous epidural anesthesia for the labor and delivery. Which statement made by Mrs. Langford indicates to the nurse that she needs more teaching?

○ 1. "I may need to be catheterized if I can't empty my bladder."

○ 2. "I may get a 'spot' of suprapubic pain."

○ 3. "I could have a shivering episode."

○ 4. "I could get a headache if I don't lie flat."

**354.** The nurse explains the external fetal monitor to Mrs. Langford. Which statement made by Mrs. Langford indicates that she understands how the monitor will be positioned and attached?

○ 1. "You'll apply a metal plate to my upper thigh."

○ 2. "You'll attach a small catheter to a pressure device."

○ 3. "You'll place an ultrasonic device across my abdomen."

○ 4. "You'll connect small wires to an electrocardiogram pad."

**355.** Mrs. Langford receives a continuous epidural anesthetic during labor. She complains of nausea, and the nurse notes that her blood pressure has dropped 30 mm Hg. In addition to having someone notify the physician, the nurse should also

○ 1. place the patient in the Trendelenburg position.

○ 2. decrease the rate of the intravenous infusion.

○ 3. turn the patient onto her left side.

○ 4. check the placement of the epidural catheter.

**356.** During assessment of Mrs. Langford's labor, the nurse notes on the fetal heart rate monitor that decelerations are occurring, beginning early in the contracting phase with the onset of the contraction and recovering at the end of the contraction. The nurse would be correct in interpreting this pattern as

○ 1. early decelerations.

○ 2. late decelerations.

○ 3. mild variable decelerations.

○ 4. severe variable decelerations.

**357.** Mrs. Langford delivers a 4-pound, 4-ounce baby girl who is assessed to be term, small for gestational age. Mrs. Langford asks the nurse what problems her baby might have. The nurse bases her answer on knowledge that newborns who are small for gestational age are subject to

○ 1. respiratory problems.

○ 2. no particular problems.

○ 3. problems with heat loss.

○ 4. sucking difficulties.

**358.** Baby Girl Langford's care continues in the newborn nursery after Mrs. Langford has been discharged home. When she visits Mrs. Langford at home, the nurse finds her crying. Mrs. Langford tells the nurse, "I'm a failure. I can't even have a healthy baby." Which of the following statements by Mrs. Langford indicates that the nurse's interventions were appropriate and successful?

○ 1. "I appreciate your listening to me talk about my feelings."

○ 2. "I know my baby is normal, just a little small."

○ 3. "I understand that all mothers go through a period of 'the blues' after childbirth."

○ 4. "I'll go to the nursery to see how my daughter is really doing."

**359.** Mrs. Langford visits her daughter in the hospital. When she tells the nurse she has not chosen a name for her baby, the nurse *correctly* interprets this as the mother's

○ 1. grief response to having a less-than-perfect baby.

○ 2. obsessiveness with choosing the perfect name.

○ 3. need for a few more suggestions for names.

○ 4. desire for a male child.

**360.** Mr. and Mrs. Langford name their daughter Alice. The nurse's observation of which behavior would indicate that Mr. and Mrs. Langford are ready to learn about caring for Alice at home?

○ 1. The increasing frequency of the parent's visits to see Alice.

○ 2. The decline in the parents' expressions of fear about taking Alice home.

○ 3. The parents' increasing involvement in Alice's care.

○ 4. The decline in the number of questions that the parents ask about Alice's condition.

# CORRECT ANSWERS AND RATIONALES

Numbers appear in parentheses following the rationales. The numbers identify textbooks listed in the references at the end of Part V, where correct answers can be verified.

**271.** 1. In addition to recurrent apnea and increased $PaCO_2$, other early manifestations of patent ductus arteriosus include bounding peripheral pulses, pericardial hyperactivity, a continuous murmur, and widening pulse pressure. Although most diagnostic of patent ductus arteriosus, the murmur may be absent in premature infants or neonates. (40)

**272.** 4. In fetal life, the ductus arteriosus connects the pulmonary artery to the aorta and shunts oxygenated blood directly into the systemic circulation, bypassing the uninflated lungs. (40)

**273.** 1. Functional closure of the ductus arteriosus occurs at or shortly after birth. Smooth muscles in its vessel walls constrict when exposed to increased oxygen tension. (40)

**274.** 4. An electrocardiogram is least likely to be useful in confirming the diagnosis of patent ductus arteriosus because an electrocardiogram is usually normal. A chest x-ray usually demonstrates left atrial and ventricular enlargement. Cardiac catheterization is associated with risks and may be unnecessary because of characteristic radiographic findings. An echocardiogram is helpful because it demonstrates an increased left atrial to aortic ratio. (40)

**275.** 4. Patent ductus arteriosus occurs in 32% of preterm infants born prior to 36 weeks gestational age. It is almost twice as common in female infants as in male infants and is one of the most common cardiac anomalies. Although patent ductus arteriosus is a common complication of severe respiratory disease in preterm infants, it is unknown whether it contributes to the development of respiratory disease, or vice versa. (25, 40)

**276.** 2. Indomethacin (Indocin) inhibits prostaglandin synthesis; prostaglandins keep the ductus arteriosus patent. Thus, the administration of indomethacin, a prostaglandin inhibitor, has been successful in constricting the ductus. (25, 40)

**277.** 1. Sodium and potassium values should be monitored closely. Indomethacin (Indocin) is associated with transient renal dysfunction and hyponatremia. Furosemide (Lasix) is associated with dilutional hyponatremia and hypokalemia. Hypokalemia increases the risk of digitalis toxicity. (25, 26, 40)

**278.** 4. Once the patent ductus arteriosus closes, the associated pulmonary and circulatory problems resolve. Activity and fluids are not limited. There is no need to count the patient's pulse. Parents need to be reassured that the problems have been cured. (26)

**279.** 4. In myasthenia gravis, the nerve impulse fails to pass to skeletal muscle at the myoneural junction. The common early symptoms are ptosis of the eyelids and diplopia. Sensation and reflexes are not altered. Muscles do not atrophy. (21)

**280.** 2. In myasthenia gravis, major respiratory complications can result from weakness in the muscles of breathing and swallowing. There is danger of aspiration, respiratory infection, and respiratory failure. Providing a safe environment and emotional support are secondary goals. Pain is not a problem with myasthenia gravis. (21)

**281.** 1. Extreme muscle weakness is present in both cholinergic and myasthenic crisis. In cholinergic crisis, IV edrophonium chloride (Tensilon), a cholinergic agent, does not improve muscle weakness; in myasthenic crisis, muscle weakness decreases after the administration of Tensilon. The muscarinic effects of pyridostigmine bromide (Mestinon) overdosage cause respiratory embarrassment, abdominal cramps, and excessive salivation in cholinergic crisis. (21)

**282.** 3. With a well-managed regimen, a patient with myasthenia gravis should be able to control symptoms, maintain a normal life-style, and achieve a normal life expectancy. Myasthenia gravis can be controlled, not cured. Episodes of increased muscle weakness should not occur if treatment is well managed. (28)

**283.** 2. Hypertension is associated with aneurysm, and antihypertensive medications are used to control arterial blood pressure. Anticoagulants, diuretics, and corticosteroids are not the drugs of choice for patients who are hypertensive and have aneurysms. (6)

**284.** 2. Encouraging the patient to have input into decisions (for example, where to put his personal belongings) gives him a sense of control. Orienting him to his room and ensuring that he will have continuity of care are important to quality patient care, but do not address the loss of environmental control. No data suggest that a referral to the psychiatric clinical nurse specialist is indicated. (8)

**285.** 4. An abdominal aneurysm is resected and replaced with a Dacron or Teflon graft. Saphenous veins are not large enough for this use. Cadaver transplants are not viable. (6, 23, 28)

**286.** 2. Acknowledging the patient's anxiety invites further exploration of his comment. Telling the patient that the surgeon has performed the procedure many times, that everyone is anxious the morning of surgery, or that he can cancel surgery neither provides reassurance nor validates the patient's feelings. (8)

**287.** 1. Veal, broccoli, and white bread are low in cholesterol and saturated fats. Eggs, bacon, cheese, and ice cream are not recommended on diets low in cholesterol and saturated fats. French bread, an English muffin, chicken, and strawberries are allowed on such a diet. (7, 18)

**288.** 1. Bone-marrow aspiration and microscopic cell examination are essential for a diagnosis of leukemia and differentiation between acute lymphocytic leukemia (ALL) and acute nonlymphocytic (myelogenous) leukemia (ANLL). Although a complete blood count provides information about the number of white and red blood cells, it does not give enough information to make a differential diagnosis. A lumbar puncture is performed after the diagnosis is made to determine the presence of central nervous system involvement. Chest x-rays are done to detect the presence of the disease in organs other than the bone marrow. (35, 40)

**289.** 2. Because the MMR (measles, mumps, rubella) contains live viruses, administering it to a child whose immune system is compromised could result in an overwhelming infection. Administering it 3 months after termination of chemotherapy allows the immune system time to recover so that it can respond when challenged with a vaccination. Giving the immunization in divided doses to a child with a compromised immune system could cause infection. (40)

**290.** 4. The most important prognostic factors in determining long-term survival for children with acute lymphoid leukemia are the initial white blood count and patient's age at diagnosis. These factors are followed by histologic type of disease and sex. (40)

**291.** 1. Jaw pain in a patient receiving vincristine sulfate (Oncovin) can indicate neurotoxicity and must be reported to the physician immediately. Neurotoxicity may necessitate cessation of the vincristine sulfate. Fever, urinary retention, and anorexia are less serious side effects than neurotoxicity. (17, 40)

**292.** 1. Encouraging a child to select meals from the hospital menu may enhance the child's intake. By age 6, most children have strong food preferences and are likely to eat better when they can choose foods they like. Children receiving chemotherapy need a high-protein, high-calorie diet, but their food

intake may be decreased by anorexia, pain, and taste alterations. Between-meal snacking is encouraged to increase caloric intake. These children rarely have dietary restrictions and may enjoy food from home. Eating with other children provides a social outlet that often encourages a better nutritional intake. (40)

**293.** 3. Administering the antiemetic medication *before* beginning chemotherapy and then routinely around the clock helps prevent nausea. Evidence suggests that giving chemotherapy at bedtime, together with a sedative, reduces nausea and vomiting. Keeping a child receiving chemotherapy n.p.o. does not reduce nausea. (40)

**294.** 4. Propantheline bromide (Pro-Banthine) is an anticholinergic agent. Anticholinergic agents (previously known as parasympatholytic agents) inhibit or block the activity of the parasympathetic nervous system. The most common side effects of such agents are blurred vision and dryness of the mouth. Other side effects include urinary retention, tachycardia, and constipation. (22)

**295.** 2. Rupture of a diverticulum causes peritonitis by the release of intestinal contents (chemicals and bacteria) into the peritoneal cavity. The inflammatory response of the peritoneal tissue produces severe abdominal rigidity and pain, diminished intestinal motility, and retention of intestinal contents (air, fluid, and stool). (21)

**296.** 1. During the acute stage of diverticulitis, a low-fiber diet is usually prescribed. Bran cereals and unpeeled apples are not low-fiber foods. (7, 37, 42)

**297.** 3. A high-fiber diet is prescribed to increase the bulk of the stool so that it moves through the colon at a normal rate. The high-fiber diet also reduces pressure in the intestine by preventing distention of the intestinal wall and the formation of more diverticula. Foods increased on high-fiber diets include bran, whole-grain cereals and breads, and legumes such as dried peas and beans. Fat is not restricted with either diverticulosis or diverticulitis. (7, 21, 37, 42)

**298.** 4. Presbycusis, the sensorineural hearing deficit of the elderly, involves the loss of the ability to perceive tones of higher frequency (pitch). Communication can be improved by accentuating consonants (the high-pitched components of speech), lowering the pitch of the voice, and speaking at a moderate rate. Overarticulating words does not facilitate communication. (21, 23)

**299.** 3. The external fetal monitor works by ultrasound. It monitors the fetal heart rate and periodic changes, but not the true r-r interval of the fetal heart rate, which is the baseline variability. The baseline variability can be assessed only through internal monitoring with application of a scalp electrode. The external contraction monitor works via a pressure transducer placed across the mother's abdomen. It displays the frequency and duration of contractions, but not the true intensity or quality; that requires an internal pressure device, because maternal tissues lie between the pressure transducer and the uterus. (38)

**300.** 2. Intravenous analgesics should be given during three to five contractions. The contractions restrict blood flow to the fetus, possibly resulting in more maternal tissue uptake and less fetal uptake. Theoretically, there is more fetal uptake of intravenous analgesics when they are given between contractions and in a bolus. Furthermore, a bolus of some analgesics may cause maternal vomiting. Giving the analgesic butorphanol tartrate (Stadol) via piggyback in solution is not recommended. (4)

**301.** 2. According to Emmanuel Friedman, protracted active-phase labor in a primigravida is one in which the cervix fails to dilate at least 1.2 cm per hour for 2 hours. Since the patient in this situation was 4 centimeters dilated when admitted, she is in the active phase of labor. To make a dysfunctional labor assessment, the nurse first should identify the patient's phase of labor, then determine if the patient meets the Friedman criteria for progress. Prolonged latent-phase labor occurs in the latent phase, from about 1 to 4 cm of dilatation, and lasts longer than 20 hours in the primigravida. Prolonged deceleration-phase labor lasts longer than 3 hours in the primigravida when the patient is dilated 8 to 10 cm. Secondary arrest of dilatation means that cervical dilatation has ceased for an hour in the active phase of labor. Multiparas have different criteria for progress. (4)

**302.** 1. Variable decelerations occur in 50% of labors and are due to some type of cord involvement, the most common being cord compression between the fetus and maternal pelvis. This often can be alleviated by a maternal position change. If the condition worsens, oxygen may be administered according to protocol. It is essential to notify the physician and chart the observations. (8)

**303.** 3. Nasopharyngeal secretions are increased with a cesarean delivery because the infant has not had the benefit of the squeezing action of a vaginal birth, which helps remove secretions from the nasopharynx. The infant may have decreased muscle tone from general anesthesia. Difficulty with nipple grasping has been reported after forceps deliveries due to compression of the face, resulting in edema, but this phenomenon does not occur with cesarean births. High-pitched cries are symptoms of neuro-

logic involvement and do not directly relate to a cesarean section. (27)

**304.** 4. When a father cannot be present at a cesarean birth, or does not want to be, the nurse can facilitate his involvement in the birthing and attachment process by having him hear the baby's first cry, letting him carry the infant to the nursery, or having him accompany the nurse as the baby is being transported to the nursery. (27)

**305.** 1. *Immediate* treatment of burns involves cooling the area with cool water. This decreases skin temperature and halts continuing direct thermal injury. After 10 minutes, saturated clothing and towels should be removed and replaced with clean, dry linens. This prevents excessive heat loss and contamination and exposure to air, which can cause increasing discomfort. No medication or ointments are applied. (25, 39)

**306.** 4. Most parents are stressed and anxious in emergency situations. However, with the help of the staff, parents can usually control their feelings enough to help the child through the experience. (39)

**307.** 3. A dramatic alteration in circulation ("burn shock") occurs in the immediate post-burn period. Cardiac output drops dramatically; this is attributed to a circulating myocardial depressant factor that directly affects the contractility of the heart muscle. The metabolic rate in burned patients is greatly accelerated, as is oxygen consumption. Hematocrit increases as fluid loss leads to hemoconcentration. (40)

**308.** 2. Accurate measurement of urinary output is essential to monitor fluid replacement and to assess renal function. Isotonic fluids are usually administered in the first 24 hours to expand extracellular volume. Because heat is lost through the burn wound, a heat lamp may be needed to keep the patient warm. Analgesics are important, but should be given intravenously rather than intramuscularly. The intravenous route provides maximum pain relief and prevents pooling of the medication due to poor circulation. (39)

**309.** 1. The goal of nursing care in the acute phase of burn care is to prevent burn shock. The acute phase, also called the resuscitative, emergent, or metabolic phase, includes the first 24 to 48 hours. Obtaining baseline information, controlling bacterial growth in the wound, and assessing the burn wound are all emphasized in the acute phase, but preventing burn shock is the goal. (40)

**310.** 2. The greatest threat to life in the management phase of a burn is infection: wound infection, generalized sepsis, and bacterial pneumonia. Contractures and Curling ulcer are complications of this phase, but shock is the primary danger of the acute or emergent phase. (40)

**311.** 2. Full-thickness burns are serious injuries in which all skin layers are destroyed. Lack of pain sensation at the wound edges is characteristic of full-thickness burns. Because the blood supply is destroyed, blanching and bleeding are absent. Blisters characterize partial-thickness burns and do not occur in full-thickness burns. (40)

**312.** 2. Toddlers are in Erikson's stage of autonomy and should be allowed some independence. Giving them the opportunity to assist with their care will promote their autonomy. Crying and temper tantrums, common during this age, should be expected and handled appropriately. A child in the management phase of a burn should be encouraged to move to prevent contractures. Play and games should be encouraged to prevent regression and depression. (40)

**313.** 3. Silver sulfadiazine (Silvadene cream) is bactericidal for up to 48 hours. It is easy to apply and absorbs slowly, and it is painless when applied. (40)

**314.** 3. Parents are encouraged to stay with the child during the dressing change so they can support the child and learn the procedure. Because dressing changes are painful, medication is given 30 minutes before the procedure. The child should know that it is all right to cry when the treatment hurts. Dressings should be changed in a clean environment. Painful procedures should not be done in the child's room because the room should be a "safe" environment. (40)

**315.** 1. It is *most important* that meals should *not* be scheduled immediately after a dressing change because most children are usually physically and emotionally exhausted. Parents should be encouraged to bring the child's favorite food from home. Children usually eat better when they can feed themselves and when they eat in an atmosphere that is as much like home as possible. Nourishing snacks are provided between meals. (40)

**316.** 1. Mesh grafts may be covered with an occlusive dressing or may be exposed. Wet dressings may be applied over the graft and kept moist with normal saline, antimicrobial agents, or silver nitrate. The moist dressings are covered with dry gauze. Plastic wraps are not used because the heat and moisture they generate cause maceration. (40)

**317.** 4. A daily bath should be followed by the application of lubricating cream or ointments. Water is a good place for exercises, and healed burn wounds are unaffected by salt, fresh, or pool water. Sunscreens should be used because they protect the wound from the sun. (26)

**318.** 4. It is important to determine whether abuse is occurring in order to provide appropriate nursing care and support for the patient. Many patients are hesitant to talk about abuse and need help to do so. It is important for nurses to ask directly about abuse when it is suspected; however, challenging confrontation may alienate the patient and make her less willing to talk about her situation. The nurse is not legally required to report abuse of adults to social services, unless they are considered vulnerable adults. (3)

**319.** 1. The nurse must consider the patient's safety. The nurse's expression of concern for her safety may help the patient validate her fears and choose to take action. Telling her to leave her husband is inappropriate advice-giving. The idea of leaving the marriage may be so overwhelming that it may push the patient away from the nurse as a support person. Talking to the patient about changing her behavior or reducing family stress are forms of victim-blaming. They reinforce the message that the patient is responsible for the abuse, the same message she is probably getting from the abuser and others. (3)

**320.** 2. Violence is never acceptable to victims; this myth condones the use of violence. Often an episode of battering is followed by a period of pleasant relations between the partners, during which the woman may hope that the violence will never happen again. She may stay in the relationship for that reason. Women are conditioned to be responsible for the family's well-being, and this is often a motivation for the woman to stay in a relationship. A woman's lack of job skills and financial resources also may cause her to stay. Many women are injured or killed when they try to leave a violent relationship. (3)

**321.** 4. Lack of religious affiliation in both partners correlates with the highest rate of spouse abuse. In family violence, the abuser and victim have some sort of power imbalance (for example, strength, physical size, or role in the family). The victim is usually weaker than the abuser and does not have equal rights in the family. Families in which domestic abuse occurs are often socially isolated, and lack of support systems often affects the victim's ability to escape the cycle of abuse. (3, 16)

**322.** 3. Assessing the patient's level of danger is a prerequisite to intervention, which usually requires a multidisciplinary approach. A woman is more open to change and more receptive to professional intervention during a crisis. At other times, it is easier for her to deny the problem and maintain usual patterns of interaction. The patient cannot control the batterer, only her responses to the batterer and to her situation. (3, 16)

**323.** 2. Battering is a major cause of injury to women and accounts for 15% to 20% of all homicides. Although battering occurs in all socioeconomic groups, it may seem more common in members of lower socioeconomic groups because they are more likely to use emergency-room services. Pregnant women are frequent victims of battering. (3, 16)

**324.** 3. Referral to a parenting education program is the most appropriate referral at this time, since the woman in this item is expressing problems with parenting. (3, 16)

**325.** 4. Caregiver behaviors that decrease a victim's fears and anxieties include moving slowly around the child, keeping the child near the center of activity, using night lights, and avoiding loud noises. (3, 16, 40)

**326.** 2. Computed tomography (CT), also called CT scanning and computerized axial tomography (CAT), uses x-rays and a special scanner. This procedure provides information about the geography and characteristics of tissue structures within solid organs. Pneumoencephalography, in which air is injected into the lumbar space, permits accurate localization of brain lesions. Ultrasound, which demonstrates the position, form, and function of anatomic structures, uses high-frequency sound waves. Radioactive iodine is used in the diagnosis and treatment of thyroid gland problems. (11)

**327.** 4. In a dissecting aneurysm, hemorrhage into a vessel wall dissects the wall. A false aneurysm is a pulsating hematoma resulting from a clot on the outside of the vessel. A fusiform aneurysm, which is spindle-shaped, involves the entire circumference of the arterial wall. A saccular aneurysm, which takes the form of a sac attached to the side of the artery, involves only part of the circumference of the artery. (28)

**328.** 1. Asking the patient to express her fears encourages her to do so and avoids making assumptions about what is bothering her. Clichés, false reassurance, and vague advice should be avoided. (8, 16, 28)

**329.** 4. Checking the operative site every 15 minutes would help detect early hemorrhage, as would checking the patient's vital signs every 15 minutes. Measuring abdominal girth and monitoring urinary output would also provide helpful information about the patient's status, but frequent monitoring of vital signs is most helpful in detecting early hemorrhage. (8, 28)

**330.** 1. The nurse should accompany the family into the patient's room to provide them with support. She should allow the family time alone with the patient, once they have seen the body initially and have asked any questions. The family need not wait for the priest to see the patient, nor does the physician need to be with them. (29)

**331.** 3. Patients admitted on involuntary commitment must remain hospitalized for the time allotted for the evaluation. If the treatment team completes the evaluation in less than the allotted time, they may decide to discharge the patient or they may institute further commitment procedures. Patients cannot sign themselves out of the hospital during this period, nor can family members release them. (31)

**332.** 1. Ambivalence is the presence of strong, conflicting attitudes or feelings toward an object, person, goal, or situation. Autistic thinking involves attributing personal and private meanings to words and situations. Associative looseness is characterized by simultaneous expression of unrelated, or only slightly related, ideas or thoughts. Auditory hallucinations are hearing sounds, words, or voices not experienced by others. (16, 36)

**333.** 1. An idea of reference is a person's view that other people recognize that he or she has an important characteristic or power. Thought insertion is the individual's belief that others, or a specific other, can put thoughts into the patient's mind. A visual hallucination is the sight of objects or persons not based in reality. A neologism is a word or language that has meaning only to the individual. (16, 36)

**334.** 4. Delusions of grandeur provide the patient with an exaggerated sense of self-esteem that is unrelated to the patient's actual achievements. Other, less grandiose, religious delusions may provide comfort or meaning for the patient. Delusions of persecution are frequently related to safety issues. Delusions may also be related to sexual issues. (16, 36)

**335.** 3. When a patient refuses medication, the nurse must discover the reason for the refusal; unwanted side effects are frequently the reason. A patient cannot legally be forcibly medicated unless he is a danger to himself or others. Lying to a patient about a medication is neither appropriate nor ethical. (16, 36)

**336.** 2. Extrapyramidal symptoms frequently result from the administration of antipsychotic medications; haloperidol (Haldol) is associated with a high incidence of severe extrapyramidal reactions. Other side effects associated with haloperidol include blurred vision, dry mouth, urinary retention, and rash. Haloperidol is associated with a low incidence of sedation and a low incidence of cardiovascular effects at therapeutic dosages. Euphoria is not associated with haloperidol. Patients taking lithium should be monitored for lithium toxicity. (1, 16, 17)

**337.** 1. When determining the patient's readiness for discharge, the nurse should give priority to assessing the patient's medication knowledge. Assessing her activity level, her ability to be employed, and her understanding of her disease are important, but not as important as assessing her medication knowledge. (16, 36)

**338.** 1. Knowledge of the history and course of a patient's illness enables the nurse to identify stressors or situations that contribute to a recurrence of psychosis. In turn, this knowledge enables the nurse to develop a care plan aimed at maintaining the patient's stability. The patient's goals are important but will be much more achievable if future psychosis is prevented. (16, 36)

**339.** 4. Medication noncompliance is a primary cause of exacerbation in chronic mental illnesses. Of the issues listed in this item, it should be addressed first; other issues can be addressed as stabilization of the patient is maintained. (16, 36)

**340.** 2. The nurse can most effectively monitor the patient's compliance with medication therapy by administering the medication herself. Education may or may not affect the patient's compliance with medication therapy. Long-term commitment is unnecessarily restrictive and would be difficult legally. Participation in a partial hospitalization program may be a desirable referral but would only indirectly affect the patient's compliance with medication therapy. (16, 17, 36)

**341.** 3. Only patients have the power and authority to allow people not directly involved in their care to view their medical records. Only a patient has the right to provide information to support persons. (31)

**342.** 1. Hallmark clinical manifestations of multiple sclerosis include weakness and fatigue, incoordination, and paresthesias. Muscle weakness and severe generalized fatigue are characteristic of myasthenia gravis, but incoordination and paresthesias are not. Parkinson's disease is characterized by impaired movement, muscle rigidity, "pill-rolling" of the fingers, and resting tremor. Amyotrophic lateral sclerosis is characterized by fatigue, awkwardness of fine finger movements, and muscle wasting. (6)

**343.** 3. An ataxic gait is an unsteady, uncoordinated walk in which the patient uses a wide base of support. A patient with a spastic gait walks with the legs held together and moves stiffly; the toes seem to drag and catch. A waddling gait involves exaggerated alternation of lateral trunk movements with

an exaggerated elevation of the hip. A hemiplegic gait involves flexion of the hip because of foot-drop and circumduction of the leg. (2, 28)

**344.** 3. The diagnosis of potential for injury related to weakness and muscle dysfunction incorporates both upper and lower motor weakness. Impaired physical mobility does not reflect upper extremity weakness. No information is provided in this item to indicate problems with self-concept or activity intolerance. (8)

**345.** 2. A wide base of support will provide stability. Short, shuffling steps make walking difficult for the patient with multiple sclerosis and increase the chance of falling. No information is provided in the item that indicates a walker is needed. A heel-toe gait is effective for patients with Parkinson's disease. (6)

**346.** 4. Adrenocorticotrophic hormone (ACTH) is prescribed by some physicians to relieve the symptoms of multiple sclerosis. Diphenhydramine hydrochloride (Benadryl) and Levodopa are used to treat Parkinson's disease. Neostigmine bromide (Prostigmin) is used in the treatment of myasthenia gravis. (6, 17, 23)

**347.** 2. Patients with multiple sclerosis may have a sense of optimism and euphoria, particularly during remissions. Euphoria is characterized by mood elevation with an exaggerated sense of well-being. Inappropriate laughter and giddiness, slurring of words when excited, and visual hallucinations and giddiness are uncharacteristic of euphoria. (6, 28)

**348.** 1. The goal is to promote urinary continence; an indication that this goal has been met is that the patient is continent 24 hours a day. A patient's self-report that her bladder control is improved may indicate that the goal has been attained, but 24-hour-a-day continence is a more definite indication that the goal has been met. Monitoring for urinary retention and complying with the drinking and voiding schedule are important but do not reflect achievement of the stated goal. (6, 28)

**349.** 2. Multiple sclerosis is characterized by exacerbations that are often associated with physical and mental fatigue. Multiple sclerosis is not necessarily confining and does not dictate a sedentary lifestyle. The disease is chronic and progressive. While good health habits may help stabilize the patient's condition, they will not alter the course of the disease. Mechanical aids will be prescribed as the patient's situation warrants. (6, 28)

**350.** 4. Fatigue, emotional lability, and loss of self-esteem and self-worth are some of the problems that may interfere with sexual activity for patients with multiple sclerosis and their partners. Resting before intercourse will help relieve some fatigue. Spasms of the adductor thigh muscles in women can make intercourse difficult, and these spasms do not respond to treatment with lubricants or stimulants. Perineal tightening exercises do not decrease problems that interfere with sexual activity for patients with multiple sclerosis. Hot baths should be avoided because they can increase weakness. (6, 28)

**351.** 4. By asking the patient to tell her more about how she is feeling, the nurse is not making any assumptions about what is troubling the patient. The nurse should acknowledge the patient's feelings and encourage her to discuss them. (8, 16)

**352.** 2. The patient in this item is a class II cardiac patient; according to the New York Heart Association, the class II cardiac patient has no symptoms at rest and has only minor activity limitations. The patient should get adequate rest and limit strenuous activity. The class III cardiac patient is comfortable at rest but experiences excessive fatigue, palpitations, or dyspnea with less than ordinary physical activity. The patient with class III cardiac disease has moderate to marked limitation on physical activity. The class IV cardiac patient has symptoms of cardiac insufficiency or of the anginal syndrome at rest and with any physical activity. This patient may be on bed rest for all or part of a pregnancy. (30)

**353.** 4. Headache is not a side effect of epidural anesthesia because the dura mater is not entered. Epidural anesthesia is associated with problems of bladder emptying due to decreased sensations to void. Shivering can occur due to heat loss caused by increased peripheral blood flow. A "spot" of suprapubic pain occasionally occurs with epidural anesthesia for reasons not clearly understood. (27)

**354.** 3. In external electronic fetal monitoring, the ultrasonic device is placed across the mother's abdomen at the point where the fetal heart rate signal is loudest. In internal fetal monitoring, after the catheter is properly placed by the physician it is taped securely to the mother's inner thigh. A pressure catheter is used with internal uterine contraction monitoring and the device is attached to a pressure transducer on the monitor. Electrocardiogram pads are not used with fetal monitoring. (30, 38)

**355.** 3. Hypotension is a common side effect of epidural anesthesia because of its sympathetic blocking action. Nausea is an early symptom of hypotension. Placing the patient on her left side may increase blood return to the heart by alleviating pressure of the uterus and fetus on the vena cava. The physician may decide to increase the intravenous infu-

sion rate. It is the physician's responsibility to determine correct placement of the epidural catheter. The patient is not placed in the Trendelenburg position because the level of anesthesia could ascend and suppress respirations. Furthermore, the vena cava would still be compressed with the patient in the Trendelenburg position. (30)

**356.** 1. Early decelerations are the mirror image of a contraction, beginning with the contraction, dipping to a nadir at the peak of the contraction and ending with the contraction. Late decelerations begin at least 15 seconds after the beginning of the contraction, reach a nadir about the end of the contraction, and return to baseline at least 15 seconds after the recovery of the contraction. All types of variable decelerations are jagged at the onset, dropping abruptly from the baseline. Variable decelerations may or may not be related to the contraction. Early decelerations are due to head compression, late decelerations to uteroplacental insufficiency, and variable decelerations to cord compression. (38)

**357.** 3. Small-for-gestational-age or intrauterine growth retardation newborns have problems with heat loss because their small size implies a high surface-area-to-volume ratio, with attendant excessive heat loss. Diminished subcutaneous fat deposits because of defective maternal transport of nutrients, defective placental transfer of nutrients, or defective utilization of nutrients by the fetus are indirect causes but do not themselves influence thermoregulation. Sucking difficulties and respiratory distress syndrome due to immature lungs are problems of the preterm newborn. The term, small-for-gestational-age newborn has mature organs of diminished size. (27)

**358.** 1. The patient in this item expresses a need to discuss her feelings. By encouraging the patient to do so, the nurse does not make any assumptions about what is bothering the patient. (27)

**359.** 1. Families who deliver what they perceive as a less-than-perfect infant spend a period of time working through their grief. This process requires them to come to terms with the loss of the conceptualized ideal infant and the reality or gain of the less-than-perfect real infant. One of the manifestations of non-acceptance of the baby, or premature grieving of the death of a baby, is the parents' failure to name the baby. (27, 30)

**360.** 3. The parents' increased involvement in caretaking responsibilities for the sick newborn indicates their readiness for teaching. Parents will still verbalize feelings of grief and insecurity and concern for the newborn's health. However, they will demonstrate attachment behaviors as well. (27, 30)

## *REFERENCES FOR PART V*
## *Postreview Comprehensive Tests*

1. Baer CL, Williams BR. Clinical Pharmacology and Nursing. Springhouse, PA: Springhouse, 1988.
2. Bates B. A Guide to Physical Assessment. 4th ed. Philadelphia: JB Lippincott, 1987.
3. Beck DM, Rawlins RP, Williams SR. Mental Health-Psychiatric Nursing: A Holistic Life-Cycle Approach. 2nd ed. St. Louis: CV Mosby, 1988.
4. Bobak IM, Jensen MD. Essentials of Maternity Nursing: The Nurse and the Childbearing Family. 2nd ed. St. Louis: CV Mosby, 1987.
5. Brunner LS, Suddarth DS. The Lippincott Manual of Nursing Practice. 3rd ed. Philadelphia: JB Lippincott, 1983.
6. Brunner LS, Suddarth DS. Textbook of Medical-Surgical Nursing. 6th ed. Philadelphia: JB Lippincott, 1988.
7. Burtis G, Davis J, Martin S. Applied Nutrition and Diet Therapy. Philadelphia: WB Saunders, 1988.
8. Carpenito LJ. Nursing Diagnosis: Application to Clinical Practice. 2nd ed. Philadelphia: JB Lippincott, 1987.
9. Christian JL, Gregor JL. Nutrition for Living. 2nd ed. Menlo Park: Benjamin/Cummings, 1988.
10. Clark JB, Queener SF, Karb VG. Pharmacological Basis of Nursing Practice. St. Louis: CV Mosby, 1986.
11. Fischbach F. A Manual of Laboratory Diagnostic Tests. 3rd ed. Philadelphia: JB Lippincott, 1988.
12. Flynn JBM, Heffron PB. Nursing—From Concept to Practice. 2nd ed. Norwalk: Appleton & Lange, 1988.
13. Govoni LE, Hayes JE. Drugs and Nursing Implications. 5th ed. New York: Appleton-Century-Crofts, 1985.
14. Green M, Harry J. Nutrition in Contemporary Nursing Practice. 2nd ed. New York: John Wiley & Sons, 1987.
15. Guzzetta CE, Dossey BM. Cardiovascular Nursing: Bodymind Tapestry. St. Louis: CV Mosby, 1984.
16. Haber J, Hoskins PP, Leach AM, Sideleau BV. Comprehensive Psychiatric Nursing. New York: McGraw-Hill, 1987.
17. Hahn AB, Oestreich SJK, Barkin RL. Mosby's Pharmacology in Nursing. 17th ed. St. Louis: CV Mosby, 1986.
18. Kneisel CR, Ames SW. Adult Health Nursing, A Biopsychosocial Approach. Reading, MA: Addison-Wesley, 1986.
19. Kozier B, Erb G. Fundamentals of Nursing. 3rd ed. Reading, MA: Addison-Wesley, 1987.
20. Kozier B, Erb G. Techniques in Clinical Nursing. 2nd ed. Reading, MA: Addison-Wesley, 1987.
21. Lewis SM, Collier IC. Medical-Surgical Nursing: Assessment and Management of Clinical Problems. 2nd ed. New York: McGraw-Hill, 1987.
22. Loebl S, Spratto GR. The Nurse's Drug Handbook. New York: John Wiley, 1986.
23. Luckmann J, Sorensen K. Medical-Surgical Nursing, A Psychophysiologic Approach. 3rd ed. Philadelphia: WB Saunders, 1987.
24. Malasanos L, Barkauskas V, Stoltenberg-Allen K. Health Assessment. 3rd ed. St. Louis: CV Mosby, 1986.
25. Marlow DR, Redding BA. Textbook of Pediatric Nursing. 6th ed. Philadelphia: WB Saunders, 1988.
26. Mott SA, Fazekas NF, James SR. Nursing Care of Children and Families, A Holistic Approach. 3rd ed. Menlo Park: Addison-Wesley, 1988.
27. Olds SB, London ML, Ludewig PA. Maternal Newborn Nursing, A Family-Centered Approach. 3rd ed. Menlo Park: Addison-Wesley, 1988.
28. Phipps WJ, Long BC, Woods NF. Medical-Surgical Nursing Concepts and Clinical Practice. 3rd ed. St. Louis: CV Mosby, 1987.
29. Potter PA, Perry AG. Fundamentals of Nursing: Concepts, Process, and Practice, St. Louis: CV Mosby, 1985.
30. Reeder SJ, Martin LL. Maternity Nursing: Family, Newborn, and Women's Health Care. 17th ed. Philadelphia: JB Lippincott, 1987.
31. Rinas J, Clyne-Jackson S. Professional Conduct and Legal Concerns in Mental Health Practice. Norwalk: Appleton-Lange, 1988.
32. Servonsky J, Opas SR. Nursing Management of Children. Boston: Jones & Bartlett, 1987.
33. Skidmore-Roth L. Nursing Drug Reference. St. Louis: CV Mosby, 1988.
34. Smith S, Duell D. Clinical Nursing Skills. 2nd ed. Los Altos: National Nursing Review, 1988.
35. Smith M, Goodman J, Ramsey N. Child and Family: Concepts of Nursing Practice. New York: McGraw-Hill, 1987.
36. Stuart GW, Sundeen SF. Principles and Practice of Psychiatric Nursing. 3rd ed. St. Louis: CV Mosby, 1987.
37. Suitor CW, Crowley MF. Nutrition: Principles and Application in Health Promotion. 2nd ed. Philadelphia: JB Lippincott, 1984.
38. Tucker SM. Pocket Guide to Fetal Monitoring. St. Louis: CV Mosby, 1988.
39. Waechter EH, Phillips J, Holoday B. Nursing Care of Children. 10th ed. Philadelphia: JB Lippincott, 1985.
40. Whaley LF, Wong DL. Nursing Care of Infants and Children. 3rd ed. St. Louis: CV Mosby, 1987.
41. Whitney EN, Cataldo CB, Rolfes SR. Understanding Normal and Clinical Nutrition. 2nd ed. St. Paul: West Publishing Company, 1987.
42. Zeman FJ, Ney DM. Applications of Clinical Nutrition. Englewood Cliffs: Prentice-Hall, 1988.

# appendix

For further information about NCLEX-RN, write to the National Council of State Boards of Nursing, Inc.:

National Council of State Boards of Nursing, Inc.
676 North St. Clair   Street
Suite 550
Chicago, Illinois 60611
(312) 787-6555

For information about the dates, requirements, and specifics of writing the examination in your state, contact the appropriate state board of nursing. The address and telephone number for each state board of nursing are provided below.

**ALABAMA**
Board of Nursing
Suite 203, 500 East Boulevard
Montgomery, Alabama 36117
*(205) 261-4060*

**ALASKA**
Board of Nursing
Div. of Occupational Licensing
P.O. Box D-LIC
Juneau, Alaska 99811
*(907) 465-2544*

**ARIZONA**
Board of Nursing
5050 North 19th Ave.
Suite 103
Phoenix, Arizona 85015
*(602) 255-5092*

**ARKANSAS**
State Board of Nursing
Univ. Tower Bldg.
Suite 800, 1123 S. Univ. Ave.
Little Rock, Arkansas 72204
*(501) 371-2751*

**CALIFORNIA**
Board of Registered Nursing
1030 13th St. Suite 200
Sacramento, California 95814
*(916) 322-3350*

**COLORADO**
Board of Nursing
1560 Broadway, Suite 670
Denver, Colorado 80202
*(303) 894-2430*

**CONNECTICUT**
Department of Health Services
Nurse Licensure
150 Washington Street
Hartford, Connecticut 06106
*(203) 566-1032/1036*

**DELAWARE**
Board of Nursing
Margaret O'Neill Building
Federal & Court Streets
Dover, Delaware 19901
*(302) 736-4522*

**DISTRICT OF COLUMBIA**
Nurses Examining Board
614 H Street, N.W., Rm 923
Washington, D.C. 20001
*(202) 727-7468*

**FLORIDA**
Board of Nursing
Suite 504, 111 E. Coastline Drive
Jacksonville, Florida 32202
*(904) 359-6331*

**GEORGIA**
Board of Nursing
Suite 400, 166 Pryor Street, S.W.
Atlanta, Georgia 30303
*(404) 656-3943*

**HAWAII**
Board of Nursing, Licensing Br.
Box 3469
Honolulu, Hawaii 96801
*(808) 548-4100*

**IDAHO**
Board of Nursing
500 S. 10th St., Suite 102
Boise, Idaho 83720
*(208) 334-3110*

**ILLINOIS**
Dept. of Professional
  Regulation
320 W. Washington Street
Springfield, Illinois 62786
*(217) 785-0800*

**INDIANA**
State Board of Nursing
Health Professions Bureau
One American Sq. Suite 1020,
  Box 82067
Indianapolis, Indiana 46282
*(317) 232-2960*

**IOWA**
Board of Nursing
1223 East Court
Des Moines, Iowa 50319
*(515) 281-3255*

**KANSAS**
State Board of Nursing
900 S.W. Jackson
Suite 551 S.
Topeka, Kansas 66601
*(913) 296-4929*

**KENTUCKY**
Board of Nursing
Suite 430, 4010 Dupont Circle
Louisville, Kentucky 40207
*(502) 897-5143*

**LOUISIANA**
Board of Nursing
Room 907, 150 Baronne Street
New Orleans, Louisiana 70112
*(504) 568-5464*

**MAINE**
Board of Nursing
295 Water Street
Augusta, Maine 04330
*(207) 289-5324*

**MARYLAND**
Board of Nursing
201 W. Preston Street
Baltimore, Maryland 21201
*(301) 225-5880*

**MASSACHUSETTS**
Board of Registration in Nursing
Room 1519, 100 Cambridge Street
Boston, Massachusetts 02202
*(617) 727-9961*

**MICHIGAN**
Board of Nursing
P.O. Box 30018
Lansing, Michigan 48909
*(517) 373-1600*

**MINNESOTA**
Board of Nursing
2700 University Ave. W. #108
St. Paul, Minnesota 55114
*(612) 642-0567*

**MISSISSIPPI**
Board of Nursing
239 N. Lamar, Suite 401
Jackson, Mississippi 39201-1311
*(601) 354-7349*

**MISSOURI**
Board of Nursing
Box 656, 3523 N. Ten Mile Drive
Jefferson City, Missouri 65102
*(314) 751-2334*

**MONTANA**
Board of Nursing
1424 9th Avenue
Helena, Montana 59620-0407
*(406) 444-4279*

**NEBRASKA**
Board of Nursing
P.O. Box 95007, Dept. of Health
Bureau of Examining Boards
Lincoln, Nebraska 68509
*(402) 471-2115*

**NEVADA**
Board of Nursing
Suite 116, 1281 Terminal Way
Reno, Nevada 89502
*(702) 786-2778*

**NEW HAMPSHIRE**
N.H. Board of Nursing
Div. of Public Health
6 Hazen Dr.
Concord, New Hampshire 03301
*(603) 271-2323*

**NEW JERSEY**
Board of Nursing, Room 319
1100 Raymond Boulevard
Newark, New Jersey 07102
*(201) 648-2490*

**NEW MEXICO**
Board of Nursing
4125 Carlisle, N.E.
Albuquerque, New Mexico 87107
*(505) 841-6524*

**NEW YORK**
Board of Nursing State Ed. Dept.
Cultural Education Center
Albany, New York 12230
*(518) 474-3843/4*

**NORTH CAROLINA**
Board of Nursing
P.O. Box 2129
Raleigh, North Carolina 27602
*(919) 782-3211*

**NORTH DAKOTA**
Board of Nursing
919 S. 7th St., Suite 504
Bismarck, North Dakota 58504-5881
*(701) 224-2974*

**OHIO**
Board of Nursing
77 South High Street, 17th Floor
Columbus, Ohio 43266-0316
*(614) 466-3947*

**OKLAHOMA**
Board of Nurse Registration and
Nursing Education
2915 Classen Blvd. Suite 524
Oklahoma City, Oklahoma 73106
*(405) 525-2076*

**OREGON**
Board of Nursing
1400 S.W. 5th Avenue, Rm. 904
Portland, Oregon 97201
*(503) 229-5653*

**PENNSYLVANIA**
Board of Nursing
Box 2649
Harrisburg, Pennsylvania 17105-2649
*(717) 783-7142*

**RHODE ISLAND**
Board of Nurse Registration
and Nursing Education
75 Davis Street, Rm. 104
Providence, Rhode Island 02908
*(401) 277-2827*

**SOUTH CAROLINA**
Board of Nursing
Suite 102, 1777 St. Julian Place
Columbia, South Carolina 29204
*(803) 737-6594*

**SOUTH DAKOTA**
Board of Nursing, Suite 205
304 South Phillips Avenue
Sioux Falls, South Dakota 57102
*(605) 335-4973*

**TENNESSEE**
Board of Nursing
283 Plus Park Boulevard
Nashville, Tennessee 37217-5407
*(615) 367-6232*

**TEXAS**
Board of Nurse Examiners
P.O. Box 140466
Austin, Texas 78714
*(512) 835-4880*

**UTAH**
Board of Nursing
Division of Professional Licensing
160 E. 300 South, Box 45802
Salt Lake City, Utah 84145
*(801) 530-6733*

**VERMONT**
Board of Nursing
26 Terrace Street
Montpelier, Vermont 05602
*(802) 828-2363*

**VIRGINIA**
Board of Nursing
1601 Rolling Hills Dr.
Richmond, Virginia 23229
*(804) 662-9909*

**WASHINGTON**
Board of Nursing
Division of Professional Licensing
Box 9649
Olympia, Washington 98504
*(206) 753-2206*

**WEST VIRGINIA**
Board of Examiners
Room 309, Embleton Building
922 Quarrier Street
Charleston, West Virginia 25301
*(304) 348-3596*

**WISCONSIN**
Board of Nursing
P.O. Box 8935
Madison, Wisconsin 53708
*(608) 266-3735*

**WYOMING**
Board of Nursing
Barrett Bldg. 4th Floor
2301 Central Ave.
Cheyenne, Wyoming 82002
*(307) 777-7601*